636.4
S978   Swine nutrition.
2001

DATE DUE

OCT 0 9 2006

SECOND EDITION
SWINE NUTRITION

SECOND EDITION

SWINE NUTRITION

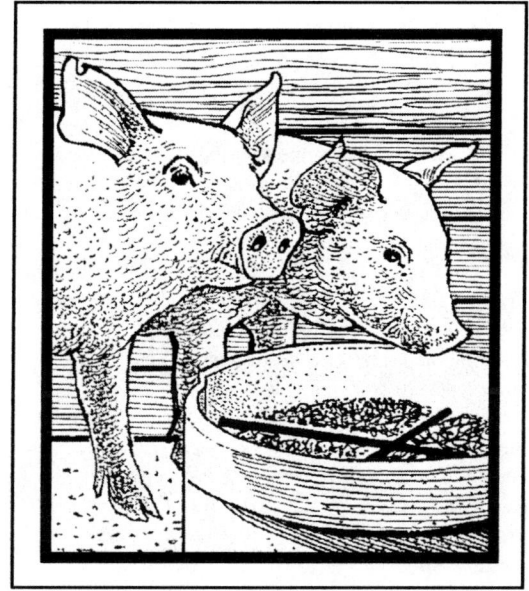

edited by
Austin J. Lewis
L. Lee Southern

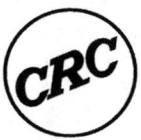

CRC Press
Boca Raton   London   New York   Washington, D.C.

Library of Congress Cataloging-in-Publication Data

Swine nutrition / edited by Austin J. Lewis and L. Lee Southern.—2nd ed.
    p. cm.
Includes bibliographical references.
ISBN 0-8493-0696-5 (alk. paper)
    1. Swine—Nutrition. 2. Swine—Feeding and feeds. I. Lewis, Austin J. II. Southern, Lincoln Lee, 1955-

SF396.5 .S95 2000
636.4′0852—dc21   0049395
                                                                                 CIP

This book contains information obtained from authentic and highly regarded sources. Reprinted material is quoted with permission, and sources are indicated. A wide variety of references are listed. Reasonable efforts have been made to publish reliable data and information, but the author and the publisher cannot assume responsibility for the validity of all materials or for the consequences of their use.

Neither this book nor any part may be reproduced or transmitted in any form or by any means, electronic or mechanical, including photocopying, microfilming, and recording, or by any information storage or retrieval system, without prior permission in writing from the publisher.

All rights reserved. Authorization to photocopy items for internal or personal use, or the personal or internal use of specific clients, may be granted by CRC Press LLC, provided that $.50 per page photocopied is paid directly to Copyright Clearance Center, 222 Rosewood Drive, Danvers, MA 01923 USA. The fee code for users of the Transactional Reporting Service is ISBN 0-8493-0696-5/01/$0.00+$.50. The fee is subject to change without notice. For organizations that have been granted a photocopy license by the CCC, a separate system of payment has been arranged.

The consent of CRC Press LLC does not extend to copying for general distribution, for promotion, for creating new works, or for resale. Specific permission must be obtained in writing from CRC Press LLC for such copying.

Direct all inquiries to CRC Press LLC, 2000 N.W. Corporate Blvd., Boca Raton, Florida 33431.

Trademark Notice: Product or corporate names may be trademarks or registered trademarks, and are used only for identification and explanation, without intent to infringe.

Visit the CRC Press Web site at www.crcpress.com

© 2001 by CRC Press LLC

No claim to original U.S. Government works
International Standard Book Number 0-8493-0696-5
Library of Congress Card Number 00-049395
Printed in the United States of America   2 3 4 5 6 7 8 9 0
Printed on acid-free paper

Dedication

This second edition of *Swine Nutrition* is dedicated to Elwyn R. Miller and Duane E. Ullrey.

Elwyn and Duane were faculty members at Michigan State University for many years and were colleagues and mentors of many of the contributors to this book. They remain personal friends of numerous swine nutritionists throughout the world. The first edition of *Swine Nutrition* was Elwyn's dream, and the editors and authors of the second edition are proud to continue that dream into the 21st century.

Both Elwyn and Duane made outstanding contributions to swine nutrition and both received the Morrison Award, the highest award given by the American Society of Animal Science, for their contributions to science. But, more than that, Elwyn and Duane served as exceptional role models to a whole generation of swine nutritionists.

Preface

Huge changes in swine production practices have occurred since the publication of the first edition of *Swine Nutrition*. Most significant has been the major consolidation of the swine industry that occurred during the 1990s. This consolidation has caused an unfortunate shift in public perceptions of pig production and focused considerable attention on issues such as soil and water pollution and odor production. Much has been learned about feeding practices that minimize pollution and odor. Changes in the swine industry have caused other changes in feeding practices. A new edition of the NRC *Nutrient Requirements of Swine* has been published, which has emphasized the value of computer models of pig growth and reproduction, and there is also a considerable amount of new data about nutrient requirements and availability of nutrients.

This new edition of *Swine Nutrition* retains the same general structure as the first edition, but it has been almost completely rewritten. Every chapter has undergone major revision, in most cases by authors different from those who contributed to the first edition. Some topics have been reduced in length or eliminated, and new topics have been added. The additions include chapters on the general characteristics of the U.S. swine industry, environmental pollution and odor control, pork quality, gene expression, and feeding of developing and adult boars. *Swine Nutrition, Second Edition* remains a book that is designed to serve as a text in advanced swine nutrition courses and as a comprehensive reference for anyone seeking information about any aspect of swine nutrition.

Most of the authors of chapters in the first edition were active or former members of the NCR-42 Regional Committee on Swine Nutrition. This tradition has been continued in the second edition and 14 of the 42 chapters have an author who is or was a member of NCR-42. However, a major portion of the current edition (six chapters) is contributed by members of another regional committee, the S-288 (formerly S-145) Committee on Sow Reproductive Efficiency. Authorship has by no means been restricted to the two committees and various other experts from the United States, Canada, and Western Europe have contributed chapters. Sadly, one of the authors died during the preparation of the book. Dr. E. T. Kornegay (a member of S-288) was a devoted and productive swine nutritionist and is much missed by those of us who knew and worked with him.

This second edition, like any book, would not have been possible but for the help of many people. The publisher, CRC Press, initiated the idea of a second edition. John Sulzycki, senior editor, has been supportive throughout and has been very understanding about the difficulties in bringing a multiauthored book such as this to fruition. Christine Andreasen, project editor, turned a collection of individual manuscripts into a coherent book. With care and dedication, she "created a silk purse from a collection of sows' ears"! The two regional research committees backed the project from the start and provided much of the authorship. Amy Guzik spent a lot of time checking and correcting reference citations in the initial drafts of many of the chapters. Lee Southern was an outstanding co-editor and was a pleasure to work with from the initial planning stages to the end of the project. Whenever my enthusiasm waned, Lee was always there to pick up the slack. Finally, I am deeply grateful to my wife, Nancy, for her sustained support of this and all my endeavors.

Austin J. Lewis

Editors

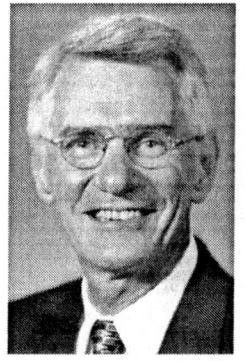

Austin J. Lewis is a professor of animal science in the Department of Animal Science at the University of Nebraska, Lincoln. He received his B.S. in agriculture (1967) from the University of Reading, England and his Ph.D. (1971) in applied biochemistry and nutrition from the University of Nottingham, England.

Dr. Lewis teaches undergraduate and graduate courses in animal nutrition and a graduate course on protein nutrition. Most of his research has focused on the amino acid nutrition of swine, and this has included investigations of the amino acid requirements of all classes of swine as well as the bioavailability of amino acids. Dr. Lewis was a co-editor of the first edition of *Swine Nutrition* and also a co-editor of *Bioavailability of Nutrients for Animals*. He has served the *Journal of Animal Science* as a member of the editorial board, as editor of the Nonruminant Nutrition section, and as editor-in-chief. In addition, he served as a member of the subcommittees responsible for the two most recent revisions of the *NRC Nutrient Requirements of Swine* and as a member of the Board on Agriculture, Committee on Animal Nutrition.

Dr. Lewis has published many refereed journal papers, abstracts, and other reports on the nutrition of swine. He received the Gamma Sigma Delta Research Award at the University of Nebraska in 1987 and the American Feed Industry Association Nutrition Award in 1988.

L. Lee Southern is a professor of animal science in the Department of Animal Science at Louisiana State University, Baton Rouge. He received his B.S. (1977) and M.S. (1979) in animal science from North Carolina State University, Raleigh and his Ph.D. (1983) in animal science from the University of Illinois, Urbana-Champaign.

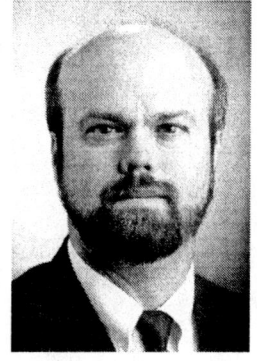

Dr. Southern teaches courses for undergraduate or graduate credit in animal nutrition and in swine production, management, and nutrition. His research interests are in the areas of trace mineral and amino acid nutrition of swine and poultry and in nutritional factors that affect meat quality. Dr. Southern has served as associate editor of *Poultry Science*, as a member of the editorial board of the *Journal of Animal Science*, and as editor of the Nonruminant Nutrition section of the *Journal of Animal Science*. He is currently president of the Southern Section, American Society of Animal Science, a member of the Board on Agriculture, Committee on Animal Nutrition, and a member of the Publications Committee for the *Journal of Animal Science*.

Dr. Southern is author or co-author of numerous refereed journal articles, abstracts, and technical publications. He has been awarded one patent for his research in poultry. In 1997, Dr. Southern received the American Feed Industry Nonruminant Nutrition Award. He also has received the LSU Phi Kappa Phi Award for Outstanding Research by Non-tenured Faculty, the First Mississippi Corporation Award of Excellence for Outstanding Work in the Louisiana Agricultural Experiment Station, the Gamma Sigma Delta Research Award of Merit, and in 1998, the Tipton Team Research Award in Recognition of Excellence in Research. Dr. Southern also has been named to the Gamma Sigma Delta Teaching Merit Honor Roll in 1995, 1997, 1998, and 1999.

Contributors

Debra K. Aaron, Ph.D.
Department of Animal Sciences
University of Kentucky
Lexington, Kentucky

Olayiwola Adeola, Ph.D.
Department of Animal Science
Purdue University
West Lafayette, Indiana

Nathan Augspurger, M.S.
Department of Animal Sciences
University of Illinois
Urbana, Illinois

Michael J. Azain, Ph.D.
Department of Animal and Dairy Science
University of Georgia
Athens, Georgia

David H. Baker, Ph.D.
Department of Animal Sciences
University of Illinois
Urbana, Illinois

Keith C. Behnke, Ph.D.
Department of Grain Science and Industry
Kansas State University
Manhattan, Kansas

Eric P. Berg, Ph.D.
Department of Animal Science
University of Missouri
Columbia, Missouri

Stephen H. Birkett, Ph.D.
Department of Animal and Poultry Science
University of Guelph
Guelph, Ontario
Canada

Joel H. Brendemuhl, Ph.D.
Department of Animal Science
University of Florida
Gainesville, Florida

Michael C. Brumm, Ph.D.
Haskell Agricultural Laboratory
University of Nebraska
Concord, Nebraska

Christopher C. Calvert, Ph.D.
Department of Animal Sciences
University of California
Davis, California

Scott D. Carter, Ph.D.
Animal Science Department
Oklahoma State University
Stillwater, Oklahoma

Lee I. Chiba, Ph.D.
Department of Animal and Dairy Sciences
Auburn University
Auburn, Alabama

Tilford R. Cline, Ph.D.
Department of Animal Sciences
Purdue University
West Lafayette, Indiana

David A. Cook, Ph.D.
Cargill Animal Nutrition Center
Elk River, Minnesota

Thomas D. Crenshaw, Ph.D.
Department of Animal Sciences
University of Wisconsin
Madison, Wisconsin

Gary L. Cromwell, Ph.D.
Department of Animal Sciences
University of Kentucky
Lexington, Kentucky

Stanley E. Curtis, Ph.D.
Department of Animal Sciences
University of Illinois
Urbana, Illinois

Craig S. Darroch, Ph.D.
Department of Agriculture
 and Natural Resources
University of Tennessee
Martin, Tennessee

Cornelis F. M. de Lange, Ph.D.
Department of Animal and Poultry Science
University of Guelph
Guelph, Ontario
Canada

C. Robert Dove, Ph.D.
Department of Animal and Dairy Science
University of Georgia
Coastal Plain Experiment Station
Tifton, Georgia

Michael Ellis, Ph.D.
Department of Animal Sciences
University of Illinois
Urbana, Illinois

Jeffery Escobar, M.S.
Department of Animal Sciences
University of Illinois
Urbana, Illinois

Richard C. Ewan, Ph.D.
Department of Animal Science
Iowa State University
Ames, Iowa

George C. Fahey, Jr., Ph.D.
Department of Animal Sciences
University of Illinois
Urbana, Illinois

Vincent M. Gabert, Ph.D.
Department of Animal Sciences
University of Illinois
Urbana, Illinois

H. Rex Gaskins, Ph.D.
Departments of Animal Sciences
 and Veterinary Pathobiology
University of Illinois
Urbana, Illinois

Christine M. Grieshop, Ph.D.
Department of Animal Sciences
University of Illinois
Urbana, Illinois

Harold W. Gonyou, Ph.D.
Prairie Swine Centre, Inc.
Saskatoon, Saskatchewan
Canada

Joe D. Hancock, Ph.D.
Department of Animal Sciences and Industry
Kansas State University
Manhattan, Kansas

Virgil W. Hays, Ph.D.
Department of Animal Sciences
University of Kentucky
Lexington, Kentucky

Gretchen Myers Hill, Ph.D.
Department of Animal Science
Michigan State University
East Lansing, Michigan

Gilbert R. Hollis, Ph.D.
Department of Animal Sciences
University of Illinois
Urbana, Illinois

Karen L. Houseknecht, Ph.D.
Animal Health Discovery Research
Pfizer, Inc.
Groton, Connecticut

Rodney W. Johnson, Ph.D.
Department of Animal Sciences
University of Illinois
Urbana, Illinois

Lee J. Johnston, Ph.D.
West Central Research and Outreach Center
University of Minnesota
Morris, Minnesota

Henry Jørgensen, Ph.D.
Department of Animal Nutrition
 and Physiology
Danish Institute of Agricultural Sciences
Tjele, Denmark

Bas Kemp, Ph.D.
Wageningen Institute of Animal Sciences
Wageningen University and Research Centre
Wageningen, The Netherlands

E. T. Kornegay, Ph.D. (Deceased)
Department of Animal and Poultry Sciences
Virginia Polytechnic Institute
  and State University
Blacksburg, Virginia

Jean Le Dividich, Ph.D.
INRA
Station de Recherches Porcines
St. Gilles, France

Xin Gen Lei, Ph.D.
Department of Animal Science
Cornell University
Ithaca, New York

Austin J. Lewis, Ph.D.
Department of Animal Science
University of Nebraska
Lincoln, Nebraska

Donald C. Mahan, Ph.D.
Department of Animal Sciences
The Ohio State University
Columbus, Ohio

Charles V. Maxwell, Jr., Ph.D.
Animal Science Department
University of Arkansas
Fayetteville, Arkansas

Phillip S. Miller, Ph.D.
Department of Animal Science
University of Nebraska
Lincoln, Nebraska

Jess L. Miner, Ph.D.
Department of Animal Science
University of Nebraska
Lincoln, Nebraska

Alva D. Mitchell, Ph.D.
Agricultural Research Service
U.S. Department of Agriculture
Beltsville Agricultural Research Center-East
Beltsville, Maryland

Patrick C. H. Morel, Ph.D.
Institute of Food, Nutrition, and Human Health
Massey University
Palmerston North, New Zealand

Robert O. Myer, Ph.D.
North Florida Research and Education Center
University of Florida
Marianna, Florida

Jean Noblet, Ph.D.
INRA
Station de Recherches Porcines
St. Gilles, France

Charles M. Nyachoti, Ph.D.
Department of Animal Science
University of Manitoba
Winnipeg, Canada

Jack Odle, Ph.D.
Department of Animal Science
North Carolina State University
Raleigh, North Carolina

Fredric N. Owens, Ph.D.
DuPont Specialty Grains
Johnson, Iowa

John F. Patience, Ph.D.
Prairie Swine Centre, Inc.
Saskatoon, Saskatchewan
Canada

Wilson G. Pond, Ph.D.
Department of Animal Science
Cornell University
Ithaca, New York

Duane E. Reese, Ph.D.
Department of Animal Science
University of Nebraska
Lincoln, Nebraska

Brian T. Richert, Ph.D.
Department of Animal Sciences
Purdue University
West Lafayette, Indiana

Alan S. Robertson, Ph.D.
Animal Health Discovery Research
Pfizer, Inc.
Groton, Connecticut

Thomas E. Sauber, Ph.D.
DuPont Specialty Grains
Johnson, Iowa

Armin M. Scholz, Ph.D.
Ludwig-Maximilians-University Munich
Oberschleissheim, Germany

Nicoline M. Soede, Ph.D.
Wageningen Institute of Animal Sciences
Wageningen University and Research Centre
Wageningen, The Netherlands

Jerry W. Spears, Ph.D.
Department of Animal Science
North Carolina State University
Raleigh, North Carolina

Philip A. Thacker, Ph.D.
Department of Animal Science
University of Saskatchewan
Saskatoon, Saskatchewan
Canada

Nathalie L. Trottier, Ph.D.
Department of Animal Science
Michigan State University
East Lansing, Michigan

Eric van Heugten, Ph.D.
Department of Animal Science
North Carolina State University
Raleigh, North Carolina

Jaap Van Milgen, Ph.D.
INRA
Station de Recherches Porcines
St. Gilles, France

Martin W. A. Verstegen, Ph.D.
Wageningen Institute of Animal Sciences
Wageningen University and Research Centre
Wageningen, The Netherlands

Trygve L. Veum, Ph.D.
Department of Animal Sciences
University of Missouri
Columbia, Missouri

Douglas M. Webel, Ph.D.
United Feeds
Sheridan, Indiana

Diane Wray-Cahen, Ph.D.
Division of Life Sciences
U.S. Food and Drug Administration
Rockville, Maryland

Jong-Tseng Yen, Ph.D.
Meat Animal Research Center
U.S. Department of Agriculture
Clay Center, Nebraska

Ruurd T. Zijlstra, Ph.D.
Prairie Swine Centre, Inc.
Saskatoon, Saskatchewan
Canada

Contents

General Characteristics of Swine

Chapter 1
Of Pigs and People 3
Wilson G. Pond and Xin Gen Lei

Chapter 2
General Characteristics of the U.S. Swine Industry 19
Gilbert R. Hollis and Stanley E. Curtis

Chapter 3
Anatomy of the Digestive System and Nutritional Physiology 31
Jong-Tseng Yen

Chapter 4
Protein, Fat, and Bone Tissue Growth in Swine 65
Cornelis F. M. de Lange, Stephen H. Birkett, and Patrick C. H. Morel

Nutrient Utilization by Swine

Chapter 5
Energy Utilization in Swine Nutrition..85
Richard C. Ewan

Chapter 6
Fat in Swine Nutrition 95
Michael J. Azain

Chapter 7
Nonstarch Polysaccharides and Oligosaccharides in Swine Nutrition 107
Christine M. Grieshop, Duane E. Reese, and George C. Fahey, Jr.

Chapter 8
Amino Acids in Swine Nutrition..131
Austin J. Lewis

Chapter 9
Bioavailability of Amino Acids in Feedstuffs for Swine 151
Vincent M. Gabert, Henry Jørgensen, and Charles M. Nyachoti

Chapter 10
Calcium, Phosphorus, Vitamin D, and Vitamin K in Swine Nutrition 187
Thomas D. Crenshaw

Chapter 11
Sodium, Potassium, Chloride, Magnesium, and Sulfur in Swine Nutrition 213
John F. Patience and Ruurd T. Zijlstra

Chapter 12
Trace and Ultratrace Elements in Swine Nutrition 229
Gretchen Myers Hill and Jerry W. Spears

Chapter 13
Vitamin A in Swine Nutrition 263
Craig S. Darroch

Chapter 14
Selenium and Vitamin E in Swine Nutrition 281
Donald C. Mahan

Chapter 15
Water-Soluble Vitamins in Swine Nutrition 315
C. Robert Dove and David A. Cook

Chapter 16
Bioavailability of Minerals and Vitamins 357
David H. Baker

Chapter 17
Water in Swine Nutrition 381
Philip A. Thacker

Factors That Influence Swine Nutrition

Chapter 18
Antimicrobial and Promicrobial Agents 401
Gary L. Cromwell

Chapter 19
Performance-Enhancing Substances 427
Diane Wray-Cahen

Chapter 20
Feed Intake in Growing-Finishing Pigs 447
Michael Ellis and Nathan Augspurger

Chapter 21
Use of Ingredient and Diet Processing Technologies (Grinding, Mixing, Pelleting, and Extruding) to Produce Quality Feeds for Pigs 469
Joe D. Hancock and Keith C. Behnke

Chapter 22
Effects of Facility Design on Behavior and Feed and Water Intake 499
Michael C. Brumm and Harold W. Gonyou

Chapter 23
Thermal Environment and Swine Nutrition 519
Jean Noblet, Jean Le Dividich, and Jaap Van Milgen

Chapter 24
Nutrition and Immunology of Swine 545
Rodney W. Johnson, Jeffery Escobar, and Douglas M. Webel

Chapter 25
Mycotoxins and Other Antinutritional Factors in Swine Feeds 563
Eric van Heugten

Chapter 26
Intestinal Bacteria and Their Influence on Swine Growth...585
H. Rex Gaskins

Chapter 27
Swine Nutrition and Environmental Pollution and Odor Control 609
E. T. Kornegay and Martin W. A. Verstegen

Chapter 28
Swine Nutrition, the Conversion of Muscle to Meat, and Pork Quality 631
Eric P. Berg

Chapter 29
Nutrient Effects on Gene Expression 659
Jess L. Miner, Alan S. Robertson, and Karen L. Houseknecht

Applied Feeding of Swine

Chapter 30
Feeding Neonatal Pigs 671
Trygve L. Veum and Jack Odle

Chapter 31
Feeding the Weaned Pig 691
Charles V. Maxwell, Jr. and Scott D. Carter

Chapter 32
Feeding Growing-Finishing Pigs 717
Tilford R. Cline and Brian T. Richert

Chapter 33
Feeding Gilts during Development and Sows during Gestation and Lactation 725
Nathalie L. Trottier and Lee J. Johnston

Chapter 34
Feeding of Developing and Adult Boars 771
Bas Kemp and Nicoline M. Soede

Feedstuffs Included in Swine Diets

Chapter 35
Cereal Grains and By-Products for Swine 785
Thomas E. Sauber and Fredric N. Owens

Chapter 36
Protein Supplements 803
Lee I. Chiba

Chapter 37
Miscellaneous Feedstuffs 839
Robert O. Myer and Joel H. Brendemuhl

Techniques in Swine Nutrition Research

Chapter 38
Swine Modeling 867
Phillip S. Miller and Christopher C. Calvert

Chapter 39
Statistical Techniques for the Design and Analysis
of Swine Nutrition Experiments 881
Debra K. Aaron and Virgil W. Hays

Chapter 40
Digestion and Balance Techniques in Pigs 903
Olayiwola Adeola

Chapter 41
Techniques for Measuring Body Composition of Swine 917
Alva D. Mitchell and Armin M. Scholz

Chapter 42
Blood Sampling and Surgical Techniques...961
Jong-Tseng Yen

Index 985

Part I

General Characteristics of Swine

1   Of Pigs and People

Wilson G. Pond and Xin Gen Lei

CONTENTS

I. Historical Perspective...3
   A. Pig Domestication 3
   B. Demographic Relationships 4
II. Anatomical and Physiological Similarities 6
   A. Gastrointestinal System..6
   B. Body Composition 7
   C. Comparative Nutrient Requirements of Pigs and Humans 7
III. The Pig as a Model in Biomedical Research..9
   A. General Considerations..9
   B. Nutrition 9
   C. Physiology and Pathophysiology...9
IV. Clinical Applications in Humans of Knowledge Derived with the Pig.................10
   A. Genetic Engineering...10
   B. Xenotransplantation 10
   C. Phytase and Mineral-Related Metabolic Disorders...10
   D. Recombinant DNA–Derived Products 11
V. Pork in the Human Diet...11
   A. Pork Composition 12
   B. Pork Acceptability..12
   C. Societal Issues..14
      1. Animal Well-Being..14
      2. Antibiotic Resistance 14
      3. Environmental Stability...14
VI. Summary 15
References 15

I. HISTORICAL PERSPECTIVE

A. PIG DOMESTICATION

The time and place of the domestication of the pig is lost in history. Evidence (Towne and Wentworth, 1950; Mellen, 1952; Porter, 1993) indicates that ancestors of the modern pig lived in what is now China, Mesopotamia, Iraq, Persia, Africa, and Europe 6000 to 9000 years ago. The modern pig, which supplies pork throughout the world, remains genetically diverse. The contemporary pig in the United States, whose ancestry probably includes the European wild pig and the Far Eastern pig, has an appearance far different from that of the contemporary Chinese pig (Figure 1.1). Present-day wild pigs of Africa (giant forest hog, warthog, bushpig), Asia (babirusa, pygmy hog, Javanese warty pig, Sulawesi warty pig, bearded pig), and Europe

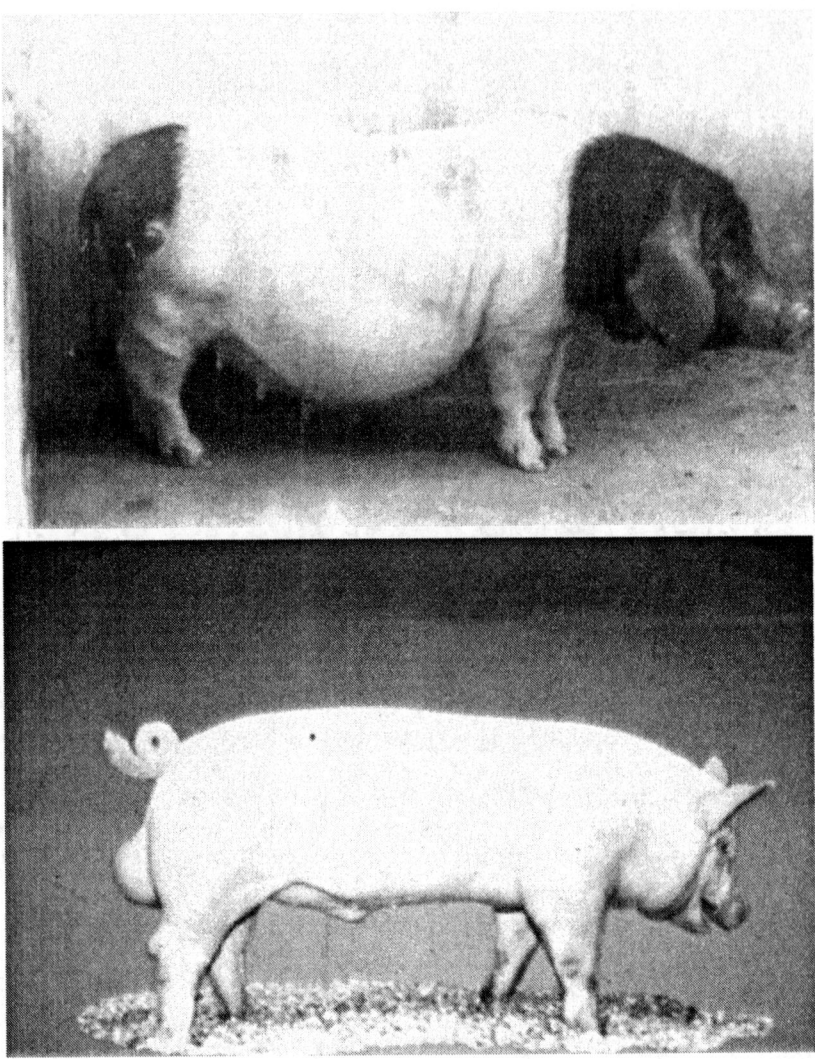

FIGURE 1.1 (Top): Contemporary Chinese Jinhua gilt, Zhejiang Province, China (courtesy of the late Larry Young); (Bottom): Contemporary Yorkshire boar, United States.

(Eurasian wild boar) presumably resemble their very early ancestors (Porter, 1993). Such a diverse germ plasm would be expected when one considers the results of thousands of years of natural selection and, more recently, the application of Mendelian genetic principles by animal breeders. Changes in traits such as body type and size, pork composition, and nutritional requirements depend on this genetic diversity.

B. Demographic Relationships

The partnership between pigs and humans throughout history has thrived because of the ability of the pig to respond favorably to widely different environments and to the changing needs and desires of humans. This plasticity must continue to be an essential attribute of the pig if this valuable historic partnership is to be sustained.

The pig converts low-quality plant and animal products and by-products to food and is an efficient storage depot for fat, proteins, vitamins, and minerals which, taken separately, would be very expensive. Pigs traditionally have been scavengers, and in early domestication they were raised as a means of utilizing food wastes. In many parts of the world, they still perform that function and, as such, are an intregal part of the culture in developing countries where they are held in high esteem.

In the United States, corn and soybean producers often can market their crops through swine at a greater profit than would be available by selling them as cash crops. Profitability of pork production based on this method of marketing grain and other surplus feed resources and by-products has been for many years, and continues to be, an alternative among farmers.

The global demand for pork continues to grow. The extent of pork production and consumption in various countries is shown in Tables 1.1 and 1.2, respectively. The United States, Denmark, Canada, Poland, and China were the top pork-exporting countries and Japan, Russia, United States, Hong Kong, and Korea were the top pork-importing countries in 1997 (USDA, 1998b).

The strong demand for pork worldwide has been made possible by dramatic increases in grain and other crop yields in response to scientific and technical advances in crop production technology, as well as to increased growth and standard of living in many regions of the world. Animal protein demand in economically developing countries increases as household incomes rise.

Pork consumption now accounts for more than 40% of annual total world consumption of meat, exceeding that of any other source (beef, lamb, poultry, fish, and other animals). The total world slaughter of more than 1 billion pigs in 1997 (Table 1.1) was produced for a total human population of nearly 6 billion. The world human population is projected to nearly double to approximately 10 billion during the first 50 years of the new millenium. The prospect of doubling pork production during the next 50 years to accommodate the increased demand for pork represents a challenge whose outcome will depend not only on sustained per capita demand for

TABLE 1.1
Pork Production in Various Countries in 1997

Country	Weight[a] (thousands of metric tons, carcass wt)	Inventory (thousands of pigs)	Slaughter (thousands of pigs)
China	42,500	457,130	560,000
United States	7,835	56,141	91,961
Germany	3,570	24,283	38,500
Spain	2,320	18,631	28,980
France	2,186	14,968	25,470
Denmark	1,625	11,081	21,120
Poland	1,600	17,697	21,400
Brazil	1,540	31,369	20,865
Russia	1,500	19,500	29,149
Italy	1,417	8,100	12,000
Netherlands	1,366	14,253	15,200
Japan	1,273	9,809	16,960
Canada	1,255	12,301	15,300
Belgium-Luxembourg	1,036	7,108	11,258
Taiwan	1,012	10,698	11,701
Total European Union	16,175	115,700	187,589
Total World	80,874	792,303	1,032,715

[a] Note that the ranking of countries based on the number of pigs slaughtered and the weight of pork produced annually differs from the ranking based on inventory (number on hand at a particular time). This discrepancy reflects differences in "extraction rate," the ratio of the number of pigs marketed per year to the inventory. For example, in the United States, the ratio is 1.6, whereas in Denmark the ratio is 1.9, in China it is 1.2, and in Brazil it is 0.7.

Source: USDA Foreign Agricultural Service.

TABLE 1.2
Per Capita Pork Consumption in Various Countries in 1997

Country	Weight (kg)	Country	Weight (kg)
Denmark	67.4	Singapore	31.4
Spain	55.8	Canada	30.1
Hong Kong	55.3	United States	28.5
Germany	53.1	United Kingdom	24.7
Hungary	41.0	Korea	19.2
Taiwan	38.1	Australia	18.2
Poland	37.8	Japan	16.4
Sweden	36.0	Russian Federation	13.2
France	34.8	Mexico	10.2
China	34.1	Brazil	9.2

Source: USDA Foreign Agricultural Service.

pork, but also on constraints on natural resources and environmental stability. The outcome will depend on forces within agriculture and on economic, environmental, social, and other forces extrinsic to agriculture and pork production.

II. ANATOMICAL AND PHYSIOLOGICAL SIMILARITIES

Many anatomical and physiological similarities between humans and pigs have been documented (Bustad and McClellan, 1966; Pond and Houpt, 1978; Roberts and Dodds, 1982; Stanton and Mersmann, 1986; Tumbleson, 1986; Tumbleson and Schook, 1996; Pond and Mersmann, 2000). Among the anatomical and physiological similarities most relevant to the use of the pig as a model animal for biomedical research are those of the skin (Monteiro-Riviere, 2000) kidney (Terris, 1986; Argenzio and Monteiro-Riviere, 2000) cardiovascular (Stanton and Mersmann, 1986; Gootman, 2000; Mersmann and Pond, 2000); gastrointestinal systems and nutritional requirements (Miller and Ullrey, 1987; Burrin, 2000; Yen, 2000), and body composition (Mitchell et al., 2000). Comparisons of the gastrointestinal system, body composition, and nutrient requirements of pigs and humans are described briefly in this section.

A. Gastrointestinal System

The general architecture of the gastrointestinal tracts of the pig and human is similar. Notable differences are the higher proportion of cardiac mucosa lining the stomach of the pig, as compared with the human (Yen, 2000), and the presence of a cecum in the pig, as compared with only a vestige, the appendix, in the human. The digestive functions of each of the segments of the gastrointestinal tract of both species are similar; qualitatively, amylolytic, lipolytic, and proteolytic activities are similar, and the secretions of each organ, including the stomach, small intestine, and pancreas, are comparable (Yen, 2000). Even the endocrine and paracrine control of gastrointestinal tract growth, motility, and overall function appear to be similar, particularly with respect to peptide hormones, some of which are found both in the brain and intestine (e.g., cholecystokinin). Both pigs and humans are able to use some plant fiber as a source of energy because of anaerobic fermentation of the fiber and production of volatile fatty acids in the large intestine. Volatile fatty acids absorbed into the portal vein may contribute more than 20% of the maintenance energy requirement of pigs (Yen, 2000).

Based on the current knowledge of many parallels between pigs and humans regarding gastrointestinal tract function, it is not surprising that the pig is widely used as a model animal for nutrition and digestive physiology in biomedical research (Tumbleson, 1986; Tumbleson and Schook, 1996). Details of gastrointestinal tract physiology in the pig are available (Moran, 1982; Yen, 2000; Burrin, 2000).

B. Body Composition

The adult human and pig are similar in body composition, and both species tend to become obese during adulthood if eating is not restrained. Thus, the pig is a favorable model for human obesity; furthermore, the propensity to obesity in both species offers the advantage of using pigs to study lipid metabolism in animals of contrasting body fat to lean ratios. Detailed information on growth and body composition in pigs is provided in Chapters 4 and 41.

The newborn pig contains <2% body fat, in contrast to the full-term human infant with an average fat content of 10%. The newborn pig resembles the low-birth-weight human infant in fat content. Therefore, the pig is increasingly used as a model for studies of alimentation of premature infants.

Mersmann (1986) reviewed lipid metabolism in pigs and pointed out important differences between pigs and humans. The primary site of fatty acid biosynthesis is adipose tissue in pigs and the liver in humans. Lipoprotein structure is similar in pigs and humans, but metabolism may differ because pigs must transport lipids from adipose tissue, where fatty acids are synthesized, to the liver, where lipoproteins are synthesized. Lipolysis in adipose tissue is stimulated by β-adrenergic agonists and inhibited by α-adrenergic agonists. The specificity of these agonists for control of lipolysis is different in pigs and humans. The pig does not have α-adrenergic inhibition of lipolysis; this represents a distinct species difference in the metabolism of lipids. Despite these differences, the pig serves as an excellent animal model for humans leading a sedentary life and tending toward excessive energy intake.

A wide range of body types occurs in pigs, as in humans. Contemporary pigs bred for leanness represent the major segment of the pig population in the United States. In contrast, some strains of pigs have been selectively bred for their small body size (Panepinto, 1996) whereas other small types (e.g., Yucatan) evolved naturally. Some pigs tend toward obesity (e.g., Ossabaw); still others have been selcted for low or high backfat thickness over many generations (Hetzer and Harvey, 1967). Ferrell and Cornelius (1984) determined the changes in body composition of pigs representing contemporary and obese (Hetzer and Harvey, 1967) body types from age 4 to 24 weeks. These data are summarized in Table 1.3. Fat accumulated in the bodies of obese pigs much more rapidly than in lean contemporary pigs (obese pigs contained 46.5% fat at age 24 weeks as compared with 25.4% for lean pigs). Human infants compare well with 4-week-old pigs in body fat content (obese, 13.3%; contemporary, 9.7%) and normal adults humans are similar to 24-week-old contemporary pigs, whereas obese adult humans are similar to 24-week-old obese pigs. Direct measurements of body composition in living humans, of course, are not feasible, but estimates based on indirect procedures indicate that highly trained athletes contain about 9% fat, whereas sedentary obese males may contain 40 to 50% or more fat; females in all categories are slightly fatter. Davidson et al. (1979) listed the normal chemical composition of a man weighing 65 kg as 17.0% protein, 13.8% fat, 1.5% carbohydrate, 6.1% minerals, and 61.6% water. This information was compiled from actual analysis of several cadavers. For studies of pig nutrition, a knowledge of genetic background of the animal is important because interactions exist between nutrition and genetic background as related to body composition. A similar relationship probably exists in humans, although it is not well documented.

C. Comparative Nutrient Requirements of Pigs and Humans

The nutrient requirements of the pig resemble nutrient requirements of humans more than those of any other nonprimate mammal. The literature is replete with information on nutrient

TABLE 1.3
Least-Squares Means for Live Weight, Empty Body Weight, and Weight of Gross Chemical Empty Body Components

Type	Age (wk)	Number of Pigs	Total Weight	Empty Body Component (kg)				
				Water	Fat	Nitrogen	FFOM[a]	Ash
Obese	4	4	4.56	3.08	0.61	0.09	0.72	0.15
	8	3	9.78	6.53	1.39	0.19	1.76	0.33
	12	6	24.8	14.4	5.82	0.61	3.90	0.71
	18	6	50.5	25.2	16.7	1.17	7.25	1.38
	24	6	87.8	34.4	40.8	1.70	10.5	2.05
Contemporary	4	5	7.75	5.38	0.75	0.20	1.34	0.28
	8	6	13.3	9.31	1.36	0.34	2.19	0.40
	12	6	31.3	20.6	4.47	0.81	5.38	0.88
	18	6	63.2	37.9	12.2	1.80	11.1	1.96
	24	6	81.9	44.9	20.8	2.22	13.7	2.47
Standard Error			0.79	0.47	0.33	0.020	0.13	0.026

[a] FFOM = fat-free organic matter.

Source: From Ferrell, C. L., and Cornelius, S., *J. Anim. Sci.*, 58:903, 1984. With permission.

requirements of the pig (Pond and Maner, 1974; Cunha, 1977; Moran, 1982; Pond et al., 1991; Miller et al., 1991; Burrin, 2000). In addition, the National Research Council (National Research Council, 1998a) regularly publishes new information on quantitative nutrient requirements of the pig and nutrient requirements are discussed in Chapters 5 to 17 and 30 to 34. Recommended daily allowances of all nutrients known to be required by humans are continually updated by committees and panels of experts representing human nutrition (National Research Council, 1998b).

There is nearly complete agreement between humans and pigs in the list of dietary requirements for nutrients, although the quantitative requirements for individual nutrients differ between the two species (e.g., protein and amino acid requirements expressed as percentages of the dry diet are higher in growing pigs than in humans because of the higher growth rate of the pig). Exceptions include (1) vitamin C, which is an absolute dietary requirement for humans but for which there is evidence that the young piglet may respond favorably to a dietary source under some conditions, and (2) a possible difference, still inconclusive, between humans and pigs in a dietary requirement for the vitamins inositol and para-amino-benzoic acid.

The list of required mineral elements for both pigs and humans may increase as more highly sensitive instrumentation and more complete control of environmental contamination (plastic instead of metal cages and utensils; highly purified air, water, and feed) become available. Many mineral elements, including aluminum, arsenic, bromine, tin, nickel, cadmium, and lead found in animal tissues, have no known metabolic function. Their significance in practical swine feeding and in human nutrition remains unknown. Most are of more concern as toxic elements than as possible required nutrients. Others, including vanadium and silicon, are required for specific functions in some animal species but have not yet been shown to be required by pigs (National Research Council, 1998a). Others, such as chromium, which affects glucose metabolism and body composition in pigs, usually have not been listed as required nutrients for swine or humans. Choline, although known to function as a methyl donor and in other metabolic conversions, was only recently identified as an essential nutrient for humans.

Overall, the similarity between pigs and humans in the list of known required nutrients provides strong support for the use of the pig as an animal model in human nutrition research.

III. THE PIG AS A MODEL IN BIOMEDICAL RESEARCH

A. GENERAL CONSIDERATIONS

The use of the pig in biomedical research of nutrition and metabolic diseases has increased dramatically during the past decade. Publication of the proceedings of two recent symposia on the use of swine in biomedical research (Tumbleson, 1986; Tumbleson and Schook, 1996) underscores the extent of this trend. Examples of chronic human diseases with nutritional implications in which the pig is widely used as an animal model are: atherosclerosis, hypertension, cerebrovascular arteriosclerosis, gastric ulcers, obesity, alcoholism, osteoporosis, diabetes, certain types of cancer, and kwashiorkor/marasmus.

Briefly highlighted is the use of the pig to study one group of chronic diseases, cardiovascular disease, which may invoke a greater appreciation of the importance of swine in biomedical research. The role of nutritional factors in cardiovascular disease is interrelated with age, gender, genetics, exercise, drugs, and psychosocial conditions; the pig has been used to study each of these interrelationships. Reviews of the use of the pig in studying nutritional components of human cardiovascular disease are numerous (Pond, 1982; Roberts and Dodds, 1982; Stanton and Mersmann, 1986; Tumbleson, 1986, Vol. 3; Pond and Mersmann, 1996; Tumbleson and Schook, 1996).

B. NUTRITION

Probably the most actively studied aspect of pig biology is nutrition because of its impact on pork production efficiency. The neonatal pig has been widely used as a model for studying nutrient requirements and digestive function in human infants. Examples include the role of colostrum in intestinal tract functional development (Burrin et al., 1995; 1997); the role of insulin-like growth factor I (IGF-I) in intestinal growth and digestive function (Donovan et al., 1996); the development of intestinal transport and brush border hydrolases (Buddington et al., 1996); changes in intestinal structure and function induced by enteric pathogens (Chandra et al., 1996; Gomez et al., 1996; Krakowka and Eaton, 1996) and nutrient functional interactions (Reeds and Odle, 1996). The physiologic and developmental effects of infant protein-energy malnutrition, a major nutritional problem worldwide, have been addressed using the baby pig as a model (Pond et al., 1996, Jahoor et al., 1999). Neonatal pigs are also used to monitor amino acid metabolism and gastrointestinal function during total parenteral nutrition (TPN) (Ball et al., 1996) and brain cholesterol accretion and behavior during dietary cholesterol deprivation (Schoknecht et al., 1994a; Boleman et al., 1998). The role of maternal malnutrition during early or late pregnancy on intrauterine growth retardation, placental and fetal metabolism, and subsequent growth and development of the offspring in humans has been studied with the pig model (Schoknecht et al., 1994b; Wu et al., 1998). The pig has been used extensively to study the role of diet composition and genetic background on atherogenesis (Roberts and Dodds, 1982; Pond and Mersmann, 1996; Hackman et al., 1996; Graf et al., 1998).

Finally, the valuable contributions to knowledge of human nutrition made over many years by agricultural scientists engaged in swine nutrition research aimed at improved efficiency of pork production often have not received adequate recognition in human nutrition. The intensified use of the pig by contemporary investigators in medical environments validates the long-established contributions of the pig to progress in human nutrition.

C. PHYSIOLOGY AND PATHOPHYSIOLOGY

The pig is used increasingly as the animal model of choice in renal, respiratory, enterohepatic, and cardivascular research. Recent pig research to advance knowledge of normal and abnormal function of these organ systems was summarized by Brown and Terris (1996). Current knowledge of the excretory (Argenzio and Monteiro-Riviere, 2000); respiratory (Ackerman, 2000); enterohepatic

(Yen, 2000); and cardiovascular (Gootman, 2000) systems and of hematology and blood clinical chemistry (Mersmann and Pond, 2000) in the pig has been assembled (Pond and Mersmann, 2000).

IV. CLINICAL APPLICATIONS IN HUMANS OF KNOWLEDGE DERIVED WITH THE PIG

A. Genetic Engineering

Most transgenic studies in mammals have been done in the laboratory mouse (Scarpelli et al., 1991; Wagner and Theuring, 1993). Yet, during the past decade, gene transfer in pigs has been shown to be an effective model system for human disease (Pursel et al., 1996). Pigs expressing growth hormone transgenes have morphologic similarities to those of humans with acromegaly (Pursel et al., 1996). Muscle IGF-I concentration is increased in pigs carrying human IGF-I transgene (Pursel et al., 1996). Transgenic pigs with a defective rhodopsin gene are available as models to study the human disorder retinitis pigmentosa (Petters, 1994). Pursel et al. (1996) predicted that as knowledge of the regulation of transgenes expands, transgenic pigs will be produced in which growth modifiers "can be turned on and off as desired." Other modulators of metabolism in normal and abnormal states may be provided in swine in which transgenes are expressed for clinical application in humans as genetic engineering technology advances (see Recombinant DNA–Derived Products later in this section).

B. Xenotransplantation

The pig is receiving serious attention as a potential source of human organ replacement in the light of severe shortages of human organ donors. Pigs are considered to be the most acceptable source of organs for xenotransplantation because of their size, availability, and limited risk of zoonosis (Lin and Platt, 1996; Gonzalez-Stawinski et al., 2000). The greatest barrier to transplanting pig organs into humans is the immunological rejection of the transplanted organ. Hyperacute rejection and acute vascular xenograft rejection must be overcome to clear the way for routine xenotransplantation. Some investigators engaged in xenotransplantation research in pigs are relatively confident that heart, liver, kidney, and perhaps other organ transplants from pigs to humans will become a clinical reality early in the 21st century through strategies to overcome immunological and physiological hurdles, including the genetic engineering of pigs for this purpose.

C. Phytase and Mineral-Related Metabolic Disorders

Recent interest in phytase depicts another excellent example of interactions among pigs, people, and the environment. Physiologically, pigs and people do not produce phytases (myo-inositol-hexokisphosphate phosphohydrolases) (Wodzinski and Ullah, 1996) and are, therefore, unable to utilize phosphorus of plant sources that are mainly in the form of phytate (myo-inositol-hexokisphosphate) (Reddy et al., 1982). Without other sources of available dietary phosphorus, both humans and pigs would develop rickets in young growing subjects and osteomalacia in adults. Although supplemental calcium phosphate, a nonrenewable source of inorganic phosphorus, effectively meets the nutritional needs of pigs, the excretion of the underutilized dietary phytate phosphorus raises serious environmental concerns (Coffey, 1996). Excessive phosphorus in animal manure may aggravate eutrophication of bodies of water due to soil runoff of phosphorus. In many parts of the world, phosphorus concentrations in manure applied to arable land are now (or will be) strictly regulated.

Attempts to use phytase added to the feed to improve phytate phosphorus utilization were made in the 1960s (Nelson et al., 1968). Because of the anticipated high phytase production cost relative to that of inorganic phosphorus, the potential for phytase was not fully explored (Lei et al., 1993b;

Cromwell et al., 1993) until the last decade. The renewed interest in phytase was driven by the heightened awareness of phosphorus and nitrogen pollution of the environment in the intensive animal production areas. Many experiments have been done to determine the effectiveness, appropriate level, and optimal dietary conditions for supplemental microbial phytase (see Chapter 27 for details). The relatively high cost and inability to resist heat denaturation of phytase in feed pelleting remain two major practical limitations for the use of current commercial phytase. Active research in selecting and engineering more effective and thermostable phytases is being carried out by the academic and private sectors (Pasamontes et al., 1997; Han et al., 1997). Alternatively, certain plant feeds can be used as a phytase source (Han et al., 1997; 1998). Plant breeders are trying to develop low-phytate variants (Raboy, 1998).

The profound potential impact of phytase research in swine nutrition on human health needs to be fully recognized. The effectiveness of microbial phytase in improving phytate phosphorus and calcium utilization in pigs may be adopted to prevent and treat rickets, osteomalacia, or osteoporosis in humans. Equally important, in many developing countries, excessive dietary intake of phytate causes growth retardation and anemia in children and/or childbearing women, because of the chelation of dietary phytate with zinc and iron. Despite many years of efforts by human nutritionists to develop effective supplements, these problems have not been eradicated. The effectiveness of microbial phytase in improving phytate-bound zinc (Lei et al., 1993a) and iron (Stahl et al., 1999) in pigs may provide an innovative approach to tackle these problems.

D. Recombinant DNA–Derived Products

Recombinant DNA techniques have shaped modern biology dramatically. Although these techniques have been relatively underused in swine science, there are examples of successful application. As discussed above, biotechnology has facilitated the development of the commercial phytase that may be used to prevent mineral element malnutrition in humans. Another example is the recognition and identification of a porcine stress syndrome gene associated with halothane sensitivity (Christian, 1974; Smith and Bampton, 1977) and the identification of a mutation in the gene (Fujii et al., 1991) followed by development of a DNA probe to screen for carriers of the gene. In addition, recombinantly derived porcine somatotropin has been tested in many experiments and shown to be effective in partitioning nutrients to increase lean tissue growth (National Research Council, 1994; Etherton and Bauman, 1998). Although its commercial use has not been approved by the U.S. Food and Drug Administration, research in swine with this product of recombinant DNA technology has provided valuable information on regulation of protein and lipid metabolism, which may be relevant to human obesity.

Several groups are mapping the pig genome (Rothschild and Ruvinsky, 1998; Rohrer, 2000). Although the initial interests focus on economically important traits, the data may provide information useful for the study of genetic similarity and diversity between pigs and humans. Another powerful technique with great potential use is the development of gene knockout (gene deletion) pigs to study function and regulation of gene expression *in vivo*. Numerous types of gene knockout mice have been generated to study basic biology and medicine (Cheng et al., 1998). With greater physiological similarities to humans, gene knockout pigs may be a better models for these purposes if current technical obstacles such as establishment of embryonic stem cells can be overcome.

V. PORK IN THE HUMAN DIET

Pork is an excellent source of many nutrients not supplied abundantly by plant materials. It contains large amounts of vitamins and trace mineral elements, and its amino acid balance is much superior to that of most plant proteins. One might consider the pig as an efficient storage depot for fat, including essential fatty acids, and for protein, vitamins, and mineral elements. If one were to purchase each of the nutritional components of pork, i.e., vitamins, amino acids, and minerals, off the shelves of a health food store, the cost of the nutrients provided in a 3-oz chop would be prohibitive.

Pork enjoys good acceptance by consumers worldwide, as discussed earlier in this chapter. The role of the pig as a scavenger in many places and as a family food bank or cash (piggy) bank in many cultures speaks clearly in favor of its survival as an important food source for the foreseeable future. Some argue that pork production cannot be sustained in a world in which the pig competes directly with humans for food. This argument notwithstanding, there are aesthetic, ecological, and nutritional grounds for the pig to survive and flourish.

A. Pork Composition

The chemical composition of pork from pigs of 15 to 20 years ago was described (USDA, 1983). The fat content of pork has declined dramatically since the 1980s, as reflected by increases in protein and decreases in fat percentages in retail carcasses (even at much higher contemporary carcass weights), decreased backfat, and decreased kilocalories per 100 g of retail carcass (National Pork Producers Council, 1998/99).

The USDA Nutrient Database for Standard Reference Release 12 (USDA, 1998a) contains detailed information on composition of raw, cooked, and processed pork and pork products. The nutrient content of fresh pork loin from contemporary pigs is described in Table 1.4. Note the low fat and cholesterol content of pork from modern swine compared with values reported 15 years ago. Cooking reduces the water content so that percentages of protein, fat, and ash are increased appreciably.

In addition to variations in composition related to processing and cooking, there may be variations associated with biological factors such as age, sex, nutritional background, and genetic makeup of the animal. Interactions between and among these factors are not well understood or documented. These and other incompletely explored variables related to pork composition provide opportunities and challenges in swine research, including research in nutrition. Consumers are keenly interested in nutritional attributes and liabilities of food products, and the knowledge to be gained through research related to nutritional factors affecting pork composition will be particularly valuable. Some of these issues are addressed in other chapters (e.g., Chapter 28).

Pork is notable among animal products in its high content of thiamin and unsaturated fatty acids. It is similar to lean beef, lamb, and poultry meat in cholesterol and total fat.

B. Pork Acceptability

In addition to the high nutritive value of pork discussed previously, there are other considerations. The acceptability of pork in relation to other meats depends on aesthetic, economic, cultural, and religious constraints. Variations in palatability factors such as tenderness, juiciness, color, aroma, and flavor are less with pork than with beef and lamb so that differences in age, breed, and environment have a relatively minor effect on pork quality. Color, firmness, and water-holding capacity are included in a general appraisal of quality ranging from pale, soft, and exudative (PSE) to dark, firm, dry (DFD) pork; the most desirable is between these extremes. The amount of intermuscular fat is rather constant and no differences have been noted between PSE and normal muscle in their percentages of protein, fat, and water. The pale color and excessive exudation of PSE pork detracts from its marketability in the retail store.

Other detracting influences on pork acceptability are the boar odor problem and trichinosis. Meat from mature boars has an objectionable odor and flavor when cooked, because of the presence of fat-soluble testosterone derivatives, among them, 5-α-androstenone. Because boars grow faster, require less feed per unit body weight, and produce leaner carcasses than castrated males, it would be advantageous to producers and consumers if boar odor could be removed without castration. Technologies to accomplish this goal are being explored. If these technologies reach commercial

TABLE 1.4
Nutrient Content of Fresh Pork Loin, Separable Lean and Fat

Nutrient	Units	Value per 100 g	Nutrient	Units	Value per 100 g
Water	g	66.920	Fatty acids, mono.	g	5.610
Energy	kcal	198.000	16:1	g	0.360
Energy	kJ	828.000	18:1	g	5.140
Protein	g	19.740	20:1	g	0.090
Lipid	g	12.580	22:1	g	0.000
Carbohydrate	g	0.000	Fatty acids, poly.	g	1.340
Fiber	g	0.000	18:2	g	1.110
Ash	g	0.960	18:3	g	0.090
Minerals			18.4	g	0.000
Calcium	mg	18.000	20:4	g	0.080
Iron	mg	0.790	20:5	g	0.000
Magnesium	mg	21.000	22:5	g	0.000
Phosphorus	mg	197.000	22:6	g	0.000
Potassium	mg	356.000	Cholesterol	mg	63.000
Sodium	mg	50.000	Amino acids		
Zinc	mg	1.740	Tryptophan	g	0.224
Copper	mg	0.056	Threonine	g	0.891
Manganese	mg	0.011	Isoleucine	g	0.910
Selenium	µg	33.200	Leucine	g	1.572
Vitamins			Lysine	g	1.766
Vitamin C (ascorbic acid)	mg	0.600	Methionine	g	0.524
Thiamin	mg	0.901	Cystine	g	0.248
Riboflavin	mg	0.248	Phenylalanine	g	0.785
Niacin	mg	4.580	Tyrosine	g	0.676
Pantothenic acid	mg	0.723	Valine	g	1.064
Vitamin B-6	mg	0.472	Arginine	g	1.245
Folate	µg	5.000	Histidine	g	0.770
Vitamin B-12	µg	0.530	Alanine	g	1.158
Vitamin A	IU	7.000	Aspartic acid	g	1.814
Vitamin A	RE	2.000	Glutamic acid	g	3.044
Vitamin E	ATE	0.290	Glycine	g	1.019
Lipids			Proline	g	0.838
Fatty acids, sat.	g	4.360	Serine	g	0.815
4:0	g	0.000			
6:0	g	0.000			
8:0	g	0.000			
10:0	g	0.010			
12:0	g	0.010			
14:0	g	0.160			
16:0	g	2.720			
18:0	g	1.420			

Source: USDA Nutrient Database for Standard Reference, Release 12, Nutrient Data Laboratory, Agricultural Research Service, Beltsville Human Nutrition Research Center, Riverdale, MD 20737. Available at http://www.nal.usda.gov/fnic/foodcomp/Data/index.html.

application, there will be a need for further quantification of the nutritional requirements of boars for meat production.

The persistence of the parasite, *Trichinella spiralis*, has been a detriment to the consumption of pork everywhere. This is still true despite the fact that in the United States the number of reported human cases of trichinosis has declined to a few cases annually. Nevertheless, the perception of a threat of infection from eating undercooked pork persists disproportionately to its actual importance. *Trichinella* organisms are destroyed by heating pork to an internal temperature of 77°C, by freezing it for 20 days at −15°C or by gamma irradiation, a procedure recently approved for use in the United States.

C. Societal Issues

In an increasingly large and urbanized population less familiar with agriculture, the role of animal agriculture, including pork production, in society is being challenged. Issues of particular concern in pork production include animal well-being, food safety, and environmental stability. Food safety concerns include the threat of pork contamination with pathogenic strains of organisms such as *Salmonella, Escherichia coli*, and *Campylobacter*. The industry is addressing these concerns aggressively by developing control measures at the farm, in pork slaughter and processing facilities, and in wholesale and retail handling. The recent approval in the United States of the use of gamma irradiation to destroy pathogens before pork reaches the consumer will have a further beneficial effect on food safety. The long-standing effectiveness of subtherapeutic levels of antibiotics fed to swine to improve growth and reproductive performance is undergoing continued scrutiny. Concerns have been raised for many years, and have recently escalated, over the consequences of the development of strains of pathogens with resistance to antibiotics used in swine feeding. These three issues, animal well-being, antibiotic resistance, and environmental stability, are addressed briefly here.

1. Animal Well-Being

Pork producers and research scientists using the pig as an animal model are acutely aware of, and sympathetic toward, the public concerns for the well-being of animals used in food production and research (Ewing et al., 1998). They recognize the need for greater acquisition and application of knowledge to ensure that pigs are treated humanely and afforded an environment conducive to their well-being. Federal, state, and institutional animal care guidelines are in use in research laboratories and on farms to achieve this end. Continuous dialogue and education to maintain the public trust is a critical ongoing commitment to assure the well-being of pigs.

2. Antibiotic Resistance

Antibiotics have been added to pig diets at subtherapeutic levels for more than 50 years to improve growth and reproductive performance. Improvements of 3 to 10% in performance of pigs fed antibiotics have been sustained over the entire 50 years, representing data on thousands of pigs in hundreds of research settings (NRC, 1998a). Yet, continual challenges are levied to ban the use of antibiotics in pig feeds because of the development of strains of pathogenic organisms resistant to specific antibiotics. Such resistance poses a potential human health threat; however, clear evidence of a relationship between antibiotic resistance and human health remains unavailable. Several countries prohibit the use of antibiotics in pig diets; if a similar ban were imposed in the United States, the cost of pork production would be increased appreciably. As in any decision regarding safety and health issues, risk–benefit relationships must be assessed. The ultimate action will be based on economic and human health perceptions and considerations and will most certainly affect pork prices and consumption. These issues are discussed in detail in Chapter 18.

3. Environmental Stability

The trend toward large, intensive pork production units in the United States has been accompanied by public concerns about air, water, soil, and general environmental pollution. Such concerns have led to litigation, tightened regulations on new and expanded pork production facilities, and ultimately to shifts in geographic location of U.S. pork production units and a movement toward large, extensive, low-cost production facilities located on large land areas in the High Plains and arid Southwest.

Globally, the increased demand for pork (discussed earlier in the chapter) requires increases in feed resources whose production has the potential to change cropping patterns and land use. Disruption of environmental stability brought about by such shifts must be addressed and curtailed.

VI. SUMMARY

Pigs and humans have lived in partnership for centuries. The pig is able to respond favorably to widely different environments and to the changing needs of humans. The pig contributes to society in two important ways: (1) as a major human food resource worldwide and (2) as an animal model in biomedical research. This introductory chapter describes domestication, demographic relationships between pigs and people, anatomical and physiological similarities, the pig as a model animal in biomedical research and in clinical applications in humans, and as pork as human food. Finally, the chapter addresses societal issues concerning animal well-being, food safety, including antibiotic resistance, and environmental stability in relation to the use of the pig in food production.

REFERENCES

Ackerman, M. R. 2000. The respiratory tract. In *Biology of the Domestic Pig*, Pond, W. G., and H. J. Mersmann, Eds., Cornell University Press, Ithaca, NY, chap. 10.

Argenzio, R. A., and N. Monteiro-Riviere. 2000. Excretory System. In *Biology of the Domestic Pig*, Pond, W. G., and H. J. Mersmann, Eds., Cornell University Press, Ithaca, NY, chap. 13.

Ball, R. O., J. D. House, L. J. Wykes, and P. B. Pencharz. 1996. A piglet model for neonatal amino acid metabolism during total parenteral nutrition. In *Advances in Swine in Biomedical Research*, Tumbleson, M. E., and L. B. Schook, Eds., Plenum Press, New York, chap. 63, p. 713.

Boleman, S. L., T. L. Graf, H. J. Mersmann, D. R. Su, L. P. Krook, J. W. Savell, Y. W. Park, and W. G. Pond. 1998. Pigs fed cholesterol neonatally have increased cerebrum cholesterol as young adults, *J. Nutr.*, 128:2498.

Brown, D. R., and J. M. Terris. 1996. Swine in physiological and pathophysiological research. In *Advances in Swine in Biomedical Research*, Tumbleson, M. E., and L. B. Schook, Eds., Plenum Press, New York, chap. 2, p. 5.

Buddington, R. K., C. Malo, and H. Zhang. 1996. Prenatal and perinatal development of intestinal transport and brush border hydrolases in pigs. In *Advances in Swine in Biomedical Research*, Tumbleson, M. E., and L. B. Schook, Eds., Plenum Press, New York, chap. 66, p. 757.

Burrin, D. G. 2000. Nutrient requirements and metabolism. In *Biology of the Domestic Pig*, Pond, W. G., and H. J. Mersmann, Eds., Cornell University Press, Ithaca, NY, chap. 7.

Burrin, D. G., T. A. Davis, S. Ebner, P. A. Schoknecht, M. L. Fiorotto, P. J. Reeds, and S. McAvoy. 1995. Nutrient independent and nutrient dependent factors stimulate protein synthesis in colostrum-fed newborn pigs, *Pediatric Res.*, 37:593.

Burrin, D. G., T. A. Davis, S. Ebner, P. A. Schoknecht, M. L. Fiorotto, and P. J. Reeds. 1997. Colostrum enhances the nutritional stimulation of vital organ protein synthesis in neonatal pigs, *J. Nutr.*, 127:1284.

Bustad, L. K., and R. O. McClellan. 1966. *Swine in Biomedical Research*, Pacific Northwest Laboratory, Richland, WA.

Chandra, G., M. Oli, B. W. Petschow, and R. K. Buddington. 1996. Changes in pig intestinal structure and functions and resident microbiota induced by acute secretory diarrhea. In *Advances in Swine in Biomedical Research*, Tumbleson, M. E., and L. B. Schook, Eds., Plenum Press, New York, chap. 67, p. 769.

Cheng, W.-H., Y-S. Ho, B. A. Valentine, D. A. Ross, G. F. Combs, Jr., and X. G. Lei. 1998. Cellular glutathione peroxidase is the mediator of body selenium to protect against paraquat lethality in transgenic mice, *J. Nutr.*, 128:1070.

Christian, L. L. 1974. Halothane test for PSS-field application. In *Proc. Amer. Assoc. Swine Practioners Conf.*, Des Moines, IA, 6–13.

Coffey, M. T. 1996. Environmental challenges as related to animal agriculture-swine. In *Nutrient Management of Food Animals to Enhance and Protect the Environment*, E. T. Kornegay, Ed., Lewis Publishers, Boca Raton, FL, pp. 29–39.

Cromwell, G. L., T. S. Stahly, R. D. Coffey, H. J. Monenque, and J. H. Randolph. 1993. Efficacy of phytase in improving the bioavailabilty of phosphorus in soybean meal and corn–soybean meal diets for pigs, *J. Anim. Sci.*, 71:1831.

Cunha, T. J. 1977. *Swine Feeding and Nutrition*, Academic Press, New York.

Davidson, S., R. Passmore, J. F. Brock, and A. S. Tresswell. 1979. *Human Nutrition and Dietetics*, 7th ed., Churchill-Livingstone, New York.

Donovan, S. M., V. M. Houle, M. H. Monaco, E. A. Schroeder, Y. Park, and J. Odle. 1996. The neonatal pig as a model to study insulin-like growth factor mediated intestinal growth and function. In *Advances in Swine in Biomedical Research*, Tumbleson, M. E., and L. B. Schook, Eds., Plenum Press, New York, chap. 64, p. 733.

Etherton, T. D., and D. E. Bauman. 1998. Biology of somatotropin in growth and lactation of domestic animals, *Physiol. Rev.*, 78:745.

Ewing, S. A, D. C. Lay, Jr., and E. von Borell. 1998. *Farm Animal Well-Being*, Prentice-Hall, Upper Saddle River, NJ.

Ferrell, C. L., and S. Cornelius. 1984. Estimation of body composition of pigs, *J. Anim. Sci.*, 58:903.

Fujii, J., K. O. F. Otsu, F. Zorzato, S. de Leon, V. K. Khanna, J. Weiler, P. J. O'Brien, and D. H. MacLennan. 1991. Identification of a mutation in the porcine ryanodine receptor that is associated with malignant hyperthermia, *Science,* 253:448.

Gomez, G. G., E. J. Rozhon, R. A. Goforth, and O. Thirakoune. 1996. An experimental rotaviral enteritit model with neonatal pigs. In *Advances in Swine in Biomedical Research*, Tumbleson, M. E., and L. B. Schook, Eds., Plenum Press, New York, chap. 69, p. 811.

Gonzalez-Stawinski, G. V., S. S. Lin, and J. L. Platt. 2000. Xenotransplantation. In *Biology of the Domestic Pig,* Pond, W. G. and H. J. Mersmann, Eds., Cornell University Press, Ithaca, NY.

Gootman, P. M. 2000. The cardiovascular system. In *Biology of the Domestic Pig,* Pond, W. G., and H. J. Mersmann, Eds., Cornell University Press, Ithaca, NY.

Graf, T. L., S. L. Boleman, L. P. Krook, D. R. Su, H. J. Mersmann, J. L. Savell, and W. G. Pond. 1998. Effect of neonatal dietary cholesterol deprivation on plasma lipids and early atherogenesis in pigs with genetically high or low plasma cholesterol, *Nutr. Res.*, 18:1615.

Hackman, A. M., W. G. Pond, H. J. Mersmann, W. W. Wong, L. P. Krook, and S. Zhang. 1996. Obese pigs fed a high cholesterol diet from birth to 2 months are less susceptible than lean pigs to atherosclerosis, *J. Nutr.*, 126:564.

Han, Y. M., F. Yang, A. G. Zhou, E. R. Miller, P. K. Ku, M. G. Hogberg, and X. G. Lei. 1997. Supplemental phytases of microbial and cereal sources improve dietary phytate phosphorus utilization by pigs from weaning through finishing, *J. Anim. Sci.*, 75:1017.

Han, Y. M., K. R. Ronneker, W. G. Pond, and X. G. Lei. 1998. Addition of wheat middlings, microbial phytase, and citric acid to corn–soybean meal diets for growing pigs may replace inorganic phosphorus supplementation, *J. Anim. Sci.*, 76:2649.

Han, Y. M., D. B. Wilson, and X. G. Lei. 1999. Expression of an *Aspergillus niger* phytase (phyA) in *Saccharomyces cerevisiae*, *Appl. Environ. Microbiol.*, 65:1915.

Hetzer, H. O., and W. R. Harvey. 1967. Selection for high and low fatness in swine, *J. Anim. Sci.*, 26:1244.

Jahoor, F., L. Wykes, M. Del Rosario, M. Frazer, and P. J. Reeds. 1999. Chronic protein undernutrition and an acute inflammatory stimulus elicit different protein kinetic responses in plasma but not in muscle of piglets, *J. Nutr.*, 129:693.

Krakowka, S., and K. A. Eaton. 1996. *Helicobacter pylori* infection in gnotobiotic piglets: a model of human gastric bacterial disease. In *Advances in Swine in Biomedical Research*, Tumbleson, M. E., and L. B. Schook, Eds., Plenum Press, New York, chap. 68, p. 779.

Lei, X. G., P. K. Ku, E. R. Miller, D. E. Ullrey, and M. T. Yokoyama. 1993a. Supplemental microbial phytase improves bioavailability of dietary zinc to weanling pigs, *J. Nutr.*, 123:1117.

Lei, X. G., P. K. Ku, E. R. Miller, and M. T. Yokoyama. 1993b. Supplementing corn–soybean meal diets with microbial phytase improves phytate phosphorus utilization by weanling pigs, *J. Anim. Sci.*, 71:3359.

Lin, S. S., and J. L. Platt. 1996. Immunologic advances towards clinical xenotranplantation. In *Advances in Swine in Biomedical Research*, Tumbleson, M. E., and L. B. Schook, Eds., Plenum Press, New York, chap. 16, p. 147.

Mellen, I. M. 1952. *The Natural History of the Pig*, Exposition Press, New York.

Mersmann, H. J. 1986. Lipid metabolism in swine. In *Swine in Cardiovascular Research*, Stanton, H. C., and H. J. Mersmann, Eds., CRC Press, Boca Raton, FL, Vol. 1, chap. 6, p. 75.

Mersmann, H. J., and W. G. Pond. 2000. Hematology and blood serum constituents. In *Biology of the Domestic Pig*, Pond, W. G., and H. J. Mersmann, Eds., Cornell University Press, Ithaca, NY, chap. 12.

Miller, E. R., and D. E. Ullrey. 1987. The pig as a model for human nutrition, *Annu. Rev. Nutr.*, 7:361.

Miller, E. R., D. E. Ullrey, and A. J. Lewis. 1991. *Swine Nutrition*, Butterworth-Heinemann, Boston, MA.

Mitchell, A. D., A. M. Scholz, and H. J. Mersmann. 2000. Growth and body composition. In *Biology of the Domestic Pig*, Pond, W. G., and H. J. Mersmann, Eds., Cornell University Press, Ithaca, NY, chap. 6.

Monteiro-Riviere, N. 2000. Integument. In *Biology of the Domestic Pig*, Pond, W. G., and H. J. Mersmann, Eds., Cornell University Press, Ithaca, NY, chap. 14.

Moran, E. T., Jr. 1982. *Comparative Nutrition of Fowl and Swine: The Gasrointestinal Systems*, Office of Educational Practice, University of Guelph, Guelph, Ontario, Canada.

National Pork Producers Council. 1998/99. *Pork Facts*, National Pork Producers Council, Des Moines, IA.

National Research Council. 1994. *Metabolic Modulators: Effects on the Nutrient Requirements of Food-Producing Animals*, National Academy Press, Washington, D.C.

National Research Council. 1998a. *Nutrient Requirements of Swine*, 10th ed., National Academy Press, Washington, D.C.

National Research Council. 1998b. *Recommended Nutrient Allowances for Humans*, National Academy Press, Washington, D.C.

Nelson, T. S., T. R. Shieh, R. J. Wodzinski, and J. H. Ware. 1968. The availability of phytate phosphorus in soybean meal before and after treatment with a mold phytase, *Poult. Sci.*, 47:1842.

Panepinto, L. 1996. Miniature swine breeds used worldwide in research. In *Advances in Swine in Biomedical Research*, Tumbleson, M. E., and L. B. Schook, Eds., Plenum Press, New York, chap. 60, p. 681.

Pasamontes, L., M. Haiker, M. Wyss, M. Tessier, and A. P. G. M. van Loon. 1997. Gene cloning, purification, and characterization of a heat-stable phytase from the fungus *Aspergillus fumigatus*, *Appl. Environ. Microbiol.*, 63:1696.

Petters, R. M. 1994. Transgenic livestock as genetic model systems for human diseases, *Reprod. Fertil. Dev.*, 6:643.

Pond, W. G. 1982. Nutrition and heart disease: the pig as an experimental model. In *Pig Model for Biomedical Research*, Roberts, H. R., and W. J. Dodds, Eds., Pig Research Institute of Taiwan, Miaoli, Taiwan, Republic of China, p. 43.

Pond, W. G., and K. A. Houpt. 1978. *Biology of the Pig*, Cornell University Press, Ithaca, NY.

Pond, W. G., and J. H. Maner. 1974. *Swine Production in Temperate and Tropical Environments*, W. H. Freeman, San Francisco, CA.

Pond, W. G., and H. J. Mersmann. 1996. Genetically diverse pig models in nutrition research related to lipoprotein and cholesterol metabolism. In *Advances in Swine in Biomedical Research*, Tumbleson, M. E., and L. B. Schook, Eds., Plenum Press, New York, chap. 72, p. 843.

Pond, W. G., and H. J. Mersmann. 2000. *Biology of the Domestic Pig*, Cornell University Press, Ithaca, NY.

Pond, W. G., J. H. Maner, and D. L. Harris. 1991. *Pork Production Systems*, Van Nostrand Reinhold, New York.

Pond, W. G., K. J. Ellis, H. J. Mersmann, J. P. Heath, L. P. Krook, D. G. Burrin, M. A. Dudley, and H.-P. Sheng. 1996. Severe protein deficiency and repletion alter body and brain composition and organ weights in infant pigs, *J. Nutr.*, 126:290.

Porter, V. 1993. *Pigs: A Handbook to the Breeds of the World*, Cornell University Press, Ithaca, NY.

Pursel, V. G., M. B. Solomon, and R. J. Wall. 1996. Genetic engineering of swine. In *Advances in Swine in Biomedical Research*, Tumbleson, M. E., and L. B. Schook, Eds., Plenum Press, New York, chap. 19, p. 189.

Raboy, V. 1998. Low phytic acid grain crops. *Proc. Cornell Nutr. Conf. for Feed Manufacturers*, Cornell University, Ithaca, NY, pp. 158–165.

Reddy, N. R., S. K. Sathe, and D. K. Salunkhe. 1982. Phytates in legumes and cereals, *Adv. Food Res.*, 28:1.

Reeds, P., and J. Odle. 1996. Pigs as models for nutrient functional interaction. In *Advances in Swine in Biomedical Research*, Tumbleson, M. E., and L. B. Schook, Eds., Plenum Press, New York.

Roberts, H. R., and W. J. Dodds, Eds. 1982. *Pig Model for Biomedical Research*, Pig Research Institute of Taiwan, Miaoli, Taiwan, Republic of China.

Rohrer, G. A. 2000. Genetics. In *Biology of the Domestic Pig,* Pond, W. G., and H. I. Mersmann, Eds., Cornell University Press, Ithaca, NY, chap. 4.

Rothchild, M. F., and A. Ruvinsky. 1998. *The Genetics of the Pig*, CAB International, New York.

Scarpelli, D. G., G. Migaki, and J. M. Pletcher. 1991. Transgenic animal models in biomedical research, *Symposium Proceedings*, National Institutes of Health, Bethesda, MD, 1–114.

Schoknecht, P. A., S. Ebner, W. G. Pond, S. Zhang, V. McWhinney, W. W. Wong, P. D. Klein, M. Dudley, J. Goddard-Finegold, and H. J. Mersmann. 1994a. Dietary cholesterol supplementation improves growth and behavioral response of pigs selected for genetically high or low serum cholesterol, *J. Nutr.*, 124:305.

Schoknecht, P. A., G. R. Newton, D. E. Weiss, and W. G. Pond. 1994b. Protein restriction in early pregnancy alters fetal and placental growth and allantoic fluid proteins in swine, *Theriogenology,* 42:217.

Smith, C., and P. R. Brampton. 1977. Inheritance of reaction to halothane anesthesia in pigs, *Genet. Res. Camb.*, 29:287.

Stahl, C. H., Y. M. Han, K. R. Ronneker, W. A. House, and X. G. Lei. 1999. Phytase improves iron bioavailability for hemoglobin synthesis in young pigs, *J. Anim. Sci.*, 77:2135.

Stanton, H. C., and H. J. Mersmann. 1986. *Swine in Cardiovascular Research*, Vols. I and II, CRC Press, Boca Raton, FL.

Terris, J. M. 1986. Swine as a model in renal physiology and nephrology: an overview. In *Swine in Biomedical Research*, Vol. 3, Tumbleson, M. E., Ed., Plenum Press, New York, p. 1673.

Towne, C. W., and E. N. Wentworth. 1950. *Pigs from Cave to Cornbelt*, University of Oklahoma Press, Norman, OK.

Tumbleson, M. E. 1986. *Swine in Biomedical Research*, Vols. 1, 2, and 3, Plenum Press, New York.

Tumbleson, M. E., and L. C. Schook. 1996. *Advances in Swine in Biomedical Research*, Vols. I and II, Plenum Press, New York.

USDA. 1983. Composition of Foods. Pork Products. Agricultural Handbook No. 8–10. Consumer Nutrition Division, Human Nutrition Information Service, USDA, Washington, D.C.

USDA. 1998a. Nutrient Database for Standard Reference Release 12. Nutrient Data Laboratory, Beltsville Human Nutrition Center, Agricultural Research Service, Riverdale, MD.

USDA. 1998b. World Pork Production. Foreign Agricultural Service, USDA, Washington, D.C.

Wagner, E. F., and F. Theuring. 1993. *Transgenic Animal as Model Systems for Human Diseases*, Schering Foundation Workshop 6, Springer-Verlag, New York, pp. 1–151.

Wodzinski, R. J., and A. H. J. Ullah. 1996. Phytase, *Adv. Appl. Microbiol.*, 42:263.

Wu, G., W. G. Pond, S. P. Flynn, T. L. Ott, and F. W. Bazer. 1998. Maternal dietary protein deficiency decreases nitric oxide synthase and ornithine decarboxylase activities in placenta and endometrium of pigs during early gestation, *J. Nutr.*, 128:2395.

Yen, J. T. 2000. Digestive system. In *Biology of the Domestic Pig,* Pond, W. G., and H. J. Mersmann, Eds., Cornell University Press, Ithaca, NY, chap. 8.

2 General Characteristics of the U.S. Swine Industry

Gilbert R. Hollis and Stanley E. Curtis

CONTENTS

I.   The Past 19
II. The Present 20
III. The Future 23
IV. Carcass Variables 24
V.   Production Systems 24
    A.   Farrowing Facilities 25
    B.   Nursery Facilities 27
    C.   Growing-Finishing Facilities 27
    D.   Breeding Facilities 28
    E.   Gestation Facilities 29
References 30

I. THE PAST

Pigs were traditionally kept in the United States as an adjunct to a crop production enterprise, used to add value to corn when corn prices were down. Very little effort was made to improve the genetic base, optimize productivity, or foster consumer acceptance of pork as a commodity in its own right. Pork production was heavily concentrated in the Midwestern Corn Belt states because of the readily available supply of feeds. Pork producers generally managed farrow-to-finish units; the pigs were bred, born, and raised to market weight in one group on one operation.

From the late 1880s through the late 1940s, consumer demand for lard was so strong that pork producers obliged consumers by raising relatively fat hogs. During World Wars I and II, pork went to war, providing the basis for "C" and "K" rations for soldiers in the field. The fat derived from the pig also went into the making of nitroglycerine for use in explosives.

The end of World War II brought great changes in the pork industry. The market for lard and other by-products of fat from hogs started to decline, and consumers began thinking more about health and diet, increasing the demand for leaner meat. In the early 1950s, U.S. pork producers concentrated their efforts on developing a leaner hog that would meet the demand for pork lower in cholesterol and fat.

Approximately 100,000 pork producers are in business today (Figure 2.1) compared with nearly 3,000,000 in 1950. Farms have grown in size. Over 80% of the hogs are grown on farms producing 1000 or more hogs per year, and over half are grown on farms producing 2000 or more. These operations, which are often very sophisticated technologically, are still predominantly individual family farms.

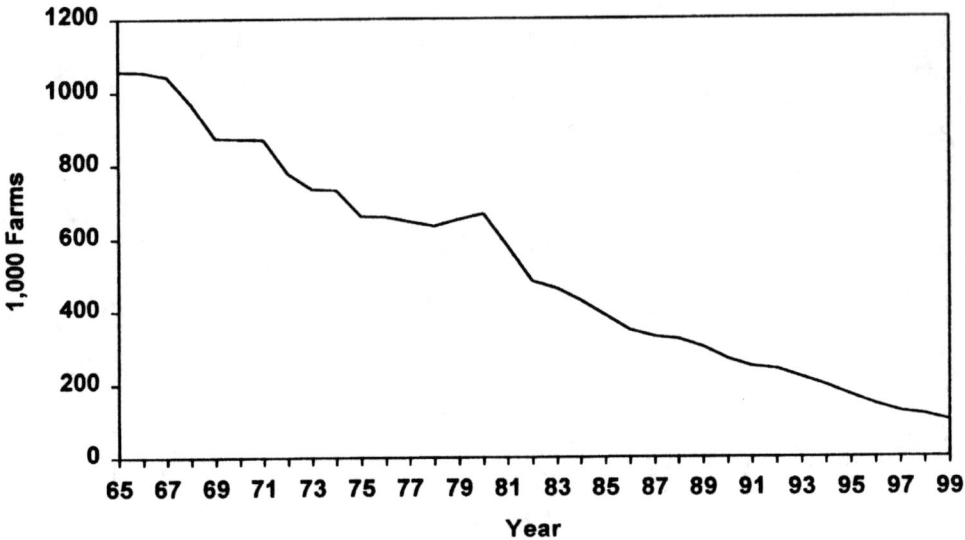

FIGURE 2.1 The number of hog operations has declined steadily since 1944. The greatest losses occurred from 1944 to 1964 when nearly 1.1 million pork producers left the industry. This reduction was caused by the post-war economic boom, which created a mass exodus from agricultural jobs to generally higher-paying manufacturing jobs. (From NASS, 1999.)

II. THE PRESENT

During the 1980s and 1990s, pork production expanded in regions outside the Midwest, particularly in the Southeastern Coastal and High Plains states. At the same time, major technological developments were occurring in the industry. Breeding programs were developed that resulted in pigs with the genetic capability for increased reproductive efficiency and lean muscle growth (with resulting increases in feed efficiency). These programs captured economies of scale and developed pig-raising methods that controlled diseases, thereby improving productive efficiency. Further, production practices are no longer limited to farrow-to-finish operations.

Today's swine industry has evolved from generalized to specialized. The large majority of hogs are still produced in the north central states (Table 2.1). However, the 11 states composing the north central region lost 10.3% of the 1998 breeding herd during 1999. North Carolina and Oklahoma continue to be the fastest growing states in total hog numbers. In 1990 North Carolina had only 5% of the U.S. breeding herd but now has over 14.9% and is second only to Iowa in level of production. Arkansas, Colorado, Oklahoma, and Pennsylvania — considerably less important hog states than North Carolina — have shown strong growth in the last 2 years, but account for a little more than half of the North Carolina herd (NASS, 1999a).

As the number of hog farms has decreased (Figure 2.1), farm size has grown as further economies of scale have been sought (Figure 2.2). The number of large farms has grown exponentially, to the extent that most of the marketplace is now controlled by farms producing more than 2000 head per year (Figures 2.3 and 2.4). Specialized operations came into being, and segregated early weaning (SEW) and multisite production schemes were adopted to increase production efficiency, both biologically and financially (see Production Systems section). Segregated early weaning improved herd health and enabled producers to customize feeding programs. These kinds of specialized operations include breeding, farrowing, nursery, and growing-finishing units (Figure 2.5). More recently, as the industry has sought to reduce production costs and improve overall profitabiity, the concept of wean-to-finish buildings has been adopted.

TABLE 2.1
Location of Hogs: Top 10 States

	Dec. 1, 1999 Inventory	
State Rank	State	Total Breeding Inventory (thousand)
1	Iowa	1160
2	North Carolina	1000
3	Minnesota	560
4	Illinois	420
5	Missouri	410
6	Nebraska	390
7	Indiana	370
8	Oklahoma	310
9	Colorado	210
10	Ohio	170
	Total — All States	6244

Source: National Agricultural Statistics Service (NASS, 1999a), Agricultural Statistics Board, U.S. Department of Agriculture.

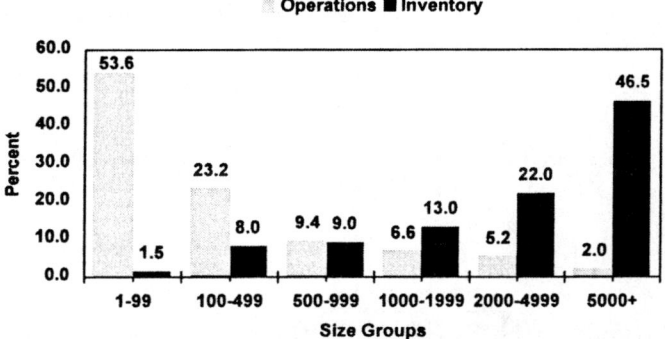

FIGURE 2.2 U.S. hog farms by size group. As the number of hog operations declined, the industry has moved to larger-scale production. Changes have occurred primarily in the largest and smallest groups of producers. The largest operations have gained the greatest market share and the very smallest are showing the greatest loss. This figure shows that in 1999, 2.0% of all hog farms produced 46.5% of U.S. hogs, whereas 86.2% of all hog farms produced 18.5% of U.S. hogs. The remaining 35.0% of the U.S. hogs were produced by 11.8% of all hog farms. (From NASS, 1999.)

Feed is the major production input to the swine production system, representing over 65% of all production expenses. The average whole-herd feed-efficiency (kilograms of live weight gain per kilogram of feed) for the U.S. swine industry is 0.28, and continues to decrease (Figure 2.6). This figure includes the feed fed to the boars and sows. Some U.S. herds now have whole-herd feed-efficiencies greater than 0.33.

The U.S. pork industry has experienced unprecedented growth and change in the 1990s. More pork was produced and more hogs slaughtered in 1998 than ever before, reaching 18.69 billion pounds and 101.028 million animals, respectively (NASS, 1999b). This led to the lowest average market prices for hogs, in December, 1998, since 1972, so total production numbers probably will decline in the short-term future.

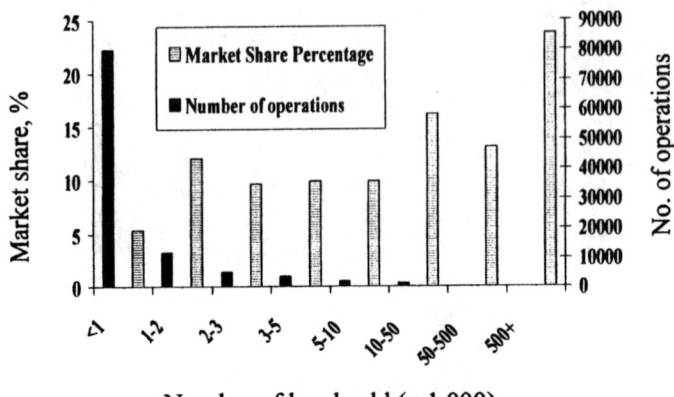

FIGURE 2.3 Estimated number of operations and share of U.S. slaughter 1997, by size category. Consolidation of the U.S. pork industry has occurred for the last 10 years. However, the changes are occurring in the largest and smallest groups of producers. The largest operations are gaining the greatest market share and the very smallest are showing the greatest loss. In 1997, 145 firms producing 50,000 hogs or more a year marketed approximately 36.9 million head. This compares with 16 million head from 66 firms in that size class in 1994. Another 51.7 million hogs (58%) were marked by an estimated 23,400 operations selling 1000 to 49,999 head a year. The remaining 5% of the hogs were marketed by approximately 80,000 farms selling fewer than 1000 hogs annually based on USDA estimate of the number of farms with hogs. (From Lawrence et al., Staff paper 311, Department of Economics, Iowa State University, Ames, 1998.)

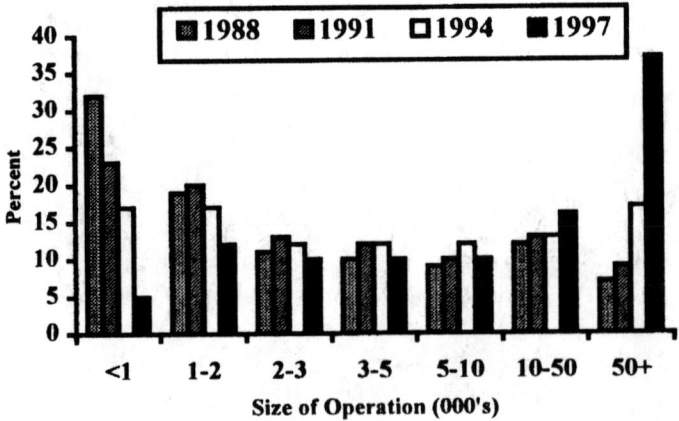

FIGURE 2.4 U.S. hogs produced by size of operation. The trend to fewer and larger operations has accelerated in the past 10 years. Over the last 10 years the share of hogs produced by firms marketing 50,000 head or more has increased from 7% in 1998 to 37% in 1997. During this same period operations marketing fewer than 1000 head dropped from 32 to 5%. (From Lawrence et al., Staff paper 311, Department of Economics, Iowa State University, Ames, 1998.)

General Characteristics of the U.S. Swine Industry

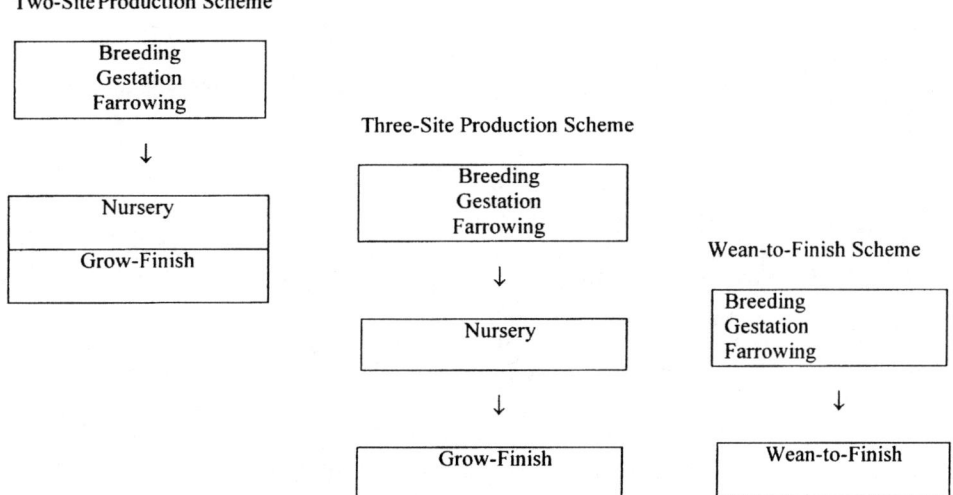

FIGURE 2.5 Production schemes. Production schemes are of three types: (1) two-site, (2) three-site, and (3) wean-to-finish.

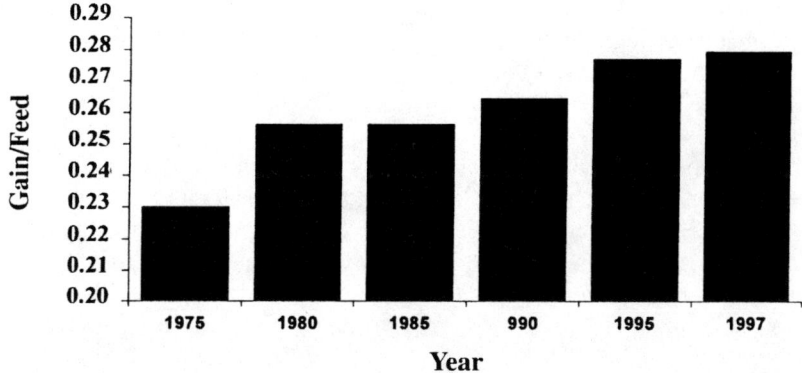

FIGURE 2.6 Gain per kilogram of feed has also improved over the years. Much of this can be attributed to improved genetics, improved nutritional programs, especially for early-weaned pigs, phase feeding, and separate-sex feeding. Since feed represents 60 to 65% of the cost of production, this improvement in feed efficiency provides more opportunity for profit. (From Holden, P. J., personal communication, 1999.)

Farm receipts from hogs place the industry in fourth or fifth position among all farm commodities. Annual farm sales usually exceed $11 billion, whereas the retail value of pork exceeds $30 billion. Pork production and processing is responsible for over $66 billion of economic activity. Through direct, indirect, and induced effects, it supports over 760,000 full-time-equivalent jobs and generates $23 billion in personal income in the United States (Lawrence, 1995).

III. THE FUTURE

The U.S. swine industry is undergoing a paradigm shift as it strives to remain competitive in a global economy. Pork production may no longer need to be located where the resource base or infrastructure has traditionally been located. Any such major shift will have important implications. Alternatively, legislative initiatives regarding environmental standards and legislation attempting to control who may produce pork may drive industry trends. In addition, the issues of what areas of the United States will welcome the swine industry in the future may become critical.

The challenge to colocate animal and crop production to achieve long-term nutrient balance is a likely national goal. Pressure to reduce livestock production near urban centers could result in pig breeding and finishing operations located in the states peripheral to the Midwest corn belt, with feeder pigs then being moved to the grain centers for growing and finishing.

An example of a production practice that might well occur would be the development of vertically coordinated operations; multiple businesses owned by proprietors, partners, or public or private corporations coordinated in a linked chain to meet consumer needs at the lowest possible cost of production. An example of production steps taken in such a business would be (1) breeding and farrowing units; (2) weaned piglets transferred to separate nursery sites; (3) feeder pigs moved to separate growing-finishing units; and (4) finished pigs weighing about 120 kg transported to market. In some cases, vertically coordinated businesses might also include meat processing and marketing steps.

The global market offers tremendous growth potential for U.S. pork producers. Pork is the meat of choice, with an approximately 43% share of the world meat protein market. The U.S. pork industry is steadily increasing its share of this world market, exporting about 5.6% of its production in 1996 after becoming a net exporter in 1995 for the first time since 1952. With many of the world's most cost-efficient producers, the U.S. pork industry is poised to capture even more of the global pork business as trade barriers fall under terms of the North American Free Trade Association (NAFTA) and General Agreements on Trade and Tarriffs (GATT).

Long-term, many other forces are converging to shape the future structure of the U.S. swine industry. They include obsolescence of facilities and the resulting need to recapitalize. Management transfer is also occurring, brought about by the aging of many pork producers. The question is the extent to which the next generation will be interested in being engaged in the pork production business.

Some industry experts now discuss a scenario where 50 pork production firms would produce the majority of the U.S. product by 2010. Some of these may be large-scale cooperative structures, with thousands of individual operations, all tied to a branded-product marketing approach. Others may be corporate integrators. They would represent dramatic shifts away from the traditional spot-market system of hog marketing to an agreement-based system, and would facilitate alignment of pork production with brand labels.

IV. CARCASS VARIABLES

Compared with the pig of 1940s, today's pig features a carcass with 50% less fat. Pigs then averaged 7.3 cm of backfat compared with less than 2.3 cm today. Today's pig yields a pork loin with 77% less fat and 53% fewer calories. Most cuts of pork contain less than 200 kcal per 85 g cooked serving.

Consumers, and consequently packers, prefer lean pork. U.S. pork producers are raising leaner, more heavily muscled pigs to satisfy these demands. Significant improvements were made in carcass leanness, especially during the 1990s (Table 2.2). This leaner pork is the result of new pork production technology, including the use of superior genetics. Virtually all market pigs are produced by crossing purebred breeds or synthetic lines to take advantage of heterosis.

V. PRODUCTION SYSTEMS

Swine can be raised in a variety of production environments, including (1) environmentally controlled buildings where pigs reside; (2) open-front buildings that permit the pigs to go outside; and (3) outside (pasture) production. The reader is referred to the *Swine Care Handbook* published by the National Pork Producers Council (1999) and the *Pork Industry Handbook* (1999) published

TABLE 2.2
Changes in Muscling (Loin Eye Area) and Carcass Backfat, 1956–1999

Year	Loin Eye Area (cm^2)	Backfat (cm)	Average Slaughter Weight (kg)
1956	26.2	3.61[a]	98.4
1960	28.8	3.56[a]	96.3
1966	32.0	3.23[a]	98.4
1970	34.2	2.97[a]	99.8
1975	34.2	3.17[a]	107.0
1980	29.6	2.64[b]	96.6
1985	30.2	2.92[b]	103.0
1990	31.8	2.79[b]	104.3
1995	43.2	1.80[b]	109.1
1999	42.1	1.48[b]	108.2

[a] Average of 3 measurements (first rib, last rib, last lumbar).
[b] Tenth rib backfat measurement.

Source: Hormel Farmer and *National Barrow Show*™ magazines. With permission.

jointly by USDA and Purdue University. They are excellent sources of information on pork production systems.

The majority of production occurs in three kinds of production systems: (1) farrow-to-finish systems that involve all stages of production, from breeding through finishing to market weights of 113 to 120 kg; (2) farrowing to nursery systems that produce and sell or contract 18- to 27-kg feeder pigs to growing-finishing farms; and (3) farrowing-to-weaning systems that sell or contract 4.5- to 7-kg pigs to nursery-growing-finishing operations (wean-to-finish).

The farrow-to-finish system involves breeding and farrowing sows, and then feeding the pigs until they reach market weight. The entire production period takes 10 to 11 months, including over 4 months for breeding and gestation plus about 6 months to raise the pigs to market weight. Of the three systems, farrow-to-finish has the greatest long-term market potential and flexibility. Farrow-to-finish operations require the most capital and labor, and they require a long-term commitment.

The farrow-to-nursery system involves breeding and farrowing sows, raising the pigs to 18 to 27 kg, and then selling or contracting them to a growing-finishing operation. It results in fewer facility requirements than farrowing-to-finishing systems, less operating capital, and less feed and manure to be handled. It provides a good foundation for increasing the number of sows or expanding into a farrowing-to-finishing operation. These producers are at the mercy of a volatile feeder pig market. This volatility may necessitate farrowing sows in groups to increase the number of pigs available during periods of high demand.

The farrowing-to-weaning system involves breeding and farrowing sows, and then the pigs are weaned directly into a house where they remain until slaughter (wean-to-finish). An apparent benefit of this production system is the elimination of the stress from moving and mixing pigs.

A. Farrowing Facilities

Choices available for farrowing facilities range from A-frame huts on pasture to environmentally controlled central farrowing units with slotted floors. Adequate environments for sows and pigs can be provided in many ways. A higher level of management is required with central farrowing systems than with pasture operations. With central farrowing, however, the labor requirement is reduced.

Critical design factors of a farrowing system include (1) comfort for pigs and sow; (2) protection of pigs from crushing by the sow; and (3) cleanliness of the farrowing-nursing area (Stanislaw and Muehling, 1997). Sows can farrow in pens, crates, or huts. Pens and huts allow the sow to move around freely, but they may result in higher newborn pig death loss because the sow may accidentally crush her pigs (McGlone and Blecha, 1987; Stevermer, 1991). Traditional farrowing crates allow the sow to stand, lie, eat, and drink, but not to turn around.

Pens: A typical farrowing pen measures 1.52 × 2.13 m. Pigs are provided a protected area of approximately 0.74 m^2, and supplemental heat is provided as needed. Penned sows typically crush more pigs than sows in crates (McGlone and Morrow-Tesch, 1987), but guard rails minimize crushing of pigs.

Crates: Relatively small farrowing-crate design differences can affect the health and performance of the animals (Curtis et al., 1989). The farrowing crate typically measures 1.52 × 2.13 m, with the sow zone about 0.61 × 2.13 m. The floors are typically slotted under or to the rear of the sow zone, allowing quick, efficient removal of excreta, thus keeping floor and equipment dry. Floors may be solid or partially or totally slotted. Acceptable types of perforated floors include metal, woven-metal, plastic-coated-metal, metal bars, fiberglass, concrete, and combinations of these. The floor should have a nonabrasive, nonporous, slip-resistant surface (Fritschen and Muehling, 1986), and it should be constructed to be free of exposed materials or projections to prevent injury to the legs, feet, or hooves of sows and pigs.

Huts: When farrowing takes place in outside huts, special care is taken to minimize the impact of a variable environment on both sow and pigs. For summer farrowing, the huts provide a cool, shady area, and they are designed to be opened for maximum airflow. For winter farrowing, they are sheltered from prevailing winds, and they are made relatively airtight to retain the sow's body heat. Adequate dry bedding is provided during cold weather. The farrowing huts are located in naturally well-drained areas, on a concrete slab, or on a mounded area of crushed stone or other coarse material. Hut locations are rotated to lessen exposure to disease agents and parasites. Hut design and size affect performance (Honeyman and Roush, 1995).

Pigs produced per litter (Figure 2.7 and Table 2.3) have steadily increased since 1924. Much of this can be attributed to improved physical facilities, adaptation of new technology, and genetics. The number of pigs produced per litter was 5.32 in 1924 and 8.79 in 1999, an increase of over 3.4 pigs. This is a phenomenal improvement and contributes significantly to a lower cost of production per pig.

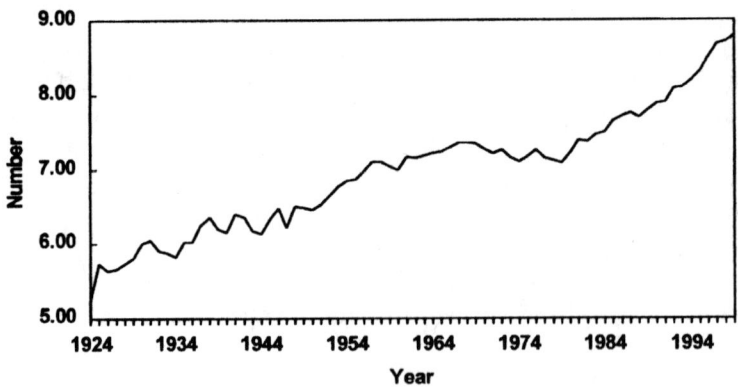

FIGURE 2.7 U.S. average annual pigs per litter has steadily increased since 1924. Much of this can be attributed to improved physical facilities, adaptation of new technology, and genetics. The number of pigs produced per litter was 5.32 in 1924 and 8.79 in 1999, an increase of over 3.4 pigs. This is a phenomenal improvement and contributes significantly to a lower cost of production per pig. (From NASS, 1999.)

TABLE 2.3
Annual Pigs per Litter, U.S., 1924–1999

Year	Pigs/Litter	Year	Pigs/Litter	Year	Pigs/Litter	Year	Pigs/Litter
1924	5.24	1943	6.17	1962	7.15	1981	7.39
1925	5.73	1944	6.13	1963	7.19	1982	7.38
1926	5.64	1945	6.32	1964	7.22	1983	7.47
1927	5.66	1946	6.47	1965	7.24	1984	7.50
1928	5.73	1947	6.21	1966	7.29	1985	7.65
1929	5.80	1948	6.50	1967	7.36	1986	7.72
1930	6.00	1949	6.48	1968	7.36	1987	7.76
1931	6.04	1950	6.45	1969	7.35	1988	7.70
1932	5.90	1951	6.52	1970	7.27	1989	7.79
1933	5.88	1952	6.64	1971	7.21	1990	7.88
1934	5.82	1953	6.76	1972	7.26	1991	7.90
1935	6.02	1954	6.85	1973	7.16	1992	8.08
1936	6.02	1955	6.86	1974	7.10	1993	8.10
1937	6.24	1956	6.97	1975	7.17	1994	8.19
1938	6.35	1957	7.10	1976	7.26	1995	8.31
1939	6.19	1958	7.10	1977	7.15	1996	8.50
1940	6.14	1959	7.04	1978	7.12	1997	8.68
1941	6.39	1960	6.99	1979	7.09	1998	8.71
1942	6.35	1961	7.17	1980	7.22	1999	8.79

Source: National Agricultural Statistics Service (NASS) Agricultural Statistics Board, U.S. Department of Agriculture.

B. NURSERY FACILITIES

A warm, dry, draft-free environment, and proper nutrition are essential to achieving optimum performance of weanling pigs. Weaning usually takes place at 2 to 4 weeks of age, and pigs typically stay in a nursery until they are 8 to 12 weeks old.

A 4-week-old piglet requires an environmental temperature of at least 26°C (Table 2.4). Nurseries in the northern United States are equipped with supplemental heating. Weaned pigs residing outdoors are provided with shelter. Pigs in nursery houses are protected from drafts at air speeds over 15.2 m/min. Thermometers are used to record highest and lowest temperatures to manage temperature fluctuations in nursery environments. Nursery rooms are managed on an all-in, all-out basis, and thoroughly cleaned and disinfected between groups of pigs.

A typical pen in an environmentally controlled nursery house holds 10 to 20 pigs. Floor area recommendations are 0.18 to 0.23 m² each for pigs from 4.5 to 14.0 kg and 0.28 to 0.37 m² each for pigs from 14.0 to 27.0 kg. Floors in nurseries are designed to be smooth, nonporous, and easy to clean and disinfect. Most nursery systems use slotted floors to reduce cleaning labor. Drier floors can be maintained on slotted floors than on solid floors.

C. GROWING-FINISHING FACILITIES

In environmentally controlled housing, the typical growing and finishing pen is rectangular and holds 15 to 40 pigs. Penning materials are sturdier than those used in nurseries because of the pigs' destructive rooting and chewing. Overcrowding of pigs lessens their opportunity to eat, drink, and rest (Tables 2.5 and 2.6). Aggressive behavior may be more frequent in crowded facilities with large group sizes (McGlone and Newby, 1994).

TABLE 2.4
Recommended Thermal Conditions for Swine

Type and Weight (lactating sow and litter)	Preferred Range[a] (15–27°C for sow; pigs have 32°C creep area)	Lower Intervention[b] (10°C for sow)	Upper Intervention[c] (32°C for sow)
Prenursery, 5 to 15 kg	27 to 32°C	15°C	35°C
Nursery, 15 to 35 kg	18 to 27°C	5°C	35°C
Growing, 35 to 70 kg	15 to 24°C	–4°C	35°C
Finishing, 70 to 100 kg	10 to 24°C	–15°C	35°C
Sows or boars	15 to 24°C	–15°C	32°C

[a] Adapted from NRC (1981); DeShazer and Overhults (1982); Hahn (1985).
[b] Bedding, supplemental heat, or other environmental modification is recommended when air temperatures approach the lower intervention points.
[c] Except for brief periods above these air temperatures, some form of cooling should be provided when temperatures approach upper intervention points.

Although many flooring materials are acceptable, total or partial concrete slats are widely adopted for slotted floors. Concrete slats 10 to 20 cm wide, with spacing of about 2.54 cm between slats, is the typical design.

Finishing systems are designed to minimize mixing of pigs to reduce the incidence of fighting and to avoid the production losses that follow fights (Tan et al., 1991; Stookey and Gonyou, 1994). Typically, the growing-finishing production system is operated on an all-in, all-out basis, with cleaning and disinfection of facilities between groups.

Breeding and gestation housing systems in use in the United States today vary in design in terms of feeding methods, breeding methods, and number of sows grouped together. Planned mating schedules, organized mating procedures, and effectively designed breeding facilities are aids to achieve high reproductive efficiency.

D. Breeding Facilities

Three mating options are (1) pen mating; (2) hand mating; and (3) artificial insemination. Pen mating occurs in a pen at least 2.4 m wide that provides 1.86 m² per sow or 1.58 m² per gilt. Pen mating in outside lots is achieved in group sizes of 30 or fewer.

With hand mating, the sow is usually mated in a special mating pen, but may be mated in the sow's or boar's pen. Mating typically takes place in a 2.4 × 2.4 m pen. Careful consideration for flooring surface in mating pens is essential during planning and construction. In breeding pens with an area of solid concrete, floors are made slip-resistant by applying a rough finish, or by placing grooves or 2.54-cm diamond-pattern cuts in the concrete (Levis et al., 1989). With hand mating indoors, absorbent substances or rubber mats are placed on the floor to provide better footing.

Artificial insemination is a breeding option that has gained in popularity. It allows producers to introduce new genetics without some of the disease risks associated with introduction of live boars, and artificial insemination decreases the time and cost of mating. It also allows use of semen from older, larger boars to inseminate young gilts or small sows.

E. GESTATION FACILITIES

Sow gestation systems used in the United States allow sows to be housed either individually or in groups. Some producers house sows in individual crates, which protect from aggression. The size of most gestation crates prevents sows and gilts from turning around, but one concept is a "turn-around" crate (McFarlane et al., 1988). Other indoor alternatives used include large group pens equipped with feeding stalls, or a limited number of sows in a group pen (Barnett et al., 1992). Many producers successfully keep breeding animals in lots or pastures with portable housing. Recommended areas for breeding sows and boars are listed for the different production systems (see Table 2.5). Individual gestation crates typically measure 0.61 × 2.13 × 1.01 m high. Individual stalls for boars are typically 0.61 × 2.13 × 1.16 m high, but larger stalls are provided for very large boars.

TABLE 2.5
Floor Area Recommended for Swine in Totally Enclosed Housing[a]

Stage of Production	Area (m^2)[b]
Litter and lactating sow, pen (depending on sow size and age of litter)	2.9 to 3.2/pen
Litter and lactating sow, sow portion of stall[c]	0.85 to 1.3/stall
Growing pigs	
5–14 kg	0.16 to 0.23/pig
14–27 kg	0.28 to 0.37/pig
27–45 kg	0.46/pig
45–68 kg	0.56/pig
68 kg to market	0.74/pig
Adults[d]	1.3 to 1.5/adult

[a] Close observation and professional judgment in modern facilities may allow higher stocking densities without interfering with the pigs' welfare. Production practices, such as group size, ventilation equipment and rate, and type of floors (partial vs. total slats), have an effect on proper stocking densities. Research is ongoing to study space requirements for different production systems.
[b] Group area allowances for growing pigs.
[c] Stall size: minimum width 56 cm; minimum length 2.1 m. Young adult females may be housed in stalls 2 m long.
[d] Based on market weight of 110 kg. Additional space may be required for heavier pigs. For large boars or sows, more floor area is needed.

Source: Adapted from MWPS (1983) and Fritschen and Muehling (1986).

TABLE 2.6
Space Recommendations for Pigs in Buildings with Outside Apron

	Space per Pig (m^2)	
Stage of Production	Inside	Outside
Growing-finishing pigs	0.56	0.56
Sows	1.0–1.1	1.0–1.1
Boars	3.7	3.7

Source: Adapted from Fritschen and Muehling (1986).

REFERENCES

Barnett, J. L., P. H. Hemsworth, G. M. Cronin, E. A. Newman, T. H. McCallum, and D. Chilton. 1992. Effects of pen size, partial stalls and method of feeding on welfare-related behavioral and physiological responses of group-housed pigs, *Appl. Anim. Behav. Sci.*, 34:207.

Curtis, S. E., R. J. Hurst, T. M. Widowski, R. D. Shanks, A. H. Jensen, H. W. Gonyou, D. P. Bane, A. J. Muehling, and R. P. Kesler. 1989. Effects of sow-crate design on health and performance of sows and piglets, *J. Anim. Sci.*, 67:80.

DeShazer, J. A., and D. G. Overhults. 1982. Energy demand in livestock production. In *Proc. 2nd Int. Livest. Environ. Symp.*, American Society of Agriculture, St. Joseph, MI, 17.

Fritschen, R. D., and A. J. Muehling. 1986. Space Requirements for Swine. PIH-55, Pork Industry Handbook. Cooperative Extension Service, University of Illinois, Urbana.

Hahn, G. L. 1985. Managing and housing of farm animals in hot environments. In *Stress Physiology in Livestock, Vol. II: Ungulates*, Yousef, M. K., Ed., CRC Press, Boca Raton, FL, chap. 11.

Holden, P. J. 1999. Personal communication. (Data taken from several years of Iowa State University Swine Enterprise Records.)

Honeyman, M. S., and W. Roush. 1995. Pig crushing mortality by hut type in outdoor farrowing. Iowa State University Pub. ASL-R1389.

Lawrence, J.D. 1995. Pork production cost and benefits: economic and environmental benefits. In *Proceedings of the 1995 National Pork Producers Lending Conference*, pp. 94–105.

Lawrence, J., G. Grimes, and M. Hayenga. 1998. Production and Marketing Characteristics of U.S. Pork Producers, 1997–1998. Staff paper 311, Department of Economics, Iowa State University, Ames.

Levis, D. G., D. R. Zimmerman, A. Hogg, D. E. Reese, M. C. Brumm, and W. T. Ahlschwede. 1989. Swine reproductive management. EC89-212, Cooperative Extension Service, University of Nebraska, Lincoln.

McFarlane, J. M., K. E. Boe, and S. E. Curtis. 1988. Turning and walking by gilts in modified gestation crates, *J. Anim. Sci.*, 66:326.

McGlone, J. J., and F. Blecha. 1987. An examination of the behavioral, immunological and reproductive traits in four management systems for sows and piglets, *Appl. Anim. Behav. Sci.*, 18:269.

McGlone, J. J., and J. Morrow-Tesch. 1987. Productivity and behavior of sows in level vs. sloped farrowing pens and crates, *J. Anim. Sci.*, 68:82.

McGlone, J. J., and B. E. Newby. 1994. Space requirements for finishing pigs in confinement: behavior and performance while group size and space vary, *Appl. Anim. Behav. Sci.*, 39:331.

MWPS (Midwest Plan Service). 1983. *Swine Housing and Equipment Handbook*, Midwest Plan Service, Iowa State University, Ames.

NASS (National Agricultural Statistics Service). 1998. *Hogs and Pigs Report*, Dec. 1, 1998.

NASS (National Agricultural Statistics Service). 1999a. *Hogs and Pigs Report*, Dec. 1, 1999.

NASS (National Agricultural Statistics Service). 1999b. Livestock slaughter. Bulletin Mt An 1-2-1 (99).

NPPC (National Pork Producers Council). 1999. *Swine Care Handbook*, NPPC, Des Moines, IA.

NRC. 1981. *Effects of Environment on Nutrient Requirements of Domestic Animals*, National Academy Press, Washington, D.C.

Pork Industry Handbook, 1999. Agricultural Communication Service, Media Distribution Center, Purdue University, Lafayette, IN.

Stanislaw, C. M., and A. J. Muehling. 1997. Swine Farrowing Units. PIH-10, Pork Industry Handbook. Cooperative Extension Service, University of Illinois, Urbana.

Stevermer, E. J. 1991. Swine Enterprise Record. ASB:EJS-185. Iowa State University, Ames.

Stookey, J. M., and H. W. Gonyou. 1994. The effects of regrouping on behavioral and production parameters in finishing swine, *J. Anim. Sci.*, 72: 2804.

Tan, S. S. L., D. M. Shackleton, and R. M. Beames. 1991. The effect of mixing unfamiliar individuals on the growth and performance of finishing pigs, *Anim. Prod.*, 52:201.

3 Anatomy of the Digestive System and Nutritional Physiology*

Jong-Tseng Yen

CONTENTS

I. Anatomy and Histology of the Porcine Digestive System 32
    A. The Mouth and Salivary Glands 32
    B. The Pharynx and Esophagus 34
    C. The Stomach 34
    D. The Liver 34
    E. The Pancreas 34
    F. The Small Intestine 36
    G. The Large Intestine 38
II. Secretions of the Porcine Digestive System 38
    A. Salivary Secretion 38
    B. Gastric Secretion 39
    C. Bile Secretion 40
    D. Pancreatic Exocrine Secretion 42
    E. Small Intestine Wall Secretion 45
III. Digestion, Fermentation, and Absorption of Carbohydrate 46
    A. Oral Digestion of Starch 46
    B. Carbohydrate Digestion and Fermentation in the Stomach 46
    C. Gastric Emptying 47
    D. Carbohydrate Digestion in the Small Intestine 47
        1. Luminal Digestion 47
        2. Mucosal Digestion 48
    E. Absorption of Small Intestinal Carbohydrate Digestion Products 49
    F. Microbial Activity in the Small Intestine 49
    G. Large Intestinal Digestion and Fermentation 49
    H. Absorption of Gut Volatile Fatty Acids 50
IV. Protein Digestion and Absorption 51
    A. Gastric Digestion of Protein 51
    B. Digestion of Protein in the Small Intestine 52
        1. Luminal Digestion 52
        2. Mucosal Digestion 52
    C. Bacterial Digestion of Protein in the Large Intestine 52
    D. Absorption of Products of Protein Digestion 53

---

* The contents of this publication do not necessarily reflect the views or policies of the U.S. Department of Agriculture, nor does mention of trade names, commercial products, or organizations imply endorsement from the U.S. Government.

V.	Digestion and Absorption of Fat	54
	A. Gastric Fat Digestion	54
	B. Fat Digestion and Absorption in the Small Intestine	54
	C. Digestion and Absorption of Fat in the Large Intestine	55
VI.	Water and Electrolyte Absorption	55
	A. Small Intestine Absorption	55
	B. Large Intestine Absorption	56
VII.	Antibody Absorption by Neonatal Enterocytes	56
VIII.	Measurements of Nutrient Digestion and Absorption	56
References		57

The digestive system is the doorway through which nutrients, electrolytes, and fluids enter the body. The digestive tract also provides a protective barrier against entrance of toxic substances and infectious agents. The porcine digestive system comprises the mouth, the pharynx, the esophagus, the stomach, small and large intestines, and several accessory glands (Figure 3.1). The small intestine consists of duodenum, jejunum, and ileum, and the large intestine is composed of cecum, colon, and rectum. The accessory glands of the porcine digestive system are the salivary glands, the liver, and the pancreas that release their secretions into the alimentary lumen.

This chapter offers a short overview of the anatomy of the digestive system and the nutritional physiology in pigs. It is a rearranged and abridged version of a book chapter published recently (Yen, 2000) in a monograph on the biology of the domestic pig edited by Pond and Mersmann (2000).

I. ANATOMY AND HISTOLOGY OF THE PORCINE DIGESTIVE SYSTEM

Several textbooks on the anatomy of domestic animals (Sisson, 1975; Schummer et al., 1979; Dyce et al., 1996) have described and illustrated the detailed structural anatomy of the porcine digestive system. Moran (1982) has reviewed the histology of the digestive system of pigs. Short descriptions of the anatomy and histology of the porcine pancreas have also been provided by Low and Zebrowska (1989) and Cranwell (1995). Liebler et al. (1992) have described briefly the histology of the porcine small and large intestines. The morphology of the mucosa of pig's large intestine has also been reported by Low and Zebrowska (1989). Schantz et al. (1996) have discussed the anatomy and histology of the porcine gastrointestinal tract as compared with that of the human.

A. THE MOUTH AND SALIVARY GLANDS

The pig has a long oral cavity. The length of a pig's oral cavity varies with the breed. The upper lip is short and thick and is blended with the snout. The lower lip is small and pointed. The pig has an elongated and narrow tongue. The porcine oral cavity is lined by a simple stratified squamous epithelium.

Saliva is secreted from three major salivary glands: the parotid glands, the mandibular (submaxillary) glands, and the sublingual glands, plus a number of minor glands (labial, lingual, buccal, and palatine glands) found in the mouth. The parotid and mandibular glands each have major ducts draining their secretions into the oral cavity. The sublingual glands have numerous openings through the mouth floor just ventrolateral to the tongue. The minor glands in the mucous membrane also have many excretory ducts emptying into the oral cavity.

The full complement of permanent teeth in the pig is three pairs of incisors, one pair of canines, four pairs of premolars, and three pairs of molars, upper and lower, for a total of 44 teeth. Pigs are not born with their entire complement of teeth, but accrue the teeth progressively with age. At birth, a pig has eight deciduous teeth, including four incisors and four canines. The full permanent dentition of a pig is acquired when it is at least $1\frac{1}{2}$ years of age.

Anatomy of the Digestive System and Nutritional Physiology

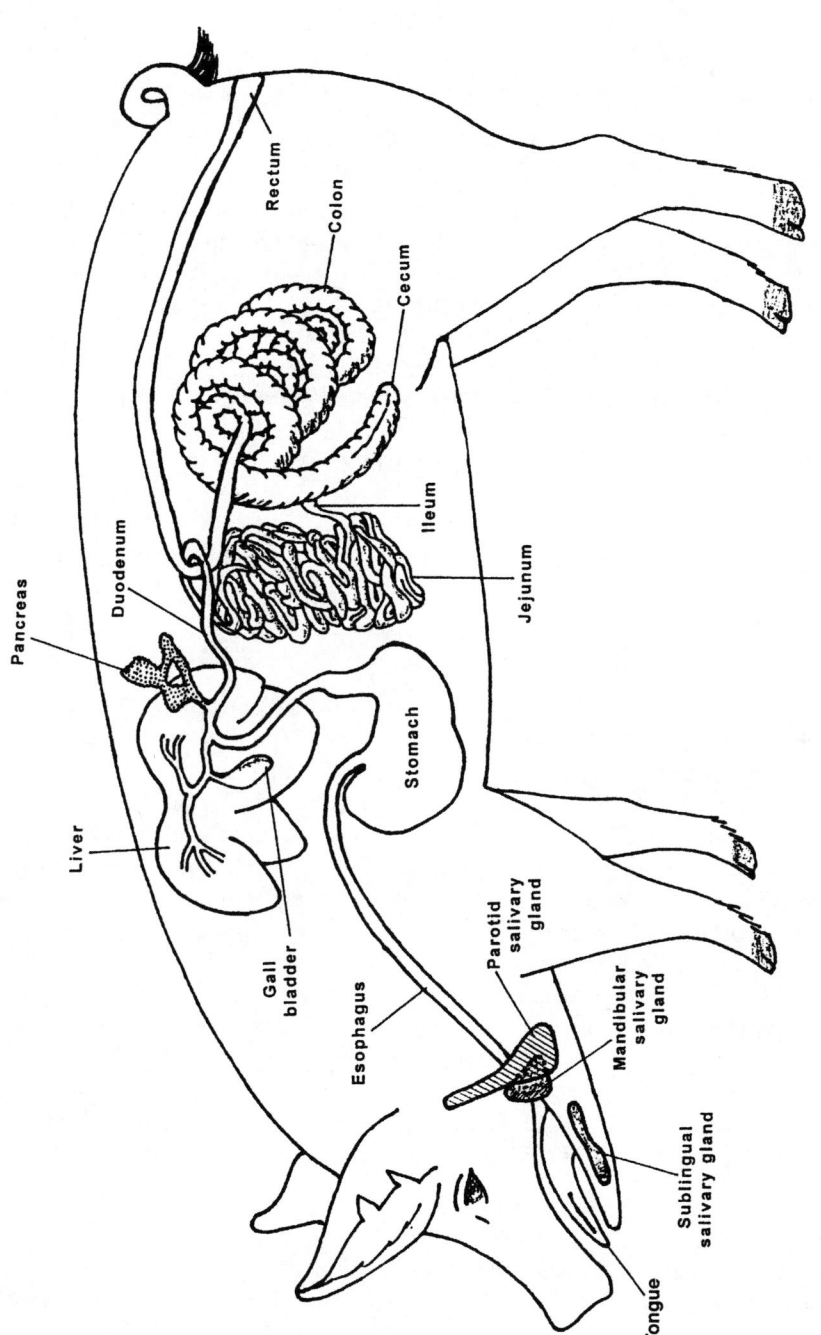

FIGURE 3.1 Diagram of the digestive system of the pig. (Adapted from Sisson, 1975; Shummer et al., 1979; and Moran, 1982.)

B. The Pharynx and Esophagus

The pharynx of the pig is long and narrow, and extends to the level of the second cervical vertebra. The short and straight esophagus originates from the caudal border of the caudal pharyngeal constrictors. The esophagus is lined with stratified squamous epithelium, beneath which are tubuloacinar mucous glands. Esophageal glands are abundant and packed closely in the cranial half of the esophagus but occur in reduced number in the caudal half of the esophagus. From the esophagus through the rectum, feed bolus manipulation in the pig is wholly involuntary.

C. The Stomach

The stomach of the pig is compartmentalized into four distinct mucosal regions that differ in appearance and structure. The esophageal region (pars esophagea) is nonglandular and it is an extension of the esophagus into the stomach proper. Adjacent to the esophageal region is the cardiac gland region, which occupies about one third of the total luminal surface area and is pale gray in color. The fundic (proper gastric) gland region has a brownish red, mottled appearance, and it also lines one third of the stomach, lying between the cardiac and pyloric regions. The pale-looking pyloric gland region is the last region of the stomach before entry into the small intestine.

The cardiac glands have mucous cells that elaborate mucus, proteases, and lipase. Three types of secretory cells exist in fundic glands and each produce a separate secretion. The three fundic secretory cells are mucous neck cells that elaborate mucus and proteases, parietal (oxyntic) cells that produce HCl, and chief cells that secrete proteases. Mucous neck cells and chief cells, but not parietal cells, are also found in pyloric glands. However, the predominant cell in pyloric glands is the mucous-secreting cell.

D. The Liver

The porcine liver has four principal lobes — left lateral, left medial, right medial, and right lateral lobes, along with a small quadrate lobe and a caudate process. The functional units of the liver are lobules. The basic structure of a pig's hepatic lobule is presented in Figure 3.2. The lobules are composed of plates of hepatocytes interdigitated between anastomotic hepatic sinusoids. The plates and sinusoids are arranged radially around a central vein. Kupffer cells and endothelial cells line portions of the hepatic sinusoids and serve as a part of the body's reticuloendothelial system. Located in the peripheral interlobular connective tissue are the portal triads that include a hepatic portal vein, a hepatic artery, and an interlobular bile duct. Afferent blood from the portal vein and hepatic artery flows centrally in the hepatic sinusoids. Bile produced by hepatocytes drains peripherally into bile canaliculi formed by hepatocytes and then through ducts of Hering to the interlobular bile ducts in the portal triad. The interlobular bile ducts merge to form larger intrahepatic ducts. The latter become the extrahepatic biliary system that includes the hepatic bile duct, which divides into a cystic duct connecting to the gallbladder, and a common bile duct connecting to the duodenum. The common bile duct opens into the duodenum at 2 to 5 cm from the pyloric sphincter on the major duodenal papilla (sphincter of Oddi).

E. The Pancreas

The porcine pancreas is composed of a large left lobe and a small right lobe connected by a centrally placed body which surrounds the portal vein. The pig has only the accessory pancreatic duct. The duct leaves the right lobe of the pancreas and terminates at the minor duodenal papilla in the descending duodenum 20 to 25 cm distal to the pylorus.

The pancreas is a mixed exocrine and endocrine organ. The exocrine pancreatic components are the acinus and the duct system. The acinus represents 95% of the exocrine pancreatic tissue and is composed of acinar cells that produce and store various pancreatic enzymes and zymogens.

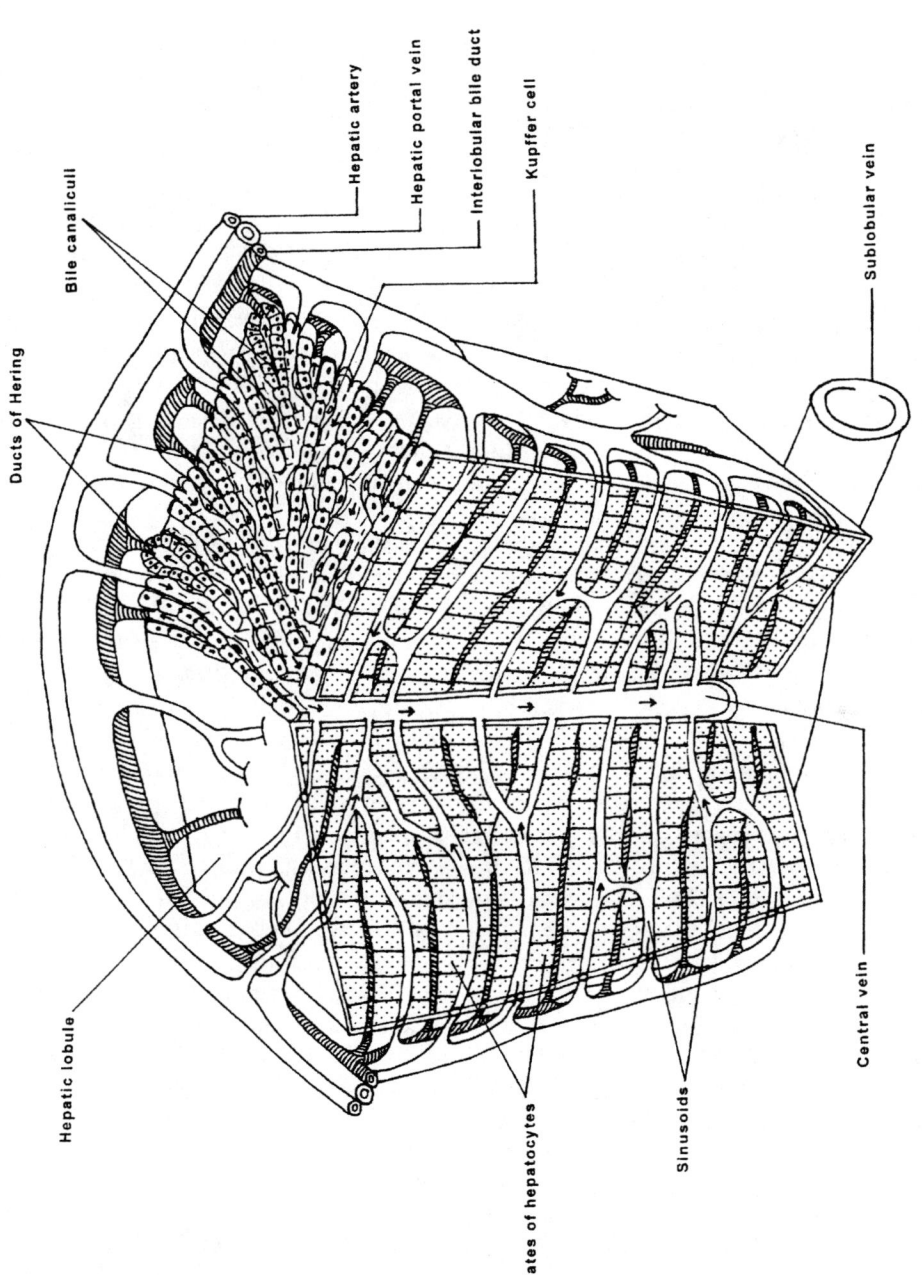

FIGURE 3.2 Basic structure of a pig's liver lobule. (Adapted from Schummer et al., 1979; Moran, 1982; Banks, 1986; and Herdt, 1992.)

When stimulated, the acinar cells release enzymes and zymogens into the acinus lumen for transport to the duodenum through the duct system. The centroacinar cells and cells lining the intercalated and intralobular ducts contribute water, bicarbonate, and other electrolytes to pancreatic juice.

The endocrine constituents of the pancreas are located in the islets of Langerhans and account for <5% of the fresh weight of the organ. The islets are distributed uniformly throughout the exocrine acinar tissue. Encapsulated in the islets are four major endocrine cells: glucagon-synthesizing A cells, insulin-synthesizing B cells, somatostatin-synthesizing D cells, and pancreatic polypeptide-synthesizing PP cells.

F. THE SMALL INTESTINE

The small intestine consists of duodenum, jejunum, and ileum. In the fully grown pig, the small intestine is 16 to 21 m long, of which 4 to 5% is duodenum, 88 to 91% jejunum, and 4 to 5% ileum. The small intestine of newborn pigs is 2 to 4 m in length. The proportion of duodenum in the neonate is similar to that in the adult, but the differentiation of jejunum and ileum is not clear.

The duodenum is the location where digesta from the stomach mixes with secretions of the intestine, liver, and pancreas. Bile is ducted into the duodenum on a major papilla 2 to 5 cm from the stomach pylorus, and pancreatic juice enters the intestine on a minor papilla 12 to 20 cm posterior to bile entry. The jejunum is long and comprises a large number of small loops. The ileum can be identified from jejunum by its slightly thicker muscular coats and junction with the large intestine. Although there are distinctive morphological features among the duodenum, jejunum, and ileum, they share many common features.

As illustrated in Figure 3.3a, the wall of the small intestine consists of four major layers: the mucosa, the submucosa, the muscularis, and the serosa. The mucosal layer is composed of three sublayers, namely, the muscularis mucosa, the lamina propria, and the epithelium. The muscularis mucosa comprises two thin sets of muscles. The inner muscle runs longitudinally along the length of the intestine and the outer muscle encircles the intestine to produce transient intestinal folds called Kerchring's valves (plicae circulares). The lamina propria is composed of blood vessels, free lymphocytes, lymph nodules (Peyer's patches), and neurons loosely held together by connective tissues. The lamina propria supports the structure of the epithelial layer and nourishes the epithelium.

The epithelial layer is a continuous sheet of single-layered epithelial cells and covers the fingerlike villi and their surrounding crypts of Lieberkuhn, to form the luminal surface of the intestine (Figure 3.3b). The length of villi increases from duodenum to mid-jejunum and then decreases through the terminal ileum. There are three types of epithelial cells on the villus surface: columnar absorptive cells, goblet cells, and enteroendocrine cells. They all originate from the stem cells located at the base of the crypts. The apical membrane covers the enterocyte surface facing the intestinal lumen and contains the microvilli (Figure 3.3c). The remaining part of enterocyte plasma membrane not facing the gut lumen is termed the basolateral membrane.

The enterocytes migrate from the crypts to the tip of the villi and are shed into the lumen. During that migration process, enterocytes undergo both structural and functional maturation, which includes a period of rapid elongation of the microvilli. When enterocytes migrate over the basal third of the villi, their structural differentiation is completed and their digestive function (carbohydrase and peptidase activity) begins. The absorptive function of enterocytes starts to develop when enterocytes reach the upper to midlevel of the villi and it continues to increase until enterocytes are sloughed at the tip of the villi.

Microvilli increase the apical surface of the enterocytes by about 14- to 40-fold. In addition to this significant amplification of digestive-absorptive surface area by microvilli, the available cross-sectional area of the intestinal tract is increased three times first by the circular folds of Kerchring and then tenfold more by the villi. This structural organization amplifies the effective surface area per unit intestinal length by a factor of 420 to 1200 and improves the efficiency for digestion and absorption dramatically.

Anatomy of the Digestive System and Nutritional Physiology

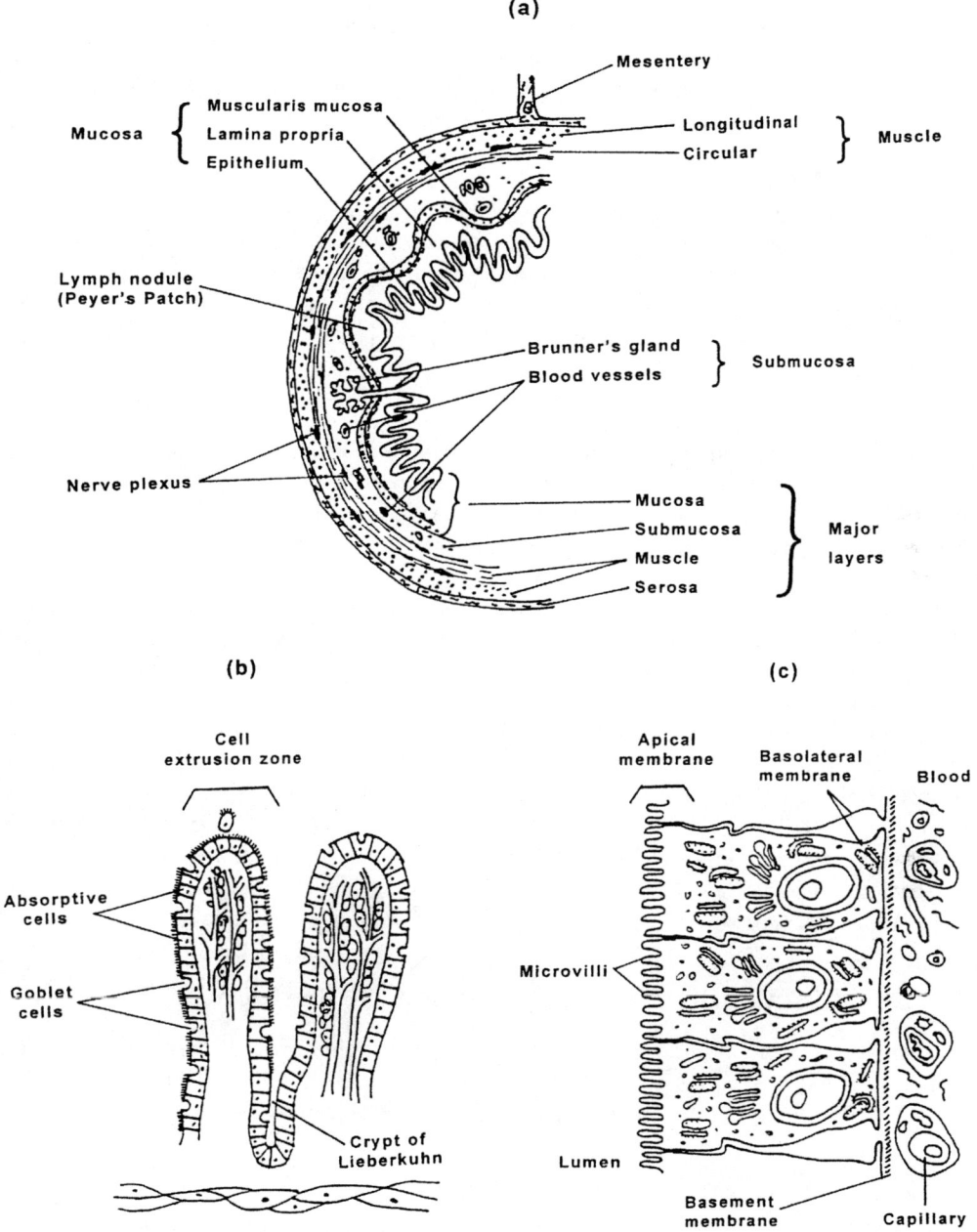

FIGURE 3.3 Structure of (a) the intestinal wall, (b) the intestinal epithelium, and (c) enterocytes. (Adapted from Moran, 1982 and Herdt, 1992.)

Goblet cells in the epithelial layer increase in number from the proximal jejunum toward the distal ileum and they secrete a viscous mucus. The enteroendocrine cells of the epithelial layer release hormones that are involved in the regulatory processes of the cellular renewal system. Enterocytes at the surface of the villi are renewed continuously. In young pigs, the epithelium is replaced by new epithelium approximately every 3 to 4 days.

The submucosal layer of the intestinal wall is a loose connective tissue arrangement that holds together the larger blood vessels, lymphatic vessels, and neural complexes. The submucosa of the first few centimeters of the duodenum is heavily endowed with intestinal submucosal glands (Brunner's glands). The number of Brunner's glands decreases thereafter, and few can be found 50 cm posterior to the pyloric sphincter. Brunner's glands secrete a copious alkaline fluid that is ducted from the submucosa through the muscularis mucosa and toward openings between epithelial cells in the villus crypts.

The muscular layer of the intestinal wall is similar to the muscularis mucosa and contains two fiber arrangements, except that the longitudinal fibers are outer to the lumen and the circular ones are inner. The circular muscle is associated with peristalsis.

The outermost layer of the intestinal wall is the serosa, which has a squamous epithelium that forms the supporting mesentery containing the connective tissue, large blood vessels, and nerves.

G. The Large Intestine

Compared with most nonruminant omnivores, pigs have a short cecum and long colon. The large intestine of the fully grown pig averages 3.5 to 6 m in length with the first 7 to 8% as cecum. The cecum is a cylindrical blind sac located at the proximal end of the colon. The length of the colon in adult pigs is only 25% of the length of the small intestine but the colon has a physical capacity similar to the entire small intestine. The colon comprises three parts that are termed the ascending, transverse, and descending colons from ileum to rectum, respectively. The first part of the ascending colon presents four complete turns that spiral toward the center of the coil and is termed the centripetal colon. A central flexure permits the spirals to reverse and 3.5 turns of the ascending colon go out from the coil center giving the centrifugal colon. The rectum is embedded in fat and widens to form ampulla recti before it ends at the anal canal.

The mucosal membrane of both cecum and colon has no villi but has some small projections of short columnar epithelium with a striated border containing microvilli. The microvilli of colonic enterocytes do not contain digestive enzymes. Numerous goblet cells intersperse the columnar cells and secrete sulfated carbohydrate–protein complex to act as a lubricant. The rectum has a simple structure of columnar epithelial cells interspersed with a few goblet cells. The anus has no mucosal cells. The epithelial turnover rate of colonic mucosa of the pig is 4 to 8 days.

II. SECRETIONS OF THE PORCINE DIGESTIVE SYSTEM

Porcine salivary glands, stomach, liver, pancreas, and intestine produce large volumes of their respective digestive secretions for digesting dietary nutrients. Synthesis and secretion of these digestive fluids is controlled by endocrine as well as intrinsic and extrinsic events.

A. Salivary Secretion

Saliva moistens feed, lubricates the esophagus, and starts the digestion of starch. Saliva is a mixture of water, mucus, and α-amylase, and it also contains lysozyme and immunoglobulin A to protect against diseases. Kidder and Manners (1978) indicated that the specific gravity, dry matter, and amylase activity dropped as the rate of salivary secretion increased. The volume or duration of salivary secretion was observed to vary in response to feed and other stimulants in the mouth. A dry cereal mixture produced greater stimulation of secretion than did diluted hydrochloric, lactic, formic, or acetic acid. Corring (1980a) found both volume and total amylase activity of the entire porcine saliva rose with increased levels of feed intake. He further suggested that the ratio of total salivary amylase to total pancreatic amylase was about 1 to 250,000 in those pigs during the 5-h period after feed ingestion. This implies that salivary amylase plays an insignificant role in starch digestion in comparison with the pancreatic enzyme.

The control of salivary secretion is by the autonomic nervous system (Moran, 1982; Argenzio, 1993a). The quantity and consistency of salivary secretion is determined by the type of nerve stimulated.

B. Gastric Secretion

The action of salivary amylase on carbohydrate continues in the esophageal and cardiac gland regions of the stomach and stops in the fundus of the stomach when the pH falls below 3.6. The low pH also creates a barrier to microbial passage into the intestine. Hydrochloric acid, various proteolytic enzymes, and small amounts of gastric lipase are the principal digestive secretions produced by the stomach in pigs.

The control of gastric acid secretion has been reviewed by Low (1990) and Argenzio (1993a). Phases of gastric acid secretion involve cephalic stimulation, gastric distention and chemical stimulation, and intestinal stimulation and inhibition. Mechanisms regulating gastric acid secretion in these processes involve a complex interplay of neural, hormonal, and nutritional stimuli and are mediated by histamine (paracrine), gastrin (endocrine), and acetylcholine (neurocrine), which act directly on the porcine parietal cell. Nutritional factors affecting gastric acid secretion in pigs include feeds of various chemical and physical composition, and physical factors such as meal size and particle size (Low, 1990).

The ontogeny of HCl secretion in pigs during the prenatal, postnatal, and postweaning periods has been reviewed recently by Cranwell (1995). In newborn pigs, gastric acid secretion responds to histamine and its analog histalog, pentagastrin, carbachol (a stable acetylcholine analog), and feeding. Compared with newborns, the gastric capacity to secrete acid in response to pentagastrin or histalog is greater for pigs at 1 to 2 weeks of age. Pentagastrin-stimulated acid output per unit of stomach weight increases fivefold during the first postnatal week and rises sevenfold overall up to 5 weeks of age. The relationship between maximal output of gastric acid and body weight in pigs from birth to 5 to 6 weeks of age is positively linear.

The four principal gastric proteases of the pig are pepsin A (also known as pepsin or pepsin II), pepsin B (parapepsin I), gastricsin (pepsin C, pepsin I, or parapepsin II), and chymosin (rennin). All are produced in the gastric mucosa of the pig. All the gastric proteases are secreted as zymogens that require a pH-dependent conformational change for their conversion into active enzymes (Foltmann et al., 1995). Cranwell (1995) indicated that gastric protease secretion was stimulated by histalog and pentagastrin in nursing pigs and by gastrin-releasing peptide (GRP), carbachol, and electrical stimulation of vagus nerve in weaned pigs.

Development of gastric proteases in pigs has also been reviewed recently by Cranwell (1995). During the week after birth, the levels of prochymosin in the fundic mucosa drop quite rapidly but it remains the dominant zymogen until 3 to 4 weeks of age after which it is gradually replaced by pepsinogen A. In the weeks before and after birth, pepsinogen A occurs in the fundic mucosa only in traces. Tissue concentration of pepsinogen A rises gradually until 3 weeks of age and more rapidly thereafter. Progastricsin exists in trace quantities during the first week after birth and subsequently has a developmental pattern similar to pepsinogen A. Only trace amounts of pepsinogen B are presented in the fundic tissue before birth. The concentration of pepsinogen B increases from 1 week after birth and reaches a peak at approximately 3 to 5 weeks of age and then levels off. From 4 to 5 weeks of age, pepsinogen A becomes the predominant zymogen in the fundic tissue of the stomach.

Prochymosin, pepsinogen A, progastricsin, and pepsinogen B are also present in the pyloric region of the stomach in fetal and nursing pigs at concentrations that are much lower than that in the fundic region. The ontogenic pattern of these zymogens in the pyloric region is similar to that in the fundic region. In weaned pigs (52- to 66-day-old), the combined concentrations of pepsinogen A and progastricsin in the pyloric mucosa was only 1 to 4% of that in fundic mucosa, and the level of pepsinogen B was extremely small.

The cardiac region of the stomach of fetal and nursing pigs contains prochymosin at a level that is lower than that in the fundic or pyloric region. Pepsinogen A, progastricsin, and pepsinogen B are rarely found in the cardiac mucosa.

The developmental patterns of pepsinogen A and progastricsin during the nursing and postweaning periods are reflected in measurements of the degree of protein digestion in the stomach and the general proteolytic activity in the gastric mucosa and gastric secretion of pigs, which are low before animals are 3 to 4 weeks old and then increase rapidly thereafter, as shown in the studies reviewed by Moughan et al. (1992).

In addition to HCl and proteases, the cardiac region of the stomach also secretes gastric lipase. The relative and specific activities of gastric lipase rise in response to increases in the level of dietary lipid in miniature pigs (Armand et al., 1992). The total lipase activity in stomach tissue of newborn pigs was about 3% of that in the pancreas (Newport and Howarth, 1985), but it was found to be only 1/600 of that in the pancreas in pigs weaned at 4 weeks of age (Jensen et al., 1997). The cardiac region of porcine stomach produces a limited amount of alkaline secretion with cation composition similar to that of plasma (Kidder and Manners, 1978).

In pigs, there is a basal gastric secretion that continues throughout the 24 h, with a greater rate during the day than the night, and the volume of gastric secretion is affected by the nature and quantity of the diet (Kidder and Manners,1978; Corring, 1980a). In 40-kg pigs equipped with a reentrant cannula immediately distal to the bile duct and fed diets with either barley and soybean meal (A) or casein and starch (B), the values of 24-h gastric secretion were calculated to be 8 and 4 l for diets A and B, respectively (Zebrowska et al., 1983). More-detailed information on the mechanisms controlling gastric secretion in the pig and other species are available in reviews by Holst et al. (1993), Lloyd (1994), and Parsons (1996).

C. Bile Secretion

Kidder and Manners (1978) and Moran (1982) have provided information concerning the composition of pig bile. Bile obtained from bile-duct cannulated pigs contains Na, K, Cl, bicarbonate, and several organic constituents and has a pH of 7.43 to 7.91. The main organic components of pig bile are bile salts, phospholipids, cholesterol, mucus, and bile pigments that are excretory waste products. Bile salts and phospholipids are substances relevant to digestive function. The ratio of total bile salt to total phospholipid concentration in pig bile is 9 to 1 (Coleman et al., 1979).

Bile salts are bile acids conjugated with glycine or taurine and they aid in the emulsification of fat to facilitate absorption. Conjugated bile acids are deconjugated and altered chemically to some extent by the bacteria in the lower small intestine. The altered and unaltered bile acids are reabsorbed in the lower small intestine and transported by the portal vein to the liver. These reabsorbed bile acids and some newly synthesized bile acids are then conjugated and secreted into the bile again. This enterohepatic recirculation provides a means of coping with demand, because daily bile acid use by the pig far exceeds its capacity for synthesis.

Pig bile comprises seven conjugated bile acids. The three principal bile acids are hyodeoxycholic, hyocholic, and chenodeoxycholic acids and they are conjugated mainly with glycine but to some extent with taurine. The hyocholic acid is unique to the bile of pigs and is produced from hydroxylation of chenodeoxycholic acid. The chenodeoxycholic acid is synthesized *de novo* from cholesterol in the liver by the hepatocytes. Reduction of hyocholic acid by the bacteria in the intestine yields hyodeoxycholic acid. Porcine bile contains little or no cholic acid, which is a major component of the bile of most other mammals. Lecithin, a phospholipid in the bile, can be hydrolyzed in the intestine by pancreatic phospholipase to lysolecithin for micellar dispersion of the products of fat digestion.

In addition to providing bile acids needed for fat digestion and absorption, bile also provides bicarbonate as a buffer for neutralization of acidic chyme entering the duodenum from the stomach. Bile further offers an excretory route for certain endogenous waste products. Bilirubin, a major end product of normal red blood cell turnover, is produced by Kupffer cells lining the lobule sinusoid and transported to the hepatocyte for conjugation. Conjugated bilirubin is secreted into the bile, converted to urobilinogen, then to urobilin and sterobilin in the intestine, and expelled from the body through defecation. Urobilin and sterobilin give feces its characteristic brown color. Some urobilin is absorbed and subsequently excreted by the kidney to give urine its yellowish color. Many drugs and toxins are metabolized in the liver and their metabolites are excreted as components of the bile.

The secretion of bile by the hepatocytes in pigs is continuous but can be increased by the presence of bile salts, secretin, or cholecystokinin (CCK) in the blood (Kidder and Manners, 1978). Although bile is secreted by hepatocytes continuously, its need for fat digestion is only intermittent. When little or no feed is present in the duodenum, the sphincter of Oddi is closed and bile coming from the hepatic bile duct is diverted into the gallbladder. In the gallbladder, bile is concentrated and its volume is reduced. The presence of fat-containing feed in the duodenum elicits the release of CCK from gut endocrine cells to cause relaxation of the sphincter of Oddi, contraction of the gallbladder, and the passage of gallbladder bile into the duodenum. Moran (1982) has ascribed the regulation of the bile movement to intramural plexus coordination more than to CCK. The use of CCK by the animal to evacuate bile rapidly into the intestine happens only when the gastric digesta contains high levels of fat.

The total bile flow during a 24-h period in 60-kg pigs averages 38 ml/kg body weight (Laplace and Ouaissi, 1977) and was 46 ml/kg body weight in 45-kg pigs (Juste et al., 1979). In both studies, bile collected from bile duct cannula was pumped continuously and directly into the duodenum and the sphincter of Oddi was not allowed to control bile flow. Using reentrant catheters in the common bile duct of pigs to allow both the gallbladder to store bile continuously and to modify its composition and the sphincter of Oddi to regulate bile flow into the duodenum, Sambrook (1981) found that total bile volume was 48 ml/kg body weight for a typical European pig diet containing barley, wheat offal, and fish meal, and was 30 ml/kg body weight for a semipurified diet containing starch, sucrose, casein, corn oil, and cellulose. In pigs fitted with a fistula in the common bile duct and a reentrant fistula in the proximal duodenum equipped with an apparatus to reinfuse the secreted bile at a rate reflecting the secretion rate, the 24-h bile secretion rate of 43-kg pigs was 35 ml/kg body weight in animals fed a wheat–casein–fish meal diet and 59 ml/kg body weight in those fed the wheat–casein–fish meal diet supplemented with 40% of wheat bran (Payne et al., 1989).

Bile secretion responds to dietary changes in pigs. The secretion rate of bile acids increased dramatically but that of bile phospholipids and cholesterol rose moderately in pigs when dietary fat content was changed from a low (2%) to medium (10%) level (Juste et al., 1983). Raising dietary fat content to a high level (20%) does not cause bile acid output to increase further but it produces additional increases in the bile output of phospholipids and cholesterol. The degree of saturation of dietary long-chain triglycerides has no effect on the secretion rates of bile acids and phospholipids, but it increases both the secretion rate and concentration of bile cholesterol (Juste et al., 1986). The relationships among bile acids, phospholipids, and cholesterol during secretion into the bile of the pig are thus dependent on the level and nature of dietary fat. This varying effect of dietary fat on the secretion rate of individual bile components may influence bile saturation with cholesterol and result in the formation of cholesterol gallstones. Surprisingly, the cholesterol saturation index of the bile in pigs has been lowered slightly by raising the fat content of the diet (Juste et al., 1985). As pointed out by Desport et al. (1997), the pig has a relatively high efficiency in converting free cholesterol to cholesteryl esters and bile acids in the liver, as well as having its main bile acids hydrophilic rather than hydrophobic, as are the human principal bile acids. Pigs, therefore, spontaneously form cholesterol supersaturated bile or cholesterol calculi as do humans.

The effect of dietary fiber on bile secretion in pigs has also been studied. Feeding pigs for 5 days a diet containing 40% wheat bran, which produced a diet that contained 5% dietary crude fiber, 21% neutral detergent fiber, and 6% acid detergent fiber, caused an increase in bile flow rate with no change in bile cholesterol concentration but a reduction in total bile acid level and resulted in an overall increased secretion in both total bile acids and bile cholesterol (Payne et al., 1989). In another study, Valette et al. (1989) observed that the flow rates of bile and total bile salts were increased after the third day of feeding a 40% wheat bran diet. However, the inclusion of wheat bran in the diet did not change the concentration of total bile acid in the bile. The increased bile flow rate and total bile acid output were maintained in a steady state throughout the remaining 5-day feeding period. These two studies indicate that a high-fiber diet seems to have a choleretic effect on pigs and that the effect is established progressively over a period of several days before reaching a plateau. Little is known about the influence of dietary fiber on bile secretion of phospholipids. More-detailed information regarding nutritional control of bile secretion in pigs and humans has been reviewed by Corring et al. (1989).

D. Pancreatic Exocrine Secretion

The primary functions of exocrine pancreatic secretion are (1) to supply enzymes for the luminal digestion of carbohydrate, fat, and protein and (2) to neutralize the acidity of chyme entering the duodenum and create a suitable intraluminal pH for the action of digestive enzymes. Porcine pancreatic juice as it enters the duodenum contains an organic composite dissolved in an alkaline electrolyte fluid. The concentrations of bicarbonate, chloride, sodium, and potassium in the pancreatic juice of the pig have been summarized (Kidder and Manners, 1978). The organic component of the pancreatic juice is composed of numerous enzymes, proenzymes, and peptides that act as enzyme cofactors and inhibitors.

The pancreas of the pig produces four major classes of digestive enzymes: proteases, carbohydrases, lipases, and nucleases. All proteases and phospholipase A_2 are secreted as proenzymes, whereas α-amylase, chitinase, triacylglycerol lipase, cholesterol esterase, and ribonuclease I are secreted as active enzymes. Enterokinase elaborated by the duodenal mucosa converts most of trypsinogen to trypsin, which activates the remaining trypsinogen, chymotrypsinogen, and procarboxypeptidases A and B as well as proelastase.

The pattern of porcine pancreatic enzymes changes considerably during both the fetal and neonatal periods, as well as at weaning. Ontogeny of pancreatic enzymes in fetal, and pre- and postweaning pigs has been reviewed by Cranwell (1995). At 65 days of gestation, α-amylase, chymotrypsins A and B, elastase II, carboxypeptidase A, and carboxylesterase appear in the pancreas of the fetal pig. Anionic trypsin is presented in fetal pancreas at day 75 of gestation. After birth and before weaning at 4 to 6 weeks of age, cationic trypsin, chymotrypsin C, protease E, and pancreatic ribonuclease appear gradually. Cationic trypsin increases markedly after weaning at 4 to 6 weeks of age, whereas anionic trypsin decreases with age and is present in only trace amounts by 7 to 8 weeks of age. Elastase I begins to appear at 5 weeks of age.

Comprehensive information on postnatal changes in the pancreatic content of several enzymes in pigs from birth to 6 to 8 weeks of age have been generated by Corring et al. (1978), Lindemann et al. (1986), and Owsley et al. (1986), and summarized by Cranwell (1995). When the results are expressed as the increment in total enzyme content of the pancreas per unit body weight and as a function of that in non-nursed pigs at birth, the relative quantities of trypsin remain constant during the first 4 weeks and then increase considerably at 6 to 8 weeks of age as a result of increase in trypsin activity in pancreatic tissue. In the study of Corring et al. (1978) the increase in trypsin coincided with the time when pigs had a 260% increase in dry matter intake compared with that at 4 weeks of age, and in studies by Lindemann et al. (1986) and Owsley et al. (1986) the increase in trypsin happened 2 weeks after weaning when pigs were consuming substantial amounts of solid food. This pattern of trypsin development in the pancreatic tissue corresponds with the findings on pancreatic trypsin secretion reported by Pierzynowski et al. (1990; 1993b) who observed low trypsin output in both pre- and postprandial secretions in pigs nursing sows for up to 4 to 5 weeks of age, and substantially high output of pancreatic trypsin in those pigs after weaning at 4 to 6 weeks of age.

The pattern of development of chymotrypsin is different from that of trypsin. The relative quantities of chymotrypsin increase 1.5- to 3.3-fold up to weaning at 4 weeks of age. There is a sharp drop for 1 week after weaning and then a return to quantities equal to or greater than those immediately before weaning in the subsequent 2 to 4 weeks. The high relative quantities of chymotrypsin during the 2- to 4-week postweaning period of pigs are caused primarily by increased size of the pancreas and by raised enzyme activity in the pancreas.

The developmental pattern of amylase resembles that of chymotrypsin (i.e., an increase in enzyme activity throughout the nursing period followed by a decline during the week after weaning and a recovery to levels similar to or higher than those immediately before weaning in the subsequent 2 to 4 weeks). However, the size of relative increase in pancreatic amylase is substantial and is in the order of 80- to 180-fold compared with less than fourfold for chymotryspin. This large increase in amylase content is partially caused by the extremely low level of amylase occurring in the pancreas at birth. Increasing age rather than changing the nature and quantity of feed received by the pig apparently is the primary factor in the development of pancreatic amylase in pigs, because significant increases in the relative amounts of pancreatic amylase (Lindemann et al., 1986) and in specific activities of CCK-stimulated pancreatic secretion (Harada et al., 1988) happen in pigs having no access to creep feed.

Pancreatic lipase also undergoes a large relative increase during the first 4 weeks after birth. This postnatal increase of lipase seems to be associated with increased intake of lipid from the milk because sow's milk contains 5 to 7% fat (Klobasa et al., 1987), and its production and subsequent consumption by the nursing pig increases during the first 3 to 4 weeks of lactation (Elsley, 1970). This contention is further supported by the findings that the relative quantities of lipase declined after weaning to predominantly carbohydrate and protein diets at 3 to 4 weeks of age (Lindemann et al., 1986; Cera et al., 1990).

In the early postweaning period, development of pancreatic trypsin and chymotrypsin activities is affected by the source of dietary protein. Makkink et al. (1994) showed that skim-milk powder produced the greatest stimulation of trypsin synthesis and secretion at day 3 after weaning and that soybean-protein concentrate was the strongest stimulant for the synthesis and secretion of both trypsin and chymotrypsin at day 6 postweaning. However, at day 10 postweaning, the effect of dietary protein source on the activities of trypsin and chymotrypsin had disappeared. It is clear that age of the pig and the nature of the diet are two major factors that affect the ontogenesis of the pancreas and pancreatic enzymes in the pig. In addition to age and diet, hormones such as corticosteroids have been observed to stimulate the development of pancreatic amylase (Bainter and Németh, 1982; Chapple et al., 1989a,b,c; Kreikemeier et al., 1990; Sangild et al., 1994) and trypsin (Sangild et al., 1994) in nursing pigs.

Pancreatic secretion of alkaline electrolyte fluid and enzymes is regulated physiologically by the autonomic nervous system and the gastrointestinal hormones secretin and CCK and their interactions as well as by the paracrine effects of peptide-secreting pancreatic islet cells and perhaps a number of circulating peptide hormones. The primary hormonal regulator for acinar cells is CCK, and secretin is the primary hormonal regulator for duct cells. However, maximum stimulation of both acinar and duct cells happens when cell surface receptors for CCK, secretin, and acetylcholine are all occupied. Therefore, CCK and secretin together elicit a potentiation of enzyme and bicarbonate output by the pancreas. Detailed information about mechanisms of neurocrine, endocrine, and paracrine control of exocrine pancreatic secretion is provided in publications by Holst (1985), Solomon (1987), and Go et al. (1993).

A negative feedback mechanism mediated through the release of secretin and CCK from the duodenum to control exocrine pancreatic secretion in pigs has been postulated. Corring (1974) found that excluding the entrance of pancreatic juice into the duodenum increased the volume of the pancreatic secretion fivefold and doubled the protein output. Reintroduction of the pancreatic juice into the duodenum suppressed the secretion to its original level. It was further observed that only reintroduction into the duodenum, but not the jejunum or the ileum, was effective in producing this negative feedback response and that infusion of trypsin into the duodenum mimicked this effect of duodenal reintroduction of the pancreatic juice. The proteolytic enzyme fraction of the juice seemed to be the relevant component to elicit a negative feedback control of exocrine pancreatic secretion. Ihse and Lilja (1979) also demonstrated that the negative feedback control of pancreatic secretion in pigs occurred when trypsin but not amylase was introduced into the duodenum. Based on the profile of gastrointestinal hormones, Corring et al. (1985) suggested that secretin may be an important regulator in the negative feedback control of pancreatic secretion. When pancreatic juice was not returned to pigs, secretin concentration in portal and peripheral blood increased significantly but blood concentrations of CCK, gastrin, somatostatin, vasoactive intestinal peptide (VIP), and pancreatic polypeptide were unchanged. Recently, Pierzynowski et al. (1993a) reported that peripheral intravenous injection of CCK into the jugular vein produced no pancreatic secretary response, whereas local injection of CCK into gastroduodenal arterial circulation resulted in increased secretion of pancreatic juice and output of total protein and trypsin in the pig. The data indicate the existence of an indirect stimulation of the exocrine pancreas by CCK through a mechanism mediated locally in the duodenum.

Pancreatic exocrine secretion comprises a basal secretion and a meal-induced postprandial secretion (Solomon, 1987). The basal secretion occurs when all ingested feed has emptied from the stomach and has been digested and absorbed by the small intestine. The meal-induced postprandial secretion occurs during ingestion of feed, and its digestion and absorption. The meal-induced postprandial pancreatic secretion probably is the net result of four phases of secretion: cephalic, gastric, intestinal, and circulatory phases. Mechanisms mediating cephalic and gastric phases of pancreatic secretion are still poorly understood (Solomon, 1987; Go et al., 1993). The existence of a basal preprandial secretion and a meal-induced postprandial secretion produces a continuous pancreatic secretion in pigs (Corring, 1980a). Pancreatic secretion exhibits a biphasic circadian rhythm in young pigs fed three times a day (Thaela et al., 1995).

During the first 4 to 5 postnatal week when pigs were nursed by the sow, the preprandial basal outflow of pancreatic juice was found to be 0.5 ml/kg/h, the total protein output was 1 mg/kg/h, and trypsin activity was 0.2 U/kg/h (Pierzynowski et al., 1990). No postprandial secretory response to feeding from suckling the sow could be detected. Weaning at 4 to 5 weeks of age caused the preprandial basal outflow of pancreatic juice to increase to about 1 to 2 ml/kg/h, the total protein output to 4 to 8 mg/kg/h, and trypsin activity to 2 to 4 U/kg/h during the period of 5 and 13 weeks of age. During this postweaning period, the ingestion of solid feed produced a more than twofold increase in the postprandial pancreatic juice outflow, the total protein output, and trypsin activity. Pierzynowski et al. (1993b) further observed that preprandial pancreatic secretion rates of lipase, co-lipase, and carboxylester lipase in pigs 1 to 2 or 3 to 4 weeks after weaning at 4 or 6 weeks of age were similar to the preweaning values. Postprandial specific activities of these enzymes after weaning were not higher than those before weaning, although postprandial pancreatic output of these enzymes was increased after weaning.

Information regarding older pig's responses in secretion of pancreatic enzymes to feed ingestion and feeding frequency has been summarized by Makkink and Verstegen (1990) and the responses to changes in diet composition have been reviewed by Low and Zebrowska (1989) and Corring et al. (1989). In 40-kg pigs, a sharp rise in outflow of pancreatic juice and the output of total protein and activities of chymotrypsin, trypsin, and amylase in pancreatic secretion occurs after each meal. The enzyme activities peak at 3 h after the meal and remain elevated for up to 5 to 7 h postprandially. For 30-kg pigs, increasing the frequency of feeding from once daily to 3 or 12 times a day raises outflow of pancreatic juice and amylase secretion but does not significantly increase the output of total protein, trypsin, chymotrypsin, lipase, or colipase (Hee et al., 1988; Botermans et al., 1997).

According to Corring (1980b), the amounts of pancreatic enzymes secreted in pigs under normal physiological conditions are sufficient to digest about ten times the quantity of feed typically ingested. Nevertheless, dramatic modification in the pancreatic secretion of pigs has been induced by dietary changes (Corring et al., 1989). Feeding a protein-rich diet to 40-kg pigs results in increased trypsin and chymotrypsin activities in the pancreatic secretion, with chymotrypsin being more responsive to the dietary change (Corring, 1980a). In addition to the level of protein intake, the type of protein source may also affect the secretion of pancreatic proteolytic enzymes in pigs. Valette et al. (1992) found that ingestion of a casein diet produced higher total activities of trypsin, chymotrypsin, carboxypeptidase B, and amylase in pancreatic secretion than did a rapeseed diet in pigs. However, Pöhland et al. (1993) observed no differences in the volume of pancreatic juice secreted and total activities of trypsin, chymotrypsin, and amylase among pigs fed a diet based on cornstarch and soybean meal, cornstarch and canola meal, or 94% of wheat or barley as the primary feed ingredients. Feeding a fat-rich and a starch-rich diet produces, respectively, increased lipase and amylase activities of pancreatic juice (Ozimek et al., 1985; Corring and Chayvialle, 1987). However, Gabert et al. (1996) showed that exocrine pancreatic secretions of lipase and co-lipase in growing pigs were not affected by feeding diets containing 15% oil with different fatty acid composition (fish oil, rapeseed oil, or coconut oil). Flores et al. (1988) reported that replacing 7% of starch with pectin in a cornstarch-based diet produced a decrease in pancreatic secretion of α-amylase but had no effect on the outflow of pancreatic juice and the total secretion of trypsin, chymotrypsin, and lipase in pigs.

Corring and Chayvialle (1987) observed no significant changes in plasma levels of CCK and secretin in pigs fed a starch- or fat-rich diet, although the dietary change yielded significantly higher amylase and lipase activities in the pancreatic juice. The findings suggest that CCK and secretin are not major hormonal regulators in the nutritional control of the amylase and lipase secretion from the exocrine pancreas in pigs.

Molecular aspects of nutritional controls of the synthesis of exocrine pancreatic enzyme in pigs have been explored by Le Huerou-Luron et al. (1993) and Lhoste et al. (1993). It is clear that the mechanisms whereby dietary components alter the expression of specific enzymes occur at the gene level (transcription), the mRNA level (processing, extranuclear transport, cytoplasmic stability, or translation efficiency), and the protein stability level.

E. SMALL INTESTINE WALL SECRETION

The small intestine produces significant amounts of secretions to buffer the contents from the stomach and to lubricate bolus movement. Secretions of the small intestine originate from Brunner's glands in the submucosa and goblet cells at the villus surface. The alkaline and viscous secretion of Brunner's glands is more prominent than that of goblet cells and is released to buffer the very acid chyme as it leaves the stomach. According to Kidder and Manners (1978), the rate of duodenal secretion of Brunner's glands in pigs increases on feeding and the secretion is mediated by neurohormonal stimuli. The mucus secreted by goblet cells is viscous and is a good lubricant for bolus movement. Goblet mucin also blends into the glycocalyx that encases the microvilli and forms a viscous coating to trap molecules near the apical membrane of the enterocytes. The glycocalyx, the mucus layer, and the unstirred water layer near the intestinal surface form a diffusion barrier through which nutrients must pass before entering the enterocytes. The mucous further covers the epithelial layer and prevents the adhesion of noxious intraluminal substances including pathogenic microorganisms.

In addition to the secretion of Brunner's glands and that of goblet cells, the lumen of small intestine also receives bile and pancreatic secretions. In spite of the simultaneous processes of secretion and absorption, there is a net secretion of fluid into the lumen in the proximal half of the small intestine. Horszcaruk et al. (1974) found that the volume of net secretion varied considerably and averaged 300 to 400 ml/m of jejunum/24 h. Total amount of juice secreted into the lumen of the small intestine over a 24-h period in 70-kg pigs was estimated to be about 6 l. Buraczewska (1979) reported that daily secretion of endogenous N into the proximal small intestine of 70-kg pigs was approximately 1 g/m, and 0.5 g/m in the distal part. Assuming the length of the small intestine was 18 m, the daily N secretion into the whole small intestine would be about 15 g.

However, substantial quantities of this endogenous N are digested and absorbed along the small intestine (Low and Zebrowska, 1989). In 45-kg pigs fitted with a permanent cannula in the pancreatic duct and the bile duct and fed a casein diet, 1.85 and 1.82 l of the pancreatic juice and bile, respectively, were secreted into the duodenum per day and would provide an additional 3.6 g of endogenous N (1.9 and 1.7 g of N through pancreatic secretion and bile, respectively) to the lumen of the small intestine (Corring et al., 1990).

III. DIGESTION, FERMENTATION, AND ABSORPTION OF CARBOHYDRATE

The principal dietary carbohydrates for the pig are starch, sugars (such as di- and monosaccharides), and fiber (nonstarch polysaccharides). Starch is a glucose-containing polysaccharide. There are two chemical forms of starch, known as amylose and amylopectin. Amylose consists of a long, unbranched chain of α-1,4-glucosyl units, whereas amylopectin contains α-1,6 branching linkages. The primary dietary disaccharides are lactose and sucrose. Crude fiber for typical feedstuffs is 50 to 80% cellulose, 20% hemicellulose, and 10 to 50% lignin. The use of dietary fiber by the pig is through fermentation and not by direct digestion, because fiber is not subject to hydrolytic action by mammalian enzymes.

A. Oral Digestion of Starch

Ingested starch is first attacked by salivary α-amylase in the mouth. The optimal pH for salivary α-amylase is 6.7, and the hydrolytic products are a mixture of oligosaccharides. Compared with that of pancreatic α-amylase, starch digestion by salivary α-amylase in the pig is very insignificant.

B. Carbohydrate Digestion and Fermentation in the Stomach

In the nonglandular esophageal region and the glandular cardiac zone of the stomach, the gastric pH is maintained above 5.0 by saliva and secretions from the cardiac region, allowing a continuous activity of salivary α-amylase and bacterial fermentation of carbohydrates. Lack of evidence for glucose absorption from carbohydrate digestion in the stomach of pigs has been voiced by Low (1989), because no ^{3}H could be detected in the peripheral blood following administration of labeled 3-O-methyl D-glucose into the stomach of anesthetized pigs with ligated esophageal and pyloric sphincters. Furthermore, no active transport of glucose could be demonstrated in isolated gastric mucosa *in vitro*.

Kidder and Manners (1978), Sambrook (1980), and Ratcliffe (1985) have reviewed gastric fermentation in the pig. Lactic acid produced from lactose fermentation by gastric microflora comprises 80 to 100% of organic acids in the stomach of the suckling pig. Gastric fermentation of lactose plays an important role in the regulation of gastric pH in the young pig. Gastric HCl production occurs in pigs from 1 day after birth but with no significant quantities until 24 days of age. It was found that only 3 of 20 suckling pigs and none of the pigs weaned at 2 days of age were secreting HCl by day 10 after birth and that there was a negative correlation between lactic acid level and pH as well as a positive correlation between pH and number of *Escherichia coli* in the stomach. The production of lactic acid by the microflora in the stomach may inhibit HCl secretion or supplement the limited HCl secretory capacity of the stomach in the young pig. Nevertheless, gastric bacterial fermentation contributes significantly to maintaining the low gastric pH in young pigs. The low pH of the stomach is important for the formation of milk clots in suckling pigs and in the denaturation of protein in general.

Compared with that in pigs consuming only milk, the level of lactic acid in the stomach was lower in pigs after the provision of creep feed. Whereas lactic acid represents 80 to 100% of total organic acids in the stomach of suckling pigs, it only accounts for 50% of total gastric organic acids in older pigs consuming cereal diets. Gastric fermentation in pigs varies with types of dietary carbohydrate. More fermentation occurs in the stomach of pigs when they receive cooked rather than raw potato. On the other hand, exchanging potato starch for cornstarch reduces gastric fermentation. Feeding pigs a diet containing 64% molasses makes the stomach the primary organ of fermentation and produces more volatile fatty acids (VFA) than lactic acid. Some large dietary particles have been found to be retained in the stomach for up to 60 h in 176-kg pigs. This prolonged retention in the stomach could allow substantial fermentation of the dietary fibrous components to proceed. Ratcliffe (1991) has indicated that digesta in the stomach may have low acidity for several hours after feeding to allow microbial growth and inhibit gastric emptying with concomitant gastric fermentation. Feeding a high-fiber rather than a low-fiber diet significantly increases total viable counts of anaerobic bacteria in the stomach content of 7-month-old pigs (Jensen and Jørgensen, 1994). As summarized by Kidder and Manners (1978), the concentrations of lactic acid and VFA in the stomach of pigs increases progressively after feeding and these organic acids are present primarily in the uppermost layer of the stomach in pigs.

C. Gastric Emptying

A primary function of the stomach is mixing, storage, and controlled emptying of small portions of the ingested feed into the duodenum. Physiological and nutritional aspects of gastric emptying in pigs have been described by Low and Zebrowska (1989) and Low (1990). Gastric emptying of liquids is a function of the pressure gradient between the stomach and the duodenum, whereas that of solids takes place when their particle size has been reduced to ≤2 mm. Those solids that cannot be broken down to a sufficiently small size are emptied and swept to the distal small intestine during fasting periods through the migrating myoelectric complex (MMC). The rate of gastric emptying in pigs is most rapid in the first hour after a meal. The postprandial initial rate of gastric emptying rises with increasing size of meal dry matter or volume of water given with the meal. The rate of porcine gastric emptying is also influenced by the particle size, viscosity, and osmolarity of the diet as well as dietary components including lipids, proteins, amino acids, sugars, starch, and nonstarch polysaccharides.

D. Carbohydrate Digestion in the Small Intestine

Once the chyme enters the duodenum, it is mixed with bile, pancreatic juice, and duodenal secretions. All these secretions are alkaline and raise the pH of the chyme out of the range of pepsins (2.0 to 3.5) and into the range of the pancreatic enzymes. The small intestine is the principal digestive and absorptive site of soluble carbohydrate in the pig. Small intestinal digestion includes a luminal phase and a mucosal phase. In the lumen of the small intestine, the macromolecules are hydrolyzed to short-chain polymers by enzymes originating from salivary glands, gastric glands, and, particularly, the pancreas. The products of luminal digestion are further hydrolyzed into monomers by enzymes located at the brush border or in the cell body of enterocytes lining the intestinal mucosa. Detailed information on nutrient digestion in the small intestine of the pig has been reviewed by Kidder and Manners (1978) and Moran (1982). Cranwell (1995) has reviewed digestion of carbohydrate in the small intestine of the neonatal pig.

1. Luminal Digestion

Pancreatic α-amylase is the only active carbohydrase in the intestinal lumen. The luminal-phase digestion of carbohydrate is mainly enzymatic hydrolysis of starch. Kidder and Manners (1978) have indicated that the products of starch digestion in the lumen of pigs include maltose, maltotriose, and α-limit dextrin, as well as traces of glucose. The maltose, maltotriose, and α-limit dextrin of luminal starch digestion and ingested disaccharides such as lactose and sucrose are further degraded into monosaccharides through brush border digestion.

Carbohydrates such as dietary fiber and physiologically resistant starch that are not digested in the small intestine pass into the large intestine where they are exposed to a large population of microflora for fermentation. Additionally, dietary fiber exerts considerable effects on digestive secretions in pigs. Significantly higher outputs of gastric, biliary, and pancreatic secretions are found in pigs fed a high-fiber diet than in those on a low-fiber diet (Dierick et al., 1989). Some dietary fibers also increase the viscosity of the meal, lengthen the retention time in the small intestine, and increase endogenous N secretion. Mechanical erosion of the mucosal surface by dietary fiber leads to increased loss of endogenous materials. A reduction of nutrient digestion generally occurs when fiber is added to the diet (Eggum, 1995), because of the factors listed above and the fact that some nutrients are adsorbed to the fiber particles and carried to the large intestine.

2. Mucosal Digestion

Brush border digestion of carbohydrate involves ingested disaccharides and the oligosaccharide products of starch digestion by salivary and pancreatic α-amylase (Alpers, 1987). Enterocytes in the mucosal layer of the small intestine produce six carbohydrases that are incorporated into the luminal membrane and transported to the tip of the brush border in the mature cells (Kidder and Manners, 1978; Alpers, 1987; Herdt, 1992; Argenzio, 1993b). These carbohydrases are lactase, trehalase, and four maltases (sucrase, isomaltase, maltase II, and maltase III).

Ingested lactose is hydrolyzed by lactase to glucose and galactose. The concentration of lactase in the intestinal mucosa is very high in the very young pigs and decreases with age. Compared with that at birth, the lactase activity at 24 h after birth is threefold higher and coincides with rapid intestinal growth in the suckling pigs (Zhang et al., 1997). The specific activity of lactase remains high during the first 7 to 10 days after birth (Sangild et al., 1991). Lactase activity is highest in the proximal part and lowest in the distal part of the small intestine in newborn and 1-day-old pigs (Buddington and Malo, 1996), but is more evenly distributed along the intestine at 6 to 10 days of age (Cranwell, 1995). In suckling pigs, the lactase activity drops considerably during the second to fifth weeks of age, and then remains constant or declines gradually to 8 weeks of age. This decline in the specific activity in lactase with age is offset by the increase in small intestinal weight. Therefore, the total lactase activity in the small intestine of the suckling pig remains fairly constant.

Ingested sucrose is hydrolyzed by sucrase to glucose and fructose. Ingested trehalose is broken down by trehalase to two α-glucose molecules. Maltose and maltotriose from luminal digestion of starch are hydrolyzed very rapidly to glucose by all the maltases. The α-limit dextrins are hydrolyzed rapidly by isomaltase and slowly by maltase II and III to yield glucose. The residual oligosaccharides of the limit dextrins may then be acted on by α-amylase or maltases or both. An α-limit dextranase which is a specific α-1,4-oligosaccharidase with a superior capacity to hydrolyze terminal 1,4-bonds in limit dextrins also occurs in the duodenal and jejunal regions of pig small intestine.

At birth, little maltase activity and little or no sucrase activity were present in the small intestine (Buddington and Malo, 1996). According to Cranwell (1995), the specific activities of maltase and sucrase in pigs' small intestine rise rapidly from 1 week of age, reach a peak at 10 to 16 days after birth, and then level off at about 3 weeks of age. From 3 to 4 to 6 to 8 weeks of age, maltase and sucrase activities either remained constant or increased gradually. The total maltase and sucrase activities in the small intestine rise over eightfold from 10 to 20 days of age in pigs fed milk-replacer diets from 2 to 20 days of age, whereas total maltase and sucrase activities in the small intestine of suckling pigs rise 26-fold and 14-fold, respectively, from 1 to 8 weeks of age. The distribution patterns of maltase and sucrase activities along the small intestine in suckling pigs at 6 to 7 days of age are similar for both enzymes and are greater in the upper to mid-jejunum than in the distal portion of the small intestine. In 2- to 4-week-old pigs, the distribution of sucrase is similar to that of 6-day-old pigs. Maltase activity changes with age from being predominantly in the proximal half of the small intestine at 1 week of age to distribute evenly along the intestine at

2 to 3 weeks of age and then to being predominantly in the mid-region of the intestine (from 10 to 15% to 80 to 90% along the small intestine) at 5 to 8 weeks of age.

Weaning produces significant changes in the carbohydrases of the small intestine. Compared with suckling pigs of similar age, pigs weaned at 3 or 5 weeks of age have significantly lower sucrase, lactase, and isomaltose activities at 5 days after weaning. However, maltase II and III activities at 5 days after weaning increase in pigs weaned at 5 weeks of age but not in those weaned at 3 weeks of age. By 11 days after weaning, sucrase activity has recovered partially to the preweaning level but lactase activity continues to drop. In addition to influencing the specific enzyme activities, weaning also causes changes in the intestinal morphology. In pigs weaned at 3 or 5 weeks of age, a reduction in villus height and cessation of growth of small intestine occur during the 3 days following weaning. These detrimental effects of weaning are more severe in the 3- than 5-week-old pigs and are caused by the reduced feed intake associated with weaning.

Kidder and Manners (1980) have determined the level and distribution of brush border carbohydrases in the small intestinal mucosa of pigs from 3 weeks to 1500 days of age. From 2 weeks after weaning up to 200 days of age the activities of brush border carbohydases, with the exception of lactase, increase continuously. After 200 days of age sucrase and isomaltase activities continue to increase, but maltase II and III and trehalase activities level off.

E. Absorption of Small Intestinal Carbohydrate Digestion Products

Glucose, galactose, and fructose are the primary end products of carbohydrate digestion and are absorbed by the mature enterocytes lining the upper third of the intestinal villi. Absorption takes place in the duodenum and jejunum and is usually complete before the chyme arrives at the ileum. Glucose and galactose are absorbed by a two-stage process (Thorens, 1993; Wright, 1993). Glucose and galactose are initially transported into the enterocyte against their concentration gradient by a Na-dependent glucose cotransporter (SGLT 1) located in the apical brush border and then are released into the blood by a facilitated sugar transporter (GLUT2) located on the basolateral membrane. Fructose is absorbed first by a Na-independent brush border fructose transporter (GLUT5) and then is released out of the enterocyte into the blood by GLUT2, as are glucose and galactose. Because of the simultaneous active transport of Na, the absorption of glucose and galactose is very rapid and efficient compared with that of fructose, which is determined by its concentration gradient from gut to blood.

F. Microbial Activity in the Small Intestine

Gut microorganisms may adhere to dietary particles, particularly fibrous components. Because of the rapid passage of digesta through the small intestine, fermentation of dietary fiber in the small intestine of the pig may be limited. However, the microbial activity in the small intestine can still have substantial implications for the degradation of some carbohydrates that are not digested by host carbohydrases. The review by Low (1989) shows that significant disappearance of the nonstarch polysaccharides from fibrous ingredients, such as rutabagas (swedes), wheat bran, and beet pulp, occurs anterior to the terminal ileum, possibly as a result of microbial activity. This largely microbial activity is associated with substantial production of VFA. Experiments in pigs with ileorectal anastomoses have shown that up to 70% of the uronic acids and 40% of the arabinose from diets containing sugar beet pulp are degraded within the small intestine.

G. Large Intestinal Digestion and Fermentation

About 30 to 60% of total gastrointestinal content of the pig resides in the large intestine where it is retained for 20 to 38 h as compared with 0 to 6 h in the stomach and 2 to 6 h in the small intestine (Low and Zebrowska, 1989). This extended retention time in the large intestine provides ample time for bacterial digestion of carbohydrate.

Dietary carbohydrates that escape digestion in the small intestine of pigs pass through ileocecal valve and into the large intestine where they are digested and fermented by the microflora. Many reviews have been published regarding the digestion and absorption of dietary nutrients in the large intestine of pigs (Kidder and Manners, 1978; Rérat, 1978; Mason, 1980; Agricultural Research Council, 1981) and the specific aspects of dietary fiber digestion (Low, 1985; Varel and Yen, 1997) and VFA production and absorption (Argenzio, 1982; Yen, 1997) in the large intestine of pigs. The role of the microorganisms in digestion that occurs in the large intestine in the pig has been reviewed by Ratcliffe (1985; 1991). Moughan et al. (1992) have summarized the development of microflora in the large intestine of newborn and suckling pigs. Function and regulation of the gastrointestinal microbiota of the pig has been reviewed by Conway (1994). More information regarding intestinal bacteria and their influence on the nutrition of the pig is also provided in Chapter 26.

Although dietary fiber and physiologically resistant starch (Englyst, 1989), which are not readily digested by host enzymes, are the primary substrates for microbial digestion and fermentation in the large intestine, all organic substances entering the large intestine are potential substrates for fermentation. The fiber is degraded by the activity of microbial species that produce cellulases, hemicellulases, pectinases, and other enzymes (Varel and Yen, 1997). The degree of fermentation depends primarily upon the source of dietary fiber and on the presence of nitrogen, minerals, and vitamins, which are essential for the overall nutrition of the microbial populations residing in the hindgut.

In addition to VFA, which are the most important products of microbial fermentation, various gases including methane are also produced in the large intestine. Methanogenesis, however, accounts for a minimal loss of digestible energy in pigs. In 20- to 120-kg growing pigs, Christensen and Thorbek (1987) estimated that methane energy production was equal to 1.2% of daily gross energy intake for cereal-based diets. Müller and Kirchgessner (1985a,b) observed that methane production from alfalfa meal and pectin represented 2.2 and 9.0% of gross energy intake in 184-kg sows, respectively. Robinson et al. (1989) reported that methane production occurred only in the colon and in half of the cecal samples in 80- to 120-kg pigs fed a corn–soybean meal diet. Significantly more methanogenic, sulfate-reducing and total anaerobic bacteria were found in the colon than the cecum in pigs that were fed a corn–soybean meal diet for 4, 8, or 11 weeks beginning at 8 weeks of age and 18 kg body weight (Butine and Leedle, 1989). In 7-month-old pigs weighing 128 kg, Jensen and Jørgensen (1994) observed that pigs fed a low-fiber wheat starch–barley diet produced methane at a rate of 1.4 l/day, compared with 12.5 l/day for pigs fed a high-fiber diet containing barley, pea fiber, and pectin.

As indicated in the review by Varel and Yen (1997), depending on the source of fiber, the number of cellulolytic bacteria in the colon of pigs may increase by prolonged feeding of high-fiber diets. In contrast to a twofold increase in cellulolytic bacteria from feeding diets containing 40 and 96% of alfalfa meal, no increase in cellulolytic activity was seen when a 20% corncob diet was fed to sows. Overall, the number of cellulolytic bacteria represents 10% of the culturable flora when high-fiber diets are fed and it is 6.7 times greater in adult than growing pigs.

H. Absorption of Gut Volatile Fatty Acids

VFA or short-chain fatty acid (SCFA) are the primary products of the bacterial fermentation in the gut and account for 98% of all organic acids occurring in the large intestine of pigs (Clemens et al., 1975). The average concentration of VFA in the large intestine of pigs is about 150 to 250 mM (Clemens et al., 1975; Kidder and Manners, 1978; Argenzio, 1982; Low, 1985; Ratcliffe, 1991; Rérat, 1996).

The predominant VFA is acetic acid, followed by propionic and butyric acids, and their proportions may vary according to many dietary factors including level and source of dietary fiber and the ratio of enzymatically degradable carbohydrates to crude fiber (Low, 1985; Kirchgessner and Muller, 1991; Breves and Stück, 1995; Rérat, 1996). As indicated in the review by Yen (1997), VFA are readily absorbed from the intestine and used in the intermediary metabolism in the intestinal tissues, the liver, and throughout the peripheral tissues. Studies with cecal infusion of carbohydrates and VFA have shown that <1 to 2% of infused energy is excreted as VFA in the feces of pigs (Kirchgessner and Muller, 1991). The net absorption of gut VFA into hepatic portal blood in pigs has been quantified by measuring portoarterial concentration differences and blood flow in the portal vein (Rérat et al., 1987; Yen et al., 1991). Based on literature estimates of the energy requirement of pigs, Rérat et al. (1987) calculated that absorbed VFA could contribute 20% of the maintenance energy requirement in 60-kg pigs when the measurement was conducted after a 24-h fast and 30% of the maintenance requirement when the fast lasted only 12 h. By placing the portoarterial-catheterized pig in an open-circuit calorimeter, Yen et al. (1991) were able to determine simultaneously the whole-body heat production and net portal absorption of VFA during the 12-h postprandial period after a 24-h fast in 37-kg pigs. With a whole-body heat production of 2.70 kcal/h/kg body weight, the VFA absorbed into the portal vein had a potential to contribute 24% of energy for the whole-body heat production if all of the absorbed VFA were combusted to CO_2. However, it should be realized that the energetic efficiency of absorbed VFA in the intermediary metabolism of pigs may be only 68% (Kirchgessner and Muller, 1991).

As pointed out by Argenzio (1981), rapid absorption of VFA by colonic mucosa facilitates colonic absorption of Na and water. Therefore, the microbial production of VFA in the large intestine not only salvages dietary organic matter that was not digested in the small intestine, it also enhances absorption of Na and water, a primary function of the large intestine.

IV. PROTEIN DIGESTION AND ABSORPTION

The general pattern of protein digestion and absorption is similar to that of carbohydrate digestion and absorption, in that macromolecular proteins are broken down into oligopeptides and then to amino acids, dipeptides, and tripeptides before being absorbed into the enterocyte.

A. Gastric Digestion of Protein

Digestion of ingested protein begins in the stomach through the action of gastric proteases and HCl. Pepsins secreted as inactive pepsinogens are the principal hydrolytic enzymes in the stomach of growing and adult pigs, although chymosin secreted as prochymosin is also important for the suckling pig (Low and Zebrowska, 1989; Low, 1990). Under the acidic condition of the stomach, pepsinogens are converted to pepsins by autocatalytic catalysis. The conversion occurs slowly at pH 5 to 6 but very rapidly at pH 2. The pepsins each have two pH optima, one about pH 2 and the other near 3.5. At pH 2, the relative values of general proteolytic activity for porcine pepsin A, pepsin B, and gastricsin are 100, 1, and 70, respectively (Cranwell, 1995). Proteolytic activity of these gastric proteases declines above pH 3.5 and is absent above pH 6.0. Pepsin A hydrolyzes only peptide bonds between L-amino acids, with greater preference for those with aromatic side chains, followed by glutamic acid, and then cysteine or cystine.

Chymosin is the most important protease in the immediate postnatal period of the pig (Cranwell, 1995). Pig chymosin is mainly a milk-clotting enzyme with limited general proteolytic activity. Chymosin acts specifically against casein of milk protein and clots milk without further proteolytic breakdown of peptide bonds. It allows peptides, growth factors, and immunoglobulins present in colostrum and milk to pass into the small intestine without being degraded. Clotting of milk plays a role in the control of gastric emptying and the development of the stomach in the suckling pig.

As described in the reviews by Low and Zebrowska (1989) and Low (1990), gastric digestion of proteins in pigs can be affected markedly by various sources of proteins and their processing treatments. Studies with 28-day-old pigs killed 1 h postprandially showed that gastric proteolysis of bovine milk proteins was slower than that of fish protein, isolated soybean protein, or whey-supplemented milk and that heat-damaged milk protein was less readily digested than undamaged protein. In older, conscious, growing pigs fitted with a duodenal cannula cranial to the pancreatic duct, gastric proteolysis during the 12-h postprandial period was found to be less rapid for a semipurified diet based on casein than for a cereal diet supplemented with soybean meal. The rate of gastric proteolysis during the 4-h postprandial period in growing pigs with gastric cannulas, however, was not influenced by different types of nonstarch polysaccharides.

Low (1989) indicated that there was no evidence for amino acid absorption in the stomach of pigs, because no ^{14}C could be detected in the peripheral blood following administration of labeled amino acids into the stomach of anesthetized pigs with ligated esophageal and pyloric sphincters. Furthermore, no active transport of amino acids could be demonstrated in isolated gastric mucosa *in vitro*.

B. Digestion of Protein in the Small Intestine

Similar to that of carbohydrate, small intestinal digestion of protein also comprises both luminal and muscosal phases.

1. Luminal Digestion

In the lumen of the small intestine, large molecular proteins are broken down by pancreatic proteases to release neutral and basic amino acids as well as oligopeptides. Unlike amylase, the pancreatic proteases secreted into the intestinal lumen are in the form of proenzymes. The pancreatic proenzymes consist of a group of endopeptidases including trypsinogen, chymotrypsinogen, and proelastase and a group of exopeptidases comprising procarboxypeptidases A and B. Trypsinogen is activated to trypsin in the duodenum by enterokinase, a duodenal brush border enzyme that is stimulated by trypsinogen and released from the membrane by the action of bile acids (Alpers, 1987). The trypsin then activates more trypsinogen autocatalytically as well as the other pancreatic proenzymes. Luminal digestion of protein by active pancreatic enzymes produces amino acids and considerable amounts of oligopeptides. Friedrich (1989) has suggested that the active pancreatic enzymes can only release a maximum of 25% of amino acids in free form and that 80% of α-amino nitrogen in the jejunum and ileum are in peptide form. Further hydrolysis of oligopeptides occurs at the brush border.

2. Mucosal Digestion

The final stages of protein digestion in the small intestine are carried out by a wide array of brush border and cytoplasmic peptidases in the enterocyte (Alpers, 1987; Argenzio, 1993b). The number of brush border and cytoplasmic peptidases identified in the enterocyte is large and is growing continuously (Alpers, 1987; Friedrich, 1989). Oligopeptides of more than three amino acids are hydrolyzed extracellularly by brush border peptidases. Tripeptides and dipeptides are broken down by both brush border and cytoplasmic peptidases (Alpers, 1987) or are absorbed intact and transported into the circulation (Friedrich, 1989). The occurrence and location of the peptidase in enterocytes has been described by Alpers (1987). The literature regarding transport steps of peptide absorption is provided by Friedrich (1989).

C. Bacterial Digestion of Protein in the Large Intestine

Microflora in the small intestine of pigs can use N from dietary nitrogenous compounds and urea diffused into the lumen as well as enzymatic secretions of the host, mucin, and sloughed epithelial cells for incorporation into bacterial cells. However, the impact of small intestinal microorganisms on host protein metabolism in the pig is small, as evidenced by the similar degree of protein digestion in the small intestine of germ-free and conventional pigs (Salter, 1984).

Anatomy of the Digestive System and Nutritional Physiology

The 20- to 38-h retention times of digesta in the large intestine of the pig provides ample time for bacterial digestion of protein. Many reviews have been published regarding the digestion and absorption of protein in the large intestine of pigs (Kidder and Manners, 1978; Rérat, 1978; Mason, 1980; Agricultural Research Council, 1981), and the specific aspects of dietary nitrogenous metabolism (Mason, 1984; Low and Zebrowska, 1989).

Between 2 to 15 g of N enter the cecum daily in pigs weighing 30 to 50 kg (Zebrowska, 1982). A considerable portion (40 to 60%) of this N is present as protein of dietary, endogenous, and bacterial origin, and the remaining portion is present as peptides, free amino acids, urea, ammonia, and others. The endogenous protein contains relatively high levels of proline and glycine as well as serine and threonine that constitute a large proportion of the mucoproteins, pancreas secretions, and bile acids. The flow of N entering the large intestine is influenced by the composition of dietary N, the type of dietary fiber, and the rate of fiber passage (Mason, 1984). The wall of the large intestine supplies N in the form of urea, mucins, and sloughed epithelial cells that account for one quarter of the N entering the lumen of the large intestine of pigs.

The microflora in the large intestine of pigs are capable of degrading most of exogenous and endogenous nitrogenous compounds through the deamination and decarboxylation of all amino acids, urea hydrolysis, and microbial protein synthesis (Low and Zebrowska, 1989; Ratcliffe, 1991). The end products of large intestinal digestion of nitrogenous compounds are ammonia, amines, VFA, and microbial amino acids. The ammonia is used by many porcine intestinal microflora as the primary or preferential N source for the synthesis of bacterial amino acids (Takahashi et al., 1980). Approximately 3 to 6 g of bacterial N are excreted in pig feces per kilogram of dry matter intake and it constitutes about 60 to 80% of the fecal N in the pig (Low and Zebrowska, 1989). The amino acid composition of the fecal nitrogenous compounds is remarkably similar to that of fecal bacteria isolated from pigs and is largely independent of diet. The magnitude of microbial protein synthesis in the large intestine of pigs is not limited by the nitrogenous supply, but rather is affected by the quantity and nature of carbohydrates entering the hind gut (Low and Zebrowska, 1989; Ratcliffe, 1991). Infusion of carbohydrate into the cecum increases bacterial protein excreted in the feces of pigs. Likewise, increasing levels of fiber as straw, oatfeed, or sugarbeet pulp increase fecal N output in pigs. Substitution of cornstarch with raw potato starch results in more undigested starch entering the large intestine and increased fecal and bacterial N outputs. Incorporation of lactulose into the diets of pigs produces a 70% increase in fecal N. Replacement of a portion of cereal with nonstarch polysaccharide such as grass meal, partly hydrolyzed straw meal, or pure straw cellulose and pectin also raises fecal and bacterial N excretion in pigs.

D. Absorption of Products of Protein Digestion

The products of luminal and mucosal digestion of protein are transported across the brush border membrane and into the enterocytes by several specialized transport mechanisms (Kidder and Manners, 1978; Herdt, 1992). The reviews by Alpers (1987), Friedrich (1989), Rérat and Corring (1991), and Kilberg et al. (1993) have covered the transport systems for amino acids and peptides in mammals. There are two Na-independent facilitated transport systems for neutral amino acids and cationic or basic amino acids. Additionally, at least four different Na-dependent active systems exist to transport most neutral amino acids, two amino acids (proline and hydroxyproline), two neutral amino acids (phenylalanine and methionine), and two acidic amino acids (glutamate and aspartate). Cysteine and cystine are taken up by a different Na-dependent transport system. A substantial amount of protein is absorbed into the enterocytes as intact dipeptides and tripeptides.

The transport systems for intact dipeptides and tripeptides are different from those for amino acids, but the number of specific peptide transfer systems is still unclear (Alpers, 1987; Friedrich, 1989; Webb et al., 1992). There is no evidence for intact transport of tetrapeptides (Silk et al., 1985; Friedrich, 1989). It is estimated in the hamster that about 90% of intact peptides entering the cell are hydrolyzed to free amino acids in the cytoplasm of the enterocyte and the remaining

10% of peptides can diffuse across the basolateral membrane into the blood (Gardner, 1984). In pigs, all the peptides seem to be hydrolyzed in the cytoplasm and no intact peptide appears in the portal blood (Rérat and Corring, 1991).

After absorption, amino acids are degraded, metabolized to other amino acids, incorporated into proteins in the intestinal wall, or released unchanged into the portal blood. Various segments of the small intestine have different absorptive capacities for products of protein digestion. In pigs weighing 50 to 75 kg, Buraczewska (1981a,b,c) found that the proximal small intestine absorbed the least N from amino acid solutions compared with the middle and distal small intestine, which absorbed similar quantities of N. The rates of amino acid absorption varied among different amino acids and depended on the concentration of amino acids in the solution. With protein hydrolyzates containing both amino acids and peptides, the disappearance from the lumen of the intestinal loop was faster for the peptide fraction than for the amino acid fraction.

Ammonia produced from microbial urea hydrolysis moves freely between the intestine and body fluids, and is the primary nitrogenous compound absorbed from the large intestine. The rate of ammonia absorption in the large intestine is dependent on the luminal pH. The quantity of ammonia available for absorption also depends on the relative rate of ammonia incorporation into microbial protein. According to Low and Zebrowska (1989), absorption of intact amino acids from bacterial, endogenous, or dietary sources in the large intestine of pigs is much more limited and probably of little nutritional significance to the pig. Studies with infusion of radiolabeled isoleucine and lysine into the cecum of 35-kg pigs show no incorporation of labeled amino acids into body proteins other than colonic wall. However, microbial lysine has recently been observed to be absorbed and incorporated into body protein by 18-kg pigs (Torrallardona et al., 1993). The absorbed lysine has been estimated to approximate the maintenance needs of the pig and to represent a not insignificant quantity (Fuller, 1994).

V. DIGESTION AND ABSORPTION OF FAT

Dietary fats are composed primarily of triglycerides and some phospholipids, sterols, and sterol esters. Fats do not dissolve in water. To subject dietary fat to the actions of water-soluble, hydrolytic enzymes in the gastrointestinal tract, fats must be emulsified.

A. Gastric Fat Digestion

Digestion of dietary fats is initiated in the stomach. Dietary fats are warmed to body temperature and subjected to the intense mixing, agitating, and sieving actions of the distal stomach. These distal-stomach actions break fat globules up into droplets that pass into the small intestine for further emulsification and eventual enzymatic hydrolysis. Although the digestion of fat is dependent primarily on pancreatic enzymes secreted into the duodenum, gastric lipase also plays a major role in the hydrolysis of triglycerides in the stomach of the young pig. The gastric lipase of newborn and 16-day-old milk-fed pigs was found to hydrolyze 25 to 50% of dietary lipid to diglycerides, monoglycerides, and free fatty acids (Newport and Howarth, 1985; Chiang et al., 1989).

B. Fat Digestion and Absorption in the Small Intestine

Digestion of triglycerides in the lumen of the small intestine involves bile emulsification of lipid droplets released from the stomach, hydrolysis of emulsified particles by the combined action of pancreatic lipase and colipase, and micelle formation of the end products of lipase digestion with bile acids and phospholipids (Kidder and Manners, 1978; Shiau, 1987; Herdt, 1992; Argenzio, 1993b). The end products of lipase hydrolysis of each triglyceride are two free nonesterified fatty acids and a monoglyceride. Phospholipids and sterols are hydrolyzed by pancreatic phospholipase and cholesterol esterase, respectively, to yield nonesterified fatty acids, lysophospholipids, and cholesterol.

Monoglycerides and fatty acids resulting from luminal lipid digestion are combined with bile acids and phospholipids to form micelles that are small negatively charged, water-soluble aggregates (Kidder and Manners, 1978; Sambrook, 1980; Shiau, 1987; Herdt, 1992; Argenzio, 1993b). The micelles diffuse through the gut lumen to the brush border of the mucosal cells and allow the lipids to diffuse across the apical membrane of the enterocyte and into the cell.

After absorption into the enterocyte, the long-chain monoglycerides are reesterified with the long-chain fatty acids to diglycerides, which are further esterified to triglycerides (Kidder and Manners, 1978; Herdt, 1992). The resynthesized triglycerides are then associated with cholesterol, cholesterol esters, phospholipids, and various apoproteins to form chylomicrons, which are in turn transported across the intestine into the lymph. The short-chain fatty acids, however, pass directly into the portal blood without being esterified. Fat absorption occurs along the whole length of the small intestine up to 30 cm cranial to the ileocecal valve in 50- to 60-kg pigs. Absorption is slight immediately caudal to the pylorus but very intense at the end of the duodenum and the proximal two thirds of the jejunum-ileum.

The metabolism of lipids in the pig is also affected by microflora of the small intestine (Ratcliffe, 1985). The presence of microflora in the small intestine reduces the digestibility of dietary fat as observed in 90-kg pigs fed diet without or with antibiotic supplements to suppress gut microflora. The microflora in the small intestine increase biohydrogenation of unsaturated fatty acids, resulting in a decreased proportion of unsaturated fatty acids and increased proportion of stearic acid that is less well absorbed. The primary bile acids secreted into the small intestine of the pig are deconjugated by intestinal lactobacilli to form secondary bile acids that are less active in forming micelles and are less well absorbed. More bile acids are excreted in the feces of 6-week-old conventional pigs compared with germ-free animals.

C. Digestion and Absorption of Fat in the Large Intestine

Mason (1980) has indicated that more total lipid is excreted in the feces than is passed through the terminal ileum in pigs fed a typical cereal-based diet, suggesting a synthesis or secretion of lipid within the large intestine of pigs. During the passage through the large intestine, unsaturated fatty acids are hydrogenated by the gut microflora. Cholesterol, dietary sterols, bile acids, and other lipids are also altered extensively by the microflora in the large intestine (Ratcliffe, 1985; 1991). Cholesterol is reduced by hindgut microflora to coprostanol, coprostanone, and cholesterone (Maxwell and Stewart, 1995). Conjugated bile acids entering the cecum and colon are hydrolyzed by the gut microflora, primarily *Bacteroides* spp., to release free bile acids. Some of free bile acids may adsorb to fibrous material and reduce micelle formation. Microbial degradation of triglycerides yields free long-chain fatty acids and VFA. The free unsaturated fatty acids may then be hydrogenated by gut microflora before forming calcium soaps. The assimilation and alteration of fat by the hindgut microflora and the endogenous secretion of fat within the large intestine secretion make it challenging to assess and interpret the digestibility of lipids from fecal samples.

VI. WATER AND ELECTROLYTE ABSORPTION

Large volumes of digestive secretions are delivered into the digestive tract. Reabsorption of water and electrolyte from these digestive secretions is a critical function of the intestine.

A. Small Intestine Absorption

Beside digesting and absorbing dietary carbohydrate, protein, and fat, the small intestine also absorbs water- and fat-soluble vitamins, minerals, and large amounts of water of both dietary and endogenous origin. Substantial quantities of fluids are secreted by the gastrointestinal tract and its accessory glands into the intestinal lumen for the processes of digestion and absorption. These fluids are reabsorbed by the enterocytes and returned to the enterosystemic circulation to preserve the extracellular volume and arterial pressure. In pigs weighing 50 to 75 kg, the capacity of fluid absorption increased along the length of the small intestine, and the quantities of fluid absorbed during a 24-h period were 1 to 2 l/m and 4 to 5 l/m length for the proximal and distal small intestine, respectively (Buraczewska, 1981a). Most of the fluid transport in the small intestine of the pig is by passive diffusion via the intercellular passage and little is by active transport via epithelial cells (Liebler et al., 1992).

B. LARGE INTESTINE ABSORPTION

The ileum and the proximal large intestine of pigs secrete large quantities of alkaline fluid to facilitate microbial digestion. Substantial quantities of this fluid and associated electrolytes are reabsorbed by the surface epithelium along the length of the colon, particularly in the proximal 40% of the colon (Mason, 1980). In 40-kg pigs, 3.2 l of water is absorbed daily in the large intestine of animals fed a cereal–fish meal diet and 1.0 l of water is absorbed in animals fed a low-fiber casein semipurified diet (Low et al., 1978). Addition of 6% cellulose to a semipurified diet containing 3% cellulose increases the flow of water through the ileum and anus of pigs by threefold (Partridge, 1978). Thus, the higher the dietary fiber content and the less digestible the diet, the more water is cycled through the digestive tract and subsequently absorbed in the large intestine of pigs. Within the first one third of the colon in the pig, the dry matter of digesta increases from 13 to 20% and within the remaining two thirds up to 25% (Liebler et al., 1992). Colonic absorption of water is a passive process that couples with active electrolyte transport. A close relationship occurs between the movement of water and sodium in the digestive tract of pigs (Partridge, 1978). Sodium and magnesium are absorbed efficiently in the large intestine. Information on colonic electrolyte transport and its regulation in the pig has been reviewed briefly by Liebler et al. (1992).

VII. ANTIBODY ABSORPTION BY NEONATAL ENTEROCYTES

As indicated by Pond and Houpt (1978), the transfer of antibodies from the sow to her pigs *in utero* is prevented by the six layers of the pig's epitheliochorial placenta, and neonatal pigs are born with little or no passive immunity. Fortunately, enterocytes in all but the most proximal regions of the small intestine of neonatal pigs are capable of absorbing colostral antibodies by endocytosis before intestinal closure at 18 to 36 h of life (Weström et al., 1984; Bainter, 1986). The intestinal closure in pigs is due to a reduced transfer of the internalized macromolecules into the blood and not caused by a decrease in the endocytotic capacity of the enterocytes or a higher degradation rate within the cells (Ekström and Weström, 1991). Only prenatally produced fetal-type enterocytes have the ability for intestinal uptake and transfer of macromolecules, and they are replaced completely during the first 19 postnatal days by adult-type enterocytes that are capable of digesting and absorbing nutrients (Smith, 1988).

VIII. MEASUREMENTS OF NUTRIENT DIGESTION AND ABSORPTION

Disappearance of a nutrient from the digestive lumen has been used as a criterion for the digestion and absorption of that nutrient in pigs. The primary method to quantify nutrient disappearance from the gut in pigs is to measure the disappearance of ingested nutrients through the end of the ileum. Values obtained in this manner are termed ileal digestibility values. For determining ileal digestibility value, several methodologies have been developed to intercept digesta before they reach the cecum of pigs. These techniques include T cannulation of the terminal ileum, reentrant cannulation between the ileum and cecum, post-ileo-cecal-valve reentrant cannulation between the ileum and colon, postvalvular T-cecum cannulation, steered ileocecal-valve cannulation, and ileorectal anastomosis. Surgical procedures for these techniques have been described briefly in Chapter 42.

Digestive secretions and desquamated mucosal cells add considerable quantities of endogenous protein to the lumen of the small intestine during the passage of feed through the gastrointestinal tract. The endogenous protein is only partly digested and absorbed in the small intestine. To obtain the true ileal digestibility of protein and amino acids in a feed, the endogenous nitrogen loss should be considered. However, because of the difficulty in quantifying endogenous protein and amino acid output, most of ileal digestibility measurements of protein and amino acids have apparent digestibility. Information on apparent and true ileal digestibility of amino acids in some feed ingredients commonly used by pigs has been compiled for formulating swine diets (NRC, 1998). This issue of apparent vs. true digestibility of amino acids is discussed in Chapter 9.

The review by Batterham (1994) shows that a substantial portion of ileal digestible lysine in some feed ingredients, such as cottonseed meal or other heat-damaged protein meals, seems to be absorbed in a form that is not efficiently utilized by the pig for optimum growth, suggesting that apparent ileal lysine digestibility values of these feed ingredients overestimate their nutritive potential. The measurement of uptake into the hepatic portal blood of amino acids and other end products of intestinal degradation of nutrients, rather than of their disappearance from the digestive lumen, would be a better measurement of the digestion and absorption of feeds in pigs. This requires the quantification of arteriovenous differences (systemic arterial blood to portal venous blood) in concentration to be multiplied by the rate of blood flow in the portal vein (Rérat et al., 1980). Methodologies to measure simultaneously the portal blood flow rate and portoarterial concentration differences in end products of intestinal digestion and absorption in pigs have been developed and these are summarized in Chapter 42. It should be realized that such uptake measurements apply only to substances that are absorbed and transported into the portal vein, but not to compounds such as long-chain fatty acids that are transported into the lymphatic system. Furthermore, because a portion of absorbed substances is metabolized by the gut wall, the quantity appearing in the portal blood represents only the net uptake into the portal vein and not the entire amount of absorption.

REFERENCES

Agricultural Research Council. 1981. *The Nutrient Requirements of Pigs*, Commonwealth Agricultural Bureaux, Slough, U.K.

Alpers, D. H. 1987. Digestion and absorption of carbohydrates and proteins. In *Physiology of the Gastrointestinal Tract*, Vol. II, 2nd ed., Johnson, L. R., Ed., Raven Press, New York, 1469.

Argenzio, R. A. 1981. Short-chain fatty acids and the colon, *Dig. Dis. Sci.*, 26:97.

Argenzio, R. A. 1982. Volatile fatty acid production and absorption from the large intestine of the pig. In *Digestive Physiology in the Pig*, Laplace, J. P., T. Corring, and A. Rérat, Eds., Proc. 2nd International Seminar, Jouy-en-Josas, Versailles, INRA, Paris, France, 207.

Argenzio, R. A. 1993a. Secretory functions of the gastrointestinal tract. In *Duke's Physiology of Domestic Animals*, 11th ed., Swenson, M. J., and W. O. Reece, Eds., Comstock Publishing Associates, Cornell University Press, Ithaca, NY, 349.

Argenzio, R. A. 1993b. Digestion and absorption of carbohydrate, fat, and protein. In *Duke's Physiology of Domestic Animals*, 11th ed., Swenson, M. J., and W. O. Reece, Eds., Comstock Publishing Associates, Cornell University Press, Ithaca, NY, 362.

Armand, M., P. Borel, P. H. Rolland, M. Senft, M. André, H. Lafont, and D. Lairon. 1992. Adaptation of gastric lipase in mini-pigs fed a high-fat diet, *Nutr. Res.*, 12:489.

Bainter, K. 1986. *Intestinal Absorption of Macromolecules and Immune Transmission from Mother to Young*, CRC Press, Boca Raton, FL.

Bainter, K., and A. Németh. 1982. The effect of triiodothyronine-prednisolone treatment on the development of digestive enzymes in the suckling pig, *Arch. Tierernähr.*, 32:229.

Banks, W. J. 1986. *Applied Verterinary Histology*, 2nd ed., Williams & Wilkins, Baltimore, MD.

Batterham, E. S. 1994. Ileal digestibilities of amino acids in feedstuffs for pigs. In *Amino Acids in Farm Animal Nutrition*, D'Mello, J. P. F., Ed., CAB International, Edinburgh, U.K., 113.

Botermans, J. A. M., J. Svendsen, L. Karlsson, M. Sörhede, I. Matsson, and S. G. Pierzynowski. 1997. The effects of feeding frequency and competition at feeding on pancreatic exocrine secretion in the pig. In *Digestive Physiology in Pigs*, Laplace, J. P., C. Fevrier, and A. Barbeau, Eds., EAAP Publ. No. 88:604, St. Malo, France.

Breves, G., and K. Stück. 1995. Short-chain fatty acids in the hindgut. In *Physiological and Clinical Aspects of Short-Chain Fatty Acids*, Cummings, J. H., J. L. Rombeau, and T. Sakata, Eds., Cambridge University Press, Cambridge, U.K., 73.

Buddington, R. K., and C. Malo. 1996. Intestinal brush-border membrane enzyme activities and transport functions during prenatal development of pigs, *J. Pediatr. Gastroenterol. Nutr.*, 23:51.

Buraczewska, L. 1979. Secretion of nitrogenous compounds in the small intestine of pigs, *Acta Physiol. Pol.*, 30:319.

Buraczewska, L. 1981a. Absorption of amino acids in different parts of the small intestine in growing pigs. 1. Absorption of free amino acids and water, *Acta Physiol. Pol.*, 32:419.

Buraczewska, L. 1981b. Absorption of amino acids in different parts of the small intestine in growing pigs. 2. Effect of addition of certain amino acids on absorption of different amino acids from hydrolysed casein, *Acta Physiol. Pol.*, 32:429.

Buraczewska, L. 1981c. Absorption of amino acids in different parts of the small intestine in growing pigs. 3. Absorption of constituents of protein hydrolysates, *Acta Physiol. Pol.*, 32:569.

Butine, T. J., and J. A. Z. Leedle. 1989. Enumeration of selected anaerobic bacterial groups in cecal and colonic contents of growing-finishing pigs, *Appl. Environ. Microb.*, 55:1112.

Cera, K. R., D. C. Mahan, and G. A. Reinhart. 1990. Effect of weaning, week postweaning and diet composition on pancreatic and small intestinal luminal lipase response in young swine, *J. Anim. Sci.*, 68:384.

Chapple, R. P., J. A. Cuaron, and R. A. Easter. 1989a. Effect of glucocorticoids and limiting nursing on the carbohydrate digestive capacity and growth rate of piglets, *J. Anim. Sci.*, 67:2956.

Chapple, R. P., J. A. Cuaron, and R. A. Easter. 1989b. Response of digestive carbohydrases and growth to graded doses and administration frequency of hydrocortisone and adrenocorticotropic hormone in nursing piglets, *J. Anim. Sci.*, 67:2974.

Chapple, R. P., J. A. Cuaron, and R. A. Easter. 1989c. Temporal changes in carbohydrate digestive capacity and growth rate of piglets in response to glucocorticoid administration and weaning age, *J. Anim. Sci.*, 67:2985.

Chiang, S.-H., J. E. Pettigrew, S. D. Clarke, and S. G. Cornelius. 1989. Digestion and absorption of fish oil by neonatal piglets, *J. Nutr.*, 119:1741.

Christensen, K., and G. Thorbek. 1987. Methane excretion in the growing pig, *Br. J. Nutr.*, 57:355.

Clemens, E. T., C. E. Stevens, and M. Southworth. 1975. Sites of organic acid production and pattern of digesta movement in the gastrointestinal tract of swine, *J. Nutr.*, 105:759.

Coleman, R., S. Iqbal, P. P. Godfrey, and D. Billington. 1979. Composition of several mammalian biles and their membrane-damaging properties, *Biochem. J.*, 178:201.

Conway, P. L. 1994. Function and regulation of the gastrointestinal microbiota of the pig. In *VIth International Symposium on Digestive Physiology in Pigs*, EAAP Publ. No. 80:231.

Corring, T. 1974. Regulation of pancreatic secretion by negative feedback in the pig, *Ann. Biol. Anim. Biochim. Biophys.*, 14:487.

Corring, T. 1980a. Endogenous secretions in the pig. In *Current Concepts of Digestion and Absorption in Pigs*, Low, A. G., and I. G. Partridge, Eds., National Institute for Research in Dairying, Reading, U.K., 136.

Corring, T. 1980b. The adaptation of digestive enzymes to the diet: its physiological significance, *Reprod. Nutr. Dev.*, 20:1217.

Corring, T., and J. A. Chayvialle. 1987. Diet composition and the plasma levels of some peptides regulating pancreatic secretion in the pigs, *Reprod. Nutr. Dev.*, 27:967.

Corring, T., A. Aumaitre, and G. Durand. 1978. Development of digestive enzymes in the piglet from birth to 8 weeks. I. Pancreas and pancreatic enzymes, *Nutr. Metab.*, 22:231.

Corring, T., J. A. Chayvialle, C. Simoes-Nunes, and J. Abello. 1985. Regulation of pancreatic secretion by negative feedback and plasma gastro-intestinal hormones in the pig, *Reprod. Nutr. Dev.*, 25:439.

Corring, T., C. Juste, and E. F. Lhoste. 1989. Nutritional regulation of pancreatic and biliary secretions, *Nutr. Res. Rev.*, 2:161.

Corring, T., W. B. Souffrant, B. Darcy-Vrillon, G. Gebhardt, J. P. Laplace, and A. Rérat. 1990. Exogenous and endogenous contribution to nitrogen fluxes in the digestive tract of pigs fed a casein diet. I. Contributions of nitrogen from the exocrine pancreatic secretion and the bile, *Reprod. Nutr. Dev.*, 30:717.

Cranwell, P. D. 1995. Development of the neonatal gut and enzyme systems. In *The Neonatal Pig, Development and Survival*, Varley, M. A., Ed., CAB International, U.K., 99.

Desport, J. C., C. Juste, B. Beaufrere, and T. Corring. 1997. The pig as a model in clinical investigation of the exocrine pancreatic insufficiency and of cholesterol crystallization from bile. In *Digestive Physiology in Pigs*, Laplace, J. P., C. Fevrier, and A. Barbeau, Eds., EAAP Publ. No. 88, St. Malo, France, 17.

Dierick, N. A., I. J. Vervaeke, D. I. Demeyer, and J. A. Decuypere. 1989. Approach to the energetic importance of fibre digestion in pigs. I. Importance of fermentation in the overall energy supply, *Anim. Feed Sci. Technol.*, 23:141.

Dyce, K. M., W. O. Sack, and C. J. G. Wensing. 1996. *Textbook of Veterinary Anatomy*, 2nd ed., W. B. Saunders, Philadelphia, PA.

Eggum, B. O. 1995. The influence of dietary fibre on protein digestion and utilization in monogastrics, *Arch. Anim. Nutr.*, 48:89.

Ekström, G. M., and B. R. Weström. 1991. Cathepsin B and D activities in intestinal mucosa during postnatal development in pigs. Relation to intestinal uptake and transmission of macromolecules, *Biol. Neonate*, 59:314.

Elsley, F. W. H. 1970. Nutrition and lactation in the sow. In *Lactation*, Falconer, I. R., Ed., Butterworths, London, U.K., 393.

Englyst, H. 1989. Classification and measurement of plant polysaccharides, *Anim. Feed Sci. Technol.*, 23:27.

Flores, C. A., P. M. Brannon, S. A. Bustamante, J. Bezerra, K. T. Butler, T. Goda, and O. Koldovsky. 1988. Effect of diet on intestinal and pancreatic enzyme activities in the pig, *J. Ped. Gastroenterol. Nutr.*, 7:914.

Foltmann, B., K. Harlow, G. Houen, P. K. Nielsen, and P. Sangild. 1995. Comparative investigations on porcine proteases and their zymogens. In Takahashi, K., Ed., *Proceedings of the 5th International Conference on Aspartic Proteases*, Plenum Press, New York, 41.

Friedrich, M. 1989. Physiology of intestinal digestion and absorption. In *Protein Metabolism in Farm Animals. Evaluation, Digestion, Absorption, and Metabolism*, Bock, H.-D., B. O. Eggum, A. G. Low, O. Simon, and T. Zebrowska, Eds., Oxford University Press, Oxford, U.K., 218.

Fuller, M. F. 1994. Amino acid requirements for maintenance, body protein accretion and reproduction in pigs. In *Amino Acids in Farm Animal Nutrition*, D'Mello, J. P. F., Ed., CAB International, Edinburgh, U.K., 155.

Gabert, V. M., M. S. Jensen, H. Jørgensen, R. M. Engberg, and S. K. Jensen. 1996. Exocrine pancreatic secretions in growing pigs fed diets containing fish oil, rapeseed oil or coconut oil, *J. Nutr.*, 126:2076.

Gardner, M. L. G. 1984. Intestinal assimilation of intact peptides and proteins from the diet — a neglected field, *Biol. Rev. Camb. Philos. Soc.*, 59:289.

Go, V.L.W., E. P. DiMagno, J. D. Gardner, E. Lebenthal, H. A. Reber, and G. A. Scheele. 1993. *The Pancreas: Biology, Pathobiology and Disease*, 2nd ed., Raven Press, New York.

Harada, E., H. Kiriyama, E. Kobayashi, and H. Tsuchita. 1988. Postnatal development of biliary and pancreatic exocrine secretion in piglets, *Comp. Biochem. Physiol.*, 91A:43.

Hee, J., W. C. Sauer, and R. Mosenthin. 1988. The effect of feeding of frequency on the pancreatic secretions in the pig, *J. Anim. Physiol. Anim. Nutr.*, 60:249.

Herdt, T. 1992. Digestion and absorption: the nonfermentative processes. In *Textbook of Veterinary Physiology*, Cunningham, J. G., Ed., W. B. Saunders, Philadelphia, PA, 286.

Holst, J. J. 1985. The neuro-endocrine control of the digestive processes. In *Proceedings of the 3rd International Seminar on Digestive Physiology in the Pig*, Just, A., H. Jørgensen, and J. A. Fernandez, Eds., Beretning Statens Husdyrbrugsforsøg No. 580, Copenhagen, Denmark, 17.

Holst, J. J., T. N. Rasmussen, P. Schmidt, and S. S. Poulsen. 1993. Transmitters in the control of gastrin and acid secretion in the pig stomach. In *Gastrin*, Walsh, J. H., Ed., Raven Press, New York, 243.

Horszcaruk, F., L. Buraczewska, and S. Buraczewski. 1974. Amount and composition of intestinal juice collected from isolated intestinal loops in pigs, *Rocz. Nauk Roln.*, 95(B-4):69.

Ihse, I., and P. Lilja. 1979. Effects of intestinal amylase and trypsin on pancreatic secretion in the pig, *Scand. J. Gastroenterol.*, 14:1009.

Jensen, B. B., and H. Jørgensen. 1994. Effect of dietary fiber on microbial activity and microbial gas production in various regions of the gastrointestinal tract of pigs, *Appl. Environ. Microbiol.*, 60:1897.

Jensen, M. S., S. K. Jensen, and K. Jakobsen. 1997. Development of digestive enzymes in pigs with emphasis on lipolytic activity in the stomach and pancreas, *J. Anim. Sci.*, 75:437.

Juste, C., T. Corring, and Ph. Breant. 1979. Biliary secretion in the pig: rate of output and response to feeding, *Ann. Biol. Anim. Biochim. Biophys.*, 19:119.

Juste, C., Y. Demarne, and T. Corring. 1983. Response of bile flow, biliary lipids and bile acid pool in the pig to quantitative variations in dietary fat, *J. Nutr.*, 113:1691.

Juste, C., T. Corring, and Y. Demarne. 1985. Effect of the lipid diet on bile saturation with cholesterol in pig, *Reprod. Nutr. Dev.*, 25:815 (abstr.).

Juste, C., Y. Demarne, and T. Corring. 1986. Effect of level and source of dietary lipid on the biliary secretion in the growing pig, *Reprod. Nutr. Dev.*, 26:1191 (abstr.).

Kidder, D. E., and M. J. Manners. 1978. *Digestion in the Pig*, Scientechnica, Bristol, U.K.

Kidder, D. E., and M. J. Manners. 1980. The level and distribution of carbohydrases in the small intestine mucosa of pigs from three weeks of age to maturity, *Br. J. Nutr.*, 43:141.

Kilberg, M. S., B. R. Stevens, and D. A. Novak. 1993. Recent advances in mammalian amino acid transport, *Annu. Rev. Nutr.*, 13:137.

Kirchgessner, M., and H. L. Muller. 1991. Energy utilization via hindgut fermentation in pigs. In *Digestive Physiology of the Hindgut*, Kirchgessner, M., Ed., Verlag Paul Parey, Hamburg, Germany, 41.

Klobasa, F., E. Werhahn, and J. E. Butler. 1987. Composition of sow milk during lactation, *J. Anim. Sci.*, 64:1458.

Kreikemeier, K. K., D. L. Harmon, and J. L. Nelssen. 1990. Influence of hydrocortisone acetate on pancreas and mucosal weight, amylase and disaccharidase activities in 14-day-old pigs, *Comp. Biochem. Physiol.*, 97A:45.

Laplace, J. P., and M. A. Ouaissi. 1977. Bile excretion in the pig. Influence of the meals and possible function of Oddi's sphincter receptors to control the choledochus flow rate, *Ann. Zootech.*, 26(4):595.

Le Huerou-Luron, I., E. Lhoste, C. Wicker-Planquart, N. Dakka, R. Toullec, T. Corring, P. Guilloteau, and A. Puigserver. 1993. Molecular aspects of enzyme synthesis in the exocrine pancreas with emphasis on development and nutritional regulation, *Proc. Nutr. Soc.*, 52:301.

Lhoste, E. F., M. Fiszlewics, A.-M. Gueugneau, C. Wicker-Planquart, A. Puigserver, and T. Corring. 1993. Effects of dietary proteins on some pancreatic mRNAs encoding digestive enzymes in the pig, *J. Nutr. Biochem.*, 4:143.

Liebler, E. M., J. F. Pohlenz, and S. C. Whipp. 1992. Digestive system. In *Diseases of Swine*, 7th ed., Leman, A. D., B. E. Straw, W. L. Mengeling, S. D'Allaire, and D. J. Taylor, Eds., Iowa State University Press, Ames, IA, 12.

Lindemann, M. D., S. G. Cornelius, S. M. El Kandelgy, R. L. Moser, and J. E. Pettigrew. 1986. Effect of age, weaning and diet on digestive enzyme levels in the piglet, *J. Anim. Sci.*, 62:1298.

Lloyd, K. C. K. 1994. Gut hormones in gastric function, *Baillière's Clin. Endocrinol. Metab.*, 8:111.

Low, A. G. 1985. The role of dietary fibre in digestion absorption and metabolism. In *Proceedings of the 3rd International Seminar on Digestive Physiology in the Pig*, Just, A., H. Jørgensen, and J. A. Fernandez, Eds., Beretning Statens Husdyrbrugsforsøg No. 580, Copenhagen, Denmark, 157.

Low, A. G. 1989. Research into the digestive physiology of pigs. In *Nutrition and Digestive Physiology in Monogastric Farm Animals*, van Weerden, E. J., and J. Huisman, Eds., Purdoc, Wageningen, The Netherlands, 1.

Low, A. G. 1990. Nutritional regulation of gastric secretion, digestion and emptying, *Nutr. Res. Rev.*, 3:229.

Low, A. G., and T. Zebrowska. 1989. Digestion in pigs. In *Protein Metabolism in Farm Animals. Evaluation, Digestion, Absorption and Metabolism*, Bock, H.-D., B. O. Eggum, A. G. Low, O. Simon, and T. Zebrowska, Eds., Oxford University Press, Oxford, U.K., 53.

Low, A. G., I. E. Sambrook, and J. T. Yoshimoto. 1978. Studies on the true digestibility of nitrogen (N) and amino acids in growing pigs, EAAP 29th Annual Meeting, Stockholm, Sweden.

Makkink, C. A., and M. W. A. Verstegen. 1990. Pancreatic secretion in pigs, *J. Anim. Physiol. Anim. Nutr.*, 64:190.

Makkink, C. A., G. P. Negulescu, Q. Guixin, and M. W. A. Verstegen. 1994. Effect of dietary protein source on feed intake, growth, pancreatic enzyme activities and jejunal morphology in newly-weaned piglets, *Br. J. Nutr.*, 72:353.

Mason, V. C. 1980. Role of the large intestine in the processes of digestion and absorption in the pig. In *Current Concepts of Digestion and Absorption in Pigs*, Low, A. G., and I. G. Partridge, Eds., The National Institute for Research in Dairying, Reading, England, 112.

Mason, V. C. 1984. Metabolism of nitrogenous compounds in the large gut, *Proc. Nutr. Soc.*, 43:45.

Maxwell, F. J., and C. S. Stewart. 1995. The microbiology of the gut and the role of probiotics. In *The Neonatal Pig, Development and Survival*, Varley, M. A., Ed., CAB International, Edinburgh, U.K., 155.

Moran, E. T., Jr. 1982. *Comparative Nutrition of Fowl and Swine. The Gastrointestinal Systems*, E. T. Moran, Jr., Guelph, Canada.

Moughan, P. J., M. J. Birtles, P. D. Cranwell, W. C. Smith, and M. Pedraza. 1992. The piglet as a model animal for studying aspects of digestion and absorption in milk-fed human infants, *World Rev. Nutr. Diet.*, 67:40.

Müller, H. L., and M. Kirchgessner. 1985a. Effect of lucerne meal on energy metabolism in sows, *Z. Tierphysiol. Tierernähr. Futtermittelkd.*, 54(4):206.

Müller, H. L., and M. Kirchgessner. 1985b. Utilization of energy from pectin by sows, *Z. Tierphysiol. Tierernähr. Futtermittelkd.*, 54(1):14.

Newport, M. J., and G. L. Howarth. 1985. Contribution of gastric lipolysis to the digestion of fat in the neonatal pig. In *Proceedings of the 3rd International Seminar on Digestive Physiology in the Pig*, Just, A., H. Jørgensen, and J. A. Fernandez, Eds., Beretning Statens Husdyrbrugsforsøg No. 580, Copenhagen, Denmark, 143.

NRC. 1998. *Nutrient Requirements of Swine*, 10th ed., National Academy Press, Washington, D.C.

Owsley, W. F., D. E. Orr, and L. R. Tribble. 1986. Effects of age and diet on the development of the pancreas and the synthesis and secretion of pancreatic enzymes in the young pig, *J. Anim. Sci.*, 63:497.

Ozimek, L., W. C. Sauer, and G. Ozimek. 1985. The response of the secretion and activity of pancreatic enzymes to the quality and quantity of fat. In *Proceedings of the 3rd International Seminar on Digestive Physiology in the Pig*, Just, A., H. Jørgensen, and J. A. Fernandez, Eds., Beretning Statens Husdyrbrugsforsøg No. 580, Copenhagen, Denmark, 146.

Parsons, M. E. 1996. Control of gastric secretion, *Proc. Nutr. Soc.*, 55:251.

Partridge, I. G. 1978. Studies on digestion and absorption in the intestines of growing pigs. 3. Net movement of mineral nutrients in the digestive tract, *Br. J. Nutr.*, 39:527.

Payne, D., C. Juste, T. Corring, and C. Fevrier. 1989. Effects of wheat bran on bile secretion in the pig, *Nutr. Rep. Int.*, 40:761.

Pierzynowski, S. G., B. R. Weström, J. Svendsen, and B. W. Karlsson. 1990. Development of exocrine pancreas function in chronically cannulated pigs during 1–13 weeks of postnatal life, *J. Pediatr. Gastroenterol. Nutr.*, 10:206.

Pierzynowski, S. G., H. Mårtensson, B. R. Weström, B. Ahrén, K. Uvnäs-Moberg, and B. W. Karlsson. 1993a. Cholesystokinin (CCK 33) can stimulate pancreatic secretion by a local intestinal mechanism in the pig, *Biomed. Res.*, 14:217.

Pierzynowski, S. G., B. R. Weström, C. Erlanson-Albertsson, B. Ahrén, J. Svendsen, and B. W. Karlsson. 1993b. Induction of exocrine pancreas maturation at weaning in young developing pigs, *J. Pediatr. Gastroenterol. Nutr.*, 16:287.

Pöhland, U., W. B. Souffrant, W. C. Sauer, R. Mosenthin, and C. F. M. de Lange. 1993. Effect of feeding different diets on the exocrine pancreatic secretion of nitrogen, amino acids and enzymes in growing pigs, *J. Sci. Food Agric.*, 62:229.

Pond, W. G., and K. A. Houpt. 1978. *The Biology of the Pig*, Comstock Publishing Associates, Cornell University Press, Ithaca, NY.

Pond, W. G., and H. J. Mersmann. 2000. *The Biology of the Domestic Pig*, Cornell University Press, Ithaca, NY.

Ratcliffe, B. 1985. The influence of the gut microflora on the digestive processes. In *Proceedings of the 3rd International Seminar on Digestive Physiology in the Pig*, Just, A., H. Jørgensen, and J. A. Fernandez, Eds., Beretning Statens Husdyrbrugsforsøg No. 580, Copenhagen, Denmark, 245.

Ratcliffe, B. 1991. The role of the microflora in digestion. In *In Vitro Digestion for Pigs and Poultry*, Fuller, M. F., Ed., CAB International, Edinburgh, U.K., 19.

Rérat, A. 1978. Digestion and absorption of carbohydrates and nitrogenous matters in the hindgut of the omnivorous nonruminant animal, *J. Anim. Sci.*, 46:1808.

Rérat, A. 1996. Chronology of VFA absorption according to the nature of carbohydrate intake in the pig, *Repr. Nutr. Dev.*, 36:3.

Rérat, A., and T. Corring. 1991. Animal factors affecting protein digestion and absorption. In *Digestive Physiology in Pigs*, EAAP Publ. No. 54. Purdoc, Wageningen, The Netherlands, 5.

Rérat, A., M. Fiszlewicz, A. Giusi, and P. Vaugelade. 1987. Influence of meal frequency on postprandial variations in the production and absorption of volatile fatty acids in the digestive tract of conscious pigs, *J. Anim. Sci.*, 64:448.

Rérat, A., P. Vaugelade, and P. Villiers. 1980. A new method for measuring the absorption of nutrients in the pig: critical examination. In *Current Concepts of Digestion and Absorption in the Pig*, Low, A. G., and I. G. Partridge, Eds., National Institute for Research in Dairying, Reading, U.K., 177.

Robinson, J. A., W. J. Smolenski, M. L. Ogilvie, and J. P. Peters. 1989. In vitro total-gas, CH_4, H_2, volatile fatty acid, and lactate kinetics studies on luminal contents from the small intestine, cecum, and colon of the pig, *Appl. Environ. Microbiol.*, 55:2460.

Salter, D. N. 1984. Nitrogen metabolism. In *The Germ-Free Animal in Biomedical Research*, Coates, M. E., and B. E. Gustafsson, Eds., Laboratory Animals Ltd., London, U.K., 235.

Sambrook, I. E. 1980. Digestion and absorption of carbohydrate and lipid in the stomach and the small intestine of the pig, In *Current Concepts of Digestion and Absorption in Pigs*, Low, A. G., and I. G. Partridge, Eds., Proc. National Institute for Research in Dairying, Reading, England, 78.

Sambrook, I. E. 1981. Studies on the flow and composition of bile in growing pigs, *J. Sci. Food Agric.*, 32:781.

Sangild, P. T., P. D. Cranwell, H. Sørensen, K. Mortensen, O. Norén, L. Wetteberg, and H. Sjöström. 1991. Development of intestinal disaccharidases, intestinal peptidases and pancreatic proteases in suckling pigs. The effects of age and ACTH treatment. In *Digestive Physiology in Pigs*, EAAP Publ. No. 54, Pudoc, Wageningen, The Netherlands, 73.

Sangild, P. T., B. Weström, A. L. Fowden, and M. Silver. 1994. Developmental regulation of the porcine exocrine pancreas by glucocorticoids, *J. Pediatr. Gastroenterol. Nutr.*, 19:204.

Schantz, L. D., K. Laber-Laird, S. A. Bingel, and M. M. Swindle. 1996. Pigs. In *Essentials of Experimental Surgery: Gastroenterology*, Jensen, S. L., H. Gregersen, F. Moody, and M. H. Shokouh-Amiri, Eds., Harwood Academic Publishers, New York, 26/1.

Schummer, A., R. Nickel, and W. O. Sack. 1979. *The Viscera of the Domestic Mammals*, 2nd ed., Springer-Verlag, New York.

Shiau, Y.-F. 1987. Lipid digestion and absorption. In Johnson, L. R., Ed., *Physiology of the Gastrointestinal Tract*, Vol. II, 2nd ed., Raven Press, New York, 1527.

Silk, D. B. A., G. K. Grimble, and R. G. Rees. 1985. Protein digestion and amino acid and peptide absorption, *Proc. Nutr. Soc.*, 44:63.

Sisson, S. 1975. Porcine digestive system. In *The Anatomy of the Domestic Animals*, 5th ed., Getty, R., Ed., W. B. Saunders, Philadelphia, PA.

Smith, M. W. 1988. Postnatal development of transport function in the pig intestine, *Comp. Biochem. Physiol.*, 90A:577.

Solomon, T. E. 1987. Control of exocrine pancreatic secretion. In *Physiology of the Gastrointestinal Tract*, 2nd ed., Johnson, L. R., Ed., Raven Press, New York, 1173.

Takahashi, M., Y. Benno, and T. Mitsuoka. 1980. Utilization of ammonia nitrogen by intestinal bacteria isolated from pigs, *Appl. Environ. Microbiol.*, 39:30.

Thaela, M.-J., S. G. Pierzynowski, M. S. Jensen, K. Jakobsen, B. R. Weström, and B. W. Karlsson. 1995. The pattern of the circadian rhythm of pancreatic secretion in fed pigs, *J. Anim. Sci.*, 73:3402.

Thorens, B. 1993. Facilitated glucose transporters in epithelial cells, *Annu. Rev. Physiol.*, 55:591.

Torrallardona, D., C. I. Harris, E. Milne, and M. F. Fuller. 1993. Contribution of intestinal microflora to lysine requirements in non-ruminants, *Proc. Nutr. Soc.*, 52:153A (abstr.).

Valette, P., T. Corring, C. Juste, and F. Levenez. 1989. Short-term effects of wheat bran incorporation into the diet on bile secretion in the pig, *Nutr. Rep. Int.*, 40:1059.

Valette, P., H. Malouin, T. Corring, L. Savoie, A. M. Gueugneau, and S. Berot. 1992. Effects of diets containing casein and rapeseed on enzyme secretion from the exocrine pancreas in the pig, *Br. J. Nutr.*, 67:215.

Varel, V. H., and J. T. Yen. 1997. Microbial perspective on fiber utilization by swine, *J. Anim. Sci.*, 75:2715.

Webb, K. E., Jr., J. C. Matthews, and D. B. DiRienzo. 1992. Peptide absorption: a review of current concepts and future perspectives, *J. Anim. Sci.*, 70:3248.

Weström, B. R., J. Svendsen, B. G. Ohlsson, C. Tagesson, and B. W. Karlsson. 1984. Intestinal transmission of macromolecules (BSA and FITC-labelled dextrans) in the neonatal pig. Influence of age of piglet and molecular weight of markers, *Biol. Neonate*, 46:20.

Wright, E. M. 1993. The intestinal Na⁺/glucose cotransporter, *Annu. Rev. Physiol.*, 55:575.
Yen, J. T. 1997. Oxygen consumption and energy flux of porcine splanchnic tissues. In *Digestive Physiology in Pigs*, Proc. EAAP Publ. 88, Institut National de la Recherche Agronomique, Paris, France, 260.
Yen, J. T. 2000. Digestive system. In *The Biology of the Domestic Pig*, Pond, W. G., and H. J. Mersmann, Eds., Cornell University Press, Ithaca, New York, chap. 8.
Yen, J. T., J. A. Nienaber, D. A. Hill, and W. G. Pond. 1991. Potential contribution of absorbed volatile fatty acids to whole-animal energy requirement in conscious swine, *J. Anim. Sci.*, 69:2001.
Zebrowska, T. 1982. Nitrogen digestion in the large intestine. In *Digestive Physiology in the Pig*, Laplace, J. P., T. Corring, and A. Rérat, Eds., Institut National de la Recherche Agronomique, Paris, France, 225.
Zebrowska, T., A. G. Low, and H. Zebrowska. 1983. Studies on gastric digestion of protein and carbohydrate, gastric secretion and exocrine pancreatic secretion in the growing pig, *Br. J. Nutr.*, 49:401.
Zhang, H., C. Malo, and R. K. Buddington. 1997. Suckling induces rapid intestinal growth and changes in brush border digestive functions of newborn pigs, *J. Nutr.*, 127:418.

4 Protein, Fat, and Bone Tissue Growth in Swine

Cornelis F. M. de Lange, Stephen H. Birkett, and Patrick C. H. Morel

CONTENTS

I. Introduction 65
II. Chemical and Physical Body Composition 66
III. Growth Patterns for the Whole Body and Body Components.........................68
    A. Directly Measure Weight of Body Components at Regular Time Intervals.............71
    B. Combine Average Growth Rate with a Standard Growth Curve Shape for Body Components...71
    C. Use Growth Models to Fit Growth Curves of Body Components to Observed Body Weight Gains 72
IV. Determinants of Body Weight Gain and Body Composition 72
    A. Pig Genotype..72
        1. Maintenance Energy and Nutrient Requirements — Basal Metabolic Rate ...73
        2. The Pig's Upper Limit to Body Protein Deposition (PDmax) 74
        3. Relationship between Energy Intake over Maintenance and Body Protein Deposition 74
        4. Voluntary Feed Intake 76
        5. Relationships between Chemical and Physical Body Components 77
    B. Nutrient and Energy Intake..77
        1. Intake of Lysine and Other Essential Amino Acids 77
        2. Energy Intake 77
    C. Environmental Stresses 78
V. Summary 78
References 78

I. INTRODUCTION

As outlined in the previous chapters, the essence of pork production is to convert nutrients supplied by a range of feedstuffs into high-quality pork products. This conversion encompasses relationships between nutrient intake and chemical body composition and between chemical and physical body composition of growing pigs. In terms of physical body composition, the amount of muscle tissue and its distribution are of prime concern; these are the main determinants of the amount and quality of pork that can be derived from the pig's carcass. Relationships between nutrient intake and chemical and physical body composition influence pork quality as well as the efficiency of pork production, and these relationships are affected by a range of factors associated with nutrition, pig genotype, environment, and stage of growth. An understanding of these relationships, and of factors affecting them, is required to identify means to manipulate pork quality and production efficiencies.

This chapter discusses the chemical and physical body composition of growing pigs. Moreover, patterns of growth for the whole body and body components are addressed. Finally, some of the main factors that affect body weight gain and its composition are presented.

II. CHEMICAL AND PHYSICAL BODY COMPOSITION

Gut fill represents the difference between empty body weight and live body weight and is approximately 5% of live body weight (ARC, 1981; Stranks et al., 1988). The four main chemical constituents in the pig's empty body are water, protein, lipid, and ash (Table 4.1). The pig's body contains only minor amounts of carbohydrates, which largely represent glycogen stores in the liver and muscle. For estimates of the whole-body mineral composition the reader is referred to ARC (1981), Rymarz (1986), and Hendriks and Moughan (1993). The main body tissues in growing pigs are muscles or lean tissue, fat, visceral organs, bones, and skin (Table 4.2). The other tissues, including nervous, lymphatic, and vascular tissue, and blood contribute <10% to empty body weight in growing and finishing pigs.

TABLE 4.1
Chemical Composition (%) of the Empty Body of Pigs at Various Live Body Weights (BW)

	Birth	7 kg	25 kg	Market Weight (approximately 110 kg; extremes)	
				Fat pigs	Lean pigs
Water	77	66	69	48	64
Protein	18	16	16	14	18
Lipid	2	15	12	35	15
Ash	3	3	3	3	3

Source: Derived from McMeekan (1940), Richmond and Berg (1971a), de Greef et al. (1994), Whittemore (1993), Bikker et al. (1995; 1996a,b), and Coudenys (1998).

TABLE 4.2
Physical Composition (%) of the Empty Body of Growing Pigs[a]

Sex/Genotype	Muscle	Visceral Organs[b]	Fat Tissue	Bone	Skin
Male					
Synthetic line	51.1	15.4	12.4	8.7	3.4
Pietrain	54.2	12.8	14.0	7.5	3.0
Large White	43.8	17.6	15.5	8.7	4.2
Female					
Large White	45.2	16.0	17.1	8.2	3.6
Castrates					
Large White	43.3	16.4	17.9	8.4	3.6
Meisham	27.8	16.7	28.1	7.2	7.4

[a] Adjusted to a mean empty body weight of 47.2 kg; derived from Quiniou and Noblet, 1995.
[b] Includes hair and blood.

The main protein tissues in the pig's body are lean tissue and visceral organs (gastrointestinal tract, liver, kidneys, spleen, heart, lungs, and reproductive tract). In market-weight pigs, between 45 and 60% of the total body protein mass is present in lean tissue, while approximately 15% of body protein is present in visceral organs (Rook et al., 1987; de Greef et al., 1994; Bikker et al., 1995, 1996a,b; Coudenys, 1998). Dissected lean tissue contains approximately 20% crude protein, 8% lipid, and 70% water; the remainder represents ash and some glycogen (de Greef et al., 1994; Bikker et al., 1995; 1996a,b; Coudenys, 1998). Visceral organs generally contain slightly less protein and water and slightly more lipid than lean tissue (Coudenys, 1998). Body water is thus closely associated with protein present in lean tissue and visceral organs. Given this association, body water mass can be predicted from body protein mass with a reasonable accuracy using allometric relationships: body water mass (kg) = A × (body protein mass; kg)$^{0.855}$, where the parameter A varies between 4.9 and 5.4 for different pig genotypes (ARC, 1981; de Greef, 1995; Emmans and Kyriazakis, 1995). Because body ash mass and bone tissue are related to lean tissue, body ash mass can be predicted from body protein mass as well: body ash mass (kg) = 0.20 × body protein mass (kg) (ARC, 1981; Moughan et al., 1990; Hendriks and Moughan, 1993; de Greef, 1995). Given the associations among body protein, water, and ash, most of the variation in chemical body composition between different groups of pigs can be attributed to variation in body lipid content (see Table 4.1). In a similar manner, body fat tissue content is the main contributor to variation in physical body composition (see Table 4.2).

Even though the amount of lean tissue in market-weight pigs varies considerably, the distribution of lean tissue among the primal cuts does not differ substantially between groups of pigs (Richmond and Berg, 1971b; Gu et al., 1992b; OPCAP, 1996; Coudenys, 1998). Generally, approximately 25, 29, 14, 11, and 13% of lean tissue in the pig's body is present in the loin, ham, Boston butt, picnic, and belly, respectively (Gu et al., 1992b). The remainder represents muscles that are present in the neck, head, and lower parts of the legs. Only in Pietrain pigs does the lean tissue distribution differ substantially from that in other main pig genotypes. Because of double muscling in the loin and hind limb, a larger proportion of total body lean tissue mass is present in the loin and ham primal cuts in this pig genotype (Swatland, 1994). It should be noted that the definition of lean tissue and methods used to estimate carcass lean tissue content may differ between packing plants, pig breeding organizations, and research institutions.

Approximately 70% of body lipid mass is present in dissectable fat tissue (Rook et al., 1987; de Greef et al., 1994; Bikker et al., 1995, 1996a,b; de Greef, 1995). Body fat tissues serve as energy stores and can be divided into three main categories: fat associated with muscles (intra and intermuscular fat; intramuscular fat is also referred to as marbling), subcutaneous fat, and abdominal fat. Because of the low value of fat tissue to the meat processing industry and the consumer, it is in the pork producers' interest to minimize body fat content in market pigs and the subcutaneous fat and abdominal fat content in particular. Moreover, it requires approximately four times the amount of energy to produce 1 kg of fat tissue as compared with producing 1 kg of lean tissue. It should, however, be noted that some marbling is required for optimal palatability of pork products. In pigs, both the body fat tissue distribution (Jones et al., 1980; Rook et al., 1987; OPCAP, 1996) and total body fat tissue content can be manipulated (de Greef et al., 1994; Bikker et al., 1995, 1996a,b; Gu et al., 1992b; Thomke et al., 1995). For example, there are clear differences between pig genotypes in the degree of marbling — it is generally higher in Duroc pigs than in Landrace or Yorkshire pigs — even though differences in subcutaneous and abdominal fat content between pigs of different genotypes may be small (OPCAP, 1996). Furthermore, according to Rook et al. (1987) the distribution of fat tissues in the pig's body can be altered through genetic selection. Variation in energy intake is an important determinant of variation in total body fat tissue contents and distribution within pig genotypes (Campbell et al., 1985; Campbell and Taverner, 1988; de Greef et al., 1994; Bikker et al., 1995, 1996a,b; Quiniou et al., 1996a; Coudenys, 1998).

Visceral organs are essential for ingestion, digestion, and metabolism of dietary nutrients; supplying nutrients and oxygen to the various tissues; and removal of waste products from the pig's body. Yet, visceral organs contribute little to the value of market pigs to the meat processing industry and the consumer. Moreover, visceral organs contribute to approximately 50% of whole-body energy expenditure and whole-body protein turnover in growing pigs (Yen, 1997). Therefore, these organs contribute to the inefficiency of converting dietary nutrients into pork products. Because energy expenditure and protein turnover in visceral organs is closely related to the size of these organs (Nyachoti, 1998), and because there seems to be variation in the size of visceral organs among groups of pigs (Quiniou and Noblet, 1995; Table 4.2), some consideration should be given to means to manipulate visceral organ size. Some of the factors that are known to influence visceral organ size are pig genotype, live body weight, feeding level, and diet composition (Koong et al., 1983; Quiniou and Noblet, 1995; Bikker et al., 1996a; Nyachoti, 1998).

Bone tissue supports the pig's body (Swatland, 1994). Moreover, bone tissue growth and mineralization determine dietary requirements of calcium and phosphorus (ARC, 1981; Hendriks and Moughan, 1993). In particular in breeding swine, bone tissue should be considered carefully because the integrity of bone tissue is one of the determinants of longevity.

For a detailed discussion about the structure and significance of the other tissues in swine, including skin and hair; nervous, lymphatic, and vascular tissue; blood and reproductive organs, the reader is referred elsewhere (Swatland, 1994). Obviously, these tissues have important functions in the pig's body. However, these tissues represent only a small proportion of live body weight. As a result, growth of these tissues has only minor influences on dietary nutrient requirements.

III. GROWTH PATTERNS FOR THE WHOLE BODY AND BODY COMPONENTS

For the development of effective multiple-phase feeding programs for growing and finishing pigs, changes in both the composition and rate of body weight gain with increasing live body weight should be considered. Moreover, for determining the optimum slaughter weight, changes in body composition around the time of slaughter should be estimated. The latter determines the rate and cost of producing marginal increments in body and carcass weight, as well as marginal changes in carcass value. These aspects of growth are known to vary considerably between groups of pigs (Moughan and Verstegen, 1988; Schinckel, 1994; Black et al., 1995; Fuller et al., 1995; Quiniou and Noblet, 1995; Quiniou et al., 1996ab, Schinckel and de Lange, 1996). Growth curves should thus be established for individual growing-finishing pig units. In addition, the factors that determine body weight gain, and lean tissue growth in particular, should be determined at the various stages of growth. The latter may lead to an identification of means to improve the efficiency and rate of lean tissue growth and carcass quality.

There are three segments to a typical growth curve (Figure 4.1). During the early stages of growth, generally up to about 50 kg live body weight, the daily growth rate increases. Between approximately 50 and 80 kg live body weight the daily growth rate is relatively constant. Thereafter, the daily growth rate starts to decline gradually toward zero when the pig's mature live body weight has been reached. Usually, pigs are slaughtered between 70 and 130 kg live body weight.

Growth curves for individual body components can be derived when estimates of body composition are combined with whole-body growth curves (Rook et al., 1987; Gu et al., 1992b; Schinckel and de Lange, 1996). With increasing live body weight, the body lipid content increases at the expense of body protein content and associated water and ash (Figure 4.2). This coincides with gradual increments in the contribution of fat tissue and reductions in the contribution of lean tissue and visceral organs to empty body weight (Figure 4.3).

In terms of body components, the rates of body protein and lipid deposition, and lean tissue growth, are of prime importance. Body protein deposition is the single largest factor determining dietary amino acid requirements. Furthermore, body protein and lipid deposition account for approximately two thirds of the total dietary energy requirements for growing and finishing pigs (NRC, 1998). Lean tissue growth is of interest because it represents the growth of the valuable body components.

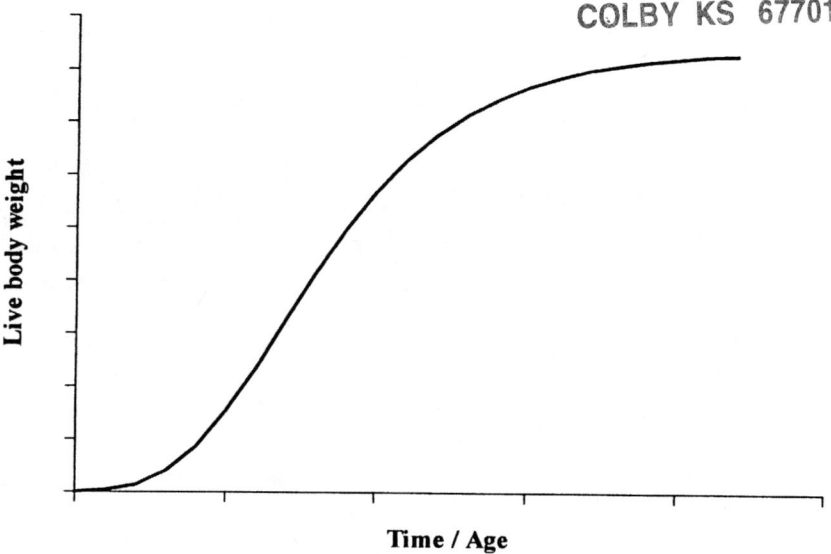

FIGURE 4.1 Typical growth curve of growing-finishing pigs.

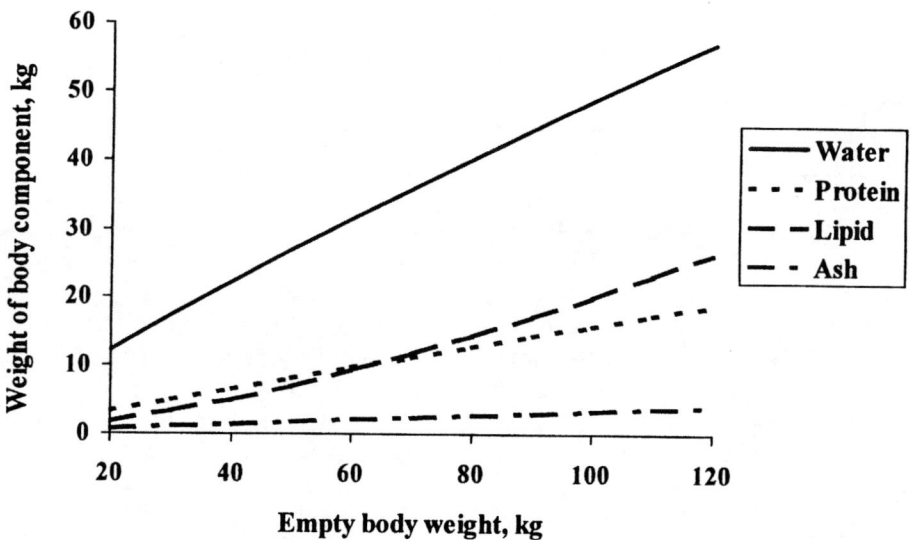

FIGURE 4.2 Typical changes in chemical body composition with increasing body weight. (Derived from ARC, 1981; de Greef et al., 1994; Whittemore, 1993; and Coudenys, 1998.)

Lean tissue growth curves can be converted to body protein growth curves, and vice versa, if assumptions are made about the protein content of lean tissue and the contribution of lean tissue to whole-body protein. For example, NRC (1998) suggests that 100 g of body protein deposition is equivalent to 255 g of fat-free lean tissue gain. Relationships such as these should be used with caution. As mentioned earlier, the definition of lean tissue may vary, and partitioning of body protein mass between lean tissue and other physical body components differs between groups of pigs. Moreover, feeding levels and diet composition influence this partitioning (de Greef et al., 1994; Bikker et al., 1995, 1996a,b; Coudenys, 1998).

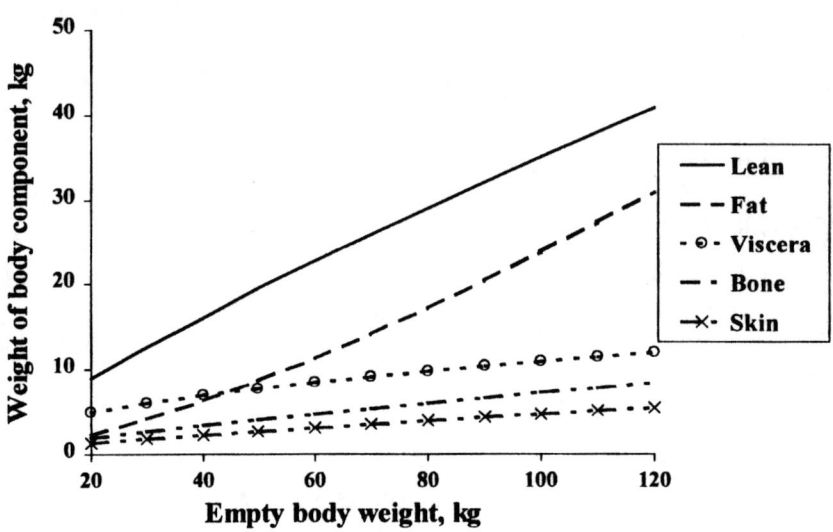

FIGURE 4.3 Typical changes in physical body composition with increasing body weight. (Derived from Richmond and Berg, 1971a; Gu et al., 1992b; Whittemore, 1993; and Coudenys, 1998.)

When using mathematical functions to represent growth patterns for the whole body or specific body components, it is important to note that body weight gain is the composite of growth of different chemical and physical body components, and that different factors determine growth at various stages. As a result, it is often not appropriate to use mathematical functions with only two or three parameters, such as these described by Gompertz, Taylor, Richards, and Bridges (Black et al., 1995; Schinckel and de Lange, 1996). Instead, rather complex mathematical functions that include more than three parameters are required (Black et al., 1986, 1995; Koops and Grossman, 1991; Schinckel and de Lange, 1996; Thompson et al., 1996; NRC, 1998). Moreover, adjustments of allometric relationships (A × BW^b) to more complex augmented allometric relationships (A × BW^b × $[c - BW]^d$) are often needed to relate body protein mass or body lipid mass to live body weight (Walstra, 1980; Wagner, 1992; Schinckel and de Lange, 1996). The effects of slight differences in fit of these mathematical functions on generated body protein or body lipid deposition curves can be very substantial (Schinckel and de Lange, 1996).

Rather than fitting complex mathematical functions, it is simpler and more appropriate to represent the relevant biological concepts underlying growth as mathematical functions. These "biological" mathematical functions include relationships between the pig's upper limit to daily body protein deposition (PDmax) or lean tissue growth potential and the stage of maturity, constraints on body lipid to protein deposition ratios, maintenance energy and nutrient requirements, and growth responses to changes in nutrient intake. These "biological" mathematical functions are generally much simpler and can be combined with observed or anticipated nutrient intake levels to represent growth patterns for the whole body and specific body components (Moughan and Verstegen, 1988; Ferguson and Gous, 1993). For example, in growing pigs when energy intake limits body protein deposition the pattern of body protein deposition varies with energy intakes. For these pigs, body protein deposition can be represented based on an assumed constant upper limit to body protein deposition, constraints on body lipid to body protein deposition ratios, and observed energy intake levels (Figure 4.4). There is increasing evidence that this approach is appropriate in growing pigs when energy intake limits body protein deposition (Moughan and Verstegen, 1988; Möhn and de Lange, 1998). Some of these concepts will be addressed in further detail in the next section.

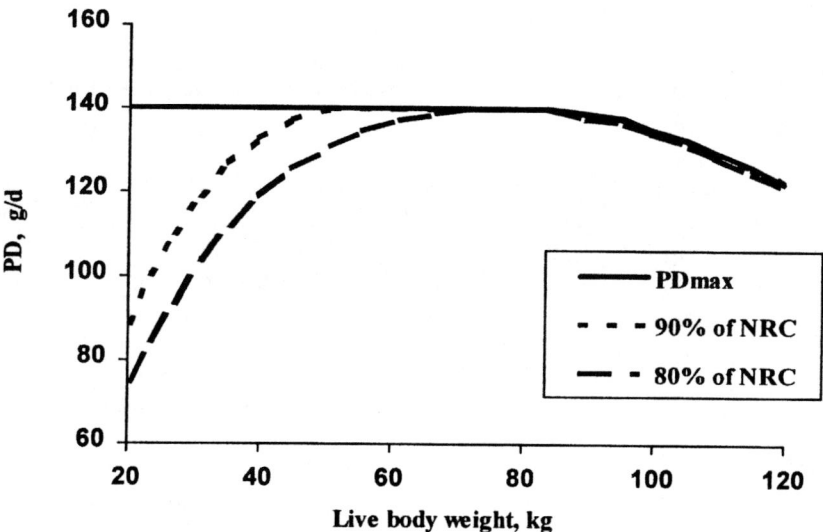

FIGURE 4.4 Estimated body PD and the animals PDmax in growing-finishing pigs that are fed at two levels of energy intake (80 or 90% of daily voluntary energy intake according to NRC, 1998). (Estimates were generated with a dynamic model that simulates growth in the pig; PPGM, 1997.)

The three practical methods to establish growth curves for body components in growing-finishing pigs are discussed in the following sections.

A. Directly Measure Weight of Body Components at Regular Time Intervals

To establish a growth curve by relating live body weight to time, measurements should be made on at least 40 pigs. On these pigs, make real-time ultrasound (or equivalent) measurements at least at four, preferably five, different live body weights that are equally spread out over the entire body weight range. This is to estimate body composition at each of these live body weights (Wagner, 1992; Schinckel and de Lange, 1996). Relate weight of body components to time using appropriate mathematical functions. Alternatively, mathematical functions may be used to relate live body weight to time and combined with mathematical functions that relate body composition to live body weight (Schinckel and de Lange, 1996). This is the preferred method for establishing growth curves for body components. The main sources of error when this method is used are the inaccuracies of the ultrasound measurements and the prediction of body composition from ultrasound (or equivalent) measurements at the various live body weights. Relationships between ultrasound measurements and body composition differ among lines of pigs (Rook et al., 1987; Wagner, 1992; Gu et al., 1992a; Hicks et al., 1998). These differences require that body composition is determined in a subsample of these pigs to calibrate real-time ultrasound measurements for each line of pigs.

B. Combine Average Growth Rate with a Standard Growth Curve Shape for Body Components

First, calculate average growth rates for body components from the estimated body composition at initial and final live body weight, or carcass composition in the case of lean tissue growth curves, and the number of days required to grow pigs from initial to final live body weight. Then, combine the average growth rate with a standard growth curve shape for that particular body component to establish growth curves. Given the minor variation in body composition of pigs <30 kg live body weight and the lack of sensitivity to errors in estimates of initial body composition, it may be assumed that body composition at initial live body weight is constant. This is the easiest method and is used by NRC (1998) to generate lean tissue growth curves for estimating nutrient requirements of growing-finishing pigs. This is also the least preferred method because it ignores differences in the shape of growth curves for body components between different groups of pigs (Schinckel et al., 1996). This method is further complicated by differences in relationships between carcass measurements and actual carcass lean contents among pig genotypes (Rook et al., 1987; Wagner, 1992; Gu et al., 1992a; Hicks et al., 1998: Swensen et al., 1998). Estimation of the amount of lean in the carcass may be improved by dissecting out one of the prime cuts such as the loin (Gu et al., 1992a; Swensen et al., 1998).

C. Use Growth Models to Fit Growth Curves of Body Components to Observed Body Weight Gains

First, establish a growth curve, based on at least four equally spread data points that relate live body weight to time with observations from at least 40 pigs per data point. Then, combine this information with an actual feed intake curve and run this through a dynamic pig growth model. Next, adjust the protein deposition curve "inside" the model to fit a predicted growth curve to the actual growth curve. This approach is very sensitive to estimates of maintenance energy requirements and feed intake. The basic principle is that energy intake in excess of maintenance requirements can only be used for either body protein deposition and associated body water and ash deposition, or body lipid deposition. Moreover, it is implied that the energetic efficiencies of using energy intake above maintenance requirements for body protein and body lipid deposition are known and constant (de Lange and Schreurs, 1995). When this method is used, both body protein and body lipid deposition patterns are generated.

Combinations of these three methods may also be used (Moughan, 1995; de Lange and Schreurs, 1995).

IV. DETERMINANTS OF BODY WEIGHT GAIN AND BODY COMPOSITION

Observed body weight gains and body compositions are the result of interactions between many factors that are associated with the pig's genotype, nutrition, or environment. The maximum rate and efficiency of body weight gain, and more specifically of lean tissue growth, is determined by the pig's genotype. However, because of nutritional or environmental constraints, pigs under commercial conditions usually achieve <75% of their genetic potential (Ellis et al. 1983; Jorgensen et al., 1985; Williams, 1994; Black et al., 1995). In this section, the three main factors that determine body weight gains and body composition are discussed: pig genotype, nutrient and energy intake, and environmental stresses.

A. Pig Genotype

Pig genotypes can be characterized based on five aspects of nutrient partitioning for growth: (1) maintenance energy and nutrient requirements (or basal metabolic rate); (2) the pigs' upper limit to body protein deposition (PDmax); (3) relationship between energy intake over maintenance and body protein deposition; (4) voluntary feed intake; and (5) relationships between chemical and physical body components. In this section, these aspects are discussed briefly. For a more detailed discussion the reader is referred elsewhere (Moughan and Verstegen, 1988; Black et al., 1986; 1995; Ferguson and Gous, 1993; Schinckel and de Lange, 1996; de Lange and Coudenys, 1996).

1. Maintenance Energy and Nutrient Requirements — Basal Metabolic Rate

Maintenance energy and nutrient requirements represent the amount of dietary energy and essential nutrients that pigs require to maintain live body weight and body composition. Maintenance requirements contribute to approximately one third of total energy requirements in growing pigs (Black and de Lange, 1995; NRC, 1998). In comparison, maintenance requirements contribute only 10 to 15% to total amino acid requirements in growing pigs (Moughan, 1995; NRC, 1998). Major energy-demanding processes that contribute to maintenance requirements include those associated with blood flow, respiration, muscle tone, ion balance, tissue turnover, animal activity, ingestion of feed, excretion of waste products, and utilization of dietary nutrients (Black and de Lange, 1995). Because estimates of maintenance energy and nutrient requirements are confounded by diet composition, it is more appropriate to characterize pig genotypes in terms of basal metabolic rates (Tess et al., 1983; Black and de Lange, 1995). However, no solid estimates of basal metabolic rates in pigs are available because it requires that energy expenditure and changes in body composition be determined in pigs that have been fasted for considerable time (van Milgen et al., 1998). Traditionally, energy requirements for maintenance have been related to live body weight using allometric mathematical functions (ARC, 1981; NRC, 1998). However, studies such as those conducted by Koong et al. (1983), Henken et al. (1991), Noblet et al. (1991), and van Milgen et al. (1998) indicate that such relationships only explain part of the variation of maintenance energy requirements that are observed between different groups of pigs that are managed under similar environmental conditions (Table 4.3). In addition to live body weight, the main factor that is likely to explain differences in maintenance energy requirements among different pig genotypes is animal activity (Henken et al., 1991; van Milgen et al., 1998). Animal activities associated with feeding and animal interactions can account for 20% or more of maintenance energy requirements (Halter et al., 1980; Verstegen et al., 1987). The distribution and energy requirements of major tissue groups (muscle, fat, visceral organs) in the pig's body should be considered as well. Because fat tissue is metabolically a relatively inactive tissue, maintenance energy requirements are lower in fat pigs than in lean pigs. For this reason maintenance energy requirements are better expressed relative to body protein mass than live body weight (Whittemore, 1983; 1993). It should, however, be noted that energy requirement per kilogram of protein in visceral organs is much larger than that in muscle tissue (Yen, 1997). Recent studies suggest that there is considerable variation in the size of visceral organs between groups of pigs (Koong et al., 1983; de Greef et al., 1994; Bikker et al. 1996a;

TABLE 4.3
Estimated Maintenance Energy Requirements in Different Genotypes and Sexes of Pigs

Sex/Genotype	Metabolizable Energy Requirements for Maintenance (kJ/kg $BW^{0.60}$)
Males	
Synthetic line	1048
Pietrain	899
Large White	974
Females	
Large White	1004
Castrates	
Large White	1004
Meisham × Large White	995
Meisham	874
Standard Error	56

Source: Derived from Noblet et al. (1991).

Quiniou and Noblet, 1995; van Milgen et al., 1998). Indications are that at least some of the variation in visceral organ size is determined by pig genotype. The latter may explain some of the variation in maintenance energy requirements among pig genotypes (see Tables 4.2 and 4.3).

2. The Pig's Upper Limit to Body Protein Deposition (PDmax)

In growing-finishing pigs PDmax varies between 90 and 160 g/day (Carr et al., 1977; Moughan and Verstegen, 1988; Thompson et al., 1996). However, in entire males of some modern pig genotypes PDmax may exceed 200 g/day (de Greef et al. 1994; van Lunen and Cole, 1998; Weatherup et al., 1998). This variation indicates that considerable improvement can be made in PDmax, and associated lean growth potentials via genetic selection.

For reasons outlined earlier, it is important that the changes in PDmax with changes in live body weight be determined in various pig genotypes. When establishing PDmax curves, it should be confirmed that body protein deposition rates that have been determined over the various live body weight ranges are indeed PDmax. The latter can be achieved by confirming that a change in the environment or the dietary supply of the first limiting nutrient does not alter the observed body protein deposition rate. It is often difficult to confirm that a change in the environment does not influence observed rates of body protein deposition or to determine the extent to which the pig's PDmax is reduced by environmental stresses. For this reason, Moughan et al. (1995) introduced the term *operational PDmax* which represents the PDmax that pigs can achieve under specific, practical conditions. Depending on the environment to which pigs are exposed, the operational PDmax may thus vary for a particular pig genotype.

PDmax curves in different pig genotypes are likely to follow a predictable pattern. One view is that PDmax is largely constant up to approximately 80 to 90 kg live body weight (Moughan and Verstegen, 1988; Moughan, 1995; Quiniou et al., 1995; 1996a; Möhn and de Lange, 1998) and that mathematical equations such as the Gompertz function can be used to represent the decline in PDmax as pigs approach maturity (Figure 4.4). An alternative view, suggested by Whittemore et al. (1988) and Ferguson and Gous (1993), is that PDmax is a function of mature body protein mass at all stages of growth. They suggest that the Gompertz function may be used to represent both increases and decreases in PDmax, at early stages of growth and as animals approach maturity respectively, and that PDmax is highest at intermediate live body weights. The latter view seems to be inconsistent with observations that PDmax at early stages of growth is as high as that at intermediate live body weights (Moughan, 1995; Quiniou et al., 1995; Möhn and de Lange, 1998). Available information suggests that there is considerable variation between different pig genotypes in the pattern of decline in PDmax (Thompson et al., 1996).

PDmax is highest in entire males, intermediate in gilts, and lowest in castrates. During the growing-finishing phase, the difference in PDmax between gilts and castrates is approximately 5% but varies between 2 and 15% (Moughan and Verstegen, 1988; Stranks et al., 1988; Thompson et al., 1996). This difference seems to vary with pig genotypes. The difference in PDmax seems to be small up to about 30 kg live body weight and increases with increasing live body weight. The decline in PDmax with increasing live body weight tends to start at a lower live body weight in castrates than in gilts (Thompson et al., 1996). Typically, PDmax is 20 to 30% higher in entire males than in castrates (Moughan and Verstegen, 1988; van Lunen and Cole, 1998).

3. Relationship between Energy Intake over Maintenance and Body Protein Deposition

The generalized relationship between energy intake and body protein deposition is represented in Figure 4.5. Over a given live body weight range, and assuming that no other nutrients limit body protein deposition, body protein deposition increases linearly with energy intake until PDmax is reached (Campbell and Taverner, 1988; Bikker et al., 1995; 1996a,b; Quiniou et al., 1995; 1996a). Further increases in energy intake increase the rates of body lipid deposition only. The latter results

Protein, Fat, and Bone Tissue Growth in Swine

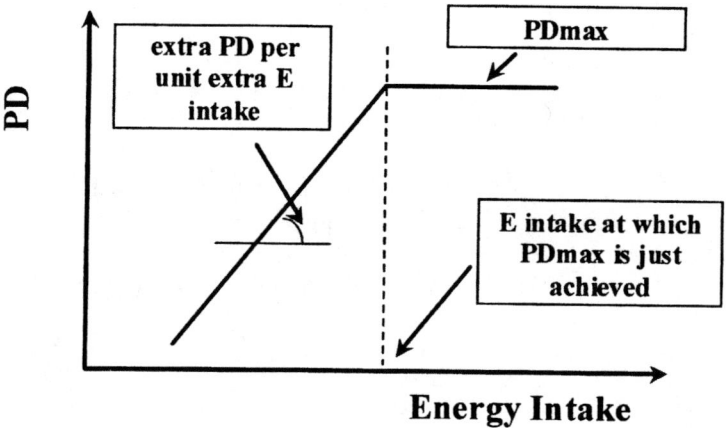

FIGURE 4.5 Generalized relationship between energy intake and body protein deposition (PD) in growing pigs.

in a fatter carcass and poorer feed efficiency. The energy intake level at which PDmax is just reached generally indicates the point at which the efficiency of pork production is maximized.

Information that is available about the relationship between energy intake and body protein deposition indicates that the energy intake level at which PDmax is just reached varies considerably among different pig genotypes (Möhn and de Lange, 1998; some data are presented in Figure 4.6). In some modern pig genotypes, energy intake is insufficient to reach PDmax even when they are allowed *ad libitum* access to feed and when they reach 90 to 100 kg live body weight (Large White × Landrace (A) boars and hybrid gilts, Figure 4.6). Yet, in other pig genotypes, PDmax can be reached at relatively low energy intake levels (Large White × Pietrain boars in Figure 4.6). These differences can largely be attributed to variation in the increase in body protein deposition per unit increase in energy intake (i.e., the "slope" of the linear relationship between energy intake and body protein deposition in Figures 4.5 and 4.6). This variation in the "slope" is largely due to differing amounts of essential body lipid that different pig genotypes deposit, even when energy

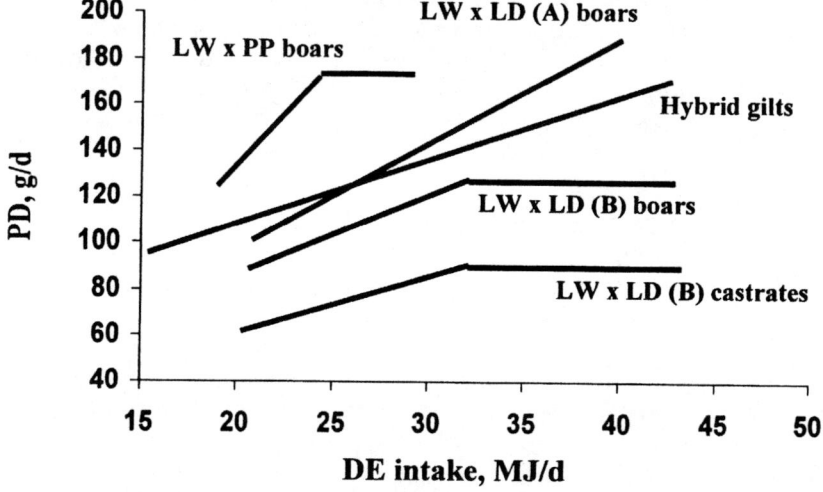

FIGURE 4.6 Relationship between DE intake and body PD in different pig genotypes between approximately 40 and 90 kg BW. LW: large white; PP: Pietrain; LD: Landrace. (Derived from Campell and Taverner, 1988; de Greef et al., 1994; Quiniou et al., 1995; and Bikker et al., 1996a.)

intake limits lean growth. This "slope" can be represented in different ways. Black et al. (1986; 1995) and NRC (1998) have used empirical linear relationships between energy intake and body protein deposition. Alternatively, constraints on the minimum ratio of increments in body lipid deposition to increments in body protein deposition, combined with estimates of the energy requirements per unit of body protein and body lipid deposition, can be used (de Greef et al., 1994; Bikker et al., 1995, 1996a,b; Quiniou et al., 1996a).

Live body weight effects, previous nutrition, and differences in maintenance energy requirements among different pig genotypes further complicate the relationship between energy intake and body protein deposition (Black et al., 1995). For example, the "slopes" in Figures 4.5 and 4.6 likely decline with increasing live body weight (Black et al., 1995; NRC, 1998). The latter implies that pigs get fatter when they grow heavier, even when energy intake limits body protein deposition, and that increasing amounts of energy intake over maintenance are required to maintain the body protein deposition constant with increases in live body weight.

Carefully planned performance studies are needed to characterize properly the effects of energy intake on body protein deposition in the different pig genotypes. Current protocols suggest that representative groups of pigs should be exposed to a minimum of three energy intake levels, two of which should be lower than that required to reach PDmax. Rates of body protein deposition need to be determined over the various live body weight ranges to relate body protein deposition to energy intake at the various live body weights (de Greef et al., 1994; Bikker et al., 1995; 1996a,b; Quiniou et al., 1995; Coudenys, 1998). Furthermore, pigs should be adjusted to energy intake levels before the first measurements are made. Quiniou et al. (1995) and Möhn and de Lange (1998) demonstrated that when energy intake restriction is first imposed, energy intake is preferentially used to support body protein deposition rather than body lipid deposition, apparently until the body protein and body lipid mass have been adjusted to a new equilibrium.

4. Voluntary Feed Intake

Both ARC (1981) and NRC (1998) suggested empirical relationships between live body weight and *ad libitum* daily intake of digestible energy (DE) indicating that diet DE content and live body weight are two of the main factors determining voluntary feed intake in pigs.

However, tremendous differences (20 to 30%) in voluntary feed intake have been observed among different pig genotypes that are managed under similar conditions and fed similar diets (Forbes et al., 1989; Schinckel, 1994). The relationship between voluntary feed intake of barrows and gilts also seems to differ among pig genotypes; it may vary between 3 and >10% (Schinckel, 1994). The difference in voluntary feed intake between these two genders tends to increase with increasing live body weight (NRC, 1998).

An approach to understanding voluntary feed intake in different groups of pigs is to recognize that voluntary feed intake is driven by the pig's requirements for nutrients, and that feed intake is reduced because of various constraints imposed on the animal (Black et al., 1986; Emmans and Kyriazakis, 1989). These constraints relate to diet characteristics (bulk density, nature and rate of digestion of fiber, water-holding capacity, nutrient and antinutrient contents), environment (thermal, social, physical, presence of disease-causing organisms), and the pig's physical capacity to ingest feed. Important first steps in characterizing voluntary feed intake in different pig genotypes are to determine the pig's potential of body protein and body lipid deposition in a nonlimiting environment (Ferguson and Gous, 1993), and the pig's physical capacity to ingest feed (Emmans and Kyriazakis, 1989; Black, 1995). As PDmax continues to increase, through genetic selection, voluntary feed intake is more likely to limit expression of PDmax at increasingly higher live body weights. These factors and others that affect feed intake are discussed in detail in Chapter 20.

5. Relationships between Chemical and Physical Body Components

The data presented in Table 4.2 indicate that there are differences between pig genotypes in physical body composition at similar live body weight. These differences coincide with differences in chemical body composition and suggest that the partitioning of both body protein and lipid mass over the various physical body components differs among pig genotypes (Rook et al., 1987; Quiniou and Noblet; 1995; Quiniou et al., 1996a,b). The latter has consequences for relating body protein deposition rates to lean tissue growth in the various pig genotypes and the conversion of dietary nutrients into edible body components. Unfortunately, limited information is available on this aspect of nutrient partitioning in the various pig genotypes.

B. Nutrient and Energy Intake

Suboptimal intakes of essential nutrients and energy will limit pigs from expressing their PDmax. For this reason, practical pig diets are generally overfortified with the relatively inexpensive nutrients, vitamins, and minerals. Furthermore, close attention should be paid to dietary levels of energy, lysine, and the other essential amino acids, and to daily feed intakes when managing growing-finishing pigs.

1. Intake of Lysine and Other Essential Amino Acids

Pigs with higher body protein deposition rates require larger quantities of dietary lysine and other essential amino acids (NRC, 1998). In fact, body protein deposition rate is the main determinant of dietary amino acid requirements. Failure to meet required amino acid intakes will result in reductions in body protein deposition rates and in associated carcass quality and efficiencies of pork production. The relationships between amino acid intake and pig performance are addressed in more detail elsewhere in this book (Chapters 8, 31, and 32).

2. Energy Intake

Energy intake can have important effects on body weight gain and chemical body composition, as well as the partitioning of body protein over the various physical body components (Table 4.4).

Observed feed intake levels and, as a result, energy intake levels differ substantially among growing-finishing pig units. This reflects the many factors, associated with the animal (live body weight, genotype, sex, health status), the feed (ingredient composition and quality, freshness, processing, water), or the environment (stocking density, effective environmental temperature,

TABLE 4.4
Distribution of Total Body Protein in Lean Tissue and Visceral Organs in Pigs at ~85 kg BW and Fed at Two Levels of Energy Intake

	Feeding Level	
	2.2 × Maintenance	3.7 × Maintenance
Percentage of whole body protein present in:		
Lean tissue	57.6	52.4
Visceral organs	12.5	16.0
Composition of lean tissue		
Protein (%)	20.2	19.1
Lipid (%)	7.9	10.3

Source: Derived from Bikker et al. (1996a,b).

feeder design and management), that affect observed feed and energy intake levels (Forbes et al., 1989). Given this variability, feed intake curves should be established for individual growing-finishing pig units and some of the main factors that are known to affect feed intake should be monitored (Forbes et al., 1989; Moughan et al., 1995; Schinckel and de Lange, 1996; NRC, 1998).

Under commercial conditions energy intake above maintenance often does not increase in pigs >60 kg live body weight. Observed increases in feed intake with increasing live body weight are often barely sufficient to satisfy the pig's increasing maintenance energy requirements. As a result, observed declines in body protein deposition rates as pigs approach market weight may be a reflection of a lack of energy intake over maintenance and not of declines in PDmax with increasing live body weight (Figure 4.4).

C. Environmental Stresses

The last few years have witnessed growing awareness of the negative effects of environmental stresses on body protein deposition. Stocking arrangements (Chapple, 1993), extreme environmental temperatures (Verstegen et al., 1987; Henken et al., 1991), and disease-causing organisms (Williams, 1994) can prevent pigs from expressing their PDmax. Researchers have reported that body protein deposition rates may be reduced by as much as 30% as a result of exposure to disease-causing organisms (Williams, 1994; Black et al., 1995). Environmental stresses will affect the animals' expression of PDmax, as well as maintenance energy and nutrient requirements and the relationship between energy intake and body protein deposition. The effect of the environment on pigs is discussed further in Chapters 22 and 23.

V. SUMMARY

For the development of effective feeding strategies for growing pigs estimates of whole-body nutrient deposition rates are required, particularly for protein and lipid. Moreover, effects of live body weight, pig genotype, environmental conditions, and nutrient intake on body protein and lipid deposition, as well as their distribution over the main tissues in the pig's body, should be characterized. In this chapter the chemical and physical body composition of growing pigs are discussed, including means to characterize nutrient and tissue accretion in individual groups of pigs. The main factors that are known to influence the rate and composition of body weight gain in pigs are addressed as well.

REFERENCES

Agricultural Research Council (ARC). 1981. *The Nutrient Requirements of Pigs*, Commonwealth Agricultural Bureaux, Slough, U.K.

Bikker, P., V. Karabinas, M. W. A. Verstegen, and R. G. Campbell. 1995. Protein and lipid accretion in body components of growing gilts (20 to 45 kilograms) as affected by energy intake, *J. Anim. Sci.*, 73:2355.

Bikker, P., M. W. A. Verstegen, B. Kemp, and M. W. Bosch. 1996a. Performance and body composition of finishing gilts (45 to 85 kilograms) as affected by energy intake and nutrition in earlier life. I. Growth of the body and body components, *J. Anim. Sci.*, 74:806.

Bikker, P., M. W. A. Verstegen, B. Kemp, and M. W. Bosch. 1996b. Performance and body composition of finishing gilts (45 to 85 kilograms) as affected by energy intake and nutrition in earlier life. II. Protein and lipid accretion in body components, *J. Anim. Sci.*, 74:817.

Black, J. L. 1995. Modelling energy metabolism in the pig — critical evaluation of a simple reference model. In *Modelling Growth in the Pig*, Moughan, P. J., M. W. A. Verstegen, and M. I. Visser-Reyneveld, Eds., Wageningen Pers, Wageningen, The Netherlands, 59.

Black, J. L., and C. F. M. de Lange. 1995. Introduction to principles of nutrient partitioning for growth. In *Modelling Growth in the Pig*, Moughan, P. J., M. W. A. Verstegen, and M. I. Visser-Reyneveld, Eds., Wageningen Pers, Wageningen, The Netherlands, 33.

Black, J. L. R. G. Campbell, I. H. Williams, K. J. James and G. T. Davies. 1986. Simulation of energy and amino acid utilization in the pig, *Res. Dev. Agric.*, 3:121.

Black, J. L., G. T. Davies, H. R. Bray, and R. P. Chapple. 1995. Modelling the effect of genotype, environment and health on nutrient utilization. In *Proc. of the IVth International Workshop on Modelling Nutrient Utilization in Farm Animals*, Danfaer, A. and P. Lescoat, Eds., National Institute of Animal Science, Tjele, Denmark, 85.

Campbell, R. G., and M. R. Taverner. 1988. Genotype and sex effects on the relationship between energy intake and protein deposition in growing pigs, *J. Anim. Sci.*, 66:676.

Campbell, R. G., M. R. Taverner, and D. M. Curic. 1985. Effects of sex and energy intake between 48 and 90 kg live weight on protein deposition in growing pigs, *Anim. Prod.*, 40:497.

Carr, J. R., K. N. Boorman, and D. J. A. Cole. 1977. Nitrogen retention in pigs, *Br. J. Nutr.*, 37:143.

Chapple, R. P. 1993. Effect of stocking arrangements on pig performance. In *Manipulating Pig Production IV*, Batterham, E. S., Ed., Australasian Pig Science Association, Attwood, Victoria, Australia, 87.

Coudenys, K. T. 1998. The Effect of Body Weight and Energy Intake on the Physical and Chemical Body Composition in Growing-Finishing Pigs. M.Sc. thesis, Department of Animal and Poultry Science, University of Guelph, Guelph, Ontario, Canada.

de Greef, K. H. 1995. Prediction of growth and carcass parameters. In *Modelling Growth in the Pig*, Moughan, P. J., M. W. A. Verstegen, and M. I. Visser-Reyneveld, Eds., Wageningen Pers, Wageningen, The Netherlands, 151.

de Greef, K. H., M. W. A. Verstegen, B. Kemp, and P. van der Togt. 1994. The effect of body weight and energy intake on the composition of deposited tissue in pigs, *Anim. Prod.*, 58:263.

de Lange, C. F. M., and K. T. Coudenys. 1996. Interactions between nutrition and the expression of performance potentials in grower-finisher pigs. In *Proc. 1996 National Swine Improvement Federation Conference*. National Swine Improvement Federation, North Carolina State University, Raleigh, NC, 36.

de Lange, C. F. M., and H. W. E. Schreurs. 1995. Principles of model application. In *Modelling Growth in the Pig*, Moughan, P. J., M. W. A. Verstegen, and M. I. Visser-Reyneveld, Eds., Wageningen Pers, Wageningen, The Netherlands, 187.

Ellis, M, W. C. Smith, R. Henderson, C. T. Whittemore, R. Laird, and P. Phillips. 1983. Comparative performance and body composition of control and selected line Large White pigs. 3. Three low feeding scales for a fixed time, *Anim. Prod.*, 37:253.

Emmans, G. C., and I. Kyriazakis. 1989. The prediction of the rate of food intake in growing pigs. In *Voluntary Food Intake of Pigs*, Forbes, J. M., M. A. Varley, T. L. J. Lawrence, H. Davies, and M. C. Dikethly, Eds., The Occasional Publication of the British Society of Animal Production, no. 13. pp. 110.

Emmans, G. C., and I. Kyriazakis. 1995. A general method for predicting the weight of water in the empty bodies of pigs, *Anim. Sci.*, 61:103.

Ferguson, N. S., and R. M. Gous. 1993. Evaluation of pig genotypes. 1. Theoretical aspects of measuring genetic parameters, *Anim. Prod.*, 56:233.

Forbes, J. M., M. A. Varley, T. L. J. Lawrence, H. Davies, and M. C. Dikethly, Eds. 1989. *The Voluntary Food Intake of Pigs*, Occasional Publication of the British Society of Animal Production, no. 13.

Fuller, M. F., M. F. Franklin, R. McWilliam, and K. Pennie. 1995. The response of growing pigs, of different sex and genotype, to dietary energy and protein, *Anim. Sci.*, 60:291.

Gu, Y., A. P. Schinckel, T. G. Martin, J. C. Forrest, C. H. Kuei, and L. E. Watkins. 1992a. Genotype and treatment biases in estimation of carcass lean of swine, *J. Anim. Sci.*, 70:1708.

Gu, Y., A. P. Schinckel, and T. G. Martin. 1992b. Growth, development and carcass composition in five genotypes of swine, *J. Anim. Sci.*, 70:1719.

Halter, H. M., C. Wenk, and A. Schurch. 1980. Effect of feeding level and feed composition on energy utilization, physical activity and growth performance of piglets. In *Energy Metabolism*, Mount, L. E., Ed., Butterworths, London, 195.

Hendriks, W. H., and P. J. Moughan. 1993. Whole-body mineral composition of entire male and female pigs depositing protein at maximal rates, *Livest. Prod. Sci.*, 33:161.

Henken, A. M., W. van der Hell, H. A. Brandsma, and M. W. A. Verstegen. 1991. Differences in energy metabolism and protein retention of limit-fed growing pigs of several breeds, *J. Anim. Sci.*, 69:1443.

Hicks, C., A. P. Schinckel, J. C. Forrest, J. T. Akridge, J. R. Wagner, and W. Chen. 1998. Biases associated with genotype and sex in prediction of fat-free lean mass and carcass value in hogs, *J. Anim. Sci.*, 76:2221.

Koong, L. J., J. A. Nienaber, and H. J. Mersmann. 1983. Effects of plane of nutrition on organ size and fasting heat production in genetically lean and obese pigs, *J. Nutr.*, 113:1626.

Koops, W. J., and M. Grossman. 1991. Applications of a multiphasic growth function to body composition of pigs, *J. Anim. Sci.*, 69:3265.

Jones, S. D. M., R. J. Richmond, M. A. Price, and R. G. Berg. 1980. Effect of breed and sex on the patterns of fat deposition and distribution in swine, *Can. J. Anim. Sci.*, 60:223.

Jorgensen, J., J. A. Fernandez, H. Jorgensen, and A. Just. 1985. Anatomical and chemical composition of female pigs and barrows of Danish Landrace related to nutrition, *Z. Tierphysiol. Tierernähr. Futtermittelkd.*, 54:253.

McMeekan, C. P. 1940. Growth and development in the pig, with special reference to carcass quality characteristics, *J. Agric. Sci.*, 30:276.

Möhn, S., and C. F. M. de Lange. 1998. The effect of energy intake on body protein deposition in a defined population of gilts between 25 and 70 kg body weight, *J. Anim. Sci.*, 76:124.

Moughan, P. J. 1995. Modelling protein metabolism in the pig — critical evaluation of a simple reference model. In *Modelling Growth in the Pig*, Moughan, P. J., M. W. A. Verstegen, and M. I. Visser-Reyneveld, Eds., Wageningen Pers, Wageningen, The Netherlands, 103.

Moughan, P. J., and M. W. A. Verstegen. 1988. The modelling of growth in the pig, *Netherl. J. Agric. Sci.*, 36:145.

Moughan, P. J., W. C. Smith, and E. V. J. Stevens. 1990. Allometric growth of chemical body components and several organs in the pig (20–90 kg liveweight), *N.Z. J. Agric. Res.*, 33:77.

Moughan, P. J., R. T. Kerr, and W. C. Smith. 1995. The role of simulation models in the development of economically-optimal feeding regimens for the growing pig. In *Modelling Growth in the Pig*, Moughan, P. J., M. W. A. Verstegen, and M. I. Visser-Reyneveld, Eds., Wageningen Pers, Wageningen, The Netherlands, 209.

National Research Council (NRC). 1998. *Nutrient Requirements of Swine*, 10th rev. ed., National Academy Press, Washington, D.C.

Noblet, J., C. Karege, and S. Dubois. 1991. Influence of growth potential on energy requirements for maintenance in growing pigs. In *Energy Metabolism in Farm Animals*, Wenk, C., and W. Boessinger, Eds., Gruppe, Zurich, Switzerland, 107.

Nyachoti, C. M. 1998. Significance of Endogenous Gut Protein Losses in Growing Pigs, Ph.D. thesis, Department of Animal and Poultry Science, University of Guelph, Guelph, Ontario, Canada.

OPCAP, Ontario Pork Carcass Appraisal Project. 1996. *Proc. National Swine Improvement Federation Conference*, National Swine Improvement Federation, North Carolina State University, Raleigh, NC, 160.

PPGM, Purina Pork Growth Model. 1997. A biological model that represents nutrient partitioning for growth in the pig and that includes cost-benefit analyses — developed by the international pig growth modelling group — University of Guelph, Canada; Massey University, New Zealand; Wageningen Agricultural University, The Netherlands; Agribrands International.

Quiniou, N., and J. Noblet. 1995. Prediction of tissular body composition from protein and lipid deposition in growing pigs, *J. Anim. Sci.*, 73:1567.

Quiniou, N., J. Noblet, J. van Milgen, and J. Y. Dourmad. 1995. Effect of energy intake on performance, nutrient and tissue gain and protein and energy utilization in growing boars, *Anim. Sci.*, 61:133.

Quiniou, N., J.-Y. Dourmad, and J. Noblet. 1996a. Effect of energy intake on the performance of different pig types from 45 to 100 kg body weight. 1. protein and lipid deposition, *Anim. Sci.*, 63:277.

Quiniou, N., J.-Y. Dourmad, and J. Noblet. 1996b. Effect of energy intake on the performance of different pig types from 45 to 100 kg body weight. 2. tissue gain, *Anim. Sci.*, 63:289.

Rao, D. S., and K. J. MacCracken. 1991. Effect of energy intake on protein and energy metabolism of boars of high genetic potential for lean growth, *Anim. Prod.*, 52:499.

Richmond, R. J., and R. T. Berg. 1971a. Tissue development in swine as influenced by liveweight, breed, sex and ration, *Can. J. Anim. Sci.*, 51:31.

Richmond, R. J., and R. T. Berg. 1971b. Muscle growth and distribution in swine as influenced by liveweight, breed, sex and ration, *Can. J. Anim. Sci.*, 51:41.

Rook, A., M. Ellis, C. T. Whittemore, and P. Phillips. 1987. Relationships between whole-body composition chemical composition, physical dissected carcass parts and backfat measurements in pigs, *Anim. Prod.*, 44:263.

Rymarz, A. 1986. Chemical body composition of growing pigs. Ca, P, K, Na and Mg contents in the body, *Pigs News Info.*, 7:177.

Schinckel, A. P. 1994. Nutrient requirements of modern pig genotypes. In *Recent Advances in Animal Nutrition*, Garnsworthy, P. C., and D. J. A. Cole, Eds., University of Nottingham Press, Nottingham, U.K. pp 133.

Schinckel, A. P., and C. F. M. de Lange. 1996. Characterization of growth parameters needed as inputs for pig growth models, *J. Anim. Sci.*, 74:2021.

Schinckel, A. P., P. V. Proeckel, and E. M. Einstein. 1996. Prediction of daily protein accretion rates of pigs from estimates of fat-free lean gain between 20 and 120 kilograms live weight, *J. Anim. Sci.*, 74:498.

Stranks, M. H., B. C. Cooke, C. B. Fairbarn, N. G. Fowler, P. S. Kirby, K. J. MacKracken, C. A. Morgan, F. G. Palmer, and D. G. Peers. 1988. Nutrient allowances for growing pigs, *Res. Dev. Agric.*, 5:71.

Swatland, H. J. 1994. *Structure and Development of Meat Animals and Poultry*, Technomic, Lancaster, PA.

Swensen K., M. Ellis, M. S. Brewer, J. Novakofski, and F. K. McKeith. 1998. Pork carcass composition: II. Use of indicator cuts for predicting carcass composition, *J. Anim. Sci.*, 76:2405.

Tess, M. W., G. L. Bennett, and G. E. Dickerson. 1983. Simulation of genetic changes in life cycle efficiency of pork production, *J. Anim. Sci.*, 56:336.

Thomke, S., T. Alaviuhkola, A. Madsen, F. Sundstol, H. P. Mortensen, O. Vangen, and K. Anderson. 1995. Dietary energy and protein for growing pigs. 2. Protein and fat accretion and organ weights of animals slaughtered at 20, 50, 80 and 110 kg live weight, *Acta Agric. Scand. Sect. A. Anim. Sci.*, 45:54.

Thompson, J. M., F. Sun, T. Kuczek, A. P. Schinckel, and T. S. Stewart. 1996. The effect of genotype and sex on the patterns of protein accretion in pigs, *Anim. Sci.*, 63:265.

Van Lunen, T. A., and D. J. A. Cole. 1998. Growth and body composition of highly selected boars and gilts, *Anim. Sci.*, 67:107.

Van Milgen, J., J. F. Bernier, Y. Lecozler, S. Dubois, and J. Noblet. 1998. Major determinants of fasting heat production and energetic costs of activity in growing pigs of different body weight and breed/castration combination, *Br. J. Nutr.*, 79:1.

Verstegen, M. W. A., A. M. Henken, and W. van der Hell. 1987. Influence of some environmental, animal and feeding factors on energy metabolism in growing pigs. In *Energy Metabolism in Farm Animals, Effects of Housing, Stress and Disease*, Verstegen, M. W. A., and A. M. Henken, Eds., Kluwer Academic Publishers, Hingham, MA, 70.

Wagner, J. R. 1992. Genotype and Sex Biases in the Estimation of Pork Carcass Composition, M.Sc. thesis, Purdue University, West Lafayette, IN.

Walstra, P. 1980. Growth and Carcass Composition from Birth to Maturity in Relating Feeding Level and Sex in Dutch Landrace Pigs, Ph.D. thesis, Wageningen Agricultural University, Wageningen, The Netherlands.

Weatherup, R. N., V. E. Beattie, B. W. Moss, D. J. Kilpatrick, and N. Walker. 1998. The effect of increasing slaughter weight on the production performance and meat quality of finishing pigs, *Anim. Sci.*, 67:591.

Whittemore, C. T. 1983. Development of recommended energy and protein allowances for growing pigs, *Agric. Syst.*, 11:159.

Whittemore, C. T. 1993. *The Science and Practice of Pig Production*, Longman Group, Essex, U.K.

Whittemore, C. T., J. B. Tullis, and G. C. Emmans. 1988. Protein growth in pigs, *Anim. Prod.*, 46:437.

Williams, N. H. 1994. Impact of genetic and environmental factors on the growth of the young pig, *Proc. Am. Assoc. Swine Pract.*, Chicago, IL, 185.

Yen, J. T. 1997. Oxygen consumption and energy flux of porcine splanchnic tissues, *Proceedings of the VIIth International Symposium on Digestive Physiology in Pigs*, St. Malo, France, EAAP Publ. No. 88, 260.

Part II

Nutrient Utilization by Swine

5 Energy Utilization in Swine Nutrition

Richard C. Ewan

CONTENTS

I. Introduction 85
II. Energy Evaluation of Feed Ingredients 87
III. Efficiency of Energy Utilization 88
    A. Growth 88
    B. Gestation 89
    C. Lactation 89
IV. Nutrient-to-Energy Ratios 89
V. Factors Affecting Energy Utilization 90
    A. Feed Composition 90
    B. Predicting Energy Concentrations from Chemical Composition 90
    C. Environment 90
VI. Energy Requirements of Pigs 91
    A. Maintenance 91
    B. Growth 91
    C. Gestation 92
    D. Lactation 92
References 93

I. INTRODUCTION

Feed accounts for about two thirds of the cost of producing market-weight swine. Through the years, efforts have been made to optimize feed efficiency so that feed costs might be minimized. Such efforts depend on knowledge of nutrient availability in feed ingredients and the requirements of the pig for those nutrients for various physiological states.

The total digestible nutrient (TDN) system allows comparisons, roughly equivalent to digestible energy concentration, between feed ingredients. TDN is the sum of digestible protein, digestible ether extract, and digestible carbohydrate. Ether extract is multiplied by 2.25 to adjust for the greater energy concentration of fat. The system has been criticized because it gives protein the same weight as carbohydrates, and, because it is the sum of several digestibility measurements, the errors associated with each of the individual measurements reduce the accuracy of the value.

Although the TDN system was used for many years, it has gradually been replaced by measures of energy to describe the value of feed ingredients. The heat of combustion is the maximum amount of energy that is available for use by animals and is defined as gross energy (GE). The GE concentration of a feed ingredient is dependent on the proportions of carbohydrate, fat, protein, minerals, and water present in the ingredient. Water and minerals contribute no energy, whereas carbohydrates provide 3.7 (glucose) to 4.2 (starch) kcal/g. Protein provides 5.6 kcal/g and fat, 9.4 kcal/g. If the composition of a feed is known, GE can be predicted fairly accurately. Measurement of GE is generally done with an adiabatic bomb calorimeter.

The utilization of the energy of a feed by the pig is illustrated in Figure 5.1. Digestible energy (DE) is the GE of the feed minus the heat of combustion of the fecal material (FE). Indigestible energy is a major variable in evaluation of feed ingredients. Digestible energy is the energy that is available for utilization by the pig and NRC (1998) use DE to predict feed intake of the pig. Metabolizable energy (ME) is DE minus the heat of combustion of the urine (UE) and of gases produced in the intestinal tract. Energy losses in the urine are small and generally associated with the excretion of nitrogenous products of metabolism. Energy lost as gas is generally <1% of GE intake of pigs and is often ignored. In complete feeds fed to pigs, ME is about 96% of DE but will decrease as the protein content of the diet increases. Metabolizable energy was used by NRC (1998) as the basis for predicting potential performance of pigs.

Metabolizable energy is divided further into net energy (NE) and heat increment (HI). HI is the heat produced by the digestion and metabolism of nutrients and by fermentation in the intestinal tract. Normally, HI is waste energy, but HI can be used to maintain body temperature. The remaining energy is first used to meet the requirement for maintenance (NE_m). The NE_m includes the energy needed to sustain life and to maintain body temperature. If the supply of NE is greater than the energy required for maintenance, it is used for production (NE_p). Productive processes include the synthesis of new tissue (protein and fat), fetal development and milk synthesis. Heat production (HP) is the sum of the HI and the energy of maintenance (NE_m).

In nutrition, the joule (J) is the basic unit used for energy in most of the world and the calorie (cal) is used in the United States. A joule is 10^7 erg, where 1 erg is the amount of energy expended in accelerating a mass of 1 g by 1 m/s. A calorie is the amount of energy required to raise the temperature of 1 g of water from 16.5 to 17.5°C and is equivalent to 4.184 J. Both joules and calories are more commonly expressed in multiples of 1000 so that a kilocalorie is 10^3 cal and a megacalorie is 10^6 cal or 1000 kcal. Corresponding units for the joule are kilojoule and megajoule. The basic unit that will be used in this chapter is the kilocalorie.

In European countries, energy systems were developed that were related to the energy content of a common feed ingredient and expressed as feeding units (e.g., the Scandinavian feed unit). These have been reviewed by Henry et al. (1988), but they have generally been replaced by systems based on the joule.

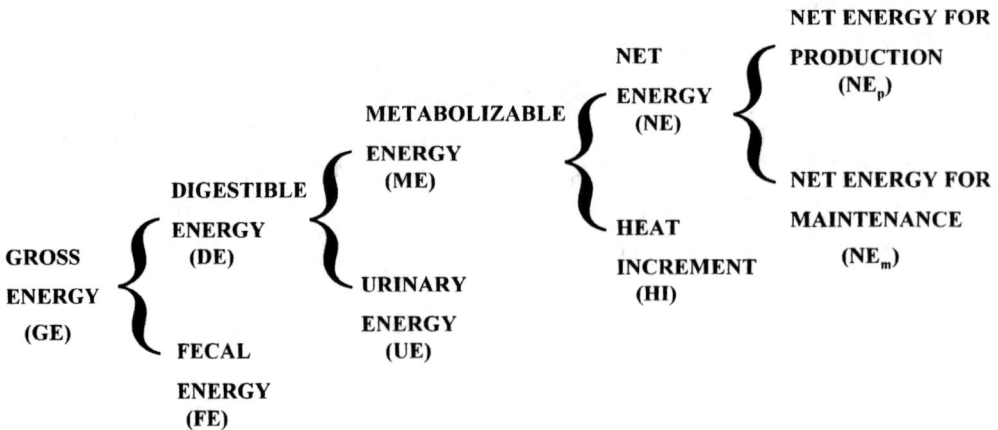

FIGURE 5.1 Utilization of energy by pigs.

II. ENERGY EVALUATION OF FEED INGREDIENTS

Pigs are normally fed diets containing several ingredients, complicating the determination of energy values of individual ingredients. The determination of DE and ME of a diet fed to pigs requires the completion of a metabolism study with collection of feces and urine. The energy content of the diet, feces, and urine is determined and DE (GE − FE) and ME (DE − UE) can be calculated. These types of metabolism studies are described in more detail in Chapter 40.

Further evaluation to determine NE requires a measurement of retained energy or of HP. Energy retention can be determined in a comparative slaughter experiment in which the energy content of pigs slaughtered at the start of the experiment is subtracted from the energy content of the pigs at the end of the experiment to determine the retained energy. Retained energy can also be determined by carbon–nitrogen balance in which nitrogen gain is attributed to protein gain and carbon retention after subtraction of the carbon in the protein gain is attributed to fat deposition. Retained energy is then calculated by applying standard values for the energy concentrations of fat and protein.

Direct or indirect calorimetry can be used to measure HP. In direct calorimetry, the HP of the pig is measured by physical methods and requires complex equipment. Indirect calorimetry uses measurement of oxygen uptake, expired carbon dioxide, and methane loss. These measures are used with standard conversion factors to give HP (Brouwer, 1965).

The maintenance requirement of the pig is necessary to complete the evaluation of NE. The maintenance requirement is generally expressed as an exponential function of body weight (often referred to as "metabolic weight"). The exponent that is generally used is 0.75 (Kleiber, 1965) but values from 0.56 (Breirem, 1939) to 1.0 (Kielanowski, 1972) have been suggested. Noblet et al. (1999) reported the results from a total of 177 energy balances from seven groups of pigs that varied by genotype and/or sex and ranged in weight from 20 to 107 kg. The results of factorial analysis in which the exponent for body weight was estimated indicated that an exponent of 0.6 provided a better fit to the data than if the exponent were fixed at 0.75. Noblet et al. (1999) suggested that maintenance requirements were underestimated with the use of the exponent 0.75 in comparison with the use of 0.60 as the exponent. The underestimation was greatest at 20 kg (approximately 30%) and decreased to small differences at 110 kg.

With the measurement of RE either by comparative slaughter or by carbon–nitrogen balance, the maintenance requirement can be estimated from the regression of ME intake and RE (ME intake = a + b RE; Figure 5.2). In this relationship with both ME intake and RE expressed per unit of metabolic weight, the intercept is a measure of NE_m and the regression coefficient is a measure of

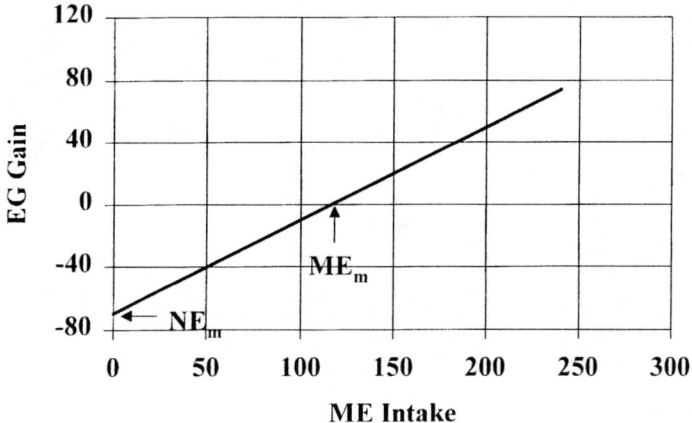

FIGURE 5.2 Estimation of maintenance requirements from daily energy gain (EG gain in $kcal/BW^{0.75}$) and daily metabolizable energy intake (ME_I in $kcal/BW^{0.75}$).

the efficiency of conversion of ME to RE. The maintenance requirement in terms of ME is the intercept divided by the efficiency.

With direct or indirect calorimetry, the HP of the conscious animal in a fasting state is used as the maintenance requirement. This is based on the assumption that HI is zero in the fasted state so the relationship, HP = HI + NE_m, becomes HP = NE_m. The length of fast has to be standardized because HP declines as the length of the fast increases.

To determine the energy value of individual ingredients in a mixed diet, some means of partitioning the energy among the ingredients is necessary. In short-term studies, diets containing essentially one ingredient have been used, but this is not satisfactory for long-term studies and may be confounded by nutrient excesses or deficiencies. Substitution of one ingredient for another and observing the change in energy values has been used. Regression techniques are used to determine the values at 100% intake of each individual component (Kromann et al., 1976). In some studies, a basal diet is fed at a constant level and the individual ingredient is fed in addition to the basal diet to determine the response to additional energy from the test ingredient (Diggs et al., 1965).

Surgically prepared pigs have been used to introduce ingredients in nylon bags into the duodenum. The bags allow digested nutrients to diffuse out but retain the undigested residue. Recovery of the bag allows measurement of the nutrient concentration of the residue. This technique has been used with protein (Sauer et al., 1983) and may provide an alternative to conventional metabolism studies for DE estimates.

Suggested values for GE, DE, ME, and NE of ingredients normally used in swine diets have been reported by NRC (1998).

III. EFFICIENCY OF ENERGY UTILIZATION

A. GROWTH

Growth or an increase in body mass results from accumulation of protein, fat, and ash and the associated energy. The deposition of 1 g of protein increases energy stores by 5.6 kcal whereas 1 g of fat results in the storage of 9.4 kcal of energy. The total cost of deposition of fat (FD) and protein (PD) can be estimated from one of the following relationships with FD and PD in g:

$$\text{ME intake} = a + b\,\text{FD} + c\,\text{PD} \tag{5.1}$$

$$NEp = b\,\text{FD} + c\,\text{PD} \tag{5.2}$$

A summary of estimates of the regression coefficients of these relationships by ARC (1981) resulted in the conclusion that the coefficient for protein was 10.5 kcal/g and for fat was 12.8 kcal/g. These values correspond to efficiencies of utilization of 0.53 for protein (k_p) and 0.73 for fat (k_f). Similar values of 10.6 kcal/g of protein and 12.5 kcal/g of fat were used by NRC (1998). Noblet et al. (1999) reported values of 12.9 kcal/g of protein and 11.2 kcal/g of fat. The energy lost as heat during protein synthesis is much greater than the biochemical cost of protein synthesis (Millward et al., 1976). Protein turnover or the need to synthesize enough protein to equal the protein degraded plus the protein retained is one cause of the lower efficiency of PD compared with FD.

The efficiency of energy utilization by the pig is determined by the amounts of fat and protein that are deposited in the gain. The deposition of 1 g of protein is accompanied by the deposition of about 4 g of water and results in deposition of 5 g of tissue. Thus, the energy required per gram of tissue gain is 1.12 kcal. The deposition of 1 g of fat is associated with the deposition of about 0.2 g of water so that the energy required per gram of tissue gain is 7.83 kcal. The deposition of fat therefore requires more energy per unit of tissue gain than does protein. The composition of daily gain changes from primarily protein and minimal fat by the young pig to a maximum of protein and increasing amounts of fat by the finishing pig. Thus, the energy requirements per unit of gain increase during the growth period.

B. GESTATION

During gestation, energy is required for the maintenance of the sow, some growth of the sow, and development of the conceptus (fetus and maternal tissue). Development of the conceptus takes priority and will develop at the expense of maternal tissue if nutrient intake is severely restricted (Walach-Janiak et al., 1986). Beyer et al. (1994) reported from a comparative slaughter experiment in which sows were fed three energy levels during three reproductive cycles that the total weight gain of the uterus, uterine fluids, products of conception, and mammary tissue was 22.8 kg and was not affected by energy level or parity. The gain of protein (2.46 kg), fat (0.46 kg), and energy (19.94 Mcal) was not affected by energy intake. Maternal weight gain was dependent on the amount of energy consumed. Nutrient demands for the conceptus are greatest during the last third of gestation when fetal growth is at a maximum. Energy intake of the sow during gestation is restricted to prevent excessive growth and fattening (Verstegen et al., 1987).

Close et al. (1985) have reported that the efficiency of energy utilization for protein retention (k_p) by the pregnant gilt was 0.69 and for fat deposition (k_f) was 0.88. The efficiency of protein deposition was greater in pregnant gilts than in nonpregnant littermate gilts (0.49). They also reported that the efficiency of energy deposition in the reproductive tissue was 0.72. Their study allowed partitioning of the energy deposition between maternal and conceptus energy gain, and they concluded that the efficiency of maternal gain was 0.87 and of conceptus gain was 0.72.

C. LACTATION

During lactation, after maintenance requirements are met, nutrients are utilized for milk production. If insufficient energy is available, energy will be mobilized from the maternal tissues to sustain milk production and weight loss will occur. Generally, lactating sows are allowed *ad libitum* access to feed, and feed intake will determine whether weight is gained or lost during lactation. Noblet and Etienne (1986) reported that restriction of energy intake reduced milk yield slightly but the concentration of fat, energy, and nitrogen in the milk from energy-restricted gilts was greater than in the milk from gilts fed a high level of energy.

Noblet and Etienne (1987) have reported that the efficiency of utilization of dietary energy for milk production was 0.72 and that the efficiency of utilization of energy from body stores for milk production was 0.88. They concluded that the overall efficiency of energy storage during pregnancy and mobilization during lactation was similar to the efficiency of utilization of dietary energy for milk production.

IV. NUTRIENT-TO-ENERGY RATIOS

Nutrient-to-energy ratios may be important because the pig, as other animals, eats to satisfy a demand for energy so that the actual amount of feed consumed depends on the energy density of the diet fed. Protein is the nutrient that is most frequently adjusted as energy density is changed, but the same logic can be applied to all nutrients. Nutrient requirements as established by the NRC (1998) are not, however, expressed per unit of energy, so that optimal nutrient to calorie ratios must be derived from the recommendations for energy density and the concentration of other nutrients. For protein, the current recommendations (NRC, 1998) decrease from 70 g/Mcal of DE for the 7.5-kg pig to 45 g/Mcal of DE for the 80-kg pig. The values for lysine decrease from 3.95 g/Mcal of DE for the 7.5-kg pig to 2.18 g/Mcal of DE for the 80-kg pig.

V. FACTORS AFFECTING ENERGY UTILIZATION

A. Feed Composition

Amino acids absorbed in excess of the demands for protein synthesis are deaminated. The nitrogen is excreted as urea, and the carbon skeleton is metabolized to yield energy. Energy is required for the synthesis of urea, and urea also contains 2.52 kcal/g (5.45 kcal/g of nitrogen). Thus, the energy in diets containing excess protein or protein with improper ratios of amino acids is utilized less efficiently than energy in diets that contain adequate amounts of balanced protein. Diets that contain inadequate amounts of balanced protein limit protein retention and result in energy being diverted to fat synthesis.

Addition of fat to diets increases energy density and results in a reduction in feed intake to maintain a constant DE intake. Fatty acids are liberated during digestion and are absorbed. They are generally deposited as fat and increase the efficiency of energy utilization. Added fat also has a lower heat increment than carbohydrate and can be beneficial at high environmental temperatures by maintaining energy intake to support maximal growth rate (Stahly and Cromwell, 1979). In pigs weaned at 3 weeks of age, additional fat is not well utilized for 10 to 14 days after weaning and can result in depression of growth rate (Cera et al., 1988a,b). Further information about the effects of various fats is provided in Chapter 6.

Feed ingredients that contain fiber result in a reduction in energy density. Pigs have a limited ability to utilize fiber, and feed intake increases in an attempt to maintain a constant DE intake. The digestive tract enlarges to accommodate a larger volume of feed, and the rate of passage of ingesta increases, resulting in a small reduction in digestibility of nutrients. Fiber is indigestible and passes to the cecum and large intestine. The cecum and large intestine have a microbial population that is similar to that in the rumen, and fiber is degraded with the production of volatile fatty acids (VFA). It has been estimated that VFA production may provide as much as 30% of the maintenance energy requirement (Rerat et al., 1987). Digestibility of energy increases slightly with increased body weight and in sows fed at restricted feed intakes (Noblet and Shi, 1993). These issues are discussed in Chapter 7.

B. Predicting Energy Concentrations from Chemical Composition

Gross energy concentrations of feed ingredients can be predicted fairly accurately from chemical composition of the ingredient (Ewan, 1989). Selected equations for predicting DE, ME, and NE from reports of Ewan (1989), Noblet and Perez (1993), and Noblet et al. (1994) were reported by NRC (1998). The equations for predicting DE concentrations reflect the positive effects of fat concentrations and the negative effects of fiber components. Prediction of ME from DE is primarily influenced by protein concentrations, with increased protein concentrations decreasing ME concentrations. Predictions of NE are less accurate but reflect negative effects of ash and fiber and positive effects of fat and starch concentrations.

C. Environment

Effective environmental temperature is the major factor that affects energy utilization by the pig. The pig has an upper and lower critical temperature bounding the thermoneutral zone, and if the effective environmental temperature is above the upper critical temperature, energy is required to dissipate heat from the body. Below the lower critical temperature, energy is diverted from productive processes to provide heat to maintain body temperature. Effective environmental temperature is the temperature that the pig experiences and is influenced by air temperature, building insulation and flooring, air movement, number of pigs per pen, size of pen, and level of DE intake (NRC, 1981).

The effective environmental temperature will alter feed intake by reducing DE intake linearly as temperature increases between 5 and 30°C (NRC, 1986). Below 5°C, feed intake increases markedly, whereas above 30°C, a marked reduction in feed intake occurs. Chapter 23 provides detailed information about the effects of the thermal environment on energy and nutrient utilization.

VI. ENERGY REQUIREMENTS OF PIGS

The energy requirements of pigs have been estimated by empirical or factorial methods. The empirical method establishes the requirements based on maximizing performance in response to varying energy intake. The factorial method is based on the amount of energy required for a specific function (e.g., maintenance, growth, or milk production) and the efficiency of utilization of ME for the specific function. The empirical approach was used by NRC (1979), whereas the factorial approach was used by ARC (1981) and NRC (1988; 1998). Close and Fowler (1985) summarized the factorial approach used by ARC (1981). The following discussion describes the factorial approach with comparison to the empirical estimates of energy requirements.

A. Maintenance

Maintenance requirements have been estimated from measurements of HP following periods of fasting. The ME required for maintenance can be estimated by assuming an efficiency of conversion of energy to meet maintenance (k_m). Measurements of fasting HP vary with the length of fast, with previous nutritional history, and with the difference in activity between fasted and fed animals; it may not relate to the maintenance requirement of the normal animal.

Maintenance requirements have been estimated from the relationship between retained energy and ME intake. Maintenance requirements are calculated as the ME intake that is necessary for zero energy retention. At zero energy retention, however, the growing animal will continue to deposit protein and mobilize fat.

A third method that has been used is to determine the multiple regression between ME intake and retention of fat and protein. This relationship provides an estimate of the ME required when no fat or protein are retained and is an estimate of maintenance requirements.

ARC (1981) reported the results of the analysis of data for pigs between 5 and 90 kg and derived the following relationship for the ME requirement at maintenance:

$$172\ W^{0.63} (\text{kcal/day}) \tag{5.3}$$

The derived exponent differs from the interspecies exponent of 0.75, but if the data were constrained to the exponent of 0.75, the following relationship was obtained:

$$109\ W^{0.75}\ (\text{kcal/day}) \tag{5.4}$$

Noblet et al. (1999) estimated maintenance with exponents of metabolic weight of 0.75 and observed maintenance requirements that ranged from 104 to 125 kcal/$W^{0.75}$ for seven genetic groups of pigs. With the same data, the use of an exponent of 0.60 resulted in a range of maintenance requirements from 224 to 268 kcal/$W^{0.60}$ for the genetic groups studied.

The recommendations of the National Research Council (NRC, 1998) used a value of 110 $W^{0.75}$ kcal of DE daily or 106 $W^{0.75}$ kcal of ME daily as the maintenance requirement for all weights of pigs.

B. Growth

Energy requirements per unit of live weight gain will vary because the amounts of protein and fat in the gain will depend on the stage of growth and the available amino acids and energy. Daily protein deposition increases to a maximum at a body weight of approximately 60 kg and is

TABLE 5.1
Energy Requirements of Growing Pigs[a]

Body Weight (kg)	Daily Gain (g)			Daily ME Required (kcal)			
	ADG[b]	Protein[c]	Fat[c]	Maintenance	Protein	Fat	Total
7.5	281	47.9	50.7	480	508	634	1,622
15.0	530	82.2	127	808	871	1,585	3,264
35.0	875	123.0	258	1,525	1,307	3,219	6,051
65.0	1,057	136.0	364	2,427	1,438	4,547	8,412
100.0	1,075	122.0	430	3,352	1,298	5,380	10,031

[a] Calculated using the growth model developed by the NRC (1998) with an average lean gain growth rate of 325 g/day and equal numbers of barrows and gilts.
[b] Average daily gain.
[c] Dry matter basis.

relatively constant from 60 kg to market weight. Daily energy intake continues to increase from 60 kg to market weight so that a constant amount of energy is required for protein deposition and the additional available energy is deposited as fat. The maximum amount of protein deposition varies with genetic strain and sex, suggesting that energy requirements for growth also vary with these factors.

Recommendations of energy requirements (Table 5.1) for growth made by the NRC (1998) are based on estimates of protein deposition from the average lean gain growth rate from 20 to 120 kg of body weight. Total energy intake is estimated from body weight. The energy required for maintenance and protein deposition is subtracted from the total and the remaining energy is utilized for fat synthesis. Total energy intake can be modified by changing the inputs for temperature, and space per pig or can be modified to reflect the experience of the user.

C. Gestation

Energy intake during gestation is generally limited to control weight gain and maintain an appropriate condition of the sow. The model developed by NRC (1998) uses a desired gestation weight gain and the expected number of pigs to determine the desired energy intake. The gain of weight, energy, and protein in the products of conception (i.e., fetus and associated reproductive tissues) are considered as constants per pig in the litter. The maternal weight gain can be determined from the desired gestation weight gain and weight gain from the products of conception. Maternal weight gain is partitioned to fat and protein, and the energy intake required is determined from the sum of the energy required for maintenance, the products of conception, and the maternal gain of fat and protein. There is an option to provide the daily energy intake, and in that situation the energy requirements for maintenance and the products of conception are calculated and the remaining energy is utilized for maternal gain.

D. Lactation

Energy is required during lactation for maintenance of the sow and for production of milk. The model developed by NRC (1998) uses the maintenance requirement for the lactating sow as 106 kcal of ME/kg$^{0.75}$. Milk energy production is calculated from the litter growth rate (Noblet and Etienne, 1989) and converted to ME intake by the efficiency of producing milk GE from dietary ME of 0.72 (Noblet and Etienne, 1987). The sum of these values is the ME intake required to support lactation without a change in sow weight. If energy intake is not adequate to support lactation, the model assumes that maternal tissue is mobilized to meet the energy demand for milk production and the body weight loss is calculated.

REFERENCES

ARC. 1981. The *Nutrient Requirements of Pigs*, Agricultural Research Council, Commonwealth Agricultural Bureaux, Slough, U.K.

Beyer, M., W. Jentsch, L. Hoffmann, R. Schiemann, and M. Klein. 1994. Untersuchungen zum Energie- und Stickstoffumsatz von graviden und laktierend Saun sowie von Saugferkeln. 4. Mitteilung — Chemische Zusammensetzung und Energiegehalt der Konzeptionsprodukte, der reproduktiven Organe und der Lebendmassezunahmen oder -abnahmen bei graviden und laktierenden Sauen, *Arch. Anim. Nutr.*, 46:7.

Breirem, K. 1939. Der Energieumsatz bei den Schweinen, *Tierernährung*, 11:487.

Brouwer, E. 1965. Report of sub-committee on constants and factors. In *Energy Metabolism*, Blaxter, K. L., Ed., EAAP No. 11, Academic Press, London, 441.

Cera, K. R., D. C. Mahan, and G. A. Reinhart. 1988a. Weekly digestibilities of diets supplemented with corn oil, lard or tallow by weanling swine, *J. Anim. Sci.*, 66:1430.

Cera, K. R., D. C. Mahan, and G. A. Reinhart. 1988b. Effects of dried whey and corn oil on weanling pig performance, fat digestibility and nitrogen utilization, *J. Anim. Sci.*, 66:1438.

Close, W. H., and V. R. Fowler. 1985. Energy requirements of pigs. In *Recent Advances in Pig Nutrition*, Cole, D. J. A., and W. Haresign, Eds., Butterworths, London, 1.

Close, W. H., J. Noblet, and R. P. Heavens. 1985. Studies on the energy metabolism of the pregnant sow. 2. The partition and utilisation of metabolisable energy in pregnant and non-pregnant animals, *Br. J. Nutr.*, 53:267.

Diggs, B. G., D. E. Becker, A. H. Jensen, and H. W. Norton. 1965. Energy value of various feeds for the young pig, *J. Anim. Sci.*, 24:555.

Ewan, R. C. 1989. Predicting the energy utilization of diets and feed ingredients by pigs. In *Energy Metabolism of Farm Animals*, van der Honing, Y., and W. H. Close, Eds., EAAP Pub. 43. Pudoc, Wageningen, Netherlands, 215.

Henry, Y., H. Vogt, and P. E. Zoiopoulos. 1988. Pigs and poultry, *Livest. Prod. Sci.*, 19:299.

Kielanowski, J. 1972. Energy requirements of the growing pig. In *Pig Production*, Cole, D. J. A., Ed., Butterworths, London, 183.

Kleiber, M. 1965. Metabolic body size. In *Energy Metabolism*, Blaxter, K. L., Ed., EAAP No. 11, Academic Press, London, 427.

Kromann, R. P., J. A. Froseth, and W. E. Meiser. 1976. Interactional digestible, metabolizable and net energy values of wheat and barley in swine, *J. Anim. Sci.*, 42:1451.

Millward, D. J., P. J. Garlick, W. P. T. James, P. M. Sender, and J. C. Waterlow. 1976. In *Protein Metabolism and Nutrition*, Cole, D. J. A., et al., Eds., EAAP No. 16, Butterworths, London, 49.

Noblet, J., and M. Etienne. 1986. Effect of energy level in lactating sows on yield and composition of milk and nutrient balance of piglets, *J. Anim. Sci.*, 63:1888.

Noblet, J., and M. Etienne. 1987. Metabolic utilization of energy and maintenance requirements of lactating sows, *J. Anim. Sci.*, 64:774.

Noblet, J., and J. M. Perez. 1993. Prediction of digestibility of nutrients and energy values of pig diets from chemical analysis, *J. Anim. Sci.*, 71:3389.

Noblet, J., and X. S. Shi. 1993. Comparative digestibility of energy and nutrients in growing pigs fed ad libitum and adult sows at maintenance, *Livest. Prod. Sci.*, 34:137.

Noblet, J., J. H. Fortune, X. S. Shi, and S. Dubois. 1994. Prediction of net energy value of feeds for growing pigs, *J. Anim. Sci.*, 72:344.

Noblet, J., C. Karege, S. Dubois, and J. van Milgen. 1999. Metabolic utilization of energy and maintenance requirements in growing pigs: effects of sex and genotype, *J. Anim. Sci.*, 77:1208.

NRC. 1979. *Nutrient Requirements of Swine*, 8th ed., National Academy Press, Washington, D.C.

NRC. 1981. *Effect of Environment on Nutrient Requirements of Domestic Animals*, National Academy Press, Washington, D.C.

NRC. 1986. *Predicting Feed Intake of Food-Producing Animals*, National Academy Press, Washington, D.C.

NRC. 1988. *Nutrient Requirements of Swine*, 9th ed., National Academy Press, Washington, D.C.

NRC. 1998. *Nutrient Requirements of Swine*, 10th ed., National Academy Press, Washington, D.C.

Rerat, A., M. Fiszlewicz, A. Giusi, and P. Vaugelade. 1987. Influence of meal frequency on postprandial variations in the production and absorption of volatile fatty acids in the digestive tract of conscious pigs, *J. Anim. Sci.*, 64:448.

Sauer, W. C., H. Jorgenson, and R. Berzins. 1983. A modified nylon bag technique for determining apparent digestibilities of protein in feedstuffs for pigs, *Can. J. Anim. Sci.*, 63:233.

Stahly, T. S., and G. L. Cromwell. 1979. Effect of environmental temperature and dietary fat supplementation on the performance and carcass characteristics of growing and finishing pigs, *J. Anim. Sci.*, 49:1478.

Walach-Janiak, M., S. Raj, and H. Fandrejewski. 1986. Protein and energy balance in pregnant gilts, *Livest. Prod. Sci.*, 15:249.

Verstegen, M. W. A., J. M. F. Verhagen, and L. A. Den Hartog. 1987. Energy requirements of pigs during pregnancy: a review, *Livest. Prod. Sci.*, 16:75.

6 Fat in Swine Nutrition

Michael J. Azain

CONTENTS

I. Introduction 95
II. Physical and Chemical Properties 95
III. Fat Quality 98
IV. Specific Uses of Fat 99
V. Biological Effects..100
VI. Overview of the Pathways of Lipid Metabolism 101
VII. Effects of Fat on Performance 101
References 103

I. INTRODUCTION

In the previous edition of this book, Pettigrew and Moser (1991) emphasized the effects of dietary fat on performance of pigs at various stages of production. These observations are still of relevance to swine nutrition and are summarized below. In addition, research related to use of fat in swine nutrition published since the first edition is emphasized.

Dietary fat refers to the lipid component of the diet. Lipids are a broad class of compounds that have the common feature of being insoluble in water. Most of the time, when one refers to fat, it is actually triglycerides that are being considered. Other lipid classes such as cholesterol and other steroids, phospholipids, or free fatty acids, while of importance in the metabolism and physiology of the animal are, at best, minor components of the diet. The fat or triglyceride in a swine diet can originate as a component of the energy or protein ingredients or can be added as a relatively pure component. For example, in a typical corn–soybean meal finishing diet, approximately 60% of the fat, as determined by ether extract, is added as animal or vegetable fat and 40% is from the corn.

II. PHYSICAL AND CHEMICAL PROPERTIES

Triglycerides are composed of three fatty acids linked to glycerol through an ester bond. The fatty acids found in plants and animals are usually long hydrocarbon chains having an even number of carbons and up to three carbon–carbon double bonds. Although there are exceptions, 14 to 20 carbon chain lengths are most abundant, and are collectively referred to as long-chain fatty acids. Fatty acids have both trivial and chemical names. The major fatty acids found in pigs or that would be components of typical diets are listed in Table 6.1. The simplest fatty acid is acetic acid, a two-carbon compound that is a volatile liquid. The two most abundant chain length fatty acids in the pig are 16 and 18 carbons. Palmitate (C16:0) is generally considered the end product of lipogenesis and accounts for approximately 20 to 30% of the fatty acids in lard or in tissue depots. Stearate (C18:0) and oleate (C18:1) are the other predominant fatty acids in pork and account for 10 to 15% and 40 to 50% of the fatty acids. These two fatty acids can be sythesized from palmitate by elongation and desaturation or can be supplied in the diet. Fatty acids with carbon chain lengths from 6 to 12 are

TABLE 6.1
Typical Fatty Acids Found in Diets and Tissue Depots

Fatty Acid		Chain Length (No. Carbons: No. Double Bonds)	Melting Point (°C)
Trivial Name	**Chemical Name**		
Caprylic	Octanoate	C8:0	16.5
Capric	Decanoate	C10:0	31.4
Lauric	Dodecanoate	C12:0	44
Myristic	Tetradecanoate	C14:0	58
Palmitate	Hexadecanoate	C16:0	63
Palmitoleic	cis-9-Hexadecenoic	$C16:1^{\Delta 9}$	1.5
Stearic	Octadecanoate	C18:0	71.5
Oleic	cis-9-Octadecenoic	$C18:1^{\Delta 9}$ (cis) ω-9	16.3
Eladic	trans-9-Octadecenoic	$C18:1^{\Delta 9}$ (trans) ω-9	45
Linoleic	all-cis-9,12-octadecadienoic	$C18:2^{\Delta 9,12}$ ω-6	−5.0
α-Linolenic	all-cis-9,12,15-Octadecatrienoic	$C18:3^{\Delta 9,12,15}$ ω-3	−11.3
γ-Linolenic	all-cis-6,9,12-Octadecatrienoic	$C18:3^{\Delta 6,9,12}$ ω-6	
Arachidic	Eicosanoic	C20:0	75.4
Arachidonic	Eicosatetraenoic	$C20:4^{\Delta 5,8,11,14}$ ω-6	−49.5
Timnodionic	Eicosapentaenoate	$C20:5^{\Delta 5,8,11,14,17}$ ω-3	
Cervonic	Docosahexanoate	$C22:6^{\Delta 4,7,10,13,16,19}$ ω-3	

Source: Adapted from Kates, M., *Techniques of Lipidology: Isolation, Analysis, and Identification of Lipids*, 2nd ed., Elsevier, New York, 1986.

referred to as medium-chain fatty acids. When these chain length fatty acids are esterified to glycerol they are called medium-chain triglycerides or MCT. The physical properties of a fat are determined by its fatty acid profile. Depending on the mix of specific fatty acids, triglycerides can exist as liquids or solids at room temperature. The term *fats* is usually retained for solid forms, whereas liquids are referred to as *oils*. In general, fats derived from animal origin are solids and contain triglycerides composed of fatty acids with 16- and 18-carbon fatty acids with no or one double bond. Fats or oils of plant origin contain primarily 18-carbon fatty acids with one to three double bonds. Double bonds introduced by eukaryotic (plant, fish, avian, mammalian, etc.) enzymes are always in the *cis* configuration. If there are two or more double bonds in a fatty acid they will generally be separated by an intervening methylene group. Thus, the configuration of double bonds in α-linolenic acid is between carbons 9 and 10, 12 and 13, and 15 and 16. Carbons 11 and 13 are the intervening groups. The designation of the position of the double bonds uses either the methyl or the carboxyl end of the fatty acid chain. The Δ system numbers from the carboxyl end. In this system, α-linolenic acid is designated C $18:3^{\Delta 9,12,15}$. The n or ω numbering systems are equivalent and, with these, the position of the double bond closest to the methyl end of the fatty acid is used. α-linolenic acid would be an n-3 or ω-3 fatty acid, while gamma linolenic (C$18:3^{\Delta 6,9,12}$) would be an n-6 or ω-6 fatty acid.

Double bonds in the *trans* configuration are produced by bacteria or by hydrogenation. Thus, *trans* fatty acids will be produced in the rumen and large intestine and will be in the diet if restaurant grease containing hydrogenated vegetable fats is used. Anaerobic bacteria can produce mixed isomers containing both *cis* and *trans* double bonds and the bonds may not be methylene interrupted. Double bonds in hydrocarbon chains that are not separated by a methylene group are referred to as conjugated bonds. In particular, a series of variants of linoleic acid are receiving a great deal of attention. Conjugated linoleic acids (CLA) are a mix of eight positional isomers that includes 9/11 and 10/12 variants, with *cis/trans*, *trans/cis*, and *trans/trans* combinations (Ha et al., 1989). Dietary CLA have been shown to have anticarcinogenic properties in rodents (Ip, 1997) and to reduce body fat in several species (Park et al., 1997), including the pig (Dugan et al., 1997). The fatty acid profile of selected fat sources is shown in Table 6.2.

TABLE 6.2
Characteristics of Some Commonly Used Fat Sources[a]

Source	Fatty Acid Profile (%)								U:S Ratio[b]	Iodine No.	Metab. Energy[c]
	≤C14	C16:0	C16:1	C18:0	C18:1	C18:2	C18:3	≥C20			
Tallow	3.6	24.9	4.2	18.9	36.0	3.1	0.6	0.3	0.92	44	7680
Blended fat	0.9	15.2	1.4	10.8	51.0	17.9	1.3	1.2	2.68	79	8379
Choice white grease	2.3	21.5	5.7	14.9	41.1	11.6	0.4	1.8	1.45	60	7955
Lard	1.6	23.8	2.7	13.5	41.2	10.2	1.0	1.0	1.44	64	7950
Sow milk	3.8	26.6	12.1	3.3	33.7	18.8	1.5	0.1	1.96	—	—

[a] Fatty acid profiles from NRC (1998) and Azain (1993).
[b] Unsaturated:saturated ratio.
[c] From NRC (1998), expressed in kcal/kg.

III. FAT QUALITY

Fats are characterized by their source and quality. Most fat added to swine diets will be rendered products that are either blended fats (animal and vegetable blends) or fats from specific animal species, e.g., poultry fat and tallow. Choice white grease is the term used for rendered pork fat, but it can also consist of a beef, pork, and poultry blend. Yellow grease is primarily restaurant grease, but it can also include other sources. Fat quality is judged by the following criteria: composition, titer or hardness, color, impurities, and stability. Several of the characteristics are interrelated. Composition refers to the fatty acid profile of the sample and is generally determined using a gas chromatograph. It should also include a measure of the percentage of total fatty acids and free fatty acids. Most feed-grade fats have minimum acceptable total fatty acid value and an upper level of free fatty acid allowed. For example, an animal fat such as tallow should have a minimum of 90% total fatty acids and a maximum of 15% free fatty acids. Blended fats may contain higher levels of soap stocks and can have up to 20% free fatty acids. The limit on free fatty acids is based on a concern about the quality of the fat. Free fatty acids or soap stocks generally have the same energy value as the triglyceride forms when they are diluted in the diet, although they may be less palatable and can be corrosive to feed-handling equipment.

The chain length and degree of unsaturation of the fatty acids in a product determines the hardness and iodine value. Vegetable oils have higher degrees of unsaturation and iodine number, and are liquids at room temperature. Animal fats are more saturated, have lower iodine numbers, and are solids at room temperature. Criteria such as iodine number and hardness can be used to predict the degree of unsaturation and can substitute for knowledge of the actual fatty acid profile. Iodine number or value is a measure of the number of double bonds in a fatty acid. It is expressed as the grams of iodine absorbed per 100 g of sample. The iodine number for soybean oil, which contains >50% linoleic acid (18:2), is >100. The iodine number for tallow, which contains large amounts of the saturated fatty acids palmitate and stearate, is in the range of 40 to 45.

Titer or hardness is a measure of the temperature in degrees Celsius where a fat sample solidifies and is inversely related to iodine value. Tallow has a typical titer of 42 to 45°C and an iodine number of 43 to 45. Poultry fat has a titer of 31 to 35°C and an iodine number of 77 to 80. Lard is intermediate. These changes are largely accounted for by increased concentration of unsaturated fatty acids, such as oleate and linoleate, and lower concentrations of saturated fatty acids, such as palmitate and stearate, in poultry fat as compared with tallow.

Fat color has little to do with nutritional quality directly, but may be an indicator of the composition or source of the product. A more informative index of quality is moisture, impurities, and unsaponifiables or the MIU index. Maximum allowable moisture in most products is 1.0 to 1.5%. Moisture has no energy value and can increase the rate of fat oxidation and the development of rancidity. Impurities also generally have no energy value and can be any number of materials such as hair, bone, soil, or plastic. The upper limit on impurities is usually 0.5 to 1.0%. Unsaponifiables are lipid soluble compounds that are not hydrolyzed upon heating under alkaline conditions. Such compounds could include sterols, such as cholesterol or ergosterol, vitamins, waxes, or hydrocarbons. Some of these may have energy or other nutritional value, but should be limited to 1% of the product.

Stability of a fat is assessed by two tests that measure breakdown of the sample exposure to oxygen. The initial peroxide value measures the milliequivalents of peroxide per kilogram of sample and is a measure of the rancidity in the product. A low value (<5 meq/kg) indicates that the sample is not currently rancid. The active oxygen method test (AOM) is a measure of the potential of a sample to become rancid and is determined by bubbling air through the sample. Fat and fat-soluble vitamins in a fat product can be stabilized or made resistant to oxidative damage by the addition of antioxidants such as ethoxyquin, butylated hydroxy anisole (BHA), or butylated hydroxy toluene (BHT).

IV. SPECIFIC USES OF FAT

While dietary fat is a source of essential fatty acids, a deficiency is rarely a concern in grain-based diets. Linoleic acid was shown to be essential in the 1930s. Several fatty acids are now recognized as required (Holman, 1998). Typically, linoleic (C18:2) and arachidonic (C20:4), members of the ω-6 (or n-6) family, and linolenic (C18:3), an ω-3 fatty acid, are collectively referred to as the essential fatty acids. The NRC (1998) specifies a requirement for linoleic acid (C18:2) at 0.10% of the diet. This represents approximately 0.5 g/day for a nursing pig and 3 g/day for a finishing pig. There is no specific requirement for the ω-3 (or n-3) fatty acids series, although it is likely that they are required. These fatty acids are required in the diet because they serve as precursors for a group of compounds referred to as the eicosanoids, which have a variety of endocrine, paracrine, and autocrine functions. Animals can desaturate fatty acids to some extent, but lack the specific enzymes to add double bonds in the correct position to give rise to the essential fatty acids. In general, animals lack desaturase enzymes that introduce double bonds beyond the ninth and tenth carbons in stearate and can only introduce a double bond between an existing one and the carboxyl end of the molecule. Thus, oleate (C18:1$^{\Delta 9}$) can be formed from stearate by Δ-9 desaturase and γ-linoleate (C18:3$^{\Delta 6,9,12}$) formed from linoleate (C18:2$^{\Delta 9,12}$) by a Δ-6 desaturase. α-Linoleate (C18:3$^{\Delta 9,12,15}$) cannot be synthesized and must be in the diet. Arachidonate can be formed from linoleate by elongation and desaturation, or can be supplied in the diet. Related to the role of specific fatty acids as essential nutrients, research in rodents (Shapiro et al., 1993), chicks (Korver and Klasing, 1997), and dogs (Wander et al., 1997) suggests that the amount and ratio of n-3 to n-6 fatty acids may also play a role in immune and endocrine function.

Although essential fatty acids are critical for normal function in the animal, the primary use of fat in swine diets is as an energy source. Under practical conditions, fat will be added in the range of 0.5% to no more than 7%. Although higher levels of fat may be used under experimental conditions, these levels create problems with feed handling and are not normally used under commercial conditions. On the practical side, fat also reduces dust (Peo and Lewis, 1992; Mankell et al., 1995), which has benefit to both the pigs and the workers in facilities.

In contrast to ruminant animals, where dietary fats are saturated prior to absorption from the gastrointestinal tract, fatty acids from the diet can be directly incorporated into tissue stores in nonruminant species. Thus, it is possible to alter the fatty acid profile of pork by dietary manipulation. In recent years, there has been an effort to reduce the total amount of fat in animal products and to alter fatty acid profiles to create a healthier image for pork products. Reduction in fat has been achieved by changes in genetics and incentives for improved carcass quality. Fat composition can be altered by inclusion of unsaturated fat sources such as fish (Overland et al., 1996; Taugbol, 1993), rapeseed (Leskanich et al., 1997), and linseed oil (Romans et al., 1995a,b; Van Oeckel et al., 1996). The concern with modifying fatty acid profile of pork is that the potential human health benefits of reduced saturated and increased polyunsaturated fatty acids are quickly offset by undesirable carcass characteristics. Feeding unsaturated fat results in softer carcasses and reduced shelf-life of products due to the increased potential for rancidity. Clearly, the fatty acid profile can be altered. Leskanich et al. (1997) compared the effects of diets containing 3% tallow:soybean oil (4:1) with those of rapeseed oil:fish oil (2:1) on various characteristics of pork. They demonstrated an increase in unsaturated fatty acid content with the rapeseed:fish oil group, but also noted that TBARS (thiobarbituric acid reactive substances, a measure of the potential for oxidative damage) were higher, firmness was reduced, and there was an increase in odor detected by a trained sensory panel. These defects were minor and could be lessened by the addition of vitamin E to the diet.

Linseed oil is high in α-linolenic acid and thus is an alternative to fish oil as a source of ω-3 fatty acids. Romans et al. (1995a,b) reported on the effects of various levels of linseed (0 to 15%) and feeding durations (1 to 4 weeks) on the physical and sensory characteristics of pork. The concentrations of linolenate and its derivative eicospentanoate (C20:5 n-3) were increased in a dose- and time-dependent manner. There were defects in sensory quality of bacon products from pigs fed 10 or 15% linseed, but not those fed 5%. There were no differences detected in loin samples. In other work, feeding 5% linseed oil did not affect any sensory evaluations and resulted in significant increases in the tissue content of n-3 fatty acids (Van Oeckel et al., 1996). Myer et al. (1992) also reported a significant increase in off-flavors in bacon from pigs fed 10% canola oil, another source of n-3 fatty acids. They also reported that, as an alternative, high-oleate peanuts increased the level of unsaturated fatty acids, but did not result in sensory defects. At present, it would seem that, other than specialty markets, it is unlikely there will be widespread adoption of fat-modified pork products. The manipulation of the fatty acid composition in meat animals has been recently reviewed (Rule et al., 1995) and is also discussed in Chapter 28.

V. BIOLOGICAL EFFECTS

Comparison of the growth and performance of pigs fed diets with and without added fat demonstrates a number of properties of fat. Because of the greater energy density of fat compared with carbohydrates and proteins, one of the most pronounced effects of fat is a decrease in absolute feed intake. This effect is largely accounted for by the effect of fat on the energy density of the diet. When intakes are expressed on an energy basis, for example, the intake is similar (e.g., Azain et al., 1991; 1992)

In the digestive tract, fat has the effect of slowing passage rate. This effect is the opposite of what is seen with fiber in the diet. Because passage rate is reduced, the digestibility of other nutrients is improved. This is referred to as the "extra-caloric effect" of fat. As an example, in nursery pigs, apparent ileal digestibility of crude protein improved from 80.7 to 83.3% as fat increased from 3.2 to 12.2% in the diet (Li and Sauer, 1994). Individual amino acids showed improvements of similar magnitude. There was no change in disappearance of amino acids in the large intestine, supporting the role of passage rate in the small intestine as the basis for the improvement.

Because of their lower heat increment and greater efficiency in utilization, animals fed diets where fat has been substituted for an equivalent metabolizable energy in the form of carbohydrate will generally have greater net energy available to them. In growing pigs, this is seen as a slight increase in growth and an increase in carcass fat. The lower heat increment of fat can be an advantage in warm climates where feed intake is compromised. Several studies suggest improved performance in heat-stressed pigs fed high-fat diets (Stahly and Cromwell, 1979; Coffey et al., 1982; Stahly, 1984). In growing animals fed above maintenance, a significant portion of the fatty acids in the diet is deposited as fatty acids in adipose tissue. The process of depositing dietary fatty acids in tissue depots is energetically more efficient than the process of converting dietary carbohydrate to tissue fatty acids. Thus, there is an increase net energy in animals fed high-fat diets.

Digestibility of the fat or lipid in sow's milk is >90%. Digestibility of fat in starting diets is reduced during the first week postweaning, but increases with age and gradually returns to the 90% range by 4 to 6 weeks postweaning (Wiseman, 1984; Cera et al, 1988). Postweaning, digestibility of shorter-chain saturated or long-chain unsaturated fatty acids is better than that of long-chain saturated fatty acids (Cera et al., 1989). Cera et al. (1988) reported that digestibility of corn oil was 79% in 6-kg pigs during the first week postweaning. Digestibility improved to 89% in the fourth week postweaning. At least part of the increase in digestibility is associated with increased pancreatic lipase production during the postweaning period (Cera et al., 1990). Values for lard and tallow were 68 and 85 and 65 and 83 at week 1 and 4, respectively. Digestibility of all types of fat increased with time, but unsaturated sources were consistently more digestible. In general, as fatty acid chain length increases, digestibility is reduced. Digestibility increases as double bonds are introduced (Stahly, 1984; Desouza et al., 1995; Doreau and Chilliard, 1997). Furthermore, there are positional effects within the triglyceride molecule. Saturated fatty acids are more digestible when on the number 2 position of glycerol as compared with the 1 or 3 position (Small, 1991).

Since the fatty acid profile of sow's milk is similar to that of lard, a saturated "fat source," it is somewhat surprising that fat digestibility decreases at weaning. At least a portion of the difference in digestibility of milk fat vs. the fat provided in a starter diets can be accounted for by the form in which fat is present in milk or feed. In milk, triglycerides are present as lipid droplets enclosed in a phospholipid monolayer. This form, which is structurally similar to that of circulating lipoproteins, is likely very compatible with the formation of micelles and consequently digestion by pancreatic lipase. Fat in dry diets is not in such an easily accessible form. Studies (Desouza et al., 1995; Jones et al., 1992) examining the effect of emulsifiers such as lecithin and lysolecithin on fat digestibility in weanling pigs indicate that, in general, the emulsifiers improved fat digestibility, but have no detectable effect on growth performance. In one study (Jones et al., 1992), tallow digestibility was improved from 81% without emulsifier to 88% by the addition of lecithin as 10% of the fat in the diet. Another study examining the effect of lecithin addition on digestibility of diets containing soybean oil concluded that, although lecithin improved nitrogen and feed efficiency, it did not specifically affect fat digestibility (Overland et al., 1993).

VI. OVERVIEW OF THE PATHWAYS OF LIPID METABOLISM

De novo lipogenesis in the pig occurs primarily in adipose tissue (O'Hea and Leveille, 1969), with very little contribution of the liver. Most of the fat deposition in market pigs occurs during the finishing phase. Lipogenic enzyme levels increase with age in various fat depots in the pig (Mourot et al., 1995). In the nursery, lipid deposition is in the range of 30 to 50 g/day and is similar to that of protein deposition. In the finishing phase, lipid deposition is in the range of 250 to 450 g/day. On a typical corn–soybean meal diet with 3 to 5% added fat, at least half of the daily lipid deposition is accounted for by *de novo* lipogenesis and presumably is achieved by using glucose liberated from cornstarch as a source of carbon for lipogenesis.

Addition of fat to the diet inhibits *de novo* lipogenesis in the pig, as well as in other species (Allee et al., 1971). In nonruminant species, this results in a change in adipose tissue fatty acid composition that reflects the fatty acid profile of the diet. The only concern here is that with unsaturated fat sources such as soybean oil or fish oil, the physical properties of carcass fat can become undesirable. In rodents and other species, the degree of inhibition of lipogenesis is directly related to the degree of unsaturation in the the fat source (Herzberg and Rogerson, 1988). Thus, fish oil is more potent than corn oil, which is more potent than lard, in inhibition of lipogenesis. This does not seem to be true in the pig. Allee et al. (1971) reported that 10% dietary corn oil or tallow had similar inhibitory effects on adipose tissue lipogenesis. More recently, Smith et al. (1996) found that lipogenesis in adipose tissue of pigs fed various fatty acids was less than in the cornstarch-fed controls, palmitate was more potent than either mono- (palmitoleic/myrsoleic or oleic) or polyunsaturated (linoleic) fatty acids. Fat metabolism in the growing pig was reviewed by Farnworth and Cramer (1987).

VII. EFFECTS OF FAT ON PERFORMANCE

Addition of fat to a diet has characteristic effects on performance and carcass characteristics. These include decreased feed intake and increased palatability, growth rate, feed efficiency, and carcass fat. The magnitude of the performance changes is influenced by the stage of production. Pettigrew and Moser (1991) performed meta-analyses summarizing the effects of dietary fat in the various phases of production in the first edition of this book. Summaries for the use of fat in starting, growing-finishing, and sow diets were reported. In all three categories, the effects of added fat were categorized into studies in which the calorie:protein ratio was maintained or where it was not adjusted. Because of the increased energy density of fat (relative to protein or carbohydrate) and the ability of animals to regulate intake based on energy content of a feed, it is necessary to increase protein content to ensure adequate amino acid intake when fat is added. Although direct evidence of the effect of failure to maintain calorie:protein ratio on carcass quality and performance is limited (Allee, 1985), the practice is widely accepted.

In the starting or nursery pig (5 to 20 kg) phase, 92 studies were used in the analysis. The predominant effects of fat at this stage of production were improved feed efficiency and palatability. There was a small (approximately 10 g/day) reduction in growth rate and this was seen in studies in which the calorie:protein ratio was not maintained. In studies in which the ratio was maintained, there was no effect on growth rate. There was a more consistent reduction in intake in response to supplemental fat, with the reduction (average –50 g/day) seen in 59 of 92 studies. The response was clearer (–70 g/day) in studies with constant calorie:protein ratio. The magnitude of the reduction in intake was greater than that of gain, and thus, the gain:feed ratio was also significantly improved in pigs fed supplemental fat. There have been numerous studies investigating the effects of fat type and source on performance in the nursery published since the Pettigrew and Moser review. In general these support the observation that efficiency is improved and that the effects on intake and gain are less obvious (Tokach et al., 1995). Discrepancies among studies in their conclusions about the magnitude of the effect of fat on performance of nursery pigs are likely due to a combination of differences in the type of fat, other dietary ingredients, such as the source of protein or copper, and age or genetic background of the pigs.

In growing-finishing pigs, the main effects noted with fat supplementation are improved gain and efficiency, decreased intake, and increased carcass fat. These responses to dietary fat are independent of whether the calorie:protein ratio of the diet is adjusted. The decreased intake in older pigs is a more consistent response than in nursery pigs, particulary when the dietary fat level exceeds 3%. At less that 3% added fat, intake increased slightly with added fat. This suggests that gut capacity in nursery-age pigs, rather than energy, may have limited intake in these studies. Pettigrew and Moser (1991) reported that the increase in backfat thickness was actually greater when diets were adjusted for energy density. The increase was 0.12 ± 0.03 cm with no adjustment and 0.27 ± 0.7 with adjustment.

By far the greatest interest in the use of fat in swine diets has centered around sow nutrition. Seerley et al. (1974) observed that fat addition during late gestation resulted in improved neonatal survival. Subsequent studies suggested that this effect was most likely accounted for by greater energy stores in the pig at birth that resulted in a greater ability to sustain life until adequate nutrition was obtained from the sow (Seerely et al., 1974; Pettigrew, 1981). At birth pigs have <2% body fat and very low liver glycogen contents. Fat feeding during late gestation increases neonatal energy stores, although the changes are small and not consistent. In theory, fatty acids or ketone bodies, generated from fatty acid oxidation in the dam, cross the placenta and provide an energy source for the developing fetus. They also spare glucose use as an energy source and result in increased liver glycogen synthesis and storage. A more reproducible response to fat feeding late in gestation and lactation is an increase in the level of fat, and thus the energy density, of both colostrum and milk (Seerley et al., 1974; Pettigrew, 1981).

The pig survival response to fat in the gestation diet was only evident when litter survival rates were <80 to 85% for the control groups. At the time these studies were conducted, this was typical of the industry. By current production standards, a 90% survival rate is to be expected (USDA, 1995) and, thus, the benefits of added fat will be less obvious. The sow feeding program is a complex consideration of birth weight, survival, lactation performance, and subsequent reproductive performance. Greater energy intake during gestation, either by increasing energy density (added fat) or simply increasing intake is generally associated with reduced intake during lactation (Coffey et al., 1994; Weldon et al., 1994). Reduced energy intake during lactation leads to increased sow weight loss and days to estrus. Conversely, fat feeding during lactation is associated with reduced sow body weight and backfat losses and a decrease in the weaning-to-estrus interval (Pettigrew and Moser, 1991). In two studies examining the effect of increased lactation diet nutrient density, there was no benefit of higher nutrient density (Coffey et al., 1994; Dove and Haydon, 1994) on survival rates. In both studies, weaning weights were improved as a result of fat addition to the lactation diet. Recent work indicates that the increase in weaning weight of pigs from sows fed fat during gestation is accounted for by an increase in carcass fat of the pigs (Tilton et al., 1999). This work also suggests that, based on earlier work (Friend, 1974), an increase in fat at weaning is likely to be associated with increased fat at market weight.

REFERENCES

Allee, G. L. 1985. The interaction of dietary protein and energy on swine performance, *Proceedings of the Georgia Nutrition Conference for the Feed Industry*, 136.

Allee, G. L., D. H. Baker, and G. A. Leveille. 1971. Influence of level of dietary fat on adipose tissue lipogenesis and enzymatic activity in the pig, *J. Anim. Sci.*, 33:1248.

Azain, M. J. 1993. Effects of adding medium chain triglycerides to sow diets during late gestation and early lactation on litter performance, *J. Anim. Sci.*, 71:3011.

Azain, M. J., R. W. Seerley, J. O. Reagan, and M. K. Andersen. 1991. Effect of a high-fat diet on the performance response to porcine somatotropin (PST) in finishing pigs, *J. Anim. Sci.*, 69:153.

Azain, M. J., K. D. Bullock, T. R. Kasser, and J. J. Veenhuizen. 1992. Relationship of mode of porcine somatotropin administration and dietary fat on the growth performance and carcass characteristics of finishing pigs, *J. Anim. Sci.*, 70:3086.

Cera, K. R., D. C. Mahan, and G. A. Reinhart. 1988. Weekly digestibilities of diets supplemented with corn oil, lard or tallow by weanling swine, *J. Anim. Sci.*, 66:1430.

Cera, K. R., D. C. Mahan, and G. A. Reinhart. 1989. Apparent fat digestibilities and performance responses of postweaning swine fed diets supplemented with coconut oil, corn oil or tallow, *J. Anim. Sci.*, 67:2040.

Cera, K. R., D. C. Mahan, and G. A. Reinhart. 1990. Effect of weaning, week postweaning and diet composition on pancreatic and small intestinal luminal lipase response in young swine, *J. Anim. Sci.*, 68:384.

Coffey, M. T., R. W. Seerley, D. W. Funderburke, and H. C. McCampbell. 1982. Effect of heat increment, and level of dietary energy and environmental temperature on the performance of growing-finishing swine, *J. Anim. Sci.*, 54:95.

Coffey, M. T., B. G. Diggs, D. L. Handlin, D. A. Knabe, C. V. Maxwell, P. R. Noland, T. J. Prince, and G. L. Cromwell. 1994. Effects of dietary energy during gestation and lactation on reproductive performance of sows: a cooperative study, *J. Anim. Sci.*, 72:4.

Desouza, T. R., J. Peiniau, A. Mounier, and A. Aumaitre. 1995. Effect of addition of tallow and lecithin on the diet of weanling piglets on the apparent total tract and ileal digestibility of fat and fatty-acids, *Anim. Feed Sci. Technol.*, 52:77.

Doreau, M., and Y. Chilliard. 1997. Digestion and metabolism of dietary fat in farm animals, *Br. J. Nutr.*, 78 (Suppl. 1):S15–S35.

Dove, C. R., and K. D. Haydon. 1994. The effect of various diet nutrient densities and electrolyte balances on sow and litter performance during two seasons of the year, *J. Anim. Sci.*, 72:1101.

Dugan, M. E. R., J. L. Aalhus, A. L. Schaefer, and J. K. G. Kramer. 1997. The effect of conjugated linoleic acid on fat to lean repartitioning and feed conversion in pigs, *Can. J. Anim. Sci.*, 77:723.

Farnworth, E. R., and J. K. G. Kramer. 1987. Fat metabolism in growing swine: a review, *Can. J. Anim. Sci.*, 67:301.

Friend, D. W. 1974. Effect on the performance of pigs from birth to market weight of adding fat to the lactation diet of their dams, *J. Anim. Sci.*, 63:1073.

Ha, Y. L., N. K. Grimm, and M. W. Pariza. 1989. Newly recognized anticarcinogenic fatty acids: identification and quantification in natural and processed cheeses, *J. Agric. Food Chem.*, 37:75.

Herzberg, G. R., and M. Rogerson. 1988. Hepatic fatty acid synthesis and triglyceride secretion in rats fed fructose- or glucose-based diets containing corn oil, tallow or marine oil, *J. Nutr.*, 118:1061–1067.

Holman, R. T. 1998. The slow discovery of the importance of ω-3 essential fatty acids in human health, *J. Nutr.*, 128:427S–433S.

Ip, C. 1997. Review of the effects of trans fatty acids, oleic acid, n-3 polyunsaturated fatty acids and conjugated linoleic acid on mammary carcinogenesis in animals, *Am. J. Clin. Nutr.*, 66 (Suppl.):1523S.

Jones, D. B., J. D. Hancock, D. L. Harmon, and C. E. Walker. 1992. Effects of exogenous emulsifiers and fat sources on nutrient digestibility, serum lipids, and growth performance in weanling pigs, *J. Anim. Sci.*, 70:3473.

Kates, M. 1986. *Techniques of Lipidology: Isolation, Analysis, and Identification of Lipids*, 2nd ed., Elsevier, New York.

Korver, D. R., and K. C. Klasing. 1997. Dietary fish oil alters specific inflammatory immune responses in chicks, *J. Nutr.*, 127:2039.

Kveragas, C. L., R. W. Seerley, R. J. Martin, and W. L. Vandergrift. 1986. Influence of exogenous growth hormone and gestational diet on sow blood and milk characteristics and on baby pig blood, body composition and performance, *J. Anim. Sci.*, 63:1877.

Leskanich, C. O., K. R. Matthews, C. C. Warkup, R. C. Noble, and M. Hazzledine. 1997. The effect of dietary oil containing (n-3) fatty acids on the fatty acid, physiochemical, and organoleptic characteristics of pig meat and fat, *J. Anim. Sci.*, 75:673.

Li, D. F., R. C. Thaler, J. L. Nelssen, D. L. Harmon, G. L. Allee, and T. L. Weeden. 1990. Effect of fat sources and combinations on starter pig performance, nutrient digestibility and intestinal morphology, *J. Anim. Sci.*, 68:3694.

Li, S., and W. C. Sauer. 1994. The effect of dietary fat content on amino acid digestibility in young pigs, *J. Anim. Sci.*, 72:1737.

Mahan, D. C. 1992. Fats: do their use and value differ for weanling swine? *Proceeding of the Georgia Nutrition Conference*, 7.

Mankell, K. O., K. A. Janni, R. D. Walker, M. E. Wilson, J. E. Pettigrew, L. D. Jacobson, and W. F. Wilcke. 1995. Dust suppression in swine feed using soybean oil, *J. Anim. Sci.*, 73:981.

Mourot, J., M. Kouba, and P. Peiniau. 1995. Comparative study of *in vitro* lipogenesis in various adipose tissues in the growing pig (*Sus domesticus*), *Comp. Biochem. Physiol.*, 111B:379.

Myer, R. O., D. D. Johnson, D. A. Knauft, D. W. Gorbet, J. H. Brendemuhl, and W. R. Walker. 1992. Effect of feeding high-oleic-acid peanuts to growing-finishing swine on resulting carcass fatty acid profile and on carcass and meat quality characteristics, *J. Anim. Sci.*, 70:3734.

NRC. 1994. *Nutrient Requirements of Poultry*, 9th ed., National Academy Press, Washington, D.C.

NRC. 1998. *Nutrient Requirements of Swine*, 10th ed., National Academy Press, Washington, D.C.

O'Hea, E. K., and G. A. Leveille. 1969. Significance of adipose tissue and liver as sites of fatty acid synthesis in the pig and the efficiency of utilization of various substrates for lipogenesis, *J. Nutr.*, 99:338.

Overland, M., O. Taugbol, A. Haug, and E. Sundstol. 1996. Effect of fish-oil on growth performance, carcass characteristics, sensory parameters, and fatty acid composition in pigs, *Acta Agric. Scand.*, 46:11.

Overland, M., M. D. Tokach, S. G. Cornelius, J. E. Pettigrew, and J. W. Rust. 1993. Lecithin in swine diets. 1: Weanling pigs, *J. Anim. Sci.*, 71:1187.

Park, Y. K. J. Albright, W. Liu, J. M. Storkson, M. E. Cook, and M. W. Pariza. 1997. Effect of conjugated linoleic acid on body composition in mice, *Lipids*, 32:853.

Peo, E. R., and A. J. Lewis. 1992. Use of inedible fats in swine diets for dust control, Fats and Proteins Research Foundation, Publ. 232.

Pettigrew, J. E. 1981. Supplemental fat for peripartal sows: a review, *J. Anim. Sci.*, 53:107.

Pettigrew, J. E., and R. L. Moser. 1991. Fat in swine nutrition. In *Swine Nutrition*, Miller, E. R., D. E. Ullrey, and A. J. Lewis, Eds., Butterworth-Heinemann, Stoneham, MA, chap. 8.

Romans, J. R., R. C. Johnson, D. M. Wolf, G. W. Libal, and W. J. Costello. 1995a. Effects of ground flaxseed in swine diets on pig performance and on physical and sensory characteristics and omega-3 fatty acid content of pork: I. Dietary level of flaxseed, *J. Anim. Sci.*, 73:1982.

Romans, J. R., D. M. Wolf, R. C. Johnson, G. W. Libal, and W. J. Costello. 1995b. Effects of ground flaxseed in swine diets on pig performance and on physical and sensory characteristics and omega-3 fatty acid content of pork. II. Duration of 15% dietary flaxseed, *J. Anim. Sci.*, 73:1987.

Rule, D. C., S. B. Smith, and J. R. Romans. 1995. Fatty acid composition of muscle and adipose tissue of meat animals. In *The Biology of Fat in Meat Animals: Current Advances*, Smith, S. B. and D. R. Smith, Eds., American Society of Animal Science, Champaign, IL.

Seerley, R. W., T. A. Pace, C. W. Foley, and R. D. Scarth. 1974. Effect of energy intake prior to parturition on milk lipids and survival rate, thermostability and carcass composition of piglets, *J. Anim. Sci.*, 38:64.

Shapiro, A.C., D. Wu, and S. N. Meydani. 1993. Eicosanoids derived from arachidonic and eicosapentaenoic acids inhibit T-cell proliferative response, *Prostaglandins*, 45:229.

Small, D. M. 1991. The effects of glyceride structure on absorption and metabolism, *Annu. Rev. Nutr.*, 11:413.

Smith, D. R., D. A. Knabe, and S. B. Smith. 1996. Depression of lipogenesis in swine adipose tissue by specific dietary fatty acids, *J. Anim. Sci.*, 74:975.

Stahly, T. S. 1984. Use of fats in diets for growing pigs. In *Fats in Animal Nutrition*, Wiseman, J., Ed., Butterworths, London, 313.

Stahly, T. S., and G. L. Cromwell. 1979. Effect of environmental temperature and dietary fat supplementation on the performance and carcass characteristics of growing and finishing swine, *J. Anim. Sci.*, 49:1478.

Taugbol, O. 1993. Omega-3 fatty acid incorporation in fat and muscle tissues of growing pigs fed supplements of fish oil, *J. Vet. Med.*, 40:93.

Tilton, S. L., P. S. Miller, A. J. Lewis, D. E. Reese, and P. M. Ermer. 1999. Addition of fat to the diets of lactating sows: I. Effects on milk production and composition and carcass composition of the litter at weaning, *J. Anim. Sci.*, 77:2491.

Tokach, M. D., J. E. Pettigrew, L. J. Johnston, M. Overland, J. W. Rust, and S. G. Cornelius. 1995. Effect of adding fat and (or) milk products to the weanling pig diet on performance in the nursery and subsequent grow-finish performance, *J. Anim. Sci.*, 73:3358.

USDA. 1995. Swine '95. Part I: Reference of 1995 Swine Management Practices, Animal and Plant Health Inspection Service, Veterinary Services, Washington, D.C.

Van Oeckel, M. J., M. Casteels, N. Warnants, L. Van Damme, and Ch. V. Boucque. 1996. Omega-3 fatty acids in pig nutrition: implications for the intrinsic and sensory quality of the meat, *Meat Sci.*, 44:55.

Wander, R. C., J. A. Hall, J. L. Gradin, S. H. Du, and D. E. Jewell. 1997. The ratio of dietary (n-6) to (n-3) fatty acids influences immune system function, eicosanoid metabolism, lipid peroxidation and vitamin E status in aged dogs, *J. Nutr.*, 127:1198.

Weldon, W. C., A. J. Lewis, G. F. Louis, J. L. Kovar, M. A. Giesemann, and P. S. Miller. 1994. Postpartum hypophagia in primiparous sows: I. Effects of gestation feeding level on feed intake, feeding behavior, and plasma metabolite concentrations during lactation, *J. Anim. Sci.*, 72:387.

Wiseman, J. 1984. Assessment of the digestible and metabolizable energy of fats for non-ruminants. In *Fats in Animal Nutrition*, Wiseman, J., Ed., Butterworths, London, 277.

7 Nonstarch Polysaccharides and Oligosaccharides in Swine Nutrition

Christine M. Grieshop, Duane E. Reese, and George C. Fahey, Jr.

CONTENTS

I. What Are Nonstarch Polysaccharides and Oligosaccharides?...108
II. How Are Nonstarch Polysaccharides Quantified?..108
III. How Are Oligosaccharides Quantified?...109
IV. What are the Nonstarch Polysaccharide and Oligosaccharide Concentrations of Selected Ingredients in Swine Feeds?...109
V. Digestion of Nonstarch Polysaccharides and Oligosaccharides by Swine.........................110
    A. Effects of Nonstarch Polysaccharides on Gastrointestinal Tract Characteristics....112
    B. Effects of Nonstarch Polysaccharides on Gastric Emptying and Rate of Passage...112
    C. Fermentation of Nonstarch Polysaccharides and Oligosaccharides in the Swine Gastrointestinal Tract..112
    D. Energy Value of VFA..113
VI. Nonstarch Polysaccharide and Oligosaccharide Effects on Dietary Nutrient Metabolism....114
    A. Glucose..114
    B. Lipids...114
    C. Protein...114
    D. Minerals..115
VII. Nonstarch Polysaccharide Effects on Growth Performance and Body Composition of Growing Swine..115
VIII. Nonstarch Polysaccharide Interactions with Ambient Temperature.................................116
IX. Nonstarch Polysaccharide Interactions with Antibiotics...117
X. Nonstarch Polysaccharide and Oligosaccharide Effects on Health of Swine....................117
XI. Nonstarch Polysaccharide Effects on Sows..117
    A. Effects of Nonstarch Polysaccharides on Reproductive Performance.....................118
    B. Effects of Nonstarch Polysaccharide Source on Reproductive Performance..........121
    C. Effects of Nonstarch Polysaccharides on Sow Behavior..121
XII. Practical Considerations in Feeding Nonstarch Polysaccharides......................................122
    A. Diet Formulation and Feeding Management..122
    B. Possible Physical Limitations to Feeding High-Nonstarch Polysaccharide Diets..123
XIII. Effects of Nonstarch Polysaccharides on Ammonia Emission..123
XIV. Summary..124
References..124

I. WHAT ARE NONSTARCH POLYSACCHARIDES AND OLIGOSACCHARIDES?

Nonstarch polysaccharides (NSP) can comprise up to 90% of the cell wall of plants (Selvendran and Robertson, 1990). The most abundant plant cell wall NSP include cellulose, hemicelluloses, and pectins. A smaller group of NSP — fructans, glucomannans, and galactomannans — serve as storage polysaccharides within the plant. Mucilages, β-glucans, and gums are also examples of NSP. Unlike starch, which is hydrolyzed by pancreatic amylase to glucose, NSP are not hydrolyzed by mammalian enzymes; rather, they are fermented by the gastrointestinal tract microflora.

The physiological impact of individual NSP is dependent on the sugar residues present and the nature of linkages between these residues. Cellulose and β-glucans are linear 1-4 β-linked glucose polymers. Mixed linkage β-glucans contain 1-3 linkages interspersed with 1-4 linkages. Cellulose occurs in tightly bound aggregates (microfibrils) in plants. Hemicelluloses contain a monosaccharide backbone of xylan, galactan, or mannan, and side chains of arabinose or galactose. Pectin is a polymer of galacturonic acid containing side chains of other sugars such as glucose, galactose, and rhamnose. Pectins also contain methoxy groups ($-OCH_3$) that are metabolized by gastrointestinal tract microflora almost completely to methane gas.

In contrast to NSP, oligosaccharides (OS) generally contain only 3 to 9 monosaccharide units. They may have similar or different monosaccharides, various linkage structures, and may be linear or branched chain. Like NSP, OS are not hydrolyzed by mammalian enzymes, but are fermented by the gastrointestinal tract microflora. Fructo-oligosaccharides (FOS) are a mixture of primarily fructose units linked by β-2-1-glucosidic bonds. As will be discussed later, FOS are preferentially used by bifidobacteria in the large intestine. α-Galacto-oligosaccharides (GOS) consist of 1, 2, or 3 units of galactose linked via α-1-3 bonds and bound to a terminal sucrose. The GOS — raffinose, stachyose, and verbascose — are of particular concern to the swine industry because they are poorly utilized by young pigs. Soybean meal, a major dietary ingredient for swine, contains high concentrations of GOS.

Lignin is not a polysaccharide but rather a high-molecular-weight polymer composed of phenylpropane residues formed by condensation of the aromatic alcohols, cinnamyl, guaiacyl, and syringyl alcohols (Southgate, 1993). The lignin content of swine feeds is typically low, with cereal and oilseed fibers usually having only a few percent lignin (Dreher, 1999). Lignin is not considered a functional dietary ingredient and is essentially indigestible by swine.

II. HOW ARE NONSTARCH POLYSACCHARIDES QUANTIFIED?

Since the introduction of the Weende system of proximate analysis of feeds in which carbohydrates were quantified as either crude fiber or nitrogen-free extract, several highly specific methods have been developed to determine the fiber, and specifically the NSP, content of swine feeds. The development of an accurate analytical method for quantifying NSP is difficult due to the complexity and diversity of the polysaccharides involved.

Two general approaches have been used to quantify the dietary fiber content of feedstuffs: gravimetric analysis and monomeric component analysis. Gravimetric analysis involves the chemical or enzymatic solubilization of dietary protein, starch, and fat, followed by weighing of the insoluble residue. The crude fiber analysis (AOAC, 1984) is an example of a gravimetric analysis. It is based on the sequential extraction of feeds with diethyl ether, dilute acid, and dilute alkali. Although the crude fiber value is still reported for most commercially available swine feeds, it is not an accurate estimation of total NSP since the recoveries of cellulose, hemicelluloses, and lignin average only 50 to 80%, 20%, and 10 to 50%, respectively (Van Soest and McQueen, 1973).

Refinement of gravimetric analyses and the need to delineate the form of fiber present in a feedstuff led to the development of detergent methods of fiber analysis. The two forms of detergent fiber are neutral detergent fiber (NDF), which includes cellulose, hemicelluloses, and lignin, and acid detergent fiber (ADF), which includes cellulose and lignin. The difference between the NDF and ADF fractions is an estimate of the hemicelluloses in a feed. Although the detergent methods of fiber analysis are great improvements compared with the crude fiber estimation, both underestimate the amount of total fiber in a feed due to an inability to recover soluble fiber components (e.g., pectins, mucilages, gums, and β-glucans).

Subsequent variations in the gravimetric analyses of fiber have focused on quantifying the amounts of total, soluble, and insoluble fiber in a feedstuff. The distinction between these fiber classifications is based on the chemical properties, rather than the chemical composition, of the fiber, and this distinction is important because soluble and insoluble fibers vary in their physiological effects. Soluble fibers include exudates and extracts from fruits and trees (e.g., pectins, gum arabic, and guar gum), while insoluble fibers include Solka Floc® (wood cellulose), oat fiber, and wheat bran.

Asp et al. (1983) developed an enzymatic–gravimetric method for determining fiber in which a sample is pretreated with enzymes for the digestion of starch and protein, followed by the recovery of the insoluble components via filtration and the soluble components by precipitation in ethanol. Because contamination of the sample with indigestible protein and minerals is possible, correction for these contaminants is necessary. Jeraci et al. (1989) modified the enzymatic–gravimetric procedure of Asp et al. (1983) by incorporating a urea enzymatic dialysis to assure the removal of essentially all starch.

Both Theander and Åman (1982) and Prosky et al. (1984) developed methods to analyze total dietary fiber (TDF) in a feedstuff. The Theander and Åman procedure indirectly determines the amount of TDF by quantifying the amounts of uronic acids, sugars, Klason lignin, and starch present, and then calculating the TDF as the sum of the sugars, uronic acids, and Klason lignin minus the concentration of starch. In contrast, the Prosky et al. procedure quantifies TDF directly. These assays have been further expanded to allow quantification of both soluble and insoluble dietary fiber components (Prosky et al., 1988; 1992) and refined to increase precision and decrease the complexity and time required (Lee et al., 1996).

In contrast to the gravimetric methods of fiber analyses, which assume that all residue present is fiber, component analysis quantifies the amounts of constituent sugars present in a substrate and then, via summation, determines the total NSP concentration. An example of component analysis is the Englyst and Cummings (1988) procedure, which quantifies the content of NSP in a substrate by enzymatic removal of starch followed by acid hydrolysis of the NSP to its constituent sugars. The individual sugars are subsequently quantified by gas–liquid chromatography or colorimetry (Englyst and Hudson, 1993). In comparison to the gravimetric methods of analysis, the Englyst and Hudson values are typically lower because of exclusion of lignin and resistant starch.

III. HOW ARE OLIGOSACCHARIDES QUANTIFIED?

Accurate quantification of OS in feedstuffs is difficult due to the complexity and variability of OS forms present, and the lack of availability of pure OS standards for purposes of component quantification. The general method used to evaluate these compounds involves enzymatic or chemical degradation of OS into individual components, which then are extracted using water (Campbell et al., 1997a) or aqueous-ethanol (Sánchez-Mata et al., 1998). Once extracted, the excess solvent is evaporated and the sample solubilized in water. Extracted OS can be characterized using high-performance anion-exchange chromatography (Sánchez-Mata et al., 1998), mass spectrometry (Brüll et al., 1998), or high-performance ion-exchange chromatography with pulsed electrochemical detection (Campbell et al., 1997a).

IV. WHAT ARE THE NONSTARCH POLYSACCHARIDE AND OLIGOSACCHARIDE CONCENTRATIONS OF SELECTED INGREDIENTS IN SWINE FEEDS?

Numerous factors affect the fiber content of commonly used swine feedstuffs including source of the fiber, plant variety, and processing method used to produce the ingredient. The NRC (1998) *Nutrient Requirements of Swine* publication reports the NDF and ADF concentrations of various feedstuffs. Corn grain contains 9.6% NDF and 2.8% ADF, while soybean meal (44% crude protein) contains 13.3% NDF and 9.4% ADF (NRC, 1998). Table 7.1 reports the NDF, ADF, TDF, and crude fiber concentrations of selected ingredients used in swine feeds. Certain feedstuffs used in the swine industry also contain considerable quantities of the fructosyl OS derivatives and galactosyl OS derivatives (raffinose and stachyose). Barley and wheat contain substantial amounts of both types of OS, while oats contain only the galactosyl OS (Table 7.1; Henry and Saini, 1989).

Because nutritionists are constantly seeking methods to reduce swine production costs and improve pig performance, there is interest in the utilization of "nontraditional" and by-product feedstuffs in swine diets. Many of these alternative feed sources have much higher fiber concentrations than corn or soybean meal.

One example of a nontraditional feedstuff currently used in some swine diets is alfalfa. The fiber content of alfalfa is greatly affected by stage of maturity at harvest. Alfalfa meal (dehydrated, 20% crude protein) contains 41.2% NDF and 30.2% ADF (NRC, 1998). Alfalfa is a viable feedstuff in both sow and growing pig diets, although the level of inclusion varies. Incorporation of between 10 and 60% alfalfa in growing swine diets has been reported to reduce average daily gain by up to 52%, while percentage carcass fat is decreased by up to 30%, and percentage muscle increased by up to 12% (Bohman et al., 1955; Powley et al., 1981).

Soybean hulls are another by-product feed that, because of their high fiber content, have not been included routinely in swine diets. Soybean hulls contain 43.4% crude fiber, 62.0% cell walls, 38.0% cell contents, 45.6% ADF, 42.2% cellulose, 16.4% hemicelluloses, and 3.0% lignin (Kornegay, 1978). Growing pigs fed up to 15% supplemental soybean hulls did not experience any depression in average daily gain or feed intake, although metabolizable energy intake was decreased linearly as the level of soybean hulls increased. In this experiment, the most efficient conversion ratio (kilocalories of metabolizable energy intake per unit of gain) was observed for pigs consuming diets containing 15% soybean hulls (Kornegay, 1981).

V. DIGESTION OF NONSTARCH POLYSACCHARIDES AND OLIGOSACCHARIDES BY SWINE

Not unexpectedly, the apparent digestibility of fibrous components by swine is quite variable and may range between 0 and 97% (Mitchell and Hamilton, 1933, as cited by Rérat, 1978; Poijarvi, 1944, as cited by Rérat, 1978). Addition of high NSP feedstuffs to swine diets reduces apparent digestibility of the diet (Pond et al., 1986; Moore et al., 1986b; Zhu et al., 1993). Numerous factors can affect the efficiency of digestion of NSP including source (Knudsen and Hansen, 1991), processing method (Fadel et al., 1989), and concentration in the diet (Stanogias and Pearce, 1985a; Goodlad and Mathers, 1991).

Swine lack the necessary digestive enzymes to degrade NSP and OS. Therefore, ingested NSP and OS are acted upon by anaerobic bacteria. Although it is commonly believed that digestion of NSP and OS occurs primarily in the large intestine of the pig, up to 62% of NSP disappearance has been observed in the upper intestine (Graham et al., 1986; Fadel et al., 1989). Knudsen and Hansen (1991) quantified the recovery of wheat NSP at the end of the small intestine as 82 to 104% whereas the recovery was only 64 to 66% for oat NSP, demonstrating that oats were degraded to a larger extent in the small intestine. Graham et al. (1986) demonstrated that feeding pigs a control diet containing barley, wheat, and oats alone or supplemented with 33% wheat bran or 33% beet pulp resulted in a 19.7, 10.6, and 36.8% NSP apparent ileal digestibility, respectively. The degradation products in the small intestine were similar to those in feces, leading to the assumption that the degradation process occurring in the small intestine was also microbial in nature (Graham et al., 1986).

Most NSP and OS are highly fermentable. Compounds such as H_2, CO_2, and small amounts of CH_4 gas are by-products of their bacterial degradation, along with the volatile fatty acids (VFA) such as acetate, propionate, and butyrate.

TABLE 7.1
Fiber and Oligosaccharide Concentrations in Common Feed Ingredients for Swine (as-is basis)

Feedstuff	Crude Fiber[a] (%)	Neutral Detergent Fiber[b] (%)	Acid Detergent Fiber[b] (%)	Total Dietary Fiber (%)	Total FOS[c] (mg/g)	Raffinose (mg/g)	Stachyose (mg/g)	Sucrose (mg/g)
Alfalfa meal, dehydrated, 17% CP	24.0	41.2	30.2		2.1			
Barley grain	5.0	18.0	6.2	17.3[d]	1.7	2.3[e]	0.02[e]	13.6[e]
Corn grain, yellow	2.6	9.6	2.8	9.0[f]	0.0			
Oat groats	2.5				0.1			
Sorghum grain	2.4	18.0	8.3					
Soy protein concentrate	0.1							
Soybean hulls	36.4		45[a]	86.0[f]	0.1			
Soybean meal, 44% CP	6.2	13.3	9.4		0.0	14.0[g]	52.0[g]	62.0[g]
Beet pulp		41.1[h]		56.3[h]	0.1			
Wheat, hard red winter	2.5	13.5	4.0	12.2[d]	1.3	4.7[e]	0.06[e]	7.9[e]
Wheat midds	8.2[i]	35.6	10.7	43.0[f]	4.6			

[a] NRC, 1982.
[b] NRC, 1998.
[c] FOS = fructo-oligosaccharides; Campbell et al., 1997a.
[d] Cho et al., 1999.
[e] Henry and Saini, 1989.
[f] Patil and Fahey, 1998.
[g] Kawamaru, as cited by Zuo et al., 1996.
[h] Campbell et al., 1997b, converted from dry matter basis as reported.
[i] Reported as wheat mill run, less than 9.5% fiber.

A. Effects of Nonstarch Polysaccharides on Gastrointestinal Tract Characteristics

Feeding high-fiber diets generally increases total empty gastrointestinal tract weight (Kass et al., 1980b; Stanogias and Pearce, 1985b; Anugwa et al., 1989), although Jin et al. (1994) observed no change in visceral weights due to inclusion of 10% wheat straw in growing pig diets. The variation in NSP sources used in these studies may explain the differences in results observed. Additional effects of feeding high-NSP diets include increased salivary (Arkhipovets, 1956, as cited by Low, 1989), gastric (Zebrowska et al., 1983; Dierick et al., 1989), biliary (Dierick et al., 1989), pancreatic (Partridge et al., 1982; Zebrowska and Low, 1987; Dierick et al., 1989), and possibly intestinal (Taverner et al., 1981) secretions.

Both high-NSP and high-OS diets affect intestinal epithelial cell proliferation rate as demonstrated by Jin et al. (1994) and Howard et al. (1995). Growing pigs fed diets containing 10% wheat straw had a 33 and 43% increase in rate of jejunal and colonic cell proliferation, respectively. These pigs also had 65 and 59% more jejunal and ileal cells undergoing programmed cell death, indicating that NSP had actually increased intestinal cell turnover rate (Jin et al., 1994). Width of the intestinal villus and crypt depth also were increased in pigs fed the high-NSP diet (Jin et al., 1994). Similarly, feeding neonatal pigs diets containing 3 g FOS/l formula resulted in an increased cecal epithelial cell density (44.7 vs. 41 cells/crypt) and number of labeled cecal mucosal cells (9.6 vs. 8.2 cells/crypt) (Howard et al., 1995).

In addition to the obvious impact the above-described physiological changes may have on nutrient digestion and absorption, feeding high NSP concentrations also may indirectly increase maintenance energy requirements of swine by increasing nutrient needs for visceral organ development and maintenance.

B. Effects of Nonstarch Polysaccharides on Gastric Emptying and Rate of Passage

Certain forms of NSP, such as guar gum and pectin, can increase viscosity of digesta. The effect of this physicochemical property in the digestive tract of the pig is to increase the viscosity of the digestive tract contents and increase the ability of the dry matter to retain water (Johansen et al., 1996). The addition of 40 to 60 g/kg guar gum to high-energy growing pig diets containing starch, casein, soybean oil, and tallow reduced the rate of gastric emptying 33 to 52% after feeding (Rainbird and Low, 1986a,b; Rainbird, 1986) and reduced the dry matter concentration of the digesta 27% (Rainbird, 1986).

Increased levels of NSP in swine diets also have been associated with alteration in the rate of passage of stomach contents. Schulze et al. (1995) observed an increase of 0.697 g of daily dry matter flow at the terminal ileum for every g/kg increase in dietary NDF provided by purified NDF (isolated from wheat bran), wheat bran, or sunflower hulls. These results are supported by Potkins et al. (1991) who found that inclusion of 75 to 300 g/kg of bran or oatmeal by-products in diets of growing pigs resulted in an increased rate of passage of up to 14 and 23%, respectively. Because neither of these fiber sources had a significant effect on gastric emptying or passage through the terminal small intestine, the increased rate of passage through the total digestive tract was thought to be due to differences in rate of passage through the large intestine (Potkins et al., 1991).

C. Fermentation of Nonstarch Polysaccharides and Oligosaccharides in the Swine Gastrointestinal Tract

Fermentative microorganisms are present in the highest concentration in the cecum and colon of the pig. Two of the most abundant cellulolytic species of microbes in the rumen, *Fibrobacter succinogenes* and *Ruminococcus flavefaciens*, are present in the pig large intestine (Varel et al., 1984a). Microbes in the large intestine of the pig primarily utilize the dietary plant cell wall polysaccharides, sloughed intestinal mucosa, glycoproteins from saliva, gastric juice, mucinous secretions, and a minor amount of dietary simple sugars and disaccharides (Varel, 1987). Oligosaccharides and possibly resistant starch also serve as fermentable substrates in the cecum and large intestine of the pig.

The population of microorganisms in the pig cecum and colon is affected by many dietary factors including feeding of high-NSP diets. Varel et al. (1984b) observed a 38% increase in the number and a 17% increase in the activity of cellulolytic bacteria in fecal samples from growing pigs fed a diet containing 35% alfalfa meal. Similar results were observed by Anugwa et al. (1989) who fed diets containing 40% alfalfa meal. The maximum average rate of fermentation in sows receiving either 0 or 475 g/day orally or 0, 285, 570, or 855 g/day of intracecally purified cellulose was 11 g/kg$^{0.75}$, and the true efficiency of bacterial protein synthesis was 5.2 g bacterial protein/100 g supplementary cellulose on average (Kreuzer et al., 1991).

Feeding FOS to humans (Modler et al., 1990) promotes growth of *Bifidobacterium*, but contradictory effects have been reported in swine. Houdijk et al. (1998) fed growing pigs diets supplemented with 7.5, 10, 15, or 20 g nondigestible oligosaccharide per kilogram diet and found no effect on fecal pH, but a decreased fecal DM content. Similarly, Gabert et al. (1995) observed no effect of feeding weanling pigs diets containing 0.2% transgalactosylated OS, 0.2% glucooligosaccharides, or 1% lactitol on bacterial populations in ileal digesta.

Fermentation of NSP in the cecum and colon of the pig results in the production of a mixture of VFA, primarily acetic, propionic, and butyric acids. Elsden et al. (1946) reported that the relative concentrations of individual VFA in the alimentary tract of numerous species including the pig, sheep, ox, red deer, horse, and rabbit were very similar, with acetic acid being the highest at 67%, followed by propionic acid and butyric acid at 19 and 14%, respectively. The specific concentrations of VFA in the swine cecum in this experiment were 62.1% acetic acid, 27.8% propionic acid, and 10.1% butyric acid (Elsden et al., 1946). Both the source and level of dietary NSP can affect fermentative breakdown of fibrous feedstuffs and the molar ratios of VFA produced in the colon of the pig, as demonstrated in Table 7.2.

D. Energy Value of VFA

VFA produced by microbial fermentation in the cecum and colon are rapidly absorbed (Latymer and Low, 1987) and can supply between 5 and 28% of the maintenance energy requirement of the pig (Farrell and Johnson, 1970, 1.9 to 2.7% of apparent digestible energy; Rérat et al., 1987, approximately 30% of metabolizable energy for maintenance; Imoto and Namioka, 1978, approximately 10% of metabolizable energy for maintenance; Yen et al., 1991, 23.8% of whole animal heat production; Kass et al., 1980a, 4.8 to 14% of the energy required for maintenance).

When considering VFA as an energy source for the pig, the losses of methane, hydrogen, and fermentation heat must be considered. These losses result in a lower energy value to the animal in comparison with hydrolytic digestion of carbohydrates. The efficiency of utilization of dietary energy is decreased 9 to 22% in animals fed high-NSP diets (Giusi-Perier et al., 1989; Noblet et

TABLE 7.2
Molar Proportions of Volatile Fatty Acids in Large Intestinal Digesta of Growing Pigs

Fiber Source	Amount in Diet (%)	Molar VFA Ratio			Ref.
		Acetate	Propionate	Butyrate	
Sugar beet pulp	30	0.59	0.23	0.18	Zhu et al., 1993
Wheat bran	75 g NDF/kg DM	0.68	0.17	0.12	Stanogias and Pearce, 1985c
Maize cobs	75 g NDF/kg DM	0.74	0.20	0.05	Stanogias and Pearce, 1985c
Alfalfa	52	0.71	0.22	0.07	Kennelly et al., 1981

al., 1994) due to a reduced absorption of glucose and amino-N from the small intestine and an inadequate compensatory increase in the absorption of VFA in the hindgut. These results demonstrate that the energy supplied from the fermentation of NSP is utilized at a lower efficiency than the energy supplied by nutrients digested and absorbed from the small intestine.

VI. NONSTARCH POLYSACCHARIDE AND OLIGOSACCHARIDE EFFECTS ON DIETARY NUTRIENT METABOLISM

NSPs influence absorption, metabolism, and utilization of nutrients including carbohydrates, amino acids, lipids, and minerals.

A. Glucose

Nunes and Malmlöf (1992) demonstrated that feeding 60 g/kg guar gum reduced glucose absorption by 32 and 29% compared with an unsupplemented basal diet or a diet supplemented with 150 g/kg purified cellulose, respectively. These results are supported by those of Sambrook and Rainbird (1985) who observed an approximate 25% decrease in plasma glucose concentration in pigs fed semipurified diets supplemented with 40 g/kg guar gum. On the contrary, Michel and Rérat (1998) and Leclere et al. (1993) did not observe an effect of 10 or 60 g/kg of sugar beet fiber or wheat bran on glucose absorption.

The inclusion of NSP in swine diets also affects glucose regulatory hormones. Inclusion of 40 or 60 g/kg guar gum in semipurified diets decreased peak postprandial production of insulin by 30%, gastric inhibitory polypeptide by 55%, insulin-like growth factor-1 by 58%, and glucagon by 40% (Nunes and Malmlöf, 1992).

B. Lipids

Increasing the NSP content of swine diets usually decreases the energy density and digestibility of the diet. Addition of 60 g/kg beet pulp or wheat bran decreased the postprandial plasma triacylglycerol response in growing pigs by approximately 40% (Leclere et al., 1993). Freire et al. (1998) also demonstrated that inclusion of 15% wheat bran in diets fed to 3-week-old pigs reduced total tract apparent digestibility of energy, fat, and ADF by 5, 10, and 10 percentage units, respectively. Possible mechanisms for the negative effect of NSP on lipid metabolism include partial inhibition of both lipolysis and intestinal fat absorption (Borel et al., 1989).

In an effort to assure that swine fed high-NSP diets receive adequate energy, fat has been added to the diet. Supplementation of diets containing 40% ground oats with 3% white or brown grease resulted in a 5.8% improvement in feed conversion efficiency, but the fat addition did not affect dry matter or energy digestibility (Myer and Combs, 1991).

Nonstarch polysaccharide level in swine diets also affects plasma cholesterol levels. Costa et al. (1994) fed semipurified diets supplemented with 10 g/kg cholesterol and 300 g/kg (dry matter basis) baked beans. Although unsupplemented pigs in this experiment experienced an increase over time in plasma cholesterol and triacylglycerol of 133 and 70%, respectively, consumption of baked beans reduced plasma cholesterol by 36% and triacylglycerol by 52%, although the difference in plasma cholesterol was not significant (Costa et al., 1994). These results support previous research in which a reduction in plasma cholesterol in hypercholesterolemic pigs was observed due to feeding 300 g/kg baked beans (Costa et al., 1993). Supplementation with baked beans increased conversion of cholesterol to coprostanol in the large intestine (Costa et al., 1994).

C. Protein

Increased NSP results in decreased dry matter (Kennelly and Aherne, 1980b; Mason et al., 1982; Schulze et al., 1994), nitrogen (N) (Eggum et al., 1982; Schulze et al., 1994), and amino acid digestibility (Mason et al., 1982; Den Hartog et al., 1988). Inclusion of 10% NSP to 16% crude protein cornstarch–casein diets resulted in an approximately 50% increase in fecal N excretion (Fahey et al., 1980). Nonstarch polysaccharides can decrease efficiency of N utilization by increasing secretion of endogenous N, reducing dietary N absorption, or increasing bacterial N excretion. Inclusion of 200 g NDF (isolated from wheat bran) in swine diets resulted in an increased total ileal N flow of 1.884 g/kg of dietary dry matter intake (Schultz et al., 1995). This increase was composed of 59% endogenous and 41% exogenous N (Schultz et al., 1995). These findings are in support of previous research that demonstrated that more than 50% of the ileal N in a pig is of bacterial origin (Schulze et al., 1994).

In an effort to characterize the effect of dietary NSP on N and amino acid digestibility, recent studies have focused on the effect of purified fibrous components on N utilization. For example, Lenis et al. (1996) found that diets containing 15% purified wheat bran NDF decreased ileal N digestibility from 94.1 to 88.9% and amino acid digestibilities by 2.0 to 5.5 percentage units, with the exception of cystine, alanine, and glycine, which were decreased by 18, 16, and 11 percentage units, respectively. In contrast, Li et al. (1994) observed no effect of inclusion of up to 13.3% Solka Floc® in cornstarch–soybean meal diets on either apparent ileal or fecal amino acid digestibility.

D. Minerals

The reported effects of NSP on digestion, absorption, and utilization of minerals are not consistent. Components of the polysaccharides and lignin that interact with minerals include the carboxyl group of uronic acids (i.e., hemicelluloses and pectin), carboxyl and hydroxyl groups of phenolic compounds (i.e., lignin), and the surface hydroxyl of cellulose (Kornegay and Moore, 1986). Stanogias et al. (1994) found that incorporating soybean hulls, pea hulls, maize hulls, or oat hulls to increase NDF content of semipurified diets from 69 to 367 g did not significantly affect apparent absorption of Ca, P, or Mg, but the added NDF reduced apparent absorption of Na and K by 22 to 57% and 7 to 70%, respectively. In contrast, Partridge (1978) reported that addition of 6% cellulose to a semisynthetic diet decreased large intestinal absorption of Ca, P, Mg, K, and Zn. Den Hartog et al. (1988) observed no detrimental effect of 5% pectin, 5% cellulose, or 5% ground straw on either apparent ileal or total tract digestibility of Na, K, Mg, or P. Total tract digestibility of Ca was reduced by 19% in pigs fed 5% carboxymethylcellulose (Den Hartog et al., 1988).

Although fibrous feedstuffs such as peanut hulls, oat hulls, wheat bran, and soybean hulls have been shown to decrease mineral absorption (Kornegay and Moore, 1986), the results are not consistent. Overall mineral utilization, given current feeding practices, appears to be relatively unaffected by dietary NSP source (Kornegay and Moore, 1986).

VII. NONSTARCH POLYSACCHARIDE EFFECTS ON GROWTH PERFORMANCE AND BODY COMPOSITION OF GROWING SWINE

It is generally accepted that pigs eat to meet their energy needs (NRC, 1987). That is, as the energy density of the diet decreases, voluntary feed intake increases in pigs allowed *ad libitum* access to feed. Diets high in NSP have a lower energy density than diets low in NSP (NRC, 1998). Also, microbial digestion of NSP and the utilization of VFA produced is less efficient than direct utilization of glucose by the animal. Consequently, as the concentration of fiber in the diet increases, growing pigs generally consume less digestible energy (NRC, 1987) and more feed. Feed intake may be reduced, however, when dietary crude fiber levels exceed 10 to 15% of the diet due to excessive bulk or reduced palatability (NRC, 1998). Growth rate and feed efficiency are usually depressed as fiber level in the diet increases.

Evidence exists that a pig's ability to respond to dietary energy concentration is affected by dietary NSP level. Campbell and Taverner (1986) conducted two experiments to determine the effect of dietary NSP on the pig's response to decreasing dietary energy concentration. Pigs fed high NSP (12.0% ADF) diets experienced a 13% increase in daily gain but a 10% decrease in feed intake when dietary fat was increased from 1.0 to 10.0% of the feed. In contrast, pigs fed low NSP (3.0 to 6.2% ADF) diets experienced a 30% increase in daily gain with no depression in voluntary feed intake when the energy concentration of the diet was increased from 2820 to 3609 kcal DE/kg (Campbell and Taverner, 1986). These results are supported by those of Troelsen and Bell (1963) and Baker et al. (1968) who observed reductions of 11 and 42% in feed intake due to dietary inclusions of wheat bran or cellulose, respectively. In contrast, Anugwa et al. (1989) reported a decrease in feed intake due to inclusion of 40% alfalfa meal in a corn–soybean meal finishing pig diet only during the first 17 days of a 66-day trial.

Growing pigs fed diets containing 40 or 80% alfalfa meal experienced a 32 and 100% reduction in daily gain, respectively (Pond et al., 1988; Anugwa et al., 1989). Addition of oat hulls (22%) or corn cobs (7.5 or 15%) to growing pig diets also resulted in a similar reduction in growth (Kennelly and Aherne, 1980a; Frank et al., 1983). Contrary to these results, gilts fed diets containing 7.5, 15.0, or 22.5% peanut hulls were able to maintain similar gains to gilts fed unsupplemented corn–soybean meal diets by increasing feed intake by up to 11% (Lindemann et al., 1986).

The utilization of high NSP diets for young pig has not been explored extensively because of the assumption that they cannot utilize such diets. Contrary to this belief, Longland et al. (1994) found that feeding 3-week-old pigs diets containing 15.0% sugar beet pulp resulted in no differences in voluntary feed intake, weight gain, feed conversion, or apparent digestibility of N and energy. The apparent digestibility of total NSP was greater for pigs fed diets containing sugar beet pulp (Longland et al., 1994). In addition, Watts and Moser (1979) observed that inclusion of 10 to 20% ground whole oats in weanling pig diets did not affect gain or feed efficiency.

Certain OS included in the diets of weanling pigs may improve growth performance. Schoenherr and Pollmann (1994) found that feeding between 0.025 and 0.05% of a glucan from the cell wall of *Saccharomyces cerevisiae* to weanling pig improved daily gain by 10%. Russell et al. (1996) and Howard et al. (1999) fed FOS to weanling pigs and observed an improvement in daily gain and feed efficiency. Davis et al. (1999) provided a mannan oligosaccharide to early-weaned pigs and also observed an improvement in daily gain and feed efficiency, but no improvement in immunocompetence. Addition of FOS to the diet stimulated growth of beneficial indigenous microflora in the colon of young pigs, preventing enteric colonization by pathogenic microorganisms and improving N retention (cited by Russell et al., 1996).

High-NSP diets can alter carcass composition including reduced carcass weight, length, backfat, and longissimus muscle area but increased relative weight of the liver, heart, stomach, small intestine, cecum, and colon (Pond et al., 1988). These results support the hypothesis that feeding a high-NSP diet results in an increase in the animal's maintenance requirement by increasing visceral organ weight and, therefore, repartitioning nutrients away from production of edible carcass.

VIII. NONSTARCH POLYSACCHARIDE INTERACTIONS WITH AMBIENT TEMPERATURE

The impact of high NSP diets on pig growth performance is affected by ambient temperature. Pigs housed in environments below their thermal neutral zone must increase heat production to maintain body temperature. Because diets high in fiber have a high heat increment, they should be more beneficial to pigs housed in cold rather than warm or hot environments. Stahly and Cromwell (1986) demonstrated that inclusion of 10% alfalfa meal in diets fed to pigs housed in hot (35°C) or optimal (22.5°C) environmental conditions reduced daily gain by 5 and 3% and feed efficiency by 10 and 7%, respectively. In contrast, when the pigs were housed in cold (10°C) environments, daily gain was decreased only by 1.8% and feed efficiency by 1.5% when a diet containing 10% alfalfa meal was provided (Stahly and Cromwell, 1986). Similarly, when Coffey et al. (1982) summarized data from several trials, a significant interaction between season of the year and dietary energy level for daily gain was observed. Low-energy diets containing 5% alfalfa meal or bermudagrass did not reduce gain during cool-season tests, but a linear reduction in gains resulted when low-energy diets were fed during warm seasons. Schoenherr et al. (1989) also found that the effects of thermal heat stress on sow milk energy yield and litter weight gain were aggravated by dietary fiber addition (48.5% wheat bran) and minimized by dietary fat addition (10.6% choice white grease). In contrast to these results, Jørgensen et al. (1996) observed negligible temperature–fiber interactions on energy metabolism in pigs fed fiber at either 5.9 or 26.8% of dry matter and housed at 13 vs. 23°C.

IX. NONSTARCH POLYSACCHARIDE INTERACTIONS WITH ANTIBIOTICS

The efficiency of utilization of NSP by pigs is dependent on the nature of the microbial population residing in the large intestine. It could, therefore, be assumed that supplementation with compounds such as antibiotics that alter the gut microflora would have an influence on fermentable fiber source utilization. Virginiamycin supplementation at 11 ppm improved dry matter, energy, NDF, ADF, hemicellulose, and cellulose digestibility in pigs fed diets containing 50% oats (Ravindran et al., 1984). The impact of antibiotic supplementation is dependent on the form of dietary NSP. Supplementation with 82 mg/kg salinomycin increased dietary energy retained, 1.32 vs. 1.34 MJ $(kg^{0.75}/day)$, and N digestibility, 80 vs. 86%, in pigs fed wheat bran, but salinomycin had no effect on pigs fed a diet containing 10% oat hulls (Moore et al., 1986b). Apparent N digestibility also was increased 12% in pigs fed diets containing 10.5% fiber due to supplementation of 0.7% nebacitin (Mason et al., 1982). Total fecal N excretion was reduced by 19% in these pigs (Mason et al., 1982).

Antibiotic supplementation of pigs fed high-NSP diets also may influence the absorption and utilization of numerous minerals. Addition of 11 ppm virginiamycin to pig diets containing 50% oats improved absorption and retention of Ca, P, Mg, Cu, Fe, Zn, and Mn (Ravindran et al., 1984). In contrast, salinomycin supplementation (82 mg/kg) did not affect Ca, Mg, Na, K, Zn, or Mn absorption or balance in pigs fed either 10% oat hulls or 20% wheat bran, but the salinomycin increased P absorption, but not retention, in pigs fed 20% wheat bran (Moore et al., 1986a).

X. NONSTARCH POLYSACCHARIDE AND OLIGOSACCHARIDE EFFECTS ON HEALTH OF SWINE

Dietary fiber seems to play a role in the health of swine. Watts and Moser (1979) reviewed results of several trials where ground whole oats were included in the diets of 2- to 4-week-old weaned pigs. They concluded that the optimal level of oats in the diets to minimize the chance of nutritional scours was 20 to 40%. However, Pluske et al. (1996) established that symptoms of swine dysentery in swine after experimental infection with *Serpulina hyodsyenteriae* were reduced by feeding diets low in soluble NSP, OS, and/or resistant starch. Subsequent research (Pluske et al., 1998) confirmed the role of fermentable carbohydrates (guar gum and resistant starch) entering the large intestine in the pathogenesis of swine dysentery.

XI. NONSTARCH POLYSACCHARIDE EFFECTS ON SOWS

Gestating sows are excellent candidates to receive high-NSP-containing diets. Limit-fed gestating sows derive more energy from fibrous feedstuffs than growing pigs allowed *ad libitum* access to feed. Sows have a higher fermentation capacity in the hindgut than do growing pigs. The low feeding rate and subsequent slow rate of passage results in an increased fermentation rate in sows (Shi and Noblet, 1993). Also, sows can consume more of a concentrate diet than necessary to meet their energy requirement during gestation (Weldon et al., 1994). This excess feed intake capacity can be exploited by offering sows low-energy, bulky feeds.

A. Effects of Nonstarch Polysaccharides on Reproductive Performance

Several researchers have studied the effects of NSP in sow gestation diets during the last 25 years. There are individual studies that show no change in sow reproductive performance due to added NSP in the diet, some show negative results, and others show positive results. This discrepancy makes it difficult for producers and nutritionists to decide whether to add fiber to sow gestation diets. Part of the reason for the mixed results is the large variation often observed in reproductive data. Large numbers of sows are needed per diet to detect diet effects and to avoid drawing inaccurate conclusions. For example, at least 98 sows are needed per diet to detect a 10% difference in litter size (about 1 pig/litter) between two diets 90% of the time at a statistical probability level of $P < 0.05$. Moreover, to detect a 5% difference in litter size (about 0.5 pig/litter) among diets, at least 388 sows would be required per diet (Cromwell et al., 1989). Another reason for the inconsistent results is that factors other than the elevated cell wall content of fibrous feeds may be important. For example, differences in amino acid, vitamin, and trace mineral content could exert influence.

Published reports were examined to compile a summary of the effects of added NSP in the diet during gestation. Data from sows fed control and high-fiber diets were collected. When multiple levels of the same fiber source were fed within the same study, the treatment means for all levels of added fiber were averaged to obtain one mean for sows fed the fibrous diets. Mean responses for sow and litter performance were weighted according to the number of litters in the study. The summary is shown in Tables 7.3 and 7.4. Researchers have used a variety of feedstuffs ($n = 17$) to provide additional NSP in the sow diet. The range in the amount of fibrous feedstuffs added to the diet to supply NSP is from 5.0 to 97.5% of the diet. The average amount of the NSP source in the diet was 45.4%.

Weight gain during gestation for sows fed high amounts of NSP was about 2 kg less than for sows fed low amounts of NSP (Table 7.3). Sows fed diets high in NSP may have gained less weight during gestation because of a combination of factors. In some studies, sows fed fibrous diets did not consume their allotment of feed or they were not given extra feed to compensate for the lower dietary energy density of the fibrous diets. Also, due to the negative effect of NSP on nutrient digestibility (Etienne, 1987; Girard et al., 1995), sows fed diets high in NSP possibly had fewer nutrients available for growth.

Sow weight loss and feed intake during lactation differed by 2 and 0.2 kg, respectively, between sows fed diets containing low and high amounts of NSP. The slightly reduced weight loss by sows fed the high-NSP diets and their small increase in feed intake during lactation may have been related to their lower weight gain during pregnancy. Sows that gain less weight during gestation generally consume more feed and lose less weight during lactation (Weldon et al., 1994).

Adding NSP to the sow diet during gestation seemed to improve sow longevity. A greater percentage (57 vs. 66%) of sows fed the high-NSP diets during gestation successfully completed the experiments than those fed the control diets. Of the eight studies that reported the percentage of sows that completed the experiment, a positive result was observed in four.

The number of pigs born alive and weaned seemed to be improved when NSP was added to the sow diet during gestation (Table 7.4). The number of pigs born alive and weaned was increased by 0.4 and 0.5 pigs/litter, respectively, by feeding the sow additional NSP. Pig preweaning survival rate was similar (data not shown). Average pig weight at birth and at weaning was similar for sows fed diets containing a low or a high level of NSP during gestation. Of the 19 studies included in the summary where the number of pigs born alive was reported, there were 6 in which the response to feeding fiber to sows was either negative (sows fed high-fiber diets farrowed fewer pigs than those fed a control diet) or zero. In the other 13 studies, the increase in the number of pigs born alive ranged from 0.1 to 2.3 pigs/litter.

As mentioned previously, there are factors other than NSP level in many feedstuffs (e.g., amino acids, vitamins, and trace minerals) that can exert influence on sow reproductive performance. Thus, it is difficult to infer a direct relationship between increased NSP or fiber intake during gestation and improved sow reproductive performance.

TABLE 7.3
Effects of Added NSP in the Gestation Diet on Sow Reproductive Performance

Researcher	NSP Source[b]	Dietary Level (%)	No. of Litters	Gestation Weight Gain (kg) −[c]	Gestation Weight Gain (kg) +[c]	Lactation Weight Change (kg) −[c]	Lactation Weight Change (kg) +[c]	Lactation Feed Intake (kd/d) −[c]	Lactation Feed Intake (kd/d) +[c]	Completion Rate (%)[a] −[c]	Completion Rate (%)[a] +[c]
Baker et al., 1974	Dehy	5	87	33.6	33.5	−6.0	−5.2	4.3	4.4	60.7	65.6
Thong et al., 1978	DDGS	31	64	45.9	44.5	−5.3	−2.6	4.4	3.9		
Pollmann et al., 1981	AH	50	230	26.3	16.8	−6.6	−3.4	5.0	5.1	66.0	88.6
Young and King, 1981	WhS	98	96			0.0	1.0				
Pond et al., 1985	Dehy; CCb	30	24	50.9	44.0			4.3	4.6		
Holzgraefe et al., 1986	AH/OGH	46	86	26.0	27.2			4.8	5.6	45.8	37.5
Lopez et al., 1986	PPH	60	23	33.4	33.9	−5.6	−6.2				
Mroz et al., 1986	OH	45	35	26.5	42.7	−2.1	−13.1				
Carter et al., 1987	AH; SfH	36	144	45.0	45.5	−2.2	−0.2	5.3	5.5	58.0	57.0
Hogen, 1988	AHyl	53	110	37.3	32.7	−4.4	−7.8	5.3	6.0	30.4	54.1
Lopez et al., 1988	PPH	80	58	37.1	24.4	−5.0	−2.1				
Honeyman and Zimmerman, 1990	CGF	93	193	28.0	28.0	2.0	6.5	5.6	5.9		
Mroz and Tarkowski, 1991	SM	10	24			−12.4	−15.1				
Nelson et al., 1992a	SyH	19	35	53.9	54.3	−6.3	−6.1	4.5	5.1		
Nelson et al., 1992b	AHyl	40	24	44.0	36.6	−4.9	−1.2	6.1	6.3		
Matte et al., 1994	WhB; CCb	48	61	57.6	61.0	−19.9	−22.4	5.6	5.5	70.0	68.0
Monegue and Cromwell, 1995	DDCS; CGF	60	90	36.0	40.3	−5.0	−10.8	5.4	5.1		
Ewan et al., 1996	WhSw	14	699	40.0	36.0	−4.0	−4.0	5.7	5.8	47.5	48.0
Farmer et al., 1996	OH	49	48					4.5	4.8		
Vestergaard and Danielsen, 1998	SBP; GM; WhB; OH	50	335	37.3	38.5	−8.0	−8.0	5.9	6.0	80.0	90.0
Total or average (weighted)		45	2487	37.2	35.6	−5.0	−3.1	5.4	5.6	56.5	66.3

[a] Number of females that completed the study/number assigned to each treatment.

[b] *Abbreviations:* Dehy, dehydrated alfalfa meal; DDGS, distillers dried grains with solubles; AH, alfalfa hay; WhS, wheat shorts; CCb, corn cobs; OGH, orchard grass hay; PPH, perennial peanut hay; OH, oat hulls; SfH, sunflower hulls; AHyl, alfalfa haylage; CGF, corn gluten feed; SM, sida meal; SyH, soybean hulls; WhB, wheat bran; WhSw, wheat straw; SBP, sugar beet pulp; GM, grass meal.

[c] Without (−) or with (+) added NSP in the gestation diet.

TABLE 7.4
Effects of Added NSP in the Gestation Diet on Litter Performance

Researcher	NSP Source[a]	Dietary Level (%)	No. of Litters	Live Pigs Born/Litter −[b]	Live Pigs Born/Litter +[b]	No. of Pigs Weaned/Litter −[b]	No. of Pigs Weaned/Litter +[b]	Birth Weight (kg) −[b]	Birth Weight (kg) +[b]	Weaning Weight (kg) −[b]	Weaning Weight (kg) +[b]
Baker et al., 1974	Dehy	5	87	9.7	8.4	8.4	7.3	1.4	1.4	7.0	7.2
Thong et al., 1978	DDGS	31	64	8.8	8.4	7.3	7.4	1.4	1.4	6.5	6.7
Pollmann et al., 1981	AH	50	230	11.2	11.6	7.9	9.0	1.5	1.4	3.9	3.8
Young and King, 1981	WhS	98	96	9.6	10.2	7.2	8.4	1.3	1.2	4.7	4.6
Pond et al., 1985	Dehy; CCb	30	24	8.1	9.1	7.6	8.3	1.4	1.3	6.6	6.5
Holzgraefe et al., 1986	AH/OGH	46	86	10.1	10.2	8.2	9.1	1.5	1.5	3.7	3.7
Lopez et al., 1986	PPH	60	23	8.5	10.6	6.7	6.3	1.3	1.2	5.2	5.6
Mroz et al., 1986	OH	45	35	9.5	11.8	8.0	9.9	1.5	1.6	5.9	5.9
Carter et al., 1987	AH; SfH	36	144	9.1	10.2	8.1	9.2	1.7	1.5	6.3	6.1
Hagen, 1988	AHyl	53	110	9.8	10.6	8.1	9.1	1.5	1.4	5.6	5.5
Lopez et al., 1988	PPH	80	58	10.3	10.1	7.5	7.1	1.4	1.2	5.1	4.5
Honeyman and Zimmerman, 1990	CGF	93	193	10.2	11.0	7.7	8.3	1.5	1.3	5.2	4.9
Mroz and Tarkowski, 1991	SM	10	24	10.2	9.4			1.3	1.4		
Nelson et al., 1992a	SyH	19	35	9.2	8.4	8.3	7.6	1.5	1.6	5.6	6.5
Nelson et al., 1992b	AHyl	40	24	9.3	10.2	8.5	9.3	1.5	1.5	6.7	6.4
Matte et al., 1994	WhB; CCb	48	61	8.9	9.6	9.0	9.0	1.5	1.5	6.2	6.0
Monegue and Cromwell, 1995	DDCS; CGF	60	90	10.0	10.1	9.4	8.7	1.5	1.4	6.9	7.2
Ewan et al., 1996	WhSw	14	699	9.8	10.3	8.4	9.1	1.5	1.5	7.3	7.0
Farmer et al., 1996	OH	49	48					1.2	1.3	5.5	5.8
Vestergaard and Danielsen, 1998	SBP; GM; WhB OH	50	335	10.8	10.8	9.5	9.3	1.6	1.5	8.4	8.3
Total or average (weighted)		45	2487	10.0	10.4	8.3	8.8	1.5	1.5	6.3	6.3

[a] *Abbreviations:* Dehy, dehydrated alfalfa meal; DDGS, distillers dried grains with solubles; AH, alfalfa hay; WhS, wheat shorts; CCb, corn cobs; OGH, orchard grass hay; PPH, perennial peanut hay; OH, oat hulls; SfH, sunflower hulls; AHyl, alfalfa haylage; CGF, corn gluten feed; SM, sida meal; SyH, soybean hulls; WhB, wheat bran; WhSw, wheat straw; SBP, sugar beet pulp; GM, grass meal.
[b] Without (−) or with (+) added NSP in the gestation diet.

Using wheat straw as a source of fiber may be the best method to determine if fiber intake in gestation per se, not other factors such as differences in sow nutrient intake, benefit sow reproductive performance. Wheat straw has an energy content close to zero for sows and growing pigs and is, therefore, a fairly nonfermentable source of fiber (Shi and Noblet, 1993). Ewan et al. (1996) utilized wheat straw as the source of added fiber, and the number of pigs born alive and weaned was improved by 0.5 and 0.7 pigs/litter, respectively. Sow energy and nutrient intake during gestation were not confounded with the effect of fiber in the diet. In addition, the control diet and the diet with added fiber were supplemented with folic acid and biotin, which are known to increase litter size (Lindemann and Kornegay, 1989; Thaler et al., 1989; Lewis et al., 1991). These results tend to support the concept that fiber per se in the gestation diet improves reproductive performance in sows.

There is no strong evidence to show that increasing the NSP level in the lactation diet improves sow reproductive performance. However, some producers include high-NSP-containing ingredients such as sugar beet pulp, alfalfa, oats, wheat bran, or psyllium in the sow diet to control constipation. These ingredients have a high water-holding capacity and can act as a laxative. Sows that are constipated consume less feed in lactation and may have more milking problems. Often sows are constipated because they are not given enough feed the first few days after farrowing, or they are too hot. If sows are constipated, it is recommended that they (1) be offered more feed after farrowing, (2) be allowed to exercise, or (3) have their thermal comfort improved, before adding a laxative to the diet (Reese et al., 1992; 1995).

Energy requirements during lactation are much higher than they are during gestation. Sows that are unable to maximize energy intake during lactation often lose excessive body weight and have reproductive problems. Thus, it is important to limit the amount of ingredients such as sugar beet pulp, alfalfa, oats, and wheat bran to about 10% of the diet to avoid reducing the energy density of the diet excessively (Reese et al., 1995).

B. Effects of Nonstarch Polysaccharide Source on Reproductive Performance

Establishing whether the source of the NSP is important for improved sow and litter performance would enable producers and nutritionists to make better decisions about feeding gestating sows. However, only a limited number of studies have been conducted where different sources of NSP were compared. Comparisons have been made between wheat straw and soybean hulls (Mroz and Tarkowski, 1991), alfalfa hay and prairie hay (Danielson and Noonan, 1975), alfalfa hay and alfalfa meal (Danielson and Noonan, 1975), alfalfa meal and corn cobs (Pond et al., 1985), and sugar beet pulp and a mixture of grass meal, wheat bran, and oat hulls (Vestergaard and Danielsen, 1998). These studies do not provide conclusive evidence that sow and litter performance is affected by source of NSP in the diet.

Better decisions regarding feeding fiber to gestating sows could be made if the response in sow and litter performance for each unit of additional NSP consumed were known. However, few dose titration studies have been conducted with NSP in gestation diets. Therefore, an optimal level of NSP in the diet cannot be recommended.

C. Effects of Nonstarch Polysaccharides on Sow Behavior

Recently, a significant amount of attention has been given to stereotypic behavior in sows. Stereotypic behavior is repeated behavior having no apparent purpose (Lawrence and Terlouw, 1993). According to the Commission of the European Communities (cited by Brouns et al., 1994a), stereotypic behavior is an indicator of reduced welfare of sows in individual housing systems.

Common types of stereotypic behavior observed in sows are bar biting, sham chewing, and excessive adjunctive drinking (Appleby and Lawrence, 1987; Robert et al., 1993). There are thought to be certain biological consequences to stereotypic behavior in sows, including increased metabolic rate and poorer feed conversion (Cronin et al., 1986). In addition, these sows may be more prone to the thin sow syndrome (Cariolet and Dantzer, 1984). It is possible that sow reproductive performance is impaired in sows prone to, or that exhibit, stereotypic behavior during gestation.

Researchers have linked feed restriction to the development of stereotypic behavior in gestating sows. In practice, gestating sows are given quantities of feed much lower than they are capable of consuming (Weldon et al., 1994). This leaves sows with a heightened feeding motivation, which they deal with through performing stereotypic behavior (Lawrence and Terlouw, 1993). Feeding motivation was measured in one study by providing sows either a low or high rate of feed during 3 months of gestation (Terlouw et al., 1991). Eating rate remained low and constant in the sows fed the high rate of feed, but increased in sows fed the low rate of feed as time progressed.

Attempts have been made to increase the bulk density and change the composition of the sow gestation diet to reduce hunger and feeding motivation. Sows fed a diet containing 50% unmolassed sugar beet pulp spent significantly less time licking the floor or trough, bar-biting, or sham chewing during the first 1.5 h after feeding than sows fed a conventional gestation diet (Brouns et al., 1994a). In another study (Robert et al., 1993), gilts were fed either a low-fiber diet (corn–soybean meal), a high fiber diet (wheat bran and corn cobs), or a very high fiber diet (oat hulls and oats) during two gestations. The total daily intake of major nutrients was calculated to be similar for all gilts. During both parities, the fiber-dense diets reduced the incidence of stereotypes, time spent drinking, and water intake. Gilts fed the bulky diets consumed 59% less water than those fed the corn–soybean meal diet. The authors indicated that the increased water intake by gilts fed the corn–soybean meal diet was not controlled by normal physiological mechanisms. Rather, the excessive water intake served to distend the stomach. Reduced water consumption may have positive benefits for producers when dealing with manure disposal. In addition, the authors presented evidence that feeding sows high-fiber diets to reduce feeding motivation and improve welfare is effective only if the diet meets the nutritional requirements of the sow.

Dietary sources of NSP differ in the behavioral and metabolic responses they elicit in sows. Voluntary feed intake of gestating sows provided *ad libitum* access to a diet containing a high level of unmolassed sugar beet pulp was low in comparison to those provided diets containing a high level of other fibrous feed ingredients, and more time was necessary for the sows to consume the sugar beet–based diet (Brouns et al., 1997). Adding sugar beet pulp to the gestation diet resulted in significantly different serum acetate, glucose, and insulin (Brouns et al., 1994b) and glucose and insulin (Vestergaard and Danielsen, 1998) profiles than those observed when other, less fermentable sources of NSP were included in the diet. These shifts in blood metabolite and hormone profiles probably explain the observed differences in sow feed intake and behavior when NSP were increased in the diet. In addition, feed intake and behavior will be affected by an increase in gastric distention and intestinal fill caused by consuming diets high in NSP.

Bulky diets containing a high level of NSP seem to result in a sow that is more "satisfied" after consuming a meal than one fed typical corn or milo–soybean meal diets. The same situation has been observed in breeding boars. The financial and production consequences of having more satisfied or docile breeding animals have not been examined.

XII. PRACTICAL CONSIDERATIONS IN FEEDING NONSTARCH POLYSACCHARIDES

A. Diet Formulation and Feeding Management

For optimal results when using fibrous feeds in pig diets, it is important to note some key details. Digestion coefficients of high-fiber ingredients obtained from limit-fed sows are greater than those obtained from growing pigs. In contrast, digestion coefficients of low-fiber ingredients are similar for sows and growing pigs (Shi and Noblet, 1993; Etienne, 1987). Thus, digestible and metabolizable energy values of feedstuffs are not constant, but they vary according to the physiological stage and body weight of the animal, and the feeding level. Most nutritional values for feedstuffs and diets have been measured with growing pigs (Noblet and Shi, 1993), but some information on fibrous feed ingredients for sows is available (Boyd et al., 1976; Pollmann et al., 1979; Noblet et al., 1989; Shi and Noblet, 1993). In addition, equations are available for predicting the nutritive value of sow diets using data derived from growing pigs (Noblet and Shi, 1993).

Digestion coefficients for dry matter, cell wall constituents, energy, and crude protein are reduced when fiber is added to diets (Etienne, 1987). Also, dry matter, gross energy, and fiber digestion of alfalfa hay is increased when particle size is reduced from 12.5 to 6.25 mm (Nuzback et al., 1984).

Gestating sows fed restricted quantities of a bulky diet require more time to eat their ration (Robert et al., 1993; Brouns et al., 1994a). In addition, sows fed high-fiber diets must be given more feed than sows fed high-energy diets to meet their energy requirement. Diets containing fibrous feedstuffs have a lower bulk density (kg/m^3) than simple grain–soybean meal diets. Therefore, it is necessary to increase not only the weight but also the volume of feed offered for the sow to consume a sufficient amount of nutrients. When feed is provided to sows using an automated feed-delivery system with "feed drop boxes," it is necessary to adjust the settings on the boxes so they deliver more feed when a high-fiber diet is used. Otherwise, sows will not be able to consume enough energy and other nutrients to gain an adequate amount of weight and condition during gestation. In some cases, it will not be possible to feed high-fiber diets once daily through feed-delivery systems with "feed boxes" because the boxes are too small to hold the daily feed allotment. In that case, divide the sows' daily allotment of feed by two and feed them twice daily. In feeding systems where scoops and buckets are used to handle feed, a greater volume of feed is also required.

B. POSSIBLE PHYSICAL LIMITATIONS TO FEEDING HIGH-NONSTARCH POLYSACCHARIDE DIETS

In addition to direct economic and pig performance considerations, other factors may limit the ability of producers to use fibrous feeds in pig diets. Some on-farm feed-mixing and feed-handling equipment cannot physically handle fibrous feed ingredients. Moreover, grinding and handling certain fibrous ingredients is time-consuming and dusty. The increased bulkiness of high fiber diets may cause bridging in bulk bins, feeders, and feed drop boxes. However, many of the handling and storage problems associated with high-fiber ingredients and feeds can be reduced by pelleting.

Costs associated with manure handling may increase due to the larger volume of solids produced by pigs fed high-fiber diets. Also, handling liquid manure may be more difficult because of larger, undigested feed particles and less liquid present in the slurry due to the pigs drinking less water (Lee and Close, 1987). Some producers report that the undigested portion of the hull from oats is particularly problematic to remove from manure storage devices.

XIII. EFFECTS OF NONSTARCH POLYSACCHARIDES ON AMMONIA EMISSION

In some areas of the world, ammonia emission from livestock operations is considered a threat to the environment. Urea excreted via the urine is a major source of ammonia emitted to the atmosphere. Ammonia and carbon dioxide are released from urea by the action of urease present in feces. The amount of ammonia released is primarily a function of urinary urea concentration, and the pH and temperature of the slurry (Cahn et al., 1998).

The addition of NSP to pig diets shifts how N is excreted from the body. Pigs that consume more NSP excrete less N via the urine in the form of urea and more N via the feces in the form of microbial protein. Because the N in microbial protein is more stable and less volatile than N in urea, less ammonia is emitted from the slurry (Cahn et al., 1998).

Ammonia emission from the slurry also is reduced due to the increased microbial activities in the hindgut of pigs fed diets containing NSP. When the amount of fermentable NSP in the diet is increased, VFA production increases, which lowers the pH of the feces and slurry. A lower pH is associated with lower ammonia emission. For each 100-g increase in the intake of dietary NSP, pH of the slurry decreased by about 0.12 units, and the ammonia emission from the slurry deceased by 54%. Soybean hulls were more effective at lowering pH and ammonia emission than sugar beet pulp or coconut expeller (Cahn et al., 1998).

These results provide strong evidence that manipulating the level and source of NSP in pig diets can have a significant impact on the amount of ammonia emitted from pork producing operations. However, further research is needed to verify the benefits of increasing NSP level in pig diets on ammonia emission in practical situations. More information about the potential environmental pollution problems as affected by swine nutrition is presented in Chapter 27.

XIV. SUMMARY

Due to the increasing interest by the swine industry to utilize nontraditional and by-product feeds more fully, and the fact that these feedstuffs commonly contain high levels of NSPs and oligosaccharides, a thorough understanding of these compounds is necessary. Improvements in analytical techniques enable researchers and nutritionists to characterize and quantify both the NSP and oligosaccharide contents of feed ingredients accurately. Although, as demonstrated in this chapter, NSPs can impact digestion and utilization of nutrients such as amino acids, lipids, and minerals, with proper dietary modification diets containing ingredients high in NSPs and oligosaccharides can be efficiently utilized for both the growing pig and the gestating sow.

REFERENCES

Anugwa, F. O. I., V. H. Varel, J. S. Dickson, W. G. Pond, and L. P. Krook. 1989. Effects of dietary fiber and protein concentration on growth, feed efficiency, visceral organ weights and large intestine microbial populations of swine, *J. Nutr.*, 119:879.

AOAC. 1984. *Official Methods of Analysis*, 14th ed., Association of Official Analytical Chemists, Arlington, VA.

Appleby, M. C., and A. B. Lawrence. 1987. Food restriction as a cause of stereotyped behavior in tethered gilts, *Anim. Prod.*, 45:103.

Asp, N.-G., C.-G. Johansson, H. Hallmer, and M. Siljestrom. 1983. Rapid enzymatic assay of insoluble and soluble dietary fiber, *J. Agric. Food Chem.*, 31:476.

Baker, D. H., D. E. Becker, A. H. Jensen, and B. G. Harmon. 1968. Effect of dietary dilution on performance of finishing swine, *J. Anim. Sci.*, 27:1332.

Baker, D. H., B. A. Molitoris, A. H. Jensen, and B. G. Harmon. 1974. Sequence of protein feeding and value of alfalfa meal and fish meal for pregnant gilts and sows, *J. Anim. Sci.*, 38:325.

Bohman, V. R., J. E. Hunter, and J. McCormick. 1955. The effect of graded levels of alfalfa and aureomycin upon growing-fattening swine, *J. Anim. Sci.*, 14:499.

Borel, P., D. Lairon, M. Senft, M. Chautan, and H. Lafont. 1989. Wheat bran and wheat germ: effect on digestion and intestinal absorption of dietary lipids in the rat, *Am. J. Clin. Nutr.*, 49:1192.

Boyd, R. D., T. D. Crenshaw, B. D. Moser, E. R. Peo, Jr., and D. M. Danielson. 1976. Nutritional value of the energy and nitrogen content of sun-cured alfalfa for gilts and sows, *J. Anim. Sci.*, 42:1348 (Abstr.).

Brouns, F., S. A. Edwards, and P. R. English. 1994a. Effect of dietary fibre and feeding system on activity and oral behavior of group housed gilts, *Appl. Anim. Behav. Sci.*, 39:215.

Brouns, F., S. A. Edwards, and P. R. English. 1994b. Metabolic effects of fibrous ingredients in pig diets, *Anim. Prod.*, 58:467 (Abstr.).

Brouns, F., S. A. Edwards, and P. R. English. 1997. The effect of dietary inclusion of sugar-beet pulp on the feeding behavior of dry sows, *Anim. Sci.*, 65:129.

Brüll, L., M. Huisman, H. Schols, F. Voragen, G. Critchley, J. Thomas-Oats, and J. Haverkamp. 1998. Rapid molecular mass and structural determination of plant cell wall-derived oligosaccharides using off-line high-performance anion-exchange chromatography/mass spectrometry, *J. Mass Spectrom.*, 33:713.

Cahn, T. T., A. L. Sutton, A. J. A. Aarnink, M. W. A. Verstegen, J. W. Schrama, and G. C. M. Bakker. 1998. Dietary carbohydrates alter the fecal composition and pH and the ammonia emission from slurry of growing pigs, *J. Anim. Sci.*, 76:1887.

Campbell, J. M., L. L. Bauer, G. C. Fahey, Jr., A. J. C. L. Hogarth, B. W. Wolf, and D. E. Hunter. 1997a. Selected fructooligosaccharide (1-kestose, nystose, and 1^F-β-fructofuranosylnystose) composition of foods and feeds, *J. Agric. Food Chem.*, 45:3076.

Campbell, J. M., E. A. Flickinger, and G. C. Fahey, Jr. 1997b. A comparative study of dietary fiber methodologies using pulsed electrochemical detection of monosaccharide constituents, *Sem. Food Anal.*, 2:43.

Campbell, R. G., and M. R. Taverner. 1986. The effects of dietary fibre, source of fat and dietary energy concentration on the voluntary food intake and performance of growing pigs, *Anim. Prod.*, 43:327.

Cariolet, R., and R. Dantzer. 1984. Motor activity of pregnant tethered sows, *Ann. Rech. Vet.*, 15:257.

Carter, D. I., J. D. Crenshaw, P. M. Swantek, R. L. Harrold, and R. C. Zimprich. 1987. The effect of fiber intake by gravid swine during three consecutive parities on sow and litter performance, *J. Anim. Sci.*, 65(Suppl. 1):89.

Cho, S. S., L. Prosky, and M. Dreher. 1999. Total carbohydrates and total dietary fiber content in grain-based foods (Appendix II). In *Complex Carbohydrates in Foods*, Cho, S. S., L. Prosky, and M. Dreher, Eds., Marcel Dekker, New York, 609.

Coffey, M. T., R. W. Seerley, D. W. Funderburke, and H. C. McCampbell. 1982. Effect of heat increment and level of dietary energy and environmental temperature on the performance of growing-finishing swine, *J. Anim. Sci.*, 54:95.

Costa, N. M. B., A. F. Walker, and A. G. Low. 1993. The effect of graded inclusion of baked beans (*Phaseolus vulgaris*) on plasma and liver lipids in hypercholesterolaemic pigs given a Western-type diet, *Br. J. Nutr.*, 70:515.

Costa, N. M. B., A. G. Low, A. F. Walker, R. W. Owen, and H. N. Englyst. 1994. Effect of baked beans (*Phaseolus vulgaris*) on steroid metabolism and non-starch polysaccharide output of hypercholesterolaemic pigs with or without an ileo-rectal anastomosis, *Br. J. Nutr.*, 71:871.

Cromwell, G. L., D. D. Hall, G. E. Combs, O. M. Hale, D. L. Handlin, J. P. Hitchcock, D. A. Knabe, E. T. Kornegay, M. D. Lindemann, C. V. Maxwell, and T. J. Prince. 1989. Effects of dietary salt level during gestation and lactation on reproductive performance of sows: a cooperative study, *J. Anim. Sci.*, 67:374.

Cronin, G. M., J. M. F. M. Van Tartwijk, W. Van der Hel, and M. W. A. Verstegen. 1986. The influence of degree of adaptation to tether-housing by sows in relation to behavior and energy metabolism, *Anim. Prod.*, 42:257.

Danielson, D. M., and J. J. Noonan. 1975. Roughages in swine gestation diets, *J. Anim. Sci.*, 41:94.

Davis, M. E., C. V. Maxwell, E. B. Kegley, B. Z. de Rodas, K. G. Friesen, D. H. Hellwig, and R. A. Dvorak. 1999. Efficacy of mannan oligosaccharide (Bio-Mos) addition at two levels of supplemental copper on performance and immunocompetence of early weaned pigs, *J. Anim. Sci.*, 76(Suppl. 1):63 (Abstr.).

Den Hartog, L. A., J. Huisman, W. J.G. Thielen, G. H. A. Van Schayk, H. Boer, and E. J. Van Weerden. 1988. The effect of including various structural polysaccharides in pig diets on ileal and faecal digestibility of amino acids and minerals, *Livest. Prod. Sci.*, 18:157.

Dierick, N. A., I. J. Vervaeke, D. I. Demeyer, and J. A. Decuypere. 1989. Approach to the energetic importance of fibre digestion in pigs. I. Importance of fermentation in the overall energy supply, *Anim. Feed Sci. Technol.*, 23:141.

Dreher, M. 1999. Food sources and uses of dietary fiber. In *Complex Carbohydrates in Foods*, Cho, S. S., L. Prosky, and M. Dreher, Eds., Marcel Dekker, New York, 327.

Eggum, B. O., G. Thorbek, R. M. Beames, A. Chwalibog, and S. Henckel. 1982. Influence of diet and microbial activity in the digestive tract on digestibility, and nitrogen and energy metabolism in rats and pigs, *Br. J. Nutr.*, 48:161.

Elsden S. R., M. W. S. Hitchcock, R. A. Marshall, and A. T. Phillipson. 1946. Volatile acid in the digesta of ruminants and other animals, *J. Exp. Biol.*, 22:191.

Englyst, H. N., and J. H. Cummings. 1988. Improved method for measurement of dietary fiber as non-starch polysaccharides in plant foods, *J. Assoc. Off. Anal. Chem.*, 71:808.

Englyst, H. N., and G. J. Hudson. 1993. Dietary fiber and starch: classification and measurement. In *CRC Handbook of Dietary Fiber in Human Nutrition*, Spiller, G. A., Ed., CRC Press, Boca Raton, FL, 53.

Etienne, M. 1987. Utilization of high fibre feeds and cereals by sows, a review, *Livest. Prod. Sci.*, 16:229.

Ewan, R. C., J. D. Crenshaw, T. D. Crenshaw, G. L. Cromwell, R. A. Easter, J. L. Nelssen, E. R. Miller, J. E. Pettigrew, and T. L. Veum. 1996. Effect of addition of fiber to gestation diets on reproductive performance of sows, *J. Anim. Sci.*, 74(Suppl. 1):190.

Fadel, J. G., R. K. Newman, C. W. Newman, and H. Graham. 1989. Effects of baking hulless barley on the digestibility of dietary components as measured at the ileum and in the feces in pigs, *J. Nutr.*, 119:722.

Fahey, G. C., Jr., G. R. Frank, A. H. Jensen, and S. S. Masters. 1980. Influence of various purified and isolated cell wall fibers on the utilization of certain nutrients by swine and hamsters, *J. Food Sci.*, 45:1675.

Farmer, C., S. Robert, and J. J. Matte. 1996. Lactation performance of sows fed a bulky diet during gestation and receiving growth hormone-releasing factor during lactation, *J. Anim. Sci.*, 74:1298.

Farrell, D. J., and K. A. Johnson. 1970. Utilization of cellulose by pigs and its effects on caecal function, *Anim. Prod.*, 14:209.

Frank, G. R., F. X. Aherne, and A. H. Jensen. 1983. A study of the relationship between performance and dietary component digestibilities by swine fed different levels of dietary fiber, *J. Anim. Sci.*, 57:645.

Freire, J. P. B., J. Peiniau, L. F. Cunha, J. A. A. Almeida, and A. Aumaitre. 1998. Comparative effects of dietary fat and fibre in Alentejano and Large White piglets: digestibility, digestive enzymes and metabolic data, *Livest. Prod. Sci.*, 53:37.

Gabert, V. W., W. C. Sauer, R. Mosenthin, M. Schmitz, and F. Ahrens. 1995. The effect of oligosaccharides and lactitiol on the ileal digestibility of amino acids, monosaccharides and bacterial populations and metabolites in the small intestine of weanling pigs, *Can. J. Anim. Sci.*, 75:99.

Girard, C. L., S. Robert, J. J. Matte, C. Farmer, and G. P. Martineau. 1995. Influence of high fibre diets given to gestating sows on serum concentration of micronutrients, *Livest. Prod. Sci.*, 43:15.

Giusi-Perier, A., M. Fiszlewicz, and A. Rérat. 1989. Influence of diet composition on intestinal volatile fatty acid and nutrient absorption in unanesthetized pigs, *J. Anim. Sci.*, 67:386.

Goodlad, J. S., and J. C. Mathers. 1991. Digestion by pigs of non-starch polysaccharides in wheat and raw peas (*Pisum sativum*) fed in mixed diets, *Br. J. Nutr.*, 65:259.

Graham, H., K. Hesselman, and P. Åman. 1986. The influence of wheat bran and sugar-beet pulp on the digestibility of dietary components in a cereal-based pig diet, *J. Nutr.*, 116:242.

Hagen, C. D. 1988. Alfalfa Haylage for Gestating Swine, Ph.D. dissertation, University of Minnesota, St. Paul.

Henry, R. J., and H. S. Saini. 1989. Characterization of cereal sugars and oligosaccharides, *Cereal Chem.*, 66:362.

Holzgraefe, D. P., A. H. Jensen, G. C. Fahey, Jr., and R. R. Grummer. 1986. Effects of dietary alfalfa-orchardgrass hay and lasalocid on sow reproductive performance, *J. Anim. Sci.*, 62:1145.

Honeyman, M. S., and D. R. Zimmerman. 1990. Long-term effects of corn gluten feed on the reproductive performance and weight of gestating sows, *J. Anim. Sci.*, 68:1329.

Houdijk, J. G. M., M. W. Bosch, M. W. A. Verstegen, and H. J. Berenpas. 1998. Effects of dietary oligosaccharides on the growth performance and faecal characteristics of young growing pigs, *Anim. Feed Sci. Technol.*, 71:35.

Howard, M. D., D. T. Gordon, L. W. Pace, K. A. Garleb, and M. S. Kerley. 1995. Effect of dietary supplementation with fructooligosaccharide on colonic microbiota populations and epithelial cell proliferation in neonatal pigs, *J. Pediatr. Gastroenterol. Nutr.*, 21:297.

Howard, M. D., H. Liu, J. D. Spencer, M. S. Kerley, and G. L. Allee. 1999. Incorporation of short-chain fructooligosaccharides and Tylan® into the diets of early weaned pigs, *J. Anim. Sci.*, 77(Suppl. 1):63 (Abstr.).

Imoto, S., and S. Namioka. 1978. VFA production in the pig large intestine, *J. Anim. Sci.*, 47:467.

Jeraci, J. L., B. A. Lewis, P. J. Van Soest, and J. B. Robertson. 1989. Urea enzymatic dialysis procedure for determination of total dietary fiber, *J. Assoc. Off. Anal. Chem.*, 72:677.

Jin, L., L. P. Reynolds, D. A. Redmer, J. S. Caton, and J. D. Crenshaw. 1994. Effect of dietary fiber on intestinal growth, cell proliferation, and morphology in growing pigs, *J. Anim. Sci.*, 72:2270.

Johansen, H. N., K. E. B. Knudsen, B. Sandström, and F. Skjøth. 1996. Effects of varying content of soluble dietary fibre from wheat flour and oat milling fractions on gastric emptying in pigs, *Br. J. Nutr.*, 75:339.

Jørgensen, H., X.-Q. Zhao, and B. Eggum. 1996. The influence of dietary fibre and environmental temperature on the development of the gastrointestinal tract, digestibility, degree of fermentation in the hind-gut and energy metabolism in pigs, *Br. J. Nutr.*, 75:365.

Kass, M. L., P. J. Van Soest, and W. G. Pond. 1980a. Utilization of dietary fiber from alfalfa by growing swine. II. Volatile fatty acid concentrations in and disappearance from the gastrointestinal tract, *J. Anim. Sci.*, 50:192.

Kass, M. L., P. J. Van Soest, W. G. Pond, B. Lewis, and R. E. McDowell. 1980b. Utilization of dietary fiber from alfalfa by growing swine. I. Apparent digestibility of diet components in specific segments of the gastrointestinal tract, *J. Anim. Sci.*, 50:175.

Kennelly, J. J., and F. X. Aherne. 1980a. The effect of fiber addition to diets formulated to contain different levels of energy and protein on growth and carcass quality of swine, *Can. J. Anim. Sci.*, 60:385.

Kennelly, J. J., and F. X. Aherne. 1980b. The effect of fiber in diets formulated to contain different levels of energy and protein on digestibility coefficients in swine, *Can. J. Anim. Sci.*, 60:717.

Kennelly, J. J., F. X. Aherne, and W. C. Sauer. 1981. Volatile fatty acid production in the hindgut of swine, *Can. J. Anim. Sci.*, 61:349.

Knudsen, K. E. B., and I. Hansen. 1991. Gastrointestinal implications in pigs of wheat and oat fractions. 1. Digestibility and bulking properties of polysaccharides and other major constituents, *Br. J. Nutr.*, 65:217.

Kornegay, E. T. 1978. Soybean hulls for growing, finishing swine, *Feedstuffs*, 50:24.

Kornegay, E. T. 1981. Soybean hull digestibility by sows and feeding value for growing-finishing swine, *J. Anim. Sci.*, 53:138.

Kornegay, E. T., and R. J. Moore. 1986. Dietary fiber sources may affect mineral use in swine, *Feedstuffs*, 58:36.

Kreuzer, M., U. Heindl, D. A. Roth-Maier, and M. Kirchgessner. 1991. Cellulose fermentation capacity of the hindgut and nitrogen turnover in the hindgut of sows as evaluated by oral and intracecal supply of purified cellulose, *Arch. Anim. Nutr.* (Berlin), 41:359.

Latymer, E. A., and A. G. Low. 1987. Tissue incorporation and excretion of ^{14}C in pigs after injection of [1–^{14}C]- or [2–^{14}C] propionic acid into the caecum, *Proc. Nutr. Soc.*, 43:12A.

Lawrence, A. B., and E. M. C. Terlouw. 1993. A review of behavioral factors involved in the development and continued performance of stereotypic behaviors in pigs, *J. Anim. Sci.*, 71:2815.

Leclere, C., D. Lairon, M. Champ, and C. Cherbut. 1993. Influence of particle size and sources of non-starch polysaccharides on postprandial glycaemia, insulinaemia and triacylglycerolaemia in pigs and starch digestion *in vitro*, *Br. J. Nutr.*, 70:179.

Lee, P. A., and W. H. Close. 1987. Bulky feeds for pigs: a consideration of some non-nutritional aspects, *Livest. Prod. Sci.*, 16:395.

Lee, S. C., R. Vincent, L. Prosky, and D. M. Sullivan. 1996. Evaluating an analytical method for complex carbohydrate determinations, *Cereal Foods World*, 41:64.

Lenis, N. P., P. Bikker, J. van der Meulen, J. Th. M. van Diepen, J. G. M. Bakker, and A. W. Jongbloed. 1996. Effect of dietary neutral detergent fiber on ileal digestibility and portal flux of nitrogen and amino acids and on nitrogen utilization in growing pigs, *J. Anim. Sci.*, 74:2687.

Lewis, A. J., G. L. Cromwell, and J. E. Pettigrew. 1991. Effects of supplemental biotin during gestation and lactation on reproductive performance of sows: a cooperative study, *J. Anim. Sci.*, 69:207.

Li, S., W. C. Sauer, and R. T. Hardin. 1994. Effect of dietary fibre level on amino acid digestibility in young pigs, *Can. J. Anim. Sci.*, 74:327.

Lindemann, M. D., and E. T. Kornegay. 1989. Folic acid supplementation to diets of gestating-lactating swine over multiple parities, *J. Anim. Sci.*, 67:459.

Lindemann, M. D., E. T. Kornegay, and R. J. Moore. 1986. Digestibility and feeding value of peanut hulls for swine, *J. Anim. Sci.*, 62:412.

Longland, A. C., J. Carruthers, and A. G. Low. 1994. The ability of piglets 4 to 8 weeks old to digest and perform on diets containing two contrasting sources of non-starch polysaccharide, *Anim. Prod.*, 58:405.

Lopez, F. D., C. E. White, and E. C. French. 1986. Reproductive performance of sows fed ground perennial peanut hay during gestation, University of Florida Swine Report, p. 54.

Lopez, F. D., C. E. White, and E. C. French. 1988. Reproductive performance of sows fed ground perennial peanut hay during four successive parities, University of Florida Swine Report, p. 104.

Low, A. G. 1989. Secretory response of the pig gut to non-starch polysaccharides, *Anim. Feed Sci. Technol.*, 23:55.

Mason, V. C., Z. Kragelund, and B. O. Eggum. 1982. Influence of fibre and Nebacitin on microbial activity and amino acid digestibility in the pig and the rat, *Z. Tierphysiol. Tierernähr. Futtermittelkd.*, 48:241.

Matte, J. J., S. Robert, C. L. Girard, C. Farmer, and G. P. Martineau. 1994. Effect of bulky diets based on wheat bran or oat hulls on reproductive performance of sows during their first two parities, *J. Anim. Sci.*, 72:1754.

Michel, P., and A. Rérat. 1998. Effect of adding sugar beet fibre and wheat bran to a starch diet on the absorption kinetics of glucose, amino-nitrogen and volatile fatty acids in the pig, *Reprod. Nutr. Dev.*, 38:49.

Modler, H. W., R. C. McKellar, and M. Yaguchi. 1990. Bifidobacteria and bifidogenic factors, *Can. Inst. Food Sci. Technol. J.*, 23:29.

Monegue, H. J., and G. L. Cromwell. 1995. High dietary levels of corn byproducts for gestating sows, *J. Anim. Sci.*, 73(Suppl. 1):86.

Moore, R. J., E. T. Kornegay, and M. D. Lindemann. 1986a. Effect of dietary oat hulls or wheat bran on mineral utilization in growing pigs fed diets with or without salinomycin, *Can. J. Anim. Sci.*, 66:267.

Moore, R. J., E. T. Kornegay, and M. D. Lindemann. 1986b. Effect of salinomycin on nutrient absorption and retention by growing pigs fed corn–soybean meal diets with or without oat hulls or wheat bran, *Can. J. Anim. Sci.*, 66:257.

Mroz, Z., and A. Tarkowski. 1991. The effects of the dietary inclusion of sida meal (*Malvaceae*) for gilts on the reproductive performance, apparent digestibility, rate of passage and plasma parameters, *Livest. Prod. Sci.*, 27:199.

Mroz, Z. M., I. G. Partridge, G. Mitchell, and H. D. Keal. 1986. The effect of oat hulls, added to the basal ration for pregnant sows, on reproductive performance, apparent digestibility, rate of passage and plasma parameters, *J. Sci. Food Agric.*, 37:239.

Myer, R. O., and G. E. Combs. 1991. Fat supplementation of diets containing high level of oats for growing-finishing swine, *J. Anim. Sci.*, 69:4665.

Nelson, D. A., S. M. El Kandelgy, S. G. Cornelius, and R. L. Moser. 1992a. Sows fed alfalfa haylage during gestation perform as well as control animals, *J. Anim. Sci.*, 70(Suppl. 1):71.

Nelson, D. A., M. G. Hogberg, E. R. Miller, and M. S. Allen. 1992b. Wheat straw and soybean hull additions to sow gestation diets during two consecutive parities, Michigan State University Swine Report 9210, p. 91.

Noblet, J., and X. S. Shi. 1993. Comparative digestibility of energy and nutrients in growing pigs fed *ad libitum* and adults sows fed at maintenance, *Livest. Prod. Sci.*, 34:137.

Noblet, J., J. Y. Dourmad, J. L. E. Dividich, and S. Dubois. 1989. Effect of ambient temperature and addition of straw or alfalfa in the diet on energy metabolism in pregnant sows, *Livest. Prod. Sci.*, 21:309.

Noblet, J., X. S. Shi, and S. Dubois. 1994. Effect of body weight on net energy value of feeds for growing pigs, *J. Anim. Sci.*, 72:648.

NRC. 1982. *United States–Canadian Tables of Feed Composition*, 3rd rev., National Academy Press, Washington, D.C.

NRC. 1987. *Predicting Feed Intake of Food-Producing Animals*, National Academy Press, Washington, D.C.

NRC. 1998. *Nutrient Requirements of Swine*, 10th ed., National Academy Press, Washington, D.C.

Nunes, C. S., and K. Malmlöf. 1992. Effects of guar gum and cellulose on glucose absorption, hormonal release and hepatic metabolism in the pig, *Br. J. Nutr.*, 68:693.

Nuzback, L. J., D. S. Pollmann, and K. C. Behnke. 1984. Effect of particle size and physical form of sun-cured alfalfa on digestibility for gravid swine, *J. Anim. Sci.*, 58:378.

Partridge, I. G. 1978. Studies on digestion and absorption in the intestines of growing pigs. 4. Effects of dietary cellulose and sodium levels on mineral absorption, *Br. J. Nutr.*, 39:539.

Partridge, I. G., A. G. Low, I. E. Sambrook, and T. Corring. 1982. The influence of diet on the exocrine pancreatic secretion of growing pigs, *Br. J. Nutr.*, 48:137.

Patil, A. R., and G. C. Fahey, Jr. 1998. Recent advances in canine nutrition research, *Proc. Petfood Forum Eur.*, p. 19.

Pluske, J. R., P. M. Siba, D. W. Pethick, Z. Durmic, B. P. Mullan, and D. J. Hampson. 1996. The incidence of swine dysentery in pigs can be reduced by feeding diets that limit the amount of fermentable substrate entering the large intestine, *J. Nutr.*, 126:2920.

Pluske, J. R., Z. Durmic, D. W. Pethick, B. P. Mullan, and D. J. Hampson. 1998. Confirmation of the role of rapidly fermentable carbohydrates in the expression of swine dysentery in pigs after experimental infection, *J. Nutr.*, 128:1737.

Pollmann, D. S., D. M. Danielson, and E. R. Peo, Jr. 1979. Value of high fiber diets for gravid swine, *J. Anim. Sci.*, 48:1385.

Pollmann, D. S., D. M. Danielson, M. A. Crenshaw, and E. R. Peo, Jr. 1981. Long-term effects of dietary additions of alfalfa and tallow on sow reproductive performance, *J. Anim. Sci.*, 51:294.

Pond, W. G., J. T. Yen, and V. H. Varel. 1985. Effects of level and source of dietary fiber in gestation on reproductive performance and nutrient digestibility in gilts, *Nutr. Rep. Int.*, 32:505.

Pond, W. G., K. R. Pond, W. C. Ellis, and J. H. Matis. 1986. Markers for estimating digesta flow in pigs and the effects of dietary fiber, *J. Anim. Sci.*, 63:1140.

Pond, W. G., H. G. Jung, and V. H. Varel. 1988. Effect of dietary fiber on young adult genetically lean, obese and contemporary pigs: body weight, carcass measurements, organ weights and digesta content, *J. Anim. Sci.*, 66:699.

Potkins, Z. V., T. L. J. Lawrence, and J. R. Thomlinson. 1991. Effects of structural and non-structural polysaccharides in the diet of the growing pig on gastric emptying rate and rate of passage of digesta to the terminal ileum and through the total gastrointestinal tract, *Br. J. Nutr.*, 65:391.

Powley, J. S., P. R. Cheeke, D. C. England, T. P. Davidson, and W. H. Kennick. 1981. Performance of growing-finishing swine fed high levels of alfalfa meal: effects of alfalfa level, dietary additives and antibiotics, *J. Anim. Sci.*, 53:308.

Prosky, L., N.-G. Asp, I. Furda, J. W. DeVries, T. F. Schweizer, and B. F. Harland. 1984. Determination of total dietary fiber in foods, food products and total diets: interlaboratory study, *J. Assoc. Off. Anal. Chem.*, 67:1044.

Prosky, L., N.-G. Asp, T. F. Schweizer, J. W. DeVries, and I. Furda. 1988. Determination of insoluble, soluble and total dietary fiber in foods and food products: interlaboratory study, *J. Assoc. Off. Anal. Chem. Chem.*, 71:1017.

Prosky, L., N.-G. Asp, T. F. Schweizer, J. W. DeVries, and I. Furda. 1992. Determination of insoluble and soluble dietary fiber in foods and food products: collaborative study, *J. Assoc. Off. Anal. Chem.*, 75:360.

Rainbird, A. L. 1986. Effect of guar gum on gastric emptying of test meals of varying energy content in growing pigs, *Br. J. Nutr.*, 55:99.

Rainbird, A. L., and A. G. Low. 1986a. Effect of guar gum on gastric emptying in growing pigs, *Br. J. Nutr.*, 55:87.

Rainbird, A. L., and A. G. Low. 1986b. Effect of various types of dietary fiber on gastric emptying in growing pigs, *Br. J. Nutr.*, 55:111.

Ravindran, V., E. T. Kornegay, and K. E. Webb, Jr. 1984. Effects of fiber and virginiamycin on nutrient absorption, nutrient retention and rate of passage in growing swine, *J. Anim. Sci.*, 59:400.

Reese, D. E., J. Ingalls, and C. Naber. 1992. Sow feeding management at farrowing, Nebraska Swine Report, p. 14.

Reese, D. E., R. C. Thaler, M. C. Brumm, C. R. Hamilton, A. J. Lewis, G. W. Libal, and P. S. Miller. 1995. Nebraska and South Dakota Swine Nutrition Guide, Nebraska Cooperative Extension Publication EC95–273.

Rérat, A. 1978. Digestion and absorption of carbohydrates and nitrogenous matters in the hindgut of the omnivorous nonruminant animal, *J. Anim. Sci.*, 46:1808.

Rérat, A., M. Fiszlewicz, A. Giusi, and P. Vaugelade. 1987. Influence of meal frequency on postprandial variations in the production and absorption of volatile fatty acids in the digestive tract of conscious pigs, *J. Anim. Sci.*, 64:448.

Robert, S., J. J. Matte, C. Farmer, C. L. Girard, and G. P. Martineau. 1993. High-fibre diets for sows: effects on stereotypes and adjunctive drinking, *Appl. Anim. Behav. Sci.*, 37:297.

Russell, T. J., M. S. Kerley, and G. L. Allee. 1996. Effect of fructooligosaccharides on growth performance of the weaned pig, *J. Anim. Sci.*, 74(Suppl. 1):61.

Sambrook, I. E., and A. L. Rainbird. 1985. The effect of guar gum and level and source of dietary fat on glucose tolerance in growing pigs, *Br. J. Nutr.*, 54:27.

Sánchez-Mata, M. C., M. J. Peñuela-Teruel, M. Cámara-Hurtado, C. Díez-Marqués, and M. E. Torija-Isasa. 1998. Determination of mono-, di-, and oligosaccharides in legumes by high-performance liquid chromatography using an amino-bonded silica column, *J. Agric. Food Chem.*, 46:3648.

Schoenherr, W. D., and D. S. Pollmann. 1994. New concept for feeding young pigs improves productivity, *Feedstuffs*, 66:13.

Schoenherr, W. D., T. S. Stahly, and G. L. Cromwell. 1989. The effects of dietary fat or fiber addition on yield and composition of milk from sows housed in a warm or hot environment, *J. Anim. Sci.*, 67:482.

Schulze, H., P. van Leeuwen, M. W. A. Verstegen, J. Huisman, W. B. Souffrant, and F. Ahrens. 1994. Effect of level of dietary neutral detergent fiber on ileal apparent digestibility and ileal nitrogen losses in pigs, *J. Anim. Sci.*, 72:2362.

Schulze, H., P. van Leeuwen, M. W. A. Verstegen, and J. W. O. van den Berg. 1995. Dietary level and source of neutral detergent fiber and ileal endogenous nitrogen flow in pigs, *J. Anim. Sci.*, 73:441.

Selvendran, R. R., and J. A. Robertson. 1990. The chemistry of dietary fibre: a holistic view of the cell wall matrix. In *Dietary Fibre: Chemical and Biological Aspects*, Southgate, D. A. T., K. Waldron, I. T. Johnson, and G. R. Fenwick, Eds., Royal Society of Chemistry Special Publication No. 83. Royal Society of Chemistry, Cambridge, 27.

Shi, X. S., and J. Noblet. 1993. Digestible and metabolizable energy values of ten feed ingredients in growing pigs fed *ad libitum* and sows fed at maintenance level; comparative contribution of the hindgut, *Anim. Feed Sci. Technol.*, 42:223.

Southgate, D. A. T. 1993. Food components associated with dietary fiber. In *Dietary Fiber in Human Nutrition*, Spiller, G. A., Ed., CRC Press, Boca Raton, FL, 27.

Stahly, T. S., and G. L. Cromwell. 1986. Responses to dietary additions of fiber (alfalfa meal) in growing pigs housed in a cold, warm or hot thermal environment, *J. Anim. Sci.*, 63:1870.

Stanogias, G., and G. R. Pearce. 1985a. The digestion of fibre by pigs. 1. The effects of amount and type of fibre on apparent digestibility, nitrogen balance and rate of passage, *Br. J. Nutr.*, 53:513.

Stanogias, G., and G. R. Pearce. 1985b. The digestion of fibre by pigs. 3. Effects of the amount and type of fibre on physical characteristics of segments of the gastrointestinal tract, *Br. J. Nutr.*, 53:537.

Stanogias, G., and G. R. Pearce. 1985c. The digestion of fibre by pigs. 2. Volatile fatty acid concentration in large intestine digesta, *Br. J. Nutr.*, 53:531.

Stanogias, G., G. R. Pearce, T. Alifakiotis, J. Michaelidis, and B. Pappa-Michaelidis. 1994. Effects of dietary concentration and source of fibre on the apparent absorption of minerals by pigs, *Anim. Feed Sci. Technol.*, 47:287.

Taverner, M. R., I. D. Hume, and D. J. Farrell. 1981. Availability to pigs of amino acids in cereal grains. 1. Endogenous levels of amino acids in ileal digesta and faeces of pigs given cereal diets, *Br. J. Nutr.*, 46:149.

Terlouw, E. M. C., A. B. Lawrence, and A. W. Illius. 1991. Influences of feeding level and physical restriction on development of stereotypes in sows, *Anim. Behav.*, 42:981.

Thaler, R. C., J. L. Nelssen, R. D. Goodband, and G. L. Allee. 1989. Effect of dietary folic acid supplementation on sow performance through two parities, *J. Anim. Sci.*, 67:3360.

Theander, O., and P. Åman. 1982. Studies on dietary fibre. A method for the analysis and chemical characterization of total dietary fibre, *J. Sci. Food Agric.*, 33:340.

Thong, L. A., A. H. Jensen, B. G. Harmon, and S. G. Cornelius. 1978. Distillers dried grains with solubles as a supplemental protein source in diets for gestating swine, *J. Anim. Sci.*, 46:674.

Troelsen, J. E., and J. M. Bell. 1963. A comparison of nutritional effects in swine and mice. Responses in feed intake, feed efficiency and carcass characteristics to similar diets, *Can. J. Anim. Sci.*, 43:294.

Van Soest, P. J., and R. W. McQueen. 1973. The chemistry and estimation of fibre, *Proc. Nutr. Soc.*, 32:123.

Varel, V. H. 1987. Activity of fiber-degrading microorganisms in the pig large intestine, *J. Anim. Sci.*, 65:488.

Varel, V. H., S. F. Fryda, and I. M. Robinson. 1984a. Cellulolytic bacteria from pig large intestine, *Appl. Environ. Microbiol.*, 47:219.

Varel, V. H., W. G. Pond, and J. T. Yen. 1984b. Influence of dietary fiber on the performance and cellulase activity of growing-finishing swine, *J. Anim. Sci.*, 59:388.

Vestergaard, E. M., and V. Danielsen. 1998. Dietary fiber for sows: effects of large amounts of soluble and insoluble fibers in the pregnancy period on the performance of sows during three reproductive cycles, *Anim. Sci.*, 68:355.

Watts, G., and B. D. Moser. 1979. Oats for early-weaning pigs, Nebraska Swine Report, p. 5.

Weldon, W. C., A. J. Lewis, G. F. Louis, J. L. Kovar, M. A. Giesemann, and P. S. Miller. 1994. Postpartum hypophagia in primiparous sows: I. Effects of gestation feeding level on feed intake, feeding behavior, and plasma metabolite concentrations during lactation, *J. Anim. Sci.*, 72:387.

Yen, J. T., J. A. Nienaber, D. A. Hill, and W. G. Pond. 1991. Potential contribution of absorbed volatile fatty acids to whole-animal energy requirements in conscious swine, *J. Anim. Sci.*, 69:2001.

Young, L. G., and G. L. King. 1981. Wheat shorts in diets of gestating swine, *J. Anim. Sci.*, 52:551.

Zebrowska, T., and A. G. Low. 1987. The influence of diets based on whole wheat, wheat flour and wheat bran on exocrine pancreatic secretion in pigs, *J. Nutr.*, 117:1212.

Zebrowska, T., A. G. Low, and H. Zebrowska. 1983. Studies on gastric digestion of protein and carbohydrate, gastric secretion and exocrine pancreatic secretion in the growing pig, *Br. J. Nutr.*, 49:401.

Zhu, J. Q., V. R. Fowler, and M. F. Fuller. 1993. Assessment of fermentation in growing pigs given unmolassed sugar-beet pulp: a stoichiometric approach, *Br. J. Nutr.*, 69:511.

Zuo, Y., G. C. Fahey, Jr., N. R. Merchen, and N. L. Bajjalieh. 1996. Digestion responses to low oligosaccharide soybean meal by ileally cannulated dogs, *J. Anim. Sci.*, 74:2441.

8 Amino Acids in Swine Nutrition

Austin J. Lewis

CONTENTS

I. Proteins and Nonprotein Nitrogen 132
    A. Crude and True Protein 132
    B. Use of Nonprotein Nitrogen 132
II. Essentiality of Amino Acids 133
    A. Essential and Nonessential Amino Acids 133
    B. Conditionally Essential Amino Acids 133
    C. Other Amino Acids 135
III. Amino Acid Balance (Protein Quality) 135
    A. Ideal Protein 135
        1. Balance among Essential Amino Acids 135
        2. The Essential:Nonessential Amino Acid Ratio 135
        3. Balance among Nonessential Amino Acids 136
    B. Amino Acid Disproportions 136
IV. Limiting Amino Acids in Feeds 137
    A. Cereal Grains 137
    B. Protein Supplements 138
    C. Complete Diets 139
V. Diet Formulation on the Basis of Amino Acids 139
VI. Amino Acid Bioavailability 139
VII. Amino Acid–Energy Relationships 140
VIII. Use of Crystalline Amino Acids 140
    A. Isomers and Analogs 141
        1. Lysine 141
        2. Tryptophan 141
        3. Threonine 141
        4. Methionine 141
    B. Frequency of Feeding 141
    C. Low-Protein, Amino Acid–Supplemented Diets 142
    D. Amino Acids as Nutraceuticals 142
IX. Amino Acid Requirements 143
References 143

I. PROTEINS AND NONPROTEIN NITROGEN

A. Crude and True Protein

Swine obtain most of their amino acid needs from the proteins in feedstuffs they consume. Proteins are composed of amino acids, and amino acids are released during digestion and absorption. The protein content of swine diets is generally determined by laboratory analysis. Actually, the laboratory procedure does not determine protein per se, but nitrogen (N) content. Protein is calculated from N by multiplying by 100/16 (or 6.25). This multiplication factor is used because the average N content of proteins is 16 g N/100 g protein. The protein content determined in this manner is usually referred to as *crude protein*. The term *crude* is used because there are two assumptions inherent in the conversion from N to protein that are not always valid.

The first assumption is that all proteins contain 16% N. Although the assumption is not true, the use of a single conversion factor is adequate because normal diets contain mixtures of proteins and average N contents are usually close to 16%. Furthermore, the protein requirements of swine have been established using the same set of assumptions; thus, the same basis has been used for establishing the composition of feedstuffs and the dietary requirements of swine. Other conversion factors are used for a few specialized products. For example, the conversion factor for wheat and its products is 5.70, and for milk and dairy products it is 6.38 (AOAC, 1999).

A second assumption in the conversion from N to protein is that all of the N is present in proteins. In most feedstuffs for swine, part of the N is contained in compounds other than proteins. For example, about 10% of the crude protein of corn and 13% of the crude protein of soybean meal is nonprotein nitrogen (NPN) (Van Soest and Sniffen, 1984). Thus, the term crude protein comprises true protein and NPN. The NPN sources inflate the estimate of protein content. Except for a few feedstuffs such as silages and immature root crops, however, most of the NPN is in the form of amino acids. These amino acids are assumed to have the same nutritional value as the amino acids in proteins. When necessary, the amount of true protein in a feedstuff can be determined by separating the actual protein by precipitation and then conducting a N analysis of the precipitate. However, the usual crude protein value is sufficiently accurate for most purposes in swine nutrition.

B. Use of Nonprotein Nitrogen

In addition to the forms of NPN found naturally in most feedstuffs, various simple forms of NPN, such as urea and ammonium salts, are available for addition to livestock feeds. Many simple sources of NPN are considerably cheaper than protein sources, and therefore the nutritional value of simple NPN compounds is of economic importance. To be of value, NPN must be in a form that can be converted to protein by the pig. During the 1970s, the utilization of simple forms of NPN by swine was the subject of a considerable amount of research. Most experiments examined the utilization of urea; others tested ammonium salts.

In experiments where ^{15}N-labeled urea has been administered orally (Liu et al., 1955) or added to the feed (Grimson et al., 1971), N from urea has been found in proteins of various body tissues including the liver, kidney, muscle, blood, and intestinal wall, although the amounts incorporated have been rather small. An initial step in the utilization of N from urea seems to be the hydrolysis of urea by bacterial urease in the intestine. Deguchi et al. (1978) observed that whereas ^{15}N from dietary urea was incorporated into body proteins in pigs with a normal intestinal flora, there was no such incorporation in germ-free pigs. The role of the intestinal microflora in the utilization of NPN was reviewed by Deguchi and Namioka (1989).

Results of practical feeding experiments to examine the nutritional value of urea for swine have not been encouraging. In most experiments (Hanson and Ferrin, 1955; Hays et al., 1957; Kornegay et al., 1965; Kornegay, 1972), there has been little or no benefit from the addition of urea to practical swine diets, even when the dietary protein content was relatively low. Some experiments have provided evidence of utilization of urea when crystalline amino acids were also included in the diet, but generally the benefits have been small and variable (Grimson and Bowland, 1971; Kornegay et al., 1970; Kornegay, 1972). Generally from 1 to 3% urea has been included in diets. In a paper presented as part of a symposium on feeding NPN to animals, Bock (1986) concluded that urea "cannot be an effective substitute of protein sources for feeding pigs or other nonruminants." However, in more recent research, addition of 0.62% urea to a low-protein diet seemed to improve carcass traits of finishing pigs (Chiba et al., 1995).

The nutritional value for swine of ammonium salts has also been examined; compounds tested have included diammonium phosphate, ammonium polyphosphate, and ammonium acetate. An active intestinal flora is not necessary for the utilization of ammonium salts. Deguchi et al. (1980) reported that ^{15}N from diammonium citrate was incorporated into amino acids in germ-free pigs. In one germ-free pig, ^{15}N was detected in all the amino acids of proteins; in another, ^{15}N was found in all amino acids except histidine, lysine, and threonine.

Experiments in which ammonium salts have been tested in practical diets have not produced promising results. Wehrbein et al. (1970) reported that the replacement of increasing amounts of intact protein by a mixture of ammonium salts progressively decreased performance. Subsequent experiments (Platter et al., 1973; Sokol et al., 1979; Clawson and Armstrong, 1981), some with additions of crystalline amino acids, also failed to demonstrate significant nutritional contributions from the NPN sources.

More recent research has demonstrated that in pigs fed normal diets (containing no simple forms of NPN) there is considerable recycling of urea of endogenous origin in the digestive tract (Thacker et al., 1982; 1984; Mosenthin et al., 1986). Nitrogen cycling in the gut has been reviewed by Fuller and Reeds (1998).

II. ESSENTIALITY OF AMINO ACIDS

It has been known for many years that when swine are fed diets that are deficient in protein they do not grow or reproduce normally (see reviews by Pond, 1973; Baker and Speer, 1983). Therefore, proteins were considered to be essential dietary constituents. It is now clearly recognized, however, that it is not proteins per se but their components, amino acids, that are the essential ingredients. Young pigs gain weight when fed diets containing no protein, but an appropriate mixture of amino acids (Shelton et al., 1950; Beeson et al., 1951; Mertz et al., 1952; Eggert et al., 1955; Chung and Baker, 1991). Furthermore, sows are able to maintain a normal pregnancy during the last 84 days of gestation when fed a diet that contains crystalline amino acids as the sole source of N (Easter and Baker, 1976).

A. Essential and Nonessential Amino Acids

There are 20 different amino acids that commonly occur in proteins, but not all of them are essential dietary components. Swine are able to synthesize some amino acids, and these do not need to be provided in the diet; they are referred to as *nonessential* (or dispensable) amino acids (NEAA). Other amino acids cannot be synthesized, or at least they cannot be synthesized at a rate sufficient to permit optimum growth or reproduction; they are referred to as *essential* (or indispensable; EAA). Experiments to determine which amino acids are essential, and which nonessential, were conducted in the 1940s and 1950s by researchers at Cornell and Purdue Universities. A classification based on their results is presented in Table 8.1.

B. Conditionally Essential Amino Acids

A few amino acids are essential dietary components in certain situations, but not in others. They are more difficult to classify and are sometimes referred to as *conditionally* essential amino acids.

TABLE 8.1
Nutritional Classification of Amino Acids for Swine

Essential	Ref.	Nonessential
Arginine	a,b	Alanine
Histidine	c,d	Asparagine
Isoleucine	e	Aspartic acid
Leucine	a,b,c	Cysteine
Lysine	g,h,i	Glutamic acid
Methionine	j,k,l	Glutamine
Phenylalanine	a,b,m	Glycine
Threonine	n,o	Proline
Tryptophan	p,q,r	Serine
Valine	a,b,s	Tyrosine

References: a, Beeson et al. (1951); b, Mertz et al. (1952); c, Eggert et al. (1955); d, Rechcigl et al. (1956); e, Brinegar et al. (1950a); f, Eggert et al. (1954); g, Mertz et al. (1949); h, Brinegar et al. (1950b); i, Shelton et al. (1951b); j, Bell et al. (1950); k, Shelton et al. (1951c); l, Curtin et al. (1952); m, Mertz et al. (1954); n, Beeson et al. (1953); o, Sewell et al. (1953); p, Beeson et al. (1948); q, Beeson et al. (1949); r, Shelton et al. (1951a); s, Jackson et al. (1953).

The requirement for the two sulfur amino acids (methionine and cystine) is usually met by a mixture of these amino acids. Cystine can by synthesized from methionine (but not vice versa), and, therefore, methionine can meet the total need for sulfur amino acids. Cystine can satisfy approximately 50% of the sulfur amino acid requirement (Shelton et al., 1951c; Becker et al., 1955; Mitchell et al., 1968; Baker et al., 1969b; Roth and Kirchgessner, 1989; Chung and Baker, 1992) and therefore can elicit growth responses similar to an essential amino acid.

In a similar manner, phenylalanine can be converted to tyrosine, and thus it can meet the requirement for both of the two aromatic amino acids. Tyrosine cannot be converted to phenylalanine, but it can satisfy at least 50% of the total aromatic amino acid requirement (Robbins and Baker, 1977).

Arginine is generally classified as an essential amino acid, even though swine can synthesize arginine, and arginine synthesis has been measured immediately after farrowing (Wu and Knabe, 1995). Dietary arginine is required for the growth of young pigs (Southern and Baker, 1983; Roth et al., 1994), but sows are able to synthesize arginine at a rate sufficient to meet their needs for postpubertal growth and pregnancy (Easter et al., 1974; Easter and Baker, 1976).

Histidine is classified as essential and is required during pregnancy (Easter and Baker, 1977). However, histidine does not seem to be a dietary requirement for maintenance of adult female swine (Baker et al., 1966).

The nutritional essentiality of proline has been a matter of debate since Ball et al. (1986) first reported that very young pigs (1 to 5 kg) were unable to synthesize proline rapidly enough to meet their requirements. Pigs can synthesize proline from amino acids such as arginine (Murch et al., 1996), glutamic acid (Murphy et al., 1996), and glutamine (Wu et al., 1994). However, the enzymes necessary for proline synthesis are low in young pigs (Samuels et al., 1989b), and endogenous synthesis may not be adequate to meet the metabolic needs (Samuels et al., 1989a). Feeding studies in which supplemental proline has been added to low-proline diets have yielded mixed results; no benefits from supplemental proline have been observed in some experiments (Murphy, 1992; Chung and Baker, 1993), whereas positive responses have been observed in other studies (Samuels et al., 1989a; Roth et al., 1994; Kirchgessner et al., 1995). Practical diets contain adequate amounts of proline, and proline supplementation is not necessary.

In some species, glutamine is considered to be a conditionally essential amino acid because it prevents intestinal atrophy under certain conditions (Lacey and Wilmore, 1990). Glutamine is certainly an important energy source for pig enterocytes during the suckling period (Darcy-Vrillon et al., 1994; Posho et al., 1994; Wu et al., 1995), and it seems to be a substrate for arginine, citrulline, and proline synthesis (Wu et al., 1994). Furthermore, Wu et al. (1996) reported that supplementation of a corn–soybean meal diet with 1% glutamine prevented jejunal atrophy during the first week postweaning. Any benefit of supplemental glutamine seems to be related to intestinal function, because parenteral glutamine supplementation has not been beneficial (Burrin et al., 1991; House et al., 1994). There is also a report that glutamine supplementation normalized lymphocyte function in pigs weaned at 21 days and infected with *Escherichia coli* (Yoo et al., 1997).

The elimination of glutamic acid from the diet of 14-kg pigs has been reported to decrease N accretion by 6% compared with a diet that contained glutamic acid (Roth et al., 1994).

C. Other Amino Acids

In addition to the 20 primary amino acids, other amino acids are found in the proteins of pig tissues. In particular, the connective tissues contain large amounts of hydroxyproline and hydroxylysine. However, these amino acids are formed during the synthesis of these proteins and there is no evidence that they are required in the diet. Similarly, other amino acids (e.g., ornithine, citrulline, and γ-amino-butyric acid) are present as free amino acids in fluids such as blood plasma and cerebrospinal fluid, but these are readily synthesized from other amino acids.

III. AMINO ACID BALANCE (PROTEIN QUALITY)

A. Ideal Protein

Proteins differ considerably in their nutritional value. Some, such as milk proteins, are high in nutritional value; others, such as sesame meal, are low. It is well established that the nutritional value (quality) of a protein is primarily dependent on its amino acid composition, especially the content of EAA, and on the availability of the amino acids. A protein that contains a perfect balance of amino acids, both among the EAA and between EAA and NEAA, has been described as an *ideal* protein. This concept has been discussed by numerous authors (Fuller and Wang, 1990; Cole and Van Lunen, 1994; Lewis, 1995; Baker, 1997).

1. Balance among Essential Amino Acids

Estimates of the proportions of amino acids in ideal protein for growing swine have been derived from an examination of various types of data, including the composition of pig tissue, the composition of sows' milk, and combinations of individual estimates of amino acid requirements. The validity of assuming that there is one set of ideal proportions among amino acids for all stages of growth has been questioned (Lewis et al., 1977) because it is clear that the ideal pattern for maintenance differs from the ideal pattern for synthesis of new tissue. Therefore, the overall ideal pattern will change as the proportions of maintenance and new tissue synthesis change. In addition, there are changes in the amino acid content of pig tissue as the pig grows from birth to market weight (Kyriazakis et al., 1993; Susenbeth, 1995; Mahan and Shields, 1998). The ideal patterns for maintenance, new tissue accretion, milk synthesis, and catabolism of body tissue used by the NRC (1998) models to predict amino acid requirements are presented in Table 8.2.

2. The Essential:Nonessential Amino Acid Ratio

Although the NEAA are generally considered relatively unimportant, there is evidence in rats (Frost and Sandy, 1951) and chicks (Stucki and Harper, 1961; Allen and Baker, 1974) that diets with

TABLE 8.2
Estimates of the Composition of Ideal Protein for Maintenance, Protein Accretion, Milk Synthesis, and Body Tisssue[a]

Amino Acid	Maintenance	Protein Accretion	Milk Synthesis	Body Tissue
Arginine	−200	48	66	105
Histidine	32	32	40	45
Isoleucine	75	54	55	50
Leucine	70	102	115	109
Lysine	100	100	100	100
Methionine + cystine	123	55	45	45
Phenylalanine + tyrosine	121	93	112	103
Threonine	151	60	58	58
Tryptophan	26	18	18	10
Valine	67	68	85	69

[a] Proportions of each amino acid relative to lysine.

Source: NRC *Nutrient Requirements of Swine*, 10th ed., National Academy Press, Washington, D.C., 1998. With permission.

EAA as the only source of N are used less efficiently than diets with a mixture of EAA and NEAA. Research with pigs has indicated that a relatively wide range of EAA:NEAA ratios will support good growth rates and N retentions. It seems that although a minimum EAA:NEAA ratio of approximately 50:50 is required for optimal N utilization (Wang and Fuller, 1989; Markert et al., 1993; Roth et al., 1993; Lenis et al., 1999), EAA:NEAA ratios of up to at least 70:30 promote efficient N utilization (Lenis et al., 1999). At high EAA:NEAA ratios, the surpluses of EAA are presumably used for NEAA synthesis.

3. Balance among Nonessential Amino Acids

Whether there is an optimal pattern among NEAA is unknown, but the pattern seems to be relatively unimportant. Chung and Baker (1991) reported that there was no difference in growth rate of 10-kg pigs when a complete mixture of NEAA (i.e., alanine, aspartic acid, asparagine, glutamic acid, glutamine, glycine, proline, and serine) was replaced by a mixture of glutamic acid, glycine, and proline.

B. Amino Acid Disproportions

In theory, any departure from the pattern of amino acids of ideal protein will lead to a reduction in animal performance, at least in terms of the efficiency with which dietary protein is utilized. In practice, however, swine seem to be relatively tolerant of quite wide variations in the pattern of amino acids, as long as all amino acid requirements are met. Nevertheless, if the dietary amino acid pattern deviates too far from the ideal, swine performance will be reduced. The negative effects caused by the ingestion of disproportionate amounts of amino acids have been classified into three main types: *toxicity*, *imbalance*, and *antagonism* (Harper et al., 1970).

Toxicities, characterized by the consumption of a large excess of an individual amino acid, are rare in practical swine nutrition. They would be caused only by misinformation or errors in mixing of a diet that included crystalline amino acids. Unfortunately, of the four amino acids that are currently available in a feed-grade form for growing-finishing pigs (lysine, methionine, tryptophan, and threonine), two (methionine and tryptophan) have the highest relative toxicity of the essential amino acids. In rats, the addition of 3% methionine to the diet is severely toxic (Benevenga and

Harper, 1967). The rat's requirement for sulfur amino acids is 0.60%; thus the margin of safety is rather small. Swine seem to be particularly sensitive to excess methionine (Baker, 1977; Edmonds and Baker, 1987a; Edmonds et al., 1987). In contrast, excesses of lysine (Lewis et al., 1986; Edmonds and Baker, 1987b; Edmonds et al., 1987) and especially threonine (Edmonds and Baker, 1987a; Edmonds et al., 1987) are well tolerated by young pigs.

Imbalances are also caused by excessive intake(s) of (an) amino acid(s), but usually the extent of the disproportion is less and there are no clear toxic features that are specific for the amino acid(s) involved. Imbalances are caused by the exacerbation of the deficiency of the most limiting amino acid, and they can be corrected by the appropriate addition of that amino acid. In an experiment by Wahlstrom and Libal (1974), as little as 0.2% added methionine reduced the performance of growing-finishing pigs, but this effect was alleviated by the addition of 0.2% lysine (the first limiting amino acid). In general, amino acid imbalances reduce feed intake with little or no effect on the efficiency of utilization of the first limiting amino acid (D'Mello, 1993).

Antagonisms are specific relationships between amino acids in which an excessive amount of one amino acid increases the requirement of a structurally related amino acid. There are two groups of amino acids in this category: (1) arginine and lysine and (2) leucine, isoleucine, and valine. Although there are clear examples of arginine–lysine antagonism (primarily high levels of lysine antagonizing arginine) in poultry (Austic and Scott, 1975), the situation is much less clear in swine. Corn–soybean meal diets typical of those fed throughout much of the United States contain considerable amounts of arginine, and it was suggested (Harmon, 1980) that the excess arginine may antagonize lysine, which is usually first limiting. However, experiments since that time in which the arginine content of diets has been reduced (by selecting ingredients low in arginine) have generally failed to show any improvement in swine performance (Miller et al., 1981a,b; Kelly et al., 1983; Anderson et al., 1984a). Furthermore, experiments that have examined the effects of crystalline arginine added to swine diets have also indicated that the amounts of excess arginine present in most practical diets probably cause little if any problem (Southern and Baker, 1982; Hagemeier et al., 1983; Anderson et al., 1984b). However, excessive supplements of crystalline arginine can reduce feed intake and growth rate. The potential leucine–isoleucine–valine antagonism also seems to be of minor importance in practical swine diets. Many diets (especially those based on corn) contain relatively high levels of leucine, but experiments with swine in which this antagonism between the branched-chain amino acids has been investigated indicate that it is unlikely to be a cause of reduced performance in most practical situations (Oestemer et al., 1973; Henry et al., 1976).

IV. LIMITING AMINO ACIDS IN FEEDS

In most practical swine diets, the amino acid "disproportion" of greatest concern is simply a deficiency of one or more amino acids. Feedstuffs with a high protein content are usually relatively expensive and thus there is a tendency to limit their inclusion in diets. When the dietary protein content is inadequate to meet the requirements for all essential amino acids, swine performance will be restricted. The amino acid that is present in the least amount relative to its requirement is said to be the *first-limiting amino acid*, and the extent to which it is adequate will determine animal performance. If the deficiency of this amino acid is corrected, then the amino acid next lowest in relation to its requirement (second-limiting) will dictate animal performance. Information about which amino acids are most limiting in natural feedstuffs is important in formulating swine diets.

A. Cereal Grains

Cereal grains form the basis of most swine diets throughout the world and generally supply 40 to 50% of the protein in the diets of growing-finishing pigs. Thus, the amino acid composition of cereals is of great importance. The most limiting amino acids of the common cereal grains are listed in Table 8.3.

TABLE 8.3
Limiting Amino Acids in Cereal Grains for Swine

Cereal Grain	Limiting Amino Acids		
	First	Second	Third
Barley	Lysine	Threonine	Histidine
Corn	Lysine and tryptophan		Threonine
Oats	Lysine		
Sorghum	Lysine	Threonine	Tryptophan
Triticale	Lysine	Threonine	
Wheat	Lysine	Threonine	

Source: Adapted from Lewis (1985).

It is evident that the primary amino acid limitations of all the cereals are very similar. With the exception of corn, lysine is invariably the first-limiting amino acid. The low concentration of lysine in all cereals, relative to the pig's requirement, makes it the most important amino acid in swine nutrition.

In corn, lysine and tryptophan are about equally limiting for growing pigs. Some experiments (Gallo and Pond, 1968) have indicated that lysine is first limiting, others (Baker et al., 1969a) have indicated tryptophan, whereas in yet others (Lewis et al., 1979) lysine and tryptophan have been colimiting. In terms of supporting nitrogen retention in young gravid gilts, corn is first limiting in lysine and second limiting in tryptophan (Allee and Baker, 1970).

After lysine, threonine is next in importance. Threonine is second limiting in all cereals except corn, and is third limiting in corn (Grosbach et al., 1985). There are less data about further amino acid limitations, but it seems that histidine is third limiting in barley (Fuller et al., 1979), and tryptophan is third limiting or third colimiting in sorghum and low-protein sorghum diets (Cohen and Tanksley, 1976; Purser and Tanksley, 1976; Brudevold and Southern, 1994; Ward and Southern, 1995). What is very clear in terms of practical diet formulation throughout most of the world (where swine diets are generally based on corn, sorghum, barley, or wheat) is that three amino acids — lysine, tryptophan, and threonine — are of primary importance.

B. Protein Supplements

Less is known about the amino acids that are limiting in protein supplements, because these ingredients are usually fed in combination with cereal grains and few have been examined as the sole source of protein. Nevertheless, there are certain common features that are important to consider.

Most plant protein sources are low in lysine and are probably first limiting in this amino acid. Included in this category are corn gluten meal, cottonseed meal, linseed meal, peanut meal, safflower meal, sesame meal, and sunflower meal. Because of their low lysine content, it is difficult to obtain satisfactory swine performance if these protein sources provide the only source of supplemental amino acids in a cereal-based diet.

Two plant sources of protein, soybean meal and canola meal (rapeseed meal), have higher lysine contents. Although it is unclear which amino acid is first limiting in canola meal, it has been established that methionine is first limiting in soybean meal (Berry et al., 1962; 1966). Because canola meal and soybean meal have relatively high lysine and low sulfur amino acid contents, they combine well with (or complement) amino acid patterns of cereal grains, which are low in lysine and high in sulfur amino acids.

Animal protein sources contain relatively high amounts of lysine, and they are generally superior to plant sources as supplements to cereal-based diets. The amino acid patterns of milk products (dried skim milk and dried whey) and fish products (fish meal and fish protein concentrate) are particularly good. Meat products (meat meal and meat and bone meal) are variable in composition, but they are low in tryptophan and isoleucine. Tryptophan is usually the first-limiting amino acid in practical diets containing cereals and meat meals (Luce et al., 1964; Batterham, 1970; Stockland et al., 1971; Stables and Carr, 1976; Evans and Leibholz, 1979a,b). Blood meal is very high in lysine but severely deficient in isoleucine (Becker et al., 1963). Spray-dried plasma proteins have an excellent amino acid pattern and seem to enhance feed intake of young pigs (Ermer et al., 1994; Kats et al., 1994; Angulo and Cubilo, 1998).

C. COMPLETE DIETS

Because lysine is deficient in cereal grains and many protein supplements, it is usually the first-limiting amino acid in complete diets. The primary exceptions to this are diets for young pigs that contain large amounts of animal proteins such as dried whey and spray-dried plasma proteins. The sequence of limiting amino acids in a corn–soybean meal diet for growing-finishing pigs has been evaluated in numerous experiments. The first three limiting amino acids are lysine, tryptophan, and threonine (Sharda et al., 1976; Corley and Easter, 1980; Russell et al., 1983). The fourth-limiting amino acid seems to be either methionine (Russell et al., 1983; 1986) or valine (Russell et al., 1987; Lewis and Nishimura, 1995).

V. DIET FORMULATION ON THE BASIS OF AMINO ACIDS

For many years, swine diets were formulated to satisfy crude protein requirements rather than to meet requirements for specific amino acids, and feed labeling regulations in the United States still require that the crude protein content of a feed be listed on the feed tag. With present knowledge of the amino acid requirements of swine and the amino acid composition of feedstuffs, the formulation of diets on the basis of amino acids rather than crude protein is a much more precise approach. This is especially true when a wide variety of different feedstuffs is available for consideration.

Diet formulation using computers makes it possible to consider all of the amino acids, but this is unnecessary. When only intact proteins (no crystalline amino acids) are included in diets, only the first-limiting amino acid needs to be considered; when the diet satisfies the requirement for it, the requirements for all of the other amino acids will be satisfied also. Thus, diets for growing-finishing pigs will almost always be formulated on a lysine basis. Levels of tryptophan and threonine, and possibly methionine and valine, should be checked to ensure that the requirements for these amino acids have been met. An excellent, step-by-step description of how to formulate a corn–soybean meal diet to met the lysine requirement of a 40-kg pig is given in NRC (1998). Formulation of diets for very young pigs is more complex because of the various special protein sources that are normally included.

The advent of commercial production of crystalline amino acids at prices that compare favorably with the prices of amino acids in protein supplements, such as soybean meal, has enabled important opportunities in diet formulation. The use of crystalline amino acids is described in Section VIII.

VI. AMINO ACID BIOAVAILABILITY

The amino acid composition of a feedstuff or a diet can be determined by chemical procedures, commonly acid hydrolysis followed by ion-exchange chromatography with colorimetric or fluorimetric detection of the amino acids. Chemical procedures do not, however, determine the amounts of amino acids that are available to a pig. To be "bioavailable," an amino acid must be absorbed and presented to the tissues in a form that can be used for normal metabolic functions. During the 1980s and 1990s, much effort was devoted to determining bioavailabilities, and there have been several comprehensive reviews of the subject (Tanksley and Knabe, 1984; Sauer and Ozimek, 1986;

Sibbald, 1987; Southern, 1991; Lewis and Bayley, 1995). Amino acid requirements are now expressed on an available (true ileal digestible) basis by the NRC (1998). Amino acid bioavailability is discussed in detail in Chapter 9.

VII. AMINO ACID–ENERGY RELATIONSHIPS

The voluntary intake of pigs allowed *ad libitum* access to feed is influenced by the net energy (NE) concentration of the diet. When the dietary energy concentration is low, pigs increase feed intake, and vice versa (Clawson et al., 1962; Cole et al., 1967; Chiba et al., 1991a,b). As a consequence, changes in dietary energy concentration affect intakes of nutrients, including amino acids. Therefore, if a constant intake of an amino acid is to be maintained when diets of different energy concentration are fed, the amino acid concentration, expressed as a percentage of the diet, must be adjusted.

Many of the common feedstuffs fed to swine in North America have a relatively uniform NE concentration, and the effects of energy density are minor. Some ingredients such as fats, however, have NE concentrations that are substantially greater than the majority of feedstuffs. Other ingredients such as those high in fiber contain relatively low NE concentrations. When energy concentrations differ considerably from those found in "standard" ingredients such as corn and soybean meal, then amino acid requirements (in terms of dietary concentration) will be affected.

To obviate the difficulties inherent in expressing amino acid requirements in terms of dietary concentration, some organizations (ARC, 1981; INRA, 1984) have listed requirements as grams of amino acid per unit of energy (digestible or metabolizable). Although this may be an improvement, there are difficulties with this approach also. First, amino acid concentrations themselves can influence feed intake, particularly when the levels of certain amino acids are marginal or deficient. Second, the NE values of ingredients may not be constant. For example, there is evidence in poultry that the NE value of fat is dependent on the amount added and also the age of the birds. Whether there are similar differences in swine is not certain. When feed intake is limited by other (nondietary) factors such as disease, crowding, or high temperatures, adjustments in dietary amino acid concentrations are generally not beneficial (Brumm and Miller, 1996).

In growing-finishing pigs allowed *ad libitum* access to feed, the amino acid–energy relationships are confounded by the pigs' changing amino acid and energy needs and their biological limits on feed intake at different stages. These issues, which have been explored in detail by R. G. Campbell and J. L. Black and their colleagues, were reviewed by SCA (1987) and Edwards and Campbell (1993). In the growing stage (up to approximately 50 kg) the pig's inherent capacity to deposit protein generally exceeds its ability to consume sufficient feed to satisfy its tissue requirements for protein synthesis. Consequently, during this stage there is a positive linear relationship between amino acid intake and protein deposition and amino acid requirements can be defined in relation to energy (e.g., grams of lysine per kilocalorie of NE). During the finishing stage, however, feed and therefore energy intakes exceed the needs for protein deposition and the pigs amino acid requirements for tissue synthesis are independent of energy intake. During this phase, amino acid requirements are best described on a daily intake basis.

VIII. USE OF CRYSTALLINE AMINO ACIDS

The amino acid requirements of swine can be met from intact proteins such as those contained in corn and soybean meal, or they can be provided by crystalline amino acids. Generally, it is much cheaper to use intact proteins to provide most of the amino acid needs, but crystalline sources of four amino acids (lysine, methionine, tryptophan, and threonine) are now available at prices that often merit their inclusion in swine diets. In addition to the single crystalline sources, some amino acids (e.g., lysine and tryptophan) are available as mixtures and some (e.g., lysine and methionine) are available as liquids.

A. Isomers and Analogs

Amino acids have an asymmetric (or chiral) carbon atom in their structure, and thus can exist in two forms (as D- or L-isomers). Almost all amino acids that are produced in nature exist as the L-isomer, and this is therefore the form that is usually ingested and utilized by pigs. Chemical synthesis, however, yields a racemic mixture (50% D- and 50% L-isomers), and thus it becomes important to know to what extent (if any) the D-isomers of specific amino acids can be used by swine. This topic was reviewed by Lewis and Baker (1995).

1. Lysine

As far as is known, there are no mammals that are able to utilize D-lysine. This is presumably because lysine does not participate in reversible transaminations, which are necessary for the inversion of D- to L-isomers. Consequently, it is assumed that relative to L-lysine, D-lysine has a potency of zero and DL-lysine a potency of 50%. Today, all of the major manufacturers of lysine use a fermentation process that yields lysine in the L-form, usually as the monohydrochloride (L-lysine·HCl). Feed-grade lysine contains a minimum of 98.5% L-lysine·HCl. This is equivalent to 78.8% actual lysine. Use of feed-grade lysine in the United States has increased substantially during the last 25 years, much of it being used in swine feeds.

2. Tryptophan

Different species vary greatly in their ability to utilize D-tryptophan. Pigs can utilize D-tryptophan, although not as efficiently as the L-form. Estimates with growing pigs of the biological activity of D-tryptophan relative to L-tryptophan range from 60 to 100% (Baker et al., 1971; Arentson and Zimmerman, 1985; Kirchgessner and Roth, 1985; Schutte et al., 1988). Almost all feed-grade tryptophan is now L-tryptophan (98.5% pure).

3. Threonine

There are four chemical isomers of threonine: D- and L-threonine and D- and L-allothreonine. In other species such as the rat (West and Carter, 1938), only the natural form, L-threonine, is biologically available. This is because threonine, like lysine, does not participate in transamination reactions. It is assumed that the same is true for pigs, although this has never been tested. Feed-grade threonine is in the L-form only (98.5% pure).

4. Methionine

The D-form of methionine is well utilized by most species, and pigs seem to be no exception. Reifsnyder et al. (1984) and Chung and Baker (1992) reported that DL-methionine can directly replace the L-form in meeting the methionine requirement. There is evidence, however, that D-methionine may have less potency than L-methionine in very young pigs (Kim and Bayley, 1983). Feed-grade sources of methionine are available as DL-methionine (99% pure) and as methionine hydroxy analog (a liquid that contains 88% methionine hydroxy analog). Although there is some controversy about the relative bioactivity of methionine and methionine hydroxy analog, on a molar basis they seem to be equivalent for swine (Reifsnyder et al., 1984; Chung and Baker, 1992).

B. Frequency of Feeding

The efficiency with which crystalline lysine is utilized by swine is influenced by the number of daily meals that they receive. A considerable amount of research in Australia (reviewed by Batterham, 1984) has demonstrated that pigs use crystalline lysine less efficiently when they are fed once per day than when they are fed six times per day (or, presumably, *ad libitum*). Subsequent research in the United States (Cook et al., 1983; 1985) and the United Kingdom (Partridge et al., 1985) has confirmed that crystalline lysine is used less efficiently when pigs are fed infrequently than when they are allowed *ad libitum* access to feed. The reason for the lower efficiency is presumed to be related to the rapid absorption of crystalline lysine relative to other amino acids derived from intact proteins. The differential absorption rates would be expected to be deleterious when the number of daily feedings is limited, but of little consequence for a pig that consumes numerous small meals throughout the day.

Whether the frequency of feeding affects the utilization of other crystalline amino acids is unclear, but if the effect is caused by rapid absorption, it would be expected to be a general phenomenon. In an elegant experiment with early weaned pigs (4 kg) force-fed three times daily, Sawadogo et al. (1997) found that the efficiency of tryptophan utilization was 54% for protein-bound tryptophan, but only 14% for crystalline tryptophan.

C. Low-Protein, Amino Acid–Supplemented Diets

Numerous experiments have investigated reducing the crude protein content of swine diets and fortifying these diets with crystalline amino acids. Initially, the goal of these experiments was to reduce diet cost and therefore increase profitability. More recently the emphasis has shifted toward reducing nitrogen excretion and reducing odor (Lewis, 1995). It has been calculated (Kerr and Easter, 1995) that for each one percentage unit reduction in dietary crude protein combined with amino acid supplementation, total nitrogen losses (fecal and urinary) can be reduced by approximately 8%. Low-protein, amino acid–supplemented diets also reduce undesirable gases and odor. Obrock et al. (1997) reported that reducing the crude protein content by four percentage units resulted in a 75% reduction in aerial ammonia and a 70% reduction in odor.

When the crude protein content of a diet is reduced by approximately two percentage units, and crystalline lysine (and sometimes crystalline tryptophan and threonine) is added, performance is equal to that achieved on standard, control corn–soybean meal diets. However, when attempts have been made to reduce the crude protein content by more than two percentage units, conflicting results have been obtained. Reductions of three percentage units can sometimes be achieved with no reductions in performance, but usually (although not invariably) when the protein content is reduced by four percentage units (with addition of crystalline lysine, tryptophan, threonine, and methionine), lean gain of the pigs has been reduced (Knowles et al., 1998).

The reasons for the inferior performance of pigs fed low-protein, amino acid–supplemented diets remain unclear. Factors that have been suggested as being responsible include improper balance of added amino acids, deficiencies of other essential amino acids, poor efficiency of utilization of crystalline amino acids, mineral or vitamin deficiencies, and growth-promoting factors present in intact protein sources but not crystalline amino acids.

D. Amino Acids as Nutraceuticals

A nutraceutical is a substance that may be considered a feed or part of a feed that provides pharmaceutical or health benefits. Examples of nutraceuticals for swine include copper sulfate and zinc oxide for nursery pigs and conjugated linoleic acid for finishing pigs. It has been claimed that several different amino acids have nutraceutical properties for humans. However, for swine, most attention has been focused on tryptophan. Because tryptophan is a precursor of serotonin (a neurotransmitter) and melatonin (a hormone secreted by the pineal grand) as well as the vitamin niacin it has been claimed that large supplements of tryptophan may influence pig behavior and possibly carcass traits. Although tryptophan supplementation does affect brain serotonin concentrations, only minor effects on behavior or meat quality have been reported (Meunier-Salaun et al., 1991; Seve et al., 1991; Adeola and Ball, 1992; Henry et al., 1992; 1996; Adeola et al., 1993).

IX. AMINO ACID REQUIREMENTS

Accurate estimates of the amino acid requirements of swine are of considerable economic importance, and their measurement has been an active area of research since the original determination of which amino acids are essential. Requirements are influenced by many factors, including dietary protein level, dietary energy density, environmental temperature, sex of the animal, and the criterion that is used for assessment. To deal with these complex issues, several different approaches have been taken.

Initially, estimates of amino acid requirements were based on empirical experiments in which the requirement for an individual amino acid was determined in a specific situation (e.g., the lysine requirement of gilts growing from 22 to 50 kg at 20°C). These types of experiments provided a great deal of very valuable information and became the basis for the previous editions of the National Research Council *Nutrient Requirements of Swine* publications. However, this approach does not permit extrapolation to other conditions (e.g., threonine rather lysine, 50 to 100 kg rather than 20 to 50 kg, etc.).

To increase the applicability of estimates of amino acid requirements, a different approach was taken by ARC (1981) and SCA (1987). These publications based requirement estimates on a combination of empirical estimates and factorial calculations. In the factorial approach, the amino acid needs for various functions (maintenance, growth, pregnancy, lactation) are estimated and summed. Thus, animals growing rapidly or with high milk yields have higher amino acid requirements than animals growing more slowly or with lower milk yields.

Most recently, the factorial approach has been taken a step farther with the aid of computer models. An example of this is the 10th edition of the *Nutrient Requirements of Swine* (NRC, 1998). This publication uses computer models to estimate the amino acid requirements of growing pigs and of sows during gestation and lactation. The user enters "input" data such as the weight and sex of the pig, the lean growth rate, and the environmental temperature. Then, based on equations and coefficients built into the model, the computer calculates the amino acid requirements for the specific inputs. A further advantage of this type of approach is that the requirements can easily be expressed both as a percentage of the diet and on an amount per day basis. In addition, the model also estimates requirements on both a bioavailable (digestible) basis and on a total basis. As with all computer models, the accuracy of the output depends on the accuracy and validity of the assumptions built into the model. In the case of the NRC (1998) models, a concerted effort was made to ensure that the output from the models was as consistent as possible with the estimates of requirements obtained from empirical experiments. The uses of computers in swine nutrition are discussed in more detail in Chapter 38.

REFERENCES

Adeola, O., and R. O. Ball. 1992. Hypothalamic neurotransmitter concentrations and meat quality in stressed pigs offered excess dietary tryptophan and tyrosine, *J. Anim. Sci.*, 70:1888.

Adeola, O., R. O. Ball, J. D. House, and P. J. O'Brien. 1993. Regional brain neurotransmitter concentrations in stress-susceptible pigs, *J. Anim. Sci.*, 71:968.

Allee, G. L., and D. H. Baker. 1970. Limiting nitrogenous factors in corn protein for adult female swine, *J. Anim. Sci.*, 30:748.

Allen, N. K., and D. H. Baker. 1974. Quantitative evaluation of nonspecific nitrogen sources for the growing chick, *Poult. Sci.*, 53:258.

Anderson, L. C., A. J. Lewis, E. R. Peo, Jr., and J. D. Crenshaw. 1984a. Effect of various dietary arginine:lysine ratios on performance, carcass composition and plasma amino acid concentrations of growing-finishing swine, *J. Anim. Sci.*, 58:362.

Anderson, L. C., A. J. Lewis, E. R. Peo, Jr., and J. D. Crenshaw. 1984b. Effects of excess arginine with and without supplemental lysine on performance, plasma amino acid concentrations and nitrogen balance of young swine, *J. Anim. Sci.*, 58:369.

Angulo, E., and D. Cubilo. 1998. Effect of different dietary concentrations of spray-dried porcine plasma and a modified soyprotein product on the growth performance of piglets weaned at 6 kg body weight, *Anim. Feed Sci. Technol.*, 72:71.

AOAC. 1999. *Official Methods of Analysis of AOAC International*, 16th ed., 5th Rev., AOAC International, Gaithersburg, MD.

ARC. 1981. *The Nutrient Requirements of Pigs*, 2nd ed., Commonwealth Agricultural Bureaux, Slough, England.

Arentson, B. E., and D. R. Zimmerman. 1985. Nutritive value of D-tryptophan for the growing pig, *J. Anim. Sci.*, 60:474.

Austic, R. E., and R. L. Scott. 1975. Involvement of food intake in the lysine-arginine antagonism in chicks, *J. Nutr.*, 105:1122.

Baker, D. H. 1977. *Sulfur in Nonruminant Nutrition*, National Feed Ingredients Association, West Des Moines, IA.

Baker, D. H. 1997. *Ideal Amino Acid Profiles for Swine and Poultry and Their Applications in Feed Formulation*, BioKyowa Technical Review 9, NutriQuest, Chesterfield, MO.

Baker, D. H., and V. C. Speer. 1983. Protein-amino nutrition of nonruminant animals with emphasis on the pig: past, present and future, *J. Anim. Sci.*, 57(Suppl. 2):284.

Baker, D. H., N. K. Allen, J. Boomgaardt, G. Graber, and H. W. Horton. 1971. Quantitative aspects of D- and L-tryptophan utilization by the young pig, *J. Anim. Sci.*, 33:42.

Baker, D. H., D. E. Becker, H. W. Norton, A. H. Jensen, and B. G. Harmon. 1966. Some qualitative amino acid needs of adult swine for maintenance, *J. Nutr.*, 88:382.

Baker, D. H., D. E. Becker, H. W. Norton, A. H. Jensen, and B. G. Harmon. 1969a. Lysine imbalance of corn protein in the growing pig, *J. Anim. Sci.*, 28:23.

Baker, D. H., W. W. Clausing, B. G. Harmon, A. H. Jensen, and D. E. Becker. 1969b. Replacement value of cystine for methionine for the young pig, *J. Anim. Sci.*, 29:581.

Ball, R. O., J. L. Atkinson, and H. S. Bayley. 1986. Proline as an essential amino acid for the young pig, *J. Nutr.*, 55:659.

Batterham, E. S. 1970. A nutritional evaluation of diets containing meat meal for growing pigs. 6. Amino acid and mineral-vitamin-antibiotic supplements for maize-meat meal diets, *Aust. J. Exp. Agric. Anim. Husb.*, 10:534.

Batterham, E. S. 1984. Utilisation of free lysine by pigs, *Pig News Info.*, 5:85.

Becker, D. E., A. H. Jensen, S. W. Terrill, and H. W. Norton. 1955. The methionine need of the young pig, *J. Anim. Sci.*, 14:1086.

Becker, D. E., I. D. Smith, S. W. Terrill, A. H. Jensen, and H. W. Norton. 1963. Isoleucine need of swine at two stages of development, *J. Anim. Sci.*, 22:1093.

Beeson, W. M., E. T. Mertz, and D. C. Shelton. 1948. The amino acid requirements of swine. I. Tryptophan, *Science*, 107:599.

Beeson, W. M., E. T. Mertz, and D. C. Shelton. 1949. Effect of tryptophan deficiency on the pig, *J. Anim. Sci.*, 8:532.

Beeson, W. M., E. T. Mertz, and H. D. Jackson. 1951. Effect of arginine, leucine, phenylalanine, and valine on the growth of weanling pigs, *J. Anim. Sci.*, 10:1037 (Abstr.).

Beeson, W. M., H. D. Jackson, and E. T. Mertz. 1953. Quantitative threonine requirement of the weanling pig, *J. Anim. Sci.*, 12:870.

Bell, J. M., H. H. Williams, J. K. Loosli, and L. A. Maynard. 1950. The effect of methionine supplementation of a soybean oil meal-purified ration for growing pigs, *J. Nutr.*, 40:551.

Benevenga, N. J., and A. E. Harper. 1967. Alleviation of methionine and homocystine toxicity in the rat, *J. Nutr.*, 93:44.

Berry, T. H., D. E. Becker, O. G. Rasmussen, A. H. Jensen, and H. W. Norton. 1962. The limiting amino acids in soybean protein, *J. Anim. Sci.*, 21:558.

Berry, T. H., G. E. Combs, H. D. Wallace, and R. C. Robbins. 1966. Responses of the growing pig to alterations in the amino acid pattern of isolated soybean protein, *J. Anim. Sci.*, 25:722.

Bock, H.-D. 1986. Utilization of urea in pigs, *Arch. Anim. Nutr.*, 36:285.

Brinegar, M. J., J. K. Loosli, L. A. Maynard, and H. H. Williams. 1950a. The isoleucine requirement for the growth of swine, *J. Nutr.*, 42:619.

Brinegar, M. J., H. H. Williams, F. H. Ferris, J. K. Loosli, and L. A. Maynard. 1950b. The lysine requirement for the growth of swine, *J. Nutr.*, 42:129.

Brudevold, A. B., and L. L. Southern. 1994. Low-protein, crystalline amino acid-supplemented, sorghum-soybean meal diets for the 10- to 20-kilogram pig, *J. Anim. Sci.*, 72:638.

Brumm, M. C., and P. S. Miller. 1996. Response of pigs to space allocation and diets varying in nutrient density, *J. Anim. Sci.*, 74:2730.

Burrin, D. G., R. J. Shulman, M. C. Storm, and P. J. Reeds. 1991. Glutamine or glutamic acid effects on intestinal growth and disaccharidase activity in infant piglets receiving total parenteral nutrition. *J. Parenter. Enteral Nutr.*, 15:262.

Chiba, L. I., A. J. Lewis, and E. R. Peo, Jr. 1991a. Amino acid and energy interrelationships in pigs weighing 20 to 50 kg. I. Rate and efficiency of weight gain, *J. Anim. Sci.*, 69:694.

Chiba, L. I., A. J. Lewis, and E. R. Peo, Jr. 1991b. Amino acid and energy interrelationships in pigs weighing 20 to 50 kg. II. Rate and efficiency of protein and fat deposition, *J. Anim. Sci.*, 69:708.

Chiba, L. I., H. W. Ivey, K. A. Cummins, and B. E. Gamble. 1995. Effects of urea as a source of extra dietary nitrogen on growth performance and carcass traits of finisher pigs, *Nutr. Res.*, 15:1029.

Chung, T. K., and D. H. Baker. 1991. A chemically defined diet for maximal growth of pigs, *J. Nutr.*, 121:979.

Chung, T. K., and D. H. Baker. 1992. Utilization of methionine analogs and isomers by pigs, *Can. J. Anim. Sci.*, 72:185.

Chung, T. K., and D. H. Baker. 1993. A note on the dispensability of proline for weanling pigs, *Anim. Prod.*, 56:407.

Clawson, A. J., and W. D. Armstrong. 1981. Ammonium polyphosphate as a source of phosphorus and nonprotein nitrogen for monogastrics in corn–soybean meal diets for growing rats and growing-finishing (G-F) pigs, *J. Anim. Sci.*, 52:1.

Clawson, A. J., T. N. Blumer, W. W. G. Smart, Jr., and E. R. Barrick. 1962. Influence of energy–protein ratio on performance and carcass characteristics of swine, *J. Anim. Sci.*, 21:62.

Cohen, R. S., and T. D. Tanksley, Jr. 1976. Limiting amino acids in sorghum for growing and finishing swine, *J. Anim. Sci.*, 43:1028.

Cole, D. J. A., and T. A. Van Lunen. 1994. Ideal amino acid patterns. In *Amino Acids in Farm Animal Nutrition*, D'Mello, J. P. F., Ed., CAB International, Wallingford, U.K., chap. 5.

Cole, D. J. A., J. E. Duckworth, and W. Holmes. 1967. Factors affecting voluntary feed intake in pigs. I. The effect of digestible energy content of the diet on the intake of castrated male pigs housed in holding pens and in metabolism crates, *Anim. Prod.*, 9:141.

Cook, H., G. R. Frank, D. W. Giesting, and R. A. Easter. 1983. The influence of meal frequency and lysine supplementation of a low-protein diet on nitrogen retention of young pigs, *J. Anim. Sci.*, 57(Suppl. 1):240 (Abstr.).

Cook, H., D. W. Giesting, and R. A. Easter. 1985. The influence of feeding frequency and crystalline lysine supplementation on performance of finisher pigs, *J. Anim. Sci.*, 61(Suppl. 1):319 (Abstr.).

Corley, J. R., and R. A. Easter. 1980. Lysine and tryptophan supplementation of low-protein diets for growing and finishing pigs, *J. Anim. Sci.*, 51(Suppl. 1):191 (Abstr.).

Curtin, L. V., J. K. Loosli, J. Abraham, H. H. Williams, and L. A. Maynard. 1952. The methionine requirement for the lean growth of swine, *J. Nutr.*, 48:499.

Darcy-Vrillon, B., L. Posho, M. T. Morel, F. Bernard, F. Blachier, J. C. Meslin, and P. H. Duee. 1994. Glucose, galactose, and glutamine metabolism in pig isolated enterocytes during development, *Ped. Res.*, 36:175.

Deguchi, E., and S. Namioka. 1989. Synthesis ability of amino acids and protein from non-protein nitrogen and role of intestinal flora on this utilization in pigs, *Bifidobacteria Microflora*, 8:1.

Deguchi, E., M. Niiyama, K. Kagota, and S. Namioka. 1978. Role of intestinal flora on incorporation of [15]N [nitrogen isotope] from dietary, ^{15}N-urea, and ^{15}N-diammonium citrate into tissue proteins in pigs, *J. Nutr.*, 108:1572.

Deguchi, E., M. Niiyama, K. Kagota, and S. Namioka. 1980. Incorporation of nitrogen-15 [isotope] from dietary [^{15}N] diammonium citrate into amino acids of liver and muscle proteins in germfree and specific-pathogen-free neonatal pigs, *Am. J. Vet. Res.*, 41:212.

D'Mello, J. P. F. 1993. Amino acid supplementation of cereal-based diets for non-ruminants, *Anim. Feed Sci. Technol.*, 45:1.

Easter, R. A., and D. H. Baker. 1976. Nitrogen metabolism and reproductive response of gravid swine fed an arginine-free diet during the last 84 days of gestation, *J. Nutr.*, 106:636.

Easter, R. A., and D. H. Baker. 1977. Nitrogen metabolism, tissue carnosine concentration and blood chemistry of gravid swine fed graded levels of histidine, *J. Nutr.*, 107:120.

Easter, R. A., R. S. Katz, and D. H. Baker. 1974. Arginine: a dispensable amino acid for postpubertal growth and pregnancy of swine, *J. Anim. Sci.*, 39:1123.

Edmonds, M. S., and D. H. Baker. 1987a. Amino acid excesses for young pigs: effects of excess methionine, tryptophan, threonine or leucine, *J. Anim. Sci.*, 64:1664.

Edmonds, M. S., and D. H. Baker. 1987b. Failure of excess dietary lysine to antagonize arginine in young pigs, *J. Nutr.*, 117:1396.

Edmonds, M. S., H. W. Gonyou, and D. H. Baker. 1987. Effect of excess levels of methionine, tryptophan, arginine, lysine or threonine on growth and dietary choice in the pig, *J. Anim. Sci.*, 65:179.

Edwards, A. C., and R. G. Campbell. 1993. Energy — protein interactions in pigs. In *Recent Developments in Pig Nutrition 2*, Cole, D. J. A., W. Haresign, and P. C. Garnsworthy, Eds., Nottingham University Press, Loughborough, U.K., chap 4.

Eggert, R. G., H. H. Williams, B. E. Sheffy, E. G. Sprague, J. K. Loosli, and L. A. Maynard. 1954. The quantitative leucine requirement of the suckling pig, *J. Nutr.*, 53:177.

Eggert, R. G., L. A. Maynard, B. E. Sheffy, and H. H. Williams. 1955. Histidine — an essential nutrient for growth of pigs, *J. Anim. Sci.*, 14:556.

Ermer, P. M., P. S. Miller, and A. J. Lewis. 1994. Diet preference and meal patterns of weanling pigs offered diets containing either spray-dried porcine plasma or dried skim milk, *J. Anim. Sci.*, 72:1548.

Evans, D. F., and J. Leibholz. 1979a. Meat meal in the diet of the early-weaned pig. I. A comparison of meat meal and soya bean meal, *Anim. Feed Sci. Technol.*, 4:33.

Evans, D. F., and J. Leibholz. 1979b. Meat meal in the diet of the early-weaned pig. II. Amino acid supplementation, *Anim. Feed Sci. Technol.*, 4:43.

Frost, D. V., and H. R. Sandy. 1951. Utilization of non-specific nitrogen sources by the adult protein-depleted rat, *J. Biol. Chem.*, 189:249.

Fuller, M. F., R. M. Livingston, B. A. Baird, and T. Atkinson. 1979. The optimal amino acid supplementation of barley for the growing pig. 1. Response of nitrogen metabolism to progressive supplementation, *Br. J. Nutr.*, 41:321.

Fuller, M. F., and P. J. Reeds. 1998. Nitrogen cycling in the gut, *Annu. Rev. Nutr.*, 18:385.

Fuller, M. F., and T. C. Wang. 1990. Digestible ideal protein — a measure of dietary protein value, *Pig News Info.*, 11:353.

Gallo, J. T., and W. G. Pond. 1968. Amino acid supplementation to all-corn diets for pigs, *J. Anim. Sci.*, 27:73.

Grimson, R. E., and J. P. Bowland. 1971. Urea as a nitrogen source for pigs fed diets supplemented with lysine and methionine, *J. Anim. Sci.*, 33:58.

Grimson, R. E., J. P. Bowland, and L. P. Milligan. 1971. Use of nitrogen-15 labelled urea to study urea utilization by pigs, *Can. J. Anim. Sci.*, 51:103.

Grosbach, D. A., A. J. Lewis, and E. R. Peo, Jr. 1985. An evaluation of threonine and isoleucine as the third and fourth limiting amino acids in corn for growing swine, *J. Anim. Sci.*, 60:487.

Hagemeier, D. L., G. W. Libal, and R. C. Wahlstrom. 1983. Effects of excess arginine on swine growth and plasma amino acid levels, *J. Anim. Sci.*, 57:99.

Hanson, L. E., and E. F. Ferrin. 1955. The value of urea in a low protein ration for weanling pigs, *J. Anim. Sci.*, 14:43.

Harmon, B. G. 1980. The role of amino acid balance in practical swine rations. In *Proceedings of the 41st Minnesota Nutrition Conference*, University of Minnesota, St. Paul, 132.

Harper, A. E., N. J. Benevenga, and R. M. Wohlhueter. 1970. Effects of ingestion of disproportionate amounts of amino acids, *Physiol. Rev.*, 50:428.

Hays, V. W., G. C. Ashton, C. H. Liu, V. C. Speer, and D. V. Catron. 1957. Studies on the utilization of urea by growing swine, *J. Anim. Sci.*, 16:44.

Henry, Y., P. H. Duée, and A. Rérat. 1976. Isoleucine requirement of the growing pig and leucine–isoleucine interrelationship, *J. Anim. Sci.*, 42:357.

Henry, Y., B. Sève, Y. Colléaux, P. Ganier, C. Saligaut, and P. Jégo. 1992. Interactive effects of dietary levels of tryptophan and protein on voluntary feed intake and growth performance in pigs, in relation to plasma free amino acids and hypothalamic serotonin, *J. Anim. Sci.*, 70:1873.

Henry, Y., B. Sève, A. Mounier, and P. Ganier. 1996. Growth performance and brain neurotransmitters in pigs as affected by tryptophan, protein, and sex, *J. Anim. Sci.*, 74:2700.

House, J. D., P. B. Pencharz, and R. O. Ball. 1994. Glutamine supplementation to total parenteral nutrition promotes extracellular fluid expansion in piglets, *J. Nutr.*, 124:396.

INRA. 1984. *L'alimentation des Animaux Monogastriques: Porc, Lapin, Volailles*, Institut National de la Recherche Agronomique, Paris.

Jackson, H. D., E. T. Mertz, and W. M. Beeson. 1953. Quantitative valine requirement of the weanling pig, *J. Nutr.*, 51:109.

Kats, L. J., J. L. Nelssen, M. D. Tokach, R. D. Goodband, J. A. Hansen, and J. L. Laurin. 1994. The effect of spray-dried porcine plasma on growth performance in the early-weaned pig, *J. Anim. Sci.*, 72:2075.

Kelly, K. A., T. D. Tanksley, Jr., D. A. Knabe, and K. D. Haydon. 1983. Effect of amino acid excess on growing pig performance, *J. Anim. Sci.*, 57(Suppl. 1):252 (Abstr.).

Kerr, B. J., and R. A. Easter. 1995. Effect of feeding reduced protein, amino acid-supplemented diets on nitrogen and energy balance in grower pigs, *J. Anim. Sci.*, 73:3000.

Kim, K. I., and H. S. Bayley. 1983. Amino acid oxidation by young pigs receiving diets with varying levels of sulphur amino acids, *Br. J. Nutr.*, 50:383.

Kirchgessner, M., and F. X. Roth. 1985. Biologische Wirksamkeit von DL-Tryptophan bei Mastschweinen, *Z. Tierphysiol. Tierernähr. Futtermittelkd.*, 54:135.

Kirchgessner, M., J. Fickler, and F. X. Roth. 1995. Effect of dietary proline supply on N-balance of piglets. 3. Communication on the importance of non-essential amino acids for protein retention, *J. Anim. Physiol. Anim. Nutr.*, 73:57.

Knowles, T. A., L. L. Southern, T. D. Bidner, B. J. Kerr, and K. G. Friesen. 1998. Effect of dietary fiber or fat in low-crude protein, crystalline amino acid-supplemented diets for finishing pigs, *J. Anim. Sci.*, 76:2818.

Kornegay, E. T. 1972. Supplementation of lysine, ammonium polyphosphate and urea in diets for growing-finishing pigs, *J. Anim. Sci.*, 34:55.

Kornegay, E. T., E. R. Miller, D. E. Ullrey, B. H. Vincent, and J. A. Hoefer. 1965. Influence of dietary urea on performance, antibody production and hematology of growing swine, *J. Anim. Sci.*, 24:951.

Kornegay, E. T., V. Mosanghini, and R. D. Snee. 1970. Urea and amino acid supplementation of swine diets, *J. Nutr.*, 100:330.

Kyriazakis, I., G. C. Emmans, and R. McDaniel. 1993. Whole body amino acid composition of the growing pig, *J. Sci. Food Agric.*, 62:29.

Lacey, J. M., and D. W. Wilmore. 1990. Is glutamine a conditionally essential amino acid? *Nutr. Rev.*, 48:297.

Lenis, N. P., H. T. M. van Diepen, P. Bikker, A. W. Jongbloed, and J. van der Meulen. 1999. Effect of the ratio between essential and nonessential amino acids in the diet on utilization of nitrogen and amino acids by growing pigs, *J. Anim. Sci.*, 77:1777.

Lewis, A. J. 1985. Use of synthetic amino acids in practical rations. In *Proceedings of the Carolina Swine Nutrition Conference*, North Carolina State University, Raleigh, 32.

Lewis, A. J. 1995. Ideal protein for swine: fact, fantasy, and the future. In *Proceedings of the Carolina Swine Nutrition Conference*, North Carolina State University, Raleigh, 69.

Lewis, A. J., and D. H. Baker. 1995. Bioavailability of D-amino acids and DL-hydroxy methionine. In *Bioavailability of Nutrients for Animals: Amino Acids, Minerals, and Vitamins*, Ammerman, C. B., D. H. Baker, and A. J. Lewis, Eds., Academic Press, New York, chap. 3.

Lewis, A. J., and H. S. Bayley. 1995. Amino acid bioavailability. In *Bioavailability of Nutrients for Animals: Amino Acids, Minerals, and Vitamins*, Ammerman, C. B., D. H. Baker, and A. J. Lewis, Eds., Academic Press, New York, chap. 2.

Lewis, A. J., and N. Nishimura. 1995. Valine requirement of the finishing pig, *J. Anim. Sci.*, 73:2315.

Lewis, A. J., E. R. Peo, Jr., P. J. Cunningham, and B. D. Moser. 1977. Determination of the optimum dietary proportions of lysine and tryptophan for growing pigs based on growth, food intake and plasma metabolites, *J. Nutr.*, 107:1369.

Lewis, A. J., E. R. Peo, Jr., B. D. Moser, and T. D. Crenshaw. 1979. Additions of lysine, tryptophan, methionine and isoleucine to all-corn diets for finishing swine, *Nutr. Rep. Int.*, 19:533.

Lewis, A. J., E. R. Peo, Jr., and J. D. Hancock. 1986. Effect of lysine additions in excess of the requirement on the performance of weanling pigs, *J. Anim. Sci.*, 63(Suppl. 1):271 (Abstr.).

Liu, C. H., V. W. Hays, H. J. Svec, D. V. Catron, G. C. Ashton, and V. C. Speer. 1955. The fate of urea in growing pigs, *J. Nutr.*, 57:241.

Luce, W. G., E. R. Peo, Jr., and D. B. Hudman. 1964. Effect of amino acid supplementation of rations containing meat and bone scraps on rate of gain, feed conversion and digestibility of certain ration components for growing-finishing swine, *J. Anim. Sci.*, 23:521.

Mahan, D. C., and R. G. Shields, Jr. 1998. Essential and nonessential amino acid composition of pigs from birth to 145 kilograms of body weight, and comparison to other studies, *J. Anim. Sci.*, 76:513.

Markert, W., M. Kirchgessner, and F. X. Roth. 1993. Balance studies with growing pigs to reduce N excretion. I. Optimal supply with essential amino acids, *J. Anim. Physiol. Anim. Nutr.*, 70:159.

Mertz, E. T., D. C. Shelton, and W. M. Beeson. 1949. The amino acid requirements of swine, lysine, *J. Anim. Sci.*, 8:524.

Mertz, E. T., W. M. Beeson, and H. D. Jackson. 1952. Classification of essential amino acids for the weanling pig, *Arch. Biochem. Biophys.*, 38:121.

Mertz, E. T., J. N. Henson, and W. M. Beeson. 1954. Quantitative phenylalanine requirement of the weanling pig, *J. Anim. Sci.*, 13:927.

Meunier-Salaün, M. C., M. Monnier, Y. Colléaux, B. Sève, and Y. Henry. 1991. Impact of dietary tryptophan and behavioral type on behavior, plasma cortisol, and brain metabolites of young pigs, *J. Anim. Sci.*, 69:3689.

Miller, E. R., J. Skomial, and P. K. Ku. 1981a. Nitrogen and energy balance of pigs fed corn-soy or balanced amino acid diets, *J. Anim. Sci.*, 53(Suppl. 1):255 (Abstr.).

Miller, E. R., J. Skomial, P. K. Ku, and M. G. Hogberg. 1981b. An evaluation of improving dietary amino acid balance of growing-finishing pigs, *J. Anim. Sci.*, 53(Suppl. 1):93 (Abstr.).

Mitchell, J. R., Jr., D. E. Becker, B. G. Harmon, H. W. Norton, and A. H. Jensen. 1968. Some amino acid needs of the young pig fed a semisynthetic diet, *J. Anim. Sci.*, 27:1322.

Mosenthin, R., H. Henkel, T. Mauritz-Boeck, W. C. Sauer, and L. Ozimek. 1986. Effect of microbial fermentation on nitrogen metabolism in growing pigs, *J. Anim. Sci.*, 63(Suppl. 1):281 (Abstr.).

Murch, S. J., R. L. Wilson, J. M. Murphy, and R. O. Ball. 1996. Proline is synthesized from intravenously infused arginine by piglets consuming low proline diets, *Can. J. Anim. Sci.*, 76:435.

Murphy, J. M. 1992. Effects of Nutrition and Development on Proline Metabolism in the Neonatal Piglet. M.Sc. thesis. University of Guelph, Guelph, Ontario, Canada.

Murphy, J. M., S. J. Murch, and R. O. Ball. 1996. Proline is synthesized from glutamate during intragastric infusion but not during intravenous infusion in neonatal pigs, *J. Nutr.*, 126:878.

NRC. 1998. *Nutrient Requirements of Swine*, 10th ed., National Academy Press, Washington, D.C.

Obrock, H. C., P. S. Miller, and A. J. Lewis. 1997. The effects of reducing dietary crude protein concentration on odor in swine facilities. Univ. Nebraska Swine Rep., p. 14.

Oestemer, G. A., L. E. Hanson, and R. J. Meade. 1973. Leucine-isoleucine interrelationship in the young pig, *J. Anim. Sci.*, 36:674.

Partridge, I. G., A. G. Low, and H. D. Keal. 1985. A note on the effect of feeding frequency on nitrogen use in growing boars given diets with varying levels of free lysine, *Anim. Prod.*, 40:375.

Platter, P. D., E. R. Peo, Jr., P. E. Vipperman, and P. J. Cunningham. 1973. Effect of amino acids on nonprotein nitrogen utilization by G-F swine, *J. Anim. Sci.*, 37:514.

Pond, W. G. 1973. Influence of maternal protein and energy nutrition during gestation on progeny performance in swine, *J. Anim. Sci.*, 36:175.

Posho, L., B. Darcy-Vrillon, F. Blachier, and P. H. Duee. 1994. The contribution of glucose and glutamine to energy metabolism in newborn pig enterocytes, *J. Nutr. Biochem.*, 5:284.

Purser, K. W., and T. D. Tanksley, Jr. 1976. Third and fourth limiting amino acids in sorghum for growing swine, *J. Anim. Sci.*, 43:257 (Abstr.).

Rechcigl, M., Jr., J. K. Loosli, D. J. Horsvath, and H. H. Williams. 1956. Histidine requirement of baby pigs, *J. Nutr.*, 60:619.

Reifsnyder, D. H., C. T. Young, and E. E. Jones. 1984. The use of low protein liquid diets to determine the methionine requirement and the efficacy of methionine hydroxy analogue for the three-week-old pig, *J. Nutr.*, 114:1705.

Robbins, K. R., and D. H. Baker. 1977. Phenylalanine requirement of the weanling pig and its relationship to tyrosine, *J. Anim. Sci.*, 45:113.

Roth, F. X., and M. Kirchgessner. 1989. Influence of the methionine:cystine relationship in the feed on the performance of growing pigs, *J. Anim. Physiol. Anim. Nutr.*, 61:265.

Roth, F. X., W. Markert, and M. Kirchgessner. 1993. Optimal supply of alpha-amino nitrogen for growing pigs. 2. Communication on balance studies to reduce N excretion, *J. Anim. Physiol. Anim. Nutr.*, 70:196.

Roth, F. X., J. Fickler, and M. Kirchgessner. 1994. N-balance of piglets as related to the omission of individual non-essential amino acids from the diet. 2. Communication on the importance of non-essential amino acids for protein retention, *J. Anim. Physiol. Anim. Nutr.*, 72:215.

Russell, L. E., G. L. Cromwell, and T. S. Stahly. 1983. Tryptophan, threonine, isoleucine and methionine supplementation of a 12% protein, lysine-supplemented, corn–soybean meal diet for growing pigs, *J. Anim. Sci.*, 56:1115.

Russell, L. E., R. A. Easter, V. Gomez-Rojas, and G. L. Cromwell. 1986. A note on the supplementation of low-protein, maize-soya-bean meal diets with lysine, tryptophan, threonine and methionine for growing pigs, *Anim. Prod.*, 42:291.

Russell, L. E., B. J. Kerr, and R. A. Easter. 1987. Limiting amino acids in an 11% crude protein corn–soybean meal diet for growing pigs, *J. Anim. Sci.*, 65:1266.

Samuels, S. E., H. L. M. Aarts, and R. O. Ball. 1989a. Effects of dietary proline on proline metabolism in the neonatal pig, *J. Nutr.*, 119:1900.

Samuels, S. E., K. S. Acton, and R. O. Ball. 1989b. Pyrroline-5-carboxylate reductase and proline oxidase activity in the neonatal pig, *J. Nutr.*, 119:1999.

Sauer, W. C., and L. Ozimek. 1986. Digestibility of amino acids in swine: results and their practical applications, a review, *Livest. Prod. Sci.*, 15:367.

Sawadogo, M. L., A. Piva, A. Panciroli, E. Meola, A. Mordenti, and B. Sève. 1997. Marginal efficiency of free or protected crystalline L-tryptophan for tryptophan and protein accretion in early-weaned pigs, *J. Anim. Sci.*, 75:1561.

SCA. 1987. Feeding Standards for Australian Livestock. Pigs. Standing Committee on Agriculture, CSIRO, Melbourne, Australia.

Schutte, J. B., E. J. Van Weerden, and F. Koch. 1988. Utilization of DL- and L-tryptophan in young pigs, *Anim. Prod.*, 46:447.

Sève, B., M. C. Meunier-Salaün, M. Monnier, Y. Colléaux, and Y. Henry. 1991. Impact of dietary tryptophan and behavioral type on growth performance and plasma amino acids of young pigs, *J. Anim. Sci.*, 69:3679.

Sewell, R. F., J. K. Loosli, L. A. Maynard, H. H. Williams, and B. E. Sheffy. 1953. The quantitative threonine requirement of the suckling pig, *J. Nutr.*, 49:435.

Sharda, D. P., D. C. Mahan, and R. F. Wilson. 1976. Limiting amino acids in low-protein corn–soybean meal diets for growing-finishing swine, *J. Anim. Sci.*, 42:1175.

Shelton, D. C., W. M. Beeson, and E. T. Mertz. 1950. Growth of weanling pigs on a diet containing ten purified amino acids, *Arch. Biochem. Biophys.*, 29:446.

Shelton, D. C., W. M. Beeson, and E. T. Mertz. 1951a. Quantitative DL-tryptophan requirement of the weanling pig, *J. Anim. Sci.*, 10:73.

Shelton, D. C., W. M. Beeson, and E. T. Mertz. 1951b. Quantitative L-lysine requirement of the weanling pig, *Arch. Biochem. Biophys.*, 30:1.

Shelton, D. C., W. M. Beeson, and E. T. Mertz. 1951c. The effect of methionine and cystine on the growth of weanling pigs, *J. Anim. Sci.*, 10:57.

Sibbald, I. R. 1987. Estimation of bioavailable amino acids in feedingstuffs for poultry and pigs: a review with emphasis on balance experiments, *Can. J. Anim. Sci.*, 67:221.

Sokol, L., R. L. Harrold, and C. H. Haugse. 1979. Utilization of ammonium salts by growing swine, *J. Anim. Sci.*, 49(Suppl. 1):95 (Abstr.).

Southern, L. L. 1991. Digestible Amino Acids and Digestible Amino Acid Requirements for Swine, BioKyowa Technical Review 2, Nutri-Quest, Chesterfield, MO.

Southern, L. L., and D. H. Baker. 1982. Performance and concentration of amino acids in plasma and urine of young pigs fed diets with excesses of either arginine or lysine, *J. Anim. Sci.*, 55:857.

Southern, L. L., and D. H. Baker. 1983. Arginine requirement of the young pig, *J. Anim. Sci.*, 57:402.

Stables, N. H. J., and J. R. Carr. 1976. Growth and nitrogen balance studies with growing pigs fed on diets containing normal or opaque-2 maize, meat and bone meal, and synthetic amino acids, *N.Z. J. Agric. Res.*, 19:311.

Stockland, W. L., R. J. Meade, and J. W. Nordstrom. 1971. Lysine, methionine and tryptophan supplementation of a corn-meal and bone meal diet for growing swine, *J. Anim. Sci.*, 32:262.

Stucki, W. P., and A. E. Harper. 1961. Importance of dispensable amino acids for normal growth of chicks, *J. Nutr.*, 74:377.

Susenbeth, A. 1995. Factors affecting lysine utilization in growing pigs: an analysis of literature data, *Livest. Prod. Sci.*, 43:193.

Tanksley, T. D., Jr., and D. A. Knabe. 1984. Ileal digestibilities of amino acids in pig feeds and their use in formulating diets. In *Recent Advances in Animal Nutrition–1984*, Haresign, W., and D. J. A. Cole, Eds., Butterworths, London.

Thacker, P. A., J. P. Bowland, L. P. Milligan, and E. Weltzien. 1982. Effects of graded dietary protein levels on urea recycling in the pig, *Can. J. Anim. Sci.*, 62:1193.

Thacker, P. A., W. C. Sauer, and H. Jørgensen. 1984. Amino acid availability and urea recycling in finishing swine fed barley-based diets supplemented with soybean meal or sunflower meal, *J. Anim. Sci.*, 59:409.

Van Soest, P. J., and C. J. Sniffen. 1984. Nitrogen fractions in NDF and ADF. In *Proceedings of the Distillers Feed Conference*, 39:73, Cincinnati, OH.

Wahlstrom, R. C., and G. W. Libal. 1974. Gain, feed efficiency and carcass characteristics of swine fed supplemental lysine and methionine in corn–soybean meal diets during the growing and finishing periods, *J. Anim. Sci.*, 38:1261.

Wang, T. C., and M. F. Fuller. 1989. The optimum dietary amino acid pattern for growing pigs. 1. Experiments by amino acid deletion, *Br. J. Nutr.*, 62:77.

Ward, T. L., and L. L. Southern. 1995. Sorghum amino acid-supplemented diets for the 50- to 100-kilogram pig, *J. Anim. Sci.*, 73:1746.

Wehrbein, G. F., P. E. Vipperman, Jr., E. R. Peo, Jr., and P. J. Cunningham. 1970. Diammonium citrate and diammonium phosphate as sources of dietary nitrogen for growing-finishing swine, *J. Anim. Sci.*, 31:327.

West, H. D., and H. E. Carter. 1938. Synthesis of α-amino-β-hydroxy-*n*-butyric acids. VI. Preparation of *d*- and *l*-allothreonine and nutritive value of the four isomers, *J. Biol. Chem.*, 122:611.

Wu, G., A. G. Borbolla, and D. A. Knabe. 1994. The uptake and release of arginine, citrulline and proline by the small intestine of developing pigs, *J. Nutr.*, 124:2437.

Wu, G., and D. A. Knabe. 1995. Arginine synthesis in enterocytes of neonatal pigs, *Am. J. Physiol.*, 269:R261.

Wu, G., D. A. Knabe, W. Yan, and N. E. Flynn. 1995. Glutamine and glucose metabolism in enterocytes of the neonatal pig, *Am. J. Physiol.*, 268:R334.

Wu, G. Y., S. A. Meier, and D. A. Knabe. 1996. Dietary glutamine supplementation prevents jejunal atrophy in weaned pigs, *J. Nutr.*, 126:2578.

Yoo, S. S., C. J. Field, and M. I. Burney. 1997. Glutamine supplementation maintains intramuscular glutamine concentrations and normalizes lymphocyte function in infected early weaned pigs, *J. Nutr.*, 127:2253.

9 Bioavailability of Amino Acids in Feedstuffs for Swine

Vincent M. Gabert, Henry Jørgensen, and Charles M. Nyachoti

CONTENTS

I. Introduction 152
II. Determination of Amino Acid Availabilities 153
    A. Slope-Ratio Assay 153
    B. Chemically Available Lysine 154
III. Determination of Ileal Amino Acid Digestibilities 154
    A. Definitions 154
    B. Apparent Ileal Amino Acid Digestibilities 154
    C. True Ileal Amino Acid Digestibilities 155
    D. Real Ileal Amino Acid Digestibilities 155
    E. Standardized Ileal Amino Acid Digestibilities 155
    F. *In Vitro* Amino Acid Digestibilities 155
    G. Summary 155
IV. Apparent Ileal Amino Acid Digestibilities 159
    A. Method of Determination 159
        1. Direct Method 159
        2. Difference Method 160
        3. Regression Method 160
        4. Rapid Measurement 161
    B. Analytical Considerations Related to Amino Acids 162
    C. Marker Method vs. Total Collection Method 162
    D. Selection of an Indigestible Marker 162
V. Approaches to Collecting Ileal Digesta from Swine 163
    A. Slaughter Method 163
    B. Simple T-Cannulation 164
    C. Reentrant Cannulation 164
    D. Ileo-Rectal Anastomosis 164
    E. Postvalvular T-Cecum Cannulation 165
    F. Steered Ileo-Cecal Valve Cannulation 165
    G. Comparisons between Collection Procedures 165
VI. True Ileal Amino Acid Digestibilities 166
    A. Definition and Significance 166
    B. Measurement of Endogenous Amino Acid Losses 166
        1. Protein-Free Diets 167
        2. Enzymatically Hydrolyzed Casein Method 167
        3. Low-Protein Casein Diets 167
        4. Regression Method 167

        5. Isotope Dilution Technique 168
        6. Homoarginine Method 168
VII. Factors Affecting Digestion and Endogenous Losses of Amino Acids 169
    A. Dry Matter Intake and Body Weight 169
    B. Ingredient and Feed Processing 170
    C. Level of Protein and Amino Acids in the Diet 171
    D. Source of Protein and Protein Solubility 172
    E. Level and Source of Dietary Fat 172
    F. Fiber Type, Level, and Fiber-Degrading Enzymes 173
    G. Phytate and Use of Phytase 174
    H. Trypsin Inhibitors 174
    I. Lectins 175
    J. Tannins 175
    K. Antibiotics 176
    L. Organic Acids 176
VIII. Conclusions 177
References 177

I. INTRODUCTION

Many different feedstuffs are included in diets for swine for the purpose of supplying essential amino acids (AA) and other nutrients. These feedstuffs include cereal grains such as corn, barley, sorghum, oats, rye, triticale, and wheat; vegetable protein sources such as soybean meal, cottonseed meal, peanut meal, sunflower meal, and canola meal; and animal protein by-products including fish meal, meat and bone meal, meat meal, blood meal, and spray-dried animal plasma. Protein sources are usually the most expensive component of swine diets; therefore, optimizing their use is economically important. Utilization of AA also needs to be optimized to maintain product pork quality and to reduce N excretion into the environment. The expression "bioavailability of AA" or, simply, availability refers to the amount of AA in a feedstuff that is released during protein digestion, absorbed from the small intestine, and used in maintenance (synthesis of replacement proteins), growth (e.g., muscle protein synthesis), and lactation (milk protein synthesis). A definition of bioavailability was presented by ARC (1981) and summarized by Fan (1994); it is defined as the percentage of the total amount of an AA that is not complexed with compounds that interfere with its digestion, absorption, or utilization by the pig for the purpose of maintenance or growth of new tissue. A straightforward definition of availability is that it is a term that is used to describe the supply of nutrients from the digestive tract to the body tissues (Danfær and Fernández, 1999). As defined, AA bioavailability is an abstract concept and can only be estimated and not measured directly (Fan, 1994).

    For estimation of AA bioavailability in feedstuffs for pigs, the slope-ratio assay (growth assay) is the most direct approach, and it results in a combined estimate of digestibility and postabsorptive AA utilization (Fan, 1994). Results obtained with this assay are referred to as AA availabilities (Batterham et al., 1979; 1984; Batterham, 1992; Leibholz, 1992). The assay provides an estimate of the availability of only one AA per assay. Because availabilities are affected by many dietary factors (discussed later on), availability estimates are not likely additive when used in the formulation of a complete diet. The concept of additivity is discussed later in this chapter.

    The term *AA digestibility* should not be interchanged with AA availability. AA digestibility is defined as the difference between the amount of an AA in the diet and the amount present in ileal digesta divided by the amount in the diet (Low, 1982; Sauer and Ozimek, 1986). AA digestibility is likely the most important single determinant of AA utilization in feedstuffs by pigs (Fan, 1994). However, swine nutritionists must be cautious when using heat-damaged feedstuffs in diet formulation. For these feedstuffs, AA availabilities will be much lower than ileal AA digestibilities (Batterham et al., 1990; Friedman, 1996).

When the ileal analysis method, as opposed to the fecal analyses method, is used to measure AA digestibilities, the modifying effects of bacterial metabolism on AA in the cecum and large intestine are avoided (Sauer and Ozimek, 1986). In addition, there is no absorption of AA from the cecum and large intestine (Zebrowska, 1973; Just et al., 1981). Therefore, the ileal analysis method is more sensitive and provides a more representative reflection of AA uptake than the fecal analyses method (Sauer and Ozimek, 1986). Ileal digestibilities of AA are very important in swine nutrition because of the large variability in protein quality that can be encountered between different feedstuffs and within the same feedstuff. Also, digestibilities are affected by processing, heat treatment, fiber content and type, susceptibility of proteins to digestion, and the presence of antinutritional compounds (e.g., Wiseman et al., 1991; Jansman et al., 1995; Fan et al., 1996). The digestible supply of AA in a feedstuff determines how diets will be formulated as well as the levels of essential AA that need to be supplemented to meet the AA requirements of the type of swine being fed (NRC, 1998). There are extensive table values available for apparent AA digestibilities (e.g., Sauer and Ozimek, 1986; Southern, 1991; NRC, 1998) and some true AA digestibility values have been published (Southern, 1991; NRC, 1998). In addition, standardized ileal AA digestibility values are now available (Rademacher et al., 1999). The main focus of this chapter is a discussion of issues relating to ileal AA digestibilities. These issues include the definition and determination of ileal AA digestibilities and the factors that affect ileal AA digestibilities in pigs.

II. DETERMINATION OF AMINO ACID AVAILABILITIES

A. Slope-Ratio Assay

The slope-ratio assay has been used in pigs to determine AA availability (Batterham et al., 1984; 1990; Leibholz, 1986; Batterham, 1992; Leibholz, 1992; Adeola et al., 1994; van Barneveld et al., 1994c). This section only provides a few examples of some of the extensive literature on this topic. This approach relies on the use of a basal diet supplemented with incremental levels of crystalline AA; in this example, crystalline L-lysine·HCl (Batterham et al., 1990; van Barneveld et al., 1994c). Experimental diets are set up with increasing levels of lysine (to match the same levels of crystalline lysine in the basal diet) supplied from a particular feedstuff of interest. A discussion of the statistical and the SAS programming aspects of the slope-ratio assay was presented by Littell et al. (1997). Growth rate, feed conversion efficiency (on a weight gain or on a carcass basis), daily carcass gain, or the amount of protein deposited (g/day) are measured (Batterham et al., 1984; 1990). The slope derived from the linear response variable with the test ingredient (b_t) is compared with the slope of the response variable in the basal diets supplemented with crystalline lysine (b_s), and the percentage value ($b_t/b_s \times 100$) is referred to as the availability of that particular AA (Batterham et al., 1984; Littell et al., 1997).

The slope ratio has been used to determine the availability of lysine in cottonseed meal, peanut meal, and soybean meal (Batterham et al., 1984; Adeola et al., 1994). Lysine availabilities in feedstuffs vary considerably; for example, using feed conversion efficiency on a carcass basis (carcass gain/feed intake), lysine availabilities in cottonseed meal, and soybean meal ranged from 27 to 39% and from 89 to 98%, respectively (Batterham et al., 1984; 1990). Lysine availabilities in peanut meal and field peas were 57 and 93%, respectively (Batterham et al., 1984). In studies with young pigs, Leibholz (1986) estimated lysine availabilities in a number of feedstuffs and observed the following ranges: meat meal, 86 to 88%; soybean meal, 95 to 99%; cottonseed meal, 69 to 75%; lupins, 90%; and milk, 99%. Lysine and tryptophan availabilities in various feedstuffs have been summarized by Knabe (1991).

Estimated AA availabilities are unique to the experimental situation and therefore may not be additive. AA availability estimates are influenced by experimental conditions that include the dietary balance of AA, amount of protein and energy in the diets, as well as the feedstuffs that they are supplied by Fan (1994). Other factors include the chronological appearance of AA at the tissue level, physiological state, and genotype of the pig (Fan, 1994). Batterham (1992) discussed the causes of high standard errors of availability estimates. Other considerations with using the slope-ratio method are the high cost of many diets and the large numbers of growing pigs required. The slope-ratio assay is very useful for investigating the effect of different factors, such as the severity of heat treatment, on the availability of one AA (Batterham et al., 1990; van Barneveld et al., 1994b,c). However, it is nearly impossible (cost- and time-prohibitive) to use this approach to obtain availabilities, in the same feedstuff, for several AA. The slope ratio is useful as long as the dietary level of the AA in question is limiting growth. From a diet formulation perspective, the slope-ratio assay by itself is an inadequate approach for the determination of the nutritional value of protein in a feedstuff (Fan, 1994). Therefore, to investigate the nutritional value of ingredients that are used extensively in diets for swine, there has been a great deal of interest in measuring ileal AA digestibilities.

B. Chemically Available Lysine

Instead of using the slope-ratio assay, chemical approaches also can be used to estimate lysine availability (chemically available lysine or so-called reactive lysine). One of these reactions involves subjecting a feedstuff sample to the FDNB (1-fluoro-2,4-dinitrobenzene) reaction. Lysine in the feedstuff reacts with FDNB, and the extent of the reaction can be quantified by chromatography or with an AA analyzer (Carpenter, 1960; Rao et al., 1963; Roach et al., 1967). The FDNB method has been reviewed by van Barneveld (1993). The guanidination reaction, which is used with the homoarginine method, also can be used to measure chemically available lysine (Hagemeister and Erbersdobler, 1985; Moughan and Rutherfurd, 1996; McNeilage et al., 2000). Further research is required on the application of chemical techniques to estimate AA availabilities in ingredients. From a diet formulation perspective, measurement of chemically available lysine by itself is an inadequate approach unless it is correlated to an *in vivo* response.

III. DETERMINATION OF ILEAL AMINO ACID DIGESTIBILITIES

A. Definitions

The collection of ileal digesta from pigs is necessary for the determination of ileal AA digestibilities. Many different cannulation methods can be used to prepare pigs surgically, and some of these procedures are discussed in Chapter 42. Ileal digestibilities are used to determine the digestible supply of AA. There are several terms relating to digestibility, which are defined below. Detailed mathematical formulas for calculating digestibilities are presented by Fan and Sauer (1995), Gabert et al. (1997), and Rademacher et al. (1999).

B. Apparent Ileal Amino Acid Digestibilities

Apparent ileal digestibilities can be determined by total collection of ileal digesta, or by sampling the digesta. Total collection of ileal digesta is possible by surgically fitting pigs with a reentrant cannula or by using ileo-rectal anastomosis (Low, 1982). Apparent ileal AA digestibilities are then determined by comparing the intake of the AA to the amount reaching the terminal ileum. When total collection of ileal digesta is not conducted, apparent ileal AA digestibilities are determined by comparing the concentration of AA in the diet to the concentration of AA in ileal digesta. An indigestible marker must be used if total collection is not carried out. The mobile nylon bag technique (MNBT) can also be used to measure apparent ileal AA digestibilities. This is possible if pigs are fitted with two cannulas, one in the duodenum and one at the terminal ileum (Sauer et al., 1983; Bornholdt et al., 1994) or if the ileo-rectal anastomosis technique is used (Viljoen et al., 1997). Apparent ileal digestibilities of AA are confounded by AA in ileal digesta that do not originate from the diet (i.e., endogenous AA, which are both animal and bacterial in nature; Dugan et al., 1994; Gabert et al., 1997; Lien et al., 1997a,b). The effects of several factors on apparent ileal AA digestibilities are shown in Table 9.2 and in Figures 9.2 and 9.3.

C. True Ileal Amino Acid Digestibilities

True ileal digestibilities are determined by correcting apparent ileal AA digestibilities for the level of endogenous AA in ileal digesta. There are many different approaches that can be used to measure the level of endogenous AA. These include (1) feeding a protein free diet; (2) feeding a diet containing enzymically hydrolyzed casein; (3) feeding a low protein casein diet; (4) use of the regression method; or (5) using the homoarginine method (Low, 1982; Hagemeister and Erbersdobler, 1985; Butts et al., 1991; Schmitz et al., 1991; Moughan et al., 1992b; Fan et al., 1995b; Gabert et al., 1997). True lysine digestibilities and endogenous flows of lysine ascertained using different approaches are presented in Table 9.1.

D. Real Ileal Amino Acid Digestibilities

Real ileal AA digestibilities are determined by correcting apparent ileal AA digestibilities for endogenous AA using an isotope dilution technique, which involves either labeling the pig with stable or radioactive tracers or labeling the diet by fertilizing crops with labeled fertilizers (Souffrant et al., 1986; Moughan et al., 1992a; Arentson and Zimmerman, 1995; Leterme et al., 1996; Gabert et al., 1997; Lien et al., 1997a,b). Dilution in individual AA or in one AA, if a constant composition of endogenous protein is assumed, is used to estimate the proportion of endogenous AA in ileal digesta (Table 9.1). A comparison of real ileal AA digestibilities to apparent and true ileal AA digestibilities is shown in Figure 9.1.

E. Standardized Ileal Amino Acid Digestibilities

Standardized ileal AA digestibilities are calculated by correcting apparent digestibilities for minimum endogenous AA losses using an averaged flow (g/kg dry matter intake, DMI) of endogenous AA (Rademacher et al., 1999). The endogenous AA flows used were calculated from experiments that used five different methods to estimate minimum endogenous AA losses (no effects of fiber or antinutritional compounds). The following flows (g/kg DMI) were used to generate the standardized AA digestibility values: lysine, 0.40; threonine, 0.61; methionine, 0.11; tryptophan, 0.14; and valine, 0.54 (Rademacher et al., 1999).

F. *In Vitro* Amino Acid Digestibilities

In vitro AA digestibilities can be measured by a number of different *in vitro* techniques that involve the use of various combinations of digestive enzymes and filtration steps (Boisen and Eggum, 1991; Parsons, 1991; Boisen and Fernández, 1995).

G. Summary

The number of digestibility terms is expanding. Practically, however, either the AA digestibility value is an apparent value in which endogenous levels of AA are not taken into consideration, or it is an estimate of true ileal digestibility. True ileal AA digestibilities have been corrected for endogenous AA losses. Several aspects of apparent and true ileal AA digestibilities are discussed in the following sections of this chapter. To simplify the terminology in this area, the terms *apparent* and *true* should be used and the method used to correct for endogenous AA losses should be specified.

TABLE 9.1
True Ileal Digestibilities of Lysine and Endogenous Flow of Lysine Determined Using Different Approaches in Studies with Growing Pigs[a]

Dietary Ingredients	Treatment and Level	Method of Determination	True Ileal Lysine Digestibility (%)	Endogenous Flow of Lysine (g/kg DMI)	Ref.
Protein source, cornstarch, and sucrose	Casein	HA	99.0[b]	0.59[d]	Nyachoti et al. (1997b)
	Barley		87.1[c]	1.10[d]	
	Canola meal		84.6[c]	1.43[b]	
	BCM		85.8[c]	1.30[bc]	
Protein source, cornstarch, and sucrose	Extruded FFSB	HA	95.5[bc]	1.49[cd]	Marty et al. (1994)
	Jet-sploded FFSB		95.3[c]	2.45[b]	
	Micronized FFSB		96.0[bc]	1.99[bc]	
	Roasted FFSB		94.1[c]	2.16[bc]	
	Soybean meal (48% CP)		97.7[b]	1.33[d]	
Soybean meal, cornstarch, and dextrose	Dietary level of protein (4 to 24% CP)	Regression		0.47	Fan et al. (1995b)
	4		93.2		Fan et al. (1995b)
	8		88.5		
	12		91.7		
	16		91.0		
	20		91.2		
	24		90.5		
Wheaten corn flour, 10% EHC, and sucrose	0.90 kg DMI/d	EHC		0.66	Butts et al. (1993b)
	1.45 kg DMI/d			0.63	
	1.81 kg DMI/d			0.59	
	2.17 kg DMI/d			0.53	
Cornstarch, 10% EHC (or protein free), and sucrose		EHC		0.46	Donkoh and Moughan (1999)
		Protein free		0.27	
Cornstarch, meat and bone meal, and sucrose	Dietary level of protein (8 to 16%)	Regression		0.26	Donkoh and Moughan (1999)
Casein, cornstarch, sucrose	5% casein (4.4% CP diet)	Low protein casein		0.59	Albin et al., unpublished
Barley and sucrose		^{15}N-IDT	68.3	0.67	Lien et al. (1997b)

[a] *Abbreviations:* DMI, dry matter intake; HA, homoarginine method; BCM, barley and canola meal–based diet; FFSB, full fat soybeans; EHC, enzymically hydrolyzed casein; ^{15}N-IDT, ^{15}N-leucine isotope dilution technique.

[b,c,d] Means within an experiment and true lysine digestibility or endogenous lysine flow with different letters differ ($P < 0.05$).

TABLE 9.2
Factors That Affect the Apparent Ileal Amino Acid Digestibilities of Lysine (Lys), Threonine (Thr), and Methionine (Met) in Young and Growing Pigs

Factor Studied and Type of Diet	Treatment and Level	Apparent Ileal Digestibilities (%)			Class of Swine; Ref.
		Lys	Thr	Met	
Dietary fiber					
Soybean meal, cornstarch, dextrose	No added fiber	85.0	77.9	88.0	Growing pigs; Sauer et al. (1991)
	10% Alfafloc	81.9	74.1	86.2	
	10% Barley straw	83.5	75.6	84.0	
Feed enzymes					
Complex formulation	Control, no phytase addition	81.0	73.8	76.7[d]	Growing pigs; Mroz et al. (1994)
	800 phytase units/kg	81.9	72.0	80.6[e]	
Oil addition to diets					
Soybean meal, cornstarch, dextrose	3.2% Canola oil	85.4[a]	77.8[a]	91.1	Young pigs; Li and Sauer (1994)
	6.2% Canola oil	86.8	79.1	91.9	
	9.2% Canola oil	88.6	80.4	91.7	
	12.2% Canola oil	88.6	81.4	90.8	
Heat treatment of ingredients					
Barley, fish meal, wheatstarch, corn meal[b]	10% untreated Chilean fish meal	92.0	92.0	88.0	Growing pigs; Wiseman et al. (1991)
	10% fish meal heated at 130°C for 3 h	90.0	75.0	83.0	
	10% fish meal heated at 160°C for 1.25 h	84.0	51.0	39.0	
Hull-less barley and soybean meal	Hull-less barley	56.1	55.6	63.3[d]	Young pigs; Huang et al. (1998)
	Micronized hull-less barley	63.5	65.0	73.3[e]	
Effect of tannin addition and protein solubility					
Several ingredients	Protein sources with low solubility	68.8[e]	66.6[d]	76.2[d]	Young pigs; Jansman et al. (1995)
	Low solubility and high-tannin hulls	63.4[e]	59.7[e]	68.2[d]	
	Protein sources with high solubility	85.1[c]	73.2[c]	84.0[e]	
	High solubility and high-tannin hulls	76.9[d]	62.7[de]	72.3[d]	
Trypsin inhibitors					
Cornstarch, defatted soy flour, dextrose	Defatted soy flour, not heated	45.1[d]	41.3[d]	70.0[d]	Growing pigs; Li et al. (1998)
	Autoclaved soy flour	80.2[e]	73.7[e]	89.4[e]	

continued

TABLE 9.2 (CONTINUED)
Factors That Affect the Apparent Ileal Amino Acid Digestibilities of Lysine (Lys), Threonine (Thr), and Methionine (Met) in Young and Growing Pigs

Factor Studied and Type of Diet	Treatment and Level	Apparent Ileal Digestibilities (%)			Class of Swine; Ref.
		Lys	Thr	Met	
Antibiotic inclusion in a diet containing different fractions of barley	Barley diet	78	70[d]	83[d]	Growing pigs; Just et al. (1980)
	Barley diet + nebacetine	79	76[c]	87[c]	
	Barley meal diet	80[d]	73[d]	83[d]	
	Barley meal diet + nebacetine	83[c]	81[c]	89[c]	
	Barley grits diet	85	78[d]	89[d]	
	Barley grits diet + nebacetine	84	82[c]	93[c]	

[a] Linear effect ($P < 0.05$).
[b] Amino acid digestibilities in fish meal were calculated using the difference method.
[c,d,e] Means within an experiment and lysine, threonine, and methionine digestibilities differ ($P < 0.05$).

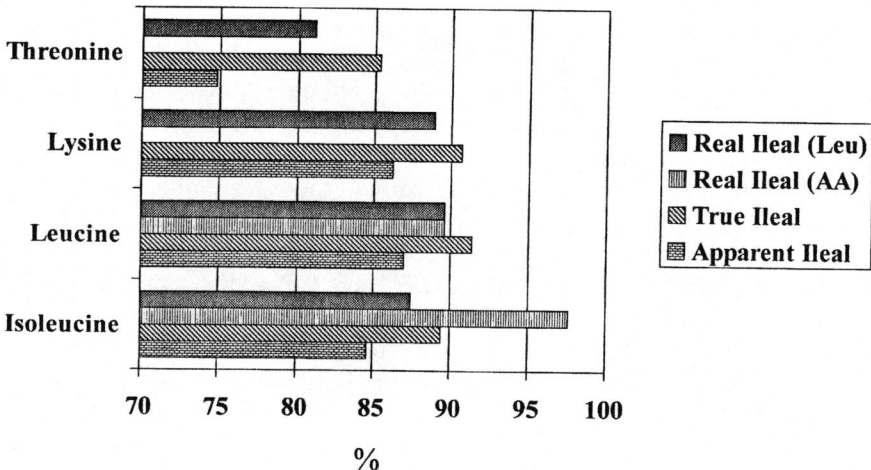

FIGURE 9.1 Comparison of apparent, real, and true ileal digestibilities for selected AA measured in growing pigs fed a wheat, fish meal, and casein–based diet (Gabert et al., 1997). Real ileal digestibilities were measured using the ^{15}N-leucine (Leu)- or the ^{15}N-AA-isotope dilution technique. True ileal AA digestibilities were calculated using the flow of endogenous AA presented by de Lange et al. (1989). Real ileal digestibilities of threonine and lysine could not be determined using the ^{15}N-AA isotope dilution technique because of the absence of enrichment in these AA.

IV. APPARENT ILEAL AMINO ACID DIGESTIBILITIES

A. Method of Determination

Apparent ileal digestibilities of AA are now known for many feedstuffs fed to growing pigs (Sauer and Ozimek, 1986; Knabe et al., 1989; Southern, 1991; NRC, 1998; Table 9.2). There are many approaches available for determining the apparent ileal digestibilities of AA. The method of determination has a large impact on the digestibility values, and care needs to be taken to ensure that the most appropriate approach is used to measure digestibility coefficients (Fan and Sauer, 1995).

1. Direct Method

The most commonly used method to determine AA digestibilities is the direct method. The direct method is used when the feedstuff of interest is the sole source of dietary protein in the diet. The direct method can be used to determine apparent ileal AA digestibilities in any feedstuff. However, recent research has shown that precautions should be taken when this method is used. The direct method should not be used with cereal grains such as corn, wheat, barley, rye, triticale, and oats because of the confounding effects of endogenous AA as discussed below (Fan and Sauer, 1995). When the direct method is used with cereal grains, diets should contain approximately 90% of the cereal grain of interest.

Artificially low apparent ileal AA digestibilities are obtained when the direct method is used with cereal grains that have a low protein content. For example, when a complete barley diet was fed by Lien et al. (1997b) and by Fan and Sauer (1995), the observed apparent lysine digestibilities were 52.7 and 54.1%, respectively. In contrast, the apparent digestibility of lysine was 61.3% when determined with the difference method (Fan and Sauer, 1995). These low digestibilities were due to a relatively large amount of endogenous protein (AA) at the end of the small intestine compared with undigested dietary protein (unabsorbed AA; Fan et al., 1994). Therefore caution must be exercised when the direct method is used. Unless the cereal grain is high in protein (greater than 18% crude protein, CP, as-is basis), which is usually only the case for hard red spring wheat, the difference or regression method should be used. The direct method for measuring apparent AA digestibilities in low-protein feedstuffs is not recommended, unless it is coupled with a technique that will estimate endogenous AA losses and allow for the determination of true AA digestibilities.

The direct method can and should be used with feedstuffs that have a relatively high protein content (at least 18% CP, as-is basis). These feedstuffs include soybean meal, soy protein concentrate, peanut meal, canola meal, peas, meat and bone meal, fish meal, spray-dried animal plasma, and many others. When the direct method is used with these feedstuffs, semipurified diets are formulated to contain these ingredients as the sole source of dietary protein.

Diets should be formulated to contain at least 17% CP, which will ensure that the dietary levels of AA exceed the threshold levels of Fan et al. (1994) for the accurate determination of apparent ileal AA digestibilities. Using 17% CP minimizes the confounding effects of endogenous AA relative to unabsorbed dietary AA. In addition, the measured apparent ileal AA digestibilities will approach true digestibilities (Fan et al., 1994).

2. Difference Method

The difference method, discussed in detail by Fan and Sauer (1995), should be used when measuring the apparent ileal digestibilities of AA in feedstuffs with a low-protein content, less than 18% CP on an as-is basis. The feedstuffs for which the difference method is most appropriate are most cereal grains. The difference method assumes that there are no associative effects (interactions) between ingredients and that apparent ileal AA digestibilities are additive (Fan and Sauer, 1995). Apparent ileal AA digestibilities have been shown to be additive; therefore, they can be used to calculate the digestible supply of AA when several ingredients are used in diets (Furuya and Kaji, 1991; Fan et al., 1993). Additivity has been demonstrated by comparing the directly determined apparent AA digestibilities in barley, wheat, and canola meal–based diets as well as in barley, wheat, and soybean meal–based diets to the calculated apparent ileal AA digestibilities (Fan et al., 1993).

Use of the difference method requires that at least two diets be prepared (Diets A and B). Diet A is a semipurified basal diet that contains one protein source such as soybean meal, canola meal, or casein, and that it is formulated to contain 17% CP (as-is basis, Fan et al., 1993). Diet B is formulated in the same way as Diet A. The feedstuff of interest (e.g., corn, barley, wheat, oats, meat and bone meal, or dried whey) is added at the expense of starch and of some of the protein source in Diet A. The two diets must contain the same level of protein (17% CP as-is basis). This approach can also be used with diets that contain three sources of protein, as in the studies of Fan et al. (1993), as long as two diets are formulated and apparent ileal AA digestibilities are measured with the direct method. The apparent ileal digestibilities of AA are measured in both diets, and the apparent ileal digestibilities of AA in the feedstuff of interest are calculated. The level of each AA supplied by the feedstuff in Diet B, the level of each AA supplied by the basal protein source in Diet B, and the apparent ileal AA digestibilities of the basal protein source measured in Diet A are used in the calculations. The difference method can be used to measure apparent ileal AA digestibilities in both low- and high-protein feedstuffs when their inclusion levels in the assay diets are relatively high (Fan and Sauer, 1995). The difference or the regression method should be used when assessing apparent ileal AA digestibilities in low-protein feedstuffs (Fan and Sauer, 1995).

3. Regression Method

The regression method allows for the determination of AA digestibilities in two feedstuffs, a basal feedstuff (such as barley) and an assay feedstuff at the same time (Fan and Sauer, 1995). The assay feedstuffs are those that cannot be included in the diet at very high levels because of concerns over palatability. Examples are canola meal, cottonseed meal, feather meal, blood meal, or meat and bone meal. Linear relationships between the apparent ileal AA digestibilities in the assay diets and the contribution of AA from the assay and basal feedstuffs are used to calculate AA digestibilities in each of the ingredients (Fan and Sauer, 1995). This method assumes that there are no associative or interactive effects between the ingredients and that digestibilities are additive (Fan and Sauer, 1995). These assumptions have been validated (Furuya and Kaji, 1991; Fan et al., 1993). To use the regression method, several assay diets (approximately three), that have increasing levels of one ingredient and decreasing levels of another ingredient, are used (Fan and Sauer, 1995). The regression method is suitable for measurement of AA digestibilities in both low- and high-protein-containing feedstuffs (Fan and Sauer, 1995).

4. Rapid Measurement

Having a quick estimate of AA digestibility in a feedstuff facilitates more accurate diet formulation and allows formulations to be updated on a regular basis. There is a great deal of interest in the development of rapid assay techniques that can be performed in the field or in the laboratory in a matter of minutes or hours. Near-infrared reflectance spectroscopy (NIRS) has been used to estimate moisture, CP, and even AA levels in feedstuffs (Degussa-Hüls AG, Hanau, Germany, personal communication; Aufrère et al., 1996; Givens and Deaville, 1999). There is interest in using NIRS to predict ileal AA digestibilities, and efforts in this area are currently under way. To use NIRS to predict digestibility, calibration curves between the NIR spectra of whole and milled grain and *in vivo* results are needed (van Barneveld et al., 1999). NIRS is by far the most rapid approach available and is in place in many commercial settings.

There are several wet chemistry approaches available, but they require more time to conduct than NIRS. The KOH test, or solubility in KOH, is used widely to predict protein quality (Parsons, 1991). A sample of feedstuff is mixed with a 0.2% (w/v) solution of KOH. A portion of the supernatant is analyzed for N content and soluble protein is calculated as a percentage of the total protein ($N \times 6.25$, Kjeldahl procedure) in the original sample (Parsons, 1991). The KOH solubility test has been used to investigate the effect of processing on soybean meal quality. There are other approaches that can be used to measure protein solubility; these include the use of 80% ethanol or trichloroacetic acid (Peiniau et al., 1996). To date, no comparisons have been made between ileal AA digestibilities obtained in pigs and KOH solubilities. Protein solubility has been shown to be an important factor that is related to AA digestibility in pigs (Jansman et al., 1995).

Various *in vitro* techniques can be used to estimate AA digestibilities. A multienzyme assay for prediction of AA digestibility was developed by Bellaver (1989). The *in vitro* systems available rely on one or more enzymes to simulate digestion. Pepsin digestion followed by pancreatin is often used (Boisen and Eggum, 1991; Boisen and Fernández, 1995). Pronase, a proteolytic enzyme, has also been used (Taverner and Farrell, 1981a). Validation of *in vitro* methods is required using correlation with values obtained *in vivo*.

The mobile nylon bag technique (MNBT) is another method that can be used to study AA digestibilities (Sauer et al., 1983). Once this method is set up, it can be used routinely to assay thousands of samples. To use the MNBT, pigs are fitted with a simple T-cannula in the duodenum and fed a commercial grower diet. Labeled rectangular nylon bags are constructed and 1 g of test ingredient is weighed and sealed inside the bag (Sauer et al., 1983). The bags are predigested *in vitro* using pepsin in a solution of HCl (Cherian et al., 1988; 1989), or they are suspended in a pig's stomach for 6 h via a gastric cannula (Leibholz, 1991). The MNBT allows the measurement of apparent fecal CP and energy digestibilities. The conditions for using this approach have been optimized (Cherian et al., 1988; 1989).

The MNBT can be used directly to determine apparent ileal AA digestibilities if the nylon bags are collected from the terminal ileum instead of being recovered from feces (Leibholz, 1991; Bornholdt et al., 1994). A postvalvular T-cecum cannula (PVTC) is surgically inserted into the cecum (van Leeuwen et al., 1991) to facilitate collection of bags from the ileum and a simple T-cannula is surgically placed into the duodenum (Sauer et al., 1983; Leibholz, 1991). Apparent ileal

AA digestibilities also can be estimated if the pigs are fitted with a duodenal cannula and prepared for the collection of ileal digesta with the ileo-rectal anastomosis technique (Viljoen et al., 1997).

B. Analytical Considerations Related to Amino Acids

Accurate measurement of ileal AA digestibilities requires accurate AA analyses, especially hydrolysis procedures (Fountoulakis and Lahm, 1998; Albin et al., 2000b,c; Smiricky et al., 2000b). To perform accurate AA analyses with ion-exchange chromatography on samples that contain chromic oxide, a common indigestible marker, special procedures may be needed (Bech-Andersen, 1979). However, the presence of chromic oxide does not interfere with AA analyses when high-pressure liquid chromatography procedures are used (Albin et al., 2000b). We have developed correction factors that can be used to adjust the concentrations of AA in soy products to 6 M HCl and 24 h of acid hydrolyses; the most common hydrolyses conditions used (Albin et al., 2000b,c; Smiricky et al., 2000b). For some AA, such as threonine, serine, and tyrosine, degradation exceeds their release from protein after a few hours of hydrolyses (Rowan et al., 1992; Fountoulakis and Lahm, 1998; Albin et al., 2000b,c; Smiricky et al., 2000b). For other AA, their release from protein is slower and longer hydrolyses times and stronger acid concentrations are needed. This is the case for valine, isoleucine, and leucine (Rudemo et al., 1980; Albin et al., 2000b,c; Smiricky et al., 2000b). In studies with various soybean products, correction factors for threonine ranged from 1.01 to 1.13, while those for valine ranged from 1.12 to 1.21 (Albin et al., 2000b). When several hydrolysis times and HCl concentrations were used for analyzing AA in soybean meal, the correction factors for lysine, threonine, and valine were 1.07, 1.07, and 1.30, respectively (Smiricky et al., 2000b). Other workers also have used correction factors before the calculation of digestibilities to obtain more accurate values (Mroz et al., 1994). More accurate measurements of AA levels in feedstuffs, as well as digestibility coefficients, will be obtained if correction factors are used.

C. Marker Method vs. Total Collection Method

The marker method is the most common approach used to ascertain ileal AA digestibilities. It relies on the use of an inert substance to account for concentration changes in AA as the meal passes through the digestive tract. As AA and other nutrients are absorbed from the small intestine, the concentration of the marker increases. Use of the total collection method to collect ileal digesta requires the surgical insertion of cannulas or use of surgical approaches that facilitate total collection.

The marker method has been compared with the total collection method for fecal digestibilities. Jørgensen et al. (1984) observed good agreement between the apparent fecal digestibilities of dry matter (DM) and CP (measured using chromic oxide, dysprosium, or total collection) in soybean meal, sunflower meal, fish meal, and meat and bone meal. However, few comparisons have been made between the marker method and the total collection method for ileal digestibilities. Sauer (1976) found good agreement between ileal DM digestibilities determined using total collection or chromic oxide when diets based on barley, corn, or wheat were fed. Similar results were reported by Zebrowska et al. (1978) in comparative studies using casein, soybean meal, and barley. Mroz et al. (1996) compared the total collection method to the use of 0.053% chromic oxide and reported fairly good agreement between the apparent ileal digestibilities of CP, which were 79 and 75%, respectively. In digestion research, the assumption has been that the marker method is as accurate as total collection and this assumption is likely correct. In most applications, the marker method requires less invasive surgical procedures, reentrant cannulation or ileo-rectal anastomosis are not required, and total collection for several days is not necessary.

D. Selection of an Indigestible Marker

Several substances can be used as markers, such as rare earth elements and insoluble forms of minerals. In swine digestion studies, the most common marker used is chromic oxide. Other markers that have been used with swine include titanium oxide, dysprosium chloride, cobalt ethylenediaminetetraacetic acid (EDTA), lanthanum, samarium, ytterbium chloride, and HCl-insoluble ash (Kennelly et al., 1980; Pond et al., 1986; Köhler et al., 1990; Jongbloed et al., 1991; Jagger et al., 1992; Gabert et al., 1997; Albin et al., 2000a). Cobalt EDTA is commonly used in diets for ruminant animals as a liquid-phase marker; however, in pigs, liquid solid separation is not usually considered to be a major concern.

The purpose of the marker is to account for changes in the concentrations of AA as digesta passes through the small intestine. The concentration of the marker increases as AA (and other nutrients) are released by digestion and are absorbed. The substance used as a marker must not be absorbed from the digestive tract, must be inert, and it must not alter digestive events. The measurement of the concentration of the marker in the diet and in digesta should be straightforward, and the marker must be able to be incorporated uniformly into the diet. Uniform mixing can be achieved by premixing the marker with the vitamin and mineral premix or part of one of the major components of the diet, such as soybean meal. A major consideration is that marker flow through the stomach and small intestine should be the same as AA flow (Jørgensen et al., 1997b).

Chromic oxide is very straightforward to assay spectrophotometrically, as chromic acid, following ashing and acid digestion (Fenton and Fenton, 1979). The level of chromic oxide used in digestion studies commonly ranges from 0.3 to 0.5% (as-is basis) of the diet (e.g., Gabert et al. 1995a; Jørgensen et al., 1997b). Limited marker comparison studies have been performed. Jagger et al. (1992) demonstrated that the marker used affects the measurement of apparent ileal AA digestibilities. When 0.5% chromic oxide (as-is) or 0.5% titanium oxide (as is) were compared in studies with growing pigs, using a barley, wheat, and soybean meal–based diet, apparent ileal lysine, threonine, and tryptophan digestibilities were 71.9 and 80.6%, 61.8 and 70.4%, and 78.7 and 83.2%, respectively (Jagger et al., 1992). In contrast, Yin et al. (2000b) reported apparent ileal lysine digestibilities of 81.9 and 80.0%, respectively, when titanium oxide or chromic oxide were used as indigestible markers. Similarly, in studies by Köhler et al. (1990) with growing pigs, ileal DM matter digestibilities were similar (range 84.9 to 86.8%) when chromic oxide, cobalt EDTA, or titanium oxide was used as the indigestible marker. When chromic oxide (0.05%, as-is basis) was compared with HCl-insoluble ash (0.05%, as-is basis), less variation was observed in the digestibility coefficients determined with chromic oxide (Jongbloed et al., 1991).

V. APPROACHES TO COLLECTING ILEAL DIGESTA FROM SWINE

There are a number of methods available for collecting ileal digesta from swine, which are discussed here in brief; for a detailed discussion of anesthetic, analgesic, and surgical procedures used in swine nutrition research, refer to Chapter 42.

A. SLAUGHTER METHOD

The slaughter method involves killing pigs by electric shock, by captive bolt followed by exanguination, or by lethal injection (Low, 1977; Prawirodigdo et al., 1998). The pigs are then dissected and ileal digesta are removed for analysis. This is a relatively simple procedure, but it is not commonly used because of cost and high pig-to-pig variation, which could decrease the sensitivity of this approach. Despite these concerns, this approach has been successfully used (Butts et al., 1993a; Prawirodigdo et al., 1998). Digestion experiments conducted in New Zealand often use the slaughter method (sodium pentobarbitone). Pigs are adapted to the diets for 9 days, fed twice daily, and on day 10, they are fed every hour for 10 h, euthanized at 10 h, and the last 20 to 25 cm of the ileum is removed and ileal digesta are flushed out with 10 ml of distilled water (Butts et al., 1993a). A large number of pigs are required to obtain an adequate number of observations. Other concerns regarding the use of this method include the fact that, when pigs are slaughtered, the intestinal contents could shift and ileal digesta may be contaminated with digesta from other parts of the digestive tract. Also, when a pig is killed, intestinal cell shedding could confound protein and AA digestibility measurements (Prawirodigdo et al., 1998).

Use of barbiturates, compared with captive bolt stunning followed by exanguination, has been shown to minimize mucosal shedding in sheep (Badawy et al., 1957; Badawy, 1964). In comparative studies, pigs were slaughtered using CO_2 stunning followed by exanguination, or had ileal digesta sampled after halothane anesthesia, or were surgically fitted with a simple T-cannula at the distal ileum (Prawirodigdo et al., 1998). Apparent ileal digestibilities of lysine and threonine were much lower in pigs that had digesta sampled by CO_2 stunning than those obtained in cannulated or halothane-anesthetized pigs (Prawirodigdo et al., 1998). Therefore, for measurement of AA digestibilities in terminal experiments, the pigs should be euthanized or anesthetized with halothane, but not killed by CO_2 or captive bolt stunning.

B. Simple T-Cannulation

Simple-T cannulation is widely used in digestion research with swine (Sauer et al., 1983). This procedure involves the surgical insertion of a "T-shaped" cannula into the distal ileum approximately 12 cm anterior to the ileo-cecal junction. The cannula can be exteriorized between the last two ribs to prevent dislodging and minimize leakage of digesta (Gabert, unpublished results). Other exteriorization sites were investigated by Horszczaruk et al. (1972). Simple T-cannulation allows multiple collections to be made from the same pig. Many different diets can be fed without blockage problems. During this procedure, the digestive tract is maintained in a normal physiological state because the small intestine is not transected and therefore the migrating myoelectric complex is maintained.

When the T-cannula approach is used, a large amount of digesta is obtained; approximately 40% of the daily flow is collected (Gabert, unpublished results). Using pigs fitted with simple T-cannulas, a 5-day adaptation to experimental diets and then 2 days of digesta collection is usually used. Digesta are collected from 0800 to 2000 hours on each day and the samples are pooled. This approach has been shown to provide a representative sample of digesta as it encompasses postprandial changes in nutrient flow (Jørgensen et al., 1997b). In addition, this collection time can be used to replace 24-h collections, which are very intensive.

C. Reentrant Cannulation

Reentrant cannulation is a procedure that involves diverting the entire flow of digesta outside the pig, and then the digesta is returned to the ileum or to the cecum (Cunningham et al., 1963; Easter and Tanksley, 1973). This procedure allows total collection of digesta and multiple sampling from the same pig. However, the use of this procedure is limited for many reasons. First, the small intestine is cut during this procedure, and, thus, the migrating myoelectric complex is interrupted and a normal physiological state in the small intestine is not maintained. Also, cannula blockage occurs when high-fiber and large-particle-sized diets are fed (Sauer and de Lange, 1992). When a blockage occurs, feed intake abruptly halts. Saline infusion into the barrel connecting the two cannulas may be necessary to maintain digesta flow (van Leeuwen et al., 1987). When reentrant cannulation is used, ileal digesta from a previous collection must be infused into the cecum while collection is occurring to maintain normal function of the cecum and large intestine. The reentrant cannulation procedure is not commonly used.

D. Ileo-Rectal Anastomosis

The ileo-rectal anastomosis (IRA) procedure (Green et al., 1987; Sauer and de Lange, 1992) was developed and is used commonly in France (Hess and Séve, 1999). The IRA procedure involves the isolation of the cecum and large intestine from the digestive tract and the surgical attachment of the ileum to the rectum; digesta is then collected from the anus. This procedure facilitates total collection of ileal digesta. Build up of fermentation gases is prevented by the insertion of a simple T-cannula into the large intestine.

The IRA procedure allows for easy collection of digesta from pigs fed high-fiber diets. However, this is a very invasive procedure and, when it is used, water intake dramatically increases and electrolytes must be added to the diet to compensate for losses of sodium, potassium, and chloride in ileal digesta (Sauer and de Lange, 1992; Redlich et al., 1997). A higher inclusion level of trace minerals may be required when the IRA method is used. There are several concerns over the use of this technique; one is the isolation of the cecum and colon, and a second is that changes occur in ileal villus length, crypt depth, and the tunica muscularis (Redlich et al., 1997). Therefore, the functional role of the small intestine changes to compensate for the missing colon, and these changes may interfere with digestive processes. When the IRA technique is used, bacterial populations in the small intestine change. Köhler et al. (1992) showed that there was a large increase in volatile fatty acid concentrations in the digesta. Cannulation of the large intestine is required when the IRA is used; thus, this method does not eliminate the necessity of having a pig with a cannula. There are also welfare concerns when the IRA method is used; digesta flows out of the anus of the pig uncontrollably after the surgery is done.

E. Postvalvular T-Cecum Cannulation

Postvalvular T-cecum cannulation (PVTC; van Leeuwen et al., 1991) is a recently developed procedure that involves the removal of the cecum and insertion of a large silicone T-cannula with a rounded flange. The cannula has an angled barrel that facilitates collection of ileal digesta. When the plug in the barrel of the cannula is removed, the ileo-cecal valve protrudes into the barrel, and digesta collection is nearly complete. Many different diets have been evaluated with this procedure and blockage problems have not been encountered (van Leeuwen et al., 1991). However, the impact of removing the cecum on intestinal physiology is not known; therefore, additional investigation on the application of this technique may be needed. This technique is commonly used in the Netherlands.

F. Steered Ileo-Cecal Valve Cannulation

Steered ileo-cecal valve (SICV) cannulation (Mroz et al., 1996) is the newest collection technique that has been developed. A silicone cannula with a large flange is inserted into the cecum, opposite the ileo-cecal valve. A stainless steel ring is secured around the outside of the ileum, a second ring is inserted into the ileum, and a nylon cord is attached to it. During periods of digesta collection, the nylon cord is pulled, and this brings the outer ring up to the barrel of the cannula and allows total collection of ileal digesta. The cord is released during times when collections are not being made. This allows the digesta to proceed into the hindgut normally. The SICV approach can be used with many different types of diets.

G. Comparisons between Collection Procedures

Donkoh et al. (1994) compared the slaughter method with simple T-cannulation and concluded that there was no effect ($P > 0.05$) of collection procedure on apparent ileal AA digestibilities. In comparative studies, apparent ileal digestibilities of AA were much lower in pigs that had digesta sampled by CO_2 stunning than in pigs that were fitted with a simple T-cannula or had digesta sampled using halothane anesthesia (Prawirodigdo et al., 1998). Zebrowska et al. (1978) compared simple T-cannulation and reentrant cannulation procedures. AA digestibilities were measured with semipurified diets and few significant differences in digestibility coefficients were reported between the two techniques. Taverner et al. (1983) did not observe any effect of collection method on the apparent ileal digestibilities of AA when simple T-cannulation and reentrant cannulation were compared. Apparent ileal CP digestibilities were higher ($P > 0.05$) when digesta was collected using a simple T-cannula than when reentrant cannulation was used in studies with pigs fed commercial-type diets (Yin et al., 1991).

Köhler et al. (1990) compared simple T, reentrant, and PVTC collection procedures and found no differences ($P > 0.05$) among the different techniques in apparent N digestibilities. In this comparative experiment, pigs were fed commercial-type and high-fiber diets (Köhler et al., 1990). In studies by Yin et al. (2000a), apparent ileal CP digestibilities were significantly higher when the PVTC method was used to collect digesta compared with the simple T-cannula. When the SICV method was compared with simple T-cannulation, apparent ileal lysine digestibilities were similar. However, the coefficients obtained by collecting samples from a simple T-cannula had higher standard deviations (Fernández et al., unpublished results). Another comparison by Leterme et al. (1990) examined simple T and IRA techniques and found few significant differences between the procedures. Simple T cannulation and the PVTC method are the most widely used procedures for collection of ileal digesta. Further research is needed to compare collection methods. Determining which technique is the "best one" depends on personal experience, duration of the experiment, type of diet fed, and animal welfare concerns. Proper management of cannulated pigs is critical, and it is seldom discussed in the literature. For example, representative samples of digesta will be obtained from a simple T-cannula if the pigs are checked on a regular basis to ensure that digesta is flowing out of the cannula. In addition, if high-fiber or coarse diets are being fed, the barrel of the cannula must be cleaned out on a regular basis, with a spoon or spatula, to ensure that sampling continues (Gabert, unpublished results).

VI. TRUE ILEAL AMINO ACID DIGESTIBILITIES

A. Definition and Significance

True ileal digestibilities of AA indicate the amount of AA actually released from dietary protein and absorbed by the small intestine. True digestibilities of AA accurately reflect how well a protein source was digested. The determination of true digestibilities allows factors that affect protein digestion to be studied. There is now more interest in defining AA requirements on a true digestible basis (NRC, 1998). To obtain true digestibilities, estimates of endogenous AA in ileal digesta are needed to remove the endogenous contribution of AA (Table 9.1; Figure 9.1). There are several approaches that can be used to estimate endogenous AA losses in ileal digesta. Each one has positive and negative attributes that must be taken into consideration before it is used. However, there are only two approaches that can be used to measure endogenous AA losses directly when commercial-type diets are fed. These two approaches are known as the isotope dilution technique and the homoarginine method. When the other approaches are used, the values obtained for endogenous AA are assumed to represent endogenous AA losses in pigs fed commercial-type diets.

B. Measurement of Endogenous Amino Acid Losses

Quantification of endogenous AA is necessary to obtain true ileal AA digestibilities. Endogenous AA are both animal and bacterial in nature and originate from pancreatic enzymes, mucin, bacterial protein, and AA from sloughed epithelial cells (Asche et al., 1989; Dugan et al., 1994; Gabert et al., 1996b; Gabert et al., 1997; Lien et al., 1997b). Amino acids, either as free AA, in peptides, or an endogenous protein, that are not reabsorbed before reaching the distal ileum and collected in ileal digesta are referred to as endogenous AA. When measured, these AA are referred to as endogenous AA losses because there is no AA absorption from the cecum and large intestine in the pig (Zebrowska, 1973; Just et al., 1981; Nyachoti et al., 1997a; Nyachoti et al., 2000).

1. Protein-Free Diets

Determining the output of AA in ileal digesta from pigs fed protein-free diets is one method of estimating the contribution of endogenous AA to total AA at the distal ileum (Table 9.1; Nyachoti et al., 1997a; Hess and Séve, 1999). However, this method is often criticized because the pig is in a catabolic state (Skilton et al., 1988). In addition, when a protein-free diet is fed, pancreatic and other digestive secretions are reduced and intestinal function may be compromised to the absence of dietary AA in the intestinal lumen (Skilton et al., 1988; Brannon, 1990; Butts et al., 1991). Therefore, when protein-free diets are fed, endogenous AA losses at the terminal ileum are underestimated (Table 9.1).

2. Enzymically Hydrolyzed Casein Method

Another approach to estimate endogenous AA is the enzymically hydrolyzed casein (EHC) method (Table 9.1). This method involves feeding pigs diets containing EHC, which has a very high digestibility, as the sole source of dietary protein (Moughan et al., 1992b). AA that are necessary for protein synthesis in the gastrointestinal tract are supplied (Alpers, 1972). This is obviously not the case when protein-free diets are fed. The technique involves the collection of ileal digesta, and the major assumption is that the feeding of EHC stimulates a representative amount of endogenous secretions and that peptides and proteins in excess of 10,000 Da represent endogenous protein secretions (Moughan et al., 1992b; Butts et al., 1993a; Donkoh and Moughan, 1999). When the EHC method is used, digesta are centrifuged and then ultrafiltered. To determine endogenous AA flow, the peptides and proteins in the retentate with a molecular weight of greater than 10,000 Da are added to the precipitate from the initial centrifugation (Donkoh and Moughan, 1999).

A major limitation of the EHC method is that it can be used only with semipurified diets that contain EHC. It can be used to investigate the effects of specific factors that affect endogenous secretions, such as fiber, tannins, trypsin inhibitors, and lectins. However, the EHC method cannot be used to evaluate the effect of feeding practical diets (for example, diets containing soybean meals processed to different extents or soybean meal containing different levels of fiber) on endogenous AA losses. The only dietary ingredients that are compatible with the EHC method are those that do not supply protein to the diet such as antinutritional compounds, cornstarch, oil, and fiber sources.

3. Low-Protein Casein Diets

We have recently adapted the use of a low-protein diet that contains 4% CP from casein (5% of the diet, as-is basis). The diet also contains cornstarch, sucrose, chromic oxide, and a mineral and vitamin premix. This approach was used to supply some AA to the pig to attempt to maintain a more physiological state as opposed to feeding a protein-free diet. Crude protein and the other endogenous AA outputs were calculated (mean ± sample standard deviation; g/kg DMI): CP, 18.92 ± 2.70; Thr, 0.74 ± 0.08; Met, 0.15 ± 0.02; Cys, 0.24 ± 0.02, and Trp, 0.17 ± 0.04 (Albin et al., unpublished results). The endogenous output of lysine is shown in Table 9.1. These estimates are within the range of values reported in the literature (de Lange et al., 1989; Gabert et al., 1997; Lien et al., 1997a,b).

4. Regression Method

Another method that can be used to estimate endogenous AA losses is known as the regression method (Table 9.1). Linear relationships between several dietary levels of AA and the amount digested is used to predict the endogenous ileal output of AA at zero AA intake (Taverner et al., 1981; Low 1982; Leibholz and Mollah, 1988; Fan et al., 1995b; Fan and Sauer, 1997). The regression method has been used in studies with cannulated pigs, as well as with the slaughter method (Leibholz, 1982).

The regression method assumes that endogenous AA losses are constant over several different inclusion levels of different ingredients, and that extrapolation to zero AA intake accurately predicts the level of endogenous AA. The regression method can be easily used to estimate endogenous ileal AA flow when commercial-type diets are fed as long as the diets are formulated to have increasing levels of CP.

5. Isotope Dilution Technique

The isotope dilution technique (IDT) involves labeling AA in the pig with ^{15}N-leucine (Souffrant et al., 1986; Gabert et al., 1997; Lien et al., 1997a,b), ^{3}H-leucine (Moughan et al., 1992a), or ^{15}N labeled diets (Leterme et al., 1996). For example, if a pig is labeled by a long infusion of ^{15}N-leucine so that a large amount of transamination occurs and several AA become enriched with ^{15}N, the amounts of endogenous CP and AA are determined by dividing the ^{15}N-enrichment in an AA in digesta by that in the same AA in the trichloroacetic acid–soluble fraction of blood plasma (Gabert et al., 1997; Lien et al., 1997a,b). This ratio is multiplied by the amount of the AA in ileal digesta (Table 9.1; Gabert et al., 1997). Alternatively, the enrichment in one AA, such as leucine, can be used and the amounts of all the other endogenous AA can be determined if a constant composition of endogenous protein is assumed (de Lange et al., 1990; Gabert et al., 1997).

The original ^{15}N-IDT of Souffrant et al. (1986) is based on enrichment in total N, and frequently overestimates the contribution of endogenous protein and AA to total protein and AA in ileal digesta due to ^{15}N-enrichment of nonprecursor N (Lien et al., 1997a,b). Real ileal digestibilities frequently exceed 100% (de Lange et al., 1990). To improve the technique, de Lange et al. (1992) determined the ^{15}N-enrichments in individual AA, namely, leucine and isoleucine, deriving the so-called ^{15}N-leucine- and ^{15}N-isoleucine-IDT, respectively. Recently, the technique has been further improved with respect to the pattern of blood sampling, analytical aspects to allow the determination of ^{15}N-enrichment in several AA, and the validity of various precursor pools (Gabert et al., 1997; Lien et al., 1997a,b). The determination of dilution in ^{15}N-enrichment in several AA led to the development of the ^{15}N-AA IDT. It is critical that blood samples are taken frequently (i.e., every hour) and not just at feeding to encompass changes in AA metabolism occurring in the postabsorptive state. The question of more frequent feeding possibly to limit differences in metabolism between the pre- and postabsorptive state is discussed by Lien (1997a,b). The improved procedures of Lien et al. (1997b) were adopted and refined by Gabert et al. (1997).

The ^{15}N-leucine- or ^{15}N-AA-IDT can be readily used to estimate endogenous AA losses in commercial-type diets, which is the major advantage of this approach (Gabert et al., 1997; Lien et al., 1997a,b). However, this technique is not commonly used because of the cost of purchasing large quantities of ^{15}N-leucine and the intensive nature of these studies. In addition, accurate measurement of isotopic enrichment in individual AA needs to be done for this approach to be used successfully.

6. Homoarginine Method

The homoarginine (HA) method is used to discriminate endogenous lysine from undigested dietary lysine in ileal digesta. The HA method involves the chemical conversion of protein-bound lysine in a guanidination reaction with O-methylisourea to HA, an AA that is not found in animal or plant proteins (Hagemeister and Erbersdobler, 1985). The usefulness of the HA method for directly determining true ileal AA digestibilities has been demonstrated in several recent studies (Schmitz et al., 1991; Marty et. al., 1994; Nyachoti et al., 1997b; Caine et al., 1998; McNeilage et al., 2000). Unlike the use of protein-free diets, low-protein casein diets or diets, containing EHC, the HA method has proved useful in estimating true ileal AA digestibilities in commercial-type diets. These include diets based on corn and soybean meal or barley and canola meal (Imbeah et al., 1996; Nyachoti et al., 1997b; McNeilage, 1998). Conditions for conducting the guanidination reaction have been investigated and optimized (Rutherfurd and Moughan, 1990; Imbeah et al., 1996; Nyachoti et al., 1997b; McNeilage, 1998).

Diets containing 50% of the converted protein are fed and the concentration of HA is determined in ileal digesta, and the digestibility of HA is calculated (Marty et al., 1994; Albin et al., 2000b). The digestibility of HA represents the true digestibility of lysine. HA is released by digestion and is absorbed from the small intestine (Schmitz et al., 1991). The endogenous flow of lysine is determined from the true and apparent lysine digestibilities (Marty et al., 1994). The endogenous contribution of the other AA is determined by using previously determined AA profiles of endogenous protein (e.g., de Lange et al., 1989; Boisen and Moughan, 1996; Gabert et al., 1997; McNeilage et al., 2000), or by using one of the previously discussed approaches to determine an endogenous profile. The HA technique also allows the evaluation of specific factors that affect the endogenous flows of AA.

It has been assumed that the HA-labeling process does not affect the digestion of the labeled diet. The authors have recently shown this by comparing apparent ileal digestibilities of AA in nonguanidinated and in guanidinated barley and canola meal–based diets. Half of the barley and half of the canola meal in the labeled diet were guanidinated. There were no differences ($P > 0.05$) in the apparent ileal digestibilities of DM, CP, or AA between the two diets (McNeilage et al., 2000). These results support the use of the HA method to determine true AA digestibilities in feedstuffs. A procedure for preparing large batches of guanidinated feedstuffs was described by Imbeah et al. (1996).

VII. FACTORS AFFECTING DIGESTION AND ENDOGENOUS LOSSES OF AMINO ACIDS

There are several factors that affect AA digestibilities and these need to be taken into consideration to interpret digestibility experiments with pigs, predict digestibilities in complete diets, and to design meaningful studies that yield useful information. Each of these factors is discussed separately; however, in most circumstances, several factors are acting at the same time.

A. DRY MATTER INTAKE AND BODY WEIGHT

The influence of feed intake (DM intake) on apparent ileal AA digestibilities has been investigated in very few studies. From a diet formulation perspective, if feed intake is an important factor, then adjustments need to be made based on feed intake under commercial conditions, to enable more accurate diet formulation on an ileal digestible AA basis. In studies by Sauer et al. (1982), growing pigs were fed 0.84, 1.26, or 1.68 kg of DM per day and there were no effects ($P > 0.05$) of DM intake on any of the apparent ileal AA digestibilities. Haydon et al. (1984) fed pigs *ad libitum*, 4.5, or 3% of their body weight (BW) per day, and they concluded that there were no effects ($P > 0.05$) of feed intake on apparent ileal AA digestibilities. The apparent ileal digestibilities of lysine in the soybean meal- and sorghum-based diet that were fed were 81.6, 79.9, and 80.1%, respectively, for *ad libitum*, 4.5 and 3% feeding levels (Haydon et al., 1984). It is clear from these two studies that feed intake (DM intake) does not significantly affect the apparent ileal digestibilities of AA in pigs.

Feed intake has been shown to affect endogenous ileal AA losses. In studies with gestating sows that were either restricted fed (average daily feed intake, ADFI, 2.0 kg) or had *ad libitum* access to feed (ADFI, 4.35 kg) endogenous loss of CP was higher ($P < 0.05$) in restricted-fed sows (Stein et al., 1999b). Endogenous losses of lysine and threonine were numerically higher in restricted-fed sows than in sows that had *ad libitum* access to feed (Stein et al., 1999b). Butts et al. (1993b) observed an increase in the endogenous ileal flow of AA, expressed in grams per day, as pigs were fed more feed. However, endogenous ileal AA losses were similar when expressed in g/kg DMI (Table 9.1; Butts et al., 1993b).

Very few studies have examined the effects of BW on apparent ileal AA digestibilities, and it is usually assumed that there are no major differences between apparent ileal AA digestibilities measured in growing or finishing pigs. Because pigs are fed more as they become heavier, BW and feed intake could have combined effects. However, when Latin square designs are used in studies with growing pigs that are 2 months or more in duration, variation due to experimental periods and pigs is removed (Fan et al., 1996; Jørgensen et al., 2000). In comparative studies between growing pigs and in gestating and lactating sows, Stein et al. (1999a) reported that there were no differences in apparent ileal lysine digestibilities in corn, barley, soybean meal, and canola meal. Some significant differences were observed between apparent ileal lysine digestibilities in meat and bone meal and in wheat between growing pigs and sows (Stein et al., 1999a). Furuya and Kaji (1992) observed few significant effects of BW, in 49- or 92-kg pigs, on endogenous ileal AA losses (expressed in g/kg DMI). However, as feed intake was increased from 0.8 to 1.2 or 1.6 kg/day in either 49- or 92-kg pigs, endogenous ileal AA losses (expressed in g/kg DMI) were decreased ($P < 0.05$) for all AA except glycine (Furuya and Kaji, 1992). In weanling pigs, BW (stage of development) is very important. In digestion studies with weanling pigs there is often an experimental period effect due to rapid digestive development and, therefore, two-period change-over designs should be used (Li and Sauer, 1994; Li et al., 1994; Gabert et al., 1995a,b; Li et al., 1996).

B. Ingredient and Feed Processing

Grinding cereal grains decreases particle size, exposes feed particles to digestive enzymes, and therefore improves the ileal digestibilities of AA and feed utilization (Sauer et al., 1977; Owsley et al., 1981). Fineness of grind (or lack of grinding) could be expected to contribute to some of the variation in AA digestibilities observed within the same feedstuff. In finely ground wheat compared to cracked wheat, Sauer et al. (1977) reported apparent ileal lysine digestibilities of 81.5 and 72.6%, respectively. Feed processing may not always improve ileal AA digestibilities. Chu et al. (1998) reported that apparent ileal AA digestibilities were decreased ($P < 0.05$) in finely-ground barley compared to course-ground barley in studies with 11-kg pigs. Partial mechanical dehulling of canola meal slightly improved ($P < 0.05$) the apparent ileal digestibility of threonine (from 72.1 to 75.5%); however, the digestibilities of the other AA were not improved by dehulling (de Lange et al., 1998).

In studies with young pigs, there was no effect of steam pelleting, expanding or expanding and pelleting on apparent ileal CP digestibilities (van der Poel et al., 1998). However, processes applied to full fat soybeans, such as extrusion, jet-sploding, micronizing and roasting, have been shown to affect ($P < 0.05$) the true ileal digestibility of lysine as well as the endogenous flow of lysine (Table 9.1; Marty et al., 1994). Micronization of hulless barley has been shown to be effective at improving ($P < 0.05$) apparent ileal digestibilities of AA in young pigs (Table 9.2; Huang et al., 1998). Conversely, in studies by Fan et al. (1995a), extrusion of full fat soybeans did not improve apparent ileal digestibilities of AA in weanling pigs compared with those determined in soybean meal. Chu et al. (1998) reported that extrusion improved apparent ileal AA digestibilities in 11-kg pigs fed barley-based diets. Supplemental lysine has been shown to be relatively stable to extrusion; apparent ileal digestibility of lysine was complete for crystalline L-lysine and L-lysine that was included in an extruded diet for growing pigs (Leibholz et al., 1986).

Processing of soy proteins improves AA digestibility in early-weaned pigs; apparent ileal lysine digestibilities in soybean meal, soy protein concentrate, and in isolated soy protein were 79.3, 88.3, and 88.2%, respectively (Sohn et al., 1994). The differences in digestibility may have been due to the presence of various antinutritional factors and carbohydrate (fiber) complexes present in soybean meal (Sohn et al., 1994).

Heat treatment is another factor that has important effects on ileal AA digestibilities. Heating soy protein products inactivates trypsin inhibitors and has very beneficial effects on ileal AA digestibility. When digestibilities measured in unheated soy flour were compared with those determined in autoclaved soy flour, a dramatic increase in apparent digestibilities of lysine and other AA were observed (Table 9.2; Li et al., 1998). In studies with growing pigs, apparent ileal digestibilities of AA were improved ($P < 0.05$) when raw soybeans were autoclaved (Herkelman et al., 1992). Heating soy flakes in a steam-jacketed cooker for 25 to 105 min at 100 to 107°C improved ($P < 0.01$) apparent ileal digestibilities of AA (Vandergrift et al., 1983). Apparent ileal AA digestibility coefficients were not affected when times greater than 25 min were used (Vandergrift et al., 1983).

Overheating can have very detrimental effects on protein digestibility. Depending on how extensive the heat damage has been, the extent to which AA digestibilities are reduced will vary. Overheating fish meal has been shown to decrease apparent ileal AA digestibilities extensively, especially for methionine (Table 9.2; Wiseman et al., 1991). When dry spring peas were overheated, the apparent ileal digestibility of lysine decreased substantially (van Barneveld et al., 1994a). Apparent ileal AA digestibilities are higher than AA availabilities in protein sources that have been excessively heat-treated, especially for lysine (Batterham et al., 1984; 1990; Batterham, 1992). This response is due to a number of factors; various compounds are formed when AA (lysine as well as several other AA) react with carbohydrate and lipid components, and some of these compounds can be absorbed but they are not necessarily available for protein synthesis (Friedman, 1996).

Maillard products are formed with lysine during heat treatment, and when the reaction progresses past the Schiff's base stage to the formation of Amadori compounds, availability of lysine in the rat decreases from 100% to zero (Friedman, 1996). A second concern is that acid hydrolyses, used to prepare samples of feed and ileal digesta for AA analyses, may break down complexes between AA and other compounds that are not available (Friedman, 1996). Therefore, ileal AA digestibilities may be overestimated. When the Maillard reaction takes place and a Schiff's base is formed, 100% of the complexed lysine is released during acid hydrolyses; however, when an Amadori compound is formed, only 40% is released (Friedman, 1996). If more advanced products are formed, none of the lysine is released (Friedman, 1996). In studies with dry peas that were either unheated or heated at 110, 135, 150, or 165°C for 15 min, van Barneveld et al. (1994a,c) measured the following apparent ileal lysine digestibilities and corresponding availabilities (in parentheses, based on daily BW gain): 75% (101%), 79% (74%), 74% (83%), 74% (59%), and 56% (16%), respectively. Therefore, heat treatment can have very dramatic effects on apparent ileal lysine digestibilities, as well as the availability of lysine.

C. LEVEL OF PROTEIN AND AMINO ACIDS IN THE DIET

Dietary AA intake influences apparent ileal AA digestibilities, and it is a factor that is responsible for a relatively large amount of variation in apparent ileal AA digestibilities (Fan et al., 1994; 1996; Fan and Sauer, 1999). The effect of the level of dietary protein (AA intake) on apparent fecal protein digestibility was first demonstrated by Eggum (1973) in experiments with rats. The apparent ileal digestibility of a particular AA or of CP increases as the level in the diet (intake) increases (Eggum, 1973; Fan et al., 1994). The reason is that the level of endogenous AA at the distal ileum continues to decrease relative to undigested dietary AA as AA intake increases (Fan et al., 1994; 1995). To obtain accurate apparent ileal digestibility measurements, the intake of AA needs to be high enough to minimize the contribution of endogenous AA compared with dietary AA in ileal digesta collected from the distal ileum (Fan et al., 1994). For example, in the studies of Fan et al. (1994), apparent digestibilities of AA in a semipurified cornstarch and soybean meal–based diet that contained 16% CP exceeded the threshold values. By setting the level of AA intake (protein level in the diet) so that measured digestibilities exceeded the threshold values (digestibilities no longer increase with increasing AA intake), and therefore reached the plateau portion of the curve, there was assurance that the digestibility coefficients were not significantly affected by the AA level (intake) in the diet. If the level of protein in the test ingredient does not exceed 16% CP, an ingredient with a higher level of protein should be used with the difference or the regression method to ensure accurate measurement of apparent ileal AA digestibilities (Fan et al., 1993; Fan and Sauer, 1995). To ensure that accurate estimates of apparent ileal AA digestibilities are obtained in growing pigs, the authors are now using semipurified and commercial diets that are formulated to contain 17% CP (as-is basis).

There is an important consideration for the calculation of apparent ileal AA digestibilities. If an AA is added to the diet, for example, if lysine is supplemented, which is assumed to be 100% digestible (Chung and Baker, 1992), then the added level of lysine must be subtracted from the level of lysine in the diet. If this is not done, apparent ileal lysine digestibility will be overestimated.

D. SOURCE OF PROTEIN AND PROTEIN SOLUBILITY

Often animal sources of protein are more digestible than plant sources of protein. In studies with early-weaned pigs, the apparent ileal digestibility of lysine was higher ($P < 0.05$) in dried skim milk (91.7%) than in soy protein concentrate (88.3%), isolated soy protein (88.2%), or soybean meal (79.3%; Sohn et al., 1994). The diets fed in these studies had a similar CP content (23.3 to 24.0%, as-is). Similar results were reported by Walker et al. (1986). Changes in the composition of plant proteins can cause changes in ileal digestibilities of AA in pigs. High-lysine barley varieties have an increased synthesis of lysine-rich endosperm proteins, known as glutelins, and a decreased synthesis of prolamin protein, known as hordein, which has a relatively low lysine content (Jørgensen et al., 1997a). Apparent ileal digestibilities of AA in the high-lysine barley cultivar Lysimax were first reported by Jørgensen et al. (1997a), and the digestibilities of lysine, threonine, and methionine were not adversely affected by the change in protein composition. The apparent ileal digestibility of lysine was slightly higher in the high-lysine barley (69.0%) compared with a normal barley variety (66.5%; Jørgensen et al., 1997a). Similar results were observed in studies with high-lysine corn; in studies with growing pigs, the apparent and true ileal digestibilities of CP did not differ ($P > 0.05$) between high-lysine corn and normal corn (Andersen et al., 2000).

The solubility of a protein in an aqueous environment, such as the gastrointestinal tract, is an important factor that can influence apparent ileal AA digestibilities. In studies with young pigs, Jansman et al. (1995) fed protein sources with an assumed low solubility (fish meal, soy protein concentrate, meat meal, potato protein, or sunflower meal) or with an assumed high solubility (casein and faba bean cotyledons). Actual solubility measurements were not made in these studies. Large differences in apparent ileal AA digestibilities were observed between diets containing low or highly soluble protein sources (Table 9.2; Jansman et al., 1995). Protein solubility, measured using KOH was discussed earlier under rapid determination of AA digestibilities. Additional research on the effect of protein solubility on apparent ileal AA digestibilities is needed.

E. LEVEL AND SOURCE OF DIETARY FAT

The level of dietary fat has been shown to affect the digestion of protein in the pig. In studies with young pigs, a significant linear effect of canola oil supplementation on apparent ileal digestibilities of lysine and threonine was observed as the level of canola oil in the diet was increased (Table 9.2; Li and Sauer, 1994). Similarly, apparent fecal CP digestibility in growing pigs was increased ($P < 0.05$) when diets were supplemented with 5, 10, 15, 20, 25, or 30% soybean oil (Jørgensen and Fernández, 2000). However, when these levels of supplementation were used with animal fat, palm oil, and a mixture of palm oil and vegetable oil, apparent fecal digestibilities of CP were not affected (Jørgensen and Fernández, 2000). The beneficial effect of canola oil or soybean oil supplementation may have been due to an effect on endogenous ileal AA losses. In recent studies with growing pigs, the authors did not observe an effect ($P > 0.05$) of supplementing 15% fish oil, rapeseed oil, or coconut oil on apparent ileal digestibility of CP (Jørgensen et al., 2000). There is a scarcity of information on the effect of fat level and source on endogenous ileal AA losses, and the effect of fat level on true AA digestibilities is not known.

F. FIBER TYPE, LEVEL, AND FIBER-DEGRADING ENZYMES

Fiber level and type can affect apparent ileal AA digestibilities by increasing endogenous AA losses. The fiber in ingredients such as barley and canola meal may be partly responsible for causing an increase in the endogenous ileal flow of lysine, compared with diets containing casein (Table 9.1; Figure 9.2; Nyachoti et al., 1997b). A large portion of the variability in apparent ileal AA digestibilities in different samples of canola meal and peas has been shown to be due to neutral detergent fiber (NDF) content. There is a negative correlation between the level of NDF and apparent ileal AA digestibilities (Figure 9.2; Fan et al., 1996; Fan and Sauer, 1999). Similar results were reported in studies with wheat (Taverner and Farrell, 1981b).

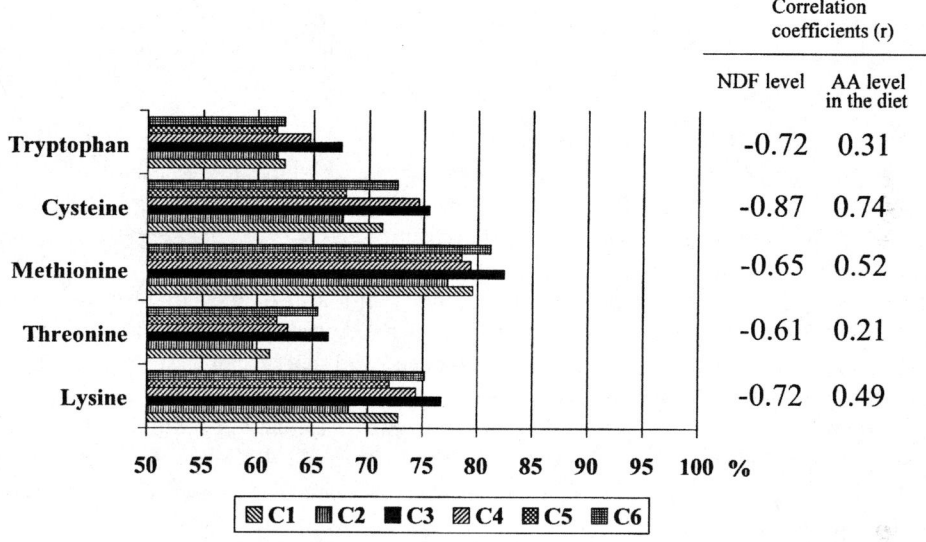

FIGURE 9.2 Selected apparent ileal AA digestibilities in samples of canola meal obtained from different canola crushers and the correlation coefficients between AA digestibilities, neutral-detergent fiber content, and the level of AA in the diet. The six canola crushers, from which the samples were obtained, are represented by C1 to C6. (Fan, M. Z. et al., *Can. J. Anim. Sci.*, 76:563, 1996. With permission.)

The effects of fiber on true AA digestibilities are not well known. Increasing levels of cellulose may increase endogenous AA losses. Li et al. (1994) showed that the addition of 4, 6, or 8% cellulose to a semipurified diet fed to weanling pigs decreased ($P < 0.05$) apparent ileal digestibilities of AA. Similar, although not significant effects, were observed when growing pigs were fed diets containing 10% alfafloc or barley straw (Table 9.2; Sauer et al., 1991). However, the addition of 3, 6, 9, or 12% wood cellulose to protein-free diets did not affect endogenous AA losses (Leterme et al., 1992). In studies with supplemental oligosaccharides and lactitol, the authors did not observe any major effects of these additives on apparent ileal AA digestibilities in weanling pigs (Gabert et al., 1995a). The potential to reduce the effects of fiber on endogenous AA losses has increased interest in supplementing fiber-degrading enzymes to diets for swine, especially young swine.

Fiber-degrading enzymes have been used successfully to improve apparent ileal AA digestibilities and/or to decrease endogenous AA losses. β-Glucanase has been used to improve ($P < 0.05$) AA digestibility in hull-less barley- and soybean meal–based diets (Figure 9.3; Li et al., 1996). Similar results were observed in studies with 11-kg pigs fed barley-based diets supplemented with β-glucanase (Chu et al., 1998). β-Glucans may increase viscosity in the intestine and, therefore, interfere with nutrient absorption (Li et al., 1996; Baidoo et al., 1998). β-Glucans and other fibrous components may also increase digestive secretions in the small intestine and therefore increase

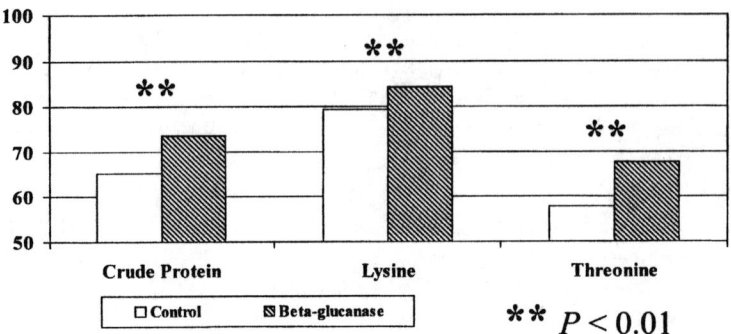

FIGURE 9.3 The effect of β-glucanase supplementation (0.2%) on selected apparent ileal AA digestibilities measured in young pigs fed hull-less barley and soybean meal–based diets. (From Li, S. et al., *J. Anim. Sci.*, 74:1649, 1996. With permission.)

endogenous AA losses (Nyachoti et al., 1997a). The apparent ileal digestibilities of AA in hulless barley were increased ($P < 0.05$) by the use of an enzyme mixture that consisted of β-glucanase and xylanase (Baidoo et al., 1998). The fecal digestibility of DM (total solids) and N were also increased ($P < 0.05$). Most of the β-glucanase activity in feed survives passage through the acidic conditions of the stomach (Baas and Thacker, 1996).

A limited number of studies have investigated the addition of fiber-degrading enzymes to corn and soybean meal based–diets. In recent experiments with growing pigs, the authors added cellulase and hemicellulase to a semipurified cornstarch soybean meal–based diet (Albin et al., 2000a). The diets (control and enzyme supplemented) were either fed dry or steeped (soaked) in water for 12 h. The dietary treatments did not affect ($P > 0.05$) the apparent ileal digestibilities of AA. A second study with growing pigs investigated the effect of supplementing cellulase, hemicellulase, xylanase, α-galactosidase, protease, and amylase to a corn and soybean meal–based diet (Smiricky et al., 2000a). The diets were either fed dry or were steeped (soaked) in water for 12 h. The apparent fecal digestibilities of DM and CP were not affected ($P > 0.05$) by the dietary treatments. As new sources of enzymes and strategies for enzyme use are developed, more research is needed on the effect of fiber-degrading enzymes on ileal AA digestibilities, as well as endogenous AA losses.

G. Phytate and Use of Phytase

The use of phytase in diets for growing pigs may improve AA absorption by reducing the association between phytate and AA. The apparent ileal digestibility of methionine was increased ($P < 0.05$) in pigs fed 800 units of phytase/kg in a diet containing corn, tapioca, soybean meal, barley, and peas (Table 9.2; Mroz et al., 1994). In a different study, supplementation of a diet for growing pigs with 900 units of phytase/kg improved the apparent ileal digestibilities of AA (Kemme et al., 1999). Supplementation of a corn and soybean meal–based diet with 500 units of phytase/kg tended to improve the apparent ileal digestibilities of lysine ($P < 0.11$, from 77.2 to 79.9%) and threonine ($P < 0.06$, from 70.5 to 74.4%) in studies with growing pigs (Johnston et al., 2000). Further research is required to investigate whether or not phytase improves apparent and true ileal AA digestibilities in pigs.

H. Trypsin Inhibitors

Trypsin inhibitors are proteins that are antinutritional compounds present in grain legumes and legume products. They interfere with the function of trypsin and chymotrypsin (Huisman and Jansman, 1991; Gabert et al., 1996a). Cereal grains, such as rye and barley, have been shown to contain trypsin inhibitors; however, they do not likely have a negative effect on protein digestion in pigs because their activity is relatively low (Sosulski et al., 1988). Growing pigs fed diets containing unheated soy flour had higher ($P < 0.05$) endogenous ileal AA losses than pigs that were fed autoclaved soy flour, suggesting that trypsin inhibitors increased endogenous secretions (Caine et al., 1998). True ileal AA digestibilities were higher ($P < 0.05$) in autoclaved soy flour than in unheated soy flour (Caine et al., 1998). The Bowman–Birk trypsin inhibitor has a high cysteine content; therefore, low apparent ileal digestibilities of cysteine may be due to the effects of this inhibitor (Fan and Sauer, 1994). Feeding raw low-trypsin-inhibitor soybeans, compared with conventional soybeans, improved ($P < 0.05$) the ileal digestibilities of AA in growing pigs (Herkelman et al., 1992). When conventional and low-trypsin-inhibitor soybeans were autoclaved, the apparent ileal digestibilities of AA in the low-trypsin-inhibitor soybeans still greatly exceeded ($P < 0.05$) those in the conventional soybeans. These results demonstrate that trypsin inhibitors interfere with the digestion of soy protein. The volume of pancreatic juice was increased in young pigs fed unheated soy flour compared with those fed autoclaved soy flour (Li, 1996). However, there was no effect ($P < 0.05$) of diet on the total activity of trypsin or chymotrypsin secreted (Li, 1996). Apparent ileal AA digestibilities determined in different pigs were severely reduced ($P < 0.05$) in unheated soy flour as opposed to autoclaved soy flour (Table 9.2; Li et al., 1998). Schulze (1994), using the ^{15}N-IDT, demonstrated that supplemental trypsin inhibitors substantially increased endogenous ileal CP losses in pigs.

Trypsin inhibitor activity is substantially reduced during heating in the desolventizer–toaster while soybeans are being processed. Soybean meal does contain some residual trypsin inhibitor activity (Huisman and Jansman, 1991), which could have a small effect on endogenous AA losses; however, this remains to be investigated. Raw soybeans contain approximately 24 mg of tryspin inhibitor activity per gram (mg of trypsin inhibited per gram) compared with soybean meal, which contains approximately 3 mg/g (Huisman and Jansman, 1991). Fan and Sauer (1999) reported that with the exception of the apparent ileal digestibility of tryptophan, no significant negative correlation coefficients were observed between the level of trypsin inhibitors in peas and apparent ileal AA digestibilities in growing pigs. Trypsin inhibitor activity can be reduced using seed germination (Schulze et al., 1997). Germination has been successfully used in studies with white kidney beans (*Phaseolus vulgaris* L.); treated beans were fed to young pigs and the apparent ileal digestibilities of AA were improved ($P < 0.05$), compared with untreated beans (Schulze et al., 1997).

I. Lectins

Lectins are glycoproteins and are also referred to as hemaglutinins (Grant and van Driessche, 1993). Glycoproteins (glycocalyx) on the surface of small intestinal enterocytes contain sugars to which lectins have affinity and, as a result, lectins bind to epithelial cells. Lectins can also bind to mucoproteins (Grant and van Driessche, 1993). When purified soybean lectins were included in diets for swine, they increased endogenous ileal CP losses, as measured at the terminal ileum using the ^{15}N-IDT (Schulze et al., 1995). These endogenous losses, likely a loss of mucus, did not seem to increase proportionally to the dietary lectin content. Lectins seem to have minor effects on true ileal CP digestibilities, but they reduce the digestibility of other nutrients as indicated by the larger flow of DM at the distal ileum in pigs fed lectins (Schulze et al., 1995). An additional effect of lectins is that they stimulate the proliferation of bacteria in the intestinal lumen (Grant and van Driessche, 1993; Schulze et al., 1995). Various feed ingredient processing procedures, such as steam treatment, autoclaving, dry roasting, and extrusion, have been shown to inactivate lectins in phaseolus beans (van der Poel, 1990). Seed germination can be used to reduce lectin content (Schulze et al., 1997). Additional research is needed to investigate the effects of lectins on apparent and true ileal AA digestibilities.

J. Tannins

Tannins are polyphenolic compounds that bind to AA and proteins (Jansman, 1993). Tannins occur in sorghum hulls as well as the hulls of faba beans (Jansman, 1993). Tannins in sorghum can adversely affect protein digestion in the pig (Cousins et al., 1981; Mitaru et al., 1984). Barley grain also has also been shown to contain tannins (Jansman, 1993); however, the effects of tannins in barley grain on ileal digestibilities of AA remain to be investigated. The apparent ileal digestibilities of CP, histidine, and threonine were reduced ($P < 0.05$) when pigs were fed diets containing dark-flowering faba beans, which have a higher tannin content than white-flowering faba beans (Mosenthin et al., 1993). However, in these studies, endogenous CP losses at the terminal ileum were not affected (Mosenthin et al., 1993). Experiments by Grala et al. (1993) demonstrated that tannins in faba beans decreased apparent ileal AA digestibilities. Supplementing diets with faba bean hulls, which had a high tannin content, also reduced the apparent ileal digestibilities of lysine, threonine, and methionine (Table 9.2; Jansman et al., 1995).

K. Antibiotics

Growth-promoting antimicrobials are used widely in swine production to improve production efficiency and to ensure that safe pork is being produced. Antimicrobials added to swine feed may exhibit their effect through a number of different mechanisms. These include (1) direct suppressive effects on microorganisms in the gastrointestinal tract, such as pathogenic *Esherichia coli* and (2) nutrient-sparing effects (Dierick et al., 1986; Yen et al., 1987). Nutrient-sparing effects are likely as a result of an increase in the amount of nutrients, such as AA and carbohydrates, absorbed from the small intestine, due to a reduction in nutrient use by bacteria for growth. The addition of the antibiotic nebacitine to diets for growing pigs increased ($P < 0.05$) the apparent ileal AA digestibilities of all AA, except for histine, isoleucine, and phenylalanine (Table 9.2; Just et al., 1980). Virginiamycin supplementation also has been shown to improve ($P < 0.05$) the apparent ileal digestibilities of AA in growing pigs (Just et al., 1985). From the limited amount of research conducted, it seems clear that antibiotic supplementation improves apparent ileal AA digestibilities. However, additional work needs to be conducted to investigate further the effects of other antibiotics on ileal AA digestibilities.

L. Organic Acids

Organic acids are used as feed additives especially in diets for weanling pigs potentially to reduce gastric pH and improve protein digestion, prevent colonization of the gastrointestinal tract by pathogenic bacteria and, depending on the acid, provide a readily available energy source to the young pig (Gabert and Sauer, 1994). However, very few studies have been conducted to investigate the effect of organic acids on ileal digestibilities of AA. the authors did not observe any effect ($P > 0.05$) of 1% formic acid on ileal AA digestibilities in weanling pigs fed semipurified fish meal diets (Gabert et al., 1995b). The high digestibility of the diet and age of the pigs may have been partly responsible for the lack of positive effects. Similarly, 0.35 or 1.3% formic acid did not affect ($P > 0.05$) apparent ileal digestibilities of OM or CP (Bolduan et al., 1988).

Mosenthin et al. (1992) observed an increase ($P < 0.04$) in the apparent ileal digestibilities of several AA when diets for growing pigs were supplemented with 2% propionic acid. Similar results were reported when diets for growing pigs were supplemented with 3% lactic acid (Kemme et al., 1999). The positive effect may have been due to a suppressive effect of propionic acid on the growth of bacteria in the small intestine (Mosenthin et al., 1992).

Fumaric acid supplementation (1, 2, or 3%) has also been shown to increase protein digestion and the apparent ileal digestibilities of AA in weanling pigs (Blank et al., 1999). However, when sodium bicarbonate was added to the diets at the expense of sucrose, a positive response was not observed (Blank et al., 1999). Supplementation with 1.5 or 3.0% fumaric acid in diets for weanling pigs did not increase the apparent ileal digestibilities of AA (Gabert and Sauer, 1995). Giesting and Easter (1991) reported no effect ($P > 0.10$) of supplementation with 2% fumaric acid on the apparent ileal digestibilities of DM and N in weanling piglets. There is some evidence in the literature that suggests that organic acid supplementation can be used to improve apparent ileal AA digestibilities in swine; however, additional research is required.

VIII. CONCLUSIONS

Ileal digestibilities of AA in feedstuffs used in diets for swine are likely the most important determinants of AA utilization. When the ileal analysis method is used, as opposed to the fecal analyses method, to measure AA digestibilities, the modifying effects of bacterial metabolism on AA in the cecum and large intestine are avoided. Ileal AA digestibilities can be defined in many ways. Ileal AA digestibilities are apparent, true, real, standardized, or *in vitro* digestibilities. Practically, however, either the AA digestibility value is an apparent value in which the endogenous contribution is not taken into consideration or it is an estimate of true digestibility. Several methods are available for determining apparent ileal AA digestibilities; these include the direct, difference, and regression methods. The choice of which method to use to measure apparent ileal AA digestibilities in feedstuffs depends on the level of protein in the feedstuff, the inclusion level of the feedstuff in the diet, as well as the palatability of the feedstuff. The marker method is routinely used in the determination of apparent ileal AA digestibilities and its use is valid. The marker used will influence ileal AA digestibility values, and the most common marker used in digestion studies with swine is chromic oxide. The concentration of this marker in diets and in ileal digesta is easily measured. Several approaches can be used to collect ileal digesta from swine. Deciding which approach is most suitable will depend on an investigator's personal experience, duration of an experiment, type of diets used, and animal welfare concerns. Several chemical or *in vitro* methods can be used to estimate quickly apparent ileal AA digestibilities, provided the measured variables are correlated to apparent ileal AA coefficients obtained *in vivo*.

To determine true ileal AA digestibilities, an accurate estimate of endogenous ileal AA losses is needed. Several approaches can be used to estimate endogenous ileal AA flows; each has several advantages and disadvantages, and there is no one ideal method of choice. The use of protein-free diets should be avoided because of the effects of not supplying AA via the lumen on the function of the gastrointestinal tract. Further refinement of methods to determine the ileal digestibilities of AA, both apparent and true, will allow more accurate measurements to be made. Many factors affect ileal AA digestibilities and these must be taken into consideration when swine diets are formulated and when ileal AA digestibilities are measured. Further research is needed on the investigation of factors that affect apparent and, especially, true ileal AA digestibilities. To facilitate this, accurate estimates of endogenous ileal AA are needed and approaches used to estimate endogenous ileal AA losses and factors that affect them need to be investigated further.

REFERENCES

Adeola, O., B. V. Lawrence, and T. R. Cline. 1994. Availability of amino acids for 10- to 20-kilogram pigs: lysine and theonine in soybean meal, *J. Anim. Sci.*, 72:2061.

Agricultural Research Council. 1981. *The Nutrient Requirements of Pigs*. Commonwealth Agricultural Bureaux, Slough, U.K.

Albin, D. M., M. R. Smiricky, J. E. Wubben, and V. M. Gabert. 2000a. The influence of fiber-degrading enzymes and steeping on the apparent ileal digestibilities of amino acids in growing pigs fed a semipurified corn starch soybean meal–based diet. Abstr. 212 presented at the Midwestern Section of ASAS and Midwest Branch ADSA 2000 Meeting, Des Moines, IA.

Albin, D. M., J. E. Wubben, and V. M. Gabert. 2000b. The effect of hydrolysis time on the determination of amino acids in samples of soybean products with ion-exchange chromatography or pre-column derivitization with phenyl isothiocyanate, *J. Agric. Food Chem.*, 48:1684.

Albin, D. M., J. E. Wubben, and V. M. Gabert. 2000c. The influence of hydrochloric acid concentration and measurement method on the determination of amino acid levels in soybean products, *Anim. Feed Sci. Tech.*, in press.

Alpers, D. 1972. Protein synthesis in intestinal mucosa: the effect of route of administration of precursor amino acids, *J. Clin. Invest.*, 51:167.

Andersen, L., J. L. Snow, P. K. Ku, H. H. Stein, M. Allen, and N. L. Trottier. 2000. Ileal starch, apparent protein, and true protein digestibility of different corn hybrids fed to growing pigs. Abstr. 201 presented at the Midwestern Section of ASAS and Midwest Branch ADSA 2000 Meeting, Des Moines, IA.

Arenston, R. A., and D. R. Zimmerman. 1995. True digestibility of amino acids and protein in pigs with ^{13}C as a label to determine amino acid secretion, *J. Anim. Sci.*, 73:1077.

Asche, G. L., A. J. Lewis, and E. R. Peo, Jr. 1989. Protein digestion in weanling pigs: effect of feeding regimen and endogenous protein secretion, *J. Nutr.*, 119:1083.

Aufrère, J., D. Graviou, C. Demarquilly, J. M. Perez, and J. Andrieu. 1996. Near infrared reflectance spectroscopy to predict energy value of compound feeds for swine and ruminants, *Anim. Feed Sci. Technol.*, 62:77.

Baas, T. C., and P. A. Thacker. 1996. Impact of gastric pH on dietary enzyme activity and survivability in swine fed β-glucanase supplemented diets, *Can. J. Anim. Sci.*, 76:245.

Badawy, A. M. 1964. Changes in the protein and non-protein nitrogen in the digesta of the sheep. In *The Role of the Gastrointestinal Tract in Protein Metabolism*, Munro, H. N., Ed., Blackwell, Oxford, U.K., 175.

Badawy, A. M., R. M. Campbell, D. P. Cuthbertson, and B. F. Bell. 1957. Changes in the intestinal mucosa of the sheep following death by humane killer, *Nature*, 180:756.

Baidoo, S. K., Y. G. Liu, and D. Yungblut. 1998. Effect of microbial enzyme supplementation on energy, amino acid digestibility and performance of pigs fed hulless barley based diets, *Can. J. Anim. Sci.*, 78:625.

Batterham, E. S. 1992. Availability and utilization of amino acids in feedstuffs for growing pigs, *Nutr. Res. Rev.*, 5:1.

Batterham, E. S., R. D. Murison, and C. E. Lewis. 1979. Availability of lysine in protein concentrates as determined by the slope-ratio assay with growing pigs and rats and by chemical techniques, *Br. J. Nutr.*, 41:383.

Batterham, E. S., R. D. Murison, and L. M. Andersen. 1984. Availability of lysine in vegetable protein concentrates as determined by the slope-ratio assay with growing pigs and rats and by chemical techniques, *Br. J. Nutr.*, 51:85.

Batterham, E. S., L. M. Andersen, D. R. Baigent, and R. E. Darnell. 1990. A comparison of the availability and ileal digestibility of lysine in cottonseed and soya-bean meals for grower/finisher pigs, *Br. J. Nutr.*, 64:663.

Bech-Andersen, S. 1979. Single-column analysis of amino acids in hydrolysates of samples containing chromic oxide, *J. Chromatogr.*, 179:227.

Bellaver, C. 1989. Estimation of Amino Acid Digestibility and Its Usefulness in Swine Feed Formulation, Ph.D. dissertation, University of Illinois, Urbana.

Blank, R., R. Mosenthin, W. C. Sauer, and S. Huang. 1999. Effect of fumaric acid and dietary buffering capacity on ileal and fecal amino acid digestibilities in early-weaned pigs, *J. Anim. Sci.*, 77:2974.

Boisen, S., and B. O. Eggum. 1991. Critical evaluation of *in vitro* methods for estimating digestibility in simple-stomach animals, *Nutr. Res. Rev.*, 4:141.

Boisen, S., and J. A. Fernández. 1995. Prediction of the apparent ileal digestibility of protein and amino acids in feedstuffs and feed mixtures for pigs by *in vitro* analyses, *Anim. Feed Sci. Technol.*, 51:29.

Boisen, S., and P. J. Moughan. 1996. Dietary influences on endogenous ileal protein and amino acid loss in the pig — a review, *Acta Agric. Scand. Sect. A. Anim. Sci.*, 46:154.

Bolduan, V. G., H. Jung, R. Schneider, J. Block, and B. Klenke. 1988. Die Wirkung von Propion- und Ameisensäure in der Ferkelaufzucht, *J. Anim. Physiol. Anim. Nutr.*, 59:72.

Bornholdt, U., R. Mosenthin, W. C. Sauer, F. Ahrens, H. Jørgensen, and B. O. Eggum. 1994. Evaluation of the "Mobile Nylon Bag Technique" for determining apparent ileal protein and amino acid digestibilities in feedstuffs for pigs. In Proceedings of the VIth International Symposium on Digestive Physiology in Pigs, Souffrant, W. B. and H. Hagemeister, Eds., EAAP publ. 80, Forschungsbereich Ernährungsphysiologie "Oskar Kellner," Dummerstorf, Germany, 118.

Brannon, P. M. 1990. Adaptation of the exocrine pancreas to diet, *Annu. Rev. Nutr.*, 10:85.

Butts, C. A., P. J. Moughan, and W. C. Smith. 1991. Endogenous amino acid flow at the terminal ileum of the rat determined under conditions of peptide alimentation, *J. Sci. Food Agric.*, 55:175.

Butts, C. A., P. J. Moughan, W. C. Smith, and D. H. Carr. 1993a. Endogenous lysine and other amino acid flows at the terminal ileum of the growing pig (20 kg bodyweight): the effect of protein-free, synthetic amino acid, peptide and protein alimentation, *J. Sci. Food Agric.*, 61:31.

Butts, C. A., P. J. Moughan, W. C. Smith, G. W. Reynolds, and D. J. Garrick. 1993b. The effect of food dry matter intake on endogenous ileal amino acid excretion determined under peptide alimentation in the 50 kg liveweight pig, *J. Sci. Food Agric.*, 62:235.

Caine, W. R., W. C. Sauer, M.W.A. Verstegen, S. Tamminga, S. Li, and H. Schulze. 1998. Guanidinated protein test meals with higher concentration of soybean trypsin inhibitors increase ileal recoveries of endogenous amino acids in pigs, *J. Nutr.*, 128:598.

Carpenter, K. J. 1960. The estimation of available lysine in animal-protein foods, *Biochem. J.*, 77:604.

Cherian, G., W. C. Sauer, and P. A. Thacker. 1988. Effect of pre-digestion factors on the apparent digestibility of protein for swine determined with the mobile nylon bag technique, *J. Anim. Sci.*, 66:1963.

Cherian, G., W. C. Sauer, and P. A. Thacker. 1989. Factors affecting the determination of protein digestibility in mobile nylon bag studies with pigs, *Anim. Feed Sci.*, 27:137.

Chu, K. S., J. H. Kim, B. J. Chae, Y. K. Chung, and I. K. Han. 1998. Effects of processing barley on growth performance and ileal digestibility of growing pigs, *Asian Aust. J. Anim. Sci.*, 11:249.

Chung, T. K., and D. H. Baker. 1992. Apparent and true amino acid digestibility of a crystalline amino acid mixture and of casein: comparison of values obtained with ileal-cannulated pigs and cecetomized cockerels, *J. Anim. Sci.*, 70:3781.

Cousins, B. W., T. D. Tanksley, Jr., D. A. Knabe, and T. Zebrowska. 1981. Nutrient digestibility and performance of pigs fed sorghums varying in tannin concentration, *J. Anim. Sci.*, 53:1524.

Cunningham, H. M., D. W. Friend, and J. W. G. Nicholson. 1963. Observations on digestion in the pigs using a re-entrant intestinal fistula, *Can. J. Anim. Sci.*, 43:215.

Danfær, A., and J. Férnandez. 1999. Developments in the prediction of nutrient availability in pigs: a review, *Acta Agric. Scand. Sect. A Anim. Sci.*, 49:73.

de Lange, C. F. M., W. C. Sauer, and W. B. Souffrant. 1989. The effect of protein status of the pig on recovery and amino acid composition of endogenous protein in digesta collected from the distal ileum, *J. Anim. Sci.*, 67:755.

de Lange, C. F. M., W. B. Souffrant, and W. C. Sauer. 1990. Real ileal protein and amino acid digestibilities in feedstuffs for growing pigs as determined with the ^{15}N-isotope dilution technique, *J. Anim. Sci.*, 68:409.

de Lange, C. F. M., W. C. Sauer, W. B. Souffrant, and K. A. Lien. 1992. ^{15}N-leucine and ^{15}N-isoleucine isotope dilution techniques versus the ^{15}N-isotope dilution technique for determining the recovery of endogenous protein and amino acids in digesta collected from the distal ileum in pigs, *J. Anim. Sci.*, 70:1848.

de Lange, C. F. M., V. M. Gabert, D. Gillis, and J. F. Patience. 1998. Digestible energy contents and apparent ileal amino acid digestibilities in regular or partial mechanically dehulled canola meal samples fed to growing pigs, *Can. J. Anim. Sci.*, 78:641.

Dierick, N. A., I. J. Vervaeke, J. A. Decuypere, and H. K. Henderickx. 1986. Influence of the gut flora and some growth-promoting feed additives on nitrogen metabolism in pigs. II. Studies *in vivo*, *Livest. Prod Sci.*, 14:177.

Donkoh, A., and P. J. Moughan. 1999. Endogenous ileal nitrogen and amino acid flows in the growing pig receiving a protein-free diet and diets containing enzymatically hydrolysed casein or graded levels of meat and bone meal, *Anim. Sci.*, 68:511.

Donkoh, A., P. J. Moughan, and W. C. Smith. 1994. Comparision of the slaughter method and simple T-piece cannulation of the terminal ileum for determining ileal amino acid digestibility in meat and bone meal for the growing pig, *Anim. Feed Sci. Technol.*, 49:43.

Dugan, M. E. R., W. C. Sauer, J. M. Dugan, Jr., and W. R. Caine. 1994. Determination of bacterial amino acid contribution to ileal digesta from pigs using ^{35}S and DAPA marker techniques, *J. Anim. Feed Sci.*, 3:149.

Easter, R. A., and T. D. Tanksley, Jr. 1973. A technique for re-entrant ileocecal cannulation of swine, *J. Anim. Sci.*, 36:1099.

Eggum, B. O. 1973. A Study of Certain Factors Influencing Protein Utilization in Rats and Pigs, D.Sc. dissertation, National Institute of Animal Science, Copenhagen, Denmark.

Fan, M. Z. 1994. Methodological Considerations for the Determination of Amino Acid Digestibility in Pigs, Ph.D. dissertation, University of Alberta, Edmonton, Canada.

Fan, M. Z., and W. C. Sauer. 1994. Amino acid and energy digestibililty in peas (*Pisum sativum*) from white-flowered spring cultivars for growing pigs, *J. Sci. Food Agric.*, 64:249.

Fan, M. Z., and W. C. Sauer. 1995. Determination of apparent ileal amino acid digestibilty in barley and canola meal for pigs with the direct, difference, and regression methods, *J. Anim. Sci.*, 73:2364.

Fan, M. Z., and W. C. Sauer. 1997. Determination of true ileal amino acid digestibility in feedstuffs for pigs with the linear relationships between distal ileal outputs and dietary inputs of amino acids, *J. Sci. Food Agric.*, 73:189.

Fan, M. Z., and W. C. Sauer. 1999. Variability of apparent ileal amino acid digestibility in different pea samples for growing-finishing pigs, *Can. J. Anim. Sci.*, 79:467.

Fan, M. Z., W. C. Sauer, and S. Li. 1993. The additivity of the apparent ileal digestible amino acid supply in barley, wheat and canola meal or soybean meal diet for growing pigs, *J. Anim. Physiol. Anim. Nutr.*, 70:72.

Fan, M. Z., W. C. Sauer, R. T. Hardin, and K. A. Lien. 1994. Determination of apparent ileal amino acid digestibility in pigs: effect of dietary amino acid level, *J. Anim. Sci.*, 72:2851.

Fan, M. Z., W. C. Sauer, and C. F. M. de Lange. 1995a. Amino acid digestibility in soybean meal, extruded soybean and full-fat canola for early weaned pigs, *Anim. Feed Sci. Technol.*, 52:189.

Fan, M. Z., W. C. Sauer, and M. I. McBurney. 1995b. Estimation by regression analysis of endogenous amino acid levels in digesta collected from the distal ileum of pigs, *J. Anim. Sci.*, 73:2319.

Fan, M. Z., W. C. Sauer, and V. M. Gabert. 1996. Variability of apparent ileal amino acid digestibility in canola meal for growing-finishing pigs, *Can. J. Anim. Sci.*, 76:563.

Fenton, T. W., and M. Fenton. 1979. An improved procedure for the determination of chromic oxide in feed and feces, *Can. J. Anim. Sci.*, 59:631.

Fountoulakis, M., and H. W. Lahm. 1998. Hydrolysis and amino acid composition analysis of proteins, *J. Chromatogr.*, 826:109.

Friedman, M. 1996. Food browning and its prevention: an overview, *J. Agric. Food Chem.*, 44:631.

Furuya, S., and Y. Kaji. 1991. Additivity of the apparent and true ileal digestible amino acid supply in barley, maize, wheat or soya-bean meal based diets for growing pigs, *Anim. Feed Sci. Technol.*, 32:321.

Furuya, S., and Y. Kaji. 1992. The effects of feed intake and purified cellulose on the endogenous ileal amino acid flow in growing pigs, *Br. J. Nutr.*, 68:463.

Gabert, V. M., and W. C. Sauer. 1994. The effects of supplementing diets for weanling pigs with organic acids: a review, *J. Anim. Feed Sci.*, 3:73.

Gabert, V. M., and W. C. Sauer. 1995. The effect of fumaric acid and sodium fumarate supplementation to diets for weanling pigs on amino acid digestibility and volatile fatty acid concentrations in ileal digesta, *Anim. Feed Sci. Technol.*, 53:243.

Gabert, V. M., W. C. Sauer, R. Mosenthin, M. Schmitz, and F. Ahrens. 1995a. The effect of oligosaccharides and lactitol on the ileal digestibilities of amino acids, monosaccharides and bacterial populations and metabolites in the small intestine of weanling pigs, *Can. J. Anim. Sci.*, 75:99.

Gabert, V. M., W. C. Sauer, M. Schmitz, F. Ahrens, and R. Mosenthin. 1995b. The effect of formic acid and buffering capacity on the ileal digestibilities of amino acids and bacterial populations and metabolites in the small intestine of weanling pigs fed semipurified fish meal diets, *Can. J. Anim. Sci.*, 75:615.

Gabert, V. M., W. C. Sauer, S. Li, M. Z. Fan, and M. Rademacher. 1996a. Exocrine pancreatic secretions in young pigs fed diets containing faba beans (*Vicia faba*) and peas (*Pisum sativum*): nitrogen, protein and enzyme secretions, *J. Sci. Food Agric.*, 70:247.

Gabert, V. M., W. C. Sauer, S. Li, and M. Z. Fan. 1996b. Exocrine pancreatic secretions in young pigs fed diets containing faba beans (*Vicia faba*) and peas (*Pisum sativum*): concentrations and flows of total, protein-bound and free amino acids, *J. Sci. Food Agric.*, 70:256.

Gabert, V. M., N. Canibe, H. Jørgensen, B. O. Eggum, and W. C. Sauer. 1997. Use of ^{15}N-amino acid isotope dilution techniques to determine endogenous amino acids in ileal digesta in growing pigs, *Acta Agric. Scand. Sect. A Anim. Sci.*, 47:168.

Giesting, D. W., and R. A. Easter. 1985. Response of starter pigs to supplementation of corn–soybean meal diets with organic acids, *J. Anim. Sci.*, 60:1288.

Giesting, D. W., and R. A. Easter. 1991. Effect of protein source and fumaric acid supplementation on apparent ileal digestibility of nutrients by young pigs, *J. Anim. Sci.*, 69:2497.

Givens, D. I., and E. R. Deavillle. 1999. The current and future role of near infrared reflectance spectroscopy in animal nutrition. A review, *Aust. J. Agric. Res.*, 50:1131.

Grala, W., A. J. M. Jansman, P. van Leeuwen, J. Huisman, G. J. M. van Kempen, and M. W. A. Verstegen. 1993. Nutritional value of faba beans (*Vicia faba* L.) fed to young pigs, *J. Anim. Feed Sci.*, 2:169.

Grant, G., and E. van Driessche. 1993. Legume lectins: physiochemical and nutritional properties. In: *Recent Advances of Research in Antinutritional Factors in Legume Seeds*, van der Poel, A. F. B., J. Huisman, and S. H. Saini, Eds., Wageningen Pers, Wageningen, The Netherlands, 219.

Green, S., S. L. Bertrand, M. J. C. Duron, and R. A. Maillard. 1987. Digestibility of amino acids in maize, wheat and barley meal, measured in pigs with ileo-rectal anastomosis and isolation of the large intestine, *J. Sci. Food Agric.*, 41:29.

Hagemeister, H., and H. Erbersdobler. 1985. Chemical labeling of a dietary protein by transformation of lysine to homoarginine: a new technique to follow intestinal digestion and absorption, *Proc. Nutr. Soc.*, 44:133A.

Haydon, K. D., D. A. Knabe, and T. D. Tanksley, Jr. 1984. Effects of level of feed intake on nitrogen, amino acid and energy digestibilities measured at the end of the small intestine and over the total digestive tract of growing pigs, *J. Anim. Sci.*, 59:717.

Herkelman, K. L., G. L. Cromwell, T. S. Stahly, T. W. Pfeiffer, and D. A. Knabe. 1992. Apparent digestibility of amino acids in raw and heated conventional and low-trypsin-inhibitor soybeans for pigs, *J. Anim. Sci.*, 70:818.

Hess, V., and B. Séve. 1999. Effects of body weight and feed intake level on basal ileal endogenous losses in growing pigs, *J. Anim. Sci.*, 77:3281.

Horszczaruk, F., T. Zebrowska, and W. Dobowolski. 1972. Trwale przetoki jelitowe do badan nad trawieniem u swin. II. Wykonoanie prostych przetok jelita cienkiego, *Roczn. Nauk Roln. Ser. B Zootech.*, 94:99.

Huang, S. X., W. C. Sauer, M. Pickard, S. Li, and R. T. Hardin. 1998. Effect of micronization on energy, starch and amino acid digestibility in hulless barley for young pigs, *Can. J. Anim. Sci.*, 78:81.

Huisman, J., and A.J.M. Jansman. 1991. Dietary effects and some analytical aspects of antinutritional factors in peas (*Pisum sativum*), common beans (*Phaseolus vulgaris*) and soyabeans (*Glycine max* L.) in monogastric farm animals. A literature review, *Nutr. Abstr. Rev. Ser. B.*, 61:901.

Imbeah, M., K. Angkanaporn, V. Ravindran, and W. L. Bryden. 1996. Investigations on the guanidination of lysine in proteins, *J. Sci. Food Agric.*, 72:231.

Jagger, S., J. Wiseman, D. J. A. Cole, and J. Craigon. 1992. Evaluation of inert markers for the determination of ileal and faecal apparent digestibility values in the pig, *Br. J. Nutr.*, 68:729.

Jansman, A. J. M. 1993. Tannins in feedsuffs for simple-stomached animals, *Nutr. Res. Rev.*, 6:209.

Jansman, A. J. M., M. W. A. Verstegen, J. Huisman, and J. W. O. van den Berg. 1995. Effects of hulls of faba beans (*Vicia faba* L.) with a low or high content of condensed tannins on the apparent ileal and fecal digestibility of nutrients and the excretion of endogenous protein in ileal digesta and feces of pigs, *J. Anim. Sci.*, 73:118.

Johnston, S. L., L. L. Southern, and L. D. Bunting. 2000. Effect of reduction of dietary calcium and phosphorus and/or phytase on the ileal digestibility of amino acids in pigs. Abstr. 204 presented at the Midwestern Section of ASAS and Midwest Branch ADSA 2000 Meeting, Des Moines, IA.

Jongbloed, A. W., J. G. M. Bakker, P. W. Goedhart, and K. F. Krol. 1991. Evaluation of chromic oxide with lower concentration and of HCl-insoluble ash as markers for measuring overall apparent digestibility of some dietary nutrients for pigs. In: *Proceedings of the 5th Int. Symp. on Digestive Physiol. in Pigs*, Verstegen, M. W. A., J. Huisman, and L. A. den Hartog, Eds., Doorwerth, Wageningen, The Netherlands. 325.

Jørgensen, H., and J. A. Fernández. 2000. Chemical composition and energy value of different fat sources for growing pigs, *Acta Agric. Scand. Sect. A Anim. Sci.*, 50 (in press).

Jørgensen, H., W. C. Sauer, and P. A. Thacker. 1984. Amino acid availabilities in soybean meal, sunflower meal, fish meal and meat and bone meal fed to growing pigs, *J. Anim. Sci.*, 58:926.

Jørgensen, H., V. M. Gabert, and B. O. Eggum. 1997a. The nutritional value of high-lysine barley determined in rats, young pigs and growing pigs, *J. Sci. Food Agric.*, 73:287.

Jørgensen, H., J. E. Lindberg, and C. Andersson. 1997b. Diurnal variation in the composition of ileal digesta and the ileal digestibilities of nutrients in growing pigs, *J. Sci. Food Agric.*, 74:244.

Jørgensen, H., V. M. Gabert, M. S. Hedemann, and S. K. Jensen. 2000. Digestion of fat does not differ in growing pigs fed diets containing fish oil, rapeseed oil or coconut oil, *J. Nutr.*, 130:852.

Just, A., W. C. Sauer, S. Bech-Andersen, H. Jørgensen, and B. O. Eggum. 1980. The influence of hind gut microflora on the digestibility of protein and amino acids in growing pigs elucidated by addition of antibiotics to different fractions of barley, *J. Anim. Physiol. Anim. Nutr.*, 43:83.

Just, A., H. Jørgensen, and J. A. Fernández. 1981. The digestive capacity of the caecum-colon and the value of nitrogen absorbed from the hind gut for protein synthesis in pigs, *Br. J. Nutr.*, 46:209.

Just, A., H. Jørgensen, and J. A. Fernández. 1985. The influence of diet composition and virginiamycin on the microbial activity, composition of fermentation products and energy deposition in growing pigs. In *Proc. 10th Symposium on Energy Metabolism of Farm Animals*, Moe, P. W., H. F. Tyrrell, and P. J. Reynolds, Eds., Rowan & Littlefield, Blue Ridge Summit, PA, 272.

Kemme, P. A., A. W. Jongbloed, Z. Mroz, J. Kogut, and A. C. Beynen. 1999. Digestibility of nutrients in growing-finishing pigs is affected by *Aspergillus niger* phytase, phytate and lactic acid levels. 1. Apparent ileal digestibility of amino acids, *Livest. Prod. Sci.*, 58:107.

Kennelley, J. J., F. X. Aherne, and M. J. Apps. 1980. Dysprosium as an inert marker for swine digestibility studies, *Can. J. Anim. Sci.*, 61:349.

Knabe, D. A. 1991. Bioavailability of amino acids in feedstuffs for swine. In *Swine Nutrition*, Miller, E. R., D. E. Ullery, and A. J. Lewis, Eds., Butterworth-Heinemann, Boston, MA, 327.

Knabe, D. A., D. C. LaRue, E. J. Gregg, G. M. Martinez, and T. D. Tanksley, Jr. 1989. Apparent digestibility of nitrogen and amino acids in protein containing feedstuffs by growing pigs, *J. Anim. Sci.*, 67:441.

Köhler, T., J. Huisman, L. A. den Hartog, and R. Mosenthin. 1990. Comparison of different digesta collection methods to determine the apparent digestibilities of the nutrients at the terminal ileum in pigs, *J. Sci. Food Agric.*, 53:465.

Köhler, T., R. Mosenthin, M. W. A. Verstegen, J. Huisman, L. A. den Hartog, and F. Ahrens. 1992. Effect of ileo-rectal anastomosis and post-valve T-caecum cannulation on growing pigs. 1. Growth performance, N-balance and intestinal adaptation, *Br. J. Nutr.*, 68:293.

Leibholz, J. 1982. The flow of endogenous nitrogen in the digestive tract of young pigs, *Br. J. Nutr.*, 48:509.

Leibholz, J. 1986. The utilization of lysine by young pigs from nine protein concentrates compared with free lysine in young pigs fed ad lib, *Br. J. Nutr.*, 55:179.

Leibholz, J. 1991. A rapid assay for the measurement of protein digestion to the ileum of pigs by the use of the mobile nylon bag technique, *Anim. Feed Sci. Technol.*, 33:209.

Leibholz, J. 1992. The availability of lysine in diets for pigs: comparative methodology, *Br. J. Nutr.*, 67:401.

Leibholz, J., and Y. Mollah. 1988. Digestibility of threonine from protein concentrates for growing pigs. 1. The flow of endogenous amino acids to the terminal ileum of growing pigs, *Aust. J. Agric. Res.*, 39:713.

Leibholz, J., R. J. Love, Y. Mollah, and R. R. Carter. 1986. The absorption of dietary L-lysine and extruded L-lysine in pigs, *Anim. Feed Sci. Technol.*, 15:141.

Leterme, P., A. Théwis, Y. Beckers, and E. Baudart. 1990. Apparent and true digestibility of amino acids and nitrogen balance measured in pigs with ileo-rectal anastomosis or T-cannulas, given a diet containing peas, *J. Sci. Food Agric.*, 52:485.

Leterme, P., L. Pirard, and A. Théwis. 1992. A note on the effect of wood cellulose level in protein-free diets on the recovery and amino acid composition of endogenous protein collected from the ileum in pigs, *Anim. Prod.*, 54:163.

Leterme, P., A. Théwis, E. Francois, P. van Leeuwen, B. Wathelet, and J. Huisman. 1996. The use of ^{15}N-labelled dietary proteins for determining true ileal amino acid digestibilities is limited by their rapid recycling in the endogenous secretions of pigs, *J. Nutr.*, 126:2188.

Li, S. 1996. Enzyme Supplementation and Exocrine Pancreatic Secretion in Pigs, Ph.D. dissertation, University of Alberta, Edmonton, Canada.

Li, S., and W. C. Sauer. 1994. The effect of dietary fat content on amino acid digestibility in young pigs, *J. Anim. Sci.*, 72:1737.

Li, S., W. C. Sauer, and R. T. Hardin. 1994. Effect of dietary fiber level on amino acid digestibility in young pigs, *Can. J. Anim. Sci.*, 74:327.

Li, S., W. C. Sauer, S. X. Huang, and V. M. Gabert. 1996. Effect of β-glucanase supplementation to hulless barley- or wheat-soybean meal diets on the digestibilities of energy, protein, β-glucans, and amino acids in young pigs, *J. Anim. Sci.*, 74:1649.

Li, S., W. C. Sauer, and W. R. Caine. 1998. Response of nutrient digestibilities to feeding diets with low and high levels of soybean trypsin inhibitors in growing pigs, *J. Sci. Food Agric.*, 76:357.

Lien, K. A., W. C. Sauer, and M. E. R. Dugan. 1997a. Evaluation of the ^{15}N-isotope dilution technique for determining the recovery of endogenous protein in ileal digesta of pigs: effect of the pattern of blood sampling, precursor pools, and isotope dilution technique, *J. Anim. Sci.*, 75:159.

Lien, K. A., W. C. Sauer, R. Mosenthin, W. B. Souffrant, and M. E. R. Dugan. 1997b. Evaluation of the ^{15}N-isotope dilution technique for determining the recovery of endogenous protein in ileal digesta of pigs: effect of dilution in the precursor pool for endogenous nitrogen secretion, *J. Anim. Sci.*, 75:148.

Littell, R. C., P. R. Henry, A. J. Lewis, and C. B. Ammerman. 1997. Estimation of the relative bioavailability of nutrients using SAS procedures, *J. Anim. Sci.*, 75:2672.

Low, A. G. 1977. Digestibility at several sites in pigs, *Proc. Nutr. Soc.*, 36:189.

Low, A. G. 1982. Digestibility and availability of amino acids from feedstuffs for pigs: a review, *Livest. Prod. Sci.*, 9:511.

Marty, B. J., and E. R. Chavez. 1995. Ileal digestibilites and urinary losses of amino acids in pigs fed heat processed soybean products, *Livest. Prod. Sci.*, 43:37.

Marty, B. J., E. R. Chavez, and C. F. M. de Lange. 1994. Recovery of amino acids at the distal ileum for determining apparent and true ileal amino acid digestibilities in growing pigs fed various heat-processed full-fat soybean products, *J. Anim. Sci.*, 72:2029.

McNeilage, E. M. 1998. Effects of Feed Enzymes and Feeding Regimens on Growth, Digestibility, Organ Weight, and Meat Quality in Finishing Pigs., M.S. thesis, University of Guelph, Ontario, Canada.

McNeilage, E. M., C. M. Nyachoti, C. F. M. de Lange, V. M. Gabert, and H. Schulze. 2000. Effect of converting lysine in barley and canola meal into homoarginine on nutrient composition and ileal amino acid digestibilities in growing pigs. In Proc. VIIIth Intl. Symposium on Digestive Physiology in Pigs, Uppsala Sweden, June 20–22, 2000, Lindberg, J. E. (Ed.) (in press).

Mitaru, B. N., R. D. Reichert, and R. Blair. 1984. The binding of dietary protein by sorghum tannins in the digestive tract of pigs, *J. Nutr.*, 114:1787.

Mosenthin, R., W. C. Sauer, F. Ahrens, C. F. M. de Lange, and U. Bornholdt. 1992. Effect of dietary supplements of propionic acid, siliceous earth or a combination of these on the energy, protein and amino acid digestibilities and concentrations of microbial metabolites in the digestive tract of growing pigs, *Anim. Feed Sci. Technol.*, 37:245.

Mosenthin, R., W. C. Sauer, K. A. Lien, and C. F. M. de Lange. 1993. Apparent, true and real protein and amino acid digestibilities in growing pigs fed two varieties of fababeans (*Vicia faba* L.) different in tannin content, *J. Anim. Physiol. Anim. Nutr.*, 70:253.

Moughan, P. J., and S. M. Rutherfurd. 1990. Endogenous flow of total lysine and other amino acids at the distal ileum of the protein- or peptide-fed rat: the chemical labeling of gelatin protein by transformation of lysine to homoarginine, *J. Sci. Food Agric.*, 52:179.

Mougan, P. J., and S. M. Rutherfurd. 1996. A new method for determining digestible reactive lysine in foods, *J. Agric. Food Chem.*, 44:2202.

Moughan, P. J., and G. Schuttert. 1991. Composition of nitrogen-containing fractions in digesta from the distal ileum of pigs fed a protein-free diet, *J. Nutr.*, 121:1570.

Moughan, P. J., P. J. Buttery, C. P. Essex, and J. B. Soar. 1992a. Evaluation of the isotope dilution technique for determining ileal endogenous nitrogen excretion in the rat, *J. Sci. Food Agric.*, 60:437.

Moughan, P. J., G. Schuttert, and M. Leenaars. 1992b. Endogenous amino acid flow in the stomach and small intestine of the young growing pig, *J. Sci. Food Agric.*, 60:437.

Mroz, Z., A. W. Jongbloed, and P. A. Kemme. 1994. Apparent digestibility and retention of nutrients bound to phytate complexes as influenced by microbial phytase and feeding regimen in pigs, *J. Anim. Sci.*, 72:126.

Mroz, Z., G. C. M. Bakker, A. W. Jongbloed, R. A. Dekker, R. Jongbloed, and A. van Beers. 1996. Apparent digestibility of nutrients with different energy density, as estimated by direct and marker methods for pigs with or without ileo-cecal cannulas, *J. Anim. Sci.*, 74:403.

NRC. 1998. *Nutrient Requirements of Swine*, 10th ed., National Academy Press, Washington, D.C.

Nyachoti, C. M., C. F. M. de Lange, B. W. McBride, and H. Schulze. 1997a. Significance of endogenous gut nitrogen losses in the nutrition of growing pigs: a review, *Can. J. Anim. Sci.*, 77:149.

Nyachoti, C. M., C. F. M. de Lange, and H. Schulze. 1997b. Estimating endogenous amino acid flows at the terminal ileum and true ileal amino acid digestibilities in feedstuffs for growing pigs using the homoarginine method, *J. Anim. Sci.*, 75:3206.

Nyachoti, M., C. F. M. de Lange, B. W. McBride, S. Leeson, and V. M. Gabert. 2000. Endogenous gut nitrogen losses in growing pigs are not caused by increased protein synthesis rates in the small intestine, *J. Nutr.*, 130:566.

Owsley, W. F., D. A. Knabe, and T. D. Tanksley, Jr. 1981. Effect of sorghum particle size on digestibility of nutrients at the terminal ileum and over the total digestive tract of growing-finishing pigs, *J. Anim. Sci.*, 52:557.

Parsons, C. M. 1991. Use of pepsin digestibility, multienzyme pH change and protein solubility assays to predict *in vivo* protein quality of feedstuffs. In *In Vitro Digestion for Pigs and Poultry*, Fuller, M. F., Ed., CAB International, Wallingford, Oxon, U.K., 105.

Peiniau, J., A. Aumaitre, and Y. Lebreton. 1996. Effects of dietary protein sources differing in solubility on total tract and ileal apparent digestibility of nitrogen and pancreatic enzyme activity in early weaned pigs, *Livest. Prod. Sci.*, 45:197.

Pond, W. G., K. R. Pond, W. C. Ellis, and J. H. Matis. 1986. Markers for estimating digesta flow in pigs and the effects of dietary fiber, *J. Anim. Sci.*, 63:1140.

Prawirodigdo, S., N. J. Gannon, R. J. van Barneveld, D. J. Kerton, B. J. Leury, and F. R. Dunshea. 1998. Assessment of apparent ileal digestibility of amino acids and nitrogen in cottonseed and soybean meals fed to pigs determined using ileal dissection under halothane anaesthesia or following carbon dioxide-stunning, *Br. J. Nutr.*, 80:183.

Rademacher, M., W. C. Sauer, and A. J. M. Jansman. 1999. *Standardized Ileal Digestibility of Amino Acids in Pigs*, Degussa-Hüls, Frankfurt, Germany.

Rao, S. R., F. L. Carter, and V. L. Frampton. 1963. Determination of available lysine in oilseed meal proteins, *Anal. Chem.*, 35:1927.

Redlich, J., W. B. Souffrant, J. P. Laplace, U. Hennig, R. Berg, and J. M. V. M. Mouwen. 1997. Morphometry of the small intestine in pigs with ileo-rectal anastomosis, *Can. J. Vet. Res.*, 61:21.

Roach, A. G., P. Sanderson, and D. R. Williams. 1967. Comparision of methods for the determination of available lysine value in animal and vegetable protein sources, *J. Sci. Food Agric.*, 18:274.

Rowan, A. M., P. J. Moughan, and M. N. Wilson. 1992. Effect of hydrolyses time on the determination of amino acid composition of diet, ileal digesta, and feces samples and on the determination of dietary amino acid digestibility coefficients, *J. Agric. Food Chem.*, 40:981.

Rudemo, M., S. Bech-Andersen, and V. C. Mason. 1980. Hydrolysate preparation for amino acid determinations in feed constituents. 5. The influence of hydrolysis time on amino acid recovery, *J. Anim. Physiol. Anim. Nutr.*, 43:27.

Rutherfurd, S. M., and P. J. Moughan. 1990. Guanidination of lysine in selected dietary proteins, *J. Agric. Food Chem.*, 38:209.

Sauer, W. C. 1976. Factors Affecting Amino Acid Availabilities for Cereal Grains and Their Components for Growing Monogastric Animals, Ph.D. dissertation, University of Manitoba, Winnipeg, Canada.

Sauer, W. C. and K. de Lange. 1992. Novel methods for determining protein and amino acid digestibilities in feedstuffs. In *Modern Methods in Protein Nutrition and Metabolism*, Nissen, S., Ed., Academic Press, San Diego, CA.

Sauer, W. C., and L. Ozimek. 1986. Digestibility of amino acids in swine: results and their practical applications. A review, *Livest. Prod. Sci.*, 15:367.

Sauer, W. C., A. Just, and H. Jørgensen. 1982. The influence of daily feed intake on the apparent digestibility of crude protein, amino acids, calcium and phosphorous at the terminal ileum and overall in pigs, *J. Anim. Physiol. Anim. Nutr.*, 48:177.

Schmitz, M., H. Hagemeister, and H. F. Erbersdobler. 1991. Homoarginine labelling is suitable for determination of protein absorbtion in miniature pigs, *J. Nutr.*, 121:1575.

Sauer, W. C., H. Jørgensen, and R. Berzins. 1983. A modified nylon bag technique for determining apparent digestibilities of protein in feedstuffs for pigs, *Can. J. Anim. Sci.*, 63:233.

Sauer, W. C., R. Mosenthin, F. Ahrens, and L. A. den Hartog. 1991. The effect of source of fiber on ileal and fecal amino acid digestibility and bacterial nitrogen excretion in growing pigs, *J. Anim. Sci.*, 69:4070.

Sauer, W. C., S. C. Stothers, and G. D. Phillips. 1977. Apparent availabilities of amino acids in corn, wheat and barley for growing pigs, *Can. J. Anim. Sci.*, 57:585.

Schulze, H. 1994. Endogenous Ileal Nitrogen Losses in Pigs, Ph.D. dissertation, Wageningen Agricultural University, Wageningen, The Netherlands.

Schulze, H., H. S. Saini, J. Huisman, M. Hessing, W. van den Berg, and M. W. A. Verstegen. 1995. Increased nitrogen secretion by inclusion of soy lectin in the diets of pigs, *J. Sci. Food Agric.*, 69:501.

Schulze, H., F. H. M. G. Savelkoul, M. W. A. Verstegen, A. F. B. van der Poel, S. Tamminga, and S. Groot Nibbenlink. 1997. Nutritional evaluation of biologically treated white kidney beans (*Phaseolus vulgaris* L.) in pigs: ileal and amino acid digestibility, *J. Anim. Sci.*, 75:3187.

Skilton, G., P. J. Moughan, and W. C. Smith. 1988. Determination of endogenous amino acid flow at the terminal ileum of the rat, *J. Sci. Food Agric.*, 44:227.

Sohn, K. S., C. V. Maxwell, L. L. Southern, and D. S. Buchanan. 1994. Improved soybean protein sources for early-weaned pigs: II. Effects on ileal amino acid digestibility, *J. Anim. Sci.*, 72:631.

Smiricky, M. R., D. M. Albin, J. E. Wubben, and V. M. Gabert. 2000a. The influence of feed enzymes and feed steeping on total tract digestibility and fecal output in growing pigs fed a corn–soybean meal diet. Abstr. 213 presented at the Midwestern Section of ASAS and Midwest Branch ADSA 2000 Meeting, Des Moines, IA.

Smiricky, M. R., J. E. Wubben, D. M. Albin, and V. M. Gabert. 2000b. The interaction between hydrolysis time and acid concentration affects the measurement of amino acids in soybean meal and ileal digesta from growing pigs. Abstr. 153 presented at the Midwestern Section of ASAS and Midwest Branch ADSA 2000 Meeting, Des Moines, IA.

Sosulski, F. W., L. A. Minja, and D. A. Christensen. 1988. Trypsin inhibitors and nutritive value in cereals, *Plant Food Hum. Nutr.*, 38:23.

Souffrant, W. B., B. Darcy-Vrillon, T. Corring, J. P. Laplace, R. Köhler, G. Gebhardt, and A. Rerát. 1986. Recycling of endogenous nitrogen in the pig (preliminary results of a collaborative study), *Arch. Anim. Nutr.*, 36:269.

Southern, L. L. 1991. Digestibile amino acids and digestible amino acid requirements for swine, BioKyowa Technical Review, No. 2.

Stein, H. H., S. Aref, and R. A. Easter. 1999a. Comparative protein and amino acid digestibilities in growing pigs and sows, *J. Anim. Sci.*, 77:1169.

Stein, H. H., N. L. Trottier, C. Bellaver, and R. A. Easter. 1999b. The effect of feeding level and physiological status on total flow and amino acid composition of endogenous protein at the distal ileum of swine, *J. Anim. Sci.*, 77:1180.

Taverner, M. R., and D. J. Ferrell. 1981a. Availability to pigs of amino acids in cereal grains. 3. A comparison of ileal availability values with faecal, chemical and enzymic estimates, *Br. J. Nutr.*, 46:173.

Taverner, M. R., and D. J. Ferrell. 1981b. Availability to pigs of amino acids in cereal grains. 4. Factors influencing the availability of amino acids and energy in grains, *Br. J. Nutr.*, 46:181.

Taverner, M. R., I. D. Hume, and D. J. Ferrell. 1981a. Availability to pigs of amino acids in cereal grains. 1. Endogenous levels of amino acids in ileal digesta and faeces of pigs given cereal diets, *Br. J. Nutr.*, 46:149.

Taverner, M. R., D. M. Curic, and C. J. Rayner. 1981b. A comparison of the extent and site of energy and protein digestion of wheat, lupin and meat and bone meal by pigs, *J. Sci. Food Agric.*, 34:122.

van Barneveld, R. J. 1993. Effect of Heating Proteins on the Digestibility, Availability and Utilisation of Lysine by Growing Pigs, Ph.D. dissertation, University of Queensland, Australia.

van Barneveld, R. J., E. S. Batterham, and B. W. Norton. 1994a. The effect of heat on amino acids for growing pigs. 1. A comparison of ileal and fecal digestibilities of amino acids in raw and heat-treated field peas (*Pisum sativum* cultivar Dundale), *Br. J. Nutr.*, 72:221.

van Barneveld, R. J., E. S. Batterham, and B. W. Norton. 1994b. The effect of heat on amino acids for growing pigs. 2. Utilization of ileal-digestible lysine from heat-treated field peas (*Pisum sativum* cultivar Dundale), *Br. J. Nutr.*, 72:243.

van Barneveld, R. J., E. S. Batterham, and B. W. Norton. 1994c. The effect of heat on amino acids for growing pigs. 3. The availability of lysine from heat-treated field peas (*Pisum sativum* cultivar Dundale) determined using the slope-ratio assay, *Br. J. Nutr.*, 72:257.

van Barneveld, R. J., J. D. Nutall, P. C. Flinn, and B. G. Osborne. 1999. Near infrared reflectance measurement of the digestible energy content of cereals for growing pigs, *J. Near Infr. Spec.*, 7:1.

van der Poel, A. F. B., J. Blonk, D. J. van Zuilichem, and M. G. van Oort. 1990. Thermal inactivation of lectins and trypsin inhibitor activity during steam processing of dry beans (*Phaseolus vulgaris* L.) and effects on protein quality, *J. Sci. Food Agric.*, 58:215.

van der Poel, A. F. B., A. Schoterman, and M. W. Bosch. 1998. Effect of expander conditioning and/or pelleting of a diet on the ileal digestibility of nutrients and on feed intake after choice feeding of pigs, *J. Sci. Food Agric.*, 76:87.

van Leeuwen, P., W. C. Sauer, J. Huisman, E. J. van Weerden, D. van Kleef, and L. A. den Hartog. 1987. Methodological aspects for the determination of amino acid digestibilities in pigs fitted with ileocecal re-entrant cannulas, *J. Anim. Physiol. Anim. Nutr.*, 58:122.

van Leeuwen, P., D. J. van Kleef, J. M. van Kempen, J. Huisman, and M. W. A. Verstegen. 1991. The post valve T-caecum technique in pigs applied to determine the digestibility of amino acids in maize, groundnut and sunflower meal, *J. Anim. Physiol. Anim. Nutr.*, 65:183.

Vandergrift, W. L., D. A. Knabe, and T. D. Tanksley, Jr. 1983. Digestibility of nutrients in raw and heated soyflakes for pigs, *J. Anim. Sci.*, 57:1215.

Viljoen, J., M. N. Ras, F. K. Siebrits, and J. P. Hayes. 1997. Use of the mobile nylon bag technique (MNBT) in combination with the ileo-rectal anastomosis technique (IRA) to determine amino acid digestibility in pigs, *Livest. Prod. Sci.*, 51:109.

Walker, W. R., C. V. Maxwell, F. N. Owens, and D. S. Buchanan. 1986. Milk versus soybean protein sources for pigs: II. Effects on amino acid availability, *J. Anim. Sci.*, 63:513.

Wiseman, J., S. Jaggert, D. J. A. Cole, and W. Haresign. 1991. The digestion and utilization of amino acids of heat-treated fish meal by growing/finishing pigs, *Anim. Prod.*, 53:215.

Yen, J. T., J. A. Nienaber, and W. G. Pond. 1987. Effect of neomycin, carbadox and length of adaptation to calorimeter on performance, fasting metabolism and gastrointestinal tract of young pigs, *J. Anim. Sci.*, 65:1243.

Yin, Y.-L., R. Hunan, H. Zhong, C.-M. Chen, and H. Dai. 1991. Influence of different cannulation techniques on the pre-caecal digestibility of protein, amino acids and cell wall constituents from diets, containing different protein meals, in pigs, *Anim. Feed Sci. Technol.*, 35:271.

Yin, Y.-L., J. D. G. McEnvoy, H. Schulze, and K. J. McCracken. 2000a. Studies on cannulation method and alternative indigestible markers and effects of food enzyme supplementation in barley-based diets on ileal and overall apparent digestibility in growing pigs, *Anim. Sci.*, 70:63.

Yin, Y.-L., J. D. G. McEvoy, H. Shulze, U. Hennig, W.-B. Souffrant, and K. J. McCracken. 2000b. Apparent digestibility (ileal and overall) of nutrients as evaluated with PVTC-cannulated or ileo-rectal anastomised pigs fed diets containing two indigestible markers, *Livest. Prod. Sci.*, 62:133.

Zebrowska, T. 1973. Digestion and absorption of nitrogenous compounds in the large intestine of pigs, *Roczn. Nauk Roln. Ser. B Zootech.*, 95:85.

Zebrowska, T., L. Buraczewska, B. Pastuszewska, A. G. Chamberlain, and S. Buraczewski. 1978. Effect of diet and method of collection on amino acid composition of ileal digesta and digestibility of nitrogen and amino acids in pigs, *Roczn. Nauk Roln. Ser. B Zootech.*, 99:75.

10 Calcium, Phosphorus, Vitamin D, and Vitamin K in Swine Nutrition

Thomas D. Crenshaw

CONTENTS

I. Interdependence of Ca, P, Vitamin D, and Vitamin K 188
    A. General Comments and Major Review References 188
    B. Requirements Driven by Physiological Functions 189
        1. Body Composition and Compartments 189
        2. Skeletal Tissue Composition and Function 191
II. Calcium 192
    A. Chemical Properties and Homeostatic Mechanisms 192
        1. Physical–Chemical Properties 192
        2. Homeostasis, Absorption, and Excretion 192
        3. Skeleton Storage and Mobilization 195
    B. Functions from Skeleton Mineralization to Cell Signal 196
    C. Requirements 197
    D. Deficiency Symptoms 197
    E. Toxicity 198
    F. Sources and Availability 198
III. Phosphorus 198
    A. Chemical Properties and Homeostatic Mechanisms 198
        1. Physical–Chemical Properties 198
        2. Absorption and Excretion 199
        3. Interference with P Absorption and Availability 199
    B. Functions 200
    C. Requirements 200
    D. Deficiency Symptoms 200
    E. Toxicity 200
    F. Sources and Availability 201
IV. Vitamin D 201
    A. Natural Forms and Derivatives 201
        1. Chemical Structures 201
        2. Absorption and Metabolic Synthesis of Active Forms 201
    B. Physiological Action 203
        1. Calcium Homeostasis, Parathyroid Hormone, and Calcitonin 203
        2. Newly Discovered Functions of Vitamin D 203
    C. Requirements 203

	D. Deficiency	204
	E. Toxicity	204
V.	Vitamin K	204
	A. Natural Forms and Derivatives	204
	1. Chemical Structures	204
	2. Absorption and Metabolic Synthesis of Active Forms	204
	B. Physiological Action	206
	1. γ-Carboxylation Reactions	206
	2. Osteocalcin	207
	C. Assessment of Vitamin K Status	207
	1. Requirements	208
	D. Deficiency	208
	E. Toxicity	209
References		209

I. INTERDEPENDENCE OF CA, P, VITAMIN D, AND VITAMIN K

A. GENERAL COMMENTS AND MAJOR REVIEW REFERENCES

Calcium and phosphorus are the most abundant mineral elements in the body. New insights into the dynamic roles for Ca and P in regulation of cellular functions have rekindled interest in these elements beyond interest in their roles of structural support. Understanding the intricate regulation of Ca and P concentrations in soft tissue and the biological pathways that sequester and mobilize these elements in skeletal tissue is fundamental to establishment of nutrient requirements. As inorganic mineral elements, neither Ca nor P is decomposed by biochemical reactions. However, elemental P is too reactive to be found free in nature; it ignites spontaneously on exposure to air. Thus, in biological systems, ortho-phosphates (PO_4) are the forms that are the base unit for metabolism. In this chapter, phosphorus (P) implies a phosphate form unless specified otherwise. Both Ca and P are classified as macrominerals along with Na, K, Cl, S, and Mg. Macrominerals are nutrients required in the diet at concentrations >100 ppm.

Throughout life, Ca and P are continuously deposited and reabsorbed from bone. Accumulation of Ca and P in skeletal tissue is interdependent, one element will not accumulate without the other. The involvement of vitamin D derivatives in regulation of Ca and P absorption and accumulation in bone is well established. Vitamin D derivatives, in coordination with parathyroid hormone (PTH) and calcitonin (CT), are involved in regulation of Ca and P homeostasis. Current evidence (Binkley and Suttie, 1995) suggests a role for vitamin K in regulation of mineralization. Vitamin K may function to prevent mineralization in soft tissue and even control mineralization in bone through post-translational carboxylation reactions with bone-specific proteins.

McDowell (1992) provided a concise 2000-year historical account of the major discoveries of nutritional benefits of minerals, including Ca and P. Summaries of research specifically focused on Ca and P nutrition in swine are provided in comprehensive reviews (Hayes, 1976; Peo, 1976; Kornegay, 1985), and a recent update of nutrient requirements was provided by NRC (1998). Information reviewed in these reports illustrate how knowledge of nutrient requirements has benefited the economics of swine production. Recent reviews on vitamin D (Jones et al., 1998; Holick, 1999) and vitamin K (Suttie, 1993; Vermeer et al., 1995) provide excellent descriptions of the physiological roles of these nutrients. The primary focus of this chapter is to provide an overview of the basic principles involved in the regulation and function of Ca and P in swine with emphasis on the role of the skeleton as a primary target and response organ. Basic principles are established and the interrelationships of these nutrients discussed in the context of meeting the nutrient requirements of swine.

B. REQUIREMENTS DRIVEN BY PHYSIOLOGICAL FUNCTIONS

Knowledge of the nutrient requirements of swine has allowed fortification of all-plant diets with minerals and vitamins so that cereal grains can serve as the main source of energy. Cereal grains are essentially devoid of Ca and, although relatively abundant in total P, the form of P is not available to nonruminant animals. Based on total ingredient costs, P is the most expensive mineral added to swine diets. The difference in costs between Ca and P is even reflected in regulatory requirements for feed labels. Feed regulations only require a minimum concentration of P to be specified on feed tags, but a minimum and maximum concentration must be specified for Ca. Without specific programming steps to prevent an overfortification of Ca, least-cost formulations will include Ca sources such as calcium carbonate instead of corn. Because of these price relationships, excess Ca is often included in swine diets, but only minimum amounts of P are included. This relationship is inverted in human nutrition. Because of the foods consumed by humans, Ca intake is often marginal and P intake is typically in excess. Costs certainly affect selection of feed ingredients for swine, but understanding the physiological functions of nutrients not supplied by the major ingredients provides the basis for successful use of the less-expensive, all-plant feed ingredients.

1. Body Composition and Compartments

Ca and P are ubiquitous in biological systems; yet these elements are highly compartmentalized with drastically different concentrations throughout the body. The majority of each element is found in skeletal tissue. Within the body, 96 to 99% of Ca is contained within the skeletal tissue. The percentage of P found in skeletal tissue (60 to 80%) is more variable than that of Ca. The variable percentage of P in skeletal tissue is not due to changes in the Ca:P ratio in bone ash, but to variation in ratios of the amounts of soft tissue relative to skeletal tissue. The concentration of P in soft tissue (lean) is nearly constant, as is the amount of P per unit of skeletal ash. Thus, changes in the percentage of total body P found in skeletal tissue are due to the absolute amounts of soft tissue and skeleton and the proportion of these tissues to each other. Assessment of the requirements for Ca and P must consider changes in skeletal storage and that skeletal storage is not directly proportional to lean growth. The ability of pigs to alter dramatically the amounts of soft tissue and skeleton is illustrated in Figure 10.1. Nearly equal weight gain was maintained in pigs fed either a control or a Ca-deficient, protein-supplemented formula, but approximately tenfold more mineral was deposited in pigs fed the control formula (Johanson et al., 1995). Thus, Ca and P requirements for soft tissue growth are independent, but have priority over requirements for skeletal growth.

A scarcity of data exists on the Ca and P distribution in skeletal and soft tissue compartments in growing swine. Nielsen (1972) found 99.1% of the Ca and 77.5% of the P in the dissected skeletal fraction of growing pigs, consistent with the distributions discussed above. In neonatal pigs 96.7% of the Ca was recovered in skeletal tissues (Schneider et al., 1997). Several reports are available (see legend for Figure 10.2) based on analysis of entire animals rather than analysis based on soft tissue and skeletal tissue compartments. These data are inconsistent and highly variable. If 98% of total-body Ca and 75% of total-body P is assumed to be present in the skeleton and skeletal ash contains a 2.2:1 ratio of Ca:P, then the Ca:P ratio in the entire carcass should be 1.65:1 and constant across age groups. The results in Figure 10.2 illustrate that the Ca:P ratio based on analysis of the entire body was not constant across the growth period. The main sources of variation undoubtedly relate to variation in the skeleton and soft tissue compartments and the differential growth of these tissues. Failure to assess the variable component of skeletal growth thwarts efforts to model requirements for Ca and P.

The differences in skeleton and soft tissue concentrations have major implications on nutrient fortification strategies. In skeletal tissue Ca and P combine in approximately a 2.2:1 ratio to form a hydroxyapatite-like compound. In soft tissue, however, the two elements have little

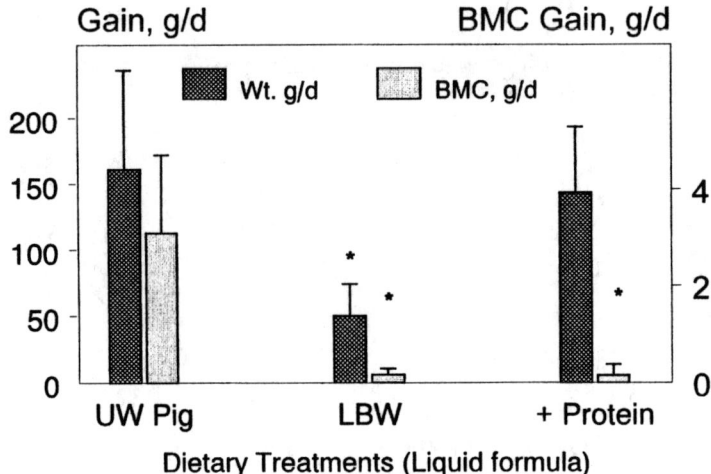

FIGURE 10.1 Soft tissue and skeletal tissue growth are independent. Compared with neonatal pigs (0 to 10 days old) fed a protein- and Ca-deficient formula (LBW), addition of a semipurified protein source (+Protein) allowed body weight gain to equal that of pigs fed a control (UW Pig) formula, but bone mineral (BMC) did not accumulate in pigs fed the Ca-deficient formula. (* Denotes difference within response criteria from control group.) (From Johanson, J. C. et al., *FASEB J.*, 9:A160, 1995. With permission.)

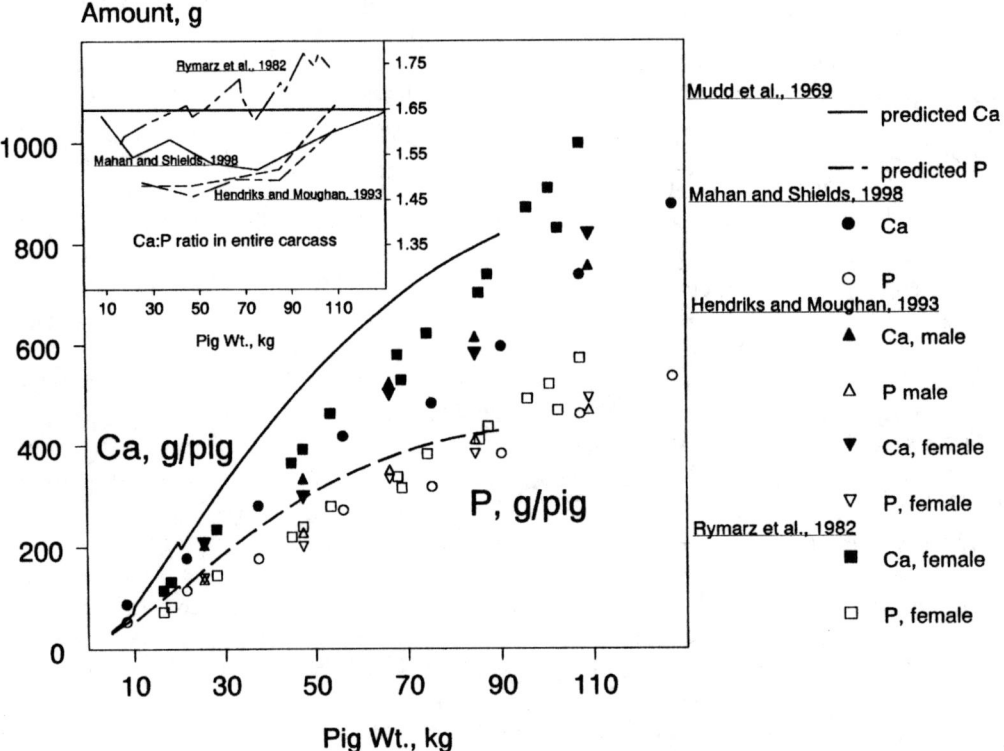

FIGURE 10.2 Ca and P accumulate in bone ash at a 2.2:1 ratio, but mineral content results based on analysis of the entire carcass are quite variable. Data were calculated from regression equations reported by Mudd et al. (1969) or at average weight intervals reported by Mahan and Shields (1998), Hendriks and Moughan (1993), and Rymarz et al. (1982). Assuming 98% of body Ca and 75% of body P is located in skeletal tissue, the Ca:P ratio in the entire animal should be constant at 1.65:1.

common function. For example, the role of P as an initiation factor for protein synthesis may be affected in animals fed diets marginally deficient in P and lean tissue gain is suppressed. Soft tissue Ca concentrations are so tightly regulated by endocrine systems that dietary deficiencies must be extreme before soft tissue accumulation is altered. Thus, marginal dietary P deficiencies will affect growth, but extreme dietary Ca deficiencies must be imposed before animal growth is compromised.

2. Skeletal Tissue Composition and Function

Bone from mature animals contains approximately 45% water, 25% ash, 20% protein, and 10% fat (Lian et al., 1999). Because fat and water content change with age and nutritional status, it is useful to describe the amount of ash as the ratio of ash relative to dry, fat-free bone. General partition of organic and inorganic fractions of bone are shown in Figure 10.3. Mineral accumulates in bone as crystals of a calcium-deficient form of hydroxyapatite ($Ca_{10}(PO_4)_6$) consisting of Ca and P in a nearly constant 2.2:1 ratio. One element will not be deposited or reabsorbed without the other. Variable amounts of carbonate, citrate, magnesium, sodium, potassium, chloride, and fluoride affect the final composition as animals age and physiological status changes. X-ray diffraction patterns of bone mineral suggest bone apatite is initially a calcium-deficient hydroxyapatite with hydrogen phosphate or carbonate groups substituting for phosphate ions (Holden et al., 1995). These substitutions may slightly alter the Ca:P molar ratio in newly formed bone crystals, but differences in ratio would not be detected by gross analysis because the greater percentage of mineral mass consists of mature crystals. Bone ash consists of 36 to 39% Ca and 17 to 19% P (Figure 10.3). The concentration of Ca and P in bone ash does not change in response to extreme shifts in nutrient intake, but the total amount of ash accumulated varies with nutrient status (Hayes, 1976). Because 96 to 99% of the body Ca is located in skeleton tissue, Ca content in the body provides a reasonably accurate index of skeletal ash content.

Before Ca and P accumulate in bone, the osteoblast cells must synthesize and accumulate an extracellular matrix composed primarily of Type I collagen and proteoglycans. The initial step in formation of a mineral crystal is not known, but when ^{45}Ca and ^{32}P are injected simultaneously, Ca apparently precedes P deposition by several hours in mineralization of skeletal tissue (Heeley and Irving, 1973). Many systemic hormones, localized growth factors, and nutrients are involved in regulation of the formation, resorption, and accumulation of the organic and inorganic matrix of bone. Full discussion of these factors is beyond the scope of this chapter and readers are referred

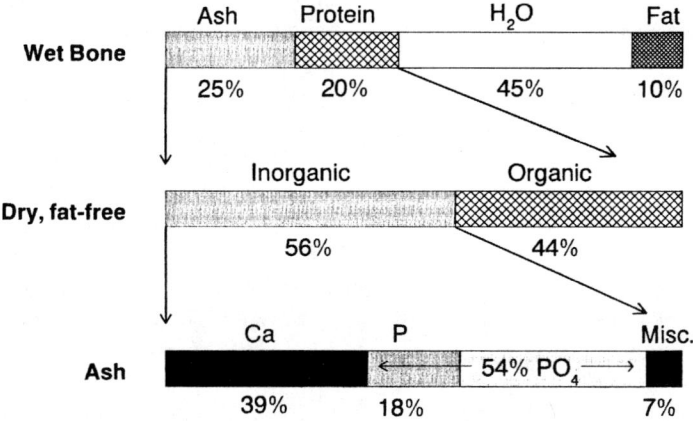

FIGURE 10.3 The percentages of mineral and ash in bone expressed as a percentage of wet bone, dry, fat-free bone, and ash. Calcium and P are a constant percentage of ash, being deposited in a 2.2:1 ratio. The amount of ash relative to organic matrix changes with nutritional status.

to current overviews by Lian et al. (1999) and Mundy (1999). Specific roles of the two major minerals, Ca and P, and the specific roles of two vitamins, D and K, will be discussed here.

II. CALCIUM

A. Chemical Properties and Homeostatic Mechanisms

The metabolism of Ca is intimately linked to that of P. Regulation of both minerals is a function of their physical–chemical properties and the intricate endocrine system that regulates these elements. The hormones most prominently involved include PTH, vitamin D, and CT.

1. Physical–Chemical Properties

After quartz (SiO_2), calcium carbonate ($CaCO_3$) is the most abundant mineral in the earth's crust. Ca composes 3.64% of the earth's crust and occurs naturally as limestone (calcium carbonate), calcium fluoride, and calcium sulfate. $CaCO_3$ is sequestered from seawater by aquatic animals to form shell and skeletal tissue. The sequestered $CaCO_3$ eventually sediments to ocean floors and forms limestone. With time and pressure, marble is formed from limestone.

Calcium, the 20th element, is an alkaline earth element that loses two electrons to form a divalent cation. The cation is strongly hydrated and, in nature, never really in a pure form, but readily forms complexes with organic and inorganic anions. Ca has a melting point of 842°C and a boiling point of 1484°C. Ca and Mg are both divalent cations, but Ca has a larger ionic radius (0.99) than Mg (0.65). Ca has a similar ionic radius as Na (0.95), but Na has only one ionic charge. These physical–chemical properties of Ca describe an element with a stronger affinity for oxygen ligands such as carboxylates, carbonyls, and phosphates than the alkali metals Na and K. Because of these properties, Ca has a unique role in biological systems. These roles can be grouped into two general areas, the ability to form complexes with proteins and the various solubilities of different phosphate salts of Ca.

In biological systems Ca forms complexes with proteins that allow reversible conformational changes in the protein and, as a result, regulates the function of the protein complex. Because Ca is a strong activator of many biological compounds, elaborate mechanisms exist to regulate Ca concentrations in body compartments. Cells have extensive mechanisms to regulate Ca binding to phosphates or proteins. Intracellular Ca is maintained at a concentration that is four times lower than extracellular Ca. Low intracellular Ca concentrations are maintained by transport proteins located on cell membranes and by calcium-binding proteins within cell cytosolic compartments. The rigid difference in intracellular and extracellular concentrations coupled with the physical–chemical properties of Ca make Ca an ideal second messenger. Intracellular Ca binds to target proteins to mediate responses even in the presence of higher concentrations of Mg, Na, and K ions. Additional roles of Ca complexes involve stabilization of protein structures, cell membranes, and extracellular matrix in skeletal tissue.

The drastically different solubilities of three calcium phosphate salts commonly found in physiological tissues are important in regulation of blood pH and bone mineralization. Primary calcium phosphate ($Ca(H_2PO_4)_2$) is highly soluble in water, but tertiary calcium phosphate ($Ca_3(PO_4)_2$) has a solubility of only slightly greater than 10^{-4} M. Approximately 85% of Ca in solution in extracellular fluid of mammals is secondary calcium phosphate ($CaHPO_4$), which has a solubility of 2×10^{-3} M. Bone contains predominately tertiary calcium phosphate, which forms hydroxyapatite crystals after precipitation. The differences in solubilities of the phosphate salts and the influence of these salts on physiological solutions are described further in Section III.A.1.

2. Homeostasis, Absorption, and Excretion

Animals have elaborate mechanisms to acquire Ca from the environment and tightly regulate Ca distribution to maintain concentrations within body compartments. Homeostatic mechanisms for

Ca are extremely complex. An increase in intracellular Ca concentrations from 10^{-7} to 10^{-5} M is lethal; yet the extracellular fluid Ca concentration is 10^{-3} M. Cell membranes form complexes with Ca in proportion to extracellular concentration. Intracellular organelles sequester Ca. The mitochondria and microsomes contain 90 to 99% of intracellular Ca.

Extracellular Ca concentration is maintained accurately and precisely (Bronner and Stein, 1995). In extracellular fluid, Ca is approximately 50% ionized, 40% bound to proteins such as albumins, and 10% complexed with citrate and phosphate ions. Protein binding is influenced by pH, with an increase in free or ionized Ca under acidosis. Ionized Ca is the reactive form. Positive or negative Ca ion loads are compensated within seconds even if these loads are imposed by intravenous infusions. Three target organs that contribute to this regulation include the intestine, kidney, and bone (Figure 10.4). Much attention has been attributed to intestinal and renal regulation, perhaps because of the relative ease of determining an apparent absorption and retention of Ca. However, bone may be of greater importance than intestinal or renal regulation of Ca because of the rate and magnitude of response by skeletal tissue to shifts in Ca concentrations (Parfitt, 1987; Talmage, 1996).

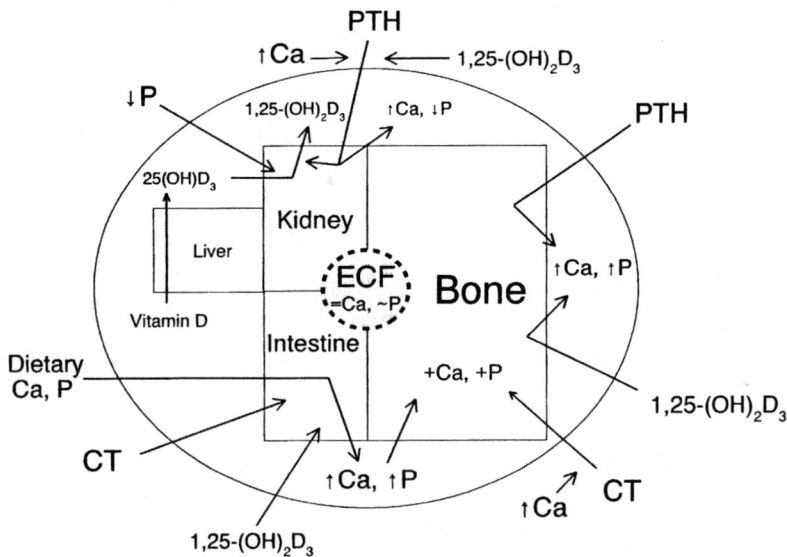

FIGURE 10.4 Regulation of Ca and P homeostasis by systemic hormones: parathyroid hormone (PTH), calcitonin (CT), and vitamin D after conversion to the active derivative 1,25-(OH)$_2$ D$_3$ in the kidney. Target tissues for hormonal action include the intestine, renal, and skeletal tissues. Immediate changes in the extracellular fluid (ECF) concentrations are shown in the larger circle with the net result being a coordinated series of regulatory steps to maintain a constant Ca (=Ca) and nearly constant (~P) concentration in ECF as illustrated in the smaller circle.

Calcium is absorbed by transcellular and paracellular routes in the intestine (Bronner, 1998). Regulation of transcellular Ca transport involves homeostatic activation of vitamin D in renal tissue and subsequent action of vitamin D on the small intestine target tissue to stimulate calcium binding protein (calbindin) synthesis (Figure 10.4). Transcellular transport, located in the proximal intestine, is saturable, is regulated by vitamin D, requires oxygen, and transports Ca against a chemical gradient. Descriptions of Ca absorption generally focus on active transport mechanisms in the upper portion (duodenum and jejunum) of the small intestine, but relatively large amounts of Ca are absorbed by passive transport in the lower small intestine and colon. Active transport is enhanced by dietary insufficiency so that the percentage of Ca absorbed by active transport mechanisms is greater than passive transport. But with abundant dietary Ca, active transport is suppressed, passive transport is enhanced, and Ca excretion is increased to maintain Ca concentrations. The paracellular process does not appear to be subject to regulation.

Bronner (1995) concluded that endogenous fecal Ca excretion was not regulated in humans. Fecal Ca excretion is a linear function of intake, whereas Ca absorption is curvilinear, consistent with a regulatory role. In humans, endogenous Ca is approximately equal to urinary Ca excretion. But, based on classical work in pigs, Besancon and Gueguen (1969) reported that urinary Ca was only about 1% of fecal Ca. Fecal Ca in pigs was approximately 20% of endogenous origin (Figure 10.5). However, the type of diet affects sites and amounts of Ca absorbed. Partridge (1978) observed net secretion of Ca in the large intestine of pigs fed semipurified diets but no net secretion in the large intestine of pigs fed natural ingredient diets. Endogenous fecal Ca excretion in rats is about ten times that of urinary Ca loss; thus, rats and pigs are similar in routes and relative percentages of Ca excretion. The relative magnitude of fecal Ca from dietary or endogenous origin is undoubtably influenced by intake relative to the requirement and to factors that might influence flux in the bone pools. As illustrated in Figure 10.5, turnover of Ca in bones of growing pigs is similar in magnitude to that of dietary intake.

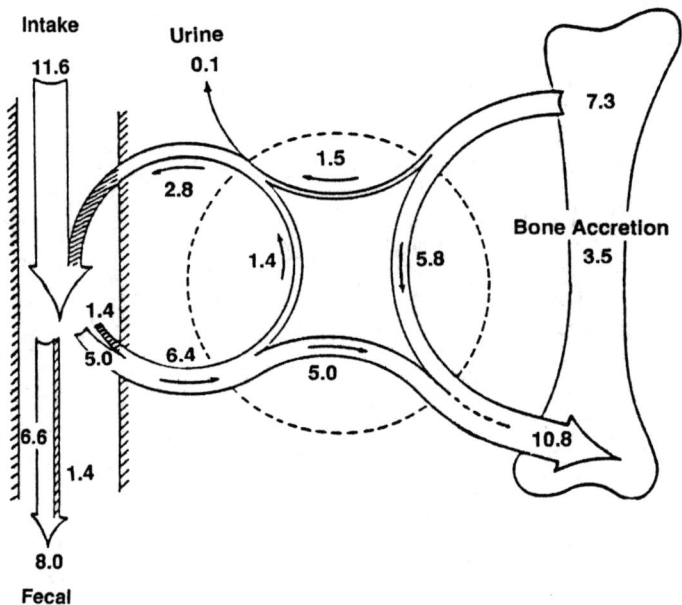

FIGURE 10.5 Calcium flux in growing pigs. Values represent grams of Ca flowing through intestine, extracellular fluid, or bone compartments. (From Besancon, P., and Gueguen, L., *Ann. Biol. Anim. Biochem. Biophys.*, 9: 537, 1969. With permission.)

In a summary of reports on Ca absorption, Kornegay (1985) concluded that only 30 to 60% of dietary Ca was absorbed by the pig and that 85 to 95% of the absorbed Ca was retained. Absorption and retention of Ca were influenced by the amount of Ca consumed, the ratio of Ca:P, pig age, and physiological demand for Ca (i.e., growth, gestation, or lactation).

The ratio of dietary Ca to P (Ca:P) affects absorption of each element. The importance of maintaining a proper Ca:P ratio is more critical if the dietary Ca or P concentration is marginal or inadequate (Hayes, 1976; Peo, 1976). If high dietary concentrations of Ca and P are fed, the ratio is not critical. The Ca:P ratio based on Ca to total P should range between 1:1 and 1.25:1 in grain–soybean meal diets for swine (NRC, 1998). Diets formulated on an available P basis should provide ratios between 2:1 and 3:1.

Other factors that may affect Ca absorption include high dietary levels of sulfates, oxalates, strontium, magnesium, or certain antibiotics. These factors are of little consequence in typical diet formulations commonly used in the swine industry.

Changes in calbindin synthesis in response to acute changes in Ca concentration are too slow to account for regulation of Ca. Likewise, similar transport mechanisms exist in the kidney, but again the responses to vitamin D are too slow to account for the short-term changes involved in Ca regulation (Parfitt, 1987; Bronner and Stein, 1995). Bronner and Stein (1995) estimated that blood must circulate 90 times in bone to clear half of a Ca load, but 900 times through the intestine, and almost 4000 times in kidneys.

3. Skeleton Storage and Mobilization

Traditional views describe the role of skeletal tissue as a mere storage pool of Ca and P in the context of homeostasis. As discussed above, careful consideration of the kinetics suggest bone is more involved than merely as a storage depot. The large surface area of bone contributes to a unique role in Ca and P homeostasis. For example, the total bone surface area of canaliculae and lucunae is 1000 to 5000 m^2 compared with 140 m^2 in lung capillaries (Baron, 1999). The bone surface is bathed in an extracellular fluid (bone fluid) found in the periosteocytic space that can exchange Ca ions with surface Ca on bone crystals in the hydration shell surrounding each crystal. Bone crystals are extremely small, 200×30 to 70 Å, compared with the 20 to 30 µm diameter of osteoblast lining cells (Green and Kleeman, 1991). The Ca concentration (0.5 mmol/l) in bone fluid is less than that of plasma (1.5 mmol/l).

In the skeleton, Ca regulation involves both cellular and noncellular reactions. Traditional descriptions of Ca regulation include long-term responses that involve control of cellular factors that stimulate cell proliferation, activation, synthesis of the extracellular protein matrix, and post-translational events that affect mineralization and resorption of bone by osteoclast cell recruitment, fusion, and activation (Figure 10.6B and C). Noncellular events involve formation and resorption of brushite, hydroxyapatite, and maturation of mineral crystals. As with intestinal transport, the cell-mediated events of bone cannot respond fast enough to explain Ca fluxes observed in response to acute shifts in the extracellular Ca concentration (Parfitt, 1987; Talmage, 1996; Bronner, 1998). But, resorption of mineral crystals and mineral ions in the hydration shell on crystal surfaces act as a Ca pool to regulate minute fluxes in Ca (Figure 10.6A). Calcium binding sites located on bone crystal surfaces are proposed as major means of minute Ca flux regulation. The binding sites are subject to hormonal regulation. Osteoblast cells that line the surface of mineralized matrix are known to change shape in response to PTH and signals from localized growth factors. The shape changes may expose bone fluid compartments to extracellular fluid and allow rapid exchange of mineral ions. Whether the rapid exchange in Ca between the bone fluid and bone mineral is due to the differences in solubilities of the Ca and P salts in the phases or the rapid changes in cell shape in response to hormonal–ligand binding (Bronner and Stein, 1995) is not clear.

The parathyroid gland is the calcium-sensing organ in the body. Within seconds, parathyroid cells respond to decreased plasma Ca concentrations by release of stored PTH (an 84-amino acid polypeptide) into circulation and by an increase in PTH gene expression. Plasma Ca increases within minutes after release of PTH by the induction of changes in target tissues. Target tissues for PTH include renal nephrons and osteoblast cells but not intestinal cells or osteoclast cells (Figure 10.4). PTH blocks renal P reabsorption and thus increases urinary P loss. PTH also indirectly increases intestinal absorption of Ca and mobilization of Ca and P from bone by effects of PTH on vitamin D metabolism. PTH stimulates 1α-hydroxylase activity in kidneys to convert 25-OH D_3 to 1,25-$(OH)_2$ D_3, which acts on intestinal target tissue to increase Ca-binding protein synthesis. In bone, PTH inhibits osteoblast cell matrix formation and promotes (through osteoblast-mediated signals) osteoclastic resorption of bone.

Elevated serum Ca also stimulates secretion of calcitonin (a 34-amino acid peptide hormone) from the thyroid C cells. Calcitonin protects against hypercalcemia and calcification of soft tissue. Calcitonin lowers plasma Ca by enhancing cellular uptake of Ca into the cytosol, enhancing renal excretion of Ca, and inhibiting resorption of bone. Calcitonin is one of only a few hormones or

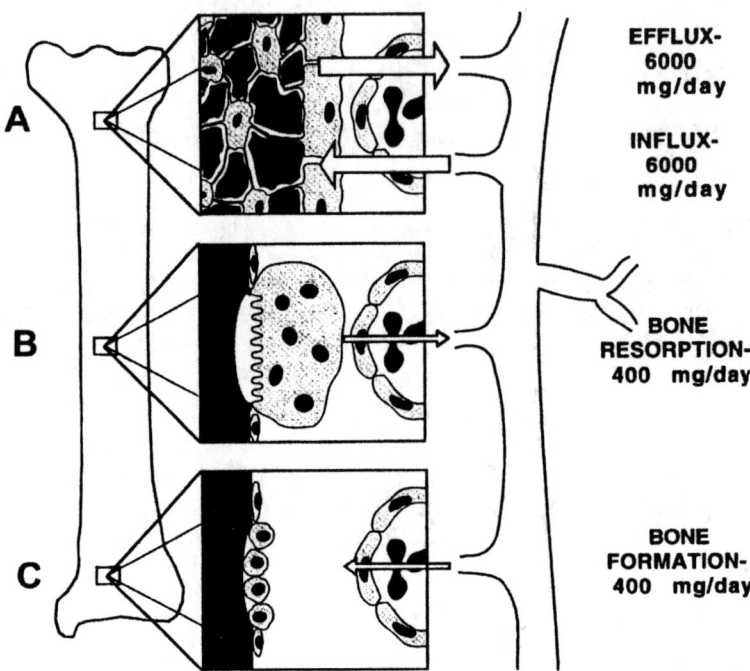

FIGURE 10.6 Modes of Ca and P flux in bone. The flux of Ca from bone in response to immediate needs of Ca in extracellular fluid (A) is an order of magnitude larger and the response is faster than can be attributed to long-term mechanisms involved in the resorption (B) and formation (C) of bone. Mechanisms involved in A are not completely understood but are thought to be under hormonal control and to involve precipitation or release of minerals from the surface of bone crystals. Most likely, some degree of regulation occurs by signals mediated by the bone lining cells. (From Talmage, R. V., in *Calcium and Phosphorus in Health and Disease*, Anderson, J. J. B., and Garner, S. C., Eds., CRC Press, Boca Raton, FL, 1996. With permission.)

growth factors that act directly on osteoclast cells. Convincing evidence is not reported to support a role for calcitonin in regulation of vitamin D hormonal levels.

B. Functions from Skeleton Mineralization to Cell Signal

The biological functions of Ca range from one of structure as an integral part of the hydroxyapatite to that of a second messenger in cell signaling. Because of the stringent regulation of extracellular Ca concentrations and the abundant reserves in skeletal tissue stores, the functional roles of Ca are not altered over a wide range of dietary Ca concentrations. Malfunctions are typically secondary, not a primary response to diet. Primary responses to diet require assessment of changes in the skeletal tissue. Response criteria used to assess dietary adequacy include measurement of the total ash content of bone or the mechanical properties of bone. The relative merits of these traits were reviewed by Crenshaw et al. (1981) and Combs et al. (1991).

Both intracellular and extracellular concentrations of Ca are tightly regulated by bidirectional Ca transport across plasma membrane of cells and even cellular organelles such as the endoplasmic reticulum, mitochondria, and the sarcoplasmic reticulum of muscle cells. These transport regulatory mechanisms and the presence of Ca-binding proteins maintain cytoplasmic ionized Ca concentration in a micromolar range compared with millimolar concentrations in the extracellular fluid compartment, allowing Ca a role as an intracellular signaling molecule.

Intracellular Ca concentration is about fourfold less than free Ca in extracellular fluid. Most intracellular Ca is located in the mitochondria and endoplasmic reticulum. External signals bind to cell surface receptors and induce the release of 1,2-diacyl glycerol or myo-inositol-1,4,5-triphosphate. These second messengers stimulate release of Ca from intracellular stores and induce Ca-mediated responses. In skeletal muscle the increase in cytosolic Ca concentration initiates muscle contraction by binding to the Ca-binding proteins, troponin C, and calmodulin. Additional functions mediated by changes in cytosolic Ca involve cell motility, membrane adhesion, nerve synaptic transmission, hormone release, and a role as a cofactor for numerous enzymes such as those involved in blood clotting and protein kinases.

C. Requirements

NRC (1998) provided estimates of Ca requirements for the entire life cycle of pigs. Controversy over which trait to use in establishing Ca and P requirements has continued for decades. Requirements certainly differ if based on amounts needed for maximum growth and reproductive traits rather than amounts required to maximize skeletal accumulation of mineral. An acceptable range (Crenshaw, 1986) is a better solution, but recent pressures from environmental concerns for P pollution have tended to decrease dietary supplementation of Ca and P to levels that compromise animal well-being. Today, attempts to establish requirements for Ca and P must balance animal well-being and economic concerns with environmental concerns (Crenshaw and Johanson, 1995; Lenis and Jongbloed, 1999).

Calcium and P requirements for swine were recently evaluated (NRC, 1998), but sufficient information was not available to allow development of a model to predict requirements for growing animals. With environmental pressures, more accurate predictions are needed. NRC (1998) provided estimates of requirements based on empirical data (which by design has to approximate the requirement but does not necessarily provide a method to predict the animal needs in a factorial model). Estimates of Ca availability are affected by experimental design and are restricted to the dietary conditions in which the determination was made. Requirements for Ca must meet the needs for maintenance, soft tissue accretion, skeletal tissue accretion, and endogenous losses. Because animals can grow soft tissue independent of the growth of skeletal tissue (see Figure 10.1), the rate of skeletal accretion must be considered a variable rather than a fixed function of growth (Crenshaw and Johanson, 1995).

D. Deficiency Symptoms

Classical symptoms of animals fed diets deficient in Ca, P, and vitamin D are well described. Animals exhibit lameness, slow gait, paralysis, rickets, and spontaneous fractures. Extreme Ca deficiencies are required to alter soft tissue growth, but marginal intake results in abnormal bone development. Growing animals fed diets deficient in either Ca or vitamin D, but with adequate P, will develop rickets. Rickets is characterized by shortened, deformed limbs as bones fail to mineralize, but the bone organic matrix and other soft tissues continue to accumulate. Often joints are enlarged and animals may experience spontaneous fractures and/or beaded ribs. Typically rickets is attributed to deficiencies of Ca or vitamin D because a marginal deficiency of P will decrease soft tissue growth in addition to bone mineralization.

Mature animals fed diets deficient in Ca or vitamin D will develop osteomalacia. Deficiencies are most commonly exhibited in sows after prolonged lactation periods or animals with high milk production performance. Posterior paralysis due to vertebrae fractures and fractures in limb bones are classical symptoms of sows that have depleted body stores for milk production when suboptimum Ca and P intake was allowed. The body mineral reserves of sows are often thought to be depleted to provide Ca and P needs of developing fetuses. However, Itoh et al. (1967) found that sows fed deficient Ca and P diets (0.30% Ca, 0.30% P) produced offspring with only about 70% as much body Ca, suggesting that the dam was not able to mobilize sufficient body stores to maintain fetal Ca levels at the same concentration as sows fed adequate (0.70% Ca, 0.50% P) diets.

Both fetal bone and soft tissue Ca concentrations were lower in fetal samples from dams fed deficient diets, but fetal plasma Ca values were equal.

E. Toxicity

High dietary concentrations of Ca depress appetite and growth rate (NRC, 1998). The effect is more severe when the Ca:P ratio is wide (Kornegay, 1985). Excessive Ca intake may also decrease P and Zn bioavailability.

F. Sources and Availability

Cereal grains and most plant protein ingredients are quite low in Ca; thus most of the requirement must be supplied by inorganic sources. In typical diets fed in the United States, approximately 25 to 50% of the inorganic Ca requirement will be supplied by sources used to meet the P requirement. The balance of the Ca requirement is typically supplied by limestone. Because of the low costs of inorganic Ca sources, little attention has been devoted to Ca availability. Particle size of limestone apparently does not affect availability (Pond et al., 1982; Ross et al., 1984). Kornegay (1985) reviewed reports on Ca availability studies in swine and concluded that only 30 to 60% of dietary Ca is absorbed by the pig. Factors such as age, sex, nutritional status, level of mineral in diet, level and form of other nutrients, health, disease, and parasite status, homeostatic control, hormone control, chelating agents, environmental factors, and feed processing all influence the actual amount of nutrient used from a single ingredient source. The time of Ca ingestion affects absorption. Ca ingested before a meal has a higher absorption than Ca ingested after a meal (Pointillart et al., 1995).

III. PHOSPHORUS

Phosphorus has more known functions than any other mineral element in the body but less is known about P homeostasis than Ca. Further research efforts are needed to develop a better understanding of P regulation. This information is especially important as concerns about environmental pollution by animal operations are added to the practical concerns of providing sufficient P for animal well-being.

A major role of P along with Ca involves mineralization of bone as discussed above. Additionally, P is located in every cell in the body with functions ranging from structural components of phospholipids in membranes to energy storage in the form of phosphate diester bonds and even osmotic balance and buffering. In proteins, phosphorylation sites are critical in activation of enzymes. Essentially every energy transfer reaction within cells involves the formation or cleavage of P bonds.

A. Chemical Properties and Homeostatic Mechanisms

1. Physical–Chemical Properties

All living matter contains P but usually in a form complexed with oxygen as a phosphate (PO_4). Pure phosphorus is too reactive to be found free in nature and ignites spontaneously when exposed to air. In nature, orthophosphates are typically found complexed with Ca and various amounts of carbonates, fluoride, and trace amounts of other elements. The primary source of P is from rock phosphate ($Ca_5(PO_4)_3F$ or $CaF_2 \cdot 3Ca_3(PO_4)_2$). Rock phosphate can be heated to form phosphoric acid, which is the primary starting material for feed and fertilizer phosphates and even food sources of P.

Phosphorus, the 15th element, has a molecular weight of 30.97. In biological systems phosphate is maintained in a ratio of dibasic (HPO_4^{-2}, mw = 95.97) to monobasic ($H_2PO_4^{-1}$, mw = 96.97) ion complexes as a function of pH, defined by the Henderson–Hasselbalch equation.

$$pH = pKa + \log(HPO_4^{-2}/H_2PO_4^{-1}) \qquad (10.1)$$

Thus, at pH 7.4 and a pKa of 6.8 for phosphates in physiological solutions, the concentration of dibasic phosphate is four times greater than the concentration of monobasic phosphate. In physiological solutions phosphates have an average molecular weight of 96.17 with a valence of 1.8 (Crenshaw, 1991).

Concentration of P in intracellular (1×10^{-4} M) and extracellular (2×10^{-4} M) fluid is less rigidly maintained than is Ca concentration. Serum P concentration varies throughout the day and is influenced by age, sex, diet, pH, and a variety of hormones (Broadus, 1999). Only about 10% of serum P is complexed with proteins; the remaining 90% is in an ionic form.

2. Absorption and Excretion

As with Ca, the major sites of P absorption are in the upper parts of the small intestine. Net secretion of P was observed in the large intestine (Partridge, 1978). Phosphate is absorbed as inorganic P from both dietary inorganic sources and from organic sources after hydrolysis by phosphatases in enterocytes (Jongbloed, 1987). Phosphate can also be absorbed as a structural part of organic compounds such as phospholipids. Phosphate absorption occurs in the small intestine by both active, saturable and passive, nonsaturable transport systems (Breves and Schroder, 1991). Phosphate absorption is stimulated by vitamin D, independent of effects of the vitamin on Ca absorption. Sodium is required for vitamin D–mediated P absorption. A vitamin D–responsive, Na–P cotransport system has been characterized in rat and rabbit small intestines. In addition a Na-independent diffusion mechanism has been described for cellular P uptake. Higher rates of active P absorption are found in jejunum than duodenum (160 vs. 40 nmol/cm^2/h) with very little absorption occurring in the ileum.

Regulation of P homeostasis is dependent on mobilization of bone reserves and the regulation of renal excretion and intestinal absorption (see Figure 10.4). Animals fed diets with marginal P concentrations increase the proportion of dietary P absorbed in the intestine, and concomitantly renal P reabsorption is increased to minimize urinary P excretion. As with the regulation of Ca, the major hormones involved are PTH, CT, and 1,25-(OH)$_2$ D$_3$. Hypophosphatemia and hyperphosphatemia are associated with increased and decreased circulating levels of 1,25-(OH)$_2$ D$_3$, respectively (Holick, 1999). Recent reports (reviewed by Econs, 1999) of studies of P wasting in humans provide limited evidence for maintenance of P homeostasis. This evidence supports a role for osteoblast cells in the production of a modifying factor that affects renal proximal tubule P transport. Cloning techniques were used to identify a phosphate-regulating gene expressed in bone and teeth.

Certain forms of P apparently play important roles in the inhibition of mineralization, especially in soft tissue. Pyrophosphate inhibits crystallization of Ca salts and formation of new hydroxyapatite crystals (Russell and Rogers, 1999). Regulation of pyrophosphate concentrations may be mediated by alkaline phosphatase. Oral administration of pyrophosphate is not effective because of hydrolysis by intestinal phosphatases. Analogs that are stable under oral administration, bisphosphonates, are currently used in treatment of osteoporosis in humans. Bisphosphonates have a high affinity for bone mineral and prevent ectopic calcification, but also inhibit resorption of hydroxyapatite by interference with osteoclast function. The family of bisphosphonates and their mode of action has recently been reviewed (Russell and Rogers, 1999).

3. Interference with P Absorption and Availability

With few exceptions, P in most inorganic sources is highly available. The inverse is true with most plant sources. The P in rock phosphate has the same availability as that of dicalcium phosphate, but rock phosphate contains high levels of fluorine, which may become toxic to animals. Orthophosphoric acid (H_3PO_4) must contain ≤100 ppm F. Phosphoric acid is produced by one of three processes: (1) furnace electrothermal reduction of phosphate rock (tricalcium phosphate fluorapatite, $3Ca_3(PO_4)_2CaF_2$) at 1540°C; (2) the pebble rock process which has a lower heat requirement (1480°C) and yields defluorinated phosphate; or (3) the wet process, which involves digestion of a slurry of phosphate rock in sulfuric acid then separation of phosphoric acid by filtration.

Animals fed raw rock phosphate develop fluorine toxicity. The P:F ratio in rock phosphate is often less than 100:1, sometimes as narrow as 15:1. Fluorine toxicity primarily affects bone because 95% of absorbed F accumulates in skeletal tissue. Although low levels of F are beneficial in human diets, F toxicity is more common than F deficiencies in animal diets. Daily supplements of 2 mg of F/100 kg body weight increased the rate of cortical bone remodeling and bone porosity compared with bone measurements from control pigs fed diets without added F (Kragstrup et al., 1989). Natural ingredients used in animal diets provide sufficient quantities of F to meet minimum requirements (Nelson, 1983).

The availability of P in most plants is low because plants store P as a phytic P. Nonruminant animals do not synthesize the phytase enzyme required for hydrolysis of phytic P. Exogenous sources of phytase enzymes offer the potential to degrade phytic P and liberate P for absorption by the animal. Phosphate bioavailability varies widely in plant feed ingredients, ranging from 10 to 60%. Variation may be partially explained by intrinsic phytase activity in some ingredients, but even with addition of exogenous phytase, availability did not exceed 60 to 70% (Weremko et al., 1997).

B. Functions

Primary functions of P include roles in mineralization of connective tissue, functional and structural component in nucleic acids, energy transport in diester phosphate bonds for such compounds as ATP, structural component of phospholipids and proteins, reactive ligand in active sites of enzymes and transport proteins, acid–base buffering, and osmotic balance. Phosphate is involved in both aerobic and anaerobic energy metabolism. Bone P serves as a reservoir to buffer changes in plasma and intracellular P.

C. Requirements

The amount of P required for maximum growth is less than that required for maximum bone mineralization or bone strength (NRC, 1998). Requirement estimates are affected by the criteria and experimental design used to determine requirement. Similarly, efforts to determine P bioavailability are limited in application to diets and concentration ranges within which the estimates are determined. As these requirements are often determined at dietary concentrations below that required for a maximum response, extrapolation to practical (higher concentrations of total P) feeding levels will likely result in less P than predicted being absorbed by the animal.

D. Deficiency Symptoms

Marginal deficiency of P will affect growth and protein deposition in animals (Vipperman et al., 1974). Certain disease states may exacerbate marginal P deficiency. Conditions involving severe diarrhea, malabsorption, or a decrease in renal P reabsorption may decrease serum, but not intracellular P levels. As discussed in Section II.D, P deficiency will affect bone development in young and mature animals.

E. Toxicity

Swine can tolerate fairly high dietary concentrations of P if the Ca:P ratio is narrow. Excess P can be detrimental if dietary Ca is marginal. Symptoms observed in animals include an increased incidence of urinary calculi, osteodystrophia fibrosa, and metastatic calcification in soft tissue (NRC, 1980).

F. Sources and Availability

In contrast to Ca, most cereal grains and plant protein ingredients used in swine diets contain modest levels of P, but the availability is poor. Most plants store P as a phytic phosphate, which is mostly unavailable to nonruminant animals. Bioavailability of phytic P from plant sources ranges from 10 to 60%. The current publication for nutrient requirements of swine lists estimates of available P from common feed ingredients (NRC, 1998). Feed processing methods such as soaking, cooking, germination, and fermentation improve P availability. These improvements are not of sufficient magnitude to be economically justified in most current feeding programs in the United States. Thus, the P requirement, like that of Ca, is commonly met by adding inorganic sources to diets. The P in most inorganic sources is considered highly available (Kornegay, 1985). Dicalcium phosphate and defluorinated phosphate are two common sources used in swine diets.

IV. VITAMIN D

A. Natural Forms and Derivatives

Vitamin D is a generic descriptor for all secosteroid compounds with cholecalciferol activity. Vitamin D_2 (ergocalciferol) and vitamin D_3 (cholecalciferol) are the two main forms of the fat-soluble vitamin. Both forms are taken up by adipose tissue for storage or by the liver for further metabolism as detailed below. The capacity for tissue storage is sufficient to support an animal for months during periods of no dietary supplement of vitamin D (Anonymous, 1991). Vitamin D provitamins are converted into intermediates and active derivatives. Conversion to the active forms occur by tightly regulated pathways. Active derivatives bind to nuclear receptors responsible for pivotal roles of Ca homeostasis and normal bone mineralization.

1. Chemical Structures

Elucidation of the role of vitamin D_3 as a precursor (Figure 10.7) to the functionally active form $1\alpha, 25$-dihydroxyvitamin D_3 ($1,25\text{-}(OH)_2\, D_3$) has allowed detailed insights into the physiological and molecular actions of this nutrient and the mechanisms of Ca and P homeostasis. An in-depth review of the physiological and molecular actions of vitamin D has recently been published (Jones et al., 1998) and a concise overview is provided by Holick (1999).

2. Absorption and Metabolic Synthesis of Active Forms

Vitamin D_3 is synthesized in skin by radiation of ultraviolet light in the 270 to 300 nm range. The ultraviolet energy induces a photochemical reaction that transforms 7-dehydrocholesterol through a series of steps to vitamin D_3. Dietary sources of either vitamin D_2 or D_3 and the vitamin D_3 synthesized in skin are activated in the liver by the same enzyme, vitamin D-25-hydroxylase, to 25-hydroxyvitamin D_2 or 25-hydroxyvitamin D_3 (25-OH D_3), respectively. The major form of vitamin D in circulation is 25-OH D_3. Pigs apparently discriminate in metabolism of the two forms of vitamin D and convert more D_3 to the 25-hydroxyvitamin than D_2 (Horst et al., 1982). Some 25-hydroxylase activity is found in extrahepatic tissues including intestine, kidney, and bone as well as the placenta during pregnancy (Holick, 1999). Circulating 25-OH D_3 is stabilized and transported by a vitamin D–binding protein. The metabolic fate of 25-OH D_3 is primarily dependent on serum Ca status. Low Ca status activates renal 1α-hydroxylase activity, whereas abundance of Ca activates 24-hydroxylase activity.

Further hydroxylation of 25-OH D_3 in the kidney by 1α-hydroxylase yields biologically active $1,25\text{-}(OH)_2\, D_3$ (Figure 10.7). The enzyme is located on the inner mitochondrial membrane of the renal proximal tubular cells. Synthesis of 25-OH D_3 is loosely regulated, but synthesis of $1,25\text{-}(OH)_2\, D_3$ is tightly regulated by serum $1,25\text{-}(OH)_2\, D_3$, Ca, and PTH. The 1α-hydroxylase

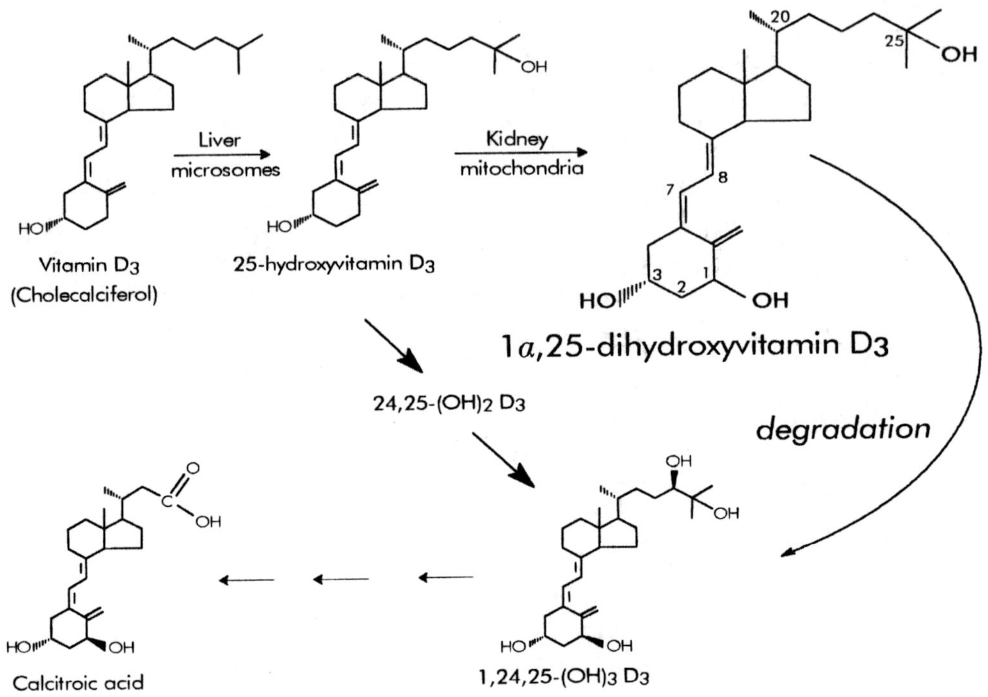

FIGURE 10.7 Pathways for activation and degradation of vitamin D. Synthesis of the active derivative, 1,25-$(OH)_2$ D_3 is regulated by PTH and serum P (see Figure 10.4). Degradation of 1,25-$(OH)_2$ D_3 involves formation of 1,24,25-$(OH)_3$ D_3, thought by some to have a metabolic role (see text), but generally assumed to be inert. (From Jones, G. et al., *Physiol. Rev.*, 78:1193, 1998. With permission.)

is induced by PTH through a cAMP/phosphatidylinositol-4,5-bisphosphate-mediated signal transduction pathway. The enzyme is downregulated by vitamin D status via a 1,25-$(OH)_2$ D_3, receptor-mediated transcriptional mechanism within 2 to 4 h after exposure to 1,25-$(OH)_2$ D_3. With the downregulation of 1α-hydroxylase is a reciprocal upregulation of 25-OH D_3-24-hydroxylase. Thus, 25-OH D_3-24-hydroxylase seems mainly to play a role of inactivation and attenuation of the biological signal inside target cells (Jones et al., 1998). The 25-OH D_3-24-hydroxylase is found in intestinal, renal, and skeletal tissues in addition to most if not all target 1,25-$(OH)_2$ D_3 tissues.

In addition to regulation of 1,25-$(OH)_2$ D_3 synthesis, degradation of this potent hormone is also regulated by apparently separate, but highly specific cytochrome P-450 enzymes (Jones et al., 1998). In degradation, 1,25-$(OH)_2$ D_3 is hydroxylated in target tissue (bone and intestine) and in the liver and kidney to an inert, water-soluble calcitroic acid (see Figure 10.7). Both 25-OH D_3 and 1,25-$(OH)_2$ D_3 undergo a 24-hydroxylation to form 24,25-dihydroxyvitamin D_3 (24,25-$(OH)_2$ D_3) and 1,24,25-trihydroxyvitamin D_3, respectively. The 24-hydroxylated derivatives are considered to be inert, first-step products of biodegradation (Jones et al., 1998; Holick, 1999), but some observations imply possible, yet undefined, roles for 24,25-$(OH)_2$ D_3 in bone formation, fracture healing, and embryonic development (Norman, 1996; Kato et al., 1998; St-Arnaud, 1999). St-Arnaud (1999) provided support for a role of 24,25-$(OH)_2$ D_3 in regulation of bone structure during embryogenesis and developmental regulation of intramembranous bone formation. This role for 24,25-$(OH)_2$ D_3 is not fully explained by current understanding of vitamin D metabolites and is potentially mediated by a receptor distinct from that of 1,25-$(OH)_2$ D_3. In contrast, animals grown for two generations with metabolically stable, fluoro-analogs of 24,25-$(OH)_2$ D_3 failed to support a role for 24,25-$(OH)_2$ D_3 in skeletal formation or maintenance of calcemia (Jones et al., 1998).

B. Physiological Action

1. Calcium Homeostasis, Parathyroid Hormone, and Calcitonin

The long-term consequence of elevated 1,25-$(OH)_2$ D_3 is to initiate Ca transport in the small intestine. In intestinal cells 1,25-$(OH)_2$ D_3 stimulates synthesis of a Ca-binding protein, calbindin D9k, but the presence of calbindin cannot solely explain Ca transport responses to 1,25-$(OH)_2$ D_3. Upregulation of Ca-binding protein has a half-life of days compared with minutes for responses observed in target tissues such as osteoblast cells. Calbindin concentrations remain elevated even after Ca absorption diminishes. Additional sites of 1,25-$(OH)_2$ D_3 action on intestinal tissue remain to be identified.

1,25-$(OH)_2$ D_3 also stimulates intestinal P absorption, independent of Ca uptake (Jones et al., 1998). Pig 1α-hydroxylase activity increased in response to decreased P intake even though serum Ca levels were maintained within normal ranges (Engstrom et al., 1985). Serum 1,25-$(OH)_2$ D_3 levels reflected the changes in 1α-hydroxylase activity.

In bone, 1,25-$(OH)_2$ D_3 stimulates osteoblast-mediated osteoclast cell formation and differentiation. Signaling mechanisms between the osteoblast and osteoclast cells have only recently been described (Yasuda et al., 1999). Osteoblast cells are stimulated to synthesize an osteoclast differentiation factor (ODF) in response to 1,25-$(OH)_2$ D_3. The ODF binds to osteoclast progenitors by a membrane-bound receptor. Also, ODF stimulated ^{45}Ca release from labeled bone in a dose-dependent manner and release was blocked by an ODF antibody.

In addition to 1,25-$(OH)_2$ D_3 cell-mediated resorption of bone, a poorly defined, but physiologically important, mechanism that mobilizes Ca and P from the bone fluid compartment, also exists (see Figure 10.6). Mobilization of Ca and P from bone requires both 1,25-$(OH)_2$ D_3 and PTH (Jones et al., 1998). The PTH-related protein (PTH-rp) does not seem to function in normal Ca homeostasis but may play a role in abnormal calcium mobilization in malignancy.

Calcitonin inhibits osteoclastic bone resorption. However, after continued exposure to exogenous therapy, the inhibitory effects are lost, apparently due to downregulation of calcitonin receptors (Mundy, 1999).

The molecular mechanisms of the hormonal action of 1,25-$(OH)_2$ D_3 are similar to those of estrogen and other steroid hormones. Target tissues have a nuclear vitamin D receptor (VDR) for 1,25-$(OH)_2$ D_3. The VDR requires interaction with a retinoic acid X receptor to form a heterodimer complex with 1,25-$(OH)_2$ D_3. Once formed, this dimer complex binds to specific response elements in promoter sequences of 1,25-$(OH)_2$ D_3 responsive genes. Further interactions of this protein–DNA complex activate transcriptional machinery inside vitamin D target cells to cause gene transcription, synthesis of messenger RNA, and translation of proteins such as osteocalcin, osteopontin, alkaline phosphatase, and calcium-binding proteins. The ultimate biological actions involve proliferation and differentiation of cells. Other actions that are not well understood involve roles in regulation of P-450-containing enzymes and apparent downregulation of PTH genes by VDR.

2. Newly Discovered Functions of Vitamin D

Several cells other than those in the classical target tissues also have receptors for 1,25-$(OH)_2$ D_3. These include nuclei of islet cells in the pancreas, keratinocytes of skin, ovarian tissue, certain neuronal tissue, promyelocytes, macrophages, and T-lymphocytes, as well as tumor cells. Functional roles for vitamin D in these cells have not been fully established (Holick, 1999).

C. Requirements

Swine do not require dietary sources of vitamin D if sufficient sunlight exposure is provided (Anonymous, 1991). Under confinement housing, dietary fortification is needed. Natural feed ingredients are limited in vitamin D or provitamin content with the exception of legume hays or animal products such as fish meals or fish oils. Vitamin D activity is lost by excessive treatment with ultraviolet light and peroxidation by free radicals formed by polyunsaturated fatty acids. Oxidative destruction is enhanced by heat, moisture, and trace elements. Economical sources of stabilized, feed-grade vitamin D_3 with 20 to 40 million units/g are available and are routinely used in swine diets. Commercial diets are routinely fortified with vitamin D levels (300 to 700 IU/kg diet) well in excess of minimum requirements (Peo, 1991).

Minimum requirements for vitamin D range from 220 to 150 IU/kg diet for pigs from 5 to 120 kg (NRC, 1998). Recommendations for breeding animals are 200 IU/kg diet. By definition one IU of vitamin D_3 is the biological activity supplied by 0.025 μg of cholecalciferol.

D. Deficiency

A deficiency of vitamin D compromises absorption and storage of Ca and P, resulting in insufficient bone mineralization. In young, growing animals, rickets develop, whereas older animals exhibit osteomalacia. Under severe deficiencies tetany may be observed. Deficiency symptoms may take 4 to 6 months to become evident (Quarterman et al., 1964) because of the tissue storage capacity.

E. Toxicity

The excess vitamin D supplementation in commercial swine diets pose no particular problem unless formulation or mixing errors occur (Peo, 1991). The practical safe upper level of vitamin D_3 is about 22,000 IU/kg diet, well above any intentional fortification level. The consequences of toxicity include slow growth, poor feed conversion, calcification of soft tissue, and death (Chineme et al., 1976; Long, 1984; Hancock et al., 1986). Weanling pigs given daily oral doses of 6250 μg of vitamin D_3 (250,000 IU D_3) exhibited poor growth and feed intake, reduced liver and bone weights, and calcification in aorta, heart, kidney, and lung tissues (Quarterman et al., 1964).

V. VITAMIN K

A. Natural Forms and Derivatives

1. Chemical Structures

Vitamin K was the last fat-soluble vitamin discovered. By definition, vitamin K is a generic descriptor for menadione, 2-methyl-1,4-naphthoquinone (vitamin K_3), and all derivatives (Figure 10.8) that exhibit antihemorrhagic activity in animals fed a vitamin K-deficient diet. Vitamin K is essential because the 1,4-naphthoquinone nucleus cannot be synthesized in mammalian cells. Menadione is not found in natural feed ingredients, but is modified systemically from derivatives found in nature. Compounds in nature with vitamin K activity can be grouped into phylloquinones, precursors synthesized by green plants and algae, and menaquinones, compounds produced by bacteria.

Menadione was synthesized almost 60 years ago (Ullrey, 1991; Suttie, 1993) and was thought at that time to have direct vitamin K activity. Now menadione is thought to be alkylated to a biologically active menaquinone by intestinal microorganisms or tissue before absorption (Suttie, 1984).

2. Absorption and Metabolic Synthesis of Active Forms

Phylloquinone is absorbed in the proximal intestine of rats by an energy-dependent process, but absorption in the distal gut is poor (Hollander, 1973). Menaquinone absorption occurs in both the proximal and distal intestine and the colon by a passive process (Hollander et al., 1976), but the efficiency of absorption is sufficient to prevent vitamin K deficiency.

Absorption of vitamin K derivatives occurs via the lymphatic system. Derivatives are incorporated into chylomicrons for transport to the liver. Absorption and transport are closely linked to

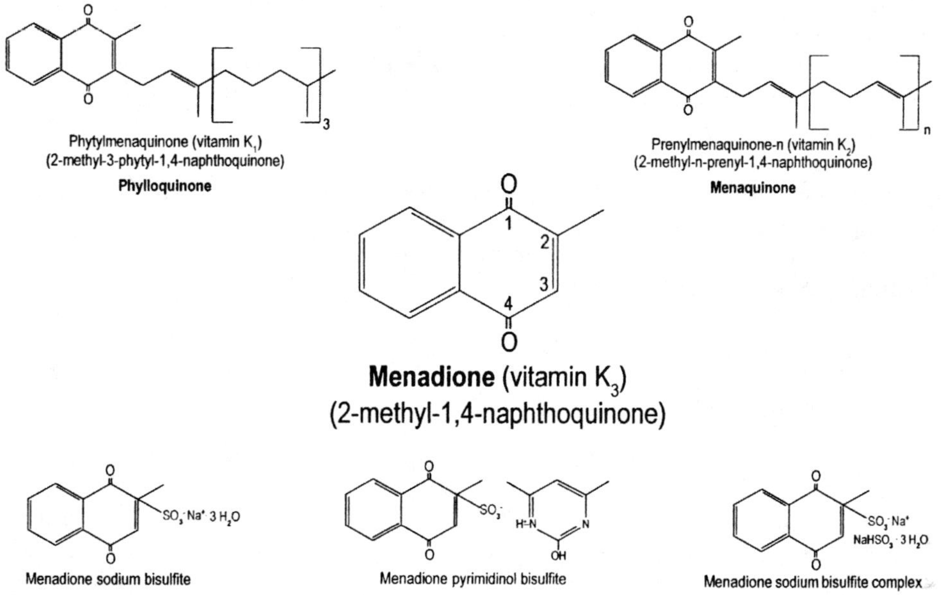

FIGURE 10.8 Precursors and active forms of vitamin K. Precursors from plants (phylloquinone) or bacteria (menaquinone) are converted to active menadione forms. Stable feed-grade forms include menadione sodium bisulfite (50% menadione), menadione sodium bisulfite complex (33% menadione), and menadione pyrimidinol bisulfite (45.5% menadione).

triglycerides and lipoproteins. Absorption of vitamin K precursors from the intestinal lumen is affected by dietary fat and dietary factors affecting stimulation of bile salt secretion and pancreatic lipase activity. Both classes of compounds (phylloquinones and menaquinones) have comparable activities after absorption, but may differ in potential for absorption because of their intestinal tract location in the native form. Precursors are converted in hepatic tissues to active forms of vitamin K.

Naturally occurring vitamin K derivatives found in green plants, and to a lesser extent in animal tissues, include phylloquinone, phytylmenaquinone, or vitamin K_1 (2-methyl-3-phytyl-1,4- naphthoquinone). A reliable database for vitamin K content of animal feed ingredients does not exist. Vegetables and fruits may contain two to ten times higher concentrations of phylloquinones (range from 1000 to 8000 μg/kg) than dairy products (10 to 500 μg/kg) and grains (3 to 70 μg/kg), but the bioavailable vitamin K from dairy products is thought to exceed that of green plants. Most precursors in plants are tightly bound to thylakoid membranes in chloroplasts (Vermeer et al., 1995) and are not readily absorbed.

Menaquinones (2-methyl-3-multiprenyl-1,4-naphthoquinone) are also compounds with vitamin K activity. The number of unsaturated isoprenoid side chains is varied and the number of chains (n) is indicated as vitamin K_2-n. Natural menaquinones produced by bacteria have from 4 to 13 side chain residues. Bacterial synthesis of menaquinones by the intestinal microflora is substantial, but absorption in the colon may be limited. Availability of microbial products to the animal is affected by the extent of coprophagy. Similarly, use of antibiotics, particularly ones that contain the methyltetrazole-thiol side chain, may alter menaquinone synthesis and perhaps even conversion to active forms in hepatic tissue (Lipsky, 1994; Vermeer et al., 1995). Unless extreme caging conditions are imposed, rats consume 60 to 80% of their feces. Estimates of fecal consumption by pigs in modern confinement housing systems are not established. Similarly, the recent adoption of medicated early-weaning practices, which include high doses of antibiotics and high levels of sanitation, merits research efforts to determine vitamin K status of these animals.

Menaquinones are found in feed ingredients of animal origin and also may be produced by menaquinone-producing bacteria on ingredients that tend to be hygroscopic. Because of a wide range of precursors and difficulties in producing a K deficiency, questions arise over recommendations concerning dietary supplementation of K.

The stability of dietary menadione is uncertain. Water-soluble derivatives of menadione have been developed. Menadione sodium bisulfite (50% menadione) is used commercially, but more stable crystals are produced in the presence of excess sodium bisulfite forming a menadione sodium bisulfite complex (33% menadione). This compound is widely used in swine and poultry feeds. A third water-soluble derivative involves the addition of dimethylpyrimidinol to the menadione sodium bisulfite complex resulting in menadione pyrimidinol bisulfite (45.4% menadione). The pyrimidinol complex is an equal or better source than menadione sodium bisulfite complex for swine and poultry (Seerley et al., 1976; Ullrey, 1991).

B. Physiological Action

1. γ-Carboxylation Reactions

Vitamin K functions as a cofactor for the formation of γ-carboxyglutamate (Gla) residues in proteins. Proteins that undergo carboxylation reactions all participate in reactions that require Ca. Carboxylation of glutamate residues increases the affinity of the protein for Ca. Figure 10.9 outlines the role of vitamin K in carboxylation of glutamate residues. Vitamin K undergoes reduction to form a biologically active hydroquinone, which acts as a cofactor for a carboxylase enzyme that adds a carboxy residue to the γ-carbon of glutamate residues in proteins resulting in the formation of a vitamin K oxide. The oxide is then reduced to vitamin K.

Numerous proteins in the body with glutamate residues undergo γ-carboxylation reactions. Most notable are proteins involved in blood clotting (prothrombin) and three proteins found mostly (but not exclusively) in bone. The bone matrix proteins include osteocalcin, matrix Gla-protein, and protein S. Osteocalcin is produced only by osteoblast cells, but matrix Gla-protein and protein

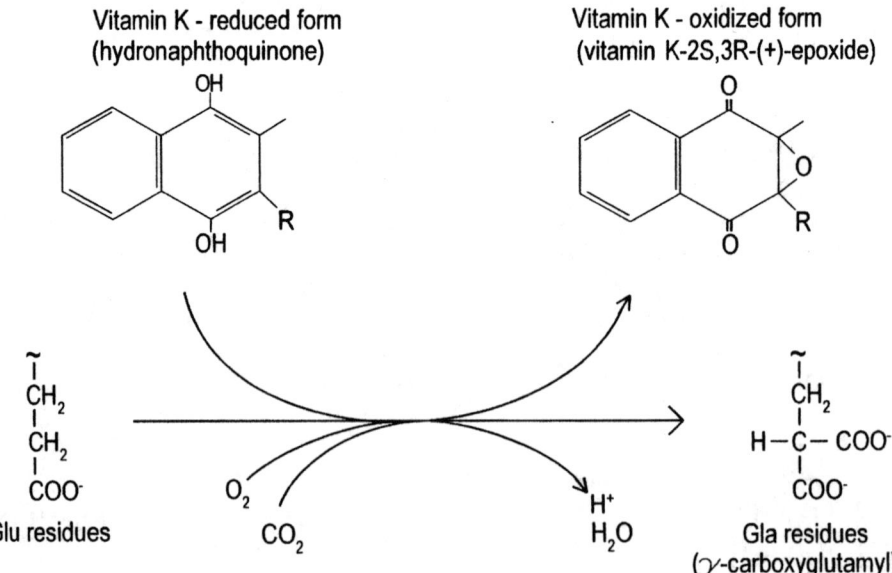

FIGURE 10.9 γ-carboxylation of glutamate residues is coupled to the oxidation of the reduced hydronaphthoquinone form to the epoxide form of vitamin K. Glutamate residues in a limited number of proteins are converted to γ-carboxyglutamate residues, which have a high binding affinity for Ca. (From Suttie, J. W., *FASEB J.*, 7:445, 1993. With permission.)

S are secreted by several cell types throughout the body. Approximately 80% of the γ-carboxylation protein residues are located in bone.

Prothrombin was the first Gla-protein characterized. A functional role of post-translational carboxylation reaction was identified in relation to clot formation. Blood coagulation is a cascade of reactions involving the conversion of fibrinogen to fibrin. Four steps in the cascade involve vitamin K–dependent activation of precursors to active proteolytic enzymes. The inactive precursors include Factors II (prothrombin), VII (proconvertin), IX (Christmas factor, plasma thromboplastin component), and X (Stuart factor). Each vitamin K–dependent step involves the formation of γ-carboxyglutamate residues that are binding sites for Ca ions.

Similar mechanisms may be involved in other proteins with Ca-binding sites. Carboxylated proteins may play pivotal roles in mineralization, but the presence of Gla residues in proteins is difficult to detect and quantitate (Hauschka et al., 1975). Assays based on immunochemical detection may not be specific for the presence and or degree of glutamate residues that are carboxylated.

2. Osteocalcin

Osteocalcin is a low molecular weight protein with three Gla residues. Osteocalcin accounts for 15 to 20% of the noncollagen protein in bone. Osteocalcin concentration is directly proportional to bone Ca content. Osteocalcin is produced by osteoblast cells during bone matrix formation and is released from matrix during resorption of bone. A small fraction of newly synthesized osteocalcin is released into circulation. Circulating osteocalcin increases after treatments known to increase bone formation (1,25-$(OH)_2$ D_3 treatment), but the concentration changes with age in humans (Binkley and Suttie, 1995). The exact role of osteocalcin in bone mineralization is not well established.

Based on the abundance of osteocalcin in bone and its association with bone Ca content, osteocalcin is used as an indirect marker of bone mineralization in human clinical trials. Elevated serum osteocalcin is generally associated with increased bone formation (Khosla and Kleerekoper, 1999). Carter et al. (1996) developed and validated a porcine radioimmunoassay (RIA) for detection of serum osteocalcin in growing swine. Serum osteocalcin and 1,25-$(OH)_2$ D_3 decreased as dietary Ca and P levels were increased, but, as expected, the amount of load withstood by bones during mechanical tests and the amount of bone ash increased as consumption of Ca and P increased.

C. Assessment of Vitamin K Status

Historically, vitamin K status has been linked to blood clotting because of the carboxylation of prothrombin. A deficiency of vitamin K results in underdecarboxylated prothrombin (also defined as descarboxy-prothrombin) which prolongs blood clotting time. Commercial kits to assess vitamin K status are based on assays of prothrombin activation. Test serum provides a source of Factors VII and X which are activated by Russell's viper venom. Under these conditions, prothrombin concentration is limiting, and the rate of clot formation is related to the amount of prothrombin in the test serum (Suttie, 1984).

A functional assay of vitamin K status is based on the presence of descarboxy-prothrombin in plasma (Lipsky, 1994). More recent understanding of carboxylated proteins and the potential for compartmentalization of liver vs. bone activity has led to suggestions that the degree of carboxylation of osteocalcin may be a more sensitive marker for vitamin K status (Binkley and Suttie, 1995). Although the exact function of osteocalcin is not defined, the extent of binding of osteocalcin to hydroxyapatite crystals is influenced by the number of carboxylated residues. Osteocalcin is associated with mineralized matrix and is a chemoattractant for osteoclast progenitor cells. Yet, carboxylated proteins are also thought to inhibit mineralization of matrix, especially in soft tissue. As such, decreases in carboxylated proteins have been linked to calcification of arterial walls and initiation of atherosclerosis plagues (Vermeer et al., 1995).

Although osteocalcin is a better marker of vitamin K status than is clotting time, detection of serum osteocalcin by immunoreactive assays may fail to distinguish vitamin K status. An assessment of the extent of carboxylation of circulating osteocalcin determined by its binding affinity for hydroxyapatite may provide a better indication of function. Binding affinity of osteocalcin has proved to be a strong predictor of subsequent hip fracture (Vermeer et al., 1995).

1. Requirements

When 1- and 2-day-old pigs were fed a purified, liquid diet containing sulfathiazole and oxytetracycline to limit intestinal microbial synthesis of vitamin K, dietary additions of 5 µg of menadione sodium phosphate/kg of body weight was sufficient to restore prothrombin clotting times to that of positive control pigs (Schendel and Johnson, 1962). Coprophagy was minimized by use of wire-bottomed cages and careful cleaning. Seerley et al. (1976) found that 1.1 mg of menadione pyrimidinol bisulfite/kg of diet prevented the hemorrhage induced in weanling pigs by the anticoagulant pivalyl. Based on prothrombin clotting time, Hall et al. (1986) concluded that 2 mg of menadione as menadione pyrimidinol bisulfite/kg of diet was needed to prevent the effects of pivalyl in growing (72-kg) pigs.

Dietary vitamin K supplements of 4 mg/kg diet improved gains in 4-kg weaned pigs compared with control pigs fed a basal diet (Neufville et al., 1973). The same level fed to sows for 3 days before farrowing and during 2 weeks of lactation resulted in no advantage in the number of pigs weaned, weight at weaning, or percent survival (Wallace et al., 1974).

Under field conditions, diets supplemented with 2 mg menadione/kg of diet prevented hemorrhage observed in pigs fed mycotoxin-contaminated feed ingredients (Muhrer et al., 1970; Osweiler, 1970; Fritschen et al., 1971). Single intramuscular injections of 3 mg of vitamin K_1 or K_2/kg body weight produced equal therapeutic responses in correction of subcutaneous hemorrhage and excessive bleeding after castration (Sasaki et al., 1985).

Bacterial synthesis of vitamin K and subsequent absorption, directly or by coprophagy, reduces or eliminates the need for supplemental vitamin K (NRC, 1998). High levels of antibiotics may decrease synthesis of vitamin K by intestinal microflora. Conclusive studies have not been conducted to determine whether supplemental vitamin K is needed for the breeding herd.

Although the reason is not understood, excessive Ca may also increase vitamin K requirements (Hall et al., 1991). Unlike other fat-soluble vitamins, liver stores of vitamin K are rapidly depleted during periods of feeding vitamin K-deficient diets (Kindberg and Suttie, 1989).

D. DEFICIENCY

Classical approaches used to assess vitamin K status have involved measurement of blood-clotting time. Blood in urine, subcutaneous hemorrhage, prolonged bleeding from the umbilicus or as a consequence of a mild trauma, and extended blood clotting time have been observed in swine (Schendel and Johnson, 1962; Fritschen et al., 1971; Brooks et al., 1973; Seerley et al., 1976; Sasaki et al., 1982).

Vitamin K antagonists, such as warfarin or dicumarol, inhibit activity of the reductase enzyme involved in the regeneration of vitamin K epoxides to the active form, hydroquinone (see Figure 10.9). Dicumarol was first discovered in investigations to identify the compound responsible for causing a hemorrhagic disease in cattle fed spoiled sweet clover hay. Several substituted hydroxycoumarins have subsequently been identified to have anticoagulant activity, as do certain substituted indandiones, alkylated naphthoquinones, pyridinols, and pryimidines (Suttie, 1984). Reports of a hemorrhagic syndrome in swine, in which blood-clotting Factors VII and X were deficient, suggested the presence of a vitamin K antagonist in moldy corn (Osweiler, 1970). The mold *Fusarium tricinctum* produces a toxin, diacetoxyscirpenol, that causes hemorrhage in rats (Gilgan et al., 1966; Bamburg et al., 1968) and swine (Clardy, 1970, as cited by Ullrey, 1991) that can be corrected by vitamin K supplementation. The vitamin K antagonists were initially used as active ingredients in rodent baits, but have found additional uses in human medicine as a therapy for coronary heart disease.

E. TOXICITY

Large excesses of vitamin K compounds are well tolerated by swine. Seerley et al. (1976) reported no signs of toxicity when 110 mg of menadione pyrimidinol bisulfite per kilogram of diet were fed for 16 weeks to weanling pigs. The toxic level of menadione seems to be at least 1000 times the dietary requirement (NRC, 1998). Some water-soluble menadiol sodium diphosphate and water-miscible formulations of phylloquinone may react with free tissue sulfhydryl groups when administered intramuscularly to neonates (Ullery, 1991). Symptoms include hemolytic anemia, hyperbilirubinemia, kernicterus, and brain damage.

REFERENCES

Anonymous, 1991. Vitamin Nutrition for Swine, Technical Publication SNW-30–91. Animal Nutrition, Hoffmann-La Roche, Nutley, NJ, p. 33.

Bamburg, J. R., N. V. Riggs, and F. M. Strong. 1968. The structures of toxins from two strains of *Fusarium tricinctum*, *Tetrahedron*, 24:3329.

Baron, R. 1999. Anatomy and ultrastructure of bone. In *Primer on the Metabolic Bone Diseases and Disorders of Mineral Metabolism*, 4th ed., Favus, M. J., Ed., Lippincott Williams & Williams, Philadelphia, PA, chap. 1.

Besancon, P., and L. Gueguen. 1969. Les principales vois metabolisme calcique chez le porc en croissance, *Ann. Biol. Anim. Biochem. Biophys.*, 9:537.

Binkley, N. C., and J. W. Suttie. 1995. Vitamin K nutrition and osteoporosis, *J. Nutr.*, 125:1812.

Breves, G., and B. Schroder. 1991. Comparative aspects of gastrointestinal phosphorus metabolism, *Nutr. Res. Rev.*, 4:125.

Broadus, A. E. 1999. Mineral balance and homeostasis. In *Primer on the Metabolic Bone Diseases and Disorders of Mineral Metabolism*, 4th ed., Favus, M. J., Ed., Lippincott Williams & Williams, Philadelphia, PA, chap. 12.

Bronner, F. 1995. Function of calcium in the mammalian organism. In *Handbook of Metal–Ligand Interactions in Biological Fluids. Bioinorganic Medicine*, Vol. 1, Berthon, G., Ed., Marcel Dekker, New York, 161.

Bronner, F. 1998. Calcium absorption — a paradigm for mineral absorption, *J. Nutr.*, 128:917.

Bronner, F., and W. D. Stein. 1995. Calcium homeostasis — an old problem revisited, *J. Nutr.*, 125:1987S.

Brooks, C. C., R. M. Nakamura, and A. Y. Miyahara. 1973. Effect of menadione and other factors on sugar-induced heart lesions and hemorrhagic syndrome in the pig, *J. Anim. Sci.*, 37:1344.

Carter, S. D., G. L. Cromwell, T. R. Combs, G. Colombo, and P. Fanti. 1996. The determination of serum osteocalcin in growing pigs and its relationship to end-measures of bone mineralization, *J. Anim. Sci.*, 74:2719.

Chineme, C. N., L. Krook, and W. G. Pond. 1976. Bone pathology in hypervitaminosis D an experimental study in young pigs, *Cornell Vet.*, 66:387.

Combs, N. R., E. T. Kornegay, M. D. Lindemann, D. R. Notter, J. W. Wilson, and J. P. Mason. 1991. Calcium and phosphorus requirement of swine from weaning to market: II. Development of response curves for bone criteria and comparison of bending and shear bone testing, *J. Anim. Sci.*, 69:682.

Crenshaw, T. D. 1986. Reliability of dietary Ca and P levels and bone mineral content as predictors of bone mechanical properties at various time periods in growing swine, *J. Nutr.*, 116:2155.

Crenshaw, T. D. 1991. Sodium, potassium, magnesium and chloride in swine nutrition. In *Swine Nutrition*, Miller E. R., D. E. Ullrey, and A. J. Lewis, Eds., Butterworth-Heinemann, Stoneham, MA, chap 11.

Crenshaw, T. D., and J. C. Johanson. 1995. Nutritional strategies for waste reduction management: minerals. In *New Horizons in Animal Nutrition and Health*, Longenecker, J. B., and J. W. Spears, Eds., Institute of Nutrition, University of North Carolina, Chapel Hill, 69.

Crenshaw, T. D., E. R. Peo, Jr., A. J. Lewis, and B. D. Moser. 1981. Bone strength as a parameter for assessing mineralization in swine: a critical review of techniques involved, *J. Anim. Sci.*, 53:827.

Econs, M. J. 1999. New insights into the pathogenesis of inherited phosphate wasting disorders, *Bone*, 25:131.

Engstrom, G. W., R. L. Horst, T. A. Reinhardt, and E. T. Littledike. 1985. Effect of dietary phosphorus levels on porcine renal 25-hydroxyvitamin D-1α - and 24R-hydroxylase activities and plasma 1,25-dihydroxyvitamin D_3 concentration, *J. Anim. Sci.*, 60:1005.

Fritschen, R. D., O. D. Grace, and E. R. Peo, Jr. 1971. Bleeding Pig Disease, Nebraska Swine Report EC71. 219:22.

Gilgan, M. W., E. B. Smalley, and F. M. Strong. 1966. Isolation and partial characterization of a toxin from *Fusarium tricinctum* on moldy corn, *Arch. Biochem. Biophys.*, 114:1.

Green, J., and C. R. Kleeman. 1991. Role of bone in regulation of systemic acid-base balance, *Kidney Int.*, 39:9.

Hall, D. D., G. L. Cromwell, and T. S. Stahly. 1986. The vitamin K requirement of the growing pig, *J. Anim. Sci.*, 63(Suppl. 1):268(Abstr.).

Hall, D. D., G. L. Cromwell, and T. S. Stahly. 1991. Effects of dietary calcium, phosphorus, calcium:phosphorus ratio and vitamin K on performance, bone strength and blood clotting status of pigs, *J. Anim. Sci.*, 69:646.

Hancock, J. D., E. R. Peo, Jr., A. J. Lewis, J. D. Crenshaw, and B. D. Moser. 1986. Vitamin D toxicity in young pigs, *J. Anim. Sci.*, 63 (Suppl. 1):268 (Abstr.).

Hauschka, P. V., J. B. Lian, and P. M. Gallop. 1975. Direct identification of the calcium-binding amino acid, γ-carboxyglutamate, in mineralized tissue, *Proc. Natl. Acad. Sci. U.S.A.*, 72:3925.

Hayes, V. W. 1976. *NFIA Literature Review on Phosphorus in Swine Nutrition*, National Feed Ingredients Association, West Des Moines, IA.

Heeley, J. D., and J. T. Irving. 1973. A comparison of histological methods for demonstrating calcification, *Calcif. Tis. Res.*, 12:169.

Hendriks, W. H., and P. J. Moughan. 1993. Whole-body mineral composition of entire male and female pigs depositing protein at maximal rates, *Livest. Prod. Sci.*, 33:161.

Holden, J. L., J. G. Clement, and P. P. Phakey. 1995. Age and temperature related changes to the ultrastructure and composition of human bone mineral, *J. Bone Miner. Res.*, 10:1400.

Holick, M. F. 1999. Vitamin D: photobiology, metabolism, mechanism of action, and clinical applications. In *Primer on the Metabolic Bone Diseases and Disorders of Mineral Metabolism*, 4th ed., Favus, M. J., Ed., Lippincott Williams & Wilkins, Philadelphia, PA.

Hollander, D. 1973. Vitamin K_1 absorption by everted intestinal sacs of the rat, *Am. J. Physiol.*, 225:360.

Hollander, D., K. S. Muralidhara, and E. Rim. 1976. Colonic absorption of bacterially synthesized vitamin K_2 in the rat, *Am. J. Physiol.*, 230:251.

Horst, R. L., J. L. Napoli, and E. T. Littledike. 1982. Discrimination in the metabolism of orally dosed ergocalciferol and cholecalciferol by the pig, rat and chick, *Biochem. J.*, 204:185.

Itoh, H., S. L. Hansard, J. C. Glenn, F. H. Hoskins, and D. M. Thrasher. 1967. Placental transfer of calcium in pregnant sows on normal and limited-calcium rations, *J. Anim. Sci.*, 26:335.

Johanson, J. C., T. D. Crenshaw, F. R. Greer, and N. J. Benevenga. 1995. Development of a neonatal pig model for assessment of calcium availability in infant formulas, *FASEB J.*, 9:A160.

Jones, G., S. A. Strugnell, and H. F. Deluca. 1998. Current understanding of the molecular actions of vitamin D, *Physiol. Rev.*, 78:1193.

Jongbloed, A. W. 1987. *Phosphorus in the Feeding of Pigs: Effect of Diet on the Absorption and Retention of Phosphorus by Growing Pigs*, Instituut voor Veevoedingsonderzoek, Lelystad, chap. 1.

Kato, A., E. G. Seo, T. A. Einhorn, J. E. Bishop, and A. W. Norman. 1998. Studies on 24R,25-dihydroxyvitamin D_3: evidence for a nonnuclear membrane receptor in chick tibial fracture-healing callus, *Bone*, 23:141.

Khosla, S., and M. Kleerekoper. 1999. Biochemical markers of bone turnover. In *Primer on the Metabolic Bone Diseases and Disorders of Mineral Metabolism*, 4th ed., Favus, M. J., Ed., Lippincott Williams & Wilkins, Philadelphia, PA.

Kindberg, C. G., and J. W. Suttie. 1989. Effect of various intakes of phylloquinone on signs of vitamin K deficiency and serum and liver phylloquinone concentrations in the rat, *J. Nutr.*, 119:175.

Kornegay, E. T. 1985. *Calcium and Phosphorus in Animal Nutrition*, National Feed Ingredients Association, West Des Moines, IA.

Kragstrup, J., A. Richards, and O. Fejerskov. 1989. Effects of fluoride on cortical bone remodeling in the growing domestic pig, *Bone*, 10:421.

Lenis, N. P., and A. W. Jongbloed. 1999. New technologies in low pollution swine diets: Diet manipulation and use of synthetic amino acids, phytase and phase feeding for reduction of nitrogen and phosphorus excretion and ammonia emission — review, *Asian-Aus. J. Anim. Sci.*, 12:305.

Lian, J. B., G. S. Stein, E. Canalis, P. G. Robey, and A. L. Boskey. 1999. Bone formation: osteoblast lineage cells, growth factors, matrix proteins, and the mineralization process. In *Primer on the Metabolic Bone Diseases and Disorders of Mineral Metabolism*, 4th ed., Favus, M. J., Ed., Lippincott Williams & Wilkins, Philadelphia, PA, chap. 3.

Lipsky, J. J. 1994. Nutritional sources of vitamin K, *Mayo Clin. Proc.*, 69:462.

Long, G. G. 1984. Acute toxicosis in swine associated with excessive dietary intake of vitamin D, *J. Am. Vet. Med. Assoc.*, 184:164.

Mahan, D. C., and R. G. Shields, Jr. 1998. Macro- and micromineral composition of pigs from birth to 145 kilograms of body weight, *J. Anim. Sci.*, 76:506.

McDowell, L. R. 1992. *Minerals in Animal and Human Nutrition*, Academic Press, San Diego, CA, p. 3.

Mudd, A. J., W. C. Smith, and D. G. Armstrong. 1969. The retention of certain minerals in pigs from birth to 90 kg live weight, *J. Agric. Sci. Camb.*, 73:181.

Muhrer, M. E., R. G. Cooper, C. N. Cornell, and R. D. Thomas. 1970. Diet related hemorrhagic syndrome in swine, *J. Anim. Sci.*, 31:1025 (Abstr.).

Mundy, G. R. 1999. Bone remodeling In *Primer on the Metabolic Bone Diseases and Disorders of Mineral Metabolism*, 4th ed., Favus, M. J., Ed., Lippincott Williams & Williams. Philadelphia, PA, chap. 4.

Nelson, T. S. 1983. Fluorine and vanadium — toxicity. In *Nutrition Institute on Minerals*, National Feed Ingredients Association, West Des Moines, IA.

Neufville, M. H., H. D. Wallace, and G. E. Combs. 1973. Vitamin K supplementation of swine diets, *J. Anim. Sci.*, 37(Suppl. 1):288.

Nielsen, A. J. 1972. Deposition of calcium and phosphorus in growing pigs determined by balance experiments and slaughter investigations, *Acta Agric. Scand.*, 22:223.

Norman, A. W. 1996. Vitamin D. In *Present Knowledge in Nutrition*, 7th ed., Ziegler, E. E., and L. J. Filer, Jr., Eds., ILSI Press, Washington, D.C., chap. 12.

NRC. 1980. *Mineral Tolerance of Domestic Animals*, National Academy Press, Washington, D.C., p. 364.

NRC. 1998. *Nutrient Requirements of Swine*, 10th ed. National Academy Press, Washington, D.C.

Osweiler, G. D. 1970. Porcine hemorrhage disease. In Proceedings of Pork Producers Day. Report AS3531, Iowa State University, Ames, IA.

Parfitt, A. M. 1987. Bone and plasma calcium homeostasis, *Bone*, 8:(Suppl. 1):S1.

Partridge, I. G. 1978. Studies on digestion and absorption in the intestines of growing pigs. 3. Net movements of mineral nutrients in the digestive tract, *Br. J. Nutr.*, 39:527.

Peo, E. R., Jr. 1976. *NFIA Literature Review on Calcium in Swine Nutrition*, National Feed Ingredients Association, West Des Moines, IA.

Peo, E. R., Jr. 1991. Calcium, phosphorus, and vitamin D in swine nutrition. In *Swine Nutrition*, Miller, E. R., D. E. Ullrey, and A. J. Lewis, Eds., Butterworth-Heinemann, Stoneham, MA, chap. 10.

Pointillart, A., C. Colin, H. C. Lacroix, and L. Gueguen. 1995. Mineral bioavailability and bone mineral contents in pigs given calcium carbonate postprandially, *Bone*, 17:357.

Pond, W. G., J. T. Yen, W. E. Wheeler, and D. A. Hill. 1982. Calcium bioavailability from limestones of differing particle size and rate of reactivity for growing nonruminants, *Nutr. Rep. Int.*, 26:1027.

Quarterman, J., A. C. Dalgarno, A. Adams, B. F. Fell, and R. Boyne. 1964. The distribution of vitamin D between the blood and the liver in the pig, and observations on the pathology of vitamin D toxicity, *Br. J. Nutr.*, 18:65.

Ross, R. D., G. L. Cromwell, and T. S. Stahly. 1984. Effects of source and particle size on the biological availability of calcium in calcium supplements for growing pigs, *J. Anim. Sci.*, 59:125.

Russell, R. G. G., and M. J. Rogers. 1999. Bisphosphonates: from the laboratory to the clinic and back again, *Bone*, 25:97.

Rymarz, A., H. Fandrejewski, and J. Kielanowski. 1982. Content and retention of calcium, phosphorus, potassium and sodium in the bodies of growing gilts, *Livest. Prod. Sci.*, 9:399.

St-Arnaud, R. 1999. Targeted inactivation of vitamin D hydroxylases in mice, *Bone*, 25:127.

Sasaki, Y., H. Kitagawa, K. Ishihara, K. Mochizuki, and H. Sano. 1982. Hemorrhagic disease in pigs associated with vitamin K deficiency, *Jpn. J. Vet. Sci.*, 44:933.

Sasaki, Y., H. Kitagawa, K. Ishihara, H. Sano, T. Mizoguchi, and K. Kajio. 1985. Therapeutic effects of vitamin K for hemorrhagic disease in pigs, *Jpn. J. Vet. Sci.*, 47:435.

Schendel, H. E., and B. C. Johnson. 1962. Vitamin K deficiency in the baby pig, *J. Nutr.*, 76:124.

Schneider, D. K., D. N. Peetz, T. D. Crenshaw, N. J. Benevenga, F. R. Greer, and S. M. Kaup. 1997. Accuracy of dissected skeletal ash and dual energy x-ray absorptiometry (DEXA) methods in neonatal pigs, *FASEB J.*, 11:A409 (Abstr.).

Seerley, R. W., O. W. Charles, H. C. McCampbell, and S. P. Bertsch. 1976. Efficacy of menadione dimethylpyrimidinol bisulfite as a source of vitamin K in swine diets, *J. Anim. Sci.*, 42:599.

Suttie, J. W. 1984. Vitamin K. In *Handbook of Vitamins*, Machlin, L. J., Ed., Marcel Dekker, New York, p. 147.

Suttie, J. W. 1993. Synthesis of vitamin K-dependent proteins, *FASEB J.*, 7:445.

Talmage, R. V. 1996. Foreword. In *Calcium and Phosphorus in Health and Disease*, Anderson, J. J. B., and S. C. Garner, Eds., CRC Press, Boca Raton, FL.

Ullrey, D. E. 1991. Vitamins A and K in Swine Nutrition. In *Swine Nutrition*, Miller, E. R., D. E. Ullrey, and A. J. Lewis, Eds., Butterworth-Heinemann, Stoneham, MA, chap. 13.

Vermeer, C., K.-S. G. Jie, and M. H. J. Knapen. 1995. Role of vitamin K in bone metabolism, *Annu. Rev. Nutr.*, 15:1.

Vipperman, P. E., Jr., E. R. Peo, Jr., and P. J. Cunningham. 1974. Effect of dietary calcium and phosphorus level upon calcium, phosphorus and nitrogen balance in swine, *J. Anim. Sci.*, 38:758.

Wallace, H. D., D. D. Thieu, and G. E. Combs. 1974. Supplementary vitamin K for sows during farrowing and lactation, Florida Agric. Exp. Station, Dept. Anim. Sci. Res. Rep. AL-1974–9.

Weremko, D., H. Fandrejewski, T. Zebrowska, I. K. Han, J. H. Kim, and W. T. Cho. 1997. Bioavailability of phosphorus in feeds of plant origin for pigs, *Asian-Aus. J. Anim. Sci.*, 10:551.

Yasuda, H., N. Shima, N. Nakagawa, K. Yamaguchi, M. Kinosaki, M. Goto, S. I. Mochizuki, E. Tsuda, T. Morinaga, N. Udagawa, N. Takahashi, T. Suda, and K. Higashio. 1999. A novel molecular mechanism modulating osteoclast differentiation and function, *Bone*, 25:109.

11 Sodium, Potassium, Chloride, Magnesium, and Sulfur in Swine Nutrition

John F. Patience and Ruurd T. Zijlstra

CONTENTS

I. Introduction 214
    A. Mineral Chemistry 215
II. General Functions 215
    A. Water Homeostasis 215
    B. Acid–Base Homeostasis 216
    C. Nutrient Digestion, Absorption, and Transport 216
    D. Signal Transduction 217
    E. Mineral–Enzyme Relationships 217
III. Chlorine 217
    A. Metabolism 217
    B. Function 217
    C. Requirements 218
    D. Deficiency 218
    E. Toxicity 218
    F. Sources 218
    G. Assay 219
IV. Magnesium 219
    A. Metabolism 219
    B. Functions 219
    C. Requirement 220
    D. Deficiency 220
    E. Toxicity 220
    F. Sources 220
    G. Assay 220
V. Potassium 220
    A. Metabolism 221
    B. Function 221
    C. Requirements 221
    D. Deficiency 221
    E. Toxicity 221
    F. Sources 221
    G. Assay 222

VI. Sodium 222
    A. Metabolism..222
    B. Function...222
    C. Requirements..223
    D. Deficiency..223
    E. Toxicity...223
    F. Sources..224
    G. Assay..224
VII. Sulfur..224
    A. Metabolism..224
    B. Function...224
    C. Requirement 225
    D. Deficiency..225
    E. Toxicity...225
    F. Sources 225
    G. Assay..225
References..225

I. INTRODUCTION

Table 11.1 illustrates the typical elemental composition of the adult mammalian body. The macrominerals, which are generally defined as those inorganic elements required in the diet of the pig in quantities greater than 100 mg/kg, follow the more abundant elements oxygen, carbon, nitrogen, and oxygen. This chapter deals with four of the six main macrominerals, the exceptions being calcium and phosphorus, which are addressed in a separate chapter.

Sulfur is included, although it clearly is unique, as compared with Na, K, Cl, and Mg. Unlike other macrominerals, S functions metabolically only as a constituent of a larger molecule, either organic compounds such as the S amino acids or chondroitin sulfate or as the sulfate or sulfite ions. All of the other minerals discussed in this chapter function at least in part in elemental form. The reactivity of S has made it a particularly difficult element to study, especially in the variable redox conditions that exist in the gastrointestinal tract.

TABLE 11.1
Typical Elemental Composition of the Adult Mammalian Body

Element	Total Body (%)
Oxygen	65.7
Carbon	17.1
Hydrogen	11.4
Nitrogen	2.9
Calcium	1.3
Phosphorus	0.7
Potassium	0.3
Sulfur	0.3
Sodium	0.1
Chlorine	0.1
Magnesium	0.05

Source: Adapted from Currie, 1988.

A. Mineral Chemistry

Table 11.2 lists the properties of the macrominerals discussed in this chapter. Sodium and K each have a valance of +1. They are alkali elements, and as such are solids at room temperature, are very reactive chemically and act as reducing agents. They also possess many of the characteristics of metals, such as electrical conductivity, reflectivity, and heat conduction. These properties take on particular importance when one considers some of the biochemical roles of these two elements.

TABLE 11.2
Properties of the Macrominerals (Excluding Calcium and Phosphorus)

Element	Atomic Number	Valence[a]	Atomic Weight (amu)	Melting Point (°C)	Boiling Point (°C)
Chlorine	17	−1	35.453	−103	−34.6
Magnesium	12	+2	24.305	650	1100
Potassium	19	+1	39.098	62.3	760
Sodium	11	+1	22.990	97.5	880
Sulfur	16	−2	32.06	119	445

[a] At physiological pH.

Magnesium has a valence of +2 and, as an alkaline earth metal, is also a good conductor of heat and electricity. It is found in free ionic form in nature only in the oceans; otherwise, it exists as such compounds as magnesite ($MgCO_3$), dolomite ($MgCO_3 \cdot CaCO_3$), magnesia (MgO), epsomite ($MgO_4S \cdot 5H_2O$), and kiersite ($MgO_4S \cdot H_2O$).

Chlorine is a halogen and easily forms a salt, such as with Na or K. As an element, it is a gas under normal conditions, but because it is a very good oxidizing agent, Cl most commonly exists in nature as the negatively charged ion, Cl^-. Sulfur is a member of group VI of the periodic table. It exists in nature in a variety of sulfide and sulfate forms.

II. GENERAL FUNCTIONS

A. Water Homeostasis

The need to maintain water homeostasis is essential to all life, since failure to maintain a constant balance of water across cell membranes disturbs many metabolic and physiological functions and ultimately leads to death. The evolution of terrestial species 400 million years ago may have placed the greatest pressure on water balance, but all aquatic species face a similar challenge.

Water fulfills an amazingly diverse array of roles in the body, including intra- and intercellular transport, thermal homeostasis, acid–base homeostasis, lubrication, and actions as a constituent of many chemical reactions. It is difficult to think of a single body function that does not involve water directly or indirectly (Patience, 1989). It is not surprising, then, that disturbance to water homeostasis can have fatal consequences.

Electrolyte balance is closely associated with water balance, so the two are often discussed together. Water typically follows electrolytes across cell membranes, so that water balance is maintained by electrolyte balance. Electrolytes, along with semipermeable cell membranes, prevent the free flow of water into and out of cells; in their absence, cellular chaos would result. By maintaining intracellular and extracellular concentrations of osmotically active compounds, such as mineral elements, water homeostasis is achieved. A typical balance of intracellular and extracellular electrolytes appears in Table 11.3. Large deviations are rare, as they are associated with pathologies that are often fatal if not corrected immediately.

TABLE 11.3
Typical Intracellular and Extracellular Electrolyte Concentrations

Electrolyte	Intracellular (mEq/l)	Extracellular (mEq/l)
Sodium	12	145
Potassium	150	5
Chloride	4	125
Bicarbonate	8	28
Protein	150	0.5

B. Acid–Base Homeostasis

Dietary undetermined anion (dUA), calculated as $[(Na + K + Ca + Mg) - (Cl + P + S_{inorganic})]$ or the simpler expression, dietary electrolyte balance (dEB), calculated as $[Na + K - Cl]$ represent in part the net acid or alkaline load contributed by the diet (Patience, 1989). The other major contributor to the acid load, under most circumstances, is likely to be oxidation of excess S amino acids (Austic and Patience, 1988). Because dUA and dEB are expressed in mEq/kg, the individual electrolytes represent only a source of electrical charges; consequently, dUA by definition is independent of the specific physiological roles of the constituent mineral elements.

By considering only the electrical charges, dUA and dEB define the net balance of fixed cations and anions present in the diet and, by extension, the presence of counterbalancing metabolizable ions responsible for maintaining electroneutrality (Brosnan and Brosnan, 1982). Dietary undetermined anion has the advantage over dEB of considering all of the fixed cations and anions that are present at levels sufficient to impact on acid–base balance. However, because the absorption of these ions varies, the true impact of dUA in a given diet is difficult to quantify precisely. Dietary electrolyte balance considers only the monovalent fixed cations and anions. Although this clearly limits its usefulness, Na, K, and Cl are the ions with the highest degree of absorption from the diet, and thus are likely to have the greatest impact on dietary acid–base homeostasis. In addition, dEB is simpler to employ commercially.

It is important to emphasize that dUA and dEB are independent of specific ion effects (Patience and Wolynetz, 1990). Although it is clearly understood that each mineral does have unique metabolic roles, many of which are discussed later in this chapter, from a nutritional perspective, this is a separate subject.

Certainly, changes in dUA or dEB affect pig performance (Patience et al., 1987a; Haydon et al., 1990; Patience and Wolynetz, 1990), nutrient metabolism (Haydon and West, 1990; Patience and Chaplin, 1997), and even excreta composition (Mroz et al., 1996).

Insufficient research has been completed to define adequately the dUA or dEB at which pig performance is maximized. While dEB above 0 mEq/kg supports maximal growth, achieving levels above 100 mEq/kg may be preferable (Patience et al., 1987a). Certainly, additional research is required on this topic.

C. Nutrient Digestion, Absorption, and Transport

While proteins are the primary mediators of nutrient absorption and transport, minerals play a varied and essential role as well. From the secretion of bicarbonate in the saliva and pancreas and hydrochloric acid in the stomach through to ion-mediated transport systems in epithelial cells lining the intestinal tract, it is clear that minerals are central to the digestion and absorption of nutrients.

The transport of nutrients across cell membranes occurs by a variety of active and passive systems. Mineral elements play a number of roles. For example, ubiquitous Na^+,K^+-ATPase not only creates a transmembrane concentration gradient, it generates an electrical gradient as well (Munck and Munck, 1994; Hediger and Rhoads, 1994). The importance of Na^+,K^+-ATPase is exemplifed by the fact that it is responsible for about one third of normal basal metabolism. There are other ATPases as well; H^+K^+-ATPase is present in acid-secreting cells and is essential to gastric acid secretion.

Once the transmembrane ion gradient has been formed, it can then be used to provide the driving force behind the movement across cell membranes of other nutrients, such as a sugar, amino acids, or another ion. The importance of the electrochemical gradient is exploited in medicine through the use of ionophores, compounds that shuttle ions across membranes and thus diminish the ionic gradient. Such compounds are routinely used as antibiotics.

D. Signal Transduction

Ion channels are present in the membrane of neurons, muscle cells, and other cells. Various stimuli cause these ion channels to open and close, resulting in a change in the transmembrane electrochemical gradient. One example is the acetylcholine receptor in neural cells. Acetylcholine is released by one neuron in response to an electrical signal, binds to the receptor on an adjacent neuron, and increases the permeability of the neural membrane to Na and K. This results in the movement of these two cations down their electrochemical gradient and depolarizes the cell membrane. Thus, the nerve impulse has been transmitted from one cell to an adjacent cell.

In addition to neural transmission, minerals play a role in endrocrine receptor binding as well. For example, S included in disulfide bonds between cysteine residues in proteins stabilizes the tertiary structure of regions of proteins involved in signal transmission. Specific examples include hormones, such as insulin and insulin-like growth factor (IGF)-I, and their receptors on cell membranes.

E. Mineral–Enzyme Relationships

Microminerals tend to play a more significant role in enzyme function than the macrominerals. Examples include Cu^{2+} in cytochrome oxidase and Zn^{2+} in carbonic anhydrase and alcohol dehydrogenase. The main exception is Mg, which is a cofactor in hexokinase, glucose-6-phosphatase, and pyruvate kinase. Potassium is a cofactor in pyruvate kinase.

III. CHLORINE

A. Metabolism

There is often confusion in using the terms *chlorine* and *chloride*. Chlorine is defined as the element, and chloride as the ion. Chlorine metabolism is closely associated with Na metabolism. During absorption in the intestine, directional fluxes of Cl follow the movement of Na across membranes under normal physiological conditions. Control of intestinal absorption of electrolytes is complex. The exact mechanism of the coupling of ions during electrogenic transport, i.e., the co-ion movement of Cl during normal Na absorption is not understood completely (Hansen and Skadhauge, 1995), although a double exchange mechanism of Cl/bicarbonate and Na/hydrogen has been proposed (Powell, 1987). Cl also seems to be transported passively down the electrical gradient through the paracellular shunt pathway (Donowitz and Welsh, 1987).

The kidneys function to maintain Cl homeostasis. Excretion of Cl is related, in part, to Na excretion. However, bicarbonate is most likely the required anion to balance excreted cation in urine (Patience et al., 1986).

B. Function

As a major anion in the body, Cl represents approximately 65% of the total anions in extracellular fluids. Together with Na and other electrolytes, Cl functions to maintain whole-body homeostasis of water and electrolytes, and acid–base balance.

Chlorine participates in many critical metabolic functions. It is the chief anion in gastric juice, causing the extreme acidity needed to cleave pepsinogen to activate pepsin and thus initiate protein digestion. In blood, erythrocytes contain an anion channel that mediates the exchange of bicarbonate for Cl, which is essential for the transport of carbon dioxide from respiring tissues to the lung. Chlorine channels are further involved in alterations of membrane potential in the central nervous system.

Control of intestinal absorption and secretion of electrolytes is complex. A specific function of Cl in the intestine is the role played in secretory diarrhea. Secretion of Cl into the intestinal lumen can be caused by activation of the immune system following the introduction of intestinal pathogens (Argenzio, 1996). In this way, the pathogens will be flushed out of the small intestine.

C. Requirements

Few experiments have been designed to determine Cl requirements specifically. The dietary Cl requirement is thus poorly defined, but is probably 0.08% maximally for the growing pig (Honeyfield and Froseth, 1985; Honeyfield et al., 1985; NRC, 1998). Similar to Na, the dietary Cl requirement for young pigs was adjusted upward to 0.25% for 3- to 5-kg pigs, to 0.20% for 5- to 10-kg pigs, and to 0.15% for 10- to 20-kg pigs. The increase was based on results by Mahan et al. (1996), indicating that weanling pigs fed diets containing dried whey or dried plasma responded to added Cl. The supporting mechanism for the response is not well understood, but might be related to insufficient gastric secretion of hydrochloric acid in pigs immediately after weaning. In the young pig, Cl requirements are considered to be linked directly to Na requirements on a weight basis (NRC, 1998). Previously, Honeyfield et al. (1985) suggested that Na and Cl should be supplied to pigs at a 1:1 molar ratio in the diet. This relationship remains and is reflected in the 0.08% Cl requirements from 20 to 120 kg for growing pigs and the 0.12 and 0.16% Cl requirement for gestating and lactating sows, respectively (NRC, 1998). Finally, Honeyfield et al. (1985) suggested that Na and Cl should be considered separately in diet formulations. Increasing dietary Cl using neutral salts such as NaCl and KCl will have no impact on acid–base balance; however, the use of acid salts, such as $CaCl_2$ would (Patience and Wolynetz, 1990; Patience and Chaplin, 1997).

D. Deficiency

Conclusive remarks regarding Cl deficiency are lacking because definitive studies separating the effects of Na and Cl deficiency are lacking (McDowell, 1992). Chlorine deficiency is thus discussed under Na deficiency.

E. Toxicity

Similar to deficiency, conclusive remarks regarding Cl toxicity are lacking because definitive studies separating the effects of Na and Cl toxicity are lacking. Chlorine toxicity is thus discussed under Na deficiency. Swine can tolerate dietary levels of NaCl up to 8%, which is equivalent to 4.8% Cl (NRC, 1980), provided they have ample access to fresh drinking water.

F. Sources

Sodium chloride (NaCl, common salt) is the predominant source of Cl. Potassium chloride (KCl) is the other source with a high concentration of Cl (NRC, 1998). Chlorine concentrations in these sources range from 47 to 59%. Although hydrochloric acid has been used to supply Cl in some experiments (Mahan et al., 1996), it is not considered routinely for diet formulation for practical and economic reasons. Chlorine generally occurs in higher concentrations than Na in most feed ingredients (NRC, 1998). Grains and their by-products contain 0.02 to 0.25% Cl, whereas animal products contain 0.3 to 3.4% Cl (NRC, 1998).

G. Assay

Unlike most other mineral elements, Cl cannot be assayed by atomic absorption spectroscopy, so that other methods are required. One of the simplest and most rapid assays employs a specific ion electrode. Difficulties in achieving a linear response by direct measurement is overcome through the use of indirect titrimetry of the unknown solution with silver nitrate. Comparison of the results against a standard curve yields excellent, repeatable results (LaCroix et al., 1970).

Chlorine may also be determined by a gravimetric method, wherein the Cl is precipitated using silver nitrate to form silver Cl (AOAC, 1984). A volumetric method is also available. Silver nitrate is added in slight excess to an aqueous solution and the excess silver is titrated with standard thiocynanate solution using alum as the indicator (Watson, 1994).

If the parent material requires ashing, great care is required as Cl is easily volatilized. To avoid such losses, the sample should be dry-ashed in the presence of calcium oxide or Na carbonate to a maximum temperature of 500°C. Retention should be verified using known standards.

IV. MAGNESIUM

Magnesium does not receive a great deal of attention in swine nutrition. Although it plays a central role in many biochemical and physiological processes, Mg deficiency rarely occurs, due to its ubiquitous presence in most common feedstuffs. It attracts much more attention in ruminant species, in part due to the metabolic disorder grass tetany. About two thirds of total-body Mg exists within the skeleton, with the remainder found in soft tissues and blood.

A. Metabolism

Magnesium appears to be absorbed from the small intestine, but not with a high degree of overall efficiency; for example, in pigs, apparent absorption in the range of 20 to 30% is typical (Patience et al., 1987b). Absorption appears to occur through two processes: a carrier-mediated system, which functions best at low concentrations, and simple diffusion. However, the degree of absorption appears to be influenced by a number of factors, including Mg status of the animal and the Mg content of the diet. Mg absorption is also impaired by calcium, phosphorus, phytate, and fatty acids.

The key site of Mg homeostasis appears to be the kidney, where tubular reabsorption conserves quantities required for skeletal growth or turnover replacement. Indeed, the kidney has the capacity to reabsorb Mg with great efficiency, so that losses under conditions of diet insufficiency are very low (Shils, 1988).

There appear to be three distinct Mg pools within the body. The extracellular pool appears to turn over most rapidly, while the intracellular pool is somewhat less dynamic. The third pool, existing within the skeleton, has a very slow turnover rate, which is not surprising.

B. Functions

After calcium and phosphorus, Mg is the most abundant mineral constituent of bone. As such, it contributes to bone strength and integrity. Magnesium is also important in nerve impulse transmission. It stabilizes the structure of ATP by acting as a ligand to the phosphate moieties. Magnesium plays a significant role in more than 300 different enzyme systems and thus participates in a huge array of reactions, including hydrolysis and transfer of phosphate groups by phosphokinases, initiation of β-oxidation of fatty acids, amino acid activation in protein synthesis, synthesis and degradation of DNA, contractility of both cardiac and smooth muscle, and in the formation of cAMP. Magnesium is known to be involved in many reactions where thiamine pyrophosphate is a cofactor.

C. Requirement

The requirement of the pig for Mg has not been well defined, in part because naturally occurring deficiency is so rare. Dietary concentrations in the range of 400 mg/kg appear adequate for the growing pig (ARC, 1981; NRC, 1998). Factorial estimates suggest that growing pigs over 50 kg require 200 mg Mg/kg or possibly less (ARC, 1981). Since most grains contain 1200 mg Mg/kg or more, and common vegetable protein sources contain double or more that of grain, a primary deficiency of Mg in the pig is unlikely. Insufficient data are available to define a requirement for the breeding herd.

D. Deficiency

Many symptoms of Mg deficiency are nonspecific, such as poor growth and anorexia. However, other signs of deficiency are more definitive and follow a particular order of appearance: hyperirratability, muscular twitching, reluctance to stand, weak pasterns, loss of equilibrium, tetany, and death (McDowell, 1992).

Serum concentration is a fair indicator of Mg status, but it only declines in severe deficiency. On the other hand, erythrocyte levels are more responsive and provide an earlier indication of marginal insufficiency. As with most minerals, urinary excretion is a more dynamic indicator of Mg status, *in situ*ations of both excessive and inadequate intake. However, this is not always easy to measure under clinical conditions.

E. Toxicity

Information on Mg toxicity in the pig is scarce. It is also difficult to study, in particular, when providing excess Mg as a sulfate begs the question whether the toxicity was from the cation or associated anion. Also, the levels of other nutrients, notably calcium and phosphorus, are also likely to affect toxic symptoms. It has been concluded that 0.3% Mg is safe for swine, although data are extremely limited (NRC, 1980).

F. Sources

Magnesium is the eighth most abundant element in the earth's crust and is rarely supplemented in commercial pig diets in North America. However, when required, common sources include Mg oxide, Mg sulfate heptahydrate (Epsom salts), and KMg sulfate. Epsom salts derive their name from Epsom, the famous English spa whose history dates back to the 17th century; Mg sulfate was the principal mineral component of the spa water.

G. Assay

Following either wet or dry ashing, Mg levels in feed are normally determined by atomic absorption spectrometry (AAS) at 285.2 nm using an air/acetylene flame (Watson, 1994). AAS is preferred over flame emission spectroscopy (FES) for Mg determinations. Gravimetric methods, using Na citrate and ammonium phosphate, are also available (AOAC, 1984). However, AAS is a much simpler technique.

V. POTASSIUM

Potassium, represented in the periodic tables by the symbol K after the Latin form *kalium*, is an important element in the nutrition of the pig. Fortunately, most practical diets exceed the K requirement of the pig, without supplementation, so deficiencies are rare. Potassium contributes to the electrolyte balance of the diet, and thus deserves additional consideration from the standpoint of acid–base homeostasis.

A. Metabolism

Potassium is readily absorbed, primarily by simple diffusion, from the upper portions of the small intestine. On the basis of slope-ratio assays, Combs and Miller (1985) reported that the K contained in both mineral supplements, such as K carbonate and K bicarbonate, and in common feedstuffs, such as corn and soybean meal, is 95% or more available.

Homeostatic mechanisms rest primarily in the kidney, which carefully controls K levels. Diarrhea impairs K absorption, resulting in the need for increased dietary intake under such conditions. Aldosterone stimulates K excretion by the renal tubules; consequently, hyperactivity of the adrenal cortex, such as that induced by stress, will lead to increased K excretion.

Avoiding K toxicity appears to be a higher priority of homeostatic mechanisms than avoiding deficiency. Since excessive extracellular K is lethal, this is not surprising.

B. Function

Potassium appears to fulfill most of the intracellular functions that Na handles in the extracellular spaces. These include osmotic regulation, water balance, and acid–base balance. While Na represents about 93% of the total extracellular cations, K represents about 75% of intracellular cations (Crenshaw, 1991). The K gradient across the plasma membrane is maintained the Na/K ATPase.

Potassium is involved in blood gas transport, and is directly responsible for about half of the carbon dioxide–carrying capacity of blood. It is involved in nerve impulse transduction and plays a critical role in cardiac function, especially in the regulation of the heart rate. In skeletal muscle, it assists in contractile processes, preventing tetany. Finally, K is a cofactor in numerous enzymes, including adenosine triphosphatase, hexokinase, pyruvate kinase, and carbonic anhydrase.

C. Requirements

Potassium is rarely supplemented in pig diets if vegetable proteins are used, as they are rich sources. NRC (1998) defines the K requirement as about 3 g/kg in the very young piglet to 1.7 g/kg in the finishing pig. ARC (1981) suggests the requirement is 2.8 g/kg, based on factorial estimates.

D. Deficiency

As stated above, K deficiency is extremely rare, and for the most part induced by feeding semi-synthetic diets. When it occurs, K deficiency is characterized by reduced appetite and poor growth rate. Because of the role of K in cardiac function, irregular electrocardiograms are observed in deficient animals (Cox et al., 1966).

E. Toxicity

Potassium toxicity is rarely reported and toxic levels are poorly defined (NRC, 1980). The toxic level for swine has been set at 3% of the diet, about ten times that required. Like Na, the likelihood of K toxicity is increased where water intake is restricted. Intravenous dosing of K as KCl results in abnormal electrocardiograms (Coulter and Swenson, 1970).

F. Sources

It is generally assumed that the K in most feedstuffs is well utilized by the pig. In addition, such supplements as KCl, K carbonate, and K bicarbonate have high biological availability (Miller, 1995). In practical diets employed in North America, K is rarely supplemented, since vegetable protein sources, such as soybean meal and canola meal, are rich in K.

G. Assay

Because K is an alkali metal, flame emission spectrometry (FES) is the method of choice. Samples may be wet or dry ashed and the absorbance is measured at 766.5 nm. Due to ionization, an ionization suppressant, such as cesium, should be used. To assay biological fluids, specific ion electrodes are often used in automated systems.

Inductively coupled argon plasma (ICP) emission spectroscopy is another alternative that is increasingly popular where economically viable. ICP has the advantage of facilitating the measurement of multiple elements in a single pass. However, AAS is favored over ICP for alkali metals.

VI. SODIUM

Although Na is easily supplemented at low cost in pig diets, the issue of Na supplementation levels remains uncertain. For example, commercially, "salt poisoning" is surprisingly common, more as a result of inadequate water than excessive salt in the diet. In addition, because most studies have employed NaCl supplementation, rather than a neutral salt, questions regarding the requirement for Na per se remain. Nonetheless, recently research has identified the need for higher levels of supplementation in the diet of the young, spurring interest in further studies on the subject.

A. Metabolism

The metabolism and directional fluxes of Na and water are strongly related. Sodium digestion has not been studied specifically in swine, probably because Na availability is high. Most Na salts are easily dissolved in water and Na ions are readily absorbed. The transport of Na across intestinal epithelium appears to be dependent upon a system of active pumps and passive leaks (Fregly, 1981). Under normal physiological conditions, Na absorption is facilitated by the energy-requiring Na/K ATPase located on the basolateral membrane of intestinal enterocytes; this pump ensures low intracellular Na concentrations and a negative transmembrane potential. These conditions allow Na to be transported across the apical membrane down its electrochemical gradient, which in turn is used to facilitate absorption of other electrolytes and nutrients with a number of cotransporters on the luminal membrane (Hansen and Skadhauge, 1995). Sodium is also simply diffused across the epithelium (Powell, 1987). Sodium absorption appears not be controlled to a specific maximum flux (Patience et al., 1987b). Thus, influx of Na can be controlled only by changes in appetite.

In contrast, the excretion of Na from the body is tightly controlled, because of the importance of water and therefore Na to the body. The kidneys function to regulate the extracellular concentration of Na by an elaborate mechanism that controls changes in glomerular filtration rate and fractional reabsorption. Sodium concentrations are monitored indirectly by a variety of systems, e.g., receptors in tissues that detect changes in fluid volume and blood pressure. Hormones, including the renin–angiotensin system, aldosterone, some prostaglandins, the kallikrein–kinin system, and natriuretic hormone work in concordance to control Na excretion to maintain Na homeostasis (Patience, 1993). Thus, Na is excreted primarily in the urine, with only small amounts lost in feces and perspiration.

B. Function

As discussed previously, Na functions to maintain whole-body homeostasis of water and electrolytes, and acid–base balance. Within the body, Na concentrations are particularly high in extracellular fluids to maintain cellular osmolarity and plasma volume. Similar to the intestine, Na is critical in cellular transport systems, due to the Na-K ATPase. The electrochemical gradient across cell membranes is controlled in part by this system and thus is critical for both active and passive transport functions and for the creation of the electrical potential required for nervous system activity and muscle contraction. Clearly, Na plays an important role throughout the body.

C. Requirements

The requirements for growing pigs less than 20 kg have been adjusted upward recently (NRC, 1998). Pigs require 0.25% Na in the diet from 3 to 5 kg, 0.20% from 5 to 10 kg, 0.15% from 10 to 20 kg, and 0.10% from 20 to 120 kg (NRC, 1998). Previously (NRC, 1988), the dietary Na requirement was assumed to be maximally 0.10% for growing-finishing pigs from birth through slaughter (Meyer et al., 1950; Alcantara et al., 1980; Honeyfield and Froseth, 1985; Honeyfield et al., 1985). The original requirement was supported further by Kornegay et al. (1991). The requirement for young pigs was adjusted upward based on results by Mahan et al. (1996), indicating that weanling pigs fed diets containing dried whey or dried plasma (both high in Na) responded to added Na. The supporting mechanism for the response is not well understood, but might be related to digestive imbalances.

The Na requirement for sows is not well defined. Cromwell et al. (1989) suggested that the existing dietary requirements (NRC, 1988) for gestating sows (0.15% Na) and lactating sows (0.20% Na) should not be lowered, which were therefore sustained (NRC, 1998). The dietary Na requirement should be higher during lactation than gestation because sow milk contains 0.3 to 0.4 g Na /kg (ARC, 1981) and considerable quantities of Na can be thus secreted with the milk.

D. Deficiency

Conclusive remarks regarding Na deficiency are lacking because definitive studies separating the effects of Na and Cl deficiency are lacking (McDowell, 1992). When a diet is deficient in NaCl, decreased performance is evident within a few days and can be observed as poor appetite, poor rate of growth, unthriftiness, and reduced feed efficiency (Cromwell et al., 1981; Cunha, 1987). Furthermore, salt-deficient pigs have been observed to keep licking their cages, presumably to satisfy a craving for salt (McDowell, 1992).

There has been considerable interest in the role of salt and, in particular, Na, as it relates to tail biting. Definitive studies of this vice are difficult, because of the infrequency and unpredictability of tail biting in a group of pigs. However, employing artificial "tails" constructed from rope, Fraser et al. (1987) reported that a primary deficiency of salt can induce tail biting. It is quite common to boost NaCl or other salt (KCl) in the face of a tail-biting outbreak. Although often effective in the short-term, failure to address the underlying cause of the tail-biting ultimately leads to its return a short time after the supplementary salt has been added to the feed.

E. Toxicity

Similar to deficiency, conclusive remarks regarding Na toxicity are lacking because definitive studies separating the effects of Na and Cl toxicity are lacking. Swine can tolerate dietary levels of NaCl up to 8%, which is equivalent to 3.2% Na (NRC, 1980), provided ample access to nonsaline drinking water. The previous dietary level to which the pig was adapted will influence the short-term response to excessive levels of Na. Signs of NaCl toxicity include increased water consumption, anorexia, weight loss, edema, nervousness, weakness, staggering, paralyses, and death (Bohstedt and Grummer, 1954; McDowell, 1992). Recent data indicate that feeding of NaCl above requirement but below toxic concentrations will increase osmolality of the diet, which might cause an increased flux of water from the intestinal mucosa into the lumen balance (Ehrlein et al., 1999). Feeding of NaCl above requirement might thus interfere with the intestinal water balance.

Salt toxicity is a misnomer resulting from the feeding of levels of salt that exceed the excretory ability of the pig due to inadequate water supply. Thus, failure of the water delivery system to deliver an adequate supply of water can cause "salt toxicity." The problem is particularly acute in weanling pigs where diets often contain high levels of whey powder and other products that may have a high salt level. Also, lethargy induced by other pathologies may reduce drinking behavior, resulting in inadequate water intake. Salt toxicity is best handled by ensuring an adequate supply of fresh water.

F. Sources

Sodium chloride (common salt) is the predominant source of Na. Other sources with high concentrations of Na include Na carbonate, Na bicarbonate, Na phosphate (mono- and dibasic), and Na sulfate (NRC, 1998). Sodium concentrations in these sources range from 13 to 43%. Most plants and plant products contain small amounts of Na in comparison with animal products (McDowell, 1992). Grains and their by-products contain 0.01 to 0.25% Na, whereas animal products contain 0.2 to 3.0% Na (NRC, 1998). Nutritionists largely ignore the contribution of Na by drinking water and major feed ingredients in diet formulation, a contribution that might be substantial (Kornegay et al., 1991). Sodium bioavailability in feed ingredients has been discussed recently (Henry, 1995). Dietary Na is assumed highly digestible and available (Peeler, 1972), in particular from the source NaCl. However, good evidence to support this assumption appears nonexistent. Apparent Na absorption ranged from 98% in a corn–soybean meal (control) diet to 94% in a corn–soybean meal diet with 0.24% supplemental NaCl (Alcantara et al., 1980).

G. Assay

Like K, another alkali metal, flame emission spectrometry (FES) is the method of choice for Na assay of feeds and ingredients. Samples may be wet or dry ashed and the absorbance is measured at 589 nm. Due to ionization, an ionization suppressant, such as K or cesium, should be used. Specific ion electrodes are often used to measure Na in automated systems applied to body fluids.

VII. SULFUR

Sulfur is rarely addressed in diet formulation the same way other nutrients are considered. Since the vast majority of S in the diet of the pig exists as methionine and cysteine, the focus of most nutritionists is on the S amino acids, rather than the element itself. Neither ARC (1981) nor AAC (1987) included it as a required nutrient. Nonetheless, S is a dietary essential and should not be overlooked, although primary S deficiency would be difficult to achieve.

A. Metabolism

Absorption of inorganic S occurs throughout the intestine, but primarily in the ileum (Dziewiatkowski, 1970), where both Na-dependent and Na-independent transporters exist (Maenz and Patience, 1997). Absorption is highly efficient in the brush border of both the intestinal tract and the kidney.

Methionine is 21.5% S and cysteine is 26.5% S. In addition to their being a constituent of proteins, these amino acids serve as precursors to other essential compounds, such as taurine and insulin.

Inorganic S has received limited attention in swine nutrition. It can be incorporated into taurine, but not into methionine or cysteine (Almquist, 1970; Henry and Ammerman, 1995).

B. Function

Unlike the other minerals included in this chapter, S does not function in elemental form; rather it is a critical component of the S amino acids (methionine, cysteine) and other important organic compounds. In proteins, the S moiety of the amino acids form disulfide linkages, which define the contour, and thus the function, of many proteins. Chondroitin is a mucoprotein and an important structural component of bone, cartilage, tendons, and walls of blood vessels. Taurine, an amino acid, is found throughout the body and is present in bile acid as the conjugate tauracholic acid. Heparin contains sulfuric acid ester groups and is responsible for blood anticoagulation.

Sulfur is included in the structure of both thiamin and biotin; however, exogenous S for *de novo* vitamin synthesis is required only for bacterial synthesis of vitamins in the lower gut. The

C. Requirement

There is no known S requirement per se for pigs. While S may be added to ruminant diets to act as a precursor to S amino acid synthesis, elemental S is of limited value in the diet of the pig. Thus, it is assumed that the excess S supplied by S amino acids is sufficient for the synthesis of S-containing compounds, such as taurine, glutathione, lapoic acid, and chondroitin sulfate (NRC, 1998). Consequently, no S requirement is defined for swine (ARC, 1981; AAC, 1985; NRC, 1998).

D. Deficiency

Little information on S deficiency can be found in the literature, primarily because so little is known about inorganic S requirements. Obviously, a deficiency in S amino acids leads to impaired performance, and the small quantity of S required for non-amino-acid nutriture is made up either by catabolized methionine and cysteine or by the small quantity of inorganic S present.

E. Toxicity

The toxicity of S depends very much on its form. Elemental S is considered one of the least toxic of elements, while hydrogen sulfide is extremely toxic. Sulfur toxicosis results in anorexia and weight loss. The toxicity of S appears to be related to the degree with which it is converted to the highly toxic hydrogen sulfide form, presumably by the intestinal microflora.

Sulfate in the drinking water acts as a highly effective laxative in swine, causing an osmotic diarrhea at high levels. However, levels of sulfate in the drinking water as high as 2650 mg sulfate/l caused no impairment in growth in newly weaned pigs, although diarrhea was reported (Fleck Veenhuizen et al., 1992; Maenz et al., 1994; Gomez et al., 1995).

F. Sources

Under typical commercial conditions, sulfate is provided in the diet by the S amino acids methionine and cysteine and other S compounds naturally present in feedstuffs. Many minerals, such as iron, copper, manganese, and zinc, may be provided in the diet as sulfates. Feedstuffs processed using sulfuric acid will contain significant quantities of S; examples include molasses and some solubles products. Sulfur is rarely supplemented in practical diets.

Limited data on the bioavailability of various sulfate sources is available in swine. Based on research with other species, it would appear that calcium sulfate, calcium sulfate dihydrate, Na sulfate, Na sulfate dihydrate, and Mg sulfate are all satisfactory sources of sulfate (Henry and Ammerman, 1995).

G. Assay

Sulfate is not an easy element to assay. Most methods are based on a gravimetric determination using barium Cl (Skoog and West, 1976).

REFERENCES

AAC. 1987. Feeding Standards for Australian Livestock: Pigs, Commonwealth Scientific and Industrial Research Organization, East Melbourne, 226 pp.

Alcantara, P. F., L. E. Hanson, and J. D. Smith. 1980. Na requirements, balance and tissue composition of growing pigs, *J. Anim. Sci.*, 50:1092.

Almquist, H. J. 1970. Sulfur nutrition of non-ruminant species. In *Sulfur in Nutrition*, Muth, O. H., and J. E. Oldfield, Eds., AVI Publishing, Westport, CT, 196.

AOAC. 1984. *Official Methods of Analysis*, Association of Official Analytical Chemists, Arlington, VA.

ARC. 1981. The Nutrient Requirements of Pigs, Commonwealth Agricultural Bureaux, Slough, U.K. 307 pp.

Argenzio, R. A. 1996. The pig as a model for studying the pathobiology of intestinal transport in infectious enteric disease. In *Advances in Swine in Biomedical Research*, Tumbleson, M. E., and L. B. Schook, Eds., Plenum Press, New York, 45.

Austic, R. E., and J. F. Patience. 1988. Undetermined anion in poultry diets: influence on acid-base balance, metabolism and physiological performance, *CRC Crit. Rev. Poultry Biol.*, 1:315.

Bohstedt, G., and R. H. Grummer. 1954. Salt poisoning of pigs, *J. Anim. Sci.*, 13:933.

Brosnan, J. T., and M. E. Brosnan. 1982. Dietary protein, metabolic acidosis and calcium balance. In *Advances in Nutritional Research*, Draper, H. H., Ed., Plenum Press, New York, 77.

Combs, N. R., and E. R. Miller. 1985. Determination of K availability in K_2CO_3, $KHCO_3$, corn and soybean meal for the young pig, *J. Anim. Sci.*, 60:715.

Coulter, D. B., and M. J. Swenson. 1970. Effects of K intoxication on porcine electrocardiograms, *Am. J. Vet. Res.*, 31:2001.

Cox, J. L., D. E. Becker, and A. H. Jensen. 1966. Electrocardiographic evaluation of K deficiency in young swine, *J. Anim. Sci.*, 25:203.

Crenshaw, T. D. 1991. Sodium, potassium, magnesium and chloride in swine nutrition. In *Swine Nutrition*, Miller, E. R., D. E. Ullrey, and A. J. Lewis, Eds., Butterworth-Heinemann, Boston, 183.

Cromwell, G. L., T. S. Stahly, and H. J. Monegue. 1981. Effects of sodium and chloride on performance of pigs, *J. Anim. Sci.*, 53(Suppl. 1):237(Abstr.).

Cromwell, G. L., D. D. Hall, G. E. Combs, O. M. Hale, D. L. Handlin, J. P. Hitchcock, D. A. Knabe, E. T. Kornegay, M. D. Lindemann, C. V. Maxwell, and T. J. Prince. 1989. Effects of dietary salt level during gestation and lactation on reproductive performance of sows: a cooperative study, *J. Anim. Sci.*, 67:374.

Cunha, T. J. 1987. *Salt and Trace Minerals*, Salt Institute, Alexandria, VA.

Currie, W. B. 1988. *Structure and Function of Domestic Animals*, Butterworths, Boston, 443 pp.

Donowitz, M., and M. J. Welsh. 1987. Regulation of mammalian small intestinal electrolyte secretion. In *Physiology of the Gastointestinal Tract*, Johnson, L. R., Ed., Raven Press, New York, 1351

Dziewiatkowski, D. D. 1970. Metabolism of sulfate esters. In *Sulfur in Nutrition*, Muth, O. H., and J. E. Oldfields, Eds., AVI Publishing, Westport, CT, 97.

Ehrlein, H., B. Haas-Deppe, and E. Weber. 1999. The sodium concentration of enteral diets does not influence absorption of nutrients but induces intestinal secretion of water in miniature pigs, *J. Nutr.*, 129:410.

Fleck Veenhuizen, M. F., G. C. Shurson, and E. M. Kohler. 1992. Effect of concentration and source of sulfate on nursery pig performance and health, *J. Am. Vet. Med. Assoc.*, 201:1203.

Fraser, D. 1987. Mineral deficient diets and the pig's attraction to blood: implications for tail-biting, *Can. J. Anim. Sci.*, 67:909.

Fregly, M. J. 1981. Sodium and potassium, *Annu. Rev. Nutr.*,1:69.

Gomez, G. G., R. S. Sandler, and E. Seal. 1995. High levels of inorganic sulfate cause diarrhea in neonatal piglets, *J. Nutr.*, 125:2325.

Hansen, M. B., and E. Skadhauge. 1995. New aspects of the pathophysiology and treatment of secretory diarrhoea, *Physiol. Res.*, 44:61.

Haydon, K. D., and J. W. West. 1990. Effect of dietary electrolyte balance on nutrient digestibility determined at the end of the small intestine and over the total digestive tract in growing pigs, *J. Anim. Sci.*, 68: 3687.

Haydon, K. D., J. W. West, and M. N. McCarter. 1990. Effect of dietary electrolyte balance on performance and blood parameters of growing-finishing swine fed in high ambient temperatures, *J. Anim. Sci.*, 68: 2400.

Hediger, M. A., and D. B. Rhoads. 1994. Molecular physiology of sodium-glucose transporters. *Physiol. Rev.*, 74:993.

Henry, P. R. 1995. Sodium and chlorine bioavailability. In *Bioavailability of Nutrients for Animals: Amino Acids, Minerals, and Vitamins*, Ammerman, C. B., D. H. Baker, and A. J. Lewis, Eds., Academic Press, San Diego, CA, 337.

Henry, P. R., and C. B. Ammerman. 1995. Sulfur bioavailability. In *Bioavailability of Nutrients for Animals*, Ammerman, C. B., D. H. Baker, and A. J. Lewis, Eds., Academic Press, San Diego, CA, 349.

Honeyfield, D. C., and J. A. Froseth. 1985. Effects of dietary sodium and chloride on growth, efficiency of feed utilization, plasma electrolytes and plasma basic amino acids in young pigs. *J. Nutr.*, 115:1366.

Honeyfield, D. C., J. A. Froseth, and R. J. Barke. 1985. Dietary sodium and chloride levels for growing-finishing pigs, *J. Anim. Sci.*, 60:691.

Kornegay, E. T., M. D. Lindemann, and H. S. Bartlett. 1991. The influence of sodium supplemenation of two phosphorus sources on performance and bone mineralization of growing-finishing swine evaluated at two geographical locations, *Can. J. Anim. Sci.*, 71:537.

LaCroix, R. L., D. R. Keeney, and L. M. Walsh. 1970. Potentiometric titration of chloride in plant tissue extracts using the chloride ion eletrode, *Commun. Soil Sci. Plant Anal.*, 1:1.

Maenz, D. D., and J. F. Patience. 1997. Presteady-state and steady-state function of the ileal brush border SO_4^{-2}-OH^- exchanger, *Biochem. Cell Biol.*, 75:229.

Maenz, D. D., J. F. Patience, and M. S. Wolynetz. 1994. The influence of the mineral level in drinking water and the thermal environment on the performance and intestinal fluid flux of newly-weaned pigs, *J. Anim. Sci.*, 72:300.

Mahan, D. C., E. A. Newton, and K. R. Cera. 1996. Effect of supplemental sodium chloride, sodium phosphate, or hydrochloric acid in starter pig diets containing dried whey, *J. Anim. Sci.*, 74:1217.

McDowell, L. R. 1992. *Minerals in Animal and Human Nutrition*, Academic Press, San Diego, CA, 524 pp.

Meyer, J. H., R. H. Grummer, R. H. Phillips, and G. Bohstedt. 1950. Sodium, chlorine, and potassium requirements of growing pigs, *J. Anim. Sci.*, 9:300.

Miller, E. R. 1995. Potassium bioavailability. In *Bioavailability of Nutrients for Animals: Amino Acids, Minerals, and Vitamins*, Ammerman, C. B., D. H. Baker, and A. J. Lewis, Eds., Academic Press, San Diego, CA, 295.

Mroz, Z., A. W. Jongbloed, K. Vreman, T. T. Cahn, J. Th. M. van Diepen, P. A. Kemme, J. Kogut, and A. J. A. Aarnink. 1996. The effect of different dietary cation-anion supplies on excreta composition and nutrient balance in growing pigs, Rep. 96-028. Institute for Animal Science and Health, Lelystad, The Netherlands, 58 pp.

Munck, L. K., and B. G. Munck. 1994. Amino acid transport in the small intestine, *Physiol. Res.*, 43:335.

NRC. 1980. *Mineral Tolerance of Domestic Animals*, National Academy Press, Washington, D.C., 577 pp.

NRC. 1988. *Nutrient Requirements of Swine*, 9th ed., National Academy Press, Washington, D.C., 93 pp.

NRC. 1998. *Nutrient Requirements of Swine*, 10th ed., National Academy Press, Washington, D.C., 189 pp.

Patience, J. F. 1989. The role of acid-base balance in amino acid metabolism, *J. Anim. Sci.*, 68:398.

Patience, J. F. 1993. The physiological basis of electrolytes in animal nutrition. In *Recent Developments in Pig Nutrition*, Cole, D. J. A., W. Haresign, and P. C. Garnsworthy, Eds., Nottingham University Press, Loughborough, England, 225.

Patience, J. F., and R. K. Chaplin. 1997. The relationship between dietary undetermined anion, acid-base balance and nutrient metabolism in swine, *J. Anim. Sci.*, 75:2445.

Patience, J. F., and M. S. Wolynetz. 1990. Influence of undetermined anion on acid-base status and performance in pigs, *J. Nutr.*, 120:579.

Patience, J. F., R. E. Austic, and R. D. Boyd. 1986. The effect of sodium bicarbonate or potassium bicarbonate on acid-base status and protein and energy digestibility in swine, *Nutr. Res.*, 6:263.

Patience, J. F., R. E. Austic, and R. D. Boyd. 1987a. Effect of dietary electrolyte balance on growth and acid-base status in swine, *J. Anim. Sci.*, 64:457.

Patience, J. F., R. E. Austic, and R. D. Boyd. 1987b. Effect of dietary supplements of sodium or potassium bicarbonate on short term macromineral balance in swine, *J. Anim. Sci.*, 64:1079.

Peeler, H. T. 1972. Biological availability of nutrients in feeds: availability of major mineral ions, *J. Anim. Sci.*, 35:695.

Powell, D. W. 1987. Intestinal water and electrolyte transport. In *Physiology of the Gastrointestinal Tract*, Johnson, L. R., Ed., Raven Press, New York, 1267.

Shils, M. E. 1988. Magnesium in health and disease, *Annu. Rev. Nutr.*, 8:429.

Skoog, D. A., and D. W. West. 1976. *Fundamentals of Analytical Chemistry*, 3rd ed., Holt, Reinhart & Winston, New York.

Watson, C. A. 1994. *Official and Standardized Methods of Analysis*, 3rd ed., Royal Society of Chemistry, Cambridge, U.K.

12 Trace and Ultratrace Elements in Swine Nutrition

Gretchen Myers Hill and Jerry W. Spears

CONTENTS

I. Introduction 230
    A. Essentiality and Toxicity 230
    B. Interactions 231
    C. Analysis 232
II. Chromium 233
    A. Metabolism 233
    B. Function 233
    C. Requirements 234
    D. Deficiency 234
    E. Toxicity 234
    F. Sources 234
III. Cobalt 234
IV. Copper 235
    A. Introduction 235
    B. Absorption 235
    C. Transport 235
    D. Functions 236
        1. Ceruloplasmin 236
        2. Amine and Diamine Oxidases 236
        3. Copper–Zinc Superoxide Dismutase 237
        4. Cytochrome c Oxidase 237
        5. Tyrosinase 238
        6. Immunity 238
        7. Growth Stimulant at Pharmacological Concentrations 238
    E. Deficiency 239
        1. Growth 239
        2. Blood 239
        3. Connective and Vascular Tissue Function 240
        4. Reproduction 240
    F. Toxicity 241
V. Iodine 241
    A. Metabolism and Function 241
    B. Requirements 241
    C. Deficiency 241
    D. Toxicity 242
    E. Sources 242

VI. Iron 242
    A. Introduction 242
    B. Absorption 242
    C. Interrelationships 243
    D. Transport 243
    E. Storage 244
    F. Requirements 244
    G. Functions 244
    H. Deficiency 245
    I. Toxicity 245
VII. Manganese 245
    A. Introduction 245
    B. Metabolism 246
    C. Function 246
    D. Requirements 246
    E. Deficiency 246
    F. Toxicity 246
    G. Sources 247
VIII. Zinc 247
    A. Introduction 247
    B. Absorption 247
    C. Transport 249
    D. Functions 250
        1. Enzymes 250
        2. Immunity 251
        3. Tissue Growth and Integrity 251
        4. Growth Stimulant at Pharmacological Concentrations 251
    E. Deficiency 251
        1. Growth and Appetite 251
        2. Reproduction 252
        3. Immunity 252
        4. Metallothionein 252
    F. Toxicity 253
IX. Other Trace Elements 253
References 254

I. INTRODUCTION

By definition, trace or microminerals are required by the body and occur in very low concentrations in the body. While iron (Fe) is considered a trace element, it is the mineral that divides macro- and microelements both by amount required and the amount stored for metabolic purposes. Interest and knowledge about the metabolism of trace and ultratrace elements and influences on their requirements have exploded in the last 25 years. The authors recognize that the function of these elements must be understood in tandem and not as individual entities.

A. ESSENTIALITY AND TOXICITY

Many elements are present in the body, but they may not meet the criterion of essentiality. To be a required nutrient, a deficiency of an element must result in a suboptimal metabolic function that affects a response variable that is prevented or reversed when adequate amounts of the element are

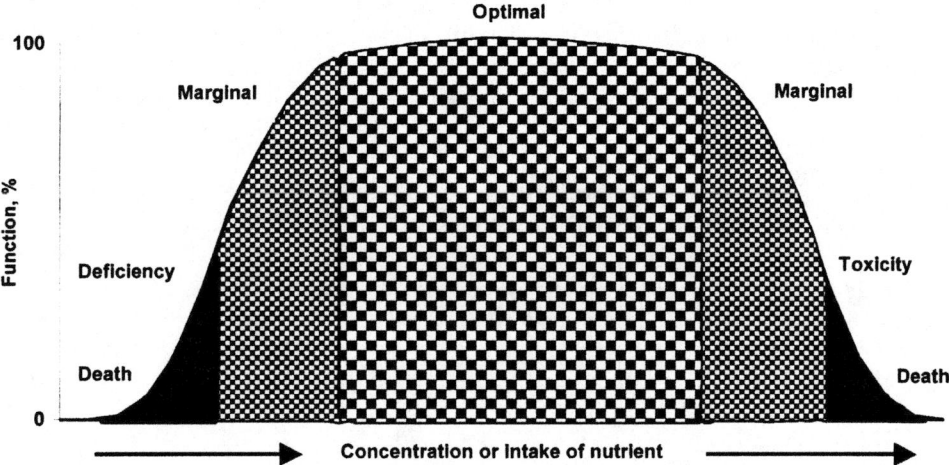

FIGURE 12.1 Dependence of biological function on tissue concentration or intake of a nutrient (From Mertz, W., The essential trace elements, *Science*, 213:1332, 1981. With permission.)

provided in the diet (Nielsen, 1984). The classic work of Underwood (1977) is a reminder that essential elements are always in all healthy tissues of living animals with concentrations being consistent between animals.

Conversely, excess of an essential or nonessential nutrient can result in toxicity and ultimately death if the body cannot prevent accumulation of the nutrient and/or its metabolic burden. These extremes are a reminder that it is balance of all nutrients that leads to normal growth, reproduction, and health and that pharmacological doses of nutrients are not within the realm of nutrient need. Mertz (1981) illustrated (Figure 12.1) that the intake of an essential nutrient was related to a metabolic function and that a deficiency or toxicity of a nutrient could result in death. It is now known that this curve is shifted when nutrient interactions occur and the distance from deficiency to toxicity is nutrient dependent.

B. INTERACTIONS

Clydesdale (1988) noted that the chemical and physical properties of minerals are a result of the configuration of their electrons, which defines the ionization potential or the energy required to remove electrons. Elements in the periodic table are arranged in order of increasing atomic number in horizontal rows. Therefore, elements with the same outermost electron configuration will be beneath one another. In the fourth period of the Periodic Table there are ten elements (scandium, titanium, vanadium, chromium, manganese, iron, cobalt, nickel, copper, and zinc) with ten electrons of the third sublevel that are filled by increasing electrons from left to right. These are the transition elements, which are known to form coordination compounds that affect bioavailability. They also have some of the biologically more important interactions.

The oxidation and reduction process where electrons are lost or gained is very important in the behavior and chemical reactions observed with trace elements. The oxidation number is increased when electrons, which are negatively charged, are lost, and the oxidation number decreases as electrons are gained. Thus, when an element donates an electron, it is a reducing agent and when it gains electrons, it is an oxidizing agent. The valence shifts that are seen as elements, especially copper (Cu) and Fe, receive or lose electrons in many enzymatic reactions are due to their ability to act as oxidizing or reducing agents.

There is a wide variation in the physical and chemical reactivity of mineral species. Hill and Matrone (1970) reported that the interaction of trace elements was due to their proximity within the periodic table and the similarities of valence electrons. They noted that when elements have similar physical and chemical characteristics, they are antagonistic in biological systems. Interactions also have been observed when elements are similar in size and number of charged electrons without identical electron configurations. Synergistic interactions of trace minerals, where elements work collaboratively toward a common goal, also have been observed, such as when nickel spares Fe. Most evidence suggests that mineral–mineral interactions are most likely to occur in the alimentary canal. Hence chemical form, valence, and concentration in the diet as well as other nutrient concentrations and dietary factors affect mineral interactions and bioavailability in the gastrointestinal tract. However, once inside the body, there are continuing opportunities for interactions to occur within tissues. The interaction of Cu and zinc (Zn) is of health as well as economic interest to the swine industry, and this interaction is discussed in the Zn section of this chapter.

C. Analysis

Since the era of minerals in the 1960s, there have been major technological advances that have enabled researchers to determine more accurately mineral concentrations and to determine more precisely biological functions, hence bioavailability. The determination of minerals is based on the destruction of organic matter in samples and the detection of often very small quantities of the element of interest.

It has been known for some time that volatilization of certain minerals occurs when the temperature exceeds 600°C; thus slow charring where the carbon is oxidized quietly and completely is essential if dry-ashing is used. If large amounts of halogens are present, losses of some metals are more likely to occur (Analytical Methods Committee, 1960).

The method of choice for organic destruction is wet-ashing, where nitric and perchloric acids of a high grade of purity are heated with the sample at increasing temperatures until the residual acid is driven off and only the ash remains. However, this is a very dangerous and expensive procedure, requiring a dedicated perchloric hood of stainless steel and a stack-to-hood washdown system. Perhaps equally dangerous are the many modifications of this method that utilize sulfuric acid, hydrogen peroxide, etc. in an attempt to destroy the organic matter, but often without the appropriate hoods or trapping systems. Documentation of these modifications to release minerals, especially from the lipid portion of the sample, has not been published. Sulfuric acid should never be used with any appreciable amounts of alkaline earth metals in the samples because insoluble sulfates absorb the trace elements and severely decrease the recovery of these elements for measurement (Analytical Methods Committee, 1960).

In recent years, utilization of microwave digestion units has advanced the sample preparation process. This technology uses a closed system containing the sample and nitric acid and extremely high temperatures. Since the advent of this method, many advances have occurred until today it may be the method of choice because of its reduced risk for laboratory personnel and the expensive perchloric hoods. The Association of Official Analytical Chemists methods books discuss many of the methods available for destruction of organic matter in mineral analysis.

Atomic absorption spectrophotometry is the most common method for determining cations in biological samples. The addition of the graphite furnace unit makes this instrument useful in determining concentrations of ultratrace elements and trace elements in samples of very limited quantity. Today, there are several instruments that may be used to determine a number of elements at one time from one sample. These include X-ray fluorescence, inductively coupled plasma spectroscopy, and neutron activation analysis. These instruments are useful in surveying for mineral interactions. Selenium (Se) has traditionally been determined by fluorescence, but it is being determined more frequently by neutron activation and hydride generation spectroscopy.

Utilization of standards, both inorganic and organic, with matching matrices is essential regardless of the technology utilized. Precautions in sample collection and storage to prevent adventitious contamination are a must in trace element analysis. Ultrapure reagents, 18-MΩ deionized water, acid-washed glassware, trace element–free syringes and pipette tips, and polypropylene materials must be utilized without compromise in trace element determinations.

II. CHROMIUM

Schwartz and Mertz (1959) reported that chromium (Cr) was an essential component of a glucose tolerance factor that corrected impaired glucose metabolism in rats fed certain diets. A Cr-containing synthetic glucose tolerance factor was later found to potentiate insulin action in pigs (Steele et al., 1977). Recent studies have indicated that Cr supplementation (as Cr picolinate) may increase carcass leanness in growing-finishing pigs and improve litter size in sows (NRC, 1997).

A. Metabolism

Chromium absorption and excretion has not been studied in swine. However, studies in rats and humans have clearly indicated that Cr is poorly absorbed. Chromium absorption in humans consuming self-selected diets ranged from 0.5 to 2.0% (Anderson and Kozlovsky, 1985). Rats consuming ^{51}Cr incorporated into kale, wheat, and eggs absorbed and retained from 1.1 to 2.3% of the dose after 9 days (Johnson and Weaver, 1986).

Absorbed Cr is excreted primarily via the urine (Offenbacher et al., 1997). Certain types of stress such as physical trauma, strenuous exercise, and lactation have been shown to increase urinary losses of Cr in humans (Anderson, 1994).

Chromium is present in tissues at very low concentrations (<1 ppm). The addition of 0.3 ppm of Cr from Cr picolinate to a corn–soybean meal diet containing 2.7 ppm Cr, increased Cr concentrations in kidney and liver but not in heart or longissimus muscle (Anderson et al., 1997a).

B. Function

Chromium functions as a potentiator of insulin action (Offenbacher et al., 1997). The active form of Cr involved in facilitating insulin function has traditionally been referred to as the glucose tolerance factor. Glucose tolerance factor was initially isolated from brewer's yeast and found to contain trivalent Cr, two molecules of nicotinic acid, glutamic acid, glycine, and cysteine (Mertz, 1992). However, the chemical identity of the biologically active form of Cr that facilitates insulin activity in the body is not known. Evidence also suggests that Cr may have a role in nucleic acid and cholesterol metabolism (Offenbacher et al., 1997).

The addition of Cr from Cr picolinate to diets of growing pigs increased glucose clearance rate following an intravenous glucose challenge (Amoikon et al., 1995). Administration of exogenous insulin resulted in a greater hypoglycemic response in pigs supplemented with Cr compared with controls (Amoikon et al., 1995). Chromium picolinate supplementation also decreased glucose and insulin concentrations 2 h post-feeding in pigs that were limit-fed (Evock-Clover et al., 1993).

Studies evaluating the effects of dietary Cr on carcass composition and performance of swine were reviewed recently (NRC, 1997). Page et al. (1993) first reported that the addition of 0.1 to 0.8 ppm of Cr, from Cr picolinate, reduced backfat and increased longissimus muscle area in growing-finishing pigs. Other studies also have shown reduced backfat (Lindemann et al., 1995; Kornegay et al., 1997; Min et al., 1997) or reduced accretion of fat and increased accretion of protein (Mooney and Cromwell, 1995; 1997) in growing-finishing pigs supplemented with Cr picolinate. Carcass responses to Cr supplementation have not been observed or at least have been inconsistent in several studies (Boleman et al., 1995; Wenk et al., 1995; Ward et al., 1997; Mooney and Cromwell, 1999). Growth and feed efficiency responses to Cr supplementation also have been highly variable (NRC, 1997). Inconsistent animal responses to supplemental Cr may relate to differences between studies relative to dietary protein content, Cr concentration, and/or Cr bioavailability of basal diets. Recent studies suggest that stress associated with inadequate pen space

(Ward et al., 1997) or lean growth potential of pigs are not major factors affecting gain or carcass responses to Cr supplementation. It is unclear if Cr affects carcass composition via increased insulin sensitivity or by some other mechanism.

Dietary Cr also may affect reproductive performance of swine. Gilts fed 0.2 ppm of Cr (from Cr picolinate) throughout growth and gestation had larger litters than controls (Lindemann et al., 1995). Litter weights were heavier for Cr-supplemented sows at birth and at 21 days of age.

C. Requirements

Chromium requirements or factors that influence Cr requirements are not well defined in swine (NRC, 1998). In studies where improvements in carcass composition have been observed, supplementing Cr (as Cr picolinate) above 0.2 ppm has not resulted in further reductions in backfat or increases in longissimus muscle area (Page et al., 1993; Lindemann et al., 1995; Min et al., 1997).

D. Deficiency

Clinical signs of Cr deficiency have not been reported in swine. Apparently, practical diets contain sufficient Cr to prevent the occurrence of severe Cr deficiency, and attempts have not been made to develop Cr deficiency in swine by feeding semipurified diets and housing animals in a controlled environment to prevent Cr exposure. Chromium deficiency has been reported in humans receiving total parenteral nutrition (Offenbacher et al., 1997). Deficiency signs included severe glucose intolerance, insulin resistance, and sudden weight loss.

E. Toxicity

Hexavalent Cr (Cr^{+6}), from occupational exposure, is very toxic and has been associated with incidence of lung cancer and dermatitis (Offenbacher et al., 1997). Trivalent Cr, the form supplemented to diets and believed to occur naturally in feeds, has a very low order of toxicity. Maximum tolerable levels for animals were set at 1000 ppm as the chloride and 3000 ppm in the oxide form (NRC, 1980). No signs of toxicity were noted in rats fed up to 100 ppm of Cr, from either Cr chloride or Cr picolinate, for 20 weeks (Anderson et al., 1997b).

F. Sources

Little is known regarding Cr concentrations in animal feedstuffs and even less is known about bioavailability of Cr from commonly used feedstuffs. A number of supplemental Cr sources have been evaluated in swine, including Cr chloride, Cr picolinate, Cr nicotinate, high Cr yeast preparations, Cr propionate, and Cr methionine. In swine studies where two or more different Cr sources have been compared at similar supplemental concentrations, few differences between Cr sources have been observed (Wenk et al., 1995; Matthews et al., 1997; van Heugten and Spears, 1997).

III. COBALT

The only known function of cobalt (Co) is as an essential component of vitamin B_{12} (Underwood, 1977). Functions and requirements of vitamin B_{12} are discussed in Chapter 15. Mammalian tissue is unable to synthesize vitamin B_{12} from Co. However, vitamin B_{12} is synthesized by microorganisms present in the intestine. Some of the vitamin B_{12} produced in the intestine may become available to swine by direct absorption from the intestine. Most of the vitamin B_{12} synthesized in the intestine is excreted and only becomes available to the animal if feces are ingested.

Anorexia, stiff-leggedness, humped back, incoordination, muscle tremors, and anemia were observed in young pigs fed 400 ppm of Co (Huck and Clawson, 1976). The addition of 0, 150, or 300 ppm Co to weanling pig diets decreased gain linearly (Kornegay et al., 1995).

IV. COPPER

A. Introduction

Many of the specifics about Cu metabolism have been learned through research with species other than the pig. In addition, no work has been published to estimate the Cu requirement of pigs weighing greater than 55 kg or the reproducing sow or boar. Details of Cu metabolism will be discussed in this chapter.

B. Absorption

The form and amount of Cu ingested, as well as other dietary components, affect the amount of Cu that is available for absorption from the small intestine. While Van Campen and Mitchell (1965) reported that Cu was absorbed from the stomach in rats, this response has not been confirmed in rats or observed in any other species. Copper is likely available as ionic Cu in the upper small intestine, because the pH there is similar to the pH that dissociates the complexes and compounds in which Cu is bound (Allen and Solomons, 1984). The binding of Cu to intestinal secretions is thought to prevent its precipitation as insoluble Cu hydroxide in the intestine, which is the primary organ of absorption. From work with several species, it would seem that from 5 to 10% of dietary Cu is absorbed unless pharmacological concentrations are fed. The amount absorbed is influenced not only by dietary concentration, but by the age, Cu status, physiological state, and species of the animal. The percent of Cu absorbed is greater when the animal is Cu deficient, or when the requirements are higher, such as during pregnancy. The absorption of dietary Cu increases as the concentration in the diet decreases; however, the quantity absorbed is actually less.

In the pig, few studies have been conducted where the actual amount of Cu absorbed was measured directly by utilizing radio or stable isotopes. Bowland et al. (1961) utilizing ^{64}Cu in a limited number of pigs, reported that 9% of 24 mg of oral cupric sulfate was absorbed, but only 4% of 185 mg was absorbed. In contrast, 2% of 20 or 125 mg of cupric sulfide was absorbed. Research where growth performance and/or hepatic uptake have been measured indicates that Cu sulfate and tribasic Cu chloride (Cromwell et al., 1998) are well utilized by the pig, but cupric sulfide and Cu oxide are not well utilized. Solubility of form would indicate that carbonate and nitrate are also absorbed by the pig. Organic Cu sources where Cu is complexed with amino acids, peptides, etc. seem to be well utilized, but the influence of the type of amino acid, configuration, or degree of polymerization is not well understood.

Absorption may be enhanced if luminal Cu is bound to absorbable ligands or presented to the brush border receptors by ligands such as citrate, gluconate, or histidine. However, it is thought that absorbed Cu enters the intestinal mucosa by simple diffusion and is controlled by mass action. The control of the amount absorbed may be by a saturable carrier on the basolateral surface (Fischer and L'Abbé, 1985). When dietary concentrations are low, it is thought that Cu is primarily transported by an active pathway with diffusion being involved when high or pharmacological concentrations of Cu are fed. If metallothionein (Mt) synthesis has been stimulated as by feeding of high or pharmacological Zn (Carlson et al.,1997), Cu will be bound by Mt and lost as the intestinal cells are sloughed. Aoyagi and Baker (1994) reported in the chick that cysteine inhibited Cu absorption when Cu was consumed in the form of sulfate, methionine, or lysine.

C. Transport

Copper absorbed from the serosal intestinal cells is carried by various components (albumin and perhaps some amino acids) of the blood to the liver and perhaps the kidneys. Recently, Bal et al. (1998) reported the presence of a high affinity binding site for Cu (II) in porcine albumin and a multimetal site binding for Cu (II), Zn (II), or Cd (II). A protein named transcuprein has been reported by Linder's laboratory (Campbell et al., 1981) to be involved in uptake from the intestine.

The liver acting as a storage organ and metabolic sink for this nutrient will utilize some Cu to make liver proteins such as ceruloplasmin, and the excess Cu will be excreted via bile in the feces.

Ceruloplasmin, which is an acute-phase reactant protein, binds 90 to 95% of the Cu in the blood. It is a single polypeptide chain (121,000 Da) with several carbohydrate side chains, and it is synthesized in the liver. Of the six to seven Cu atoms that are bound in ceruloplasmin, only one is easily removed. Ceruloplasmin delivers Cu to tissues, especially the brain and heart. Percival and Harris (1990) reported that Cu dissociates from the ceruloplasmin protein before it is taken up by cells. Receptors on the cell surface for ceruloplasmin have been reported in a number of species and organs, but none has been reported for the pig.

Utilizing information gleaned from the isolation and cloning of genes responsible for two diseases that have defects in Cu distribution (Menkes and Wilson), membrane-bound Cu-transporting ATPases (Cu-ATPases) have been reported (Vulpe, 1995). These will be important in Cu homeostasis and transmembrane transport. Membrane-bound Cu-ATPases have not been reported in the pig.

D. Functions

Copper serves many roles in the body, and often it acts as an enzyme activator, where a change in valence state is crucial.

1. Ceruloplasmin

Ceruloplasmin (Cp) is not just involved in the transport of Cu, but it is a multifaceted oxidative enzyme. Sang (1995) suggests that it has four possible roles: (1) Cu transport and homeostasis, (2) ferroxidase activity, (3) amine oxidase activity, and (4) superoxide dismutase activity. Ceruloplasmin is involved in changing the valence state of Fe so that it can bind to transferrin, and in this role it is often referred to as ferroxidase I. As an acute-phase reactant protein, Cp acts as an antioxidant, and it is involved in the inflammatory process.

Chang et al. (1975) reported that the neonatal pig had little to no Cp activity at birth and then after approximately 15 h, activity of this enzyme began to develop. Activity continued to increase until 2 to 3 weeks of age when it had reached the adult amount (Milne and Matrone, 1970). Copper-deficient pigs show no serum Cp activity (Hill et al., 1983a).

More recently, Wooten et al. (1996) reported that Cp is the primary Cu-binding protein in colostrum, term milk, and amniotic fluid, and that Cp was higher in colostrum than in more mature milk of the sow. The Cu content of colostrum and mature milk is influenced by the Zn content of the dam's diet, but is always higher in colostrum than milk at 1, 2, or 3 weeks of lactation (Hill et al., 1983b). Utilizing ^{67}Cu, newborn rats were shown to preferentially absorb Cp Cu in milk compared with ionic Cu (Wooten et al., 1996).

The secretion of Cp, as an acute-phase reactant protein, is influenced by monokines such as IL-1, IL-6, and tumor necrosis factor, prostaglandin E_1, and perhaps direct action of glucocorticoids. Confounding the use of Cp and serum Cu as Cu status indicators is the impact of estrogens, both natural as occurring during the estrous cycle or synthetic, on the increase of circulating Cp and hence serum Cu. As a result, knowledge regarding physiological state — estrus, stage of pregnancy, presence of malignant growing tumors, etc. — may be helpful in the interpretation of these parameters (Ehnis et al.,1996). Thyroxine and parathyroid hormone may influence Cp.

2. Amine and Diamine Oxidases

Amine and diamine oxidases are Cu-containing enzymes that are found in plasma, and they are believed to inactivate and catabolize active biogenic amines such as histamine, tyramine, dopamine, and serotonin (Linder, 1991). The presence of an amine oxidase in porcine cardiac tissue that is identical to that found in plasma has recently been reported by Dowling et al. (1998).

Lysyl oxidase is a Cu-requiring enzyme involved in cross-linking collagen, and it is essential for the functioning of connective tissue. Aortic ruptures were reported in Cu-deficient animals (Coulson and Carnes, 1967) before it was known that lysyl oxidase was the enzyme that was necessary to catalyze the oxidative deamination of lysine to form allysine for strong elastin and collagen. Lysyl oxidase acts on newly formed collagen, partially converted procollagen and soluble elastin and is found with connective tissue throughout the body including the skin, teeth, lungs, bone, etc. (Linder, 1991). During bone growth and mineralization when collagen and elastin are laid down in early development, it is more active. Hill et al. (1983a) reported reduced lysyl oxidase activity in young Cu-deficient pigs, but because it is one of the more difficult Cu enzymes to measure, its activity is seldom assessed.

Estrogen has been shown to increase lysyl oxidase activity in skin and bone. While Cu is necessary for sperm motility and effectiveness, testosterone also has been shown to increase lysyl oxidase release by smooth muscle cells cultured from the aorta.

Dopamine β-hydroxylase is involved in the synthesis of the sympathetic neurotransmitters norepinephrine and epinephrine, and it is found in the adrenal gland and in numerous locations in the brain (locus ceruleus, brain stem, and posterior hypothalamus). The Cu ions in this enzymatic molecule are believed to be loosely bound and the actual number is unknown. However, two Cu ions are necessary for the catalytic process for optimal activity (Klinman and Brenner, 1988). Concentration of norepinephrine is decreased in the spleen and heart of Cu-deficient pigs while the concentration of dopamine is elevated. The extent of this alteration is greater in the pig than in the rat (Schoenemann et al., 1990).

3. Copper–Zinc Superoxide Dismutase

In addition to the antioxidant properties of Cp, a Cu–Zn-containing enzyme, superoxide dismutase (SOD), is found in plasma and extracellular fluids, but it is not the same as the SOD found in mitochondria. The activity of SOD in plasma varies from species to species, and it has not been quantified in the pig.

During times when superoxide is generated in the cell, such as metabolic disturbances caused by free Fe and Cu, drugs and environmental insults, and "metabolic bursts" associated with cell killing by leukocytes, cytosolic SOD is essential to dismutase the superoxide radical to peroxide and dioxygen. The amino acid sequence shows a great deal of homology in the 11 species where it has been sequenced, and the gene for SOD in the pig is located on chromosome 9 (Bannister et al., 1987). Red blood cell SOD may be a possible indicator of Cu status (L'Abbé and Fischer, 1984).

Williams et al. (1975) were the first to confirm that SOD activity was decreased as Cu status decreased. They noted that in the red blood cell, the activity of SOD decreased at a slower rate than Cp and plasma Cu when pigs were fed a Cu-deficient diet, and they indicated that this was probably due to the life span of the red blood cell. However, they did not correlate these variables with changes in hepatic Cu. Das et al. (1987) reported that SOD activity increases during the first 10 days of life and then remains rather constant. This was not observed by Hill et al. (1999) who observed no increase in activity from 3 to 21 days of age except when pigs were anemic at 21 days of age. The SOD activity in the red blood cell on a protein basis was higher at day 21 than at 3 days of age when they were not anemic. Scholfield et al. (1990) reported a decrease in erythrocyte SOD activity when pigs were fed a Cu-deficient diet for 10 weeks.

4. Cytochrome c Oxidase

In the mitochondria, the last enzyme in the electron transport chain is cytochrome c oxidase. It reduces oxygen to water and with other enzymes of the chain allows for the formation of ATP. The activity of this Cu- and Fe-containing enzyme seems to reflect the metabolic and respiratory functions of the tissue, as well as the availability of Cu. Hill et al. (1983a) reported a decrease in cytochrome c oxidase activity in the heart and liver of Cu-deficient pigs. Biochemically, the essentially of this enzyme is clear; however, it is seldom measured in swine studies.

5. Tyrosinase

The Cu-containing enzyme, tyrosinase, is essential for melanin formation. Tyrosinase catalyzes three different reactions in the synthesis of melanin. However, the biology of pigmentation is complex with many genes in the tyrosinase family (Hearing and Tsukamoto, 1991). The melanin pigments derived from tyrosine are responsible for the color in hair, skin, and eye and they are synthesized within melanocytes, which are dependent on Cu and growth factors. Achromotrichia or the loss of color has been observed during Cu deficiency in sheep, cattle, dogs, cats, rats, guinea pigs, and rabbits, but not in pigs (Underwood, 1977).

6. Immunity

Copper is necessary for normal immune function in swine. For greater detail relative to immunity in the pig, see Chapter 24. A Cu deficiency results in greater susceptibility to disease in many species, but the impact of the deficiency in domestic vs. laboratory animals is not alike. Percival (1998) in a recent review noted that Cu is necessary for several functions in the immune system, but the direct mechanism of action is often poorly understood.

Failla's laboratory (Bala et al., 1992) reported that the impact of Cu deficiency on the immune system of young pigs was not as severe as in rats and mice. They reported that mononuclear cells isolated from the blood of Cu-deficient pigs exhibited a decreased reactivity to T-cell mitogens. Since T-cell and red blood cell numbers were not affected, it would suggest that the blastogenic responsiveness of porcine T-cells to mitogens is more sensitive to Cu status than T cell development and maturation or erythropoiesis. Thus, traditional indices of Cu deficiency, leukopenia and anemia, were not observed, but immune function was impaired. The relationship of nutrition to immunity in the livestock industry has not been well explored due to the difficulty in carrying out immunological studies with diverse genetics, nutrition, and management.

7. Growth Stimulant at Pharmacological Concentrations

Braude, as early as 1948, observed that pigs licking Cu pipes grew faster than those without access to extra Cu, and he is responsible for the first reporting of growth enhancement by pharmacological concentrations (125 to 250 ppm) of Cu (Barber et al., 1957). Copper sulfate is known to have limited antibacterial properties (see Chapter 18), and it is often used as an antifungal agent, but the mechanism for this Cu-induced growth promotion has been elusive. However, if it is acting as an antimicrobial agent, it is of interest that the addition of antibiotics produces an additive effect (Stahly et al., 1980; Roof and Mahan, 1982). Shurson et al. (1990) reported that germ-free pigs had a decreased average daily gain (ADG) and average daily feed intake (ADFI) in response to 283 ppm Cu, whereas conventionally reared pigs showed increased growth. With reduced intestinal weight and thickness, the germ-free pigs stored less hepatic Cu and Zn, but had higher Cp activity than conventionally raised pigs. From this, one might assume that high Cu needs a certain microbial population to be effective.

Most studies with pharmacological concentrations of Cu have found that 250 ppm of Cu from $CuSO_4 \cdot 5H_2O$ to be effective in growth promotion, and in some studies 125 ppm Cu was equally effective. However, higher and lower concentrations of Cu sulfate do not have this same effect.

Miller (1973) reported that the growth response to 200 ppm Cu as Cu hydroxide (Cu$[OH]_2$) was similar to that of Cu sulfate. Cromwell et al. (1989) reported that Cu oxide (CuO) not only did not improve growth performance at 125, 250, 375, or 500 ppm Cu, but it also did not increase hepatic stores of this element. Recently, this same group reported that 100 or 200 ppm Cu as tribasic chloride ($Cu_2[OH]_3Cl$) improved growth similarly to 200 ppm Cu from Cu sulfate

(Cromwell et al., 1998). Apgar et al. (1995) reported that Cu lysine did not differ from Cu sulfate as a growth promotant, and the excretion pattern for the two forms was not different (Apgar and Kornegay, 1996).

In response to environmental concerns, Miller (1973) investigated different Cu- feeding regimes in an attempt to reduce the amount of Cu in manure. He reported that lack of Cu in finishing diets did not affect performance when Cu was fed at 250 ppm in the grower phase. Anderson et al. (1991) reported that when 250 ppm Cu was fed in the diet, approximately 1300 ppm Cu was found in the manure. In a 10-year study of continual application of 325 kg Cu/ha from manure, Cu concentration in the corn ear, leaves, and grain remained within the normal range. There was no decrease in corn yield, which the researchers felt was due to the neutral soil pH decreasing Cu availability. However, seven consecutive years of fertilization of sheep pasture with swine waste slurry containing 85 ppm Cu resulted in soil Cu concentrations of 26 ppm (vs. 7 ppm when no Cu was added) and forages containing 13 ppm (Kerr and McGavin, 1991). A number of sheep died prior to a diagnosis of Cu toxicity.

Cunnane (1984) states in his review that, more than 45 years ago, Cu was shown to impair phospholipid synthesis and that, in 1964, the feeding of 250 ppm Cu resulted in an increase in the softness of backfat in market animals. Since that time, pharmacological concentrations of Cu have been shown to increase the activity of Δ^9-desaturase, and a deficiency of Cu will decrease its activity, resulting in a decreased proportion of polyunsaturated fatty acids in tissues. More recently, Dove and Haydon (1992) reported that addition of 250 ppm Cu with 5% animal fat resulted in a significant Cu by fat interaction for improving growth.

E. Deficiency

1. Growth

The extent of the reduction of Cu status and dietary Cu content as well as the length of time the diet is fed will influence the severity of the Cu deficiency. Hence, all the signs of Cu deficiency described herein will not always be present in a Cu-deficient animal. In the early work with Cu-deficient swine, Lahey et al. (1952) did not observe a severe impact on growth. However, Hill et al. (1983a) reported that weight was reduced in Cu-deficient animals to one half that of Cu-supplemented pigs in a 35-day study.

2. Blood

While Cu is known to be important in changing the valence of Fe for binding to transferrin and ferritin, it is often assumed that the anemia that results during Cu deficiency is due to this specific Cu function. However, the mode of action that results in the microcytic and hypochromic anemia in Cu deficiencies characterized by a decrease in mean corpuscular volume (MCV) and hemoglobin concentration is not known. Because heme biosynthesis and reticulocyte numbers are altered (Williams et al., 1976), hematocrit is also decreased (Lahey et al., 1952; Hill et al., 1983a).

Leukopenia, which develops in Cu-deficient animals, is due to a reduction in polymorphonuclear and mononuclear cells. However, the greatest reduction is in the polymorphonuclear fraction. Neutropenia also has been reported as a consequence of Cu deficiency in malnourished children (Cordano et al., 1968). While Bala et al. (1992) did not observe a decrease in the percentage of T cells, CD4 or CD8 cell subsets, or B cells, the expression of SLA-DQ and sla-dr class II major histocompatibility complex antigens was increased and T-cell function was decreased in Cu deficiency. This study was the first to report that the pig's immune response to Cu deficiency was different from that of the rodent response.

Bush et al. (1956) reported that the life span of the red blood cell was shortened resulting in increased turnover of red blood cells during Cu deficiency in the pig. Similar observations have been made by O'Dell and his group (Bettger et al., 1978) with rodents. While there are several theories for this alteration, due to the oxidative products that were detected in cellular membranes, it seems that the cause may be the lack of antioxidant potential due to reduced red blood cell SOD and serum Cp.

3. Connective and Vascular Tissue Function

Connective and vascular tissue health is dependent on normal collagen and elastin fibers. Because a Cu-requiring enzyme, lysyl oxidase, is the rate-limiting enzyme in the cross-linking of these fibers, Cu is essential for the maintenance and function of these tissues. Skeletal abnormalities in severely Cu-deficient pigs were observed (Teague and Carpenter, 1951; Lahey et al., 1952). Leg deformities and reduced bone length were hypothesized to be due to a reduction in the activity of lysyl oxidase. This was confirmed by Hill et al. (1983a) in young pigs with demonstrable skeletal defects. More recently, Pond et al. (1990) observed that cartilage differentiation and bone resorption were retarded in Zn-induced, Cu-deficient pigs. Lameness and severe damage to the humeral–radioulnar joint had previously been reported (Hill et al., 1983c) in Zn-induced (5000 ppm Zn), Cu-deficient sows.

Cardiac hypertrophy and weakened walls of blood vessels resulting in rupture have been reported in the pig (Shields et al., 1962; Hill et al., 1983a) as well many other species. The aorta ruptures in the ascending segment, or the initial portion of the arch. More recently, the collaborative work of Vadlamudi et al. (1993) reported that collagen cross-linking was reduced in the myocardium and bicuspid valves in Cu-deficient pigs. They hypothesized that the reduction in left ventricular collagen cross-linking may be responsible for the development of cardiac hypertrophy observed in Cu-deficient animals.

4. Reproduction

It is known that Cu is required for normal reproduction because of the extensive roles of Cu-requiring enzymes in the body. However, there is no specific loss of reproductive function during a Cu deficiency. Marginal or acute Cu-deficient sows have not been studied. However, Cu-deficient ewes produce lambs with underdeveloped brains resulting in an enzootic ataxia, which can be prevented by the administration of Cu (Hurley, 1983). Gross neural brain lesions and pups with other physical abnormalities, which often result in fetal death, have been observed when rats are fed a Cu-deficient diet (Hurley, 1983).

It has been known for some time that the transfer of Cu across the placenta assures the neonate that Cu will be available from the liver for growth. However, the mechanisms and physiological influences in the pig have not been studied. The concentration of Cu in the liver of neonatal pigs born to first parity sows is approximately 50 ppm on a wet tissue basis and may increase slightly as parity of the dam advances (Hill et al., 1983d). This is in contrast to 50-day-old pigs and second-parity sows with hepatic Cu concentrations of approximately 15 ppm (wet basis). Thus, the pig, like other mammals, has a higher hepatic Cu concentration at birth than at any other time in the life cycle if the dam's Cu status was adequate. Mas and Sarkar (1988) reported that Cu was associated with the soluble and nuclear fractions of the placenta in the rat. Metallothionein has been found in the placenta of humans and may have a role in reducing the transfer of toxic elements to the fetus (Mas and Sarkar, 1988). Placental Cu and Cd are correlated in humans, but no mechanism of interaction has been published (Kuhnert et al., 1993). McArdle and Erlich (1991) reported that the rat has a specific Cu transport system during pregnancy, which appears to mature before birth. The placenta seems to obtain Cu from both albumin and Cp for transfer to the fetus. Similar work has not been done in the pig.

Cao and Chavez (1995) fed a Cu-deficient diet (2 ppm) and a Cu-adequate diet (10 ppm) to first-parity sows throughout gestation resulting in daily Cu intakes of 4.26 and 25 mg/day. The Cu-adequate diet resulted in improved balance of Cu, Zn, and Fe. However, retention of Cu as a percentage of dietary Cu was greater in sows fed the marginally deficient diet, but the absolute amount retained was less than in the control sows. As expected, urinary Cu was not altered by dietary Cu concentrations.

F. TOXICITY

As previously discussed, high dietary Cu concentrations in swine diets stimulate growth. Similar concentrations (250 ppm) would be lethal to ruminants. Thus, swine would be considered Cu tolerant. However, 500 ppm Cu reduces gains and produces an anemia ultimately resulting in death (Combs et al., 1966; Suttle and Mills, 1966), whereas 1000 ppm is more quickly lethal (Allcroft et al., 1961). The addition of 150 ppm Zn and 150 ppm Fe reduced the observed toxic effects of 500 ppm Cu (Suttle and Mills, 1966). This is expected because there is a known interaction among Cu, Zn, and Fe.

Signs of acute Cu toxicosis observed in many species include vomiting, salivation, violent abdominal pain, convulsions, paralysis, collapse, and death (NRC, 1980).

V. IODINE

Early reports indicated the natural occurrence of iodine (I) deficiency in swine in the Northwest and Great Lakes regions of the United States where feedstuffs were produced on low-I soils (Miller, 1991).

A. METABOLISM AND FUNCTION

Iodine functions as an essential component of the thyroid hormones, thyroxine (T_4), and triiodothyronine (T_3). The thyroid hormones regulate the rate of energy metabolism in the body and are essential for growth and development in the young animal (Underwood, 1977). Triiodothyronine is three to five times more active in terms of thyroidal activity than T_4 (Underwood, 1977).

Iodine is very well absorbed from the gastrointestinal tract and a large portion of absorbed I is taken up by the thyroid gland by an energy-dependent process that can be blocked by goitrogens (Underwood, 1977). In the thyroid gland, I reacts with tyrosine residues to form the thyroid hormone precursors mono- and diiodotyrosine. Thyroid hormones are stored in the thyroid bound to thyroglobulin.

Uptake of I by the thyroid and synthesis of and release of thyroid hormones are stimulated by thyroid-stimulating hormone produced in the pituitary, which in turn is synthesized and released in response to thyrotropin-releasing hormone from the hypothalamus. Adequate circulating concentrations of thyroid hormones inhibit release of thyrotropin-releasing hormone. In humans, T_4 has been shown to be deiodinated to the more active T_3 by deiodinases in a number of tissues (Hetzel and Wellby, 1997). Deiodinase found primarily in the liver is an Se metalloenzyme (Arthur et al., 1990). Iodine is excreted largely in the urine.

B. REQUIREMENTS

Iodine requirements of all classes of swine have been estimated at 0.14 ppm (NRC, 1998). Studies in growing pigs fed a corn–soybean meal diet indicated an I requirement of between 0.086 and 0.132 ppm (Cromwell et al., 1975). Iodine requirements are poorly defined in sows. Goitrogens that are present in certain feedstuffs including rapeseed, linseed, peanuts, and soybeans increase I requirements (Underwood, 1977). The addition of 0.4 ppm of I to the diet of pregnant gilts fed 12% rapeseed meal did not prevent I deficiency in their pigs (Devilat and Skoknic, 1971).

C. DEFICIENCY

As circulating thyroid hormone concentrations decline below normal, thyroid-stimulating hormone stimulates the thyroid gland to enlarge in an attempt to trap more I. Sows fed I-deficient diets farrow hairless pigs with thickened skin and subcutaneous edema (Miller, 1991). Early mortality is extremely high in I-deficient pigs and on necropsy, the thyroid gland is enlarged and hemorrhagic. Iodine deficiency in young, growing pigs results in reduced plasma protein-bound I concentrations and increased thyroid weights (Cromwell et al., 1975). A more severe I deficiency produced by feeding goitrogens caused pigs to appear stunted, lethargic, and have shortened legs (Sihombing et al., 1974; Cromwell et al., 1975).

D. Toxicity

Swine can tolerate high dietary concentrations of I without adverse effects. Dietary I concentrations of 400 ppm reduced liver Fe concentrations but did not affect performance of growing pigs (Newton and Clawson, 1974). However, the addition of 800 or 1600 ppm of I decreased gain, feed intake, hemoglobin concentrations, and liver Fe concentrations. Feeding sows up to 2500 ppm of I during the last 30 days of gestation and lactation was not harmful to sows or their pigs (Arrington et al., 1965).

E. Sources

The I content of cereal grains and oilseed meals is highly available and is affected by the I concentration in the soil (Underwood, 1981). Iodine is generally supplemented to diets as calcium iodate or ethylenediamine dihydroiodide (EDDI). Both forms are highly available and stable in mineral supplements and diets. Iodide forms such as potassium iodide are less stable and losses can occur due to heat, moisture, light, or exposure to other minerals (Nelson, 1985).

VI. IRON

A. Introduction

Iron deficiency is the most commonly known potential mineral deficiency in swine. The rapid growth of the young pig and the low concentration of Fe in milk result in the use of hepatic Fe, which was stored *in utero*. It has long been known that without an exogenous source of Fe, young pigs will become severely Fe deficient resulting in anemia.

Iron in the body can be classified as (1) essential because it is associated with compounds that have specific physiological roles or (2) storage Fe, which seems to regulate Fe homeostasis and provide a reserve. Essential compounds include hemoglobin, in which the heme portion functions to carry Fe from the lungs to tissues, mitochrondrial Fe enzymes that are essential for oxidative production of cellular energy, and the myoglobin of muscle.

B. Absorption

The common oxidation states of Fe are Fe^{2+} and Fe^{3+}, and in an acid media they are in the hydrated form. The water molecules can be replaced by ligands, and stable and soluble complexes will be formed. As a solution becomes more basic, such as the change that occurs in the small intestine, hydrolysis occurs and hydrides are formed. At a pH greater than 3, ferric Fe is insoluble. Hence, dietary factors and components influence the form in which Fe can be found. However, in swine diets, this has not been extensively studied.

Regulation of absorption is poorly understood, partially because of the scientific reliance on the rat, which will continually accumulate Fe, unlike pigs and humans. However, it is clear that Fe absorption in mammals increases as Fe stores decrease and as erythropoiesis increases. Nonheme Fe is taken up in the ionic form primarily as ferrous Fe by receptors on the proximal intestinal mucosal cells. Iron status seems to influence this binding capacity. The valence of Fe must return to the ferric state before it will bind to membrane proteins. Transport across the mucosal cells may be by diffusion or by the use of amino acids, such as cysteine, ornithine, lysine, or histidine with Fe in the ferrous state. Ferric Fe may bind to apotransferrin, similar to plasma transferrin, within the mucosal cell for movement to and release from the basolateral membrane. Ferritin formation within the mucosal cell is highest when the body's Fe status is replete. The Fe bound to ferritin is eventually discarded as the mucosal cells are exfoliated.

Lactoferrin is a major Fe-binding protein in high concentration in sow's milk, and specific receptors for this protein are found in the neonatal pig's small intestine. While this is a low-affinity receptor, its number of binding sites is rather constant from 0 to 600 cm from the pylorus and from 0 to 20 days of age (Gíslason et al., 1994). It has been hypothesized that because the casein in sow's milk may not be well digested until the milk reaches the small intestine, the availability of lactoferrin receptors beyond where Fe is absorbed in the mature animal may allow the neonate to capture a greater portion of the Fe in sow's milk.

C. Interrelationships

Much work has been done, primarily in the rat, to evaluate the effect of dietary components on Fe availability for absorption. The Fe contained in soy products has been considered unavailable. Macfarlane et al. (1990) noted that when protein content and composition are considered, the effect differs between soy products. Pérez-Llamas et al. (1996) postulated that the effect of a protein source on the availability of Fe for absorption may be related to the amount of free amino acids and/or small peptides released during digestion. However, this may also be related to phytate, which is known to reduce Fe absorption, as discussed for Cu and Zn. Although proteins of animal origin are known to enhance Fe absorption, which may be due to their heme content or amino acid profile, dairy products are believed to decrease Fe absorption because of their high Ca content. However, Galan et al. (1991) have shown that dairy products may not be detrimental to Fe availability, as once thought. Thus, oversupplementing whey-, casein-, and dried skim milk–based diets with Fe may not be necessary.

In an outstanding review by Davis (1980), he states that the interaction between Zn, Cu, and Fe may be in the feed, lumen of the intestine, within the cells of various organs, related to the transport mechanisms, at target organs, and ultimately during catabolic processes that lead to excretion. With species differences, the influence of genetics, differing dietary sources, the presence or absence of disease, the mechanisms of the interactions are not completely understood, as discussed in the sections on Cu and Zn. Hill et al. (1983d) reported this three-way interaction in the offspring of sows fed 5000 ppm Zn. While Zn and Fe were increased in the liver, hepatic Cu was decreased. Recently, the NCR-42 Swine Nutrition Committee (Hill et al., 2000) reported an alteration in plasma Fe and Cu when pharmacological concentrations of Zn were fed to nursery pigs. Hill et al. (1983a) had previously noted that Cu-deficient pigs had decreased Zn concentrations in some tissues, whereas Fe concentration was elevated in the liver and hair.

D. Transport

Transferrin is a hepatic-synthesized glycoprotein in the plasma that transports Fe in the ferric state. The change in valence to enable binding is accomplished by enzymes that have ferroxidase activity, such as ceruloplasmin. This transport protein has two binding sites for minerals. The sites located near the C-terminus and N-terminus have high affinity for ferric Fe. However, the N-terminus site also will bind Cr, Cu, Mn, Cd, Zn, and Ni. Generally, only one third of the binding sites on the transferrin molecule are filled with Fe. If all were filled, Fe-binding capacity would be fully saturated. Transferrin receptors are located in the cell plasma membrane and are involved in the endocytosis of Fe into the cell and the exocytosis of the transferrin protein for reutilization. During an Fe deficiency, there is an increase in transferrin gene expression.

To be absorbed by the fetus, Fe must cross the trophoblasts of the placenta, which contain a large number of transferrin receptors. It seems that only the Fe crosses, thus preventing the presence of maternal proteins on the fetal side. Control of the amount of Fe, which crosses in this unidirectional system, is believed to be by the number of transferrin receptors on the apical side and the amount of ferritin within the placenta. Because high cellular Fe decreases the number of transferrin receptors, and vice versa, it seems that placental Fe availability is controlled by the Fe needs of the fetus (Harris, 1992). Thus, this feedback mechanism would make placental Fe uptake independent of the Fe status of the dam. Hence, hepatic Fe loading or deficiency would not risk the health of the offspring. Several researchers are investigating the potential of transgenic manipulation to determine if the amount of Fe stored in the neonatal pig can be increased.

E. Storage

The storage of Fe is primarily as ferritin, which has a protein shell into which Fe is deposited in the cavity. Dormant mRNAs for ferritin exist in the cytoplasm, and they can be activated to accommodate a rise in cellular Fe. Iron regulatory proteins 1 and 2 are two cytoplasmic RNA-binding proteins that prevent the message from being translated until Fe accumulates in the cell (Munro, 1993). The release of the ferritin mRNAs by the Fe binding proteins allows for ferritin to be synthesized and incoming cellular Fe to be bound. These regulatory proteins are responsive to dietary Fe, and have not been investigated in the pig.

Ferritin, like other proteins of the body, is not static but constantly turning over and providing an intracellular Fe pool. Splenic ferritin of pigs contains two fractions with equal P and Fe contents, but differing in carbohydrate content (van Gelder et al., 1996). There seems to be an equilibration between serum ferritin (glycosylated) and tissue ferritin (nonglycosylated). Another Fe storage protein is hemosiderin, which is believed to be a degradation product of ferritin. The release of Fe from hemosiderin is much slower than from ferritin.

F. Requirements

The Fe requirement of the pig was not changed in the latest revision of the NRC (1998). Most swine diets have an excess of Fe because of contamination from Ca sources and rust.

G. Functions

Although the role of Fe in heme for oxygen transport is well known, its role for transitional storage of oxygen in tissues as myoglobin and the transport of electrons in the electron transport chain should not be overlooked. The last enzyme in the electron transport chain is cytochrome a-a_3, which has one coordinate bond with Fe and a protein, and also requires Cu. Cytochromes b and c, also in the electron transport chain, pass electrons onto oxygen by changing the valence state of the Fe atom. Also, containing Fe are cytochrome b_5, which is involved in lipid metabolism, and P-450, which is involved in drug metabolism.

Myeloperoxidase, peroxidase, and catalase are also heme-containing enzymes. Catalase converts hydrogen peroxide to water; hence it is involved as an antioxidant enzyme. Although it is a ubiquitous enzyme in nature, Hill et al. (1999) recently showed that catalase was significantly higher at 21 days of age than at 7 days of age, regardless of the number of Fe injections (one vs. two). Myeloperoxidase is released into phagocytic vesicles within the neutrophil, and it also catalyzes the conversion of hydrogen peroxide to water and hypochlorate, which is used to destroy foreign materials such as bacteria. Thus, it is involved in immune system function.

Other Fe-containing enzymes include tryptophan dioxygenase, phenylalanine hydroxylase, homogentisate oxidase, xanthine dehydrogenase, xanthine oxidase, glycerol phosphate dehydrogenase, aconitase, phosphoenolpyruvate carboxykinase, ribonucleotide reductase, 4-butyrobetaine hydroxylase, and trimethyllysine hydroxylase. The diversity of function may be misleading until the ease of valence changes in electron transfers and the importance of Fe being bound to protein is remembered.

H. Deficiency

Classic descriptions of Fe deficiency in the baby pig include labored and spasmodic breathing referred to as the "thumps," loss of appetite and weight, and ultimately death (Underwood, 1977). However, this is seldom seen in commercial swine production. Pigs are given an intramuscular injection of Fe at 1 to 3 days of age in a form that will minimize tissue necrosis. The standard dose given in the industry today is 200 mg Fe (per ml or cc) as Fe dextran. Oral Fe also can be administered. However, if it is not given within 24 h of birth, gut closure may result in a greatly reduced availability (Hill et al., 1999). Access to the sow's feces and feed will also provide Fe to the young pig. Low body stores of Fe at birth and no polycythemia in the neonate reduce the opportunity for endogenous Fe sources to provide Fe for erythropoesis. Supplementary feeding or injections of Fe prior to farrowing does not alter hepatic Fe stores of the neonate.

Lemacher and Bostedt (1994) reported that 40% of newborn pigs showed latent or overt Fe deficiency at birth. Hemoglobin concentration at birth was positively correlated with weight gain in the following 3 days. Hemoglobin concentration declined by 27% and plasma Fe by 61% in untreated pigs during this time period.

Hill et al. (1999) did not show any benefit of a second Fe injection in traditionally weaned pigs. Injecting vitamin E with or without Se did not improve Fe status as measured by hemoglobin concentration in early-weaned or traditionally weaned pigs.

Of interest to researchers, the hematocrit test diagnosed anemia in up to 10% of the population that had a normal hemoglobin concentration and failed to detect anemia in up to 50% of those who had depressed hemoglobin concentrations (Graitcer et al., 1981), thus indicating that hematocrits cannot be substituted for hemoglobin in the determination of microcytic, hypochromic anemias.

The depletion of Fe from the body, when dietary Fe is not adequate or an animal has an excessive parasite load, initially results in a depletion of Fe stores, which can first be observed in the loss of Fe from the bone marrow. Plasma ferritin will drop during this time and Fe-binding capacity and absorption will be increased. Hemoglobin color and red blood cell numbers will not be altered. As the deficiency progresses, bone marrow Fe will decrease to zero, plasma ferritin will continue to decrease, as well as plasma Fe and transferrin saturation. The red blood cell will be normal. Only in a severe, prolonged Fe deficiency will red blood cells become hypochromic and microcytic. Hence, anemia is a sign of a very severe Fe deficiency, not an initial depletion.

I. Toxicity

As with many mineral toxicities, Fe toxicosis results in reduced feed intake, growth rate, and feed efficiency. Signs of a phosphorus (P) deficiency were noted in pigs fed 5102 or 7102 ppm Fe when P was present at 0.92% of the diet (Furugouri, 1972). The severity of Fe toxicity from oral doses of 200 mg Fe administered within 6 h of birth depended on the Fe source given. Dosing with ferric ammonium citrate resulted in 66% mortality by 21 days of age (Cornelius and Harmon, 1976). Limited data with other species indicate that lipid peroxidation is increased and phagocytic function is decreased in Fe toxicosis. As excessive Fe concentrations due to accidental contributions from feed mills and other ingredients occur, these negative effects on health may be of interest to the swine industry.

VII. MANGANESE

A. Introduction

Manganese (Mn) was shown to be essential for growth and fertility in rats and mice in 1931 (Underwood, 1981). Later studies clearly indicated that Mn played a critical role in formation of the organic matrix of bone.

B. Metabolism

Dietary Mn is poorly absorbed. True absorption of a single oral dose of ^{54}Mn was 0.5%, whereas apparent absorption was 1.7% in growing pigs fed a practical diet containing 42 ppm of Mn (Finley et al., 1997). Gamble et al. (1971) reported that gilts in late pregnancy absorbed 28% of an oral dose of ^{54}Mn and that Mn readily crossed the placenta. Dietary factors that may affect Mn absorption have not been studied in swine. In other species, Fe deficiency enhances Mn absorption, whereas high dietary Ca and P reduce Mn absorption (Leach and Harris, 1997). In chicks, high dietary P decreases Mn absorption to a much greater extent than high dietary Ca (Wedekind et al., 1991).

Manganese is found in low concentrations in body tissues with liver containing the highest concentrations. Absorbed Mn is excreted largely via the bile (Leach and Harris, 1997) with only small amounts excreted in the urine.

C. Function

Manganese functions as a component of the enzymes pyruvate carboxylase, mitochondrial SOD, and arginase and as an activator for a number of enzymes (Leach and Harris, 1997). Those activated by Mn include a number of hydrolases, kinases, transferases, and decarboxylases. Of the many enzymes that can be activated by Mn, only the glycosyl transferases are known specifically to require Mn. Glycosyl transferases are involved in the addition of sugar molecules to core proteins to form proteoglycans or mucopolysaccharides. Proteoglycans are found in the organic matrix component of cartilage and play an important role in the integrity of cartilage. The skeletal abnormalities observed in Mn deficiency are related to reduced proteoglycans. Evidence also suggests that Mn plays a role in pancreatic insulin synthesis, response of peripheral tissues to insulin, and in cholesterol biosynthesis (Leach and Harris, 1997).

D. Requirements

Requirements and dietary factors that may affect Mn requirements are not well defined for swine. In pigs, requirements have been estimated at 2 to 4 ppm (NRC, 1998). Feeding nursery pigs diets containing 0.4 ppm of Mn did not affect pig performance but reduced Mn concentrations in liver and kidney (Leibholz et al., 1962). Plumlee et al. (1956) reported no difference in gain or feed efficiency of growing pigs fed 0.5 or 40 ppm of Mn. However, skeletal abnormalities were noted in pigs fed the low Mn diet.

The Mn requirement for reproduction is higher than for growth. Gestating and lactating sows require approximately 20 ppm of Mn (NRC, 1998). Sows fed a basal diet containing 10 ppm of Mn had lower litter weights at birth than sows fed the basal diet supplemented with 84 ppm of Mn (Rheaume and Chavez, 1989). Christianson et al. (1989; 1990) reported heavier birth weights of pigs born to sows fed 20 ppm compared with those fed 5 ppm of Mn.

E. Deficiency

Severe Mn deficiency in growing female pigs fed a diet containing 0.5 ppm of Mn resulted in increased fat deposition and skeletal abnormalities, including shorter and thicker front legs, bowed front legs, and enlarged hocks (Plumlee et al., 1956). Irregular or complete absence of estrus was observed in Mn-deficient female pigs once they reached breeding age. At parturition, Mn-deficient females had poor udder development and gave birth to small, weak pigs that showed signs of poor balance and coordination (Plumlee et al., 1956). A marginal Mn deficiency reduced pig birth weights and delayed return to estrus in sows (Christianson et al., 1989; 1990).

F. Toxicity

Manganese is relatively nontoxic. Supplementing 500 ppm Mn to a diet containing 12 ppm of Mn reduced gain, feed intake, and caused limb stiffness in growing pigs (Grummer et al., 1950).

In 2-week-old pigs, feeding 4000 ppm of Mn for 10 weeks decreased gain; however, 400 ppm of Mn had no adverse effects (Leibholz et al., 1962).

G. Sources

Cereal grains usually contain between 5 and 40 ppm of Mn with corn being especially low (Underwood, 1981). Plant protein sources normally contain 30 to 50 ppm, whereas animal protein sources only contain 5 to 15 ppm of Mn. Manganese is generally supplemented to diets as $MnSO_4$ or MnO. Based on studies in poultry, Mn from MnO is 52 to 93% as available as $MnSO_4$ (Wong-Valle et al., 1989).

VIII. ZINC

A. Introduction

Solomons and Cousins (1984) noted that the need for Zn is related to the size of the animal and its energy consumption. Zinc functions in growth, development, reproduction, and metabolic activity, through its participation as a constituent of more than 100 metalloenzyme systems. Its role may be one of structural integrity, or it may be involved directly in the reaction at the active site. In addition, Zn seems to be involved in host defense, cytostructural, and regulatory processes, which are nonenzymatic in nature. While Zn can exist in several different valence states and is ubiquitous in the body, it is usually found as a divalent ion (Zn^{2+}). Organs of highest concentration include the bone, liver, and kidney. However, because homeostatic regulation protects the activity of many Zn enzymes during times of dietary deficiency, a good indicator of Zn status is not known.

B. Absorption

Mammalian absorption of Zn is influenced by many factors, including Zn status, age, physiological state, dietary components, health, and perhaps species. Much of this information has been gleaned from research with the rat, which differs from the pig especially due to its lack of a gall bladder.

Zinc in the intestinal tract is not only of dietary origin, but from salivary, intestinal, biliary, and pancreatic secretions. The Zn content of these endogenous secretions is reduced during Zn deficiency (Taylor et al., 1991), and Zn concentration is greatest in pancreatic secretions (Birnstingl et al., 1956).

In 1981, Jackson et al. utilizing ^{65}Zn in rats found that two mechanisms seem to control Zn absorption. One was involved when dietary Zn concentrations were below 0.24 µmol/g of diet, and the second was predominant when the rats had a normal Zn status and dietary intakes were within the normal range. This mechanism absorbs Zn in proportion to the dietary content, thus implying that Zn homeostasis is achieved through Zn excretion. The impact of very high Zn intakes was not studied. No receptor sites for a specific mechanism or carrier have been identified. The relative contribution of the duodenum, jejunum, and ileum to Zn absorption is not clear for any species. It is not known if Zn is absorbed into the enterocyte in the ionic form or if its absorption is assisted by the presence of amino acids. When ligand:Zn ratio was equal to or less than 3:1, Wapnir et al. (1983) found that L-glutamate, glycine, L-histidine, L-tryptophan, and glycylglycine simulated Zn absorption, but if the ratio was 130:1, absorption with L-histidine was much less than when the ratio was 3:1. Utilizing pig brush-border membrane vesicles, Tacnet et al. (1993) reported that a tripeptide of glycine–glycine–histidine stimulated the uptake of Zn in a dose-dependent manner as a peptide carrier system. This work in rats and pigs and may help one to understand the differing uptakes observed with some organic Zn products.

The lack of research relative to Zn absorption in swine may be because corn–soybean meal diets, typical of the U.S. swine industry, provide approximately 40 ppm Zn, which prevents parakeratosis, a classical sign of Zn deficiency (Smith et al., 1960).

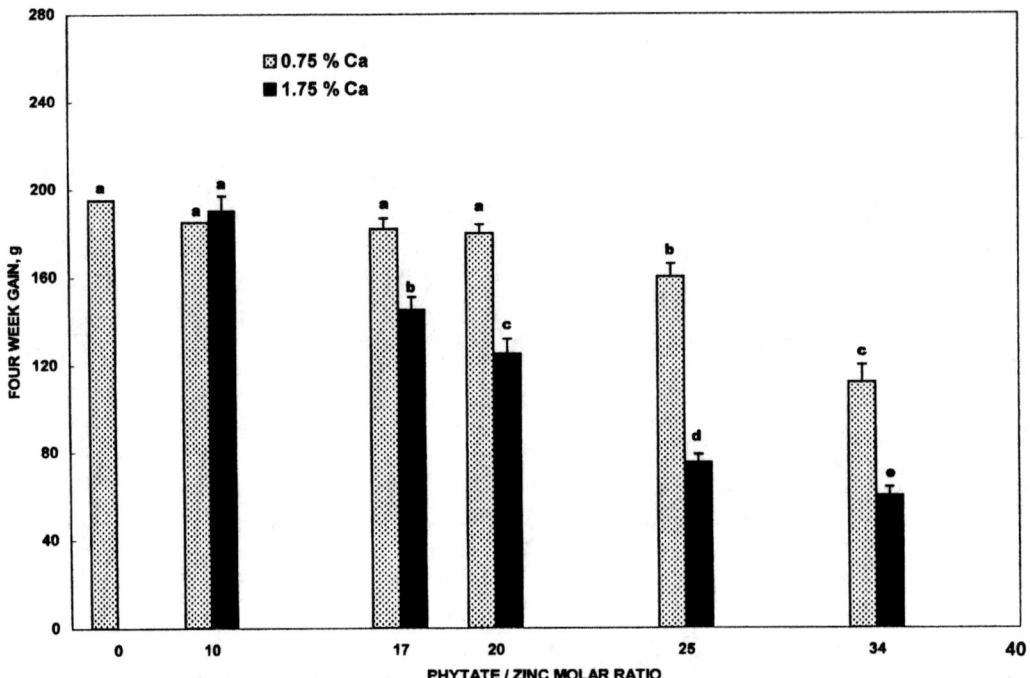

FIGURE 12.2 Effect on growth of rats of dietary phytate/zinc molar ratio in diets of constant phytate concentration (experiment 3). All diets except the comparison diet (ratio 0) contained 6.25 g phytate (approximately 9.6 mmol) per kilogram as sodium phytate. The comparison diet contained 12 ppm zinc as $ZnSO_4 \cdot 7H_2O$, which was also added to the diets to attain the respective ratios. Total zinc concentrations were 60, 36, 30, 24, and 18 ppm, respectively, for ratios 10, 17, 20, and 34. Each bar represents mean ± SE gain of seven or eight rats, and bars that do not share a common superscript differ significantly by Duncan's multiple-range test, $P < 0.05$. (From Morris and Ellis, *J. Nutr.*, 110:1037, 1980.)

The classical work of O'Dell and Savage (1960) demonstrated the impact of phytic acid on Zn requirements. Utilizing ^{65}Zn, Heth and Hoekstra (1965) reported that Ca significantly decreased the percentage of Zn absorbed while increasing femur Zn and decreasing Zn in the liver, kidney, and muscle. Morris and Ellis (1980) reported that the Zn requirement was 2.5 to 5 times greater as the phytate:Zn molar ratio increased beyond 12, but this is also influenced by the Ca content in the diet (Figure 12.2; Morris and Ellis, 1980). The interaction among Ca, Zn, and phytate is extremely important as one observes dietary Ca intakes escalating in the swine industry, whereas trace elements are being reduced in diets.

Other factors known to affect the intraluminal environment of the gastrointestinal tract are Fe, folic acid, vitamin B_6, sugars, and solutes. The three-way interaction of Zn, Cu, and Fe has become more evident in recent years, but the mechanism other than a role for metallothionein has been elusive. It has been demonstrated in humans that excessive Fe (10 or 5:1 Fe:Zn) regardless of form inhibits Zn absorption (Valberg et al., 1984). While very high Zn intakes will reduce Cu absorption, the reverse does not seem to be true.

Folic acid and Zn interact in the gut lumen of the rat (Ghishan et al., 1986) resulting in a mutual inhibition at the site of intestinal transport (mucosal to serosal transfer). Women depleted of vitamin B_6 have increased Zn absorption and retention, but serum Zn declines (Turnland et al., 1991). It is possible that the increased Zn absorbed is not biologically available so transport and enzyme activities are not altered. However, it should be kept in mind that serum Zn is a poor indicator of status except in an extreme deficiency or toxicity state.

Research with 7- to 10-day-old pigs indicates that the presence of resistant and digestible starch does not alter Zn absorption (Morais et al., 1996). Sugars with known active transport systems (glucose and galactose) reduce the appearance of Zn in the blood. However, this does not occur with passively absorbed sugars (fructose and mannitol; Chikosi et al., 1985). Steinhardt and Adibi (1984) observed that Zn absorption was stimulated by glucose and a mixture of glycylleucine but a mixture of glycine and leucine had no effect. However, Watkins et al. (1989) reported that Zn inhibited glucose uptake by reducing its affinity for its sodium–glucose co-transporter. Steinhardt and Adibi (1984) also noted that Zn inhibited the net absorption of sodium and water in the jejunum.

The above discussion has focused on the digestive tract, but Keen and Hurley (1977) reported that plasma Zn increased within 24 h following $ZnCl_3$ application to a decimated area of Zn-deficient pregnant rats. The value of this absorptive technique might be useful in disease states where the gastrointestinal tract is compromised.

The impact of physiological state on Zn absorption has not been elucidated in the pig. However, fractional Zn absorption in women was higher in lactation than in gestation, but only if the women were not taking an Fe supplement (Fung et al., 1997). Zinc concentration in milk is highest in colostrum and decreases and remains constant in week 1 to 3 of lactation (Hill et al., 1983b).

Tremblay et al. (1989) reported that sows had higher serum Zn concentrations at breeding than at weaning or 30-day postbreeding. However, Girard et al. (1996) did not observe any changes in serum Zn during gestation or lactation in first-parity sows. In second-parity sows, a higher serum Zn concentration at breeding resulted in a greater decrease in Zn concentration at week 5 and 10 than was observed for parity-one sows. This research indicates that Zn status may be affected by parity.

Advancing age is known to alter absorption of nutrients, and Zn ileal absorptive capacity is reduced 50% in aging rats (Teillet et al., 1995). Implications of this decrease for the swine industry may be limited; however as attempts are made to increase the number of parities for sows, nutrient requirements may be increased because of reduced absorptive capacity. No work has been done in this area with swine.

Wang et al. (1993) reported that dexamethasone therapy in pigs increased Zn uptake and decreased Zn efflux rate across brush border membrane vesicles. Swine producers sometimes use dexamethasone in small neonatal pigs.

C. Transport

Zinc that enters the enterocyte may be used within the cell, remain in the cell bound to metallothionein, or pass through the basolateral membrane into the plasma (Solomons and Rosenberg, 1984). Dietary pharmacological concentrations of Zn (3000 ppm) have been shown by Carlson et al. (1999) to increase the metallothionein concentration in the enterocytes of nursery pigs resulting in increased Zn bound to this protein. This Zn is lost as the cells are sloughed in the rapid turnover in the gut.

Approximately 94% of newly absorbed Zn crossing the basolateral membrane is transported by albumin (Smith et al., 1978). However, other components of transport are α-2 macroglobulin, transferrin, and immunoglobulin G. Cysteine and histidine loosely bind 2 to 8% of the Zn in circulation in a histidine–zinc–cysteine complex.

Uptake of Zn into tissues seems to be related to tissue need and storage roles of various organs. The synthesis of certain Zn-requiring enzymes may increase Zn entry or exit into organs via a Zn transporter protein described by Palmiter and Findley (1995) and called ZnT-1. McMahon and Cousins (1998) noted that the ZnT-1 rat gene seemed to be responsible for mammalian resistance to high concentrations of extracellular Zn, and they classified its role as an exporter. The Zn T-1 is believed to be associated with the plasma membrane, and it will efflux Zn in a nonsodium- and nonenergy-dependent manner when the Zn supply is elevated. The expression of ZnT-1 is high in the duodenum and jejunum of rats fed high Zn, but not in the ileum and colon. It has been found in the basolateral surface of rat enterocytes lining the villi and in renal tubular cells, but not in intestinal goblet cells or cells within the lamina propria.

Palmiter and Findley (1995) also identified a second Zn transporter protein, ZnT-2, which is shorter than ZnT-1 with only 26% homology. This transporter does not have an identified physiological role and seems to function in vesicular Zn uptake or cellular export in several organs. Another Zn transport protein, ZnT-3, is found in the brain and testis, and ZnT-4 seems to have a role in the brain and mammary glands.

Some transport proteins seem to have transport capabilities with several minerals. An example is DCT 1. Its mRNA is highest in the lining of crypts and lower villi of enterocytes and lower in villi tips. Its expression seems to increase during an Fe deficiency; yet it has a role in Zn transport. As such, this protein may have a role in the Zn–Fe interaction. Sillard et al. (1993) isolated a cysteine-rich peptide (ZF-1) from porcine intestine that is homologous to the Zn-finger motif, and it may also have a role in mineral transport.

Mobilization of Zn during times of dietary deficiency is not likely to occur from muscle, brain, lungs, and heart. Some will be released from liver and kidney, but bone Zn is very slowly mobilized and only a limited amount will be released (Zhou et al., 1993; Bobilya et al., 1994). Hence, during times of deficiency, the catabolism of Zn containing less essential metalloproteins in muscle and soft tissues may be used to provide Zn when critically needed for life. The role of the previously described transport proteins may be extremely crucial in such times.

D. Functions

Zinc has a functional role in metalloenzymes, such as Zn oxidoreductases, hydrolases, lyases, isomerases, transferases, and ligases. Other roles include gene expression, cell replication, membrane and cytoskeletal stabilization, and hormone structure.

1. Enzymes

The diversity of Zn enzymes can be illustrated by discussing a few of the better known enzymes. Carbonic anhydrase, which is found in the red blood cell, is essential for life because of its role in the disposal of carbon dioxide. As such, changes in Zn status have no effect on its presence. Hence, it is a protected enzyme.

Alkaline phosphatase contains four Zn ions per molecule with two required for activity. This enzyme has several isozymes and lacks substrate specificity for its role in hydrolyzing monoesters of phosphates from various compounds, including those involved in bone metabolism. Alkaline phosphatase is sometimes used as an indicator of Zn status because its activity decreases during Zn deficiency, but its activity is not well correlated with subtle changes in Zn status. Many factors affect the activity of alkaline phosphatase other than Zn status. These factors include fasting (Chua and Shrago, 1978), age (Long et al., 1965), storage time of serum (Long et al., 1965), feeding high levels of Zn (Hill and Miller, 1983), and the type of tissue sampled (Goode et al., 1965).

Other Zn metalloenzymes include the following. Carboxypeptidase A is secreted by the pancreas into the duodenum to digest proteins. Its activity decreases during Zn deficiency. Alcohol dehydrogenase contains four Zn ions, and it converts alcohols to aldehydes, such as retinol to retinal that is needed for vision, hence the metabolic connection between Zn and vitamin A. Its activity will change during Zn deficiency, but it does not respond to minor changes in Zn status. The Zn in δ-aminolevulinic acid dehydratase maintains the free thiols in this enzyme, which are essential for heme synthesis. The SOD enzyme, which requires two atoms of Cu and two atoms of Zn, converts the oxygen radical, superoxide, into hydrogen peroxide and oxygen. Activity of this enzyme may be more reflective of Cu status than Zn status.

Angiotensin-converting enzyme (dipeptidyl carboxypeptidase I) is often used to monitor steroid and hypertensive drug therapies. Zinc is necessary for activation of this enzyme, and feeding a Zn-deficient diet to rats for 4 days will decrease its activity by 79% (Reeves and O'Dell, 1985).

More recently, 5′-nucleotidase, a Zn-dependent enzyme, has been used as an indicator of mild Zn deficiency in humans (Meftah et al., 1991). This enzyme may be one of the important links to the observed immune insufficiency during a Zn deficiency, but it has not been measured in pigs.

2. Immunity

Zinc is essential for cell-mediated immunity and host defense. The impact of a Zn deficiency on immunity is discussed in the Zn deficiency section, and immunity is the topic of Chapter 24.

3. Tissue Growth and Integrity

Tissue synthesis requires Zn, and a moderate deficiency will impair growth within a short period of time. The role of Zn in protein synthesis includes its function in the synthesis and catabolism of nucleic acids as well as polysome conformation, recycling of thymine, catabolism of RNA, assisting in the regulation of the transcription process, and perhaps others. Zinc metalloenzymes involved in these processes include DNA and RNA polymerases, deoxythymidine kinase, deoxynucleotidyl tranferase, nucleoside phosphorylase, and reverse transcriptase.

Compensatory gain during recovery from undernutrition in the suckling period was characterized by a disproportionately high fat gain in rat pups fed marginal Zn diets (Morgan et al., 1988). However, if Zn was adequate in the diet, body composition that occurred during compensatory gain was normal.

The effect of Zn on membrane integrity and conformation may be due to its effect on protein synthesis and the activity of Zn-containing enzymes. Protection of lipids and stabilization of phospholipids and thiol groups is provided by SOD, which requires Zn and Cu, as it functions to protect against peroxidative damage.

4. Growth Stimulant at Pharmacological Concentrations

As early as 1988, European researchers reported that pharmacological concentrations of Zn provided as ZnO stimulated growth in the nursery, and they hypothesized its mode of action was the control of *Escherichia coli* scours (Holm, 1990; Poulsen, 1995). The benefit of Zn supplementation in the nursery has been documented by several researchers (Smith et al., 1997; Carlson et al., 1999; Hill et al., 2000), but the mode of action is still unknown. Jensen-Waern et al. (1998) reported that *E. coli* numbers in excreted fecal material were not altered by dietary pharmacological concentrations of Zn. However, the improvement in villus height and the increase in intestinal metallothionein concentration reported by Carlson et al. (1999) in pigs fed 3000 ppm Zn may be related to the role of Zn in protein synthesis and integrity. Feeding the weanling pig is discussed in Chapter 31.

E. Deficiency

Failure to eat, grow, reproduce, accompanied by alopecia, gross skin lesions, poor wound healing, and impaired brain development are major characteristics of Zn deficiency. Deficiency of Zn can be induced when the concentration of one or more nutrients is increased beyond the requirements. An example would be overfeeding of Ca with adequate Zn in the diet, which would decrease the Zn available for bodily functions (see Figure 12.2).

1. Growth and Appetite

As early as 1934, reduced growth as a result of feeding a Zn-deficient diet was reported in the rat (Todd et al., 1934). However, because animals fed a Zn-deficient diet have a reduced appetite, growth as an indicator of deficiency is confounded by reduced feed intake. Hence, when Zn-deficient diets are fed by researchers, additional animals should also be fed the Zn-adequate diet at the same rate of consumption as the animals fed the Zn-deficient diet. This practice is referred to as pair-feeding. The reduced appetite is because Zn is a component of gustin, a protein involved in taste acuity (Shatzman and Henkin, 1981).

The importance of Zn in normal growth is due to its function in many metalloenzymes associated with RNA, DNA, and protein synthesis. Zinc is a necessary structural component of DNA-binding proteins, which due to their shape are referred to as "Zn fingers." The configuration is a result of cysteine and histine residues being twisted and coiled in the protein. Without adequate Zn, nucleic acid synthesis is decreased, thymine is not conserved, and catabolism of RNA is altered. Also, during Zn deficiency, there is a decrease in insulin response and altered glucose tolerance in experimental animals.

2. Reproduction

Liptrap et al. (1970) reported that boars have a higher Zn requirement than barrows or gilts. However, quantitation of the Zn requirement of boars, especially during times of high semen collection, has not been reported. Atrophy of the seminiferous tubules and testicular germinal epithelium accompanied by retarded development of the testes, epididymis, prostate, and pituitary glands has been observed in Zn-deficient males in many species. When Zn is not adequate post-pubertally, damage may be irreversible (Mason et al., 1982). Wegger and Palludan (1977) found degeneration of testes, lack of spermatogenesis, and an increase in connective tissue in the Leydig cells in boars fed a Zn-deficient diet for 10 weeks.

The impact of Zn-deficient diets in the female seems to depend on age, Zn status, physiological state, and its timing, severity, and duration. Monkeys fed a Zn-deficient diet failed to conceive (Swenerton and Hurley, 1980). Wegger and Palludan (1977) noted that Zn deficiency during the last trimester of pregnancy resulted in delayed farrowing. Litter size and birth weight were not affected, but pig viability was decreased.

As with Cu, serum or plasma Zn concentration as an indicator of status during reproduction may not be valid, as previously discussed relative to parity.

3. Immunity

Zinc has a role in both the cellular and molecular mechanisms of immunity, and the effect on the immune system of a deficiency of Zn has been well studied in experimental animals. Few scientific studies are available relative to farm species (Chapter 24). In rodents, a rapid atrophy of the thymus gland, especially in the cortical area, lymphopenia, delayed hypersensitivity, and impaired T-cell helper and natural killer cell functions are all signs of compromised immune function during Zn deficiency. The Zn-deficient mouse can reconstruct the thymus gland and restore T-cell-dependent, antibody-mediated responses upon Zn repletion (Fraker et al., 1978).

Recently, Telford and Fraker (1998) have shown that Zn may induce apoptosis in some cells (B220 IgM+ B-lineage cells of bone marrow and IgM+ B-cells) of the spleen and of the immune system.

4. Metallothionein

This protein has a low molecular weight with an exceptionally high content of cysteine, no aromatic amino acids, and binds a number of elements, including Cu and Zn. Its primary role is unknown, but it is involved in mineral homeostasis in mammals. When approximately 30 ppm of hepatic Zn accumulates, hepatic metallothionein synthesis is initiated. It is thought that Zn metabolism is regulated by the synthesis of intestinal and hepatic metallothionein. The movement of Zn from mucosal cells is dependent on the amount of Zn in these cells. When Zn concentration increases, more metallothionein is synthesized, which reduces the amount of Zn that enters the plasma. Conversely, less Zn results in less metallothionein being produced, resulting in a greater proportion of mucosal Zn entering the plasma. Gallant and Cherian (1987) reported that hepatic metallothionein concentrations fluctuate in response to the Zn dietary concentrations in rats. Even though Bremner and Young (1976) isolated hepatic thioneins that bind Zn and Cu from the pig, the impact of different dietary Zn intakes on hepatic metallothionein concentrations has not been determined. However, Carlson et al. (1999) noted that intestinal and hepatic metallothionein concentrations increased in nursery pigs fed 3000 ppm Zn compared with those fed 150 ppm.

Hepatic Zn is high in the neonate, which has led researchers to investigate the role of metallothionein in placental Zn transfer. Lindsay et al. (1994) reported an increased rate of Zn transfer from the dam to the rat fetus, which is accelerated at day 18. Zinc is transferred across the placenta, and is secreted into fetal plasma, and taken up by the fetal liver, where metallothionein synthesis is stimulated.

During Zn deficiency, Blalock et al. (1988) noted a tissue-specific regulation of metallothionein gene expression in response to dietary Zn. Metallothionein mRNA is reduced in the liver when dietary Zn is deficient.

F. Toxicity

Most of the chronic toxic effects of Zn result from the induction of a Cu deficiency, whereas acute toxicity is often due to mixing errors or ingestion of an acidic feed or food prepared in a galvanized container. As with deficiency, the Zn status, age, physiological state, timing, duration, sex, and species as well as the source of the Zn all influence the occurrence and severity of Zn toxicity. The veterinary diagnostic toxicology laboratory in Ontario reported 887 cases of metal toxicosis in domestic animals, of which 49 were due to Zn, but none occurred in pigs (Hoff et al., 1998). This clearly illustrates that the occurrence of Zn toxicity is not a major problem in the swine industry, even though 90 to 95% of the nursery pigs in the United States are fed 2000 to 3000 ppm Zn.

Brink et al. (1959) determined that the level of Zn tolerance in the pig was 1000 ppm Zn when Zn was provided as carbonate, and that 2000 ppm was toxic. They observed a depression in gain, feed intake and efficiency, gastritis, severe bone and cartilage abnormalities, as well as extensive hemorrhage in the axillary spaces, ventricles of the brain, lymph nodes, and spleen. However, others fed 4000 ppm Zn as ZnO and found none of the above signs of toxicity. Hill et al. (1983c) fed 5000 ppm Zn as ZnO to gilts from 30 kg until the completion of two parities. They reported a greater number of abnormal pigs per litter and fewer and lighter-weight pigs were weaned from sows fed 5000 ppm than from sows fed an additional 0, 50, or 500 ppm supplemented Zn. The concentration of Zn in the liver, kidney, and aorta was increased, and hepatic and aortic Cu and hepatic Fe were decreased in sows fed 5000 ppm. Similar to Brink's findings, osteochondrosis was higher in sows fed 5000 ppm Zn. Clearly, the range from Zn deficiency to toxicity is very wide in the pig and dependent not only on amount consumed but also form.

IX. OTHER TRACE ELEMENTS

Research suggests that a number of other trace minerals including molybdenum (Mo), arsenic (As), boron (B), nickel (Ni), silicon (Si), and vanadium (V) are required at low concentrations (Nielsen, 1996). Many of these minerals have not been studied in swine.

Molybdenum functions as a component of the enzymes xanthine oxidase and sulfite oxidase (Nielsen, 1996). Molybdenum deficiency has been developed in pigs fed diets containing 0.02 ppm of Mo (Anke and Risch, 1989). Signs of deficiency noted were decreased growth and feed intake and impaired reproduction. No evidence is available to suggest that Mo deficiency occurs in swine fed practical diets.

Mammalian functions for the other trace minerals listed above have not been identified. Bacterial urease has been shown to be a Ni metalloenzyme. In young pigs, the addition of supplemental (5 or 25 ppm) Ni to diets containing 0.12 to 0.16 ppm of Ni did not affect growth or bacterial urease activity in the lower gut (Spears et al., 1984). However, the addition of 5 ppm of Ni to the basal diet increased liver Fe and Zn concentrations at 21 days of age.

Boron was recently studied in nursery pigs (Armstrong et al., 1999). The addition of 5 or 15 ppm of B to a corn–soybean meal–based diet containing 6.7 ppm of B did not affect performance or bone characteristics. However, feed efficiency and bone breaking strength were improved when 5 ppm of B was added to a semipurified diet containing 1.0 ppm of B.

REFERENCES

Allcroft, R. K., N. Burns, and G. Lewis. 1961. The effects of high levels of copper in rations for pigs, *Vet. Rec.*, 73:714.

Allen, L. H., and N. W. Solomons. 1984. Copper. In *Current Topics in Nutrition and Disease*, Vol. 12: *Absorption and Malabsorption of Mineral Nutrients*, Solomons, N. W., and I. H. Rosenberg, Eds., Alan R. Liss, New York, 199.

Amoikon, E. K., J. M. Fernandez, L. L. Southern, D. L. Thompson, Jr., T. L. Ward, and B. M. Olcott. 1995. Effect of chromium tripicolinate on growth, glucose tolerance, insulin sensitivity, plasma metabolites, and growth hormone in pigs, *J. Anim. Sci.*, 73:1123.

Analytical Methods Committee. 1960. Methods for the destruction of organic matter, *Analyst*, 85:643.

Anderson, M. A., J. R. McKenna, D. C. Martens, S. J. Donohue, E. T. Kornegay, and M. D. Lindemann. 1991. Long-term effects of copper rich swine manure application on continuous corn production, *Commun. Soil Sci. Plant Anal.*, 22:993.

Anderson, R. A. 1994. Stress effects on chromium nutrition of humans and farm animals. In *Biotechnology in the Feed Industry*, Lyons, T. P., and K. A. Jacques, Eds., Nottingham University, Leicestershire, 267.

Anderson, R. A., and A. S. Kozlovsky. 1985. Chromium intake, absorption and excretion of subjects consuming self-selected diets, *Am. J. Clin. Nutr.*, 41:1177.

Anderson, R. A., N. A. Bryden, C. M. Evock-Clover, and N. C. Steele. 1997a. Beneficial effects of chromium on glucose and lipid variables in control and somatotropin-treated pigs are associated with increased tissue chromium and altered tissue copper, iron, and zinc, *J. Anim. Sci.*, 75:657.

Anderson, R. A., N. A. Bryden, and M. M. Polansky. 1997b. Lack of toxicity of chromium chloride and chromium picolinate in rats, *J. Am. Coll. Nutr.*, 16:273.

Anke, M., and M. A. Risch. 1989. Importance of molybdenum in animal and man. In *6th International Trace Element Symposium*, Anke, M., W. Baumann, and H. Braunlich, Eds., Friedrich-Schiller-Universität, Jena, 303.

Aoyagi, S., and D. H. Baker. 1994. Copper-amino acid complexes are partially protected against inhibitory effects of L-cysteine and L-ascorbic acid on copper absorption in chicks, *J. Nutr.*, 124:388.

Apgar, G. A., E. T. Kornegay, M. D. Lindemann, and D. R. Notter. 1995. Evaluation of copper sulfate and copper lysine complexes as growth promoters for weanling swine, *J. Anim. Sci.*, 73:2640.

Apgar, G. A., and E. T. Kornegay. 1996. Mineral balance of finishing pigs fed copper sulfate or a copper-lysine complex at growth-stimulating levels, *J. Anim. Sci.*, 74:1594.

Armstrong, T. A., J. W. Spears, and L. F. Stikeleather. 1999. Effect of boron supplementation on bone characteristics and plasma mineral concentrations in young pigs, *J. Anim. Sci.*, 77(Suppl. 1):196 (Abstr.).

Arrington, L. R., R. N. Taylor, Jr., C. B. Ammerman, and R. L. Shirley. 1965. Effects of excess dietary iodine upon rabbits, hamsters, rats and swine, *J. Nutr.*, 87:394.

Arthur, J. R., F. Nicol, and G. J. Becket. 1990. Hepatic iodothyronine 5-deiodinase, *Biochem. J.*, 272:537.

Bal, W., J. Christodoulou, P. J. Sadler, and A. Tucker. 1998. Multi-metal binding site of serum albumin, *J. Inorg. Biochem.*, 70:33.

Bala, S., J. K. Lunney, and M. L. Failla. 1992. Effects of copper deficiency on T-cell mitogenic responsiveness and phenotypic profile of blood mononuclear cells from swine, *Am. J. Vet. Res.*, 53:1231.

Bannister, J. V., W. H. Bannister, and G. Rotilio. 1987. Aspects of the structure, function and applications of superoxide dismutase, *CRC Crit. Rev. Biochem.*, 22:111.

Barber, R. S., R. Braude, D. G. Mitchell, J. A. Rock, and J. G. Rowell. 1957. Further studies on antibiotic and copper supplements for fattening pigs, *Br. J. Nutr.*, 11:70.

Bettger, W. J., T. J. Fish, and B. L. O'Dell. 1978. Effects of copper and zinc status of rats on erythrocyte stability and superoxide dismutase activity, *Proc. Soc. Exp. Biol. Med.*, 158:279.

Birnstingl, M., B. Stone, and V. Richards. 1956. Excretion of radioactive zinc (^{65}Zn) in bile, pancreatic and duodenal secretions of the dog, *Am. J. Phys.*, 186:377.

Blalock, T. L., M. A. Dunn, and R. J. Cousins. 1988. Metallothionein gene expression in rats: tissue-specific regulation by dietary copper and zinc, *J. Nutr.*, 118:222.

Bobilya, D. J., G. L. Johanning, T. L. Veum, and B. L. O'Dell. 1994. Chronological loss of bone zinc during dietary zinc deprivation in neonatal pigs, *Am. J. Clin. Nutr.*, 59:649.

Boleman, S. L., S. J. Boleman, T. D. Bidner, L. L. Southern, T. L. Ward, J. E. Pontif, and M. M. Pike. 1995. Effect of chromium picolinate on growth, body composition, and tissue accretion in pigs, *J. Anim. Sci.*, 73:2033.

Bowland, J. P., R. Braude, A. G. Chamberlain, R. F. Glascock, and K. G. Mitchell. 1961. The absorption, distribution and excretion of labeled copper in young pigs given different quantities, as sulphate or sulphide, orally or intravenously, *Br. J. Nutr.*, 15:59.

Braude, R. 1948. Some observations on the behaviour of pigs in an experimental piggery, *Bul. Anim. Behav.*, 6:967.

Bremner, I., and B. W. Young. 1976. Isolation of (copper, zinc)-thioneins from pig liver, *Biochem. J.*, 155:631.

Brink, M. F., D. E. Becker, S. W. Terrill, and A. H. Jensen. 1959. Zinc toxicity in the weanling pig, *J. Anim. Sci.*, 18:836.

Bush, J. A., J. P. Mahoney, C. J. Gubler, G. E. Cartwright, and M. M. Wintrobe. 1956. Studies on copper metabolism XXI. The transfer of radiocopper between erythrocytes and plasma, *J. Lab. Clin. Med.*, 47:898.

Campbell, C. H., R. Brown, and M. C. Linder. 1981. Circulating ceruloplasmin is an important source for normal and malignant cells, *Biochim. Biophys. Acta*, 678:27.

Cao, J., and E. R. Chavez. 1995. Comparative trace mineral nutritional balance of first-litter gilts under two dietary levels of copper intake, *J. Trace Elem. Med. Biol.*, 9:102.

Carlson, M. S., S. L. Hoover, G. M. Hill, J. E. Link, and T. L. Ward. 1997. The impact of organic and inorganic sources of zinc supplementation on intestinal metallothionein concentration in the nursery pig, *J. Anim. Sci.*, 75 (Suppl. 1):188 (Abstr.).

Carlson, M. S., G. M. Hill, and J. E. Link. 1999. Early- and traditionally weaned nursery pigs benefit from phase-feeding pharmacological concentrations of zinc oxide: effect on metallothionein and mineral concentrations, *J. Anim. Sci.*, 77:1199.

Chang, I. C., T. Lee, and G. Matrone. 1975. Development of ceruloplasmin in pigs during the neonatal period, *J. Nutr.*, 105:624.

Chikosi, S. F., D. McMaster, and A. H. G. Lowe. 1985. Absorption and transport of zinc by the mammalian gut: influence of the presence of some sugars in the lumen, *Nutr. Res. Suppl.*, 1:259.

Christianson, S. L., E. R. Peo, Jr., and A. J. Lewis. 1989. Effects of dietary manganese levels on reproductive performance of sows, *J. Anim. Sci.*, 67(Suppl. 1):251 (Abstr.).

Christianson, S. L., E. R. Peo, Jr., A. J. Lewis, and M. A. Giesemann. 1990. Influence of dietary manganese levels on reproduction, serum cholesterol, and milk manganese concentration of sows, *J. Anim. Sci.*, 68(Suppl. 1):368 (Abstr.).

Chua, B., and E. Shrago. 1978. Effects of experimental diabetes and food intake on rat intestine and serum alkaline phosphatase, *J. Nutr.*, 108:196.

Clydesdale, F. M. 1988. Mineral interactions in foods. In *Nutrient Interactions*, Bodwell, C. E., and J. W. Erdman, Jr., Eds., Marcel Dekker, New York, chap. 3.

Combs, G. E., C. B. Ammerman, R. L. Shirley, and H. D. Wallace. 1966. Effects of source and level of dietary protein on pigs fed high-copper rations, *J. Anim. Sci.*, 25:613.

Cordano, A., R. P. Placko, and G. G. Graham. 1968. Hypocupremia and neutropenia in copper deficiency, *Blood*, 22:280.

Cornelius, S. G., and B. G. Harmon. 1976. Sources of oral iron for neonatal piglets, *J. Anim. Sci.*, 42(Suppl. 1):1350 (Abstr.).

Coulson, W. F., and W. H. Carnes. 1967. Cardiovascular studies on copper-deficient swine. IX. Repair of vascular defects in deficient swine treated with copper, *Am. J. Pathol.*, 50:861.

Cromwell, G. L., D. T. H. Schombing, and V. W. Hays. 1975. Effects of iodine level on performance and thyroid traits of growing pigs, *J. Anim. Sci.*, 41:813.

Cromwell, G. L., T. S. Stahly, and J. H. Monegue. 1989. Effects of source and level of copper on performance and liver copper stores in weanling pigs, *J. Anim. Sci.*, 67:2996.

Cromwell, G. L., M. D. Lindemann, H. J. Monegue, D. D. Hall, and D. E. Orr, Jr. 1998. Tribasic copper chloride and copper sulfate as copper sources for weanling pigs, *J. Anim. Sci.*, 76:118.

Cunnane, S. C. 1984. Essential fatty-acid/mineral interactions with reference to the pig. In *Proceedings of Easter School of Agriculture Science University of Nottingham*, Vol. 37, Butterworths, London, chap. 8.

Das, D. K., D. Flansaas, R. M. Engelman, J. A. Rousou, R. H. Breyer, R. Jones, S. Lemeshow, and H. Otani. 1987. Age-related development profiles of the antioxidative defense system and the peroxidative status of the pig heart, *Biol. Neonate*, 51:156.

Davis, G. K. 1980. Microelement interactions of zinc, copper and iron in mammalian species, *Ann. N.Y. Acad. Sci.*, 77:130.

De Rosa, G., C. L. Keen, R. L. Leach, and L. S. Hurley. Regulation of superoxide dismutase activity by dietary manganese, *J. Nutr.*, 110:795.

Devilat, J., and A. Skoknic. 1971. Feeding high levels of rapeseed meal to pregnant gilts, *Can. J. Anim. Sci.*, 51:715.

Dove, C. R., and K. D. Haydon. 1992. The effect of copper and fat addition to the diets of weanling swine on growth performance and serum fatty acids, *J. Anim. Sci.*, 70:805.

Dowling, T. G., S. Cambi, and F. Buffoni. 1998. Semicarbazide-sensitive amine oxidase in pig heart, *J. Neural Transm.*, 105 (Suppl. 52):265.

Ehnis, L. R., G. M. Hill, J. E. Link, J. B. Barber, and D. R. Hawkins. 1996. Impact of physiological state and breed on long term copper status of cattle, *J. Anim. Sci.*, 74 (Suppl. 1):182 (Abstr.).

Evock-Clover, C. M., M. M. Polansky, R. A. Anderson, and N. C. Steele. 1993. Dietary chromium supplementation with or without somatotropin treatment alters serum hormones and metabolites in growing pigs without affecting growth performance, *J. Nutr.*, 123:1504.

Finley, J. W., J. S. Caton, Z. Zhow, and K. L. Davison. 1997. A surgical model for determination of true absorption and biliary excretion of manganese in conscious swine fed commercial diets, *J. Nutr.*, 127:2334.

Fischer, P. W. F., and M. R. L'Abbé. 1985. Copper transport by intestinal brush border membrane vesicles from rats fed high zinc or copper deficient diets, *Nutr. Res.*, 5:759.

Fraker, P. J., P. DePasquale-Jardieu, C. M. Zwickl, and R. W. Luecke. 1978. Regeneration of T-cell helper function in zinc-deficient adult mice, *Proc. Nat. Acad. Sci. U.S.A.*, 75:5660.

Fung, E. B., L. D. Ritchie, L. R. Woodhouse, R. Roehl, and J. C. King. 1997. Zinc absorption in women during pregnancy and lactation: a longitudinal study, *Am. J. Clin. Nutr.*, 66:80.

Furugouri, K. 1972. Effect of elevated dietary levels of iron on iron stores in liver, some blood constituents and phosphorus deficiency in young swine, *J. Anim. Sci.*, 34:573.

Galan, P., F. Cherouvrier, P. Preziosi, and S. Hercberg. 1991. Effects of the increasing consumption of dairy products upon iron absorption, *Eur. J. Clin. Nutr.*, 45:553.

Gallant, K. R., and M. G. Cherian. 1987. Changes in dietary zinc result in specific alterations of metallothionein concentrations in newborn rat liver, *J. Nutr.*, 117:709.

Gamble, C. T., S. L. Hansard, B. R. Moss, D. J. Davis, and E. R. Lidvall. 1971. Manganese utilization and placental transfer in the gravid gilt, *J. Anim. Sci.*, 32:84.

Ghishan, F. K., H. M. Said, P. C. Wilson, J. E. Murrell, and H. L. Greene. 1986. Intestinal transport of zinc and folic acid: a mutual inhibitory effect, *Am. J. Clin. Nutr.*, 43:258.

Girard, C. L., S. Robert, J. J. Matte, C. Farmer, and G. P. Martineau. 1996. Serum concentration of micronutrients, packed cell volume, and blood hemoglobin during the first two gestations and lactations of sows, *Can. J. Vet. Res.*, 60:170.

Gíslason, J., S. Iyer, G. C. Douglas, T. W. Hutchens, and B. Lönnerdal. 1994. Binding of porcine milk lactoferrin to piglet intestinal lactoferrin receptor. In *Lactoferrin Structure and Function*, Hutchens, T. W., S. V. Rumball, and B. Lönnerdal, Eds., Plenum Press, New York, 239.

Goode, L., A. C. Warnick, and H. D. Wallace. 1965. Alkaline and acid phosphatase activity in the endometrium and ovary of swine, *J. Anim. Sci.*, 24:955.

Graitcer, P. L., J. B. Goldsby, and M. Z. Nichaman. 1981. Hemoglobins and hematocrits: are they equally sensitive in detecting anemias? *Am. J. Clin. Nutr.*, 34:61.

Grummer, R. H., O. G. Bentley, P. H. Phillips, and G. Bohstedt. 1950. The role of manganese in growth, reproduction, and lactation, *J. Anim. Sci.*, 9:170.

Harris, E. D. 1992. New insights into placental iron transport, *Nutr. Rev.*, 50:329.

Hearing, V. J., and K. Tsukamoto. 1991. Enzymatic control of pigmentation in mammals, *FASEB J.*, 5:2902.

Heth, D. A., and W. G. Hoekstra. 1965. Zinc-65 absorption and turnover in rats: a procedure to determine zinc-65 absorption and the antagonistic effect of calcium in a practical diet, *J. Nutr.*, 85:367.

Hetzel, B. A., and M. L. Wellby. 1997. Iodine. In *Handbook of Nutritionally Essential Mineral Elements*, O'Dell, B. L., and R. A. Sunde, Eds., Marcel Dekker, New York, chap. 19.

Hill, C. H., and G. Matrone. 1970. Chemical parameters in the study of *in vivo* and *in vitro* interactions of transition elements, *Fed. Proc.*, 29:1474.

Hill, G. M., and E. R. Miller. 1983. Effect of dietary zinc levels on the growth and development of the gilt, *J. Anim. Sci.*, 57:106.

Hill, G. M., P. K. Ku, E. R. Miller, D. E. Ullrey, T. A. Losty, and B. L. O'Dell. 1983a. A copper deficiency in neonatal pigs induced by a high zinc maternal diet, *J. Nutr.*, 113:867.

Hill, G. M., E. R. Miller, and P. K. Ku. 1983b. Effect of dietary zinc levels on mineral concentration in milk, *J. Anim. Sci.*, 57:123.

Hill, G. M., E. R. Miller, and H. D. Stowe. 1983c. Effect of dietary zinc levels on health and productivity of gilts and sows through two parities, *J. Anim. Sci.*, 57:114.

Hill, G. M., E. R. Miller, P. A. Whetter, and D. E. Ullrey. 1983d. Concentration of minerals in tissues of pigs from dams fed different levels of dietary zinc, *J. Anim. Sci.*, 57:130.

Hill, G. M., J. E. Link, L. Meyer, and K. L. Fritsche. 1999. Effect of vitamin E and selenium on iron utilization in neonatal pigs, *J. Anim. Sci.*, 77:1762.

Hill, G. M., G. L. Cromwell, T. D. Crenshaw, R. Dove, R. C. Ewan, D. A. Knabe, A. J. Lewis, G. W. Libal, D. C. Mahan, G. C. Shurson, L. L. Southern, and T. L. Veum. 2000. Growth promotion effects of high dietary concentrations of zinc and copper in weanling pigs, *J. Anim. Sci.*, 78:1010.

Hoff, B., H. J. Boermans, and J. D. Baird. 1998. Retrospective study of toxic metal analyses requested at a veterinary diagnostic toxicology laboratory in Ontario (1990–1995), *Can. Vet. J.*, 39:39.

Holm, A. 1990. *E. coli* associated diarrhea in weaner pigs: zinc oxide added to the feed as a preventative measure, *Proc. Int. Pig Vet. Soc.*, 154.

Huck, D. W., and A. J. Clawson. 1976. Cobalt toxicity in pigs, *J. Anim. Sci.*, 43:253 (Abstr.).

Hurley, L. S. 1983. Teratogenic effects of manganese, zinc, and copper deficiencies. In *Biological Aspects of Metals and Metal-Related Diseases*, Sarjar, B., Ed., Raven Press, New York, 199.

Jackson, M. J., D. A. Jonmes, and H. T. Edwards. 1981. Zinc absorption in the rat, *Br. J. Nutr.*, 46:15.

Jensen-Waern, M., L. Melin, R. Lindberg, A. Johannisson, L. Petersson, and P. Wallgren. 1998. Dietary zinc oxide in weaned pigs — effects on performance, tissue concentrations, morphology, neutrophil functions, and faecal microflora, *Res. Vet. Sci.*, 64:225.

Johnson, C. D., and C. M. Weaver. 1986. Chromium in kale, wheat, and eggs: intrinsic labeling and bioavailability to rats, *J. Agric. Food Chem.*, 34:436.

Keen, C. L., and L. S. Hurley. 1977. Zinc absorption through skin: correction of zinc deficiency in the rat, *Am. J. Clin. Nutr.*, 30:528.

Kerr, L. A., and H. D. McGavin. 1991. Chronic copper poisoning in sheep grazing pastures fertilized with swine manure, *J. Am. Vet. Med. Assoc.*, 198:99.

Klinman, J. P., and M. Brenner. 1988. Role of copper and catalytic mechanism in the copper monooxygenase, dopamine β-hydroxylase. In *Oxidases and Related Redox Systems*, King, T. E., H. S. Mason, and M. Morrison, Eds., Alan R. Liss, New York, 227.

Kornegay, E. T., D. Rhein-Welker, M. D. Lindeman, and C. M. Wood. 1995. Performance and nutrient digestibility in weanling pigs as influenced by yeast culture additions to starter diets containing dried whey or one of two fiber sources, *J. Anim. Sci.*, 73:1381.

Kornegay, E. T., Z. Wang, C. M. Wood, and M. D. Lindemann. 1997. Supplemental chromium picolinate influences nitrogen balance, dry matter digestibility, and carcass traits in growing-finishing pigs, *J. Anim. Sci.*, 75:1319.

Kuhnert, B. R., P. M. Kuhnert, N. Lazebnik, and P. Erhard. 1993. The relationship between placental cadmium, zinc and copper, *J. Am. Coll. Nutr.*, 12:31.

L'Abbé, M. R., and P. W. Fischer. 1984. The effects of high dietary zinc and copper deficiency on the activity of copper-requiring metalloenzymes in the growing rat, *J. Nutr.*, 114:813.

Lahey, M. E., C. J. Grubler, M. S. Chase, G. E. Cartwright, and M. M. Wintrobe. 1952. Studies on copper metabolism II. Hematologic manifestations on copper deficiency in swine, *Blood*, 7:1053.

Leach, R. M., Jr., and E. D. Harris. 1997. Manganese. In *Handbook of Nutritionally Essential Mineral Elements*, O'Dell, B. L., and R. A. Sunde, Eds., Marcel Dekker, New York, chap. 10.

Leibholz, J. M., V. C. Speer, and V. W. Hays. 1962. Effect of dietary manganese on baby pig performance and tissue manganese levels, *J. Anim. Sci.*, 21:772.

Lemacher, S., and H. Bostedt. 1994. Zur Entwicklung der Plasma-Fe-Konzentration und des Hämoglobingehaltes beim Ferkel in den ersten drei Lebenstagen und zur Bedeutung der pränatalen Anämie, *Tierärztl. Prax.*, 22:39.

Lindemann, M. D., C. M. Wood, A. F. Harper, E. T. Kornegay, and R. A. Anderson. 1995. Dietary chromium picolinate additions improve gain:feed and carcass characteristics in growing-finishing pigs and increase litter size in reproducing sows, *J. Anim. Sci.*, 73:457.

Linder, M. C. 1991. *Biochemistry of Copper*, Plenum Press, New York.

Lindsay, Y., L. M. Duthie, and J. J. McCardle. 1994. Zinc levels in the rat fetal liver are not determined by transport across the placental microvillar membrane or the fetal liver plasma membrane, *Biol. Reprod.*, 51:358.

Long, C. H., D. E. Ullrey, and E. R. Miller. 1965. Serum alkaline phosphatase in post-natal pig and effect of serum storage on enzyme activity, *Proc. Soc. Exp. Biol. Med.*, 119:412.

Liptrap, D. O., E. R. Miller, D. E. Ullrey, D. L. Whitenack, B. L. Schoepke, and R. W. Luecke. 1970. Sex influence on the zinc requirement of developing swine, *J. Anim. Sci.*, 30:736.

Macfarlane, B. J., W. B. van der Riet, T. H. Bothwell, R. D. Baynes, D. Siegenberg, U. Schmidt, A. Tal, J. R. Taylor, and F. Mayet. 1990. Effect of traditional Oriental soy products on iron absorption, *Am. J. Clin. Nutr.*, 51:873.

Mas, A., and B. Sarkar. 1988. The metabolism of metals in rat placenta, *Biol. Trace Element Res.*, 18:191.

Mason, K. E., W. A. Burns, and J. C. Smith, Jr. 1982. Testicular damage associated with zinc deficiency in pre- and postpubertal rats: response to zinc repletion, *J. Nutr.*, 112:1019.

Matthews, J. O., L. L. Southern, J. M. Fernandez, A. M. Chapa, L. R. Gentry, and T. D. Bidner. 1997. Effects of dietary chromium tripicolinate or chromium propionate on growth, plasma metabolites, glucose tolerance, and insulin sensitivity in pigs, *J. Anim. Sci.*, 75(Suppl. 1):187 (Abstr.).

McArdle, H. J., and R. Erlich. 1991. Copper uptake and transfer to the mouse fetus during pregnancy, *J. Nutr.*, 121:208.

McMahon, R. J., and R. J. Cousins. 1998. Mammalian zinc transporters, *J. Nutr.*, 128:667.

Meftah, S., A. S. Prasad, D. Lee, and G. Brewer. 1991. Ecto 5′nucleotidase (5′NT) as a sensitive indicator of human zinc deficiency, *Lab. Clin. Med.*, 115:309.

Mertz, W. 1981. The essential trace elements, *Science*, 213:1332.

Mertz, W. 1992. Chromium history and nutritional importance, *Biol. Trace Element Res.*, 32:3.

Miller, E. R. 1973. Copper in growing-finishing rations, Michigan State University Swine Report, East Lansing, MI.

Miller, E. R. 1991. Iron, copper, zinc, manganese, and iodine in swine nutrition. In *Swine Nutrition*, Miller, E. R., D. E. Ullrey, and A. J. Lewis, Eds., Butterworth-Heinemann, Boston, 267.

Milne, D. B., and G. Matrone. 1970. Forms of ceruloplasmin in developing piglets, *Biochim. Biophys. Acta*, 212:43.

Min, J. K., W. Y. Kim, B. J. Chae, I. B. Chung, I. S. Shin, Y. J. Choi, and I. K. Han. 1997. Effects of chromium picolinate on growth performance, carcass characteristics and serum traits in growing-finishing pigs, *Asian Aust. J. Anim. Sci.*, 10:8.

Mooney, K. W., and G. L. Cromwell. 1995. Effects of dietary chromium picolinate supplementation on growth, carcass characteristics, and accretion rates of carcass tissues in growing-finishing swine, *J. Anim. Sci.*, 73:3351.

Mooney, K. W., and G. L. Cromwell. 1997. Efficacy of chromium picolinate and chromium chloride as potential carcass modifiers in swine, *J. Anim. Sci.*, 75:2661.

Mooney, K. W., and G. L. Cromwell. 1999. Efficacy of chromium picolinate on performance and tissue accretion in pigs with different lean gain potential, *J. Anim. Sci.*, 77:1188.

Morais, M. A., A. Feste, R. G. Miller, and C. H. Lifschitz. 1996. Effect of resistant and digestible starch on intestinal absorption of calcium, iron, and zinc in infant pigs, *Pediatr. Res.*, 39:872.

Morgan, P. N., C. L. Keen, and B. Lönnerdal. 1988. Effect of varying dietary zinc intake of weanling mouse pups during recovery from early undernutrition on tissue mineral concentrations, relative organ weights, hematological variables and muscle composition, *J. Nutr.*, 118:699.

Morris, E. R., and R. Ellis. 1980. Effect of dietary phytate/zinc molar ratio on growth and bone zinc response of rats fed semipurified diets, *J. Nutr.*, 110:1037.

Munro, H. 1993. The ferritin genes: their response to iron status, *Nutr. Rev.*, 51:65.
National Research Council. 1980. *Mineral Tolerance of Domestic Animals*, National Academy Press, Washington, D.C.
National Research Council. 1997. *The Role of Chromium in Animal Nutrition*, National Academy Press, Washington, D.C.
National Research Council. 1998. *Nutrient Requirements of Swine*, 10th ed., National Academy Press, Washington, D.C.
Nelson, J. 1985. Bioavailability of trace mineral ingredients, In *Proc. Western Nutr. Conf.*, p. 60.
Newton, G. L., and A. J. Clawson. 1974. Iodine toxicity: physiological effects of elevated dietary iodine on pigs, *J. Anim. Sci.*, 39:879.
Nielsen, F. H. 1984. Ultratrace elements in nutrition, *Annu. Rev. Nutr.*, 4:21.
Nielsen, F. H. 1996. Other trace elements. In *Present Knowledge in Nutrition*, Ziegler, E. E., and L. J. Filer, Jr., Eds., ILSI Press, Washington, D.C.
O'Dell, B. L., and J. E. Savage. 1960. Effects of phytic acid on zinc availability, *Proc. Soc. Exp. Biol. Med.*, 103:304.
Offenbacher, E. T., F. X. Pi-Sunyer, and B. J. Stoecker. 1997. Chromium. In *Handbook of Nutritionally Essential Minerals Elements*, O'Dell, B. L., and R. A. Sunde, Eds., Marcel Dekker, New York.
Page, T. G., L. L. Southern, T. L. Ward, and D. L. Thompson, Jr. 1993. Effect of chromium picolinate on growth and serum and carcass traits of growing-finishing pigs, *J. Anim. Sci.*, 71:656.
Palmiter, R. D., and S. D. Findley. 1995. Cloning and functional characterization of a mammalian zinc transporter that confers resistance to zinc, *EMBO J.*, 14:639.
Percival, S. S. 1998. Copper and immunity, *Am. J. Clin. Nutr.*, 67 (Suppl.):1064S.
Percival, S. S., and E. D. Harris. 1990. Copper transport from ceruloplasmin: characterization of the cellular uptake mechanism, *Am. J. Physiol.*, 258:C140.
Pérez-Llamas, F., M. G. E. Diepenmaat-Wolters, and S. Zamora. 1996. *In vitro* availability of iron and zinc: effects of the type, concentration and fractions of digestion products of the protein, *Br. J. Nutr.*, 76:727.
Plumlee, M. P., D. M. Thrasher, W. M. Beeson, F. N. Andrews, and H. E. Parker. 1956. The effects of a manganese deficiency upon the growth, development, and reproduction of swine, *J. Anim. Sci.*, 15:352.
Pond, W. G., L. P. Krook, and L. M. Klevay. 1990. Bone pathology without cardiovascular lesions in pigs fed high zinc and low copper diet, *Nutr. Res.*, 10:871.
Poulsen, H. D. 1995. Zinc oxide for weanling piglets, *Acta Agric. Scand.*, 45:159.
Reeves, P. G., and B. L. O'Dell. 1985. An experimental study of the effect of zinc on the activity of angiotensin converting enzyme in serum, *Clin. Chem.*, 31:581.
Rheaume, J. A., and T. R. Chavez. 1989. Trace mineral metabolism in non-gravid, gestating and lactating gilts fed two dietary levels of manganese, *J. Trace Elem. Electrolytes Health Dis.*, 3:231.
Roof, M. D., and D. C. Mahan. 1982. Effect of carbadox and various dietary copper levels for weanling swine, *J. Anim. Sci.*, 55:1109.
Sang, Q. A. 1995. Specific proteolysis of ceruloplasmin by leukocyte elastase, *Biochem. Mol. Biol. Int.*, 37:573.
Schoenemann, H. M., M. L. Failla, and R. W. Rosebrough. 1990. Cardiac and splenic levels of norepinephrine and dopamine in copper-deficient pigs and rats, *Comp. Biochem. Physiol.*, 97C:387.
Scholfield, D. J., S. Reiser, M. Fields, N. C. Steele, J. C. Smith, S. Darcy, and K. Ono. 1990. Dietary copper, simple sugars, and metabolic changes in pigs, *J. Nutr. Biochem.*, 1:362.
Schwartz, K., and W. Mertz. 1959. Chromium (III) and the glucose tolerance factor, *Arch. Biochem. Biophys.*, 85:292.
Shatzman, A. R., and R. I. Henkin. 1981. Gustin concentration changes relative to salivary zinc and taste in humans, *Proc. Natl. Acad. Sci. U.S.A.*, 78:3867.
Shields, G. S., W. F. Coulson, D. A. Kimball, W. H. Carnes, G. E. Cartwright, and M. M. Wintrobe. 1962. Studies on copper metabolism XXXII. Cardiovascular lesions in copper-deficient swine, *Am. J. Pathol.*, 41:603.
Shurson, G. C., P. K. Ku, G. L. Waxler, M. T. Yokoyama, and E. R. Miller. 1990. Physiological relationships between microbiological status and dietary copper levels in the pig, *J. Anim. Sci.*, 68:1061.
Sihombing, D. T. H., G. L. Cromwell, and V. W. Hays. 1974. Effects of protein source, goitrogens and iodine level on performance and thyroid status of pigs, *J. Anim. Sci.*, 39:1106.
Sillard, R., H. Jörnvall, M. Carlquist, and V. Mutt. 1993. Chemical assay for cyst(e)ine-rich peptides detects a novel intestinal peptide ZF-1, homologous to a single zinc-finger motif, *Eur. J. Biochem.*, 211:377.

Smith, J. W., II, M. D. Tockach, R. D. Goodband, J. L. Nelssen, and B. T. Richert. 1997. Effects of the interrelationship between zinc oxide and copper sulfate on growth performance of early weaned pigs, *J. Anim. Sci.*, 75:1861.

Smith, K. T., M. L. Failla, and R. J. Cousins. 1978. Identification of albumin as the plasma carrier for zinc absorption by perfused rat intestine, *Biochem. J.*, 184:627.

Smith, W. H., M. P. Plumlee, and M. W. Beeson. 1960. Zinc requirements for growing swine, *Science*, 128:1280.

Solomons, N. W., and R. J. Cousins. 1984. Zinc. In *Current Topics in Nutrition and Disease*, Vol. 12: *Absorption and Malabsorption of Mineral Nutrients*, Solomons, N. W., and I. H. Rosenberg, Eds., Alan R. Liss, New York, 125.

Solomons, N. W., and I. H. Rosenberg. 1984. *Current Topics in Nutrition and Disease*, Vol. 12: *Absorption and Malabsorption of Mineral Nutrients*, Alan R. Liss, New York, 152.

Spears, J. W., E. E. Jones, L. J. Samsell, and W. D. Armstrong. 1984. Effect of dietary nickel on growth, urease activity, blood parameters and tissue mineral concentrations in the neonatal pig, *J. Nutr.*, 114:845.

Stahly, T. S., G. L. Cromwell, and H. J. Monegue. 1980. Effects of the dietary inclusion of copper and/or antibiotics on the performance of weanling pigs, *J. Anim. Sci.*, 51:1347.

Steele, N. C., T. G. Althen, and L. T. Frobish. 1977. Biological activity of glucose tolerance factor in swine, *J. Anim. Sci.*, 45:1341.

Steinhardt, H. J., and S. A. Adibi. 1984. Interactions between transport of zinc and other solutes in human intestine, *Am. J. Physiol. Gastr. Liver Physiol.*, 10:G176.

Suttle, N. F., and C. F. Mills. 1966. Studies of the toxicity of copper to pigs. I. Effects of oral supplements of zinc and iron salts on the development of copper toxicosis, *Br. J. Nutr.*, 20:135.

Swenerton, H., and L. S. Hurley. 1980. Zinc deficiency in rhesus and bonnet monkeys, including effects on reproduction, *J. Nutr.*, 110:575.

Tacnet, F., F. Lauthier, and P. Ripoche. 1993. Mechanisms of zinc transport into pig small intestine brush-border membrane vesicles, *J. Physiol.*, 465:57.

Taylor, C. M., J. R. Bacon, P. J. Aggett, and I. Bremner. 1991. Homoeostatic regulation of zinc absorption and endogenous losses in zinc-deprived men, *Am. J. Clin. Nutr.*, 53:755.

Teague, H. S., and L. E. Carpenter. 1951. The demonstration of a copper deficiency in young growing pigs, *J. Nutr.*, 43:389.

Teillet, L., F. Tacnet, P. Ripoche, and B. Corman. 1995. Effect of aging on zinc and histidine transport across rat intestinal brush-border membranes, *Mech. Ageing Dev.*, 79:151.

Telford, W. G., and P. J. Fraker. 1998. Zinc induced apoptosis in bone marrow and splenic B-lineage lymphocytes of the mouse, *Nutr. Res.*, 18:319.

Todd, W. R., C. A. Elvehjem, and E. B. Hart. 1934. Zinc in the nutrition of the rat, *Am. J. Physiol.*, 107:146.

Tremblay, G. F., J. J. Matte, C. L. Girard, and G. J. Brisson. 1989. Serum zinc, iron and copper status during early gestation in sows fed a folic acid-supplemented diet, *J. Anim. Sci.*, 67:733.

Turnland, J. R., W. R. Keyes, C. A. Hudson, A. A. Betschart, M. J. Kretsch, and H. E. Sauberlich. 1991. A stable-isotope study of zinc, copper, and iron absorption and retention by young women fed vitamin B-6 deficient diets, *Am. J. Clin. Nutr.*, 54:1059.

Underwood, E. J. 1977. *Trace Elements in Human and Animal Nutrition*, 4th ed., Academic Press, New York.

Underwood, E. J. 1981. *The Mineral Nutrition of Livestock*, Commonwealth Agricultural Bureaux, Slough, U.K.

Vadlamudi, R. K., R. J. McCormick, D. M. Medeiros, J. Vossoughi, and M. L. Failla. 1993. Copper deficiency alters collagen types and covalent cross-linking in swine myocardium and cardiac valves, *Am. J. Physiol.*, 33:H2154.

Valberg, L. S., P. R. Flanagan, and M. J. Chamberlain. 1984. Effects of iron, tin, and copper on zinc absorption in humans, *Am. J. Clin. Nutr.*, 40:536.

Van Campen, D. R., and E. A. Mitchell. 1965. Absorption of ^{64}Cu, ^{65}Zn, ^{99}Mo, and ^{59}Fe, from ligated segments of the rat gastrointestinal tract, *J. Nutr.*, 86:120.

van Gelder, W., M. I. E. Huijskes-Heins, D. Klepper, W. L. van Noort, M. I. Cleton-Soeteman, and H. G. van Eijk. 1996. Isolation and partial characterization of two porcine spleen ferritin fractions with different electrophoretic mobility, *Comp. Biochem. Physiol. Part B. Biochem. Mol. Biol.*, 115:191.

van Heugten, E., and J. W. Spears. 1997. Immune response and growth of stressed weanling pigs fed diets supplemented with organic or inorganic forms of chromium, *J. Anim. Sci.*, 75:409.

Vulpe, C. D. 1995. Cellular copper transport, *Annu. Rev. Nutr.* 15:293.

Wang, Z., S. A. Atkinson, R. F. P. Bertolo, S. Polberger, and B. Lönnerdal. 1993. Alterations in intestinal uptake and compartmentalization of zinc in response to short-term dexamethasone therapy or excess dietary zinc in piglets, *Pediatr. Res.*, 33:118.

Wapnir, R. A., D. E. Khani, M. A. Bayne, and F. Lifshitz. 1983. Absorption of zinc by rat ileum: effects of histidine and other low-molecular-weight ligands, *J. Nutr.*, 113:1346.

Ward, T. L., L. L. Southern, and T. D. Bidner. 1997. Interactive effects of dietary chromium tripicolinate and crude protein level in growing-finishing pigs provided inadequate and adequate pen space, *J. Anim. Sci.*, 75:1001.

Watkins, D. W., C. Chenu, and P. Ripoche. 1989. Zinc inhibition of glucose uptake in brush-border membrane vesicles from pig small intestine, *Pflügers Arch.*, 415:165.

Wedekind, K. J., E. C. Titgemeyer, A. R. Twardock, and D. H. Baker. 1991. Phosphorus, but not calcium, affects manganese absorption and turnover in chicks, *J. Nutr.*, 121:1776.

Wegger, I., and B. Palludan. 1977. Zinc metabolism in swine with special emphasis on reproduction. In *Trace Element Metabolism in Man and Animals* — 3, Kirchgessner, M., Ed., Institut für Ernährungsphysiologie, Technische Universität München, Freising-Weihenstephan, 428.

Wenk, C., S. Gebert, and H. P. Pfirter. 1995. Chromium supplements in the feed for growing pigs: influence on growth and meat quality, *Arch. Anim. Nutr.*, 48:71.

Williams, D. M., R. E. Lynch, G. R. Lee, and G. E. Cartwright. 1975. Superoxide dismutase activity in copper-deficient swine, *Proc. Soc. Exp. Biol. Med.*, 149:534.

Williams, D., D. Loukopoulos, G. R. Lee, and G. E. Cartwright. 1976. Role of copper in mitochondrial iron metabolism, *Blood*, 48:77.

Wong-Valle, J., C. B. Ammerman, P. R. Henry, P. V. Rao, and R. D. Miles. 1989. Bioavailability of manganese from feed grade manganese oxides for broiler chicks, *Poul. Sci.*, 68:1368.

Wooten, L., R. A. Shulze, R. W. Lancey, M. Lietzow, and M. C. Linder. 1996. Ceruloplasmin is found in milk and amniotic fluid and may have a nutritional role, *J. Nutr. Biochem.*, 7:632.

Zhou, J. R., M. M. Canar, and J. W. Erdman, Jr. 1993. Bone zinc is poorly released in young, growing rats fed marginally zinc-restricted diet, *J. Nutr.*, 123:1383.

13 Vitamin A in Swine Nutrition

Craig S. Darroch

CONTENTS

I. Characteristics and Sources of Vitamin A and Carotenoids 263
    A. Nomenclature and Occurrence..263
    B. Bioavailability of Retinoids and Carotenoids..265
        1. Biological Availability...265
        2. Stability of Vitamin A 266
        3. Determination of Vitamin A Levels and Activity............................266
II. Requirements for Vitamin A and Carotenoids 267
    A. Dietary Requirements for Swine 267
    B. Use of Vitamin A and β-Carotene in the Breeding Herd 267
III. Dietary Vitamin A and Nutrient Interactions 268
IV. Absorption, Transport, Distribution, and Metabolism of Retinoids and Carotenoids........268
    A. Absorption of Vitamin A 268
    B. Absorption of Carotenoids...269
    C. Uptake and Storage of Vitamin A by the Liver 270
    D. Retinol Binding Proteins and Transport of Vitamin A..............................271
    E. Carotenoid Storage, Transport, and Interactions.......................................271
    F. Vitamin A Metabolism...272
V. Biological Functions of Retinoids and Carotenoids 272
    A. Role of Vitamin A in Vision 272
    B. Cell Proliferation, Differentiation, and Gene Regulation 273
    C. Role of Vitamin A and β-Carotene in Reproduction 273
    D. Immunity and Health...275
VI. Retinoid and Carotenoid Deficiencies 275
    A. Clinical Symptoms in Pigs 275
    B. Effects of a Vitamin A Deficiency on Immune Function 276
    C. Reproductive Problems Associated with Vitamin A Deficiency..............276
    D. Other Factors Leading to Vitamin A Deficiency......................................276
VII. Toxicity Associated with Retinoids and Carotenoids...277
    A. Clinical Symptoms of Toxicity in Swine 277
    B. Bone Toxicity Associated with High Levels of Vitamin A......................277
References 278

I. CHARACTERISTICS AND SOURCES OF VITAMIN A AND CAROTENOIDS

A. NOMENCLATURE AND OCCURRENCE

Vitamin A is essential for vision, health, fertility, and the growth and differentiation of epithelial tissues, and it is involved in gene expression. This vitamin was first identified as a growth factor

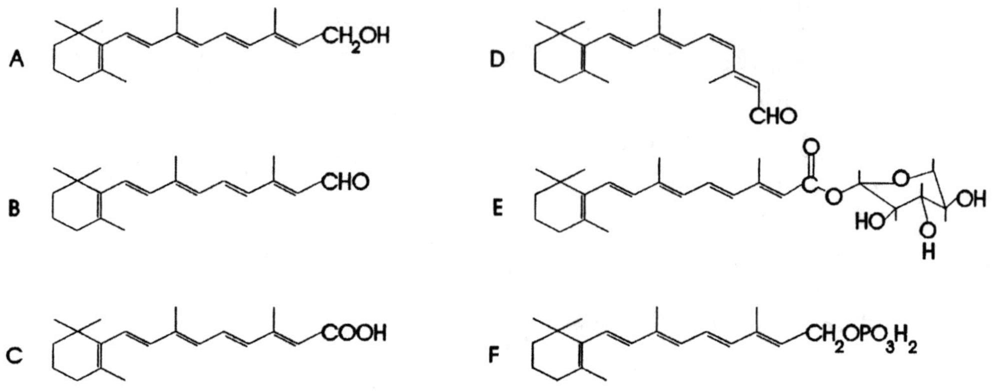

FIGURE 13.1 Chemical structures of vitamin A metabolites: (A) all-*trans* retinol, (B) all-*trans* retinaldehyde or retinal, (C) all-*trans* retinoic acid, (D) 11-*cis* retinal, (E) all-*trans* retinoyl β-glucuronide, and (F) all-*trans* retinyl phosphate.

in 1915 and its structure characterized in 1930. Vitamin A is a generic name given to chemical compounds having β-ionone derivatives that exhibit the biological activity of all-*trans* retinol (Figure 13.1).

Vitamin A, active metabolites, and synthetic analogs are commonly referred to as retinoids in the literature. The esters of all-*trans* retinol are termed retinyl esters, the aldehyde form of all-*trans* retinol is termed retinaldehyde or retinal, and the acidic form of all-*trans* retinol is termed retinoic acid (Figure 13.1). Biologically, retinal is active in vision and plays a role in reproduction, whereas retinoic acid is essential for normal growth and differentiation of cells. Other vitamin A compounds are present in the body and include retinoyl β-glucuronide in bile and retinyl phosphate, an intermediate in glycoprotein synthesis.

With the exception of whole milk and fish liver oils, feeds for swine contain little if any natural vitamin A. Plant feedstuffs, particularly green plants, contain carotenoids, which are converted to vitamin A in animals. Dehydrated alfalfa meal (20% crude protein) contains 150 mg/kg carotene and 200,000 IU/kg of vitamin A. Corn gluten meal (60% crude protein) is another relatively good source of carotene (44 mg/kg) and has some vitamin A activity (70,000 IU/kg). Other swine feedstuffs that contain ≥1 mg/kg β-carotene include beet pulp, hominy feed, oat and barley grains, distiller's grains and solubles, lentil and pea seeds, wheat bran and middlings, bakery waste, and soybeans (NRC, 1998). The amount of carotenoids in plants varies widely, depending on the time of harvest, degree of wilting, method of preservation, and length of storage.

For practical purposes, the vitamin A and carotenoid contents of swine feedstuffs are not considered in diet formulation, and 100% or more of the pig's dietary vitamin A requirement is met through supplementation. Commercially, vitamin A is available as a dry stable product used in feeds, or in an oily preparation with ≥500,000 IU/g activity that is used in liquid feed applications or as an injectable product. Injectable vitamin A is available, but is most often marketed in mixtures of fat-soluble vitamins, which include combinations of vitamins A and D or A, D, and E. Commercial forms of β-carotene are also available as a dry stable product with ≥10% active provitamin A content.

The carotenoids are usually referred to as provitamin A compounds. There are more than 600 carotenoids that have been characterized, but only about 80 have provitamin A activity. In the United States, 40 carotenoids are commonly found in human foods, and 20 to 26 carotenoids have been detected in human serum and tissues (Bertram, 1999; Cooper et al., 1999). Carotenoids are thought to play various roles in protection against cancer, cardiovascular disease, and aging. Of the active carotenoids, most have at least one unsubstituted β-ionone ring. Nutritional research has

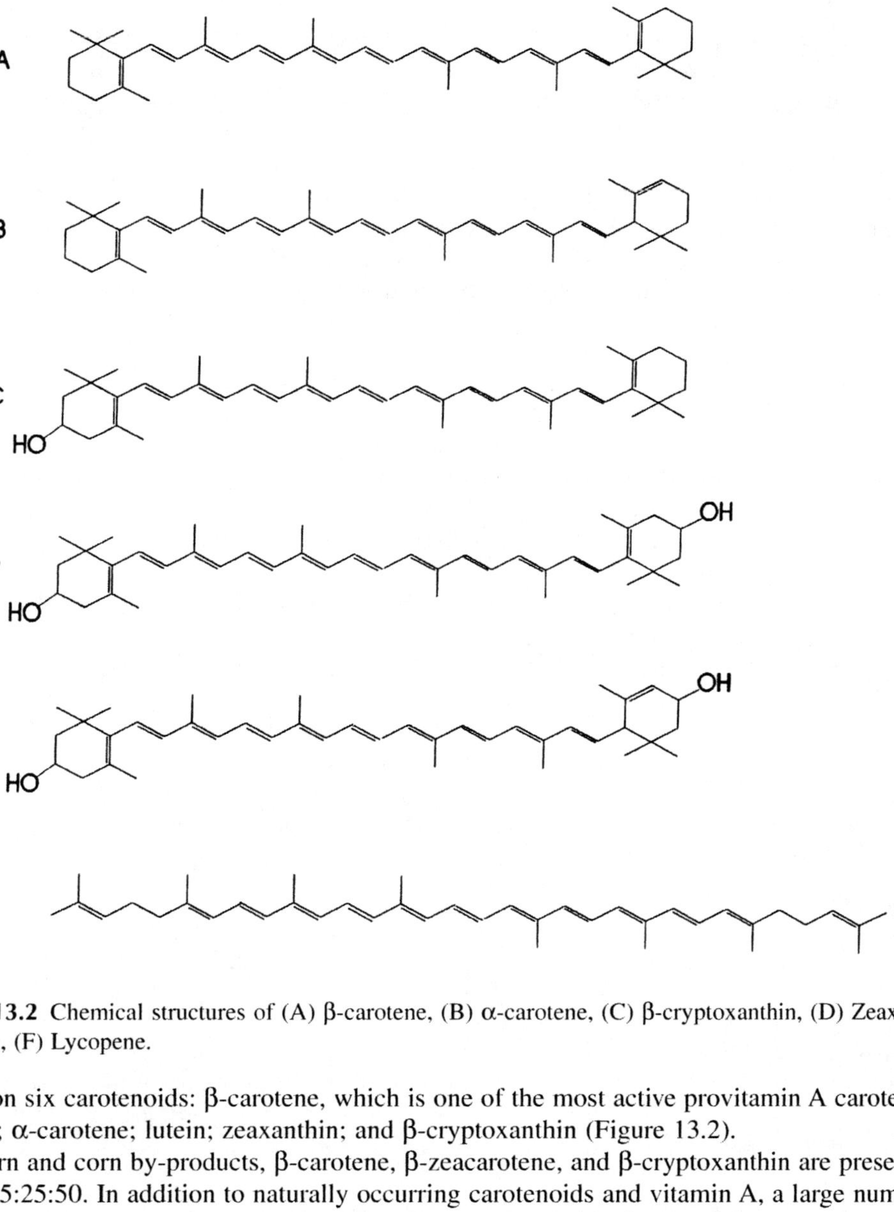

FIGURE 13.2 Chemical structures of (A) β-carotene, (B) α-carotene, (C) β-cryptoxanthin, (D) Zeaxanthin, (E) Lutein, (F) Lycopene.

focused on six carotenoids: β-carotene, which is one of the most active provitamin A carotenoids; lycopene; α-carotene; lutein; zeaxanthin; and β-cryptoxanthin (Figure 13.2).

In corn and corn by-products, β-carotene, β-zeacarotene, and β-cryptoxanthin are present in a ratio of 25:25:50. In addition to naturally occurring carotenoids and vitamin A, a large number of analogs have been synthesized and display various levels of vitamin A activity.

B. Bioavailability of Retinoids and Carotenoids

1. Biological Availability

Biological activity of vitamin A is expressed in international units (IU). For comparative purposes 1 IU of vitamin A activity equals 1 USP unit, 0.3 μg of all-*trans* retinol (international standard for vitamin A), 0.344 μg of retinyl acetate, 0.55 μg of retinyl palmitate, or 0.358 μg retinyl propionate (Behm et al., 1992). To compare different carotenoids or vitamin A compounds, activity is often expressed in terms of retinol equivalents (RE). One RE is defined as 1 μg of all-*trans* retinol. Olson (1983) reported that in the pig, 6 μg of β-carotene was equivalent to 1 μg of retinol, which gives β-carotene an RE value of 0.167. This RE value is reported several times in the literature, but there is controversy over the true value for the pig. Blair et al. (1996) assumed a vitamin A biopotency of β-carotene in young pigs of 0.2 IU/μg, which equals a RE value of 0.06, considerably lower than the value reported by Olson. The NRC (1998) recommends using RE values of 0.080 and 0.092 if converting reported feedstuff β-carotene values to retinol and retinyl acetate, respectively. One must be cautious when looking at values for carotenoids because the conversion of carotenoids of plant origin to vitamin A differs from species to species, and as carotenoid intake increases, the conversion rate falls. In addition, most plant feedstuffs contain a variety of carotenoids that have different biopotencies, and interactions between these carotenoids affect intestinal absorption, postprandial conversion to vitamin A, and effects in tissues (van den Berg, 1999). Pigs are less efficient than poultry or rats in converting carotenoids to vitamin A. Ullrey (1972) has shown that only 16% of carotenoids in corn were converted and stored as vitamin A in the liver of pigs.

2. Stability of Vitamin A

Biological activity of vitamin A in feedstuffs also relates to the chemical stability of the various forms of vitamin A and carotenoids. Vitamin A retinol has five double bonds and contains a free hydroxy group that makes it highly susceptible to oxidation. To protect vitamin A from oxidation, manufacturers emulsify it in gelatin and sugars and process it into a beadlet containing an antioxidant. Unprotected vitamin A oxidizes rapidly in feedstuffs when moisture levels exceed 12%. Moisture may exist naturally in cereals and protein supplements, may be added when high-moisture feedstuffs such as fish solubles or molasses are used in ration formulation, and moisture may be added during the processing of feedstuffs or mixed diets. Moisture levels can also rise in the diet during storage. In addition to moisture, light, acidity, and minerals that include copper, iron, manganese, zinc, and iodine present in the diet as water-soluble salts contribute to vitamin A oxidation. Elevated temperatures, moisture, friction, and pressure that accompany feed processing contribute significantly to vitamin A oxidation. Friction and pressure in pelleting and extrusion processes erode the gelatin–sugar beadlet coating exposing vitamin A to chemical oxidation, which is accelerated by high pelleting and extrusion temperatures and humidity. In feeds, polyunsaturated fatty acids (PUFA) and peroxides also contributes to vitamin A oxidation. A gram of PUFA can destroy 3000 IU of vitamin A. In practical situations, vitamin A in swine feeds and premixes is considered moderately stable and losses may vary between 0.5 and 11% per month (Anonymous, 1993). In some instances, vitamin A losses may reach 100%. This situation may occur in a swine vitamin/mineral premix stored for an extended period of time in the hot, humid summer months in the southern United States.

Bioavailability of injectable vitamin A products can also vary. Duggan et al. (1994), using a liver biopsy technique, found significant differences in the bioavailability of four commercially available injectable vitamin A, D, E sources in Charolais crossbred steers injected with an equivalent of 1,000,000 IU vitamin A measured over a 14-day period.

3. Determination of Vitamin A Levels and Activity

The amount and biological activity of natural and synthetic forms of vitamin A and carotenoids can be measured in a variety of ways. Depletion/repletion growth assays using the pig and more commonly the rat and chick give species specific values of biological activity. In these assays, growth performance, feed efficiency, health status, and tissue vitamin A levels are determined along with other specific biological traits. Sample tissues are saponified, vitamin A is extracted, and vitamin A isomers and carotenoids separated and quantitated using high-performance liquid chromatography (HPLC) and ultraviolet (UV) detection. The feed industry has used spectrophotometric and chemical (Carr–Price) methods to determine the biopotency of vitamin A, but accuracy, sensitivity, and specificity have been variable, limiting their use. These methods have been largely replaced by growth, microbiological, or analytical assays with assay variations for vitamin A and β-carotene ranging from 10 to 25% and 5 to 20%, respectively.

II. REQUIREMENTS FOR VITAMIN A AND CAROTENOIDS

A. Dietary Requirements for Swine

The NRC (1998) requirements for vitamin A for growing pigs and breeding stock are summarized in Table 13.1. Young pigs (3 to 10 kg) require about 2,200 IU vitamin A/kg diet. The vitamin A requirement for growing-finishing pigs (10 to 120 kg) falls from 1,750 to 1,300 IU/kg diet as the pig ages. Gestating and lactating sows require 7,400 and 10,500 IU of vitamin A daily, and sexually active boars need 8,000 IU daily. There can be considerable variation in reported vitamin A requirements for pigs in the literature. This relates, in part, to differences in the criteria used to establish the requirement, animal variation, and differences in housing and environmental conditions. For growing-finishing pigs the requirements can vary from 102 to 2,703 IU/kg diet.

Feed manufacturers recommend dietary vitamin A fortification levels for swine that are approximately ten times the NRC levels. These levels account for animal and environmental variation, variability in feedstuff vitamin A levels, effects of feed processing, and distribution errors in premixing and feed mixing. Blair et al. (1989; 1996) have reported that these industry levels can be tolerated by young and growing pigs (10 to 60 kg). The requirement for β-carotene has not been clearly established for pigs, but breeding sows have responded favorably to daily intakes of 400 mg from weaning until mating (Behm et al., 1992).

TABLE 13.1
The Dietary Vitamin A Requirements of Growing and Breeding Age Pigs

Type of Pig	Body Weight (kg)	Vitamin A Requirement[a]		Feed Intake[a] (g/day)	ME Intake[a] (kcal/day)
		IU/kg diet[b]	IU/day[b]		
Growing	3–5	2,220	550	250	820
	5–10	2,200	1,100	500	1,620
	10–20	1,750	1,750	1,000	3,265
	20–50	1,300	2,412	1,855	6,050
	50–80	1,300	3,348	2,575	8,410
	80–120	1,300	3,998	3,075	10,030
Gestation	120–240	4,000	7,400	1,850	6,040
Lactation	140–260	2,000	10,500	5,520	17,135
Boars	120–350	4,000	8,000	2,000	6,530

[a] NRC (1998) recommended level.
[b] 1 IU of vitamin A equals 0.344 μg retinyl acetate.

B. Use of Vitamin A and β-Carotene in the Breeding Herd

Much of the interest in the use of injectable vitamin A to improve reproductive performance stems from work of Brief and Chew (1985) and Coffey and Britt (1993) who reported increases in litter size in gilts and sows. The improved reproductive performance occurs after injection of vitamin A or β-carotene, but not after diet supplementation. Improved performance relates to an increased number of pigs born alive in first-litter gilts and multiparous sows. This increase in live pigs per litter may relate to reduced embryonic mortality and to a reduction in the number of stillborn pigs. Repeat service rate, farrowing rate, days to return to estrus after weaning, and individual pig weights were not influenced by vitamin A injection. It is apparent from a review of the literature that the timing of injection and dose and form of vitamin A are important and will influence the observed responses. Pusateri et al. (1996) did not observe an increase in litter size when 1,000,000 IU vitamin A was injected intramuscularly (i.m.) into multiparous sows at weaning, breeding, or various days throughout gestation in a commercial farrowing operation located in central Indiana. In a large regional study by the S-288 (formerly S-145) Technical Committee (Darroch et al., 1998), injection of vitamin A at weaning and again at breeding increased the number of pigs born alive but the responses were variable across stations participating in the trial.

Maternal vitamin A status directly determines the supply of vitamin A to the neonate. In a radioisotope tracer study with ewes, Donaghue (1988) showed that vitamin A in milk comes from plasma retinol bound to retinol-binding protein (RBP) and that the transfer was not regulated. Rate of transfer of vitamin A into milk was correlated to clearance of retinol from plasma in the ewes. Milk concentrations of vitamin A increased linearly with vitamin A intake, and were highest in initial milk secretions and decreased thereafter as lactation progressed. Vitamin A in ewe milk was in the form of retinyl esters.

III. DIETARY VITAMIN A AND NUTRIENT INTERACTIONS

Type and level of dietary protein may affect plasma and liver levels of vitamin A. Poiffait et al. (1988a) looked at the effects of different levels of casein and soybean meal proteins on vitamin A status in rats. When dietary protein was marginal (10% crude protein) and the vitamin A level (1.3 mg/kg) close to the animal's requirement, protein from casein increased the efficiency of vitamin A uptake from the diet compared with diets in which the dietary protein was derived from soybean meal. The authors postulated that the phosphorylated serine residues of casein protein could stimulate retinol absorption through membrane recognition. When dietary vitamin A levels were in excess of requirement (6.5 mg/kg), the source of dietary protein had no effect on the efficiency of vitamin A uptake from the diet, and hepatic retinol stores were positively correlated to dietary intake levels. Increasing dietary protein levels from 10 to 20% resulted in a decrease in hepatic retinol levels. In a second study, Poiffait et al. (1988b) supplied vitamin A in the diet in three different forms (retinol palmitate, all-*trans* retinal, and all-*trans* retinoic acid) and measured the effects of protein from casein and soybean meal on vitamin A utilization. Dietary vitamin A in the form of retinol and retinal resulted in higher levels of hepatic and plasma retinol than did retinoic acid. Compared with soybean meal protein, casein significantly increased the efficiency of utilization when dietary vitamin A was in the form of retinal and tended to improve uptake of retinol. There was no specific effect of casein protein on retinoic acid utilization.

A deficiency of dietary iron low enough to reduce growth rates in rats elevated hepatic levels of retinyl esters and retinol. The molar ratio of hepatic retinyl esters to retinol was also increased in rats fed diets deficient in iron (Rosales et al., 1999). Dietary vitamin A and β-carotene also seem to improve gastrointestinal iron absorption. This may be related to the complexing of soluble iron with vitamin A or β-carotene, preventing an interaction with phytates and polyphenols present in feedstuffs, two substances that are known to lower nutrient availability (Garcia-Casal et al., 1998). In a study comparing vitamin A, D, and E levels in 13 Finnish and 13 Floridian women of similar age, serum vitamin A levels were similar (488 ± 168 µg/l) and were unaffected by dietary vitamin A intake or differences in dietary habits (Punnonen et al., 1988). However, dietary vitamin A intakes several times the pig's requirement may affect the immune system by reducing the content of vitamin E in tissues (Hoppe et al., 1992). In a study by Blair et al. (1996), dietary vitamin A fed at levels up to 200 times the requirement for 10-kg pigs did not affect growth performance or the immune system even though serum and liver tocopherol levels were significantly reduced when the dietary vitamin A level exceeded ten times the pig's requirement.

IV. ABSORPTION, TRANSPORT, DISTRIBUTION, AND METABOLISM OF RETINOIDS AND CAROTENOIDS

A. Absorption of Vitamin A

After ingestion of feed, preformed vitamin A is released by the action of pepsin in the stomach of the pig and other proteolytic enzymes in the duodenum. Vitamin A derivatives aggregate into lipid globules that are dispersed in the intestinal lumen by conjugated bile acids. Esters of vitamin A in lipid emulsions are hydrolyzed by a pancreatic carboxyl retinyl ester hydrolase and duodenal brush border–associated retinyl ester hydrolases to retinol. Retinol is then incorporated into mixed micelles containing other fat-soluble vitamins, carotenoids, free fatty acids, monoglycerides, phospholipid and cholesteryl esters, and bile acids. The mixed micelles diffuse into the glycoprotein layer surrounding the microvilli of enterocytes and then are passively absorbed. Absorption efficiency of dietary vitamin A is usually 80 to 90% and is only reduced at high dietary levels. Variability in the efficiency of vitamin A absorption depends on endogenous factors influencing lipid digestion and absorption and the presence of dietary compounds that interfere with lipid uptake from the gastrointestinal tract. This has been demonstrated recently in pig studies evaluating the nutritional effects of Olestra®, a mixture of sucrose esters that have similar physicochemical and cooking characteristics to those of dietary fats and oils (Cooper et al., 1997a). Olestra, which is used as a zero-calorie replacement for dietary fat in human foods, does not undergo lipolysis in the gut and is not absorbed. Other lipophilic substances, including vitamin A, in the gastrointestinal tract partition into Olestra and are not available for incorporation into micelles and subsequent absorption by enterocytes. As an example of Olestra's effect on vitamin A absorption in the pig, Cooper et al. (1997b) have reported a 55 to 61% decrease in vitamin A absorption when Olestra was included in the diet at a level of 4.8%. Hypovitaminosis A can be prevented by adding extra vitamin A and/or β-carotene to the diet at levels equivalent to 0.93 μg retinyl palmitate/g Olestra (Cooper et al., 1997c). Differences in the lipophilicity of retinyl palmitate and β-carotene result in differences in their respective availabilities in diets containing Olestra.

Once absorbed, the majority of retinol is reesterified with palmitic acid in enterocytes. Coenzyme A and ATP are required for the esterification step. Esterification with phospholipids or other acyl donors may also occur. In addition, some retinol in enterocytes is oxidized to retinaldehyde and to retinoic acid. Retinyl esters along with triglycerides and phospholipid and cholesteryl esters are incorporated into chylomicrons. Chylomicrons through the process of exocytosis pass from enterocytes into the lymph and eventually enter the general blood circulation.

B. Absorption of Carotenoids

The process of digestion and absorption of carotenoids is similar to that of vitamin A and lipids, but carotenoid absorption is 40 to 60% lower, is negatively correlated to dietary level, and is dependent on the presence of bile salts. Gastric action and pancreatic lipase are needed to dissociate carotenoids and to encourage dissolution and dispersion in fat globules prior to absorption. Fatty acid esters of carotenoids require hydrolysis by pancreatic carboxylic ester hydrolase before duodenal uptake into enterocytes. Carotenoids are incorporated into mixed micelles in the same manner as retinol. Degree of carotenoid incorporation into mixed micelles relates to physicochemical properties of carotenoids and on micellar chemical composition. There is a linear increase in the rate of carotenoid uptake by enterocytes, until single oral doses of carotenoids exceed 20 to 30 mg. At higher doses, physicochemical factors of the mixed carotenoid-containing micelles may limit absorption (van den Berg, 1999). Differential absorption of carotenoids is also related to type and isomeric form, with the all-*trans* carotenoids being preferentially absorbed. The presence of 9-*cis*-β-carotene in the small intestine seems to improve the absorption of all-*trans* β-carotene.

After mucosal absorption, β-carotene and other provitamin A carotenoids are primarily converted by enterocytes into retinyl esters of vitamin A (Figure 13.3). Two proposed pathways currently exist to explain the conversion mechanism. In the first and most accepted pathway, the polyene chain of β-carotene is cleaved by β-carotene-15–15′-dioxygenase leading to the formation of two retinal molecules. This seems to be the central pathway in *in vitro* studies with pig intestinal mucosa (Nagao et al., 1996). In the second pathway, eccentric cleavage of β-carotene leads to the formation of apocarotenoids that are converted to one molecule of retinal and a variety of smaller fragments. Depending on the dietary level of β-carotene, the animal species and vitamin A status, the rate of cleavage of β-carotene is estimated to be between 20 and 75%.

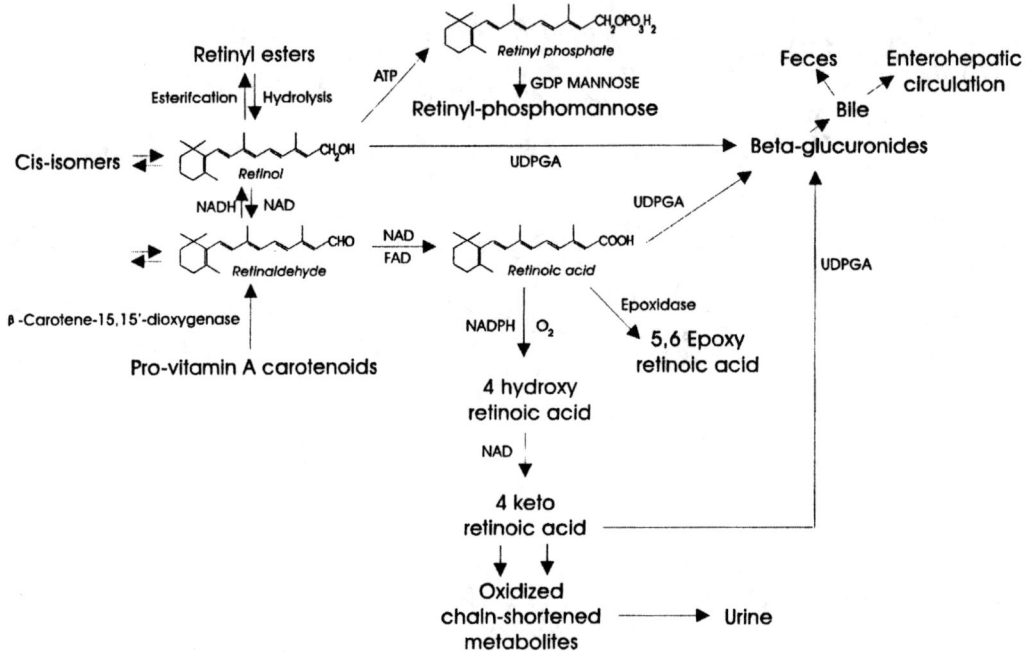

FIGURE 13.3 Metabolic and excretory pathways of vitamin A and provitamin A carotenoids.

In a manner similar to retinol, intact carotenoids and cleavage products in enterocytes are incorporated into chylomicrons and then secreted into the lymphatic system, which drains into the venous circulation.

C. Uptake and Storage of Vitamin A by the Liver

After vitamin A–containing chylomicra enter the general circulation from the lymph, they are degraded by plasma lipoprotein lipase, which reduces the triglyceride content of the chylomicra. This results in a smaller, very low density chylomicron remnant, which is removed from the circulation by parenchymal cells called hepatocytes. Hepatocytes represent 60 to 65% of liver cells and they have two plasma membrane receptors (a low-density lipoprotein receptor and an *apo-E-receptor*) that can bind chylomicron remnants. The majority of dietary vitamin A that is absorbed into the body is taken up by the liver within 4 to 6 h. Although hepatocytes function in removal of vitamin A from the circulation, most vitamin A in liver seems to be stored in perisinusoidal stellate cells, often referred to as lipocytes. As much as 90% of body vitamin A stores are in the liver. Levels of vitamin A in liver increase in a dose–response manner as the concentrations of dietary vitamin A and β-carotene increase. In pigs, liver storage levels of vitamin A increased from 56 to 89 nmol/g liver when dietary vitamin A levels increased from the NRC (1988) recommended levels to 1.6 times the NRC requirement (Cooper et al., 1997a). In lipocytes, which represent only 7% of total liver cells, the storage form of vitamin A represents a lipoglycoprotein complex consisting of 96% retinyl esters and 4% unesterified retinol. The formation of retinyl esters in lipocytes is dependent on the activity of two enzymes systems, acyl-CoA:retinol acyltransferase (ARAT) and lecithin:retinol acyltransferase (LRAT) and the presence of cellular RBP. Unesterified retinol can be oxidized to retinaldehyde and retinoic acid (see Figure 13.3). Retinoic acid binds to cellular retinoic acid–binding protein (RABP), which functions to transfer cytoplasmic retinoic acid to nuclear retinoic acid receptors. Intracellular RABP also protect cells from membrane damage sometimes caused by high levels of retinoids. Closely associated with this complex is a tightly bound retinyl ester hydrolase that hydrolyzes the retinyl esters and transfers the retinol to intracellular *apo*-RBP. In hepatocytes, retinyl palmitate hydrolase transfers retinol to *apo*-RBP. The resultant retinol–RBP complex, *holo*-RBP, is then secreted from hepatocytes and lipocytes into the plasma, where it forms a reversible 1:1 molar complex with transthyretin (prealbumin).

D. Retinol Binding Proteins and Transport of Vitamin A

The primary means by which vitamin A is physiologically transported in the blood of most species involves binding of retinol to its specific carrier, RBP. Serum RBP has a molecular weight of about 21,000 and when bound to transthyretin has a combined molecular weight of 70,000. The formation of the serum RBP–transthyretin complex seems to stabilize the interaction of retinol with RBP, reducing glomerular filtration and renal catabolism of retinol and RBP. The liver is a primary site of RBP synthesis, but several other organs, such as the kidney and other tissues, can synthesize RBP and aid in regulation of plasma retinol concentrations. In most species, 90% of serum RBP is saturated with retinol. The half-life of the *holo*-RBP-transthyretin complex in plasma is approximately 11 to 16 h. Unbound *holo*-RBP and *apo*-RBP is turned over in about 4 h. The majority of retinol taken up by the kidney is recycled to the blood. For most species, unspecific, lipoprotein-bound vitamin A in blood is only reported when an animal has hypervitaminosis A. The dog seems to be a special case, in that the majority of vitamin A in plasma is transported as retinyl esters (70%) associated with lipoproteins (Schweigert, 1988) and only 30% as retinol bound to RBP. Schweigert (1988) reported that concentrations of total vitamin A in plasma were up to ten times higher compared with other species such as the pig and that dogs were less sensitive to the negative effects of nonspecific tissue delivery of vitamin A that occurs in animals with hypervitaminosis A.

Plasma retinol levels can be used to assess vitamin A utilization by tissues. Based on kinetic tracer studies in rats (Kelley and Green, 1998), plasma retinol exchanges with tissue vitamin A in two distinct extra vascular compartments. The rate of irreversible oxidation of retinol in tissues to retinoic acid is not decreased to compensate for low dietary vitamin A levels if liver vitamin A stores are adequate. Changes in plasma retinol levels accounted for 92% of the variability in rates of irreversible retinol oxidation in tissues.

In the pig and other species, a family of RBP, distinct from serum RBP, are secreted by the uterine endometrium in response to progesterone. These uterine RBP aid in the transfer of retinol and retinoic acid from the maternal blood supply to areolae, specialized absorptive regions on the pig's placenta. In studies with pigs, the uterine RBP were only 50% saturated with vitamin A (Clawitter et al., 1990).

E. Carotenoid Storage, Transport, and Interactions

A detailed discussion of carotenoid metabolism is beyond the scope of this chapter and readers are encouraged to review articles by Ross (1993) and van den Berg (1999). In the blood and liver, chylomicrons containing carotenoids are modified by lipoprotein lipase and lipoprotein interactions. As a result, lipoproteins become the major carrier for carotenoids in the bloodstream. After a meal, very low density lipoproteins (VLDL) are a primary carrier and in a fasting state, low density lipoproteins (LDL) become the main carrier. The ratio of LDL to high density lipoproteins (HDL) uptake from the GIT may play a role in contributing to variation in tissue levels of carotenoids. The liver seems to be the main storage site for carotenoids in animals and humans. In the pig, the liver has only a limited ability to store β-carotene. In one study, pig liver β-carotene levels were only 0.04 to 0.06 µg/g liver, compared with newborn chicks that had liver β-carotene levels of 0.4 to 1.3 µg/g liver (Poor et al., 1987). There seem to be two hepatic pools of β-carotene that are affected by dietary levels of β-carotene but not vitamin A. One pool of β-carotene is lost rapidly from serum and tissues of gerbils fed a β-carotene-deficient diet, and a second pool is lost more slowly over time (Thatcher et al., 1998). Upon removal of β-carotene from the diet, liver stores of β-carotene in chicks are also lost rapidly. It seems that hepatic stores of β-carotene are not conserved for later vitamin A tissue needs even when dietary vitamin A or β-carotene is deficient.

Other tissues such as the kidney, lung, and perirenal fat accumulate carotenoids, but the amounts stored vary considerably among species and are appreciably less (up to 100 times) than liver stores. Higher levels of β-carotene in cattle corpus luteum and pineal glands suggest that there may be selective tissue uptake of carotenoids. In contrast to gastrointestinal tract absorption, tissues show a preference for *cis* isomers of carotenoids.

Carotenoid interactions can affect uptake from the gastrointestinal tract and tissues and lead to differences in tissue storage levels. Increased levels of lutein in the diet reduced the absorption of β-carotene and liver vitamin A levels. Canthaxanthin and lycopene also seem to affect β-carotene uptake and tissue storage levels. Interaction effects may be species specific. Canthaxanthin reduces β-carotene uptake in ferrets but enhances β-carotene uptake in humans. Most interactions between carotenoids have been observed in short-term, single-dose studies. Recent long-term intervention studies in humans given β-carotene supplementation have not resulted in any significant change in plasma or tissue carotenoid profiles. Non-provitamin A carotenoids such as lutein, lycopene, and xanthophylls can reduce β-carotene cleavage to retinal through competitive inhibition of β-carotene-15–15′-dioxygenase.

F. Vitamin A Metabolism

The metabolism of dietary vitamin A and provitamin A carotenoids in animal tissues to the major biologically active retinoid metabolites is depicted in Figure 13.3. There are many other retinol metabolites that display some biological activity. Retinol formed from retinyl esters can be converted in body tissues to retinal and retinoic acid through oxidative reactions. Formation of retinol from retinyl esters in the intestine involves pancreatic carboxyl ester hydrolases and brush border retinyl ester hydrolases. Once absorbed from the gastrointestinal tract, retinol can be reconverted to retinyl esters in body tissues or oxidized to retinal and retinoic acid. Conversion of retinol to retinyl esters by lecithin:retinol acyltransferase and acyl-CoA:retinol acyl transferase, or oxidation by NADH retinol dehydrogenase to retinoic acid may be influenced by presence of specific cytoplasmic retinoid-binding proteins (Ross, 1993). Central cleavage of a molecule of β-carotene or other provitamin A carotenoids in the intestine by β-carotene 15,15′-dioxygenase yields two molecules of retinal. The formation of retinoic acid from retinal is an irreversible oxidation step in retinol metabolism, and this accounts for the lower activity of retinoic acid in some tissues that specifically utilize retinal or retinol. Further oxidation of retinoic acid in tissues facilitates excretion either in bile or urine. Oxidized, polar metabolites of retinol, retinal, and retinoic acid that retain intact chains in their structures are converted into β-glucuronides, which pass into bile. Once in the bile, these glucuronides can be lost in the feces or recycled in the enterohepatic circulation. Oxidized, chain-shortened metabolites of retinoic acid display little or no biological activity and are predominantly excreted in the urine (Figure 13.3). Esterification of retinol in tissues also represents a recycling mechanism and, together with enterohepatic recycling, influences the vitamin A status of the pig. The conversion of retinol to a retinyl-phosphomannose metabolite (Figure 13.3) may relate to vitamin A roles in cell communication and differentiation. Retinyl-phosphomannose acts as a carbohydrate donor in glycoprotein synthesis, and glycoproteins play important roles in cell membrane function. Regulation of vitamin A metabolism and expression of retinoid binding proteins depends on vitamin A status, which is a function of retinoic acid production.

V. BIOLOGICAL FUNCTIONS OF RETINOIDS AND CAROTENOIDS

A. Role of Vitamin A in Vision

The role of vitamin A in vision is specifically related to all-*trans*-retinol, which is involved in the synthesis and cyclic regeneration of rhodopsin, a photoreceptor for vision at low light intensities.

In the eye, all-*trans*-retinol is oxidized to all-*trans*-retinaldehyde and then converted to 11-*cis*-retinaldehyde. Retinal then combines with opsin to form rhodopsin. When light falls on the retina, rhodopsin breaks down into opsin and all-*cis*-retinaldehyde, which reverts to all-*trans*-retinaldehyde, initiating an action potential that travels up the optic nerve. In the dark the all-*trans*-retinaldehyde is isomerized back to all-*cis*-retinaldehyde and the latter recombines with opsin to regenerate rhodopsin, resensitizing the retina to light.

B. CELL PROLIFERATION, DIFFERENTIATION, AND GENE REGULATION

Retinoids can influence hormone action at the cellular level, alter signal transduction, and affect enzyme systems within cells that lead to changes in metabolism, cell proliferation, and differentiation. In retinoid-responsive cells, retinol and retinoic acid bind to their respective cytosolic binding proteins, CRBP and CRABP, and are translocated to the nucleus, stimulating mRNA and protein synthesis in a manner characteristic of many steroid hormones.

The role of vitamin A, specifically retinoic acid, in tissue growth may involve upregulation (increased number) of cell membrane growth factor receptors for epidermal growth factor, insulin-like growth factor-I, and interleukin-1. In addition, retinoic acid may influence cell growth by altering cellular communication through modification of cell membrane gap junction permeability. Evidence to support this hypothesis has been presented in cancer studies reviewed by Bertram (1999). Retinoids and carotenoids have the ability to upregulate connexin 43 gene expression. Connexins are a family of transmembrane proteins that represent the structural element of a gap junction. In tissues, connexins function to transmit information and allow the exchange of nutrients and waste products. Tumor cells communicate poorly, and it is believed that retinoid and carotenoid induced gap junction communication allows the transfer of growth-inhibiting signals from normal cells. Related to cell metabolism, Shin and McGrane (1997) have detailed the role of retinoic acid in the upregulation of genes for two enzyme systems, phosphoenolpyruvate carboxykinase (PEPCK) and 6-phosphofructo-2-kinase/fructose-2,6-bisphosphatase, that are involved in hepatic gluconeogenesis. Without adequate vitamin A, stimulation of the PEPCK gene by food deprivation or cyclic adenosine monophosphate is inhibited. In general, retinoids influence gene expression in the following manner. Retinoic acid binds to nuclear retinoic acid receptors (RAR) that bind to retinoid responsive genes, known as retinoic acid–responsive elements. The binding of retinoic acid to RAR leads to a conformational change in the receptors. This results in the displacement of silencing elements and encourages binding of transcriptional cofactors that stimulate gene expression. The RAR not complexed with retinoic acid are believed to act as transcriptional silencers. The mechanisms by which carotenoids affect gene expression have not been elucidated but may involve oxidation to retinoid-like molecules. Evidence is emerging that suggests that carotenoids, such as lycopene (Dorgan et al., 1998) and canthaxanthin (Bertram, 1999), may also influence gene expression in ways that do not involve conversion to retinoid-like molecules.

C. ROLE OF VITAMIN A AND β-CAROTENE IN REPRODUCTION

Chew (1993) provides a good review of the roles vitamin A and β-carotene play in swine reproduction. A beneficial response in sows to supplemental vitamin A or β-carotene seems to be related to injection and not dietary fortification. However, the use of vitamin A injections to enhance reproductive performance has produced variable results that may relate to concentration, source, and stability of the injectable vitamin A; vitamin A and health status of the sow herd; animal management; and environmental conditions at the time of the trials. Reproductive benefits have been reported in studies that injected 50,000 to 1,000,000 IU of vitamin A or >200 mg β-carotene around the time of breeding. Brief and Chew (1985), Coffey and Britt (1993), and Whaley et al. (1997) have observed improvements in litter size and embryo survival in sows and gilts injected with vitamin A or β-carotene, whereas Pusateri et al. (1996) failed to see any improvement. In a large-scale regional sow study (Darroch et al., 1998), injection of vitamin A at weaning and breeding for three parities increased the number of pigs born alive, but the response was not consistent across all experimental stations participating in the trial.

Vitamin A status of the sow seems to influence the actions of retinoids and carotenoids in reproductive tissues. In sows and rats with sufficient vitamin A liver stores, supplemental retinol and retinoic acid increases ovarian progesterone secretion. Increased progesterone levels prior to ovulation have been positively correlated with oocyte maturation and embryo survival. It has been proposed that increased variation in oocyte maturation in the sow may adversely affect embryo survival. This is supported by the findings of Whaley et al. (1997), who injected vitamin A palmitate (1,000,000 IU) into gilts and studied subsequent reproductive performance. Compared with control gilts, vitamin A–treated gilts had higher progesterone concentrations in follicular fluid 24 to 28 h after onset of estrus, oocytes were more advanced developmentally, and there was less variation in the meiotic stage of development. Vitamin A injection did not affect ovulation rate, number of oocytes aspirated, or recovery rates of oocytes or embryos.

The increase in progesterone and presence of vitamin A may also positively affect the uterine environment, promoting embryo development and enhancing survival. The porcine trophoblast does not invade the uterine epithelium and relies on several uterine transport proteins during development. In the pig, the uterine endometrium secretes a family of RBP, distinct from serum RBP in response to progesterone (Adams et al., 1981) and possibly estrogen produced by the conceptus (Trout et al., 1992). Subsequent studies by Trout (1994) indicate that conceptus estrogen may not regulate uterine RBP expression at the time of trophoblast elongation. Chew et al. (1982) have shown that vitamin A and β-carotene can influence the composition of uterine secretions, but they did not specifically measure RBP. Suzuki et al. (1995) failed to modulate cellular RBP, type II in rat jejunal mucosa by feeding vitamin A or β-carotene up to 1000 times the NRC (1978) rat requirement for vitamin A of 4.2 μmol/kg. These uterine RBP, which appear to be 50% saturated, aid in the transfer of retinol and retinoic acid from the maternal blood supply to areolae, specialized absorptive regions on the pig's placenta (Clawitter et al., 1990). Secretion of porcine uterine RBP increases 390-fold between day 10 and 13 of gestation (Mahan and Vallet, 1997), a critical period in embryo development and survival. The increase in RBP may ensure delivery of retinol and other compounds to the conceptus and protect fetal tissues against oxidative reactions enhancing early embryonic survival.

Retinoic acid activity in early embryogenesis plays a key role in cell proliferation and differentiation that leads to the formation of the primitive streak and the embryonic plate. This stage in the pig occurs around day 11 to 13 of gestation and involves complex biochemical and morphological changes. Later in embryogenesis, retinoic acid acts as a morphogen, a signaling compound that controls the position and polarity of developing limb structures, face, and eye, and vitamin A has been linked to development of avian heart, embryonal circulation, and the central nervous system (Zile, 1998). In studies with mice, some alcohol (specifically alcohol dehydrogenase-IV) and aldehyde dehydrogenase enzymes prefer retinol and retinal, respectively, over ethanol and acetaldehyde, and these enzymes participate in the initiation of retinoid signaling beginning at day 7.5 of embryogenesis (Duester, 1998). Intoxicating levels of ethanol during this time period in early embryogenesis inhibit retinol oxidation, an essential step required for normal vertebrate development. Although retinol oxidation to retinoic acid is essential, high levels of retinoic acid in early stages of embryogenesis are teratogenic, producing neural tube defects that result in embryo loss, abortion, and malformations. In studies in which vitamin A–deficient pigs, rats, and guinea pigs were supplemented with retinoic acid there were increases in fetal abortions and malformations. Apgar et al. (1994; 1995) have proposed that this may relate to an increased teratogenicity of retinoic acid in vitamin A–deficient females. This could also explain the negative effect of retinoic acid supplementation on ovarian progesterone secretion in vitamin A–deficient rats.

In boars and males of other species, vitamin A is essential for spermatogenesis. Retinol can stimulate steroidogenesis and spermatogenesis, whereas retinoic acid only supports steroidogenesis. Retinoic acid receptors are present in sertoli and germ cells and are regulated by retinol.

D. Immunity and Health

Carotenoids such as lycopene are effective antioxidants and function to protect cells from free radical oxidation, which has been linked to premature aging, cancer, atherosclerosis, cataracts, and other degenerative diseases in animals and humans. Retinoids and carotenoids act as immunomodulators and influence both T- and B-cell function, induce cell differentiation, and inhibit proliferation of certain cell types. The specific effect on immune system function seems to be related to form and level of vitamin A (Chew, 1995). β-Carotene supplementation increased mitogen-induced lymphocyte proliferation in pigs and peripartum dairy cows, while vitamin A failed to produce a similar response, and retinoic acid suppressed lymphocyte proliferation. Other effects of β-carotene noted by Chew (1995) include an increase in the number of T lymphocytes, an increase in the number of mononuclear cells with natural killer cell surface markers, interleukin 2 receptors, and transferrin receptors; and an increase in natural killer cell cytotoxicity, interleukin 1, and tumor necrosis factor α. In a review of *in vitro* studies, T-cell proliferation appears to be induced by low levels and inhibited by high levels of retinyl acetate, whereas retinoic acid inhibits proliferation.

One mechanism by which vitamin A and carotenoids modulate the immune system may involve their antioxidant mode of action. β-Carotene contains many double bonds, which react with cytotoxic peroxyl radicals to render them inactive, thus protecting immune system cell membrane integrity (Chew, 1995); however, support for this mechanism in *in vivo* human studies is lacking (Cooper et al., 1999). Carotenoids may modulate the immune system by stimulating gap junction intracellular communication through expression of the gap junction protein, connexin 43 (Cooper et al., 1999). Again, the ability to stimulate intracellular communication may relate to the type and level of vitamin A or carotenoid, and to tissue type. Vitamin A may also modulate the immune system by enhancing neutrophil chemotaxis and phagocytosis (Twinning et al., 1997).

VI. RETINOID AND CAROTENOID DEFICIENCIES

A. Clinical Symptoms in Pigs

Symptoms related to a deficiency of retinoids and/or carotenoids, also referred to as hypovitaminosis A, in swine can appear when there is a deficiency of vitamin A or provitamin A carotenoids in the diet. Deficiency symptoms in pigs appear when serum vitamin A levels fall below 0.35 µmol/l (Cooper et al., 1997b). In some cases deficiency symptoms may relate to a lack of non-provitamin A carotenoids such as lycopene or canxanthanin. Deficiency symptoms can also manifest themselves, if the absorption, storage, transport, or metabolism of retinoids or carotenoids is compromised in pigs that are consuming diets that meet or exceed their vitamin A requirement.

Deficiency symptoms associated with reduced plasma vitamin A or liver storage in swine include reduced weight gain, aborted fetuses, stillbirths, debilitation, weakness and paralysis of the hind limbs, incoordination, tilting of the head, roughness of the skin, corneal opacity, eye discharge, blindness, respiratory dysfunction, and increased cerebrospinal fluid pressure. In aborted or stillborn pigs the following conditions have been observed: anophthalmia, microphthalmia, cleft palate, hare lip, and deformed hind legs. Histopathological examinations in vitamin A–deficient pigs showed vascular and granular degeneration, necrosis and lymphoid cell foci in liver, and degeneration of neurons, gliosis, and satellitosis in the cerebellum (Saini et al., 1995).

Respiratory problems in vitamin A–deficient animals may relate to altered enzyme regulation and activity. In vitamin A–deficient guinea pigs, superoxide dismutase, glutathione peroxidase activities, and glutathione levels were reduced. These compounds protect the lung from toxic oxygen free radicals. In addition, cytochrome P-450 enzymes involved in microsomal detoxification of inhaled xenobiotics were increased and this could have contributed to the pool of reactive free radicals in damaged lung tissue (Nair et al., 1988).

B. Effects of a Vitamin A Deficiency on Immune Function

A vitamin A deficiency in pigs reduces their ability to fight infections. This in part may relate to an impaired immune system. In rats, a deficiency of vitamin A increases the percentage of neutrophils that are hypersegmented and contain lower levels of cathespin G. This reduces chemotaxis of neutrophils and their ability to adhere to, phagocytize, and oxidize foreign organisms. This loss of neutrophil function can be restored by vitamin A supplementation (Twining et al., 1997). Supplementation of vitamin A can also alleviate immune system depression caused by a dietary protein deficiency. In protein-deficient mice immunized with 20 µg of cholera toxin (CT), oral retinyl acetate (1 mg) supplementation prevented the decline in intestinal mucosal levels of anti-CT specific IgA observed in untreated CT-infected mice. The authors proposed that vitamin A may stimulate Th2 cytokine production, increasing resistance to infection (Nikawa et al., 1999). Improved growth responses have also been seen in malnourished, parasitized children in undeveloped countries who were treated with vitamin A, suggesting that both vitamin A deficiency and immune system dysfunction contribute to the clinical growth retardation seen in vitamin A–deficient pigs. In vitamin A–deficient lambs, serum IgG levels were lower than in healthy lambs.

C. Reproductive Problems Associated with Vitamin A Deficiency

The vitamin A requirement for pregnancy in the rat seems to be less than that needed by the guinea pig. In a study by Gardner and Ross (1993), female rats consuming 3.6 and 8 RE/day, which is below the rats' requirement, had successful pregnancies, and litter sizes and average pup birth weights were not different from rats consuming vitamin A (80 RE/day) above their requirement. Vitamin A levels in milk were correlated closely to vitamin A levels in maternal plasma. Neonatal rats from dams fed marginal vitamin A levels had low plasma vitamin A levels and could not increase liver stores. When pups from vitamin A–deficient dams were fed marginal vitamin A diets postweaning, there was accelerated depletion of liver retinol and early clinical signs of vitamin A deficiency (ataxia, dermal changes, reduced growth, and negligible hepatic lecithin:retinol acyltransferase activity) compared with pups from dams fed adequate levels of vitamin A.

D. Other Factors Leading to Vitamin A Deficiency

Non-nutritive food additives, such as Olestra, that affect absorption of fat-soluble vitamins, reduce plasma and hepatic vitamin A levels in pigs, and may lead to classical symptoms of hypovitaminosis A, unless diets are supplemented with additional vitamin A (Cooper et al., 1997c). Similarly, disease conditions, such as cystic fibrosis in humans, which result in fat malabsorption in 85 to 90% of patients can produce severe deficiencies in fat-soluble vitamins, including vitamin A (Rust et al., 1998).

Environmental stressors that interfere with physiological functions in swine can also induce a vitamin A deficiency. For example, prolonged oxygen exposure can decrease both lung and liver levels of vitamin A. In a study by Zachman (1988) newborn rabbits were exposed to 70 to 75% oxygen for 68 h. Retinol levels in the lung and retinyl esters (palmitate and stearate) in the liver were lowered on average by 25% by the stress of an oxygen environment, but there was no significant increase in histological symptoms related to alveolar emphysema or focal atelectasis, which are suggestive of oxygen toxicity. The authors suggest possible mechanisms of action explaining the effect of oxygen on retinol may include increased oxidation in lung endothelial membranes, increased mobilization of retinol associated with a stress-mediated increase in RBP, an increase in retinyl palmitate hydrolase activity, or an increase in the conversion of retinol into other biologically active metabolites.

Increased liver activity that is typically associated with xenobiotic detoxification may lead to a deficiency of vitamin A. Polychlorinated biphenyl detoxification results in increased vitamin A utilization and subsequent reductions in liver stores (Innani et al., 1976). Mycotoxins, such as aflatoxin B_1, may produce vitamin A deficiency in pigs. Karppanen and Rizzo (1983) have correlated hypovitaminosis in various domestic livestock in Finland beginning in the early 1980s to higher endemic mycotoxin levels that have resulted from increased international commodity trading. An induced vitamin A deficiency may also increase the toxicity of xenobiotics in pigs. Aflatoxin B_1, which is suspected of inducing a vitamin A deficiency, becomes more toxic in animals with a known vitamin A deficiency, and has resulted in increased clotting times in rats, guinea pigs, and rabbits (Bassir et al., 1980). Sulfa-drug treatment can also alter vitamin A storage and distribution. Sulfomethoxypyridazine administration to rats resulted in decreased plasma vitamin A levels and increased hepatic levels, which suggests that this drug interfered with RBP transport of vitamin A between liver and blood (Bravo et al., 1977).

VII. TOXICITY ASSOCIATED WITH RETINOIDS AND CAROTENOIDS

A. Clinical Symptoms of Toxicity in Swine

Vitamin A toxicity or hypervitaminosis A is related to the dietary intake or injection of high levels of retinoids and possibly some carotenoids and to an increased sensitivity to retinoids and carotenoids in the pig. Toxicity related to an increased sensitivity to retinoids may occur in animals that are clinically deficient in vitamin A and are receiving supplements either in the diet or by injection. Frequently reported clinical symptoms of hypervitaminosis A in pigs include congenital and skeletal malformations, spontaneous fractures, internal hemorrhage, appetite and weight loss, slow growth, skin thickening, suppressed keratinization, and increased blood-clotting time. These symptoms in part are related to increased levels of free unesterified retinol in the body. Excess retinol is toxic to biological membranes through its detergent properties (Smith and Goodman, 1976). In pigs with clinical symptoms, high concentrations of serum retinyl palmitate are positively correlated to the activity of lecithin:retinol acyltransferase, one of two main enzymes involved in esterification of retinol. Accompanying increased retinyl palmitate levels are high levels of circulating triglycerides and reduced growth rates (Suzuki et al., 1995). These researchers also noted that an equivalent amount of β-carotene fed to rats did not produce the dramatic increase in retinyl palmitate.

In hypervitaminosis A, mitochondrial and lysosomal membranes are subject to labilization and altered membrane function. These effects are related to a vitamin A–induced increase in phospholipase A_2 activity. The vitamin A–induced membrane lysis can be partially prevented by oral administration of spermine, which inhibits phospholipase A_2 activity, and by sterically hindering the interaction of phospholipases with their substrates (Chandra et al., 1988). Retinoic acid may be more toxic in animals that are vitamin A deficient due to upregulation of retinoic acid receptors (McMenamy and Zachman, 1993) and retinoic acid may be more toxic in a purified diet than in a commercial diet (Thompson et al., 1964).

B. Bone Toxicity Associated with High Levels of Vitamin A

Intakes of vitamin A greater than ten times the NRC (1988) requirement for growing pigs may lead to adverse changes in bone integrity (Blair et al., 1989; Pryor et al., 1989; Blair et al., 1992). Clinical signs of osteochondrosis with swelling and pain in joints in pigs appear about 2 to 5 weeks after feeding diets high in vitamin A. Histopathological lesions relate to a focal thickening of articular or epiphyseal cartilage that may relate to a defect in chondrocyte proteoglycan metabolism. Standeven et al. (1996) have induced premature epiphyseal plate closure in guinea pigs through vitamin A supplementation. Epiphyseal plate closure was associated with an increased abundance of osteoclasts and a loss of basophilic staining in the extracellular chondrocyte matrix, which is indicative of changes in cartilage-specific proteoglycan metabolism. In general, increased osteoclast activity in periosteal and endosteal tissues leads to abnormal bone remodeling and increased bone fragility. These researchers provide evidence that bone toxicity may be associated with retinoids that specifically stimulate nuclear retinoic acid receptors as opposed to α, β, and γ retinoid receptors. In a subsequent pig study by Blair et al. (1996), the researchers did not observe any clinical signs of hypervitaminosis in young pigs fed dietary vitamin A up to 200 times the NRC (1988) requirement, and could not correlate incidences of osteochondrosis to high dietary vitamin A concentrations.

REFERENCES

Adams, K. C., F. W. Baer, and R. M. Roberts. 1981. Progesterone induced secretions of a retinol-binding protein in the pig uterus, *J. Reprod. Fertil.*, 62:39.

Anonymous. 1993. Vitamins—one of the most important discoveries of the century, In *Animal Nutrition*, 5th ed., BASF Corporation, Parsippany, NJ.

Apgar, J., T. Kramer, and J. C. Smith. 1994. Retinoic acid and vitamin A: effect of low levels on outcome of pregnancy in guinea pigs, *Nutr. Res.*, 14:741.

Apgar, J., T. Kramer, and J. C. Smith. 1995. Marginal vitamin A intake during pregnancy in guinea pigs: effect on immune parameters in neonate, *Nutr. Res.*, 15:545.

Bassir, O., A. A. Adekunle, and Z. S. C. Okoye. 1980. Effect of vitamin A deficiency on anticoagulant action of aflatoxin B_1, *Toxicon*, 18:121.

Behm, G., D. Dressler, W. Kohler, K. Küther, W. Lindner, and G. Schwarz. 1992. *Vitamins in Animal Nutrition*, Arbeitsgemeinschaft für Wirkstoffe in der Tierernährung, Bonn.

Bertram, J. S. 1999. Carotenoids and gene regulation, *Nutr. Rev.*, 57:182.

Blair, R., B. A. Burton, C. E. Doige, A. C. Halstead, and F. E. Newsome. 1989. Tolerance of weanling pigs for dietary vitamin A and D, *Int. J. Vitam. Nutr. Res.*, 59:329.

Blair, R., F. X. Aherne, and C. E. Doige. 1992. Tolerance of growing pigs for dietary vitamin A, with special reference to bone integrity, *Int. J. Vitam. Nutr. Res.*, 62:130.

Blair, R., M. Facon, R. J. Bildfell, B. D. Owen, and J. P. Jacob. 1996. Tolerance of young pigs for dietary vitamin A and β-carotene, with special reference to the immune response, *Can. J. Anim. Sci.*, 76:121.

Braude, R., A. S. Foot, K. M. Henry, S. K. Kon, S. Y. Thompson, and T. H. Mead. 1941. Vitamin A studies with rats and pigs, *Biochem. J.*, 35:693.

Bravo, M. E., F. Monckeberg, and J. Urbina. 1977. The effect of sulphomethoxypyridazine on liver and plasma levels of vitamin A in rats, *Br. J. Pharmacol.*, 60:181.

Brief, S., and B. P. Chew. 1985. Effects of vitamin A and β-carotene on reproductive performance in gilts, *J. Anim. Sci.*, 60:998.

Chandra, R., R. Beri, and U. K. Misra. 1988. Effect of spermine on membranolytic effect of vitamin A in rats, *Int. J. Vitam. Nutr. Res.*, 58:13.

Chew, B. P. 1993. Effects of supplemental β-carotene and vitamin A on reproduction in swine, *J. Anim. Sci.*, 71:247.

Chew, B. P. 1995. Antioxidant vitamins affect food animal immunity and health, *J. Nutr.*, 125:1804S.

Chew, B. P., P. H. Rasmussen, M. H. Pubols, and R. L. Preston. 1982. Effects of vitamin A and β-carotene on plasma progesterone and uterine protein secretions in gilts, *Theriogenology*, 18:643.

Clawitter, J., W. E. Trout, M. G. Burke, S. Araghi, and R. M. Roberts. 1990. A novel family of progesterone-induced, retinol binding proteins from uterine secretions of the pig, *J. Biol. Chem.*, 265:3248.

Coffey, M. T., and J. H. Britt. 1993. Enhancement of sow reproductive performance by β-carotene or vitamin A, *J. Anim. Sci.*, 71:1198.

Cooper, D. A., D. A. Berry, V. A. Spendel, A. L. Kiorpes, and J. C. Peters. 1997a. The domestic pig as a model for evaluating Olestra's nutritional effects, *J. Nutr.*, 127:1555S.

Cooper, D. A., D. A. Berry, V. A. Spendel, M. B. Jones, A. L. Kiorpes, and J. C. Peters. 1997b. Nutritional status of pigs fed Olestra with and without increased dietary levels of vitamins A and E in long-term studies, *J. Nutr.*, 127:1609S.

Cooper, D. A., D. A. Berry,, M. B. Jones, A. L. Kiorpes, and J. C. Peters. 1997c. Olestra's effect on the status of vitamins A, D and E in the pig can be offset by increasing dietary levels of these vitamins, *J. Nutr.*, 127:1589S.

Cooper, D. A., A. L. Eldridge, and J. C. Peters. 1999. Dietary carotenoids and lung cancer: a review of recent research, *Nutr. Rev.*, 57:133.

Darroch, C. S., L. I. Chiba, M. D. Lindemann, R. Dove, A. F. Harper, and E. T. Kornegay. 1998. S-145 Committee on Nutritional Systems for Swine to Increase Reproductive Efficiency. Effects of injections of high levels of vitamin A on reproductive performance in sows, *J. Anim. Sci.*, 76 (Suppl. 1):160.

Donoghue, S. 1988. Vitamin A transport in plasma of ewes during late gestation and into milk during early lactation, *Int. J. Vitam. Nutr. Res.*, 58:3.

Dorgan, J. F., A. Sowell, C. A. Swanson, N. Potischman, R. Miller, N. Schussler, and H. E. Stephenson. 1998. Relationships of serum carotenoids, retinol, alpha-tocopherol and selenium with breast cancer risk: results from a prospective study in Columbia, Missouri (United States), *Cancer Causes Control*, 9:89.

Duester, G. 1998. Alcohol dehydrogenase as a critical mediator of retinoic acid synthesis from vitamin A in the mouse embryo, *J. Nutr.*, 128:459S.

Duggan, J. B., C. R. Richardson, and K. J. Smith. 1994. Bioavailability of injectable vitamin A sources in finishing steers, *J. Anim. Sci.*, 72(Suppl. 1):187.

Garcia-Casal, M. N., M. Layrisse, L. Solano, M. A. Barón, F. Arguello, D. Llovera, J. Ramírez, I. Leets, and E. Tropper. 1998. Vitamin A and β-carotene can improve nonheme iron absorption from rice, wheat and corn by humans, *J. Nutr.*, 128:646.

Gardner, E. M., and A. C. Ross. 1993. Dietary vitamin A restriction produces marginal vitamin A status in young rats, *J. Nutr.*, 123:1435.

Hoppe, P. P., F. J. Schoner, and M. Frigg. 1992. Effects of dietary retinol on hepatic retinol storage and on plasma and tissue tocopherol in pigs, *Int. J. Vitam. Nutr. Res.*, 62:121.

Innani, S., A. Nakamura, M. Miyazaki, S. Nagayama, and E. Nishide. 1976. Further studies on the reduction of vitamin A content in livers of rats given polychlorinated biphenyls, *J. Nutr. Sci. Vitaminol.*, 22:409.

Karppanen, E., and A. Rizzo. 1983. Disturbances of vitamin A metabolism in animals, *Acta Vet. Scand.*, 24:524.

Kelley, S. K., and M. H. Green. 1998. Plasma retinol is a major determinant of vitamin A utilization in rats, *J. Nutr.*, 128:1767.

Mahan, D. C., and J. L. Vallet. 1997. Vitamin and mineral transfer during fetal development and the early postnatal period in pigs, *J. Anim. Sci.*, 75:2731.

McMenamy, K. R., and R. D. Zachman. 1993. Effect of gestational age and retinol (vitamin A) deficiency on fetal rat lung nuclear retinoic acid receptors, *Pediatr. Res.*, 33:251.

Nagao, A., A. During, C. Hoshino, J. Terao, and J. A. Olson. 1996. Stoichiometric conversion of all trans-β-carotene to retinal by pig intestinal extract, *Arch. Biochem. Biophys.*, 328:57.

Nair, C. R., M. M. Davis, and S. K. Das. 1988. Effect of vitamin A deficiency on pulmonary defense systems of guinea pig lung, *Int. J. Vitam. Nutr. Res.*, 58:375.

Nikawa, T., K. Odahara, H. Koizumi, Y. Kido, S. Teshima, K. Rokutan, and K. Kishi. 1999. Vitamin A prevents the decline in immunoglobulin A and Th2 cytokine levels in small intestinal mucosa of protein-malnourished mice, *J. Nutr.*, 129:934.

NRC. 1978. *Nutrient Requirements of Laboratory Animals*, 10th ed., National Academy Press, Washington, D.C.

NRC. 1988. *Nutrient Requirements of Swine*, 9th ed., National Academy Press, Washington, D.C.

NRC. 1998. *Nutrient Requirements of Swine*, 10th ed., National Academy Press, Washington, D.C.

Olson, J. A. 1983. Formation and function of vitamin A. In *Biosynthesis of Isoprenoid Compounds*, Porter, J. W., and Spurgeon, S. L., Eds., John Wiley & Sons, New York, 371.

Poiffait, A., E. Moustaïzis-Carpeli, T. Karisto, and J. Adrian. 1988a. Effect of soybean and casein on the vitamin A status in the rat, *Int. J. Vitam. Nutr. Res.*, 58:27.

Poiffait, A., T. Karisto, and J. Adrian. 1988b. Influence of vitamin A form and protein nature on the retinol status in the rat, *Int. J. Vitam. Nutr. Res.*, 58:33.

Poor, C. L., S. D. Miller, G. C. Fahey Jr., R. A. Easter, and J. W. Erdman, Jr. 1987. Animal models for carotenoid utilization studies: evaluation of the chick and the pig, *Nutr. Rep. Int.*, 36:229.

Pryor, W. J., A. A. Seawright, and P. J. McCosker. 1989. Hypervitaminosis A in the pig, *Aust. Vet. J.*, 45:563.

Punnonen, R., M. Gillespy, M. Hahl, T. Koskinen, and M. Notelovitz. 1988. Serum 25-OHD, vitamin A and vitamin E concentrations in healthy Finnish and Floridian women, *Int. J. Vitam. Nutr. Res.*, 58:37.

Pusateri, A. E., M. A. Diekman, and W. L. Singleton. 1996. Failure of vitamin A to alter litter size in swine when injected at breeding and various stages of gestation, *J. Anim. Sci.*, 74(Suppl. 1):247.

Rosales, F. J., J.-T. Jang, D. J. Piñero, K. M. Erikson, J. L. Beard, and A. C. Ross. 1999. Iron deficiency in young rats alters the distribution of vitamin A between plasma and liver and between hepatic retinol and retinyl esters, *J. Nutr.*, 129:1223.

Ross, C. A. 1993. Overview of retinoid metabolism, *J. Nutr.*, 123:346.
Rust, P., I. Eichler, S. Renner, and I. Elmadfa. 1998. Effects of long-term oral beta-carotene supplementation on lipid peroxidation in patients with cystic fibrosis, *Int. J. Vitam. Nutr. Res.*, 68:83.
Saini, S. S., R. S. Khehra, Ramneek, and D. V. Joshi. 1995. Hypovitaminosis A in pigs, *Indian J. Anim. Sci.*, 65:891.
Schweigert, F. J. 1988. Insensitivity of dogs to the effects of nonspecific bound vitamin A in plasma, *Int. J. Vitam. Nutr. Res.*, 58:23.
Shin, D. J., and M. M. McGrane. 1997. Vitamin A regulates genes involved in hepatic gluconeogenesis in mice: phosphoenolpyruvate carboxykinase, fructose-1,6-biphosphatase and 6-phosphofructo-2-kinase/fructose-2,6-bisphosphatase, *J. Nutr.*, 127:1274.
Smith, F. R., and D. S. Goodman. 1976. Vitamin A transport in human vitamin A toxicity, *N. Engl. J. Med.*, 294:805.
Standeven, A. M., P. J. A. Davies, R. A. S. Chandraratna, D. R. Mader, A. T. Johnson, and V. A. Thomazy. 1996. Retinoid-induced epiphyseal plate closure in guinea pigs, *Fundam. Appl. Toxicol.*, 34:91.
Suzuki, R., T. Goda, and S. Takase. 1995. Consumption of excess vitamin A, but not excess β-carotene, causes accumulation of retinol that exceeds to binding capacity of cellular retinol-binding protein, type II in rat intestine, *J. Nutr.*, 125:2074.
Thatcher, A. J., C. M. Lee, and J. W. Erdman, Jr. 1998. Tissue stores of β-carotene are not conserved for later use as a source of vitamin A during compromised vitamin A status in Mongolian gerbils (*Meriones unguiculatus*), *J. Nutr.*, 128:1179.
Thompson, J. N., J. McC. Howell, and G. A. J. Pitt. 1964. Vitamin A and reproduction in rats, *Proc. R. Soc. London Ser. B.*, 159:510.
Trout, W. E. Uterine retinol-binding protein and conceptus development in swine, *J. Anim. Sci.*, 2(Suppl. 1):339.
Trout, W. E., J. A. Hall, M. L. Stallings-Mann, J. M. Galvin, R. V. Anthony, and R. M. Roberts. 1992. Steroid regulation of the synthesis and secretion of retinol-binding protein by the uterus of the pig, *Endocrinology*, 130:2557.
Twinning, S. S., D. P. Schulte, P. M. Wilson, B. L. Fish, and J. E. Moulder. 1997. Vitamin A deficiency alters rat neutrophil function, *J. Nutr.*, 127:558.
Ullrey, D. E. 1972. Biological availability of fat-soluble vitamins: vitamin A and carotene, *J. Anim. Sci.*, 35:648.
van den Berg, H. 1999. Carotenoid interactions, *Nutr. Rev.*, 57:1.
Whaley, S. L., V. S. Hedgpeth, and J. H. Britt. 1997. Evidence that injection of vitamin A before mating may improve embryo survival in gilts fed normal or high-energy diets, *J. Anim. Sci.*, 75:1071.
Zachman, R. D. 1988. Effect of oxygen on newborn rabbit lung and liver retinol stores, *Int. J. Vitam. Nutr. Res.*, 58:17.
Zile, M. H. 1998. Vitamin A and embryonic development: an overview, *J. Nutr.*, 128(2):455S.

14 Selenium and Vitamin E in Swine Nutrition

Donald C. Mahan

CONTENTS

I.	Historical Perspective	282
II.	Soil Supply of Available Selenium	282
III.	Plant and Grain Sources of Selenium	283
IV.	Plant and Grain Sources of Vitamin E	284
V.	Commercial Sources	286
	A. Selenium	286
	B. Vitamin E	287
VI.	Absorption of Selenium and Vitamin E	289
	A. Selenium	289
	B. Vitamin E	289
VII.	Blood and Tissue Distribution	290
	A. Selenium	290
	B. Vitamin E	291
VIII.	Metabolic Roles	292
	A. Antioxidant Function	292
	1. Selenium	292
	2. Vitamin E	293
	B. Immune Function	293
	C. Arachidonic Acid and Prostaglandin Metabolism	294
IX.	Excretion	294
	A. Selenium	294
	B. Vitamin E	295
X.	Deficiency Onset and Symptoms	295
	A. Tissue Responses	295
	B. Clinical Symptoms	296
XI.	Factors that Contribute to Selenium and Vitamin E Deficiency in Swine	296
XII.	Selenium and Vitamin E in Fetal and Neonatal Pigs	297
	A. General	297
	B. Iron Toxicity	298
XIII.	Selenium and Vitamin E during the Nursing and Postnatal Period	298
XIV.	Selenium and Vitamin E during the Growing-Finishing Period	299
	A. Growth	299
	B. Effect on Pork Quality	300
XV.	Selenium and Vitamin E during Reproduction	300
	A. Sows	300
	B. Boars	303

XVI. Excesses	303
A. Selenium	303
B. Vitamin E	304
XVII. Dietary Requirements	304
References	306

I. HISTORICAL PERSPECTIVE

The recognition that selenium (Se) was an essential trace mineral in the diets of animals occurred over 40 years ago (Schwarz and Foltz, 1957). Shortly after that discovery, it was recognized that Se prevented white muscle disease in sheep (Muth et al., 1958; Oldfield et al., 1960), and liver necrosis, cardiac myopathy, and exudative diathesis in other species (NRC, 1983). It was, however, not until 1973 (Rotruck et al., 1973) that the involvement of Se as a component of the glutathione peroxidase (GSH-Px) enzyme provided biological evidence of its function in the body. Investigations into the role of Se in different production phases of all livestock species have since yielded additional findings that Se not only can affect animal performance, but also animal health.

Vitamin E has a longer nutritional history than Se, but its role in animal nutrition has not escaped controversy. In 1922, Evans and Bishop (1922a,b) identified a fat-soluble extract in wheat germ that contained an unknown antisterility factor. That extract is now known to contain several chemically related compounds, collectively termed vitamin E. The involvement of vitamin E with the antioxidant system in the body, the prevention of diseases, the immunological competence of animals, and the enhancement of the shelf life and quality of meat has greatly enlarged the original function assigned to this vitamin. Its role as an antioxidant in biological tissue is now widely accepted as the major biological function, but how and if it affects other animal systems is currently being explored.

It is now universally recognized that both Se and vitamin E are metabolic and dietary essentials. Although there is a shared relationship in their biological functions and they have common deficiency symptoms, there are dietary requirements for both nutrients that are independent of one another.

II. SOIL SUPPLY OF AVAILABLE SELENIUM

In well-aerated, alkaline soils, Se exists in an oxidized state (i.e., selenate, selenite). Selenate is the chemical form of the element that is most effectively absorbed by plants, followed by selenite. In acid or poorly aerated soils subject to excessive rain, irrigation, and leaching, Se is reduced to an insoluble form (i.e., elemental Se, selenide), unavailable for plant absorption. The liming of soils and the subsequent increase in soil pH increases the conversion of reduced Se toward the oxidized form, which increases its availability to plant tissues. Sandy soils contain very little Se because it is not readily bound to these soil particles and is thus easily leached. The more-oxidized Se forms (i.e., selenite, selenate), however, may complex with certain soil minerals, notably iron (Fe), converting oxidized Se to a reduced form (Swaine, 1955). Other soil minerals, e.g., sulfur (S), compete with selenate at the root membrane, which can affect its absorption (Mayland, 1985). Ultimately, it is the "available" soil Se (i.e., selenate) that determines its concentration in plant tissue, not the total soil Se content.

Most soils have a Se content within the range of 0.10 to 2.0 ppm. Areas in the United States and Canada that produce grains and forages low in Se content (eastern Midwestern states, southern states, northwestern states, northeastern and northwestern Canada) generally have soils that contain <0.50 ppm Se (Swaine, 1955; Cary et al., 1967; Levesque, 1974). Areas that have moderate crop Se contents (Nebraska, North and South Dakota, Montana, Wyoming, Kansas, Utah, Colorado, New Mexico) have soil Se levels that range from 2 to 10 ppm (Mayland, 1985). Most cereal grains for livestock and human consumption are grown in areas with inadequate or moderate Se soil reserves (NRC, 1983). There are, however, areas with high-Se-containing soils that produce toxicity (selenosis) conditions in livestock. "Indicator" plants (plants that selectively absorb and concentrate Se) grown on these seleniferous soils can accumulate Se in excess of 1000 ppm, whereas other plants raised in the same area contain ≤50 ppm Se. It is interesting to note that many seleniferous areas are oftentimes relatively close to areas that also produce crops that have low Se concentrations and Se deficiencies have been reported.

In some of the western sections of the United States, the leaching of Se from soils and rock has occurred after extensive mining operations. This has resulted in the subsequent transfer of Se and other heavy metals to irrigation waters and to wetland areas. The accumulation of these mineral elements in the tissues of wildlife living in these areas has frequently been detrimental to their survival. Wildlife abnormalities, reproductive defects, and high mortality rates have subsequently been reported particularly among the young in certain regions (e.g., Kesterson reservoir). Although this had initially raised concerns about the level of Se added to animal diets, subsequent investigations did not attribute these selenosis effects to supplemental Se (CAST, 1994).

Adding selenite or selenate to fertilizer has been shown to increase the Se content of grain (Pond et al., 1971; Nielsen et al., 1979). Selenate is more effectively absorbed by plants than selenite (Hupkens et al., 1977; Koivistoinen and Huttenen, 1986). Continued application of selenized fertilizer to land has, however, been controversial, but there have been no reported problems in those countries when this practice has been followed. Some soil microorganisms oxidize Se from the reduced to the oxidized state, which increases its availability to plant tissue (Sarathchandra and Watkinson, 1981). Fly ash from the coal-burning process produces a form of Se that is readily absorbed by plants (Mandisodza et al., 1979). Because of the continuous cropping systems now being widely practiced in many areas, soil pH is gradually declining and the subsequent conversion to selenate is slower than when soils were more frequently limed. High crop yields will ultimately produce grains with lower Se concentrations, exacerbating the potential deficiency. Adding animal excrement to cropland from animals fed supplemental Se (selenite) has not resulted in an increased grain Se content (CAST, 1994). This is because the Se in animal waste has been converted to a chemically reduced form in the intestinal tract, and most of the excreted Se (selenide) is not available for plant absorption.

III. PLANT AND GRAIN SOURCES OF SELENIUM

Selenium is not required for plant growth but is retained in plant tissue in proportion to the available Se content in the soil and the plants protein content. Upon absorption, Se can replace the S component of organic metabolites of the plant. Methionine synthesized by plants normally contains S, but Se can replace the S component largely forming the seleno amino acid selenomethionine. The Se-containing amino acid selenomethionine has been found to represent >50% of the total Se in plants (Olson et al.,1970; Allaway et al.,1981). The remaining Se in grains and forage is found in other organic Se analogs (Se-methylselenomethionine, selenocystine, selenocysteine, etc.), and are in water-soluble form. Consequently, the Se content of grains and forages is highly correlated with their crude protein content.

Several investigators have analyzed the Se content of grains and forages in much of the world. This information has been frequently used to explain why certain regions have livestock Se deficiencies. Figure 14.1 presents the Se content of grains and forages in the United States and Canada. The eastern corn belt and the East and West Coasts of the United States and Canada (Young et al., 1977b; NRC, 1983) are areas that have crops with low Se contents. These areas also correspond to the regions where animal deficiencies are frequently encountered. Maps illustrating the Se content of grains and forages have been developed for many other countries of the world (Oldfield, 1999).

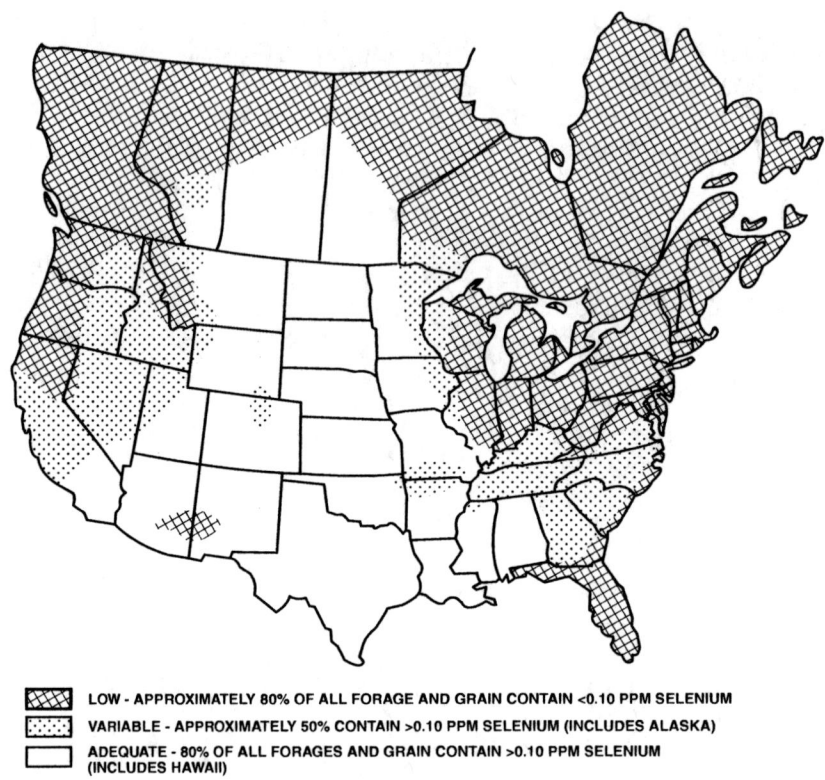

FIGURE 14.1 Regional distribution of forages and grain containing low, variable, or adequate levels of selenium in the United States and Canada. (From NRC, *Selenium in Nutrition*, National Academy Press, Washington, D.C., 1983. With permission.)

A study by Ku et al. (1972) demonstrated wide differences in loin Se contents of growing-finishing swine fed grains that were grown in various regions of the United States (Figure 14.2). Higher loin Se contents resulted when pigs consumed grains and feeds that had an indigenously higher Se content than grains from areas of low Se content (r = 0.95). This perhaps helps to explain the regional differences in the onset of the Se deficiency.

IV. PLANT AND GRAIN SOURCES OF VITAMIN E

Plants synthesize a group of fat-soluble compounds that have a similar chemical structure and have been found to be essential for animal reproduction. These compounds have collectively been termed vitamin E. They are in the free alcohol form, comprise eight isomers (four tocopherols, four tocotrienols), and chemically occur in the "D" configuration. Each grain source has been found to have a different quantity and ratio of these eight isomers. Although the eight isomers have a similar chemical structure, they have different potency responses in animals. The α-tocopherol form is the most bioactive form in animals. In the past, laboratory analyses had reported the total vitamin E (tocopherols and tocotrienols) content of grains, but with the advent of high-performance liquid chromatography (HPLC) equipment, the α-tocopherol content is now commonly reported.

The major vitamin E forms in plant and animal feed sources are presented in Table 14.1. Cereal grains and most of the oil seed protein sources contain relatively low concentrations of α-tocopherol, but generally have a higher concentration of the γ-isomer. Wheat germ oil, however, has a high

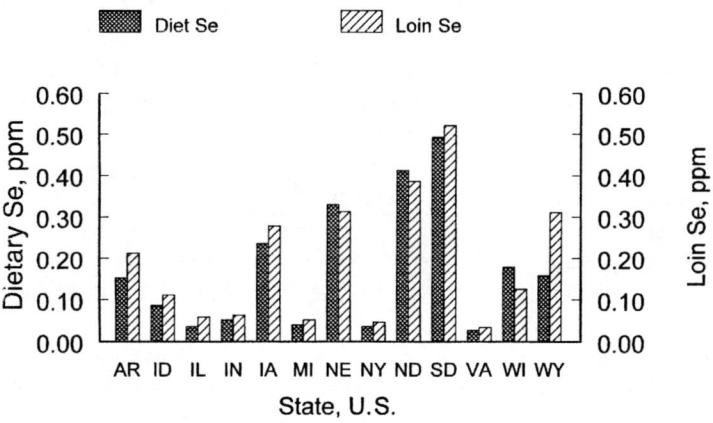

FIGURE 14.2 Effect of feeding indigenous selenium from grains raised in various regions of the United States to growing-finishing pigs on resulting loin selenium content. (From Ku, P. K. et al., *J. Anim. Sci.*, 34:208, 1972. With permission.)

TABLE 14.1
Tocopherol and Tocotrienol Concentration in Various Plant and Animal Tissue (mg/kg)

Feedstuff	Tocopherol				Tocotrienol				Total
	α	β	γ	δ	α	β	γ	δ	
Cereal grain									
Barley	6	3	0.5	—	25	—	3	—	40
Corn	6	0.3	38	2	7	—	56	0.2	60
Milo	5	—	15	—	<1	—	—	—	50
Oats	7	2	3	—	16	—	—	—	44
Wheat	10	9	—	0.08	3	—	—	—	49
Oilseed proteins									
Canola meal	13	—	5	—	—	—	—	—	25
Cottonseed meal	8	—	10	—	—	—	—	—	20
Soybean meal	2	—	14	tr	—	—	—	—	16
Sunflower meal	9	—	—	—	—	—	—	—	20
Plant oils and animal fats									
Corn oil	324	13	749	41	21	—	—	—	1148
Soybean oil	107	27	743	356	<1	—	—	—	1233
Sunflower oil	783	25	19	7	—	—	—	—	835
Tallow	16	—	—	—	—	—	—	—	18
Wheat germ oil	1330	710	—	—	—	—	—	—	2040
Lard	8	—	—	—	—	—	—	—	9
Forages									
Alfalfa, green	50	—	—	—	—	—	—	—	50
Alfalfa, hay	33–77	—	—	—	—	—	—	—	33–77
Alfalfa meal	215	—	—	—	—	—	—	—	227
Ryegrass, young	70	—	—	—	—	—	—	—	70

Source: Adapted from the data of Cort et al., 1983; Machlin, 1984; Ewan, 1989 (personal communications); NRC, 1998.

proportion of α-tocopherol. The tocotrienols are generally present in the bran and endosperm fractions of grains, whereas the tocopherols are located largely in the germ (Peterson and Wood, 1997). In animal fats (i.e., lard, tallow) the vitamin E is in the α-tocopherol form.

Almost all the vitamin E of young growing grasses and legumes is α-tocopherol. The leaves of forages are the site of α-tocopherol synthesis, notably in the chloroplasts of the leaves, whereas the β-, γ-, and δ-forms are usually found in plant tissue outside the chloroplasts (Combs, 1992). As the number of leaves decline or as the plant matures, the proportion of stalk relative to leaf increases, and the resulting α-tocopherol content of the plant declines (Robowsky and Knabe, 1970). Gestating and lactating sows fed corn–soybean meal diets without added vitamin E on pasture had higher serum α-tocopherol concentrations than sows fed the same diet in confinement (Mutetikka and Mahan, 1993). Therefore, pigs consuming growing grasses and legumes will have a higher vitamin E status than pigs raised in confinement. Consequently, under confinement conditions or when green forages are removed from the diets, vitamin E must be provided to meet the animals' requirement for this nutrient.

The biopotencies of different plant isomers using different criteria are presented in Table 14.2. Although different biological assays have been used to evaluate the efficacy of the various isomers, α-tocopherol has the highest activity of all the vitamin E forms. It is because of their differing biopotencies and ratios of isomers that standard units for vitamin E have been adopted by the U.S. Pharmacopoeia (1980). The unit is the International Unit (IU) and is equivalent to the bioactivity of 1 mg of synthetic DL-α-tocopheryl acetate, 0.909 mg DL-α-tocopherol, 0.735 mg D-α-tocopheryl acetate, or 0.671 mg D-α-tocopherol.

TABLE 14.2
Biopotencies of Natural Tocopherols and Tocotrienols Using Different Bioassays[a]

Compound	Fetal Resorption (rat)	RBC[b] Hemolysis (rat)	Myopathy Prevention (chick)	Myopathy Cure (rat)
D-α-Tocopherol	100	100	100	100
D-β-Tocopherol	25–40	15–27	12	—
D-γ-Tocopherol	1–11	3–20	5	11
D-δ-Tocopherol	1	0.3–2	—	—
D-α-Tocotrienol	28	17–25	—	28
D-β-Tocotrienol	5	1–5	—	—

[a] The γ- and δ-tocotrienols have low (<1%) biopotency.
[b] Red blood cell.

Source: Combs, G. F., Jr., *The Vitamins: Vitamin E*, Academic Press, New York, 1992, 181. With permission.

Although the indigenous vitamin E compounds within the plant or cereal grain are in the alcohol form and easily oxidized when exposed to air, the outer waxy covering of cereal grains forms a protective layer and prevents the entry of water and oxygen, which accelerates the oxidative process. Consequently, any harvesting or feed-processing method that disrupts the outer covering of grain seeds will lower its α-tocopherol content. Diseased and light-weight corns contain less tocopherol than does normal weight corn (Adams et al., 1975). Excessive heat during storage; prolonged storage of corn and grains of a high moisture content; the presence of molds; and the grinding, pelleting, and storage of complete feeds for extended times contributes to oxidation of the indigenous α-tocopherol of grains (Adams et al., 1975; Young et al., 1975).

V. COMMERCIAL SOURCES

A. SELENIUM

The Food and Drug Administration (FDA, 1987) permits manufactured premixes to contain no more than 200 mg Se/kg (90.8 mg Se/lb). Their restriction allows a supplemental level not to exceed 0.3 ppm Se provided from sodium selenite or sodium selenate (FDA, 1987). This level can, however, be supplemented to diets regardless of the natural Se indigenous in the grain. Both selenite and selenate are equally effective in swine but, because of its lower cost, sodium selenite is the form more commonly used. Sodium selenite is, however, water soluble and may be toxic to human handlers if inhaled or if it comes in contact with skin. Safety precautions are therefore recommended when individuals handle Se premixes. Other inorganic forms are less water soluble and therefore less toxic for human handlers (i.e., calcium selenite, barium selenite), but are not currently approved by FDA as a dietary supplement for swine. Calcium selenite can result in the same biological response as sodium selenite with pigs (Mahan and Magee, 1991).

Recent investigations comparing an organically produced Se-enriched yeast to sodium selenite demonstrated that the organic Se source can be an important form of Se for swine. The organic Se source may be somewhat less biopotent in terms of GSH-Px activity at low dietary Se (<0.10 ppm) levels but will result in a similar GSH-Px activity when added at the normally fortified levels of 0.3 ppm Se (Mahan et al., 1999). The bioavailability of organic Se for milk, placental Se transfer to the fetus, and the retention of Se in muscle and liver tissue in swine is substantially higher than that of sodium selenite (Mahan and Parrett, 1996; Mahan and Kim, 1996; Mahan et al., 1999, 2000). The profile of the Se-containing organic amino acids and their analogs in the Se-enriched yeast has demonstrated that a high proportion (>40%) of the Se is present as selenomethionine (Kelly and Power, 1995).

B. Vitamin E

The free alcohol forms of the various vitamin E compounds present in cereal grains and oil seed sources are readily oxidized. The indigenous vitamin E found in grain sources cannot, therefore, be depended upon for its nutritional contribution. Therefore, stabilized forms of vitamin E are commercially produced and are normally added to swine diets. There are two major types of commercial products; one uses a mixture of organic chemicals to synthetically produce vitamin E, whereas the other uses natural tocopherols and tocotrienols extracted from plant oils.

Perhaps no area of vitamin nutrition has been more confusing than the understanding and terminology used in the vitamin E area. For example "natural" vitamin E conveys the idea that the product is the natural product extracted from plant tissue. However, as indicated in Table 14.1, the major vitamin E form present in plant tissue is γ-tocopherol, which has a low biopotency for animals. Although the "natural" vitamin E product commercially produced is indeed from plant oils, it is processed in a manner that all of the tocopherols and tocotrienols are hydrogenated and methylated such that the end product has been converted to the D-α-tocopherol isomer. Thus, it is actually a "naturally derived" vitamin E product rather than just "natural."

Synthetic DL-α-tocopherol is a mixture of eight isomers all having the same α-tocopherol chromanol ring configuration, but eight isomeric differences occur in the side chain. These eight isomers result in an equimolar mixture of compounds that have a bioactivity that ranges from 21 to 100% when compared to D-α-tocopherol (Figure 14.3). Because of the different biopotencies between the "natural" and "synthetic" vitamin E sources, most of the recent scientific reports are now identifying the chemical form of the vitamin E product. The natural vitamin E product is termed D-α-tocopherol or RRR D-α-tocopherol (where R refers to the stereoisomers configuration on the side chain), whereas the synthetic vitamin E product is termed DL-α-tocopherol or all-*rac*-DL-α-tocopherol, the latter term used because the side chain contains the racemic mixture of all eight α-tocopherol isomers.

Both natural and synthetic vitamin E forms can be easily oxidized upon exposure to air, and therefore need to be stabilized to prevent their oxidative destruction. The insertion of an acetate or succinate moiety on carbon 6 of the chromanol ring of either the natural or synthetic

Name/configuration	Structure	IU/mg	Activity Compared to d-alpha
d-α-tocopherol (2R 4′R 8′R)	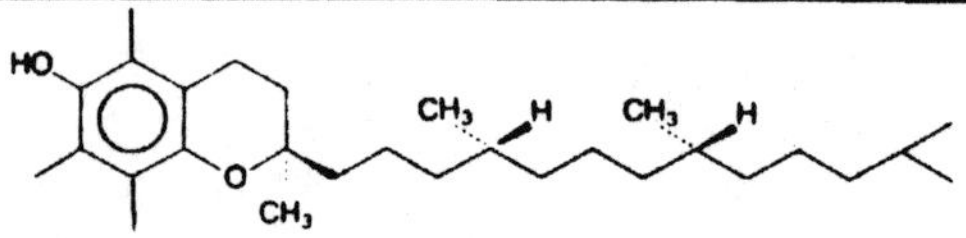	1.49	100%
l-α-tocopherol (2S 4′R 8′R)	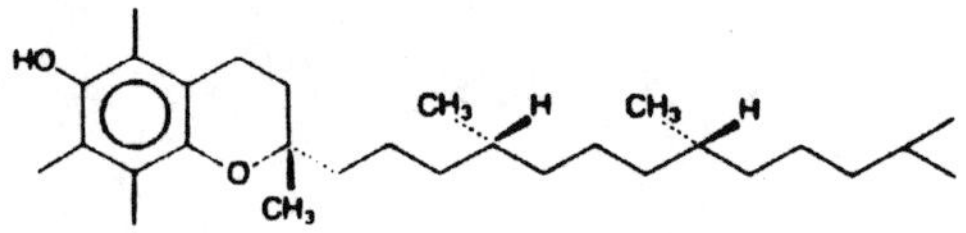	0.46	31%
2R 4′R 8′S-α-tocopherol	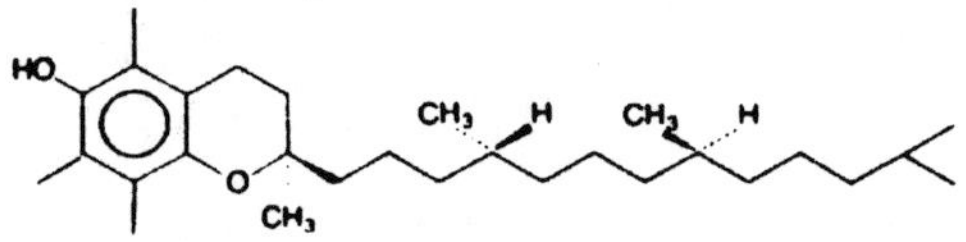	1.34	90%
2S 4′R 8′S-α-tocopherol	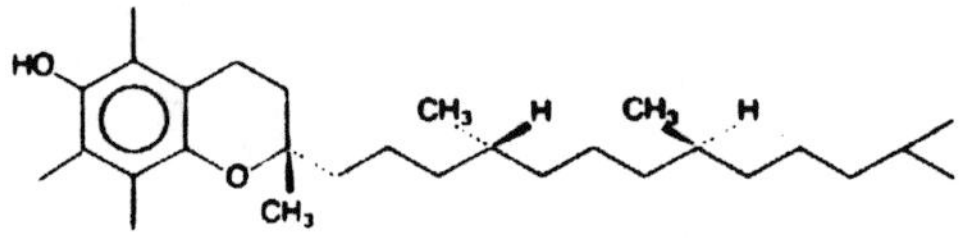	0.55	37%
2R 4′S 8′S-α-tocopherol	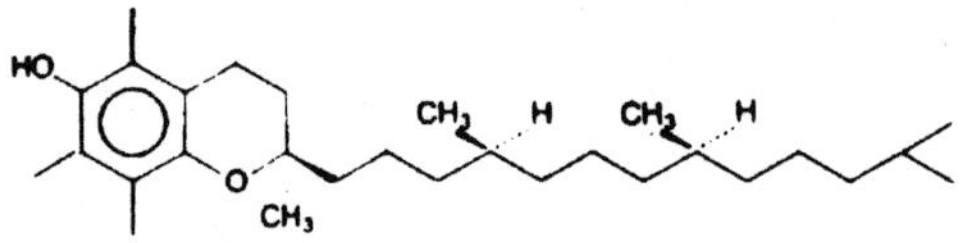	1.09	73%
2S 4′S 8′R-α-tocopherol	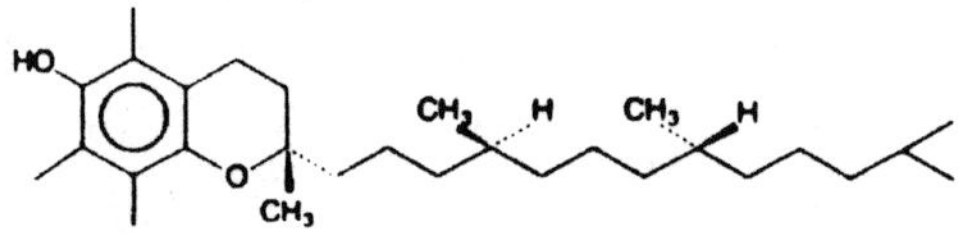	0.31	21%
2R 4′S 8′R-α-tocopherol	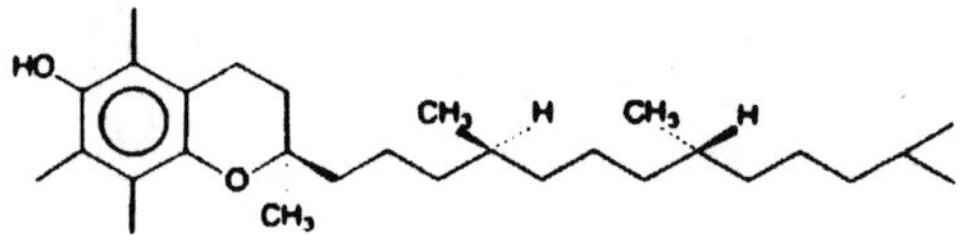	0.85	57%
2S 4′S 8′S-α-tocopherol	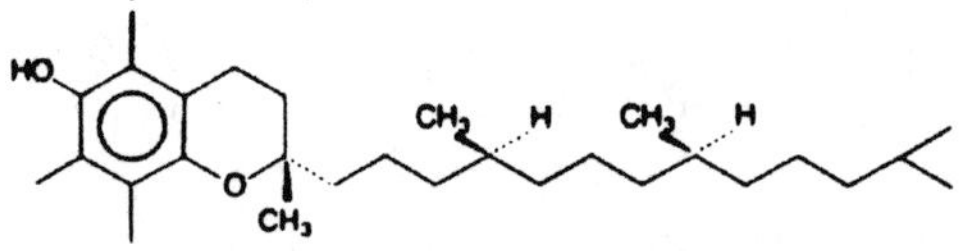	1.10	60%

FIGURE 14.3 Chemical configuration of the eight isomers of synthetic vitamin E. Note the stereoisomeric placement of CH_3 groups on the side chain; the positioning of the one closest to the chromanol ring results in the highest activity of the compound. (Courtesy of VERIS, 1998.)

source stabilizes the compound. When acetate is inserted the commercial names DL-α-tocopheryl acetate (all-*rac*-α-tocopheryl acetate) and D-α-tocopheryl acetate (RRR-α-tocopheryl acetate) are for the synthetic and naturally derived vitamin E products, respectively. The succinate form has been shown to be less biologically active than the acetate form (Jensen et al., 1999).

Commercial forms of vitamin E (DL-α-tocopheryl acetate or D-α-tocopheryl acetate) will maintain their vitamin E activity in storage or in mixed feeds until the acetate is removed from the molecule. They are, therefore, stable under normal handling and storage conditions (Dove and Ewan, 1991). Although unsaturated fatty acids, rancid fats (Obel, 1953), and certain trace minerals (i.e., Fe, Cu) will lower the indigenous tocopherol content of grains, those situations will not affect the commercial vitamin E products when in the acetylated form.

VI. ABSORPTION OF SELENIUM AND VITAMIN E

A. Selenium

The site and mechanism of how and where Se is absorbed from the intestinal tract will vary, but all of the forms normally added to the diet seem to be relatively well absorbed. Although selenide is the biologically active form of Se in the body, it is not readily absorbed. Consequently, the oxidative state of this element can affect its absorption from the intestine. The Se status of the animal does not seem to influence the absorption rate of either inorganic or organic Se compounds even when fed at high dietary levels (Kim, 1999).

Selenate absorption is sodium dependant and occurs in the brush border cells in the ileum via an active transport mechanism and competes with sulfate and other metal oxides at the absorption site (Wolffram et al., 1986; 1988). This competitiveness seems to be of minor practical importance unless the elements are ingested at toxic concentrations. In contrast, selenite absorption is sodium independent and occurs by passive diffusion in the duodenum and upper portion of the ileum (Wolffram et al., 1986).

The absorption of organic Se compounds depends completely on an active transport system. Both selenomethionine and methionine are actively absorbed and compete with each other at the same absorption site. Consequently, their absorptions are largely dependent upon the dietary ratio of the two amino acids (McConnell and Cho, 1965). The absorption of other organic seleno-compounds does not seem to be inhibited by their respective S analogs (NRC, 1983). Animal Se sources generally have a lower (<25%) absorption rate of Se than Se from plant tissue (>60%). However, Se absorption is influenced by the type of animal product being fed. For example, the absorption of Se from bovine milk is high and equivalent to that of selenite (Mathias et al., 1967), whereas Se in meat and bone meal or poultry by-products is ≤20% (Cantor et al., 1975). Overall, the organic Se seleno amino acids from grains are absorbed effectively but at a somewhat slower rate than the inorganic sources (Groce et al.,1973a). Mahan and Parrett (1996) demonstrated a higher apparent absorption of inorganic selenite compared with the organic Se source (from yeast) in growing pigs, but the retention of Se was higher when the organic form was fed.

The oxidative state of minerals can affect their absorption from the intestinal tract. Strong electronegative characteristics attract electrons from other elements, which effectively chelates and alters their absorption. It is this binding or chelating property of Se that allows it to reduce the availability and toxicity of other metals, but this in turn also reduces the availability of Se (Hill, 1975). Selenate and selenite will, however, retain their oxidative state and high bioavailability under normal feed and premix storage conditions (Groce et al., 1971; 1973a; Olson et al., 1973).

Heavy metal content in some feed sources (e.g., fish meal) and products from the biliary extract (i.e., glutathione, cysteine, heavy metals) can bind inorganic Se in the digestive tract and reduce Se absorption. The effects of heavy metals in most swine diets seem to be relatively minor unless present at high dietary concentrations. When certain heavy elements are fed at high dietary levels and the diet is moderate to low in Se content, these heavy metals can induce the Se–vitamin E deficiency (Van Vleet and Ruth, 1977; Van Vleet, 1982). Although some of these minerals and organic arsenicals have been added to swine diets, no Se deficiencies have been reported from their usage (Hitchcock et al., 1978; Thulin et al., 1985).

B. Vitamin E

Because of its fat-soluble characteristics, the absorption of natural vitamin E from grain is closely aligned with the digestion and absorption of dietary fat. The absorption of vitamin E largely depends upon bile, pancreatic juices, and the presence of dietary fat. The esters of the acetylated vitamin E forms must be hydrolyzed by pancreatic and intestinal esterases before absorption can occur.

The freed α-tocopherols thus become associated with dietary fat particles and micelles from the bile–fat interface. Vitamin E is thus passively transferred into the micelle and absorbed through the brush border cells, combined with resynthesized chylomicrons in the lymph, whereupon it is subsequently transported through the thoracic duct into the systemic circulation system. As the dietary vitamin E level increases, the total amount of vitamin E absorbed will increase but the relative amount absorbed declines. Of the natural vitamin E compounds, approximately 32% of the α-, 18% of the β-, 30% of the γ-, and <2% of the δ-tocopherol forms are absorbed (Pearson and Barnes, 1970). Overall, approximately 20 to 30% of orally ingested vitamin E is absorbed (Gallo-Torres, 1973; Chow, 1985).

Although several factors can affect the absorption of vitamin E in pigs, the principal one seems to be dietary fat. The young pig consumes sow colostrum and milk, which are high in fat and α-tocopherol concentrations. Milk fat is considered highly digestible (>95%) by the young pig. Consequently, α-tocopherol and γ-tocopherol are both present in sow milk and are highly available, as reflected by their high serum α-tocopherol concentration in the nursing pig (Malm et al., 1976; Mahan 1991; 1994). Serum α-tocopherol, however, has been found to decline rapidly upon weaning but subsequently increases within 3 to 4 weeks postweaning (Mahan and Moxon, 1980; Meyer et al., 1981). Although this suggests that commercial forms of vitamin E are not as well absorbed as those in sow milk, there are many physiological factors that are concurrently changing during the transition from consuming a liquid milk to a dry diet. It is probable that the low amount and different types of fat provided in most postweaning diets may limit the absorption of vitamin E products, particularly during the initial days postweaning. When an emulsified vitamin E source was added to the drinking water of young pigs the absorption of DL-α-tocopheryl acetate was high during the initial days postweaning (Moreira et al., 1999). Although the hydrolysis of the acetate from the vitamin E molecule may be a factor limiting the absorption of this nutrient in young pigs, it is also probable that the dietary fat source and level used in most weaned pig diets may not allow optimum absorption of vitamin E.

Polyunsaturated fats can oxidize free vitamin E in the diet and intestinal lumen and destroy its antioxidant activity (Weber, 1981). High dietary levels of vitamin A have been shown to reduce vitamin E absorption in young pigs (Ching and Mahan, 1995), but not in growing-finishing pigs (Anderson et al., 1995). It should be noted that any intestinal disease that interferes with fat digestion or with pancreatic function will affect vitamin E absorption.

VII. BLOOD AND TISSUE DISTRIBUTION

A. SELENIUM

Absorbed inorganic Se is rapidly incorporated into the erythrocyte, but within a short time some of it is released into the serum. When organic Se compounds are absorbed, the seleno amino acids or their analogs are circulated in the systemic circulatory system. Serum and plasma have similar Se concentrations and generally reflect the short-term Se status of the animal, whereas whole-blood Se values reflect the long-term status of the pig. Normal whole-blood Se values (>0.20 ppm) are higher than serum or plasma concentrations because of the higher amount of Se retained in red blood cells. Normal serum Se values are generally within the range of 0.08 to 0.15 ppm (Mahan and Moxon, 1978a; Meyer et al., 1981). When organic Se sources are fed to swine, serum Se values are somewhat higher than when inorganic Se sources are fed (Mahan and Parrett, 1996; Mahan et al., 1999).

Selenomethionine enters the body's methionine pool after absorption. It is used for GSH-Px production, but substantial amounts are also incorporated into body protein tissue. Selenomethionine remains in the tissue until protein catabolism or turnover takes place. Absorbed selenomethionine, selenocysteine, and the various Se analogs can, however, be catabolized and the released Se diverted to the body Se pool, converted to selenocysteine, or excreted.

The amount of selenium retained in body tissue reflects both the quantity and source of dietary Se being fed to the pig. The tissues of highest Se concentration in declining order are kidney > liver > glandular tissue > muscle (Groce et al., 1973b; Young et al., 1976; 1977b; Mahan and Moxon, 1978b; 1980; Kurkela and Kaantee, 1984; Kim, 1999). Because organic Se contains a high proportion of selenomethionine, the Se content of all tissue, but particularly muscle is generally higher when an organic Se source is fed (Mahan and Parrett, 1996; Mahan et al., 1999). The amount of organic Se retained in muscle reflects the relative amount of methionine and selenomethionine in the diet (Ku et al., 1972). Because of the large mass of muscle relative to other body tissue in the pig, most of the organic Se is incorporated into muscle. The liver seems to be the tissue that perhaps best reflects the animal's Se status. For example, in a deficient condition, there is a greater decline of Se from the liver relative to other tissue (Mahan et al., 1977; Peplowski et al., 1981), suggesting its mobilization is being used for the production of essential selenoproteins. In contrast, in selenosis conditions a more rapid increase in liver Se occurs relative to other tissues, suggesting that this tissue can also serve as a large storage reservoir (Mahan and Moxon, 1984; Kim, 1999). In a study with growing-finishing pigs when either inorganic or organic Se sources were fed, the liver had a similar Se concentration at 55 kg body weight, but at 105 kg, liver Se was higher when the organic Se form was fed (Mahan et al., 1999). This suggests that during early growth much of the selenomethionine was retained in the muscle and less was available for retention in other tissues, notably the liver. In contrast, when muscle tissue accretion declines during the finishing period, more selenomethionine becomes available, thus resulting in an elevated liver Se content. Replacement gilts fed an organic Se source will have a higher Se status at breeding.

B. Vitamin E

Chylomicrons formed in the brush border cells during fat absorption are transported to the thoracic duct and carried to the liver. Although some of the passively bound vitamin E within the chylomicron is released to the tissues by lipoprotein lipase or transferred to blood lipoproteins, most of the vitamin E is retained in the hepatocyte cells of the liver. A transfer protein within the liver preferentially selects the RRR-α-tocopherol isomer transferring it to other body tissue (Traber et al., 1990; Weiser et al., 1996). In these body tissues, lipoprotein lipase releases RRR-α-tocopherol from the circulating triacylglyceride for subsequent incorporation into the cell lipoprotein membrane layer. Grains contain a substantial amount of γ-tocopherol that is readily absorbed (Desai et al., 1964). The γ-tocopherol is transported to the liver, or in the case of lactating sows into milk (Mahan, 1991), and/or excreted through the bile (Desai et al., 1964). Much of the remaining synthetic α-tocopherol stereoisomers seem to be largely retained in the liver, transported in the blood (Weiser et al., 1996), or converted to a tocopherol metabolite and voided in urine (Traber et al., 1998). The major form of vitamin E transported and retained in nonhepatic tissues is therefore the RRR-α-tocopherol or D-α-tocopherol form (Weiser et al., 1996). Tissues vary in their concentration of RRR-α-tocopherol, but the major reservoir is in the liver and fatty tissues (Machlin, 1984). Tissues that have a high fat content and high lipoprotein lipase activity thus have a higher α-tocopherol content. Although vitamin E seems to be largely concentrated in the cellular membrane fractions, it has been suggested that its bioavailability from this deposit for subsequent mobilization is limited (Machlin et al., 1979). Mahan et al. (2000), however, demonstrated that older sows have a declining milk and lower adipose α-tocopherol content, suggesting that when body fat reservoirs are mobilized the sow may divert α-tocopherol from body fat stores into the milk supply. Therefore, the liver can be considered a retention and labile transfer organ for absorbed tocopherols, whereas adipose cells may also be a tissue reservoir for RRR-α-tocopherol.

Although there is a difference between the various tissues in their α-tocopherol content, all body cells contain α-tocopherol in their lipoprotein membrane layer. Plasma α-tocopherol levels in swine seem to be lower than other species (Lindberg, 1973). Blood and serum α-tocopherol were associated with blood lipoproteins, but the correlation of α-tocopherol to blood triglyceride or to cholesterol was not high in the young weanling pig (Chung et al., 1992).

VIII. METABOLIC ROLES

A. ANTIOXIDANT FUNCTION

The body has an effective defense system against oxygen-induced damage. The sequential addition of electrons to oxygen can produce a number of intermediates, some of which are toxic and can interact with cellular constituents particularly membrane lipids. These oxidants can ultimately alter and damage the membrane structure of the cell. Within the cytoplasm, both superoxide and hydrogen peroxide are produced as the result of carbohydrate and amino acid metabolism. In the presence of excess electrons, such as from iron (Fe^{3+}), the superoxide ion can initiate the formation of free radicals, thus causing oxidative damage to subcellular membranes unless the superoxide ion is converted to a nontoxic form. The cytoplasmic enzymes superoxide dismutase (SOD), catalase (CAT), and GSH-Px prevent free radical formation by converting the superoxide and hydrogen peroxide to water. If free radicals form, however, they can interact with the unsaturated fatty acids in the intracellular membranes forming a lipid free radical (R·), followed by a rearrangement of the double bonds to form a fatty acid peroxyl radical (ROO·). The peroxyl radical attracts a hydrogen ion from another unsaturated fatty acid forming a fatty acid hydroperoxide (ROOH) and another free radical (R·), thus initiating a chain reaction. Peroxidation of unsaturated fatty acid residues of phospholipids causes a change in the bonding of the cell, altering the structural integrity of the cellular or subcellular membranes. This effect is detrimental, and damage to cell integrity can result. Vitamin E can directly and rapidly contributes an H ion to this process, thus preventing the further loss of the H ion from an unsaturated fatty acid. This rapid antioxidant capability of vitamin E prevents further oxygen damage to unsaturated fatty acids by preventing the formation of hydroperoxides in the membranes. The higher the dietary level of vitamin E, the greater the α-tocopherol content in the membrane layer. In contrast, Se is a component of the GSH-Px enzyme located in the cytoplasm. This enzyme causes glutathione to lose its H ion and prevents oxidative damage from the superoxide molecule generated within the cytoplasm of the cell.

1. Selenium

Absorbed Se from sodium selenite is converted to selenide in the red blood cells and liver. Diplock et al. (1971) demonstrated that vitamin E was effective in maintaining a greater tissue pool of selenide, probably serving in an antioxidant protection role. Selenide is the active form of Se produced in the body, whereupon it is ultimately converted to selenocysteine. Selenocysteine is incorporated into various selenoproteins via the cystathionine pathway (Esaki et al., 1981), whereas selenide is incorporated into the amino acid via a cotranslational mechanism involving $HSePO_3^-$ and Ser-tRNA (Sunde, 1997). The seleno amino acid selenocysteine accounts for the biological activity of the known Se-containing enzymes of the body and cannot be replaced by cysteine. Selenocysteine cannot be extensively stored; thus a readily available supply of Se is essential to meet the animal's biological need for Se. Both organic and inorganic Se can, however, adequately supply the body's selenocysteine need. The Se in selenomethionine initially retained in body tissue can be diverted for later body use when tissue catabolism or tissue turnover occurs. Selenomethionine that is incorporated into muscle tissue and its ultimate catabolism conversion to selenocysteine, when tissue turnover occurs, may be a source of Se for the animal.

When inorganic Se is fed, the GSH-Px enzyme accounts for approximately 30 to 40% of the total body supply of Se. There are currently four known GSH-Px enzymes in the body. These enzymes reduce hydroperoxides absorbed either from the diet or generated from body metabolism. The most abundant form of GSH-Px is a cellular GSH-Px located in the cytoplasm of the cells where hydroperoxides from cellular metabolism are reduced via glutathione. A second form is localized in the cells of the intestinal tract where absorbed hydroperoxides are reduced, the third is located in the extracellular fluid or plasma (secreted in kidney and liver) where it reduces hydroperoxides esterified to phospholipids as well as free hydroperoxides, and the fourth enzyme is an intracellular phospholipid hydroperoxide GSH-Px located adjacent to subcellular membranes preventing intracellular lipid peroxidation.

Riboflavin is involved in the activity of glutathione reductase, an enzyme essential for the production of glutathione. A deficiency of riboflavin can therefore result in lowered GSH-Px activity because of the lower concentration of glutathione (Brady et al., 1979; Parsons et al., 1985).

There is an Se-dependent and an Se-independent form of GSH-Px in animal tissue (Lawrence and Burk, 1978). Meyer et al. (1981) demonstrated that the Se-dependent form in pig liver was responsive to dietary selenite, whereas the independent form was not. It has been suggested that the activity of GSH-Px is perhaps the best criterion to reflect the Se status of the pig and its requirement (Hakkarainen et al., 1978a,b; Chavez, 1979a,b). However, because GSH-Px activity increases with animal age (Mahan et al., 1999) and there is currently a wide variation in analytical values among laboratories, its use as a clinical tool to measure the pig's Se status is questionable. Workers have reported high correlations between tissue and serum GSH-Px activities when dietary Se is below or at the animals' requirement level, but when the dietary Se level exceeds the animals' requirement the correlation is lower (Meyer et al., 1981). The incorporation of Se into GSH-Px thus seems to be of high biological priority, but as the animals' requirement for Se is met more of the Se is diverted to other selenoproteins, retained in tissue, bound to tissue in a nonselective manner, or excreted.

In addition to GSH-Px, two types of iodothyronine deiodinases enzymes are located in the body that contain the selenocysteine selenoprotein chain (Berry and Larsen, 1992; Arthur and Beckett, 1994). These enzymes remove iodine [I] from the thyroid hormone thyroxine (T_4) converting it to the active form triiodothyronine (T_3). The thyroid hormone is involved in animal growth and feed utilization. Thus, a relationship exists between I and Se, whereby a deficiency of either or both can affect animal performance. A deficiency of either exacerbates the deficiency of the other.

A recent report has indicated the existence of a selenoenyzme thioredoxin reductase. This cellular enzyme maintains thioredoxin in a reduced state. Reduced thioredoxin activates the enzyme ribonucleotide reductase and stimulates DNA binding of a subunit in the transcription process that can affect cell growth.

Selenoprotein P is located in the plasma and a selenoprotein W appears to be located in muscle tissue. The function of these latter selenoproteins has yet to be clarified but probably both have antioxidant properties. It has been estimated that there may be >30 selenoproteins in the body, many as yet unidentified.

2. Vitamin E

Reactive free radicals or superoxides are normally formed by the mitochondrial electron transport system and from cytoplasmic metabolism. Vitamin E is one of the primary antioxidants in the body's oxygen-generated defense system. Because vitamin E is fat soluble, it is directly incorporated within the cell membrane, where it protects the lipoprotein layer from oxidative damage. Vitamin E prevents the formation of free radicals by contributing an H ion, thus stopping the chain reaction from free radical formation. The tocopherol molecule is subsequently oxidized to the tocopheroxyl radical, which can be converted back to α-tocopherol by either vitamin C or glutathione.

B. Immune Function

The immune response to pathogenic organisms utilizes many cell types: macrophages, B-lymphocytes, and T-lymphocytes. An interaction exists between these cells, promoting both cellular and humoral immunogenic responses. Larsen and Tollersrud (1981) demonstrated enhanced T-cell proliferation when Se or vitamin E were administered. Nockels (1979) demonstrated an increase in plaque-forming cells and demonstrated that vitamin E fed to nonimmunized hens increased the primary immune response of their progeny. Macrophages and T-lymphocytes engulf foreign antigens or organisms, killing and removing them from the body. The humoral response thus enhances the production of serum antibodies secreted by B-lymphocytes. These antibodies bind and rid the body of invading organisms.

Selenium and vitamin E seems to work synergistically in the cellular and humoral response system. Tengerdy et al. (1973) and Nockels (1979) demonstrated that the dietary level of vitamin E required for optimum immune function may be higher than the amount required for growth processes. Peplowski et al. (1981) demonstrated a humoral response in weaned pigs when either Se or vitamin E were provided in the diet or injected, but when both nutrients were given together antibody titers were higher, suggesting a synergistic relationship. Ellis and Vorhies (1976) demonstrated improved humoral responses to an *Escherichia coli* bacterin when young pigs were fed high dietary levels (110 IU/kg) of vitamin E. Other workers (Teige, 1977; Teige et al., 1977; 1978) have demonstrated that dietary Se and vitamin E were effective in enhancing the immune response in pigs. Kornegay et al. (1986) did not achieve an improvement in antibody titer by dietary inclusion of Se or vitamin E, but their pigs were probably in a good Se and vitamin E status at the start of their experiment.

Because pigs are essentially born immunologically sterile, the antibody content of colostrum is extremely important for neonatal survival. Hayek et al. (1989) demonstrated that in sows injected with Se (5 mg) or vitamin E (1000 IU) 2 weeks before farrowing higher IgM concentrations occurred in both the sow's colostrum and in the pig's serum at 20 h postfarrowing. Teige et al. (1977; 1978) and Saxegaard and Teige (1977) also suggested that swine deficient in Se and vitamin E are more susceptible to dysentery.

It has been suggested that vitamin E may have an adjuvant role in the immune response by increasing the efficiency of the immune response against an antigen (Tengerdy et al., 1973; Afzai et al., 1984).

C. Arachidonic Acid and Prostaglandin Metabolism

Arachidonic acid found in the phospholipid layer of cellular membranes is involved in the synthesis of different prostaglandins. Vitamin E stimulates the conversion of linoleic acid to arachidonic acid, a reaction that involves free radical metabolism (Diplock, 1981). Prostaglandin synthesis was found to be reduced in the testis and muscle of vitamin E–deficient animals (Chan et al., 1980). Platelet aggregation was increased and prostaglandin E inhibited under vitamin E deficiency conditions (Mustard and Packham, 1970; Lake et al., 1977). Recent research by Marin-Guzman et al. (2000b) suggests that when vitamin E was fed in excess of the animals' requirement, $PGF_{2\alpha}$ synthesis in the testis was reduced. The role of vitamin E in the synthesis of the prostaglandins may help to explain many clinical deficiency signs encountered in both growing and reproducing swine.

IX. EXCRETION

A. Selenium

Normal Se excretion in swine, as with other nonruminants, occurs mainly through the kidney and gastrointestinal tract. Intestinal bacteria convert dietary selenite and undigested organic Se into insoluble selenide to metal selenides or microbial selenoproteins, whereupon they are excreted in the feces. Most of the Se that passes through the digestive tract is reduced to the nonabsorbable selenide form. The proportion of microbial Se is higher in ruminants, but constitutes approximately 45% of total fecal Se in the nonruminant. The biliary system diverts a large portion of absorbed Se to the intestinal lumen (Olson et al., 1963; Lavender and Bagman, 1966; Whagner, 1981). As

Se intake increases, an increasing proportion of Se is voided in the urine (Mahan, 1985). Urinary Se is in the form of trimethylselenide, a reduced form of the element (Palmer et al., 1970). Growing pigs fed sodium selenite therefore excreted more Se in the urine and less in the feces than when organic Se was fed. However, approximately 20% more total Se was voided in swine excrement when the inorganic Se form was provided at various dietary levels (Mahan and Parrett, 1996). Animal feces, thus, return a large proportion of Se in the reduced Se form to the soil, but it is unavailable for plant absorption unless microbial or soil chemical oxidative processes convert it to the oxidized form.

B. Vitamin E

Because much of the dietary vitamin E is not absorbed from the intestinal tract, it is excreted via the feces, but this can vary widely depending upon the form provided and the dietary level fed. The tocopherols that pass through the intestinal tract occur from incomplete absorption, secretion from the mucosal cells into the lumen, desquamation of intestinal epithelial cell, and biliary excretion (Machlin, 1984). Of the absorbed tocopherols, some are converted to the quinone and excreted. The biliary route can excrete tocopheryl acetates and tocopherol (Machlin, 1984), but the amount is relatively small (~2.4%).

X. DEFICIENCY ONSET AND SYMPTOMS

A. Tissue Responses

Tissues that have a high growth rate probably need more Se and vitamin E than tissues with lower rates of growth. Tissues with higher polyunsaturated fatty acid contents and higher metabolic activities are also generally those tissues where the deficiency is more likely to be encountered. Extreme deficiencies can interfere with growth and feed utilization processes, whereas mild deficiencies generally have not shown this response. Both Se and vitamin E are associated with the mitochondria, thyroid hormone, and those cellular organelles where oxidative phosphorylation occurs. Deficiency signs for each nutrient cannot be separated because of their common biological functions, albeit at different locations in the cell.

When oxidative damage to cellular membranes occurs and the membranes are disrupted, the cellular contents are released into the systemic circulation. The leakage of cellular fluids results in an edema condition (exudative diathesis) and an elevated concentration of cellular enzymes (generally amino acid transferases) in the blood. These enzymes can be subsequently measured and are frequently used to confirm the deficiency (Wretlind et al., 1959; Ewan et al., 1969; Tollersrud, 1973). Some of the enzymes may indicate muscle damage, whereas others may reflect liver necrosis. Low serum Se and vitamin E concentrations generally occur prior to the elevation of these blood enzymes.

Reduced prothrombin time, increased red blood cell hemolysis, and morphological abnormalities of bone marrow cells reflect conditions deficient in Se-vitamin E (Baustad and Nafstad, 1972; Jensen et al., 1979; 1983; Bartholomew et al., 1998). Although anemia has frequently been reported with vitamin E deficiencies (Obel, 1953; Grant, 1961; Nafstad, 1965; Nafstad and Nafstad, 1968; Baustad and Nafstad, 1972), the effect has not always been encountered (Ewan et al., 1969; Fontaine et al., 1977a,b,c; Niyo et al., 1980). Because labored breathing from stress conditions also occurs in Se and vitamin E deficient swine, the condition implies a lower oxygen content in the red blood cells.

Sweeney and Brown (1972) and Lake et al. (1977) reported vascular damage in connective tissues, suggesting that Se and vitamin E may be involved in collagen and connective tissue synthesis. Although the spraddle leg condition is reported in neonatal pigs, it is possible that impairment of connective tissue development may be involved in the deficiency.

Various disease or disease-related problems are frequently associated with the Se–vitamin E deficiency. Thomlinson and Buxton (1963) presented evidence that young swine deficient in Se and vitamin E can be hypersensitive to *E. coli*, resulting in an anaphylactic reaction with signs resembling gut edema. This effect was prevented when diets were supplemented with vitamin E (Teige et al., 1973; Teige, 1977).

B. CLINICAL SYMPTOMS

Increased fluid accumulation in the pericardial sac, gut edema in intestinal membranes, and postweaning diarrhea are commonly observed clinical symptoms in swine deficient in Se–vitamin E. Clinical observations also include liver deterioration and hemorrhages (hepatosis dietetica), cardiac myopathy (weakened, thin-walled, enlarged, pale striations), hemorrhages in the auricle (mulberry heart), light-colored or pale striated muscles that are especially noticeable in the more active muscles (nutritional muscular dystrophy), and cecal and colonic hemorrhages (Grant and Thafvelin, 1958; Grant, 1961; Ewan et al., 1969; Nafstad and Tollersrud, 1970; Bengtsson et al., 1978). Tissue atrophy and Ca deposits occur in Se-deficient (white muscle disease) lambs, but the pale muscle color that occurs in deficient swine is attributed to a lack of oxygen supplied to the muscle tissues. Steatitis or the yellow discoloration of body fat, which is a commonly observed deficiency sign, seems to be associated more with vitamin E than with the Se deficiency. Gastric ulcers occur with the Se–vitamin E deficiency, but Se may be more responsible for the condition than vitamin E (Mahan et al., 1975).

It is commonly reported in commercial swine operations that the largest, fastest-growing animals seem to be more prone to the sudden death condition, which has been attributed to Se–vitamin E deficiency. This death generally occurs within 2 to 4 weeks postweaning, but is also reported with growing-finishing pigs at a lower frequency. The incidence of highest occurrence seems to be largely in areas of the United States where grain Se content is low, suggesting that the indigenous Se in grains may be important in preventing the deficiency onset.

Research workers have reported that both dietary Se and vitamin E supplementation can prevent the deficiency. Although high levels of vitamin E are frequently incorporated into diets to reduce the deficiency, the deficiency is still encountered on many swine farms.

The feeding of semipurified diets deficient in Se and vitamin E and diets containing unsaturated or rancid fats have resulted in more marked deficiency signs than when animals are fed practical-type diets (Obel, 1953; Grant et al., 1961; Lanneck et al., 1962; Ewan et al., 1969). Swine fed semipurified diets fortified with Se or vitamin E will generally demonstrate an improved growth rate and feed efficiency response (Forbes and Draper, 1957; Ewan et al., 1969; Glienke and Ewan, 1977; Adkins and Ewan, 1984), whereas when cereal grain diets are fed, animal performance is generally not improved when Se or vitamin E are added to the diet (Mahan and Moxon, 1978a,b; Nielsen et al., 1979; Meyer et al., 1981).

XI. FACTORS THAT CONTRIBUTE TO SELENIUM AND VITAMIN E DEFICIENCY IN SWINE

Field cases of the Se–vitamin E deficiency in swine began to be reported during the 1960s and early 1970s (Michel et al., 1969; Trapp et al., 1970, Van Vleet et al., 1970). It was subsequently determined that supplemental Se and vitamin E were needed either in the diet or as an injection to prevent the deficiency. The FDA (1974; 1982; 1987) subsequently approved the addition of inorganic Se to swine diets when provided as sodium selenite or sodium selenate. The addition of dietary Se and vitamin E has reduced the incidence of the deficiency, but the problem has not been eliminated. Reasons for the continued occurrence of the deficiency are currently under investigation but continue even when high dietary levels of vitamin E (>100 IU/kg) are fed. Several factors that initially caused the Se–vitamin E deficiency are identified below, as well as others that may exacerbate the current situation.

1. Swine confinement has eliminated the soil and green forages from the pig's natural diet. These components contributed major sources of Se and α-tocopherol to the diet.
2. Simplified diets (corn and soybean meal) have resulted in the elimination of many feed sources that previously contributed Se and vitamin E (e.g., alfalfa meal, meat and bone meal, etc.) to the pig's diet.
3. High oil grains and the increased incorporation of fats or fat blends (vegetable and animal fats) into modern swine diets have increased the dietary requirement for vitamin E. The presence of unsaturated fatty acids or rancid fats oxidizes the natural vitamin E content in mixed diets.
4. Higher dietary levels of some trace minerals (i.e., Cu, Fe) into mixed feeds can destroy the indigenous α-tocopherol content of grains.
5. Swine confinement has resulted in increased pig growth rates and higher metabolic activities. Consequently, dietary needs for both Se and vitamin E are higher.
6. Genetic differences may possibly affect the requirement and utilization of Se and vitamin E in swine (Jensen et al., 1979; 1984; Stowe and Miller, 1985). Lean pigs have a higher requirement for Se and vitamin E because of the increased oxygen demand of lean tissue. Leaner animals frequently have a lower feed intake, which reduces the total amount of nutrients consumed. Different colored swine hair retains Se differently, thus affecting the Se requirement of the animal (Wahlstrom et al., 1984; Kim, 1999).
7. Maintaining high-producing sows for several parities has resulted in the depletion of body stores of both Se and vitamin E. The deficiency symptoms in the progeny of older sows are thus more frequent than those of younger sows.
8. Early weaning has resulted in lower tissue storage reserves of both Se and vitamin E in the weaned pig.
9. Increased crop yields have resulted in lower Se concentrations in cereal grains.
10. Continuous cropping systems, less crop rotation, and increased irrigation has resulted in a lower soil Se content and oftentimes a lower soil pH, thus reducing available soil Se for plant absorption.
11. Storage of grains for extended periods and the presence of molds destroys the indigenous α-tocopherol content of feedstuffs.
12. Feed processing (i.e., roller mill, grinding, pelleting, extruding) will lower the α-tocopherol content of grains or oil seeds due to oxidation processes.
13. High-moisture grains have a lower α-tocopherol content due to oxidation processes.
14. The pig's ability to retain Se in several body tissues is lower when inorganic Se is fed compared with when organic Se is fed. The rapid mobilization of tissue Se from the liver for functional purposes seems to be somewhat limited.
15. Inorganic Se sources are not as effectively retained in swine tissue, deposited in fetal tissue, or incorporated into sow colostrum and milk as organic Se sources.

XII. SELENIUM AND VITAMIN E IN FETAL AND NEONATAL PIGS

A. GENERAL

The progeny of sows deficient in Se–vitamin E are weak at birth, have weakened muscles, and a reduced desire to nurse the sow, which results in higher mortality rates. The slower release of milk from the mammary tissue of deficient sows and the subsequent decline in glycogen reserves exacerbate the mortality problems in young pigs. Spraddle-legged pigs have been reported born to sows deficient in Se and vitamin E (Adams et al., 1975). This effect may be associated with inadequate collagen formation and weakened muscles.

Selenium is increasingly transferred through the placenta to the developing fetus as the dietary level fed to the sow is increased (Mahan et al., 1975; 1977). The pig at birth, however, has a total

Se body content of ≤0.10 mg (Piatkowski et al., 1979; Mahan and Watts, unpublished data). Feeding sows an organic Se source increases the neonatal Se liver content (Mahan and Kim, 1996). Whether this increase is adequate in itself to prevent the deficiency is not known. Colostrum, a rich and high-availability source of both Se and vitamin E, is generally adequate to prevent the deficiency in the neonate. High-producing sows, however, have a lower Se status as they age, and more neonatal deficiencies have been reported from older sows.

In contrast to Se, α-tocopherol is not effectively transferred across the sow's placenta and the young pig is born with low tissue concentrations of this nutrient (Mahan, 1991; 1994; Mahan et al., 2000). An exogenous source of α-tocopherol must be supplied to prevent free radical tissue damage and death in the young pig. Sow colostrum can be an excellent source of α-tocopherol, but if dietary vitamin E is not adequate during gestation or if sow tissue α-tocopherol concentrations are depleted, colostrum and later milks will have a lower α-tocopherol content. In such cases, Se and α-tocopherol can be provided by injection.

B. Iron Toxicity

British and Scandinavian workers (Lanneck et al., 1962; Tollerz and Lanneck, 1964; Patterson et al., 1967; 1969; 1971) demonstrated that neonatal pigs deficient in Se and vitamin E were sensitive to iron-dextran injections. When vitamin E and Se are deficient, pigs frequently die from an apparent Fe toxicosis condition within a few hours after Fe injection. Iron can induce myodegeneration causing peroxidative damage to muscle cells because of the increased affinity of skeletal muscle for Fe^{3+}. The injection of vitamin E, not Se, 1 day before an Fe injection seems to provide adequate protection from Fe toxicity (Tollerz and Lanneck, 1964; Tollerz, 1973). Loudenslager et al. (1986) demonstrated a decline in serum tocopherol and an increased GSH-Px activity after Fe was administered to neonatal pigs. Ullrey (1981) produced pig deaths when 8-day-old pigs from dams fed a 5% lipid diet were injected with 750 mg Fe and orally fed 5 to 10 mL of aerated cod-liver oil daily. However, Miller et al. (1973) were unable to repeat the Fe toxicity response in pigs born of sows fed corn–soybean meal diets not fortified with Se or vitamin E. These combined results suggest that when sows are deficient in Se or vitamin E, an Fe toxicity problem may occur in neonatal pigs. Neonatal pigs should therefore preferably consume colostrum prior to an Fe injection. Hill et al. (1999) demonstrated that a 200-mg injection of iron dextran in neonatal pigs did not affect GSH-Px, SOD, or CAT activities.

XIII. SELENIUM AND VITAMIN E DURING THE NURSING AND POSTNATAL PERIOD

Both Se and α-tocopherol in sow colostrum and milk are highly available to the nursing pig. Their ultimate deposition in the tissues of nursing pigs depends, however, on the Se and vitamin E status of the sow, the dietary level fed to the sow, and the length of the nursing period. Serum and liver Se content in the pig at weaning are higher after feeding organic Se to sows than if sodium selenite had been fed, but the sow's serum GSH-Px activity was similar regardless of either Se source (Mahan and Kim, 1996).

Rapid declines in serum and tissue Se and α-tocopherol concentrations occur in the weaned pig and continue to be low for 2 to 4 weeks postweaning. It is during this postweaning period that deficiency onset is most frequently encountered. Weaned pigs of a low Se status will encounter deficiency onset sooner after weaning than pigs of a higher Se status (Mahan et al., 1977). The most common symptom of the deficiency onset is the sudden death of the largest and fastest-growing pigs (Mahan et al., 1973). The presence of mulberry heart, enlarged heart, and an increased fluid content in the pericardial sac are commonly observed symptoms. It is probable that when Se and vitamin E status is low, oxidative damage occurs sooner in faster-growing pigs to those cells that have higher metabolic demands.

Meyer et al. (1981) evaluated the dietary Se requirement of 21-day-old pigs and demonstrated that the required dietary level, when expressed as ppm or mg/kg diet, was higher at 3 weeks and declined by 8 weeks of age. They demonstrated that the Se requirement for the overall period was 0.35 ppm Se. Work by Lei et al. (1998) using the GSH-Px activities of several tissues demonstrated the dietary requirement of 4-week-old pigs was approximately 0.2 ppm. Serum GSH-Px activity has been shown to increase as the pig ages (Mahan et al., 1999).

Serum and tissue α-tocopherol concentrations also decline postweaning. An exogenous source of vitamin E is therefore necessary to prevent the deficiency onset. When <20 IU vitamin E/kg diet was fed to weanling pigs, serum α-tocopherol concentrations declined during the initial weeks postweaning, whereas by 4-week postweaning serum values began to increase. Subsequent research (Moreira et al., 1999) suggested that a dietary level of 40 to 60 IU vitamin E /kg may be necessary for the weanling pig. The inclusion of an emulsifiable form of vitamin E in the drinking water increased the serum α-tocopherol content during the initial days postweaning (Moreira et al., 1999). Chung and Mahan (1995) demonstrated that naturally derived vitamin E had higher serum and tissue α-tocopherol concentrations in weanling pigs than when the synthetic form of vitamin E was added to the diet at similar IU levels. These experiments suggest that the dietary vitamin E requirement may be higher than the current NRC (1998) standard for weanling pigs.

XIV. SELENIUM AND VITAMIN E DURING THE GROWING-FINISHING PERIOD

A. GROWTH

Se–vitamin E deficiency is encountered less frequently in growing-finishing pigs than during the early postweaning period. The most common deficiency sign is the sudden death of apparently normal fast-growing pigs. Upon necropsy, there is evidence of mulberry heart, increased fluid in the pericardial sac, gastric ulcers, and pale muscles. The Se–vitamin E status of the pig at the start of the growing period can be important in the prevention of deficiency onset, but other factors may also be involved. Dietary factors that seem to precipitate deficiency onset include the feeding of grain stored for an extended time, feeding high-moisture grain (Sharp et al., 1972; Whitehair and Miller, 1985), and providing diets inadequately fortified in Se and vitamin E.

The inclusion of sodium selenite in the diets of growing-finishing pigs has resulted in serum GSH-Px activities that reach a plateau at a supplemental level of approximately 0.10 ppm Se for the growing pig (Mahan and Parrett, 1996; Mahan et al., 1999). Research with inorganic and organic Se has demonstrated similar GSH-Px activity responses. At lower dietary inclusion levels, inorganic Se generally resulted in a higher GSH-Px activity than did the organic Se source. This is because that at lower dietary inorganic Se levels, Se is primarily used for GSH-Px production, whereas some of the absorbed organic Se is deposited in body tissue with less being available for GSH-Px production.

Providing an organic Se source to growing-finishing pigs has resulted in increased tissue Se concentrations compared with sodium selenite (Mahan and Parrett, 1996; Mahan et al., 1999). Ku et al. (1973) demonstrated that when inorganic Se was added to diets with a naturally high indigenous Se content, the added inorganic Se did not further increase the tissue Se concentration. This suggests that tissue Se concentrations are affected by Se source, and when sodium selenite is added to diets where the Se level is above the pigs' requirement, no further increase in Se retention occurs.

During the finishing period, higher feed intakes and lower muscle tissue accretion results in a lower dietary Se requirement than during the growing period. The available data suggest that the supplemental level of Se needed to maximize GSH-Px activity for finishing pigs is <0.10 ppm Se (Mahan et al., 1999).

The requirement for dietary vitamin E is somewhat more difficult to assess because there is no specific biological system that requires vitamin E, except for the prevention of oxidative damage to tissue cells. Dietary fats or membrane phospholipids containing unsaturated fatty acids can, however, precipitate oxidative damage and elevate the dietary requirement for vitamin E (Drochner,

1976). Anderson et al. (1995) showed no growth or feed performance responses to dietary vitamin E levels from 0 to 150 IU/kg. They also demonstrated that high levels of vitamin A did not interfere with serum or tissue α-tocopherol concentrations. Because there was no apparent beneficial performance response to dietary vitamin E, the biological function of vitamin E seems to be principally in maintaining tissue integrity and preventing oxidative damage to cellular membranes.

B. Effect on Pork Quality

Apart from microbial contamination of the carcass postslaughter, lipid oxidation of muscle is the major reason for the loss in pork quality. In the live animal there are several defense systems for preventing oxidative damage to cells. However, upon slaughter, there are several new factors (preslaughter and slaughtering stresses, postmortem pH changes, changes in carcass temperatures, etc.) that can influence pork quality (Buckley et al., 1995). Tissue changes may occur prior to slaughter that may influence the antioxidant defense system and therefore exacerbate the amount of oxidative damage postslaughter. Fasting prior to slaughter has, however, not been shown to be detrimental to pork quality.

The prevention of cellular peroxidation is important in maintaining meat quality, generally measured by thiobarbituric acid reactive substances (TBARS), color changes, and fluid loss (drip loss) from fresh and stored meat. The tissues of greatest susceptibility to oxidative damage are those that contain polyunsaturated fatty acids. Cellular and subcellular membranes are particularly vulnerable to oxidative damage. Vitamin E is primarily a lipid antioxidant and has been shown to extend the shelf life of pork (Tagwerker, 1981), whereas Se is a more effective antioxidant in the cytoplasm of the cell. In the postmortem state, the effectiveness of SOD, CAT, and GSH-Px enzymes have questionable merit in retaining meat quality; therefore, the antioxidant role of vitamin E becomes of greater importance in maintaining meat quality (Buckley et al., 1995). Several investigators have reported that pork quality was enhanced when dietary vitamin E levels were high during the growing-finishing period (Monahan et al., 1990; 1992; 1994; Asghar et al., 1991; Buckley et al., 1995). However, when vitamin E is supplemented only during the latter part of the finishing period, tissue lipid peroxidation responses are not consistent.

Corino et al. (1999) demonstrated that high dietary levels of vitamin E (i.e., 300 IU/kg) fed during the last 60 days of the finishing period increased ground tissue α-tocopherol content with lower lipid oxidation, but there was no effect on drip loss. This is consistent with previous results showing that high dietary levels of vitamin E prevented oxidative damage to pork muscle (Monahan et al., 1990; 1992; 1994; Asghar et al., 1991; Buckley et al., 1995). Dietary vitamin E needs to be increased when vegetable oils are fed because of the presence of unsaturated fatty acids. Pork muscle is therefore more susceptible to lipid peroxidation when pigs are fed vegetable oils compared with tallow (Monahan et al., 1992; Buckley et al., 1995). Dammers et al. (1958) suggested that 40 mg of vitamin E per kilogram diet was the minimum quantity required for pork meat to have a satisfactory shelf life when diets contained added fat. A recent study by Mahan et al. (1999) indicated that sodium selenite may have a detrimental effect on drip loss and may cause an increase in muscle paleness, whereas organic Se did not affect these traits. These combined results indicate that high dietary levels of vitamin E can reduce lipid peroxidation and increase tissue α-tocopherol content, but the role of Se and other minerals (Cu, Fe) on pork quality are as yet unclear. More information about the effects on pork quality is provided in Chapter 28.

XV. SELENIUM AND VITAMIN E DURING REPRODUCTION

A. Sows

Historically, Adamstone et al. (1949) reported that vitamin E–deficient sows had a smaller litter size, which they attributed to increased embryonic deaths. Neonatal pigs exhibited muscular incoordination and necrosis of muscle fibers. Mahan et al. (1974) reported similar findings when a semipurified diet deficient in both Se and vitamin E had been fed to sows for two parities. They reported that sows deficient in Se and vitamin E had prolonged farrowing times, reduced frequency of milk letdown, and weaker progeny. Piatkowski et al. (1979), however, did not demonstrate any fetal atrophy when first-litter gilts were fed a semipurified diet low in both vitamin E and Se. Although vitamin E–Se deficiency has been reported in the neonatal pig, Se or vitamin E injections in the neonate and/or pretreatment of the sow prior to farrowing effectively reduces baby pig mortality (Van Vleet et al., 1973).

Practical diets fed to reproducing animals do not show evidence of the deficiency as readily as when semipurified diets are fed. Mahan et al. (1974) demonstrated when sows were fed corn–soybean meal diets devoid of added Se or vitamin E that a lower litter size occurred in Parity 2 but not in Parity 1. Chavez (1985) also did not demonstrate a lower litter size from gilt litters, nor did Nielsen et al. (1979) when Se and vitamin E were added to a low-Se-containing barley diet for gilts. Feeding high moisture corn has reduced litter size with poor overall reproductive performance of multiparous sows (Young et al., 1977a, c; 1978; Whitehair and Miller, 1985). It is probable that gilts have a higher body reserve of both Se and vitamin E that are at least adequate to prevent the deficiency onset during the initial parity, but with prolonged periods of depletion the nutrient deficiency manifested itself. Confined sows are also more likely to have a lower Se and vitamin E status; thus, they and their progeny are more prone to exhibit the deficiency than those that have access to pasture (Wilkinson et al., 1977a; Mutetikka and Mahan, 1993).

Most reproductive studies have not evaluated the effects of Se and vitamin E independently. Nielsen et al. (1979) used a factorial experiment and evaluated the effects of Se and vitamin E with first-parity gilts. A numerical (but nonsignificant) increase in litter size occurred when vitamin E was added at 30 IU/kg diet (total 46.5 IU/kg). Two other reports that studied supplemental dietary vitamin E levels over several parities demonstrated a litter size improvement at a dietary vitamin E level of 33 IU/kg (total 41 IU) in one experiment, and to 44 IU/kg (total 51 IU) in a second study (Mahan, 1991; 1994). Supplemental vitamin E has, therefore, generally resulted in improved reproductive performance at dietary inclusion levels of ≥40 IU/kg diet. Dietary vitamin E levels above 40 IU/kg may also be necessary to achieve improved sow health (Whitehair and Miller, 1985; Mahan, 1991; 1994; Wuryastuti et al., 1993).

Serum α-tocopherol concentration declines during the last week of gestation. Because colostrum has a high α-tocopherol content followed by a lower concentration in mature milks (Nielsen et al., 1973; Malm et al., 1976; Mahan, 1991; 1994), the decline in serum α-tocopherol is attributed to the transfer of α-tocopherol from serum to mammary tissue. Injecting α-tocopherol during late gestation increases colostrum α-tocopherol content, but the increase was greater when the natural vs. the synthetic form was administered (Chung and Mahan, 1995).

Only small increases in fetal liver α-tocopherol content occur during gestation when vitamin E is fed to sows (Mahan, 1991; 1994). Consequently, the neonate is born with a poor antioxidant status. The mammary transfer of α-tocopherol increases the plasma tocopherol concentration in pigs and can prevent the deficiency onset. Less tocopherol is transferred to sow colostrum of later parities, suggesting sow depletion of this nutrient occurs as sows get older. Studies that evaluated dietary vitamin E over several parities have shown a decline in milk α-tocopherol content as the number of parities increase (Vrzgula et al., 1980; Mahan, 1991; 1994). Because there is also a concurrent decline in sow backfat thickness with advancing parity and because adipose tissue has a high α-tocopherol content, the decline in milk α-tocopherol with age is understandable.

Gestating and lactating sows achieve maximum serum GSH-Px activity at a supplemental level of approximately 0.10 ppm Se (Mahan and Kim, 1996). The addition of Se to practical sow diets, however, has generally not improved litter size or pig birth weights, but the source and level of Se can affect the Se status of both the neonate and sow. Increasing the dietary Se intake of the sow increases placental and mammary transfer of Se, but the responses are greater when an organic Se source is fed (Mahan, 2000). Feeding organic Se to sows has resulted in increased sow tissue, colostrum, and milk Se contents. The progeny of sows fed organic Se also have a higher Se status at birth and weaning (Mahan and Kim, 1996).

Three separate studies in which 0.3 ppm Se was fed for several parities to high-producing sows demonstrated a decline in sow milk Se (Figure 14.4) and sow hair Se contents (Figure 14.5) as the number of parities increases (Mahan, 1991; 1994; Kim, 1999). These results are in agreement with the data of Mahan and Newton (1995) who demonstrated lower body Se contents in higher-producing sows after three parities compared with a lower-producing sow group. These results suggest that Se depletion occurs as sows mature and that Se depletion seems to be exacerbated with higher sow productivities.

Retained placenta is a reported sign of Se–vitamin E deficiency in dairy cattle (Julien et al., 1976), but this effect has not been demonstrated in swine. Extended parturition times, and the slower expression of milk from mammary tissue have, however, been observed in sows, implying inadequate smooth muscle contractions in both species, and possibly an inadequate prostaglandin production.

Disease conditions are often associated with Se–vitamin E deficiency during the reproductive period (Trapp et al., 1970). A high incidence of mastitis, metritis, and agalactia (MMA) occurred when sows were fed a dried high-moisture corn diet, but when the diet was supplemented with Se and vitamin E, no evidence of MMA was demonstrated (Whitehair and Miller, 1985). These results are consistent with the observations of Ringarp (1960), who reported a high MMA incidence when poor-quality feed was fed to reproducing sows. The incidence of MMA was

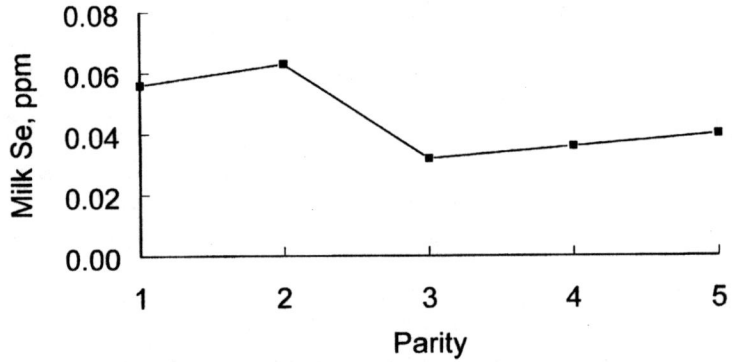

FIGURE 14.4 Sow milk selenium concentration at 21 days of lactation. All sows had been fed 0.3 ppm selenium (sodium selenite) from weaning through their reproductive cycles. Each mean represents at least 85 observations. (Compiled from the data of Mahan, 1991; 1994; Mahan et al., 1999.)

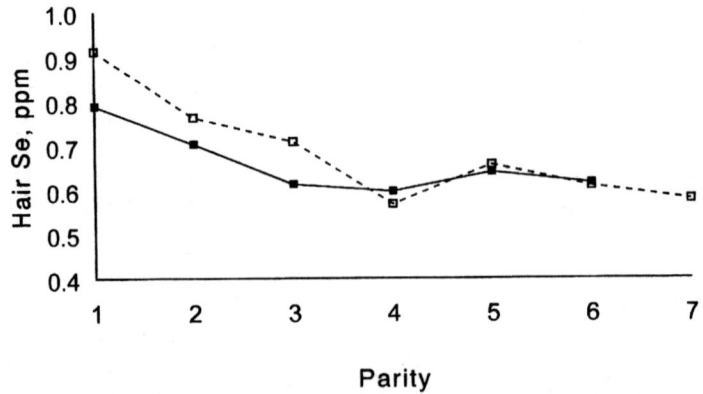

FIGURE 14.5 Sow hair selenium content by parity from two commercial farms. All sows had been fed 0.3 ppm selenium. (From Kim and Mahan, unpublished data.)

reduced when vitamin E was supplemented, and when sows were housed in a less clean environment (Mahan, 1994). Wuryastuti et al. (1993) demonstrated that the combination of Se and vitamin E was more effective than either singly in enhancing the sow's ability to produce antibodies. Hayek et al. (1989) demonstrated higher IgM in sow colostrum and milk when Se and vitamin E were administered. Although MMA is a complex disease that probably involves several factors and generally occurs during a stressful period, these results suggest that vitamin E and Se reduce the incidence of this and possibly other reproductive diseases that seem to be exacerbated under less sanitary housing conditions.

B. Boars

The adult male pig seems to be fairly resilient against nutrient insult until that nutrient becomes extremely deficient. Even when the major nutrients (i.e., protein, energy) are low, the boar continues to produce sperm, albeit of a lower quantity and quality. With the increasing use of artificial insemination in many commercial herds, the subsequent dilution of semen used for breeding purposes, and the high dependence on fewer boars, the proper nutrition of the boar to maintain high semen quality is becoming more critical.

Boars accumulate high concentrations of Se in the testes during growth and development (Marin-Guzman et al., 1997). Sperm tail abnormalities, a reduction in sperm motility, and a lower percentage of normal sperm occur when low dietary levels of Se are fed to boars, effects that are independent of vitamin E (Wu et al., 1973; Liu et al., 1982; Marin-Guzman et al., 1997). Selenium is involved in the formation of a protein surrounding the mitochondrial sheath of the sperm tail (Wu et al., 1979; Calvin et al., 1981). Marin-Guzman et al. (2000a,b) demonstrated that ATP concentration in the semen of Se-deficient boars was lower, that sperm production in the testicular cells was reduced during early spermatogenic development, and that semen from Se-deficient boars resulted in lower conception rates in gilts with fewer accessory sperm in the ovum.

Testicular degeneration has long been recognized as one manifestation of a vitamin E deficiency. The damage occurred in the germinal epithelium but was reversible in many species upon vitamin E supplementation (Mason and Maner, 1957). Marin-Guzman et al. (2000a) demonstrated that growing boars fed a semipurified diet with ≤4 mg α-tocopherol/kg diet failed to show any evidence of testicular degeneration. Brezezinska-Slebodzinska et al. (1995) demonstrated that when 1000 IU/day was fed to boars for a 7-week period lipid peroxidation of collected semen was improved. Marin-Guzman et al. (1997) demonstrated that the seminal plasma of semen contained no α-tocopherol, suggesting that the presence of this antioxidant in semen was probably associated with maintaining sperm cell membrane integrity.

XVI. EXCESSES

A. Selenium

The toxic (selenosis) level of Se depends on the chemical form of the element, animal age, and how it is administered. Elemental Se is relatively nontoxic and has a median lethal dose (LD_{50}) of 6700 ppm in rats (Cummins and Kirmura, 1971). Dimethylselenide, the principal metabolite exhaled through the lung under toxicosis conditions has a LD_{50} of 1600 ppm, while the urinary metabolite trimethylselenide has an LD_{50} of 49.4 ppm (McConnel and Portman, 1952; Obermeyer et al., 1971).

Responses to selenosis are categorized as chronic (effects over a long time period) or acute (effects within a short time period). When excess Se is administered, the body attempts to rid itself of excess Se through several channels (principally the urine, bile, lung) or by trapping it in various tissues (muscle, hair), making it biologically less available for biological purposes. The portion that overwhelms these excretion systems produces a toxic effect in various tissues.

Chronic selenosis generally occurs when diets or feedstuffs contain 5 to 20 ppm Se (Kim, 1999). Symptoms are initially characterized in growing swine by reduced growth rates and feed intakes, and later by the loss of hair and separation of the hoof at the coronary band site (Goehring et al., 1984a,b; Mahan and Moxon, 1984). The effect is more pronounced when sodium selenite is the Se source compared with organic Se (Kim, 1999).

Chronic selenosis in reproducing sows results in lower conception rates, smaller litter size, small, weaker pigs, and a higher percentage of stillbirths. In pigs nursing these sows, there is a loss of hair and separation of the hoof at the coronary band (Wahlstrom and Olson, 1959; Kim, 1999).

Acute selenosis occurs after the ingestion of large quantities of Se from seleniferous feeds, a diet containing high levels of inorganic Se, or after a large quantity of Se is injected. Acute selenosis occurred when Se was injected at ≥1.65 mg/kg body weight (Diehl et al., 1975) or fed at ≥20 mg Se/kg diet (Miller, 1938; Miller and Williams, 1940; Mahan and Moxon, 1984). Acute signs of selenosis include labored breathing, pulmonary edema, vomiting, prostration, frothing at the mouth, and abnormal staggering movements (blind staggers). Death generally occurs within hours or a few days of injection (Orstadius, 1960; Herigstad et al., 1973; Diehl et al., 1975). Ingesting large quantities of Se resulted in feed refusal, loss of weight, respiratory distress, spinal paralysis, incoordination, loss of hair, and ultimately death (Miller, 1938; Miller and Williams, 1940; Herigstad et al., 1973; Harrison et al., 1983; Mahan and Moxon, 1984). Acute selenosis is generally not a problem under most swine-feeding programs, but may occur under conditions of errors in weighing of Se premixes or misapplication of injectable Se.

Selenosis may be counteracted by administering sodium arsenate (Moxon, 1937; 1941). Wahlstrom et al. (1955; 1956) reported that organic arsenicals provide effective protection against toxic levels of Se. Arsenic compounds chelate and divert absorbed Se to the biliary system (Olson et al., 1963; Lavender and Bagman, 1966), thus increasing its clearance from the body. The organic arsenicals, arsanilic acid at 0.01% and 0.005% of 3-nitro-4-hydroxyphenylarsonic acid, in the diet are less dangerous than inorganic arsenic (Wahlstrom et al., 1955). Linseed meal provides protection against selenosis (Moxon, 1937; Wahlstrom et al., 1956), largely through its cyanogenic glucoside properties (Palmer et al., 1980).

B. Vitamin E

High dietary levels of vitamin E have not been found to be harmful to swine, even when added at the high levels currently being used in many swine diets. Feeding ≤1000 IU/ kg diet has not resulted in detrimental responses in growing swine (Mahan, unpublished data).

XVII. DIETARY REQUIREMENTS

The dietary requirements for vitamin E and Se as reflected by the various NRC committees have perhaps changed more than most other nutrients over the past three decades (Table 14.3). The NRC in 1973 did not recognize a supplemental need for Se but established the vitamin E requirement at 11 IU/kg diet for all phases of swine production. In 1979, Se 0.15 ppm Se was inserted in the NRC tables for all swine production phases while vitamin E remained at 11 IU/kg diet. In 1998, the NRC requirement for vitamin E increased to 44 IU/kg diet for reproducing animals, with Se increasing to 0.30 ppm in the nursery period. The NRC requirements are generally based on optimum growth, environmental and health conditions, and reflect the minimum requirement where optimum performance can be achieved. However, on many swine farms many environmental and health issues not present in research facilities may modify the pigs' requirements. The requirements for both Se and vitamin E, when expressed as an IU vitamin E or ppm Se level, decline during later growth periods, but they are higher during the reproductive phases (Mahan et al., 1977; Wilkinson et al., 1977b). Because the animal's requirement may be influenced by various factors, this author has attempted to include these conditions as safety margins in the recommendations in Table 14.3.

TABLE 14.3
Dietary Requirements for Selenium and Vitamin E

Production Phase	1973[a]		1979[a]		1988[a]		1998[a]		This Author[b]	
	Vitamin E (IU/kg)	Se (mg/kg)	Vitamin E (IU/kg)	Se (mg/kg)	Vitamin E (IU/kg)	Se (mg/kg)	Vitamin E (IU/kg)	Se (mg/kg)	Vitamin E (IU/kg)	Se (mg/kg)
Nursery (5 to 20 kg)	11	—	11	0.15	11	0.30	14	0.30	40	0.30
Grower (20 to 60 kg)	11	—	11	0.15	11	0.15	11	0.15	20	0.20
Finisher (60 kg to market)	11	—	11	0.15	11	0.10	11	0.15	11[c]	0.15
Gestation	11	—	10	0.15	22	0.15	44	0.15	60	0.30
Lactation	11	—	10	0.15	22	0.15	44	0.15	60	0.30

[a] Values reflect minimum standards to achieve optimum responses (NRC publications).
[b] Values reflect the author's recommendations and include safety margins.
[c] Higher levels may be justified to enhance meat quality.

REFERENCES

Adams, C. R., H. F. Eoff, and Z. R. Zimmerman. 1975. Protecting feeds from vitamin E and A deficits in light weight, moldy and blighted corn, *Roche Agreport*, 401.

Adamstone, F. B., J. L. Rider, and M. F. James. 1949. Response of swine to vitamin E-deficient rations, *Ann. N.Y. Acad. Sci.*, 52:260.

Adkins, R. S., and R. C. Ewan. 1984. Effect of selenium on performance, serum selenium concentration and glutathione peroxidase activity in pigs, *J. Anim. Sci.*, 58:346.

Afzai, M., R. P. Tengerdy, R. P. Ellis, C. V. Kimberling, and C. J. Moris. 1984. Protection of rams against epididymis by a *Brucella ovis* vitamin E adjuvant vaccine, *Vet. Immunol. Immunopathol.*, 7:293.

Allaway, W. H., E. E. Cary, and C. F. Ehlig. 1981. The cycling of low levels of selenium in soils, plants and animals. In O. H. Muth, Ed., *Selenium in Biomedicine*, AVI Publishing, Westport, CT, 273.

Anderson, L. E., Sr., R. O. Myer, J. H. Brendemuhl, and L. R. McDowell. 1995. The effects of excessive dietary vitamin A on performance and vitamin E status in swine fed diets varying in dietary vitamin E, *J. Anim. Sci.*, 73:1093.

Arthur, J. R., and G. J. Beckett, 1994. Roles of selenium in type I iodothyronine 5'-deiodinase and in thyroid hormone and iodine metabolism. In Burk, R. F., Ed., *Selenium in Biology and Human Health*, Springer-Verlag, New York, 93.

Asghar, A., J. I. Gray, E. R. Miller, P. K. Ku, A. M. Booren, and D. J. Buckley. 1991. Influence of supranutritional vitamin E supplementation in the feed on swine growth, performance and deposition in different tissues, *J. Sci. Food Agric.*, 57:19.

Bartholomew, A., D. Latshaw, and D. E. Swayne. 1998. Changes in blood chemistry, hematology, and histology caused by a selenium/vitamin E deficiency and recovery in chicks, *Biol. Trace Elem. Res.*, 62:7.

Baustad, B., and I. Nafstad. 1972. Hematologic response to vitamin E in piglets, *Br. J. Nutr.*, 28:183.

Bengtsson, G., J. Hakkarainen, L. Jonsson, N. Lannek, and P. Lindberg. 1978. Requirement for selenium (as selenite) and vitamin E (as alpha-tocopherol) in weaned pigs. I. The effect of varying alpha-tocopherol levels in a selenium deficient diet on the development of the VESD syndrome, *J. Anim. Sci.*, 46:143.

Berry, M. J., and P. R. Larsen, 1992. The role of selenium in thyroid hormone action, *Endocr. Rev.*, 13:207.

Brady, P. S., L. J. Brady, M. J. Parsons, D. E. Ullrey, and E. R. Miller. 1979. Effects of riboflavin deficiency on growth and glutathione peroxidase system enzymes in the baby pig, *J. Nutr.*, 109:1615.

Brzezinska-Slebodzinska, E., A. B. Slebodzinski, B. Pietras, and G. Wieczorek. 1995. Antioxidant effect of vitamin E and glutathione on lipid peroxidation in boar semen plasma, *Biol. Trace Elem. Res.*, 47:69.

Buckley, D. J., P. S. Morrissey, and J. I. Gray. 1995. Influence of dietary vitamin E on the oxidative stability and quality of pig meat, *J. Anim. Sci.*, 73:3122.

Calvin, H. I., E. Wallace, and G. W. Cooper. 1981. The role of selenium in the organization of the mitochondrial helix in rodent spermatozoa. In O. H. Muth, Ed., *Selenium in Biology and Medicine*, AVI Publishing, Westport, CT, 319.

Cantor, A. H., M. L. Scott, and T. Noguchi. 1975. Biological availability of selenium in feedstuffs and selenium compounds of exudative diathesis in chicks, *J. Nutr.*, 105:96.

Cary, E. E., G. A. Wieczorek, and W. H. Allaway. 1967. Reactions of selenite selenium added to soils that produce low-selenium forages, *Soil Sci. Soc. Am. Prod.*, 31:21.

CAST. 1994. Risks and Benefits of Selenium in Agriculture. Issue Paper No. 3. Supplement, 35 pp.

Chan, A. C., C. E. Allen, and P. V. J. Hegarty. 1980. Effects of vitamin E depletion and repletion on prostaglandin synthesis in semitendinous muscle of young rabbits, *J. Nutr.*, 110:66.

Chavez, E. R. 1979a. Effects of dietary selenium on glutathione peroxidase activity in piglets, *Can. J. Anim. Sci.*, 59:67.

Chavez, E. R. 1979b. Effects of dietary selenium depletion and repletion on plasma glutathione peroxidase activity and selenium concentration in blood and body tissue of growing pigs, *Can. J. Anim. Sci.*, 59:761.

Chavez, E. R. 1985. Nutritional significance of selenium supplementation in a semi-purified diet fed during gestation and lactation to first-litter gilts and their piglets, *Can. J. Anim. Sci.*, 65:497.

Ching, S., and D. C. Mahan. 1995. Interrelationship of recommended and high dietary vitamin E and vitamin A levels in the postweaning diets of pigs, *J. Anim. Sci.*, 73(Suppl.1):71 (Abstr.).

Chow, C. K. 1985. Vitamin E and blood, *World Rev. Nutr. Diet.*, 45:133.

Chung, Y. K., and D. C. Mahan. 1995. Efficacy of various injectable vitamin E forms on sow vitamin E transfer, *Korean J. Anim. Sci.*, 37:616.

Chung, Y. K., D. C. Mahan, and A. J. Lepine. 1992. Efficacy of dietary D-α-tocopherol and DL-α-tocopheryl acetate for weanling pigs, *J. Anim. Sci.*, 70:2485.

Combs, G. F., Jr. 1992. *The Vitamins: Vitamin E*. Academic Press, New York, 181.

Corino, C., G. Oriani, L. Pantaleo, G. Pastorelli, and G. Salvatori. 1999. Influence of dietary vitamin E supplementation on "heavy" pig carcass characteristics, meat quality, and vitamin E status, *J. Anim. Sci.*, 77:1755.

Cort, W. M., T. S. Vicente, E. H. Waysek, and B. D. Williams. 1983. Vitamin E content of feedstuffs determined by high performance liquid chromatography fluorescence, *J. Agric. Food Chem.*, 31:1330.

Cummins, L. M., and E. T. Kimura. 1971. Safety evaluation of selenium sulfide antidandruff shampoos, *Toxicol. Appl. Pharmacol.*, 20:89.

Dammers, J., K. Stolk, and G. Van Wieringen. 1958. The importance of vitamin E for fattening pigs, *Versl. Landbouwkd.*, 64:5.

Desai, I. D., C. K. Parekh, and M. L. Scott. 1964. Absorption of D- and L-α-tocopheryl acetates in normal and dystrophic chicks, *Biochem. Biophys. Acta*, 100:280.

Diehl, J. S., D. C. Mahan, and A. L. Moxon. 1975. Effects of single intramuscular injections of selenium at various levels to young swine, *J. Anim. Sci.*, 40:844.

Diplock, A. T. 1981. The role of vitamin E and selenium in the prevention of oxygen-induced tissue damage. In O. H. Muth, Ed., *Selenium in Biology and Medicine*, AVI Publisher, Westport, CT, 303.

Diplock, A. T., H. Baum, and J. A. Lucy. 1971. The effect of vitamin E on the oxidative state of selenium in rat liver, *Biochem. J.*, 123:721.

Dove, C. R., and R. C. Ewan. 1991. The effect of trace minerals on the stability of vitamin E in swine grower diets, *J. Anim. Sci.*, 69:1994.

Drochner, W. 1976. Current status of vitamin E research presented on the example of the vitamin E requirements and supply status of the pig, *Übers. Tierernähr.*, 4:93.

Ellis, R. P., and X. W. Vorhies. 1976. Effect of supplemental dietary vitamin E on the serologic response of swine to an *Escherichia coli* bacterin, *J. Am. Vet. Med. Assoc.*, 68:231.

Esaki, N., T. Nakamura, H. Tanaka, T. Suzuki, Y. Morino, and K. Soda. 1981. Enzymatic synthesis of selenocysteine in rat liver, *Biochemistry*, 20:4492.

Evans, H. M., and R. S. Bishop. 1922a. On the existence of a hitherto unrecognized dietary factor essential for reproduction, *Science*, 56:650.

Evans, H. M., and K. S. Bishop. 1922b. On the relations between fertility and nutrition. II. The ovulation rhythm in the rat on inadequate nutritional regimes, *J. Metab. Res.*, 1:335.

Ewan, R. C., M. E. Wastell, E. J. Bicknell, and V. C. Speer. 1969. Performance and deficiency symptoms of young pigs fed diets low in vitamin E and selenium, *J. Anim. Sci.*, 9:912.

FDA. 1974. Food additives permitted in feed and drinking water of animals: selenium. Final rule, *Fed. Regis.*, 39:1355.

FDA. 1982. Food additives permitted in feed and drinking water of animals: selenium. Final rule, *Fed. Regis.*, 47:26814.

FDA. 1987. Food Additives permitted in feed and drinking water of animals: selenium, *Fed. Regis.*, 52:21001.

Fontaine, M., V. E. O. Valli, and L. G. Young. 1977a. Studies on vitamin E and selenium deficiency in young pigs. III. Effect on kinetics of erythrocyte production and destruction, *Can. J. Comp. Med.*, 41:57.

Fontaine, M., V. E. O. Valli, and L. G. Young. 1977b. Studies on vitamin E and selenium deficiency in young pigs. IV. Effect on coagulation system, *Can. J. Comp. Med.*, 41:64.

Fontaine, M., V. E. O. Valli, L. G. Young, and J. H. Lumsden. 1977c. Studies on vitamin E and selenium deficiency in young pigs. I. Hematological and biochemical changes, *Can. J. Comp. Med.*, 41:41.

Forbes, R. M., and H. H. Draper. 1957. Production and study of vitamin E deficiency in the baby pig, *J. Anim. Sci.*, 16:1037 (Abstr.).

Gallo-Torres, H. 1973. Studies on the lymphatic absorption, tissue distribution and storage of vitamin E, *Acta Agric. Scand. Suppl.*, 19:97.

Glienke, L. R., and R. C. Ewan. 1977. Selenium deficiency in the young pig, *J. Anim. Sci.*, 45:1334.

Goehring, T. B., I. S. Palmer, O. K. Olson, G. W. Libal, and R. C. Wahlstrom. 1984a. Effects of seleniferous grains and inorganic selenium on tissue and blood composition and growth performance of rats and swine, *J. Anim. Sci.*, 59:725.

Goehring, T. B., I. S. Palmer, O. K. Olson, G. W. Libal, and R. C. Wahlstrom. 1984b. Toxic effects of selenium on growing swine fed corn–soybean meal diets, *J. Anim. Sci.*, 59:733.

Grant, C. A. 1961. Morphological and etiological studies of dietetic microangiopathy in pigs ("mulberry heart"), *Acta Vet. Scand.*, 2(Suppl. 3):1.

Grant, C., and B. Thaivelin. 1958. Selenium and hepatosis dietetica of pigs, *Nord. Vet. Med.*, 10:657.

Grant, C. A., B. Thafvelin, and A. Christell. 1961. Retention of selenium by pig tissues, *Acta Pharmacol. Toxicol.*, 18:285.

Groce, A. W., E. R. Miller, K. K. Keahey, D. E. Ullrey, and D. J. Ellis. 1971. Selenium supplementation of practical diets for growing-finishing swine, *J. Anim. Sci.*, 32:905.

Groce, A. W., E. R. Miller, J. P. Hitchcock, D. E. Ullrey, and W. T. Magee. 1973a. Selenium balance in the pig as affected by selenium source and vitamin E, *J. Anim. Sci.*, 37:942.

Groce, A. W., E. R. Miller, D. E. Ullrey, P. K. Ku, K. K. Keahey, and D. J. Ellis. 1973b. Selenium requirements in corn-soy diets for growing-finishing swine, *J. Anim. Sci.*, 37:948.

Hakkarainen, J., P. Lindberg, G. Bengtsson, and L. Johnsson. 1978a. Serum glutathione peroxidase activity and blood selenium in pigs, *Acta Vet. Scand.*, 19:269.

Hakkarainen, J., P. Lindberg, G. Bengtsson, L. Johnsson, and N. Lannek. 1978b. Requirement for selenium (as selenite) and vitamin E (as alpha-tocopherol) in weaned pigs. III. The effect on the development of the VESD syndrome of varying selenium levels in a low tocopherol diet, *J. Anim. Sci.*, 46:1001.

Harrison, L. H., B. M. Colvin, B. P. Stuart, L. T. Sangster, E. J. Gorgacz, and H. S. Gosser. 1983. Paralysis in swine due to focal symmetrical poliomalacia: Possible selenium toxicosis, *Vet. Pathol.*, 20:265.

Hayek, M. G., G. E. Mitchell, Jr., R. J. Harmon, T. S. Stahly, G. L. Cromwell, R. E. Tuckerand, and K. B. Barker. 1989. Porcine immuno globulin transfer after prepartum treatment with selenium or vitamin E, *J. Anim. Sci.*, 67:1299.

Herigstad, R. R., C. K. Whitehair, and O. K. Olson. 1973. Inorganic and organic selenium toxicosis in young swine: comparison of pathologic changes with those in swine with vitamin E-selenium deficiency, *Am. J. Vet. Res.*, 34:1227.

Hill, C. H. 1975. Interrelationships of selenium with other trace elements, *Fed. Proc.*, 34:2096.

Hill, G. M., J. E. Link, L. Meyer, and K. L. Fritsche. 1999. Effect of vitamin E and selenium on iron utilization in neonatal pigs, *J. Anim. Sci.*, 77:1762.

Hitchcock, J. P., E. R. Miller, K. K. Keahey, and D. E. Ullrey. 1978. Effects of arsanilic acid and vitamin E upon utilization of natural or supplemental selenium by swine, *J. Anim. Sci.*, 46:425.

Hupkens van der Elst, F. C. C., and J. H. Watkinson. 1977. Effect of top-dressing pasture with selenium prills on selenium concentration in blood of stock, *N.Z. J. Exp. Agric.*, 5:79.

Jensen, A. M., P. T. Jensen, K. Vinter, P. Jessen, and E. W. Skov-Jensen. 1984. Effect of perinatal mortality of a single selenium injection to sows and gilts, *Acta Vet. Scand.*, 25:436.

Jensen, P. T., V. Danielsen, and H. E. Nielsen. 1979. Glutathione peroxidase activity and erythrocyte lipid peroxidation as indices of selenium and vitamin E status in young pigs, *Acta Vet. Scand.*, 20:92.

Jensen, P. T., H. E. Nielsen, V. Danielsen, and T. Leth. 1983. Effect of dietary fat quality and vitamin E on the antioxidant potential of pigs, *Acta Vet. Scand.*, 24:135.

Jensen, S. K., R. M. Engberg, and M. S. Hedemann. 1999. All-rac-α-tocopherol acetate is a better vitamin E source than all-rac-α-tocopherol succinate for broilers, *J. Nutr.*, 129:1355.

Julien, W. E., H. R. Conrad, J. E. Jones, and A. L. Moxon. 1976. Selenium and vitamin E and the increase of retained placenta in parturient cows. II. Prevention in commercial herds with prepartum treatments, *J. Dairy Sci.*, 59:1960.

Kelly, M. P., and R. F. Power. 1995. Fractionation and identification of the major selenium compounds in selenized yeast, *J. Dairy Sci.*, 78(Suppl 1):237 (Abstr.).

Kim, Y. Y. 1999. Selenium Metabolism and Toxicity of Inorganic and Organic Selenium Sources and Levels on Growth, Reproduction and Other Mineral Nutrients in Swine, Ph.D. thesis, Ohio State University, Columbus, 149 pp.

Koivistoinen, P., and J. K. Huttunen. 1986. Selenium in food and nutrition in Finland: An overview on research and action, *Ann. Clin. Res.*, 18:13.

Kornegay, E. T., J. B. Meldrum, G. G. Schurig, M. D. Lindemann, and F. C. Gwazdauskas. 1986. Lack of influence of nursery temperature on the response of weanling pigs to supplemental vitamins C and E, *J. Anim. Sci.*, 63:484.

Ku, P. K., W. T. Ely, A. W. Groce, and D. E. Ullrey. 1972. Natural dietary selenium, alpha-tocopherol and effect on tissue selenium, *J. Anim. Sci.*, 34:208.

Ku, P. K., E. R. Miller, R. C. Wahlstrom, A. W. Groce, J. P. Hitchcock, and D. E. Ullrey. 1973. Selenium supplementation of naturally high selenium diets for swine, *J. Anim. Sci.*, 37:501.

Kurkela, P., and E. Kaantee. 1984. Effects of barley-bound organic selenium compared with inorganic selenite on selenium concentration and structure of tissues in pigs, *J. Agric. Sci. Fin.*, 56:61.

Lake, A. M., M. J. Stuart, and F. A. Oski. 1977. Vitamin E deficiency and enhanced platelet function: reversal following E supplementation, *J. Pediatr.*, 90:722.

Lanneck, N., P. Lindberg, and G. Tollerz. 1962. Lowered resistance to iron in vitamin E-deficient piglets and mice, *Nature* (London), 195:1006.

Larsen, H. J., and S. Tollersrud. 1981. Effect of dietary vitamin E and selenium on phytohaemagglutinin response of the pig lymphocytes. *Res. Vet. Sci.*, 31:301.

Lavender, O. A., and C. A. Bagman. 1966. Selenium metabolism: effect of arsenic on the excretion of selenium in the bile, *Toxicol. Appl. Pharmacol.*, 9:106.

Lawrence, R. A., and R. F. Burk. 1978. Species, tissues and subcellular distribution of non Se-dependent glutathione peroxidase, *J. Nutr.*, 108:211.

Lei, G. X., H. M. Dann, D. A. Ross, W. H. Cheng, G. F. Combs, Jr., and K. R. Roneker. 1998. Dietary selenium supplementation is required to support full expression of three selenium-dependent glutathione peroxidases in various tissues of weanling pigs, *J. Nutr.*, 128:130.

Levesque, M. 1974. Selenium distribution in Canadian soil profiles, *Can. J. Soil Sci.*, 54:63.

Lindberg, P. 1973. Plasma tocopherol in pigs, *Acta Vet. Scand. Suppl.*, 19:39.

Liu, C. H., Y. M. Chen, J. Z. Zhang, M. Y. Huang, Q. Zu, Z. H. Lu, R. X. Yin, G. Z. Zhao, D. Fang, and P. L. Zhang. 1982. Preliminary studies on influence of selenium deficiency to the developments of genital organs and spermatogenesis of infancy boars, *Acta Vet. Exotic. Sin.*, 13:73.

Loudenslager, M. J., P. K. Ku, P. A. Whetter, D. E. Ullrey, C. K. Whitehair, H. D. Stowe, and E. R. Miller. 1986. Importance of diet of dam and colostrum to the biological antioxidant status and parenteral iron tolerance of the pig, *J. Anim. Sci.*, 63:1905.

Machlin, L. J. 1984. Vitamin E. In L. J. Machlin, Ed., *Handbook of Vitamins: Nutritional, Biochemical and Clinical Aspects*, Marcel Dekker, New York, 99.

Machlin, L. J., J. Keating, J. Nelson, M. Brin, R. Filipski, and O. N. Miller. 1979. Availability of adipose tissue tocopherol in the guinea pig, *J. Nutr.*, 109:105.

Mahan, D. C. 1985. Effect of inorganic selenium supplementation on selenium retention in postweaning swine, *J. Anim. Sci.*, 61:173.

Mahan, D. C. 1991. Assessment of the influence of dietary vitamin E on sows and offspring in three parities: reproductive performance, tissue tocopherol, and effects on progeny, *J. Anim. Sci.*, 69:2904.

Mahan, D. C. 1994. Effects of dietary vitamin E on sow reproductive performance over a five parity period, *J. Anim. Sci.*, 72:2870.

Mahan, D. C. 2000. Effect of organic and inorganic selenium sources and levels on sow colostrum and milk selenium content, *J. Anim. Sci.*, 78:100.

Mahan, D. C., and Y. Y. Kim. 1996. Effect of inorganic or organic selenium at two dietary levels on reproductive performance and tissue selenium concentrations in first parity gilts and their progeny, *J. Anim. Sci.*, 74:2711.

Mahan, D. C., and P. L. Magee. 1991. Efficacy of dietary sodium selenite and calcium selenite provided in the diet at approved, marginally-toxic and supra-toxic levels to growing swine, *J. Anim. Sci.*, 69:4722.

Mahan, D. C., and A. L. Moxon. 1978a. Effect of increasing the level of inorganic selenium supplementation in the postweaning diets of swine, *J. Anim. Sci.*, 46:384.

Mahan, D. C., and A. L. Moxon. 1978b. Effects of adding inorganic or organic selenium sources to the diets of young swine, *J. Anim. Sci.*, 47:456.

Mahan, D. C., and A. L. Moxon. 1980. Effect of dietary selenium and injectable vitamin E-selenium for weanling swine, *Nutr. Rep. Int.*, 21:829.

Mahan, D. C., and A. L. Moxon. 1984. Effect of inorganic selenium supplementation on selenosis in postweaning swine, *J. Anim. Sci.*, 58:1216.

Mahan, D. C., and E. A. Newton. 1995. Effect of initial breeding weight on macro- and micro- mineral composition over a three-parity period using a high-producing sow genotype, *J. Anim. Sci.*, 73:151.

Mahan, D. C., and N. A. Parrett. 1996. Evaluating the efficacy of Se-enriched yeast and inorganic selenite on tissue Se retention and serum glutathione peroxidase activity in grower and finisher swine, *J. Anim. Sci.*, 74:2967.

Mahan, D. C., J. E. Jones, J. H. Cline, R. F. Cross, H. S. Teague, and A. P. Grifo, Jr. 1973. Efficacy of selenium and vitamin E injections in the prevention of white muscle disease in young swine, *J. Anim. Sci.*, 36:1104.

Mahan, D. C., L. H. Penhale, J. H. Cline, A. L. Moxon, A. W. Fetter, and J. T. Yarrington. 1974. Efficacy of supplemental selenium in reproductive diets on sow and progeny performance, *J. Anim. Sci.*, 39:536.

Mahan, D. C., A. L. Moxon, and J. H. Cline. 1975. Efficacy of supplemental selenium in reproductive diets on sow and progeny serum and tissue selenium values, *J. Anim. Sci.*, 40:624.

Mahan, D. C., A. L. Moxon, and M. Hubbard. 1977. Efficacy of inorganic selenium supplementation to sow diets on resulting carry-over to their progeny, *J. Anim. Sci.*, 45:738.

Mahan, D. C., T. R. Cline, and B. Richert. 1999. Effects of dietary levels of selenium-enriched yeast and sodium selenite as selenium sources fed to grower-finisher pigs on resulting performance, tissue selenium, serum glutathione peroxidase activity, and carcass characteristics, *J. Anim. Sci.*, 77:2172.

Mahan, D. C., Y. Y. Kim, and R. L. Stuart. 2000. Effects of vitamin E sources (RRR- or all-*rac*-α- tocopheryl acetate) and levels on sow reproductive performance, serum, tissue, and milk α-tocopherol contents over a five parity period, and the effects on the progeny, *J. Anim. Sci.*, 78:110.

Malm, A., W. G. Pond, E. F. Walker, Jr., M. Homan, A. Aydin, and D. Kirtland. 1976. Effect of polyunsaturated fatty acids and vitamin E level of the sow gestation diet on reproductive performance and on level of alpha tocopherol in colostrum, milk and dam and progeny blood serum, *J. Anim. Sci.*, 42:393.

Mandisodza, K. T., W. G. Pond, D. J. Lisk, D. E. Hogue, L. Krook, E. E. Cary, and W. H. Gutenmann. 1979. Tissue retention of Se in growing pigs fed fly ash or white sweet clover grown on fly ash, *J. Anim. Sci.*, 49:535.

Marin-Guzman, J., D. C. Mahan, Y. K. Chung, J. L. Pate, and W. F. Pope. 1997. Effects of dietary selenium and vitamin E on boar performance and tissue responses, semen quality and subsequent fertilization rates in mature gilts, *J. Anim. Sci.*, 75:2994.

Marin-Guzman, J., D. C. Mahan, and J. L. Pate. 2000a. Effect of dietary selenium and vitamin E on spermatogenic development in boars, *J. Anim. Sci.* (in press).

Marin-Guzman, J., D. C. Mahan, and R. Whitmoyer. 2000b. Effect of dietary selenium and vitamin E on the ultrastructure and ATP concentration of boar spermatozoa, and the efficacy of added sodium selenite in extended semen on sperm motility, *J. Anim. Sci.* (in press).

Mason, K. E., and S. I. Maner. 1957. Reversible testis damage in the vitamin E deficient hamster, *Anat. Rec.*, 127:329 (Abstr.).

Mathias, M. M., D. E. Hogue, and J. K. Loosli. 1967. Biological value of selenium in bovine milk for the rat and chick, *J. Nutr.*, 93:14.

Mayland, H. F. 1985. Selenium in soils and plants. In *Selenium Responsive Diseases in Food Animals*, Western States Vet. Conf., 5.

McConnel, R. P., and O. W. Portman. 1952. Excretion of dimethyl selenide by the rat, *J. Biol. Chem.*, 195:277.

McConnell, K. P., and G. J. Cho. 1965. Transmucosal movement of selenium, *Am. J. Physiol.*, 208:1191.

Meyer, W. R., D. C. Mahan, and A. L. Moxon. 1981. Value of dietary selenium and vitamin E for weanling swine as measured by performance and tissue selenium and glutathione peroxidase activities, *J. Anim. Sci.*, 52:302.

Michel, R. L., C. K. Whitehair, and K. K. Keahey. 1969. Dietary hepatic necrosis associated with selenium-vitamin E deficiency in swine, *J. Am. Vet. Med. Assoc.*, 155:50.

Miller, E. R., K. K. Kuan, P. K. Ku, D. E. Ullrey, R. W. Cook, C. K. Whitehair, and K. K. Keahey. 1973. Iron tolerance and E-Se status of young swine, Rep. Swine Res. 232, Michigan State University, 43.

Miller, W. T. 1938. Toxicity of selenium fed to swine in the form of sodium selenite, *J. Agric. Res.*, 56:831.

Miller, W. T., and K. T. Williams. 1940. Minimum lethal dose of selenium, as sodium selenite, for horses, mules, cattle and swine, *J. Agric. Res.*, 60:163.

Monahan, F. J., D. J. Buckley, P. A. Morrissey, P. B. Lynch, and J. I. Gray. 1990. Effect of dietary α-tocopherol supplementation on α-tocopherol levels in porcine tissues and on susceptibility to lipid peroxidation, *J. Food Sci. Nutr.*, 42F:203.

Monahan, F. J., D. J. Buckley, P. A. Morrissey, P. B. Lynch, and J. I. Gray. 1992. Influence of dietary fat and α-tocopherol supplementation in lipid oxidation in pork, *Meat Sci.*, 31:229.

Monahan, F. J., J. I. Gray, A. Asghar, A. Haug, G. M. Strasburg, D. J. Buckley, and P. A. Morrissey. 1994. Influence of diet on lipid oxidation and membrane structure in porcine muscle microsomes, *J. Agric. Food Chem.*, 42:599.

Moreira, I., D. C. Mahan, S. Ching, and T. G. Wiseman. 1999. Efficacy of vitamin E in the diets or drinking water of 2-week old weaned pigs, *J. Anim. Sci.*, 77(Suppl 1):58 (Abstr.).
Moxon, A. L. 1937. Alkali disease or selenium poisoning, *S. Dak. Agric. Exp. Sta. Bull.* No. 311.
Moxon, A. L. 1941. The influence of arsenic on selenium poisoning in hogs, *Proc. S. Dak. Acad. Sci.*, 21:34.
Mustard, J. F., and M. A. Packham. 1970. Factors influencing platelet function, adhesion, release and aggregation, *Pharmacol. Rev.*, 22:97.
Mutetikka, D. B., and D. C. Mahan. 1993. Effect of pasture, confinement and diet fortification of vitamin E and selenium on reproducing gilts and their progeny, *J. Anim. Sci.*, 71:3211.
Muth, O. H., J. E. Oldfield, L. F. Remmert, and J. R. Schubert. 1958. Effects of selenium and vitamin E on white muscle disease, *Science*, 128:1090.
Nafstad, I. 1965. Studies of hematology and bone marrow morphology in vitamin E-deficient pigs, *Pathol. Vet.*, 2:277.
Nafstad, I., and H. J. Nafstad. 1968. An electron microscopic study of blood and bone marrow in vitamin E-deficient pigs, *Pathol. Vet.*, 5:520.
Nafstad, I., and S. Tollersrud. 1970. The vitamin E-deficiency syndrome in pigs. I. Pathological changes, *Acta Vet. Scand.*, 11:452.
Nielsen, H. E., N. J. Hogaard-Olsen, W. Hjarde, and E. Leerbeck. 1973. Vitamin E content in colostrum and sow's milk and sow milk yield at two levels of dietary fats, *Acta Agric. Scand. Suppl.*, 19:35.
Nielsen, H. E., V. Danielsen, M. G. Simesen, G. Gissel-Nielsen, W. Hjarde, T. Leth, and A. Basse. 1979. Selenium and vitamin E deficiency in pigs. I. Influence on growth and reproduction, *Acta Vet. Scand.*, 20:276.
Niyo, Y., R. D. Glock, A. E. Ledet, F. K. Ramsey, and R. C. Ewan. 1980. Effects of intramuscular injections of selenium and vitamin E on peripheral blood and bone marrow of selenium-vitamin E deficient pigs, *Am. J. Vet Res.*, 41:474.
Nockels, C. F. 1979. Protective effects of supplemental vitamin E against infection, *Fed. Proc.*, 38:2134.
NRC. 1973. *Nutrient Requirements of Swine*, 7th ed., National Academy Press, Washington, D.C.
NRC. 1979. *Nutrient Requirements of Swine*, 8th ed., National Academy Press, Washington, D.C.
NRC. 1983. *Selenium in Nutrition*, rev. ed., National Academy Press, Washington, D.C.
NRC. 1988. *Nutrient Requirements of Swine*, 9th ed., National Academy Press, Washington, D.C.
NRC. 1998. *Nutrient Requirements of Swine*, 10th ed., National Academy Press, Washington, D.C.
Obel, A. L. 1953. Studies on the morphology and etiology of so-called toxic liver dystrophy (hepatosis dietetica) in swine, *Acta Pathol. Microbiol. Scand. Suppl.*, 94:1.
Obermeyer, B. D., I. S. Palmer, O. K. Olson, and A. W. Halverson. 1971. Toxicity of trimethylselenonium chloride in the rat with and without arsenic, *Toxicol. Appl. Pharmacol.*, 20:135.
Oldfield, J. E. 1999. *Selenium World Atlas*. Selenium-Tellurium Development Association. Grimbergen, Belgium, 83 pp.
Oldfield, J. E., J. R. Schubert, and O. H. Muth. 1960. Selenium and vitamin E as related to growth and white muscle disease in lambs, *Proc. Soc. Exp. Biol. Med.*, 103:799.
Olson, O. E., B. M. Schulte, E. I. Whitehead, and A. W. Halverson. 1963. The effect of selenium metabolism in rats, *J. Agric. Food Chem.*, 11:531.
Olson, O. E., C. E. Holmquist, and C. W. Carlson. 1973. The stability of inorganic selenium in premixes, *Poult. Sci.*, 52:403.
Olson, O. E., E. J. Novacek, E. I. Whitehead, and I. S. Palmer. 1970. Investigations of selenium in wheat. *Phytochemistry*, 9:1181.
Orstadius, K. 1960. Toxicity at a single subcutaneous dose of sodium selenite in pigs, *Nature*, 188:1117.
Palmer, I. S., R. P. Gunsolus, A. W. Halverson, and O. K. Olson. 1970. Trimethylselenonium ion as a general excretory product from selenium metabolism in the rat, *Biochim. Biophys. Acta*, 208:260.
Palmer, I. S., O. K. Olson, A. W. Halverson, R. Miller, and C. Smith. 1980. Isolation of factors in linseed oil meal protective against chronic selenosis in rats, *J. Nutr.*, 110:145.
Parsons, M. J., P. K. Ku, D. E. Ullrey, H. D. Stowe, P. A. Whetter, and E. R. Miller. 1985. Effects of riboflavin supplementation and selenium source on selenium metabolism in the young pig, *J. Anim. Sci.*, 60:451.
Patterson, D. S. P., W. M. Allen, D. C. Thurley, and J. T. Done. 1967. The role of tissue peroxidation in iron-induced myodegeneration of piglets, *Biochem. J.*, 104:2.
Patterson, D. S. P., W. M. Allen, S. Berrett, D. Sweasy, D. C. Thurley, and J. T. Done. 1969. A biochemical study of the pathogenesis of iron-induced myodegeneration of piglets, *Zentralbl. Vet. Med. Assoc.*, 16:199.

Patterson, D. S .P., W. M. Allen, S. Berrett, D. Sweasy, and J. T. Done. 1971. The toxicity of parenteral iron preparations in the rabbit and pig with a comparison of the chemical and biochemical responses to iron-dextrose in 2 days old and 8 days old piglets, *Zentralbl. Vet. Med. Assoc.*, 18:453.

Pearson, C. K., and M. M. Barnes. 1970. Absorption of tocopherols by small intestine loops of the rat *in vivo*, *Int. J. Vitam. Res.*, 40:19.

Peplowski, M. A., D. C. Mahan, F. A. Murray, A. L. Moxon, A. H. Cantor, and K. E. Ekstrom. 1981. Effect of dietary and injectable vitamin E and selenium in weanling swine antigenically challenged with sheep red blood cells, *J. Anim. Sci.*, 51:344.

Peterson, D. M., and D. F. Wood. 1997. Composition and structure of high-oil oat, *J. Cereal Sci.*, 26:121.

Piatkowski, T. L., D. C. Mahan, A. H. Cantor, A. L. Moxon, J. H. Cline, and A. P. Grifo, Jr. 1979. Selenium and vitamin E in semi-purified diets for gravid and nongravid gilts, *J. Anim Sci.*, 48:1357.

Pond, W. G., W. H. Allaway, E. F. Walker, Jr., and L. Krook. 1971. Effects of corn selenium content and drying temperature and of supplemental E on growth, liver selenium and blood vitamin E content of chicks, *J. Anim. Sci.*, 33:996.

Ringarp, N. 1960. Clinical and experimental investigations into a postparturient syndrome with agalactia in sows, *Acta Agric. Scand. Suppl.*, 7:140.

Robowsky, K. O., and O. Knabe. 1970. Studies on the content of alpha-tocopherol in forage grasses. 1. Effect of stage of growth upon the content of alpha-tocopherol in forage grasses, *Arch. Tierernähr.*, 20:621.

Rotruck, J. T., A. L. Pope, H. E. Ganther, A. B. Swanson, D. G. Hafeman, and W. G. Hoekstra. 1973. Selenium: biochemical role as a component of glutathione peroxidase, *Science*, 179:588.

Sarathchandra, S. U., and J. H. Watkinson. 1981. Oxidation of elemental selenium to selenite by *B. megaterism*, *Science*, 211:600.

Saxegaard, F., and J. Teige, Jr. 1977. Induction of swine dysentery with a pure culture of *Treponema hyodysenteriae* in vitamin E and selenium deficient pigs, *Acta Vet. Scand.*, 18:563.

Schwarz, K., and C. M. Foltz. 1957. Selenium as an integral part of factor 3 against dietary necrotic liver degeneration, *J. Am. Chem. Soc.*, 79:3292.

Sharp, B. A., L. G. Young, and A. A. van Dreumel. 1972. Effect of supplemental vitamin E and selenium in high moisture corn diets on the incidence of mulberry heart disease and hepatosis dietetica in pigs, *Can. J. Comp. Med.*, 36:393.

Stowe, H. D., and E. R. Miller. 1985. Genetic predisposition of pigs to hypo- and hyperselenemia, *J. Anim. Sci.*, 60:200.

Sunde, R. A., 1997. Selenium. In *Handbook of Nutritionally Essential Mineral Elements*, O'Dell, B. L., and R. A. Sunde, Eds., Marcel Dekker, New York, 493–556.

Swaine, D. J. 1955. The trace-element content of soils: Harpenden, England, *Common. Bur. Soil Sci.* (Great Britain) *Tech. Commun.*, 48:91.

Sweeney, P. R., and R. G. Brown. 1972. Ultrastructure changes in muscular dystrophy. I. Cardiac tissue of piglets deprived of vitamin E and selenium, *Am. J. Pathol.*, 68:479.

Tagwerker, F. J. 1981. Vitamins and quality of food products of animal origin, *Roche Sem*.

Tengerdy, R. P., D. L. Meyer, L. H. Lauerman, D. C. Leuker, and D. F. Nockles. 1973. Vitamin E-enhanced humoral antibody response to *Clostridium perfringens* type D in sheep, *Br. Vet. J.*, 139:147.

Teige, J., Jr. 1977. The generalized Schwartzman reaction induced by a single injection of endotoxin in pigs fed a vitamin E deficient commercial diet, *Acta Vet. Scand.*, 18:140.

Teige, J., Jr., K. Nordstoga, M. Fjolstad, and I. Nafstad. 1973. The generalized Shwartzman reaction in pigs induced by diet and single injection of disintegrated cells or partially purified endotoxin from *Escherichia coli*, *Acta Vet. Scand.*, 14:92.

Teige, J., Jr., K. Nordstoga, and J. Aurajo. 1977. Influence of diet on experimental swine dysentery. 1. Effects of vitamin E and selenium deficient diet supplemented with 6.8% cod liver oil, *Acta Vet. Scand.*, 18:384.

Teige, J., Jr., F. Saxegaard, and A. Froslie. 1978. Influence of diet on experimental swine dysentery. 2. Effects of a vitamin E and selenium deficient diet supplemented with 3% cod liver oil, vitamin E or selenium, *Acta Vet. Scand.*, 19:133.

Tengerdy, R. P., R. H. Heinzerling, G. L. Brown, and M. M. Mathias. 1973. Enhancement of the humoral immune response by vitamin E, *Int. Arch. Allergy Appl. Immunol.*, 44:221.

Thomlinson, J. R., and A. Buxton. 1963. Anaphylaxis in pigs and its relationship to the pathogenesis of oedema disease and gastro-enteritis associated with *Escherichia coli*, *Immunology*, 6:126.

Thulin, A. J., D. S. Pollman, F. Blecha, G. A. Kennedy, G. L Allee, and P. Whetter. 1985. Biological interactions of copper, selenium and vitamin E for weanling swine, *J. Anim. Sci.*, 61(Suppl. 1):74.

Tollersrud, S. 1973. Changes in the enzymatic profile in blood and tissues in pre-clinical and clinical vitamin E-deficiency in pigs, *Acta Agric. Scand. Suppl.*, 19:124.

Tollerz, G. 1973. Vitamin E, selenium (and some related compounds) and tolerance toward iron in piglets, *Acta Agric. Scand. Suppl.*, 19:184.

Tollerz, G., and N. Lannek. 1964. Protection against iron toxicity in vitamin E deficient piglets and mice by vitamin E and synthetic antioxidants, *Nature*, 201:846.

Traber, M. G., G. W. Burton, K. U. Ingold, and H. J. Kayden. 1990. RRR- and SRR- alpha-tocopherol are secreted without discrimination in human chylomicrons, but RRR-alpha-tocopherol is preferentially secreted in very low density lipoproteins, *J. Lipid. Res.*, 31:675.

Traber, M. G., A. Elsner, and R. Brigelius-Flohe. 1998. Synthetic as compared with natural vitamin E is preferentially excreted as α-CEHG in human urine: studies using deuterated α-tocopheryl acetates, *FEBS Lett.*, 437:145.

Trapp, A. L., K. Keahey, D. L. Whitenack, and C. K. Whitehair. 1970. Vitamin E–selenium deficiency in swine: differential diagnosis and nature of field problem, *J. Am. Vet. Med. Assoc.*, 157:289.

Ullrey, D. E. 1981. Vitamin E for swine, *J. Anim. Sci.*, 53:1039.

U.S. Pharmacopeia and National Formulatory. 1980. Vitamin E. In *The United States Pharmacopeia*, 20th rev., and the *National Formulatory*, 15th ed., 846.

Van Vleet, J. F. 1982. Amounts of twelve elements required to induce selenium vitamin E deficiency in ducklings, *Am. J. Vet. Res.*, 43:851.

Van Vleet, J. F., W. Carlton, and H. J. Olander. 1970. Hepatosis dietetica and mulberry heart disease associated with selenium deficiency in Indiana swine, *J. Am. Vet. Med. Assoc.*, 157:1208.

Van Vleet, J. F., and G. R. Ruth. 1977. Efficacy of supplements in prevention of selenium-vitamin E deficiency in swine, *Am. J. Vet Res.*, 38:1299.

Van Vleet, J. F., K. B. Meyer, and H. J. Olander. 1973. Control of selenium-vitamin E deficiency in growing swine by parenteral administration of selenium vitamin E preparations to baby pigs or to pregnant sows and their baby pigs, *J. Am. Vet. Med. Assoc.*, 163:452.

Van Vleet, J. F., A. H. Rebar, and V. J. Ferrans. 1977. Acute cobalt and isoproterenol cardiotoxicity in swine: protection by selenium-vitamin E supplementation and potentiation by stress-susceptible phenotype, *Am. J. Vet. Res.*, 38:991.

VERIS. 1998. *Vitamin E Abstracts*, LaGrange, IL.

Vrzgula, L., M. Prosbwa, G. Kovac, J. Blazovsky, and I. Paulikova. 1980. Dynamika selenu v krvnom sere prasnic po suplementacii krmne; davkyvitaminom E a selenom pocas gravidity, *Vet. Med.* (Prague), 25:391.

Wahlstrom, R. C., and O. K. Olson. 1959. The effect of selenium on reproduction in swine, *J. Anim. Sci.*, 18:141.

Wahlstrom, R. C., L. D. Kamstra, and O. K. Olson. 1955. The effect of arsanilic acid and 3-nitro-4-hydroxyphenylarsonic acid on selenium poisoning in the pig, *J. Anim. Sci.*, 14:105.

Wahlstrom, R. C., L. D. Kamstra, and O. K. Olson. 1956. The effect of organic arsenicals, chlortetracycline and linseed oil meal on selenium poisoning in swine, *J. Anim. Sci.*, 15:794.

Wahlstrom, R. C., T. B. Goehring, D. D. Johnson, G. W. Libal, O. K. Olson, I. S. Palmer, and R. C. Thaler. 1984. The relationship of hair color to selenium content of hair and selenosis in swine, *Nutr. Rep. Int.*, 29:143.

Weber, F. 1981. *Nutrition in Health and Disease and International Development*, Symposia from the XII International Congress of Nutrition, Alan R. Liss, New York, pp. 119.

Weiser, H., G. Riss, and A. W. Kormann. 1996. Biodiscrimination of the eight α-tocopherol stereoisomers results in preferential accumulation of the four 2R forms in tissues and plasma of rats, *J. Nutr.*, 126:2539.

Whagner, P. D. 1981. Selenium and heavy metal toxicity. In *Selenium in Biology and Medicine*, Spallholz, Ganther, M., Ed., AVI Publishing, Westport, CT.

Whitehair, C. K., and E. R. Miller. 1985. Vitamin E and selenium in swine production. In *Selenium Responsive Diseases in Food Animals*, West States Vet. Conf., 11.

Wilkinson, J. E., M. C. Bell, J. A. Bacon, and F. B. Masincupp. 1977a. Effects of supplemental selenium on swine. I. Gestation and lactation, *J. Anim. Sci.*, 44:224.

Wilkinson, J. E., M. C. Bell, J. A. Bacon, and C. C. Melton. 1977b. Effects of supplemental selenium on swine. II. Growing-finishing, *J. Anim. Sci.*, 44:229.

Wolffram, S., E. Anliker, and E. Scharrer. 1986. Uptake of selenate and selenite by isolated brush border membrane vesicles from pig, sheep and rat intestine, *Biol. Trace Elem. Res.*, 10:293.

Wolffram, S., B. Grenacher, and E. Scharrer. 1988. Transport of selenate and sulphate across the intestinal brush border membrane of pig jejunum by two common mechanisms, *Q. J. Exp. Physiol.*, 73:103.

Wretlind, B., K. Orstadius, and P. Lindberg. 1959. Transaminase and transferase activities in blood plasma and in tissues of normal pigs, *Zentralbl. Vet. Med. A.*, 6:963.

Wu, A. S. H, J. E. Oldfield, P. D. Whanger, and P. H. Weswig. 1973. Effects of selenium, vitamin E and antioxidants on testicular function in rats, *Biol. Reprod.*, 8:625.

Wu, A. S. H., J. E. Oldfield, L. R. Shull, and P. R. Cheeke. 1979. Specific effect of selenium deficiency on rat sperm, *Biol. Repro.*, 20:793.

Wuryastuti, H., H. D. Stowe, R. W. Bull, and E. R. Miller. 1993. Effects of vitamin E and selenium on immune responses of peripheral blood, colostrum, and milk leukocytes of sows, *J. Anim. Sci.*, 71:2464.

Young, L. G., A. Lun, J. Pos, R. P. Forshaw, and D. Edmeades. 1975. Vitamin E stability in corn and mixed feeds, *J. Anim. Sci.*, 40:495.

Young, L. G., J. H. Lumsden, A. Lun, J. Claxton, and D. Edmeades. 1976. Influence of dietary levels of vitamin E and selenium on tissue and blood parameters in pigs, *Can. J. Comp. Med.*, 40:92.

Young, L. G., A. G. Castell, and D. Edmeades. 1977a. Influence of dietary levels of selenium on tissue selenium of growing pigs in Canada, *J. Anim. Sci.*, 44:590.

Young, L. G., K. J. Jenkins, and D. Edmeades. 1977b. Selenium content of feedstuffs grown in Canada, *Can. J. Anim. Sci.*, 57:793.

Young, L. G., R. B. Miller, D. Edmeades, A. Lun, G. C. Smith, and G. J. King. 1977c. Selenium and vitamin E supplementation of high moisture corn diets for swine reproduction, *J. Anim. Sci.*, 45:1051.

Young, L. G., R. B. Miller, D. Edmeades, A. Lun, G. C. Smith, and G. J. King. 1978. Influence of method of corn storage and vitamin E and selenium supplementation on pig survival and reproduction, *J. Anim. Sci.*, 47:639.

15 Water-Soluble Vitamins in Swine Nutrition

C. Robert Dove and David A. Cook

CONTENTS

I. Introduction 317
II. Biotin 317
    A. History 317
    B. Structure and Nomenclature 318
    C. Metabolism 318
        1. Digestion and Absorption 318
        2. Function 318
    D. Nutritional Requirements 319
    E. Deficiency and Toxicity Signs 320
    F. Determination of Status 320
    G. Sources 320
III. Choline 320
    A. History 320
    B. Structure and Nomenclature 321
    C. Metabolism 321
        1. Digestion and Absorption 321
        2. Function 321
    D. Nutritional Requirements 321
    E. Deficiency and Toxicity Signs 322
    F. Determination of Status 322
    G. Sources 322
IV. Folate 323
    A. History 323
    B. Structure and Nomenclature 323
    C. Metabolism 323
        1. Digestion and Absorption 323
        2. Function 324
    D. Nutritional Requirements 324
    E. Deficiency and Toxicity Signs 325
    F. Determination of Status 325
    G. Sources 325
V. Niacin 325
    A. History 325
    B. Structure and Nomenclature 326

		C.	Metabolism	326
			1. Digestion and Absorption	326
			2. Function	326
		D.	Nutritional Requirements	327
		E.	Deficiency and Toxicity Signs	327
		F.	Determination of Status	327
		G.	Sources	327
	VI.	Pantothenic Acid		328
		A.	History	328
		B.	Structure and Nomenclature	328
		C.	Metabolism	328
			1. Digestion and Absorption	328
			2. Functions	328
		D.	Nutritional Requirements	329
		E.	Deficiency and Toxicity Signs	329
		F.	Determination of Status	329
		G.	Sources	330
	VII.	Riboflavin		330
		A.	History	330
		B.	Structure and Nomenclature	330
		C.	Metabolism	330
			1. Digestion and Absorption	330
			2. Function	331
		D.	Nutritional Requirements	331
		E.	Deficiency and Toxicity Signs	331
		F.	Determination of Status	332
		G.	Sources	332
	VIII.	Thiamin		332
		A.	History	332
		B.	Structure and Nomenclature	332
		C.	Metabolism	333
			1. Digestion and Absorption	333
			2. Function	333
		D.	Nutritional Requirements	333
		E.	Deficiency and Toxicity Signs	334
		F.	Determination of Status	334
		G.	Sources	335
	IX.	Vitamin B_6		335
		A.	History	335
		B.	Structure and Nomenclature	335
		C.	Metabolism	335
			1. Digestion and Absorption	335
			2. Function	336
		D.	Nutritional Requirements	336
		E.	Deficiency and Toxicity Signs	336
		F.	Determination of Status	337
		G.	Sources	337
	X.	Vitamin B_{12}		337
		A.	History	337
		B.	Structure and Nomenclature	337

	C.	Metabolism	338
		1. Digestion and Absorption	338
		2. Functions	338
	D.	Nutritional Requirements	339
	E.	Deficiency and Toxicity Signs	339
	F.	Determination of Status	339
	G.	Sources	340
XI.	Ascorbic Acid		340
	A.	History	340
	B.	Structure and Nomenclature	340
	C.	Metabolism	340
		1. Digestion and Absorption	340
		2. Function	341
	D.	Nutritional Requirements	341
	E.	Deficiency and Toxicity Signs	342
	F.	Determination of Status	342
	G.	Sources	342
References			342

I. INTRODUCTION

By using chemically defined diets, it can be shown that the pig has a dietary requirement for all of the water-soluble vitamins with the exception of ascorbic acid. In general, however, feed ingredients and microbial synthesis in the gastrointestinal tract provide sufficient quantities of vitamin B_6, thiamin, and possibly biotin to meet the pig's requirement. There is clear evidence of improved reproductive performance when choline, folic acid, and pantothenic acid are added to a corn–soybean meal diet. However, choline is clearly not required in similar diets for growing-finishing swine, while the data for folic acid and pantothenic acid are inconclusive. Vitamin B_{12}, riboflavin, and niacin, on the other hand, must be added to the diet to prevent the development of frank deficiencies.

Considerable research was conducted during the "vitamin era" between 1930 and 1955 to establish the qualitative vitamin needs of pigs. Since that time, most experiments have been directed at verification of quantitative requirements and solution of problems related to human medicine. The careful reader will no doubt conclude that there is a need for additional vitamin research. The following review provides a summary of current knowledge. Other than the vitamins discussed in this chapter and elsewhere in this text, there is no evidence that compounds having a "vitamin" function in metabolism remain to be discovered.

II. BIOTIN

A. HISTORY

At the turn of the century, a factor present in yeast and wort was discovered that was required for growth of certain strains of yeast. This factor was named "bios." Bios was later fractionated (Lucas, 1924; Lash Miller, 1924), and, still later, Kögl (1935) isolated "biotin" from one of the fractions of bios. Kögl and Tonnis (1936) subsequently isolated biotin as its crystalline methyl ester from egg yolk, and vitamin H concentrates were isolated from liver (György et al., 1937). From comparison of the physical, chemical, and biological properties, it was later shown that biotin and vitamin H were the same (György et al., 1940). du Vigneaud and co-workers (1942) established the structure of biotin, and subsequently Harris et al. (1945) were the first to synthesize biotin chemically.

B. Structure and Nomenclature

"The compound with the formula hexahydro-2-oxo-1H-thieno[3,4-d]imidazole-4pentanoic acid, formerly referred to as vitamin H or coenzyme R, should be designated biotin" (Anonymous, 1987).

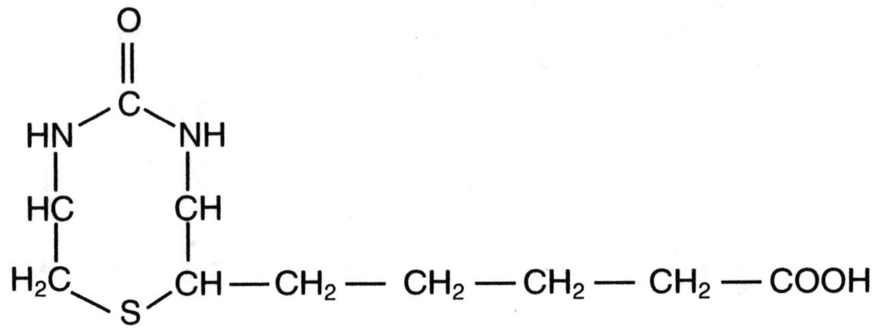

FIGURE 15.1 Biotin.

C. Metabolism

1. Digestion and Absorption

Biotin is absorbed from the small intestine by active transport at low concentrations and by simple diffusion at higher concentrations (Bowman and Rosenberg, 1987; Bowman et al., 1989; Said et al., 1989; Mock, 1990; 1996; Said and Derweesh, 1991). Biotin absorption increases with age with the active transport site in rats shifting from the ileum to the jejunum as the animal ages. A significant amount of biotin is synthesized by the flora of the colon; however, the bioavialability of colonic biotin is thought to be low (Bowman and Rosenberg, 1987; Mosenthin et al., 1990).

Neither the exact mechanism of intestinal hydrolysis of protein-bound biotin nor the relationship between the digestion of protein-bound biotin and bioavailabilty has been defined. The ratio of free biotin to protein-bound biotin varies; however, the majority of biotin in cereals and meats is thought to be protein bound (Mock, 1996). It has been postulated that biotinidase in the pancreatic juice may be responsible for the release of biotin during the luminal phase of proteolysis (Wolf et al., 1984).

2. Function

Biotin serves as the prosthetic group on enzymes involved in carboxylation reactions. All biotin enzymes present in animal tissues are dependent on adenosine triphosphate (ATP) and Mg^{2+} ions, which are required for enzyme activation via the attachment of the biotinyl moiety to the apoenzyme (Bonjour, 1984). The active site of a biotin enzyme consists of a carboxylase subsite that catalyzes the carboxylation of the biotinyl moiety, a transferase subsite that catalyzes the transfer of the carboxyl group from biotin to the substrate, and the biotinyl-carrying site. The biotin prosthetic group functions as a mobile carboxyl carrier, as it is bound to the enzyme by a flexible arm that allows it to oscillate back and forth between the carboxylase and transferase subunits (Wood and Barden, 1977).

Of the biotin enzymes known to exist, only four are found in animal tissues. These include pyruvate, acetyl-coenzyme A (CoA), propionyl-CoA, and 3-methylcrotonyl-CoA carboxylases. An extensive review of the relevant aspects of these enzymes regarding biochemical nutrition, their metabolic functions, and their regulation is offered by Achuta Murthy and Mistry (1977) and Mock (1996).

Pyruvate carboxylase, a mitochondrial enzyme, is involved in both gluconeogenesis and lipogenesis. The reaction that it catalyzes yields oxaloacetate from pyruvate and has an absolute requirement for acetyl-CoA. In combination with phosphoenolpyruvate carboxykinase, pyruvate carboxylase can achieve the formation of phosphoenolpyruvate, which is a key reaction in the production of glucose from three carbon precursors such as pyruvate, lactate, and gluconeogenic amino acids. In addition, pyruvate carboxylase is important in lipogenesis, as oxaloacetate is necessary for the translocation of acetyl-CoA from the mitochondria to the cytosol, the site of fatty acid synthesis.

Acetyl-CoA carboxylase is an essential enzyme in *de novo* synthesis of fatty acids. This enzyme catalyzes the carboxylation of acetyl-CoA to malonyl CoA, which is the first committed step in fatty acid synthesis.

Propionyl-CoA carboxylase catalyzes the carboxylation of propionyl-CoA to methyl-malonyl-CoA, which through a series of reactions can result in the synthesis of oxaloacetate. Thus, propionate, produced as the result of oxidation of odd-numbered fatty acids; degradation of branched-chain amino acids, methionine, and threonine; and fermentation in hindgut can enter into the tricarboxylic acid cycle or gluconeogenesis.

3-Methylcrotonyl-CoA carboxylase catalyzes the carboxylation of 3-methylcrotonyl CoA, an intermediate in the catabolism of leucine, to 3-methylglutaconyl-CoA, which following a series of reactions results in the production of acetyl-CoA and acetoacetate.

D. NUTRITIONAL REQUIREMENTS

Typically, supplementation of diets with biotin has produced no improvement in performance of growing pigs. Newport (1981) reported no improvement in growth rate or feed efficiency of 2- to 28-day-old pigs when a filtered skim milk diet containing approximately 10 µg biotin/kg of dry matter was supplemented with 50 µg biotin/kg of diet. Moreover, the addition of 55 to 880 µg biotin/kg of diet has been shown to have no beneficial effect on performance of nursery pigs (Peo et al., 1970; Hanke and Meade, 1971; Washam et al., 1975; Hamilton and Veum, 1986) or growing-finishing pigs (Meade, 1971; Simmins and Brooks, 1980; Easter et al., 1983; Bryant et al., 1985b; Hamilton and Veum, 1986). In contrast to these findings, Adams et al. (1967) reported an improvement in performance of nursery pigs when 110 µg biotin/kg of diet was added to a corn–milo–soybean meal diet. Peo et al. (1970) also reported a response to supplemental biotin in one trial when 440 µg/kg of diet were added.

Biotin supplementation of sow diets has been reported to reduce hoof cracks and foot pad lesions and, in general, to improve the integrity of the foot as well as to improve skin and hair coat condition (Halama, 1979; Grandhi and Strain, 1980; Misir and Blair, 1984; Webb et al., 1984; Bryant et al., 1985a,b; Simmins and Brooks, 1985). However, no improvement was observed by Bane et al. (1980), Hamilton and Veum (1984), Tribble et al. (1984), and Lewis et al. (1991). Penny and co-workers (1981) reported biotin supplementation to be ineffective in alleviating established foot lesions, but they suggested that supplementation during growth and development may be helpful.

Biotin supplements of 100 to 550 µg/kg of diet have been reported to improve reproductive performance as measured by number of pigs farrowed and weaned, litter weaning weight, and weaning to estrus interval (Brooks et al., 1977; Halama, 1979; Penny et al., 1981; Easter et al., 1983; Simmins and Brooks, 1983; Hamilton and Veum, 1984; Misir and Blair, 1984; Tribble et al., 1984; Bryant et al., 1985c; Lewis et al., 1991). However, the responses in these studies were inconsistent for the reproductive criteria measured. In addition, Grandhi and Strain (1980) and Watkins et al. (1991) reported no improvement in reproductive performance. Thus, due to the many confounding factors, it is difficult to estimate the biotin requirement for reproduction.

E. DEFICIENCY AND TOXICITY SIGNS

A biotin deficiency in swine has been produced by inclusion of large amounts of desiccated egg white in the diet (Cunha et al., 1946; Hamilton et al., 1983). This is due to the presence of avidin in raw egg white, which forms a complex with biotin in the intestinal tract, making it unavailable to the pig. A biotin deficiency has also been produced by the addition of specific sulfa drugs to a synthetic diet (Lindley and Cunha, 1946; Cunha et al., 1948; Lehrer et al., 1952), which is presumably the result of a reduction in bacterial synthesis of the vitamin in the intestinal tract. Deficiency signs that have been reported include alopecia, spasticity of the hind legs, dermatitis, skin ulcerations, a brown exudate on the skin and about the eyes, transverse cracking of the hooves, cracking and bleeding of the foot pads, diarrhea, and an inflammation of the mucous membranes of the mouth (Cunha et al., 1946; 1948; Lindley and Cunha, 1946; Lehrer et al., 1952).

Studies with swine indicate that pigs can safely tolerate levels of biotin as high as ten times the nutritional requirement, and considering that the vitamin is not well retained, the maximum tolerable level may be considerably higher (National Research Council, 1987).

F. DETERMINATION OF STATUS

Determinations of biotin in whole blood, serum, and urine have been used as indicators of biotin status (Bonjour, 1984). However, these values can be variable depending on the assay used as well as on the level of biotin intake. Misir and Blair (1986) have determined serum biotin levels indicative of various nutritional states for sows. Blood pyruvate carboxylase activity has also been investigated as an indicator of biotin status in pigs (Whitehead et al., 1980).

G. SOURCES

The supply of biotin to the pig is affected not only by the biotin content of the diet, but by the digestibility and availability of the biotin in the feed ingredients and the level of synthesis by the intestinal microflora. Sauer and co-workers (1988) determined the apparent digestibility of biotin in a number of protein supplements and cereal grains for the growing pig. Apparent digestibilities determined at the distal ileum were 55.4, 2.7, and 3.9% in soybean meal, meat and bone meal, and canola meal, respectively, and 4.8, 4.0, and 21.6% in barley, corn, and wheat, respectively. Bioavailabilities determined in the chick had previously been used to estimate the availability of biotin for the pig (Kornegay, 1986). However, in view of the findings of Sauer and co-workers, these may not be applicable as bioavailability values determined in the chick are generally higher than digestibility values determined in the pig.

III. CHOLINE

A. HISTORY

The name choline arises from the word *chole*, which is German for bile, as choline was originally isolated from bile of pigs by Strecker (1862). Strecker (1868) subsequently demonstrated that choline was the active constituent of lecithin that provides the lipotropic activity (Hershey, 1930). Best and Huntsman (1932) were the first to demonstrate the nutritional importance of choline when they reported the development of fatty livers in rats fed a low-choline, high-fat diet, which could be prevented by choline supplementation.

Choline is required by most animals in concentrations that far exceed the normal definition of a vitamin. Kuksis and Mookerjea (1984) stated emphatically that choline was not a vitamin, but a nutrient whose essentiality varies with species and conditions. Choline deficiencies have been seen in swine, particularly young swine; therefore, choline is included with the water-soluble vitamins even though it does not strictly meet the definition of a true vitamin (National Research Council, 1998).

B. Structure and Nomenclature

"The compound with formula $(CH3)_3N + CH_2CH_2OH$ should be designated choline" (Anonymous, 1987).

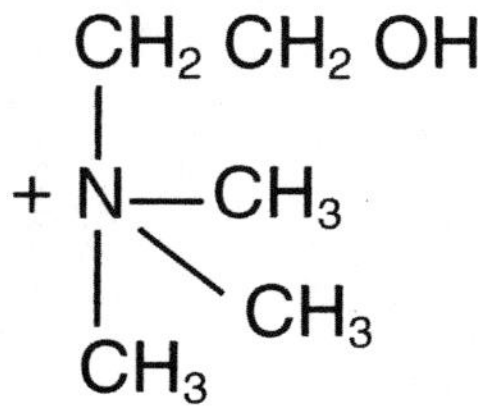

$$\overset{+}{N}\underset{CH_3}{\overset{CH_2\ CH_2\ OH}{{\vert}}}\!\!\begin{array}{c}-CH_3\\ \diagdown CH_3\end{array}$$

FIGURE 15.2 Choline.

C. Metabolism

1. Digestion and Absorption

Choline seems to be absorbed through a transport system in the small intestine that is not dependent on cellular energy (Rose, 1980). Most animals are capable of significant biosynthesis of choline (Greenberg, 1963; Lucas and Ridout, 1967); therefore, absorption from the intestine may not be critical to the animal under normal conditions. Biosynthesis of choline is the result of the decarboxylation of the amino acid serine to ethanolamine in a pyridoxal dependant reaction. Ethanolamine is then progressively methylated to form choline (Kuksis and Mookerjea, 1984). Excess dietary methionine is one of the main sources of the methyl groups used in the biosynthesis of choline (Greenberg, 1963).

2. Function

Choline is considered part of a labile methyl pool capable of contributing methyl groups for the biosynthesis of methionine and other methylated compounds, including purines and pyrimidines (Kuksis and Mookerjea, 1984). It is believed, however, that choline must first be oxidized to betaine before it can donate its methyl groups. Choline is also a precursor for acetylcholine, which is formed by reaction with acetyl-CoA by enzymatic action of choline acetylase (Freeman and Jenden, 1976). Choline is also a precursor for the *de novo* synthesis of phosphatidylcholine (Kennedy and Weiss, 1956) and sphingomyelin (Stoffel and Melzner, 1980). Thus, as a constituent of phospholipids, choline plays a role in the structure of biological membranes.

D. Nutritional Requirements

Johnson and James (1948) reported that the addition of 260 mg choline/kg to a synthetic milk diet (13% solids) that contained 0.8% methionine prevented development of a choline deficiency in 1- to 4-day-old pigs. Neumann and co-workers (1949), using the same diet and pigs of similar weight and age, determined that 1000 mg of choline/kg of dry matter were required to maximize weight gain and feed efficiency and to prevent fat infiltration of the liver and kidneys. Nesheim and Johnson (1950) later demonstrated that the addition of 0.8% methionine to this diet (1.6% total methionine) alleviated the need for supplemental choline. The investigators thus concluded that even at this early age, the pig can utilize excess methionine as a methyl donor for choline synthesis. Kroenig and Pond (1967) further supported this finding when they demonstrated in 3-week-old pigs that choline did not elicit a growth response unless methionine was limiting in the diet. Russet and co-workers (1979a,b) determined the choline requirement of pigs 3 to 8 weeks of age to be approximately 330 mg/kg of a semipurified diet (23% crude protein) in the presence of 0.31% methionine and 0.33% cystine. However, choline supplementation to corn–soybean meal or corn–isolated soybean protein diets fed to nursery, growing, and finishing pigs showed no response in weight gain (Bryant et al., 1977; Russet et al., 1979b; NCR-42 Committee on Swine Nutrition, 1980; Southern et al., 1986).

Choline supplementation of sow diets during gestation and lactation improves reproductive performance. Kornegay and Meacham (1973) reported an increase in the number of live pigs farrowed during the fifth and sixth parity when 880 mg choline/kg was added to a corn–soybean meal diet. Stockland and Blaylock (1974) fed a corn–soybean meal diet supplemented with 412 mg choline/kg to gestating and lactating sows over three parities and found an increase in pigs farrowed, farrowed alive, and weaned, as well as an improvement in conception rate. The NCR-42 Committee on Swine Nutrition (1976) reported an increase in total and live pigs born per litter, and an increase in number of pigs at 2 weeks of age, as well as a reduction in spraddle-legged pigs, upon supplementation of a corn–soybean meal diet with 770 mg of choline/kg. Luce et al. (1985) reported that gilts fed a choline-supplemented diet during gestation farrowed heavier pigs, but they observed no reduction in spraddle-legged pigs. A more recent report provided similar results when a sorghum–soybean meal diet was supplemented with 882 mg choline/kg during gestation and lactation (Maxwell et al., 1987). An increase in pig weight at day 42 and in litter weight at day 21 and day 42 were observed. Choline supplementation of lactation diets containing 8 to 10% vegetable or animal fat had no effect on lactational performance in sows (Seerley et al., 1981; Boyd et al., 1982).

E. Deficiency and Toxicity Signs

The clinical signs of a choline deficiency have been previously described (National Research Council, 1998). Gross observation reveals a reduction in weight gain, a rough hair coat, and an unsteady and staggering gait. Examination of blood samples from deficient animals indicates a reduction in red cell number and a decrease in hematocrit and hemoglobin concentrations. Upon necropsy, fat infiltration of the liver and kidney has been observed. As a result of severe choline deficiency, kidney glomeruli can become occluded due to massive fat infiltration.

Clinical signs of choline toxicity have not been observed in swine (National Research Council, 1987). Emmert (1997) reported that the addition of 10,000 mg/kg of choline had no effect on the growth response of 10-kg pigs. However, Southern et al. (1986) reported a reduction in growth when diets containing 2000 mg choline/kg were fed to nursery, growing, and finishing pigs.

F. Determination of Status

A number of blood and plasma variables have been used as indicators of choline status (Russet et al., 1979a,b), but none has been shown to be consistent. Many of the variables can be confounded by the status of other nutrients, such as methionine, folic acid, and vitamin B_{12}. Plasma choline level has been used in humans, but it has been shown to be highly reflective of dietary consumption (Hirsch et al., 1978).

G. Sources

Molitoris and Baker (1976) and Emmert and Baker (1997) determined that the bioavailability of choline in soybean meal was between 65 and 83% in the chick. No estimate is available for the bioavailability of choline in feed ingredients for the pig. Dehulled soybean meal was reported to have 2218 mg total choline/kg and 1855 mg available choline/kg (Emmert and Baker, 1997). These same authors reported that the available choline was 71% in peanut meal and 24% in canola meal compared with the 83% availability they reported for dehulled soybean meal. The phospholipid-bound choline found in most feedstuffs and unprocessed fats is thought to be well utilized (Emmert et al., 1996). However, the phospholipid-bound choline in refined oils is almost completely removed in the degumming process (Anderson et al., 1979).

IV. FOLATE

A. History

A bacterial growth factor was found in spinach leaves (Mitchell et al., 1941) that had properties similar to a factor in liver and yeast that was shown to prevent anemia in chicks (Hogan and Parrot, 1940) and monkeys (Day et al., 1945). Folic acid was subsequently isolated (Stokstad et al., 1948), and its structure was determined (Mowatt et al., 1948).

B. Structure and Nomenclature

"The term folate should be used as a generic descriptor for folic acid and related compounds exhibiting qualitatively the biological activity of folic acid" (Anonymous, 1987). "The compound, pteroylmonoglutamic acid, formerly known as vitamin B_c, should be referred to as folic acid. Folic acids and folates (plural) should be used as general terms in reference to a group of compounds based on the N-[(6-pteridinyl) methyl]-p-aminobenzoic acid skeleton conjugated with one or more L-glutamic acid residues. Related compounds exhibiting folic acid activity should be named and abbreviated in accordance with the International Union of Pure and Applied Chemistry-International Union of Biochemistry (IUPAC-IUB) Commission on Biochemical Nomenclature (1966)" (Anonymous, 1987). The terms folate, folates, folacin, and folic acid are generally considered interchangeable (Selhub and Rosenberg, 1996).

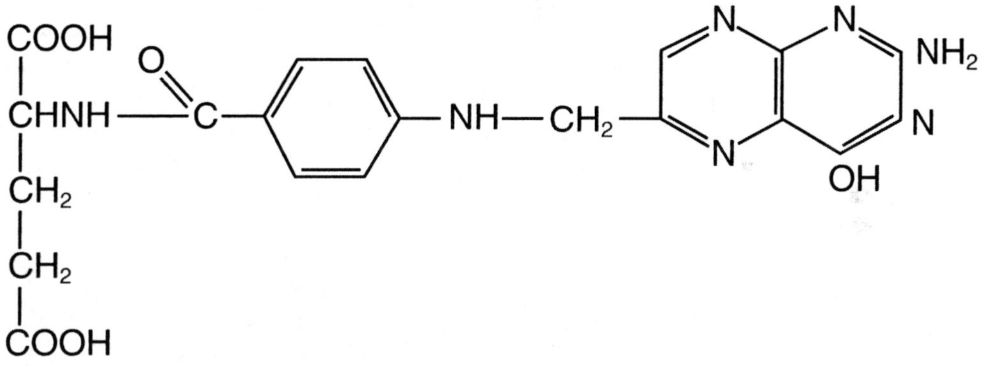

FIGURE 15.3 Folic acid.

C. Metabolism

1. Digestion and Absorption

Intestinal absorption of folates is thought to occur as the monoglutamate form. Therefore, hydrolysis of the polyglutamates to monoglutamates must occur within the absorption process (Rosenburg et al., 1987; Halstead, 1992; Mason, 1992). The brush border membrane of the small intestine of humans and pigs contains a pteroylglutamate hydrolase that has different pH requirements, and that has an increased sensitivity to inhibitors compared with the pteroylglutamate hydrolase found in the enterocyte (Reisenauer et al., 1979). The pteroylglutamate hydrolase is thought to be at least partially responsible for the hydrolysis of dietary folate polyglutamates (Reisenauer et al., 1979; Gregory et al., 1989). Intestinal transport of the monoglutamyl folates is carrier mediated and pH dependent, with an optimum pH for transport of 5.0 to 6.0 (Blair et al., 1976). Folates are also absorbed by a simple diffusion mechanism when concentrations are at pharmacological levels, or when the intestinal pH is above 6.0 (Selhub and Rosenberg, 1996). Most of the folates taken up by the intestinal brush border are reduced to tetrahydrofolic acid and then methylated to ^5N-methyl tetrahydrofolic acid (National Research Council, 1998).

2. Function

The metabolic role of folic acid coenzymes in mammalian tissues is in the transfer of single carbon moieties, such as methyl, formyl, formate, or hydroxymethyl groups. The coenzymatically active forms of the vitamin are the tetrahydro derivatives. Some of the specific reactions and the enzymes in which these coenzymes are involved are methylation of homocysteine to methionine (methionine synthetase), the interconversion of serine and glycine (serine hydroxymethyltransferase), the synthesis of purines (glycinamide ribonucleotide and 5-amino-4-imidazole-carboxamide ribonucleotide transformylases) and pyrimidines (thymidylate synthetase), and the oxidation of histidine (10-formyltetrahydrofolate dehydrogenase) and threonine (serine hydroxymethyltransferase). For a more detailed discussion of enzymatic reactions in which folic acid is involved, see Selhub and Rosenberg (1996).

D. NUTRITIONAL REQUIREMENTS

It is generally accepted that the growing pig can obtain sufficient folic acid from the common feed ingredients and from bacterial synthesis in the intestine. Johnson et al. (1948) found no response to folic acid supplementation when a synthetic milk diet, which contained 2% sulfathaladine, was fed to 4-day-old pigs, and Cunha et al. (1947) reported similar findings in 8-week-old pigs fed a synthetic diet. Moreover, Newcomb and Allee (1986) found no beneficial effect in pigs weaned at 17 to 27 days fed a corn–soybean meal–whey diet supplemented with 1.1 mg folic acid/kg. However, Lindemann and Kornegay (1986) reported an improvement in average daily gain in pigs weaned at 28 days when 0.5 mg folic acid/kg was added to the diet. The investigators noted, however, that the response was mediated through an increase in feed intake as efficiency of feed utilization was not affected. The supplementation of a corn–soybean meal diet with 200 μg folic acid/kg was shown to have no effect on growth or feed efficiency when fed during the starter, grower, or finisher phases (Easter et al., 1983).

Matte et al. (1984a) demonstrated that serum folates decreased by 50% from weaning to day 60 of gestation, and they suggested that this could indicate a possible deficiency of folic acid during midgestation. These researchers reported an increase in litter size farrowed with the administration of 15 mg folic acid intramuscularly ten times from weaning to day 60 of gestation (Matte et al., 1984b). Further research by these authors has shown an inconsistent response to dietary folates (15 mg/kg of diet) on uterine fluids and hormones, suggesting that the reproductive response to folate may be related to parity and and/or prolificacy of the sow (Matte et al., 1996; Duquette et al., 1997). Tremblay et al. (1986) found that addition of 4.3 mg supplemental folic acid/kg of diet maintained serum folates similar to those obtained with ten injections of 15 mg of folic acid administered from weaning to day 56 of gestation. Kornegay and Lindemann (1989) reported that addition of 1 mg folic acid/kg to a corn–soybean meal diet resulted in an improvement in the total number of pigs born and born live over three parities. In addition, Thaler and co-workers (1989) reported that addition of 1.65 mg folic acid/kg of diet increased the number of pigs born, born live, and alive on days 14 and 21 of lactation during a two-parity study. However, Easter et al. (1983) reported no improvement in number of pigs born or weaned when 200 μg folic acid/kg diet was added to a corn–soybean meal diet. Harper et al. (1994) found that the addition of up to 4 ppm dietary folic acid in both the gestation and lactation diets had no effect on reproductive performance, but it did increase serum folate levels.

Tremblay et al. (1989a) showed a reduction in embryonic mortality at day 30 of gestation by the addition of 5 mg folic acid/kg of diet, and an increased protein content of the fetuses from dams fed folic acid compared with control sows. Serum Zn concentrations in sows supplemented with folic acid remained constant during the first 30 days of gestation, whereas serum Zn levels decreased in control sows. Folic acid supplementation did not have any effect on serum Cu or Fe (Tremblay et al., 1989b). However, O'Conner et al. (1989) showed that supplementation of sow diets with either 25 or 125 mg/kg Fe may alter folate utilization in both sows and neonatal swine. Sows fed the lower concentration of Fe had decreased milk folate and their pigs had reduced serum and liver folate levels.

Pharazyn and Aherne (1987) showed no beneficial effect of folic acid supplementation of a wheat–barley–based diet fed during lactation. In addition, Matte and Girard (1989) reported that pigs from sows injected with 15 mg of folic acid per week from day 2 of lactation to weaning had significantly higher serum folate levels, but they observed no response in the growth rate of the pig.

E. Deficiency and Toxicity Signs

Signs of a folic acid deficiency have been previously described (National Research Council, 1998) and include a reduction in growth rate, fading hair color, macrocytic and normocytic anemia, leukopenial thrombopenia, reduced hematocrit, and bone marrow hyperplasia. It should be noted, however, that a synthetic diet containing 1 to 2% of a sulfa drug or a folic acid antagonist was necessary to produce a folic acid deficiency (Cunha et al., 1948; Heinle et al., 1948; Cartwright et al., 1949; Johnson et al., 1950).

Folic acid is generally considered to be nontoxic as no adverse effects have been reported following the ingestion of high levels of the vitamin in any of several species (National Research Council, 1987). A reversible, crystalline folic acid precipitation in the renal tubules has been observed in rats fed pharmacological doses (100 to 400 mg/kg body weight; Huguenin et al., 1978).

F. Determination of Status

The most commonly used assay for folic acid status is the direct estimation of serum and red cell folate (Longo and Herbert, 1976). However, the whole-blood deoxyuridine (dU) suppression test can be used both to determine folic acid status and to distinguish between a folic acid and a vitamin B_{12} deficiency (Das et al., 1980).

G. Sources

Folates are supplied in the diets by most natural feedstuffs. However, the folate content of natural feedstuffs is highly variable and therefore should be considered an unreliable source of the vitamin (Lindemann, 1993). The variability of folate content in feedstuffs may be due to variety, processing, or storage differences (Matte et al., 1989; Lindemann, 1993). Bacteria in the colon seem to produce a significant amount of folates; however, the contribution of bacterial folates to the animals needs is unknown and may be very low as the preferred sight of absorption is the jejunum (Halstead, 1980) and the optimal pH is between 5.0 and 6.0 (Blair et al., 1976).

The apparent digestibility of folates in feedstuffs seems to be variable. The apparent availability in wheat and barley is around 80%, whereas most of the protein feeds have folate apparent availabilities in the range of 30 to 60% (Gannon, 1991). Matte and Girard (1994) found that postprandial variations of serum pterogluglutamates was not an accurate method for the measurement of folate availability in pigs. Additional studies are needed to quantify the availability of folates in feedstuffs.

V. NIACIN

A. History

The first biochemical function of nicotinic acid was demonstrated by Warburg and co-workers when they isolated the compound from coenzyme II (NADP), and they later found that it functioned as part of a hydrogen transport system (Warburg and Christian, 1936). Shortly thereafter, Elvehjem et al. (1938) demonstrated that niacinamide was the active component of liver extracts that was successful in treating black tongue in dogs. It was also shown at this time that nicotinic acid cured pellagra in humans, the parallel of black tongue in dogs (Fouts et al., 1937; Smith et al., 1937; Spies et al., 1938).

B. Structure and Nomenclature

"The term niacin should be used as a generic descriptor for pyridine 3-carboxylic acid and derivatives exhibiting qualitatively the biological activity of nicotinamide" (Anonymous, 1987). "The compound pyridine 3-carboxylic acid, also known as niacin or vitamin PP, should be referred to as nicotinic acid. Nicotinamide is the preferred term for the compound also known as niacinamide or nicotinic acid amide" (Anonymous, 1987).

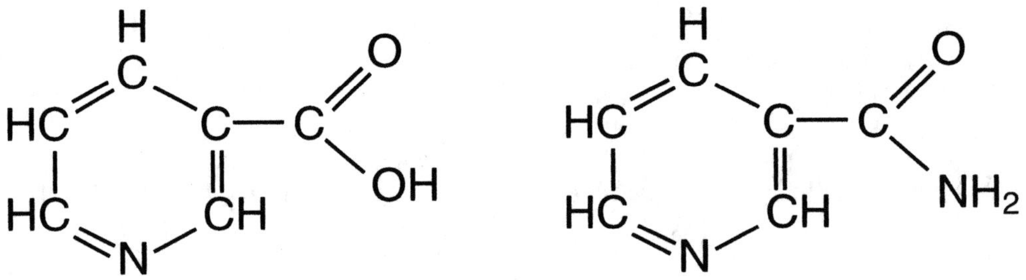

FIGURE 15.4 Nicotinic acid and nicotinamide.

C. Metabolism

1. Digestion and Absorption

Nicotinic acid and nicotinamide are rapidly absorbed from the stomach and small intestine (Bechgaard and Jespersen, 1977). A Na^+-dependent-facilitated transport occurs at low concentrations, whereas passive diffusion predominates at higher concentrations. Nicotinamide adenine dinucleotide (NAD) and NAD phosphate (NADP) are the main dietary forms of niacin and are hydrolyzed by enzymes in the intestinal mucosa to yield nicotinamide. Nicotinamide is the main form of the vitamin in blood (Jacob and Swendseid, 1996). The pig, like most mammals, can synthesize niacin from excess dietary tryptophan (Van Eys, 1991). The biosynthesis of niacin from tryptophan is affected by numerous hormonal and nutritional factors. Vitamin B_6, riboflavin, and Fe are essential cofactors for the enzymes involved in the biosynthesis of niacin, and deficiencies of these nutrients can slow the conversion process (Jacob and Swendseid, 1996).

2. Function

Nicotinamide and nicotinic acid act as precursors for the coenzymes NAD and NADP in which nicotinic acid serves as a more efficient substrate (Ijichi et al., 1966). NAD is the coenzyme for a number of dehydrogenases participating in the metabolism of fat, carbohydrate, and amino acids (Rao and Gopalan, 1984). NADP also participates in dehydrogenation reactions, particularly in the hexose monophosphate shunt.

The coenzymes of nicotinamide have also been implicated in other biological reactions such as the synthesis and repair of DNA and synthesis of protein (Honjo et al., 1971). Nicotinic acid has been reported to be a component of the glucose tolerance factor, but its function is as yet not known (Mertz, 1975).

D. Nutritional Requirements

The requirement for niacin is complicated by the presence of excess tryptophan in the diet, and by its limited availability in certain feed ingredients. With the exception of the newborn, all classes of pigs have been shown to have the ability to convert excess tryptophan to niacin (Cartwright et al., 1948; Luecke et al., 1948; Powick et al., 1948). In addition, Firth and Johnson (1956) estimated that 1 mg of niacin could be obtained from each 50 mg of tryptophan in excess of the requirement. The niacin in yellow corn, oats, wheat, and grain sorghum has been shown to be in a bound form and to be largely unavailable to the young pig (Kodicek et al., 1956; Luce et al., 1966; Harmon et al., 1969; 1970).

The dietary niacin requirement of the baby pig (1 to 8 kg) was estimated to be not >20 mg/kg of available niacin in a diet that contained the minimum amount of tryptophan necessary for normal growth (Firth and Johnson, 1956). These workers also concluded that the 2- to 3-day-old pig was unable to convert tryptophan to nicotinic acid. For growing pigs (10 to 50 kg), the niacin requirement has been estimated to be approximately 10 to 15 mg/kg of available niacin in diets containing tryptophan levels near the requirement (Braude et al., 1946; Kodicek et al., 1959; Harmon et al., 1969). Although niacin is typically added to growing-finishing diets (National Research Council, 1998), recent studies demonstrated no improvement in the performance of growing-finishing pigs (average weight, 41 to 45 kg) when corn–soybean meal diets were supplemented with niacin (Yen et al., 1978; Copelin et al., 1980). However, it has been suggested that the diets used contained tryptophan in excess of the requirement (National Research Council, 1998). No information is available on the niacin requirement of gestating or lactating sows. However, niacin supplementation to a corn–soybean meal–oat diet (14% crude protein) did not affect sow or litter performance (Ivers et al., 1989).

E. Deficiency and Toxicity Signs

Niacin deficiency signs in swine have been described previously (National Research Council, 1998) and include anorexia, reduced weight gain, vomiting, diarrhea, dry skin, dermatitis, rough hair coat, hair loss, ulcerative gastritis, buccal mucosa ulcerations, inflammation and necrosis of the cecum and colon, and normocytic anemia.

No signs of a niacin toxicity in swine have been reported. Toxicity signs such as vasodilation, nausea, vomiting, and occasional skin lesions have been reported in other animals (Robie, 1967). A level of 350 mg nicotinamide/kg of body weight is presumed safe under cases of chronic exposure (National Research Council, 1987).

F. Determination of Status

Urinary excretion of N'-methyl-nicotinamide and N'-methyl-2-pyridone-5-carboxamide has been shown to decrease during niacin deficiency (Luce et al., 1966; 1967). Determination of the activity of erythrocyte nicotinic acid mononucleotide pyrophosribosyl transferase has been used as a possible method to assess the nutritional status of niacin in swine (Arienti et al., 1982).

G. Sources

Niacin is widely distributed in most plant and animal products. Cereal grains and legumes, as well as seeds, yeast, milk, and meats are all considered to have significant concentrations of niacin. However, the niacin in many plants (including most cereal grains) may be bound and unavailable to pigs. Niacin in wheat is bound to several macromolecules and unavailable, whereas the availability of niacin in corn can be increased by pretreatment of the corn with limewater (Jacob and Swendseid, 1996).

VI. PANTOTHENIC ACID

A. History

Work by Norris and Ringrose (1930) and Ringrose et al. (1931) is generally recognized as having led to the eventual identification of pantothenic acid. These researchers observed the development of a deficiency syndrome, first called chick pellagra, after feeding a diet composed largely of casein, middlings, and yellow corn.

B. Structure and Nomenclature

"The compound N-(2,4-dihydroxy-3,3-dimethyl-l-oxobutyl)-beta-alanine, formerly known as pantoyl-beta-alanine, should be designated pantothenic acid" (Anonymous, 1987).

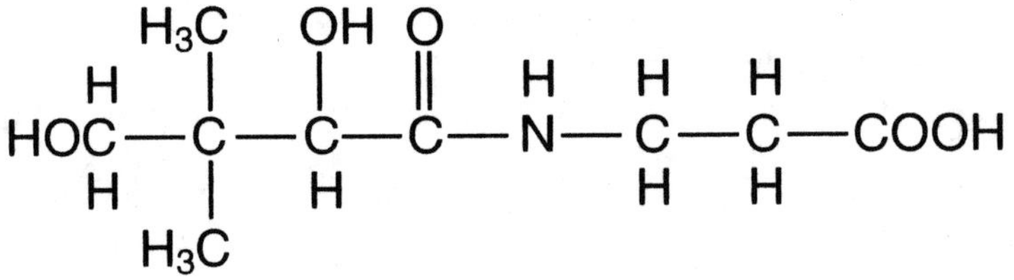

FIGURE 15.5 Pantothenic acid.

C. Metabolism

1. Digestion and Absorption

Pantothenic acid is often found in feedstuffs in the forms of CoA, acyl CoA synthetase, and acyl carrier protein (National Research Council, 1998). Coenzyme A is hydrolyzed in the intestinal lumen to pantothenic acid. Pantothenic acid crosses the intestinal lumen into the blood by a specific Na-dependent transport system at low concentrations (Fenstermacher and Rose, 1986). When pantothenic acid is present in the diet at higher concentrations, it is absorbed from the intestinal lumen by simple diffusion (Shibata et al., 1983). Pantothenic acid in the blood is cotransported with Na across the cell membrane and is converted back into CoA.

2. Functions

Pantothenic acid, in the form of pantotheine, is the functional group of the biologically active CoA, acyl carrier protein, and guanosine 5′-triphosphate (GTP) dependent acyl CoA synthetase (Olson, 1984). CoA functions as a carrier of acyl groups in enzymatic reactions involved in biological acetylations (including choline, sulfonamides, and para-aminobenzoate) and in the synthesis of fatty acids, cholesterol, sphingosine, citrate, acetoacetate, porphyrins, and sterols, as well as in the oxidation of fatty acids, pyruvate, and α-ketoglutarate (Fox, 1984; Olson, 1984). Pantothenic acid, in the form of 4′-phosphopantotheine, is incorporated into acyl carrier protein, which acts as an acyl carrier in fatty acid synthesis. It is also the prosthetic group of GTP-dependent acyl CoA synthetase, which converts succinyl CoA to GTP plus CoA (Olson, 1984). The biosynthesis of the amino acids leucine, arginine, and methionine include a pathothenate-dependent step (Plesofsky-Vig, 1996).

Pantothenate donates the acetate to the N-terminal amino acid of proteins during protein synthesis (Driessen et al., 1985).

D. Nutritional Requirements

Pantothenic acid has been shown to be highly available in barley, wheat, and soybean meal, but low in corn and grain sorghum (Southern and Baker, 1981). For this reason, synthetic pantothenic acid is typically added to all swine diets in the form of Ca-pantothenate. Because only the *d*-isomer of pantothenic acid is biologically available, the *d*-form of Ca-pantothenate has 92% activity, whereas the racemic mixture (dl) contains only 46% activity (National Research Council, 1998).

Stothers and co-workers (1955) determined the pantothenic acid requirement of baby pigs (2 to 10 kg) to be approximately 15.0 mg/kg of diet. The requirement for pigs from 5 to 50 kg has been estimated to range from approximately 4.0 to 9.0 mg/kg of diet (Luecke et al., 1953; Barnhart et al., 1957; Sewell et al., 1962; Palm et al., 1968). Estimates of the pantothenic acid requirement of growing-finishing swine (approximately 20 to 90 kg) range from approximately 6.0 to 10.5 mg/kg of diet (Catron et al., 1953; Pond et al., 1960; Davey and Stevenson, 1963; Palm et al., 1968; Meade et al., 1969; Roth-Maier and Kirchgessner, 1977).

Ullrey et al. (1955) reported that pantothenic acid at a level below 5.9 mg/kg of diet resulted in poor reproductive performance. This finding has been confirmed by Davey and Stevenson (1963) and Teague et al. (1970). In addition, Bowland and Owen (1952) reported normal reproductive performance when a barley-based diet was supplemented with 6.6 mg pantothenic acid/kg. For optimal reproductive performance, the requirement for pantothenic acid has been estimated to be 12.0 to 12.5 mg/kg of diet (Ullrey et al., 1955; Davey and Stevenson, 1963).

E. Deficiency and Toxicity Signs

The primary sign noted in pantothenic acid deficiency in growing swine is that of an abnormal gait in the hind legs referred to as "goose stepping." Hughes and Ittner (1942) confirmed that this abnormal gait was the result of a pantothenic acid deficiency. Other deficiency signs that have been observed include reduced growth, anorexia, diarrhea, dry skin, rough hair coat, alopecia, and reduced immune response (Hughes and Ittner, 1942; Wintrobe et al., 1943b; Luecke et al., 1948; 1950; 1952; Wiese et al., 1951; Stothers et al., 1955). Gestating and lactating gilts fed a diet with low levels of pantothenic acid were observed to develop fatty livers, enlarged adrenal glands, intramuscular hemorrhage, eccentric dilatation of the heart, rectal congestion, atrophic ovaries, and infantile uteri (Ullrey et al., 1955). Pigs born to the gilts that did farrow exhibited locomotor incoordination and diarrhea and had a low rate of survival.

Pantothenic acid is generally considered to be nontoxic as no adverse response to the ingestion of elevated levels of pantothenic acid has been reported in any species (Omaye, 1984).

F. Determination of Status

Clinical signs typically have been used to determine the pantothenic acid status of swine. Requirement studies have consistently used growth as the response criterion for lack of a better determinant. Luecke et al. (1950) found that blood levels of pantothenic acid seemed to be related to the levels consumed, and Owen and Bowland (1952) demonstrated that both blood and milk levels of lactating sows increased as the intake of pantothenic acid increased. However, in the latter study, the pantothenic acid level was also dependent on the day of lactation in which the sampling occurred. The CoA activity in blood as determined by the sulfanilamide acetylation test has been suggested as a possible method of assessing nutritional status (Ellestad et al., 1970).

G. Sources

Pantothenic acid is widely distributed in nature as it is essential for all forms of life (Plesofsky-Vig, 1996). Southern and Baker (1981) found that the bioavialability of pantothenic acid was low in wheat, barley, and sorghum, but higher in corn and soybean meal. Pantothenic acid is relatively stable at neutral pH; however, cooking is reported to destroy 15 to 50% of the vitamin in meat, and the processing of vegetables was associated with a loss of 37 to 78% of the vitamin (Tahiliani and Beinlich, 1991).

VII. RIBOFLAVIN

A. History

Riboflavin does not have the dramatic background associated with some of the other vitamins; rather, its discovery was the result of patient, deliberate investigation. Originally known as vitamin B_2 and also as ovoflavin, it was isolated from egg white and shown to be effective in promoting growth in rats in Kuhn's laboratory at the Wilhelm Institute for Medical Research in 1932 (Cooperman and Lopez, 1984).

B. Structure and Nomenclature

"The compound with the formula …7,8-dimethyl-10-(1'-D-ribityl)isoalloxazine, formerly known as vitamin B_2, vitamin G, lactoflavin(e), or riboflavine, is designated riboflavin" (Anonymous, 1987).

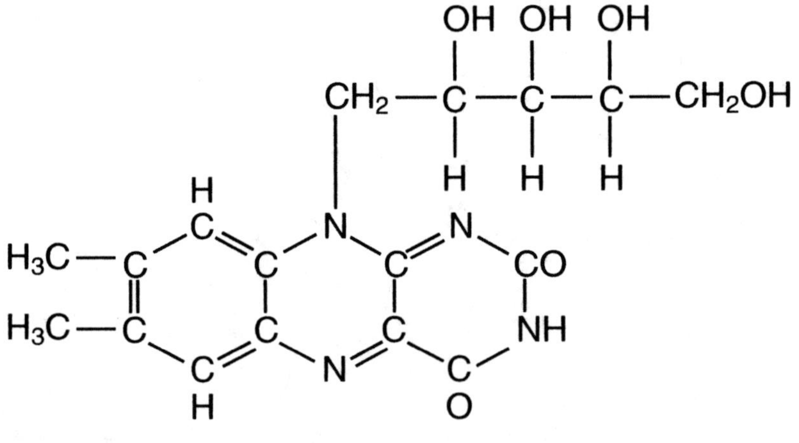

FIGURE 15.6 Riboflavin.

C. Metabolism

1. Digestion and Absorption

Dietary sources of riboflavin are mostly in the form of coenzyme derivatives and must be hydrolyzed before they can be absorbed (Rivlin, 1996). Riboflavin is absorbed by a specialized phosphorylation–dephosphorylation transport mechanism (Jusko and Levy, 1967). The process is Na dependent and involves an ATPase active transport system, which can be saturated (Rivlin, 1996). Intestinal absorption of riboflavin seems to be increased by the presence of food in the intestine (Jusko and Levy, 1967) and by decreased rate of gastric emptying (Roe, 1988). It is thought that food in the intestinal tract may decrease the rate of gastric emptying, allowing a more complete absorption of riboflavin (Rivlin, 1996).

2. Function

Riboflavin participates in metabolism as a precursor of either flavin adenine dinucleotide (FAD) or flavin mononucleotide (FMN). Both FAD and FMN are the prosthetic groups for a number of flavin-linked dehydrogenases. Examples of these enzymes are nicotinamide adenine dinucleotide (NADH) dehydrogenase, succinate dehydrogenase, xanthine oxidase, and glutathione reductase. The isoalloxazine ring of riboflavin is involved in the transfer of hydrogens in oxidation–reduction reactions. Given the role of FAD and FMN in hydrogen transfer reactions, it should be apparent that the flavoprotein enzymes are critical in the metabolism of carbohydrates, proteins, and fats. For a more-detailed discussion of the chemical, biochemical, and nutritional functions of riboflavin, see Cooperman and Lopez (1984), Rivlin (1996), or McCormick (1986; 1994).

D. Nutritional Requirements

The necessity of riboflavin in the pig's diet was first established by Hughes (1939). Subsequent work indicates a riboflavin requirement for baby pigs (2 to 20 kg) to be between 2.0 and 3.0 mg/kg in a synthetic diet (Forbes and Haines, 1952; Miller et al., 1954). Estimates of the riboflavin requirement in a synthetic diet for growing pigs have ranged from 1.1 to 2.9 mg/kg of diet (Hughes, 1940a; Krider et al., 1949; Mitchell et al., 1950; Terrill et al., 1955). Krider and co-workers (1949) and Miller and Ellis (1951) reported estimates of 1.8 to 3.1 mg riboflavin/kg for growing pigs fed a practical diet. Mitchell et al. (1950) reported that the riboflavin requirement was dependent on environmental temperature. These investigators reported that the riboflavin requirement of the growing pig was approximately 1.2 mg/kg of diet at 28°C, whereas the requirement was 2.3 mg/kg at 4°C. However, Seymour and co-workers (1968) reported no consistent interaction between riboflavin and environmental temperature.

Miller and co-workers (1953) reported that an inadequacy in riboflavin (1.1 mg/kg of diet) for reproducing swine resulted in reproductive failure. This was later confirmed by Frank et al. (1984), in that of six gilts fed 0.77 mg riboflavin/kg of diet, four gilts farrowed approximately 7 days prematurely, two had stillborn litters, and the remaining two failed to farrow by day 121 of gestation. Esch and co-workers (1981) reported that a riboflavin deficiency can lead to anestrus. The riboflavin requirement for gestating swine has been estimated to be between 6.4 and 6.6 mg/day, based on farrowing performance and erythrocyte glutathione reductase activity (Frank et al., 1984). Subsequent work by this group (Frank et al., 1988) indicates a riboflavin requirement for lactation to be 14.0 to 16.3 mg/day under an *ad libitum* feeding regimen depending on whether pig or dam erythrocyte glutathione reductase activity coefficients were used. A response to the addition of 100 mg riboflavin/day to a corn–soybean meat diet from day 4 to 10 following onset of estrus has been reported in sows (Bazer and Zavy, 1988). The supplemental riboflavin resulted in an increase in litter size, embryonic survival, and allantoic fluid volume at day 30 of gestation, as well as an increase in conception rate and more pigs at birth, day 21, and day 42 of lactation. However, other studies have failed to show improved litter size from the supplementation of high levels of riboflavin during early pregnancy (Luce et al., 1990; Tilton et al., 1991; Wiseman et al., 1991). Pettigrew et al. (1996) showed that increased levels of riboflavin for 21 days postbreeding had no effect on litter size, but may have increased farrowing percentage.

E. Deficiency and Toxicity Signs

Signs typical of riboflavin deficiency have been described previously (National Research Council, 1998), and they include a reduction in growth rate, stiffness of gait, alopecia, seborrhea, vomiting, and cataracts. Examination of pigs with severe riboflavin deficiency reveals increased blood neutrophil granulocytes, reduced immune response, discolored kidney and liver tissue, fatty liver, and degeneration of the myelin of the sciatic and brachial nerves. Females with severe deficiency also have been shown to have collapsed follicles and degenerating ova.

There is insufficient data available to estimate a maximum tolerable level of riboflavin for pigs. Seymour and co-workers (1968) found no detrimental effect when diets containing 8.8 mg riboflavin/kg of body weight were fed to 5-week-old pigs. Furthermore, riboflavin does not seem to be highly available from common feedstuffs; therefore, high levels included in the diet should not pose a hazard to pigs (National Research Council, 1987).

F. Determination of Status

Early work utilized deficiency signs, riboflavin excretion in the urine, and growth and reproductive performance as indicators of riboflavin status. However, more recently, the measurement of erythrocyte glutathione reductase (EGR), a flavin-dependent enzyme, has been widely accepted as an indicator of riboflavin status (Bamji and Sharada, 1972; Nichoalds, 1974; Prentice and Bates, 1981). Erythrocyte glutathione reductase activity is determined in the presence and absence of exogenous FAD and is expressed as a ratio, the EGR activity coefficient. This assay was validated as an indicator of riboflavin status in swine by Esch et al. (1981) and Pettigrew et al. (1996).

G. Sources

The riboflavin in feedstuffs is primarily in the form of FAD (National Research Council, 1998). The riboflavin present in a corn–soybean meal diet was estimated to be 59% bioavailable relative to crystalline riboflavin (Chung and Baker, 1990). Riboflavin photodegrades in the presence of light, and appreciable amounts of riboflavin may be lost during the processing and storage of cereal grains and feeds (Rivlin, 1996).

VIII. THIAMIN

A. History

The discovery of thiamin stems from early studies of the cause of beriberi, a disease once prevalent in many countries where the staple food was polished rice. K. Takaki, M.D., is credited with the first real breakthrough in the prevention of beriberi (Gubler, 1984). In 1885, as the surgeon general of the Japanese Navy, Takaki suggested decreasing the carbon:nitrogen ratio of the diet of crews by increasing the protein intake. Shortly thereafter, it was shown that rice bran, extracts of rice bran, or whole rice could alleviate the symptoms of the disease. Thiamin was subsequently identified as the active factor in rice bran that prevented beriberi (Jansen and Donath, 1926).

Many of the events leading to the discovery of thiamin are also considered key to the development of the present vitamin concept. Early work by Christian Eijkman and his successor, Gerrit Grijns, investigating a polyneuritis in chickens that resembled beriberi, is credited as being the first adventure in the experimental characterization of a nutritional deficiency. Additionally, it provided an animal model to study a human disorder (Gubler, 1984). In fact, the word *vitamin* was first coined in reference to thiamin when a young chemist, Casimir Funk, convinced he had isolated the active antiberiberi factor that seemed to possess an amine function, coined the name *vitamine* to refer to thiamin as an amine essential for life (Funk, 1911).

B. Structure and Nomenclature

"The compound 3-(4-amino-2-methylpyrimidin-5-ylmethyl)-5-(2-hydroxyethyl)-4methylthiazolium, formerly known as vitamin B_1, vitamin F, aneurin(e), or thiamine, should be designated thiamin" (Anonymous, 1987).

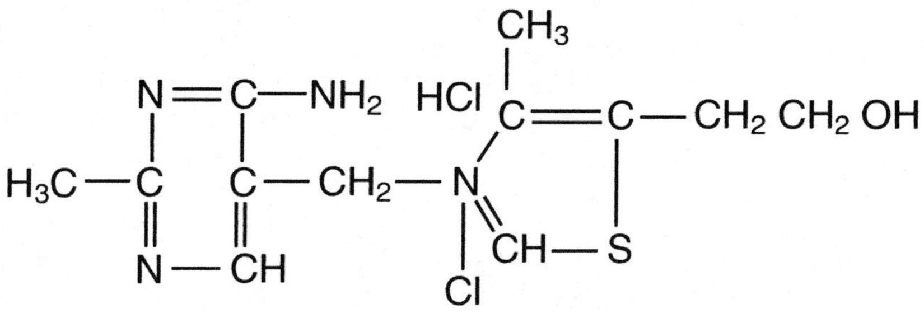

FIGURE 15.7 Thiamin hydrochloride.

C. Metabolism

1. Digestion and Absorption

Thiamin absorption takes place mostly in the jejunum of the small intestine. The thiamin phosphoesters are completely hydrolyzed by intestinal phosphatases, and thiamin is present in the lumen of the intestine in free form (Rindi, 1996). At low intestinal concentrations, active transport occurs. The pattern of *in vivo* intestinal absorption of thiamin by animal species suggests the presence of a saturable transmucosal transport (Rindi and Ventura, 1972). At concentrations less then 1 µmol/l in the intestine, thiamin is absorbed by an active carrier-mediated system that involves phosphorylation of the vitamin and it seems to be age related. At higher concentrations, a passive diffusion system seems to be active (Rindi and Ferrari, 1977; Gastaldi et al., 1992).

2. Function

The only known biologically active form of thiamin is the coenzyme thiamin pyrophosphate (TPP). Thiamin is converted to TPP by means of the enzyme thiamin pyrophosphokinase and adenosine triphosphate (Sauberlich, 1967). Thiamin, in the form of TPP, is essential for the metabolism of carbohydrates and proteins. Thiamin pyrophosphate functions as a coenzyme in the oxidative decarboxylation of ∂-ketoacids. Specifically, TPP is a coenzyme in the pyruvate dehydrogenase complex, the ∂-ketoglutarate complex, and the decarboxylation of the branched-chain ∂-ketoacids derived from the deamination of leucine, isoleucine, and valine (Gubler, 1984). Thiamin pyrophosphate also functions in the transketolase reaction of the pentose phosphate shunt, and it is believed that thiamin, in the form of thiamin triphosphate, might play a role in nerve conduction (Gubler, 1976).

D. Nutritional Requirements

Hughes (1939) demonstrated thiamin to be essential for normal growth and well-being of swine. Miller et al. (1955) estimated the thiamin requirement of baby pigs (2 to 10 kg) to be 1.5 mg/kg for a diet containing 10% fat. A requirement of 1.0 mg thiamin/kg of diet was determined for pigs weaned at 3 weeks of age and fed to 40 kg of weight (Van Etten et al., 1940; Ellis and Madsen, 1944). It has also been reported that the requirement for thiamin decreases as dietary energy from fat increases (Ellis and Madsen, 1944). Peng and Heitman (1974) reported a requirement of 1.1 mg/kg of diet to maximize weight gain and 0.85 mg/kg of diet to maximize feed intake for pigs weighing from 30 to 90 kg.

The use of erythrocyte transketolase activity as an indicator of thiamin status has also been investigated. Estimates of thiamin requirements based on this method are four times the level required to maximize weight gain (Peng and Heitman, 1973). In addition, it was shown that increasing the environmental temperature from 20 to 35°C resulted in an increase in the thiamin requirement determined by this method (Peng and Heitman, 1974). However, it has been suggested that this change may be the result of a reduction in feed intake coinciding with the elevation in environmental temperature (National Research Council, 1998).

Sulfur dioxide treatment of feed ingredients has been shown to destroy thiamin activity (Gray, 1980). Early studies investigating the thiamin requirement of pigs utilized this treatment to develop thiamin-deficient diets (Van Etten et al., 1940; Ellis and Madsen, 1944). The antimicrobial activity of sulfur dioxide has been well established (Schroeter, 1966). The possibility of feeding sulfur dioxide–treated, high-moisture grains to pigs is of interest. Gibson et al. (1987) demonstrated that 61% of the dietary thiamin in a diet containing sulfur dioxide–treated, high-moisture barley was destroyed within 7 days of mixing. Therefore, they concluded that its value in preserving swine diets based on high-moisture grains may be limited because of the rapid rate at which dietary thiamin is destroyed.

There was early interest in the use of swine to clear bracken-infested pastures due to their ability to "root" up the rhizomes (Evans et al., 1963). It was not known at the time if pigs would develop "bracken poisoning" as a result of the thiaminase enzyme contained in the plant. However, Evans and co-workers (1963) reported that the rhizomes alone, when included in a complete ration, would produce a thiamin deficiency. Another antithiamin factor, thiaminase 1, has been identified in a number of freshwater fish (Tanphaichitr and Wood, 1984). Signs of thiamin deficiency have developed in association with the feeding of moderate levels of unprocessed fish known to contain thiaminase 1 (Green et al., 1941; Krampitz and Wooley, 1944).

There is a general lack of information on the thiamin requirement for gestating and lactating sows. The early work on this subject was confounded by a deficiency of other factors that were as yet not recognized as essential (Ensminger et al., 1947). Easter et al. (1983) reported that the addition of 1.0 ppm thiamin to a corn–soybean meal diet had no effect on reproductive performance of first litter gilts.

E. Deficiency and Toxicity Signs

Hughes (1940b) noted anorexia and an associated reduction in weight gain in thiamin-deficient pigs. Similar signs were noted by Van Etten and co-workers (1940), who also noted a depression in body temperature, occasional vomiting, and a flabby heart. Other signs include bradycardia, hypertrophy of the heart, myocardial degeneration, and sudden death associated with heart failure (Wintrobe et al, 1943a; Ellis and Madsen, 1944; Heinemann et al., 1946; Miller et al., 1955). Electrocardiograms of thiamin-deficient pigs were shown consistently to exhibit arrhythmia (Miller et al., 1957b). Transketolase activity is also decreased in response to a thiamin deficiency (Peng and Heitman, 1973).

No clinical signs of thiamin toxicity have been reported for swine. Levels as high as 100 mg/kg of body weight have been fed to young pigs with no ill effects (Ellis and Madsen, 1944). In studies on acute toxicity in laboratory animals, excess thiamin seems to block nerve transmission and results in the development of clinical signs such as restlessness, epileptiform convulsions, cyanosis, and labored breathing (National Research Council, 1987). It has been suggested that levels as high as 1000 times the requirement might be safe for most species.

F. Determination of Status

Deficiency signs have been used in the past to determine the thiamin status of an animal. However, deficiency signs can be confused with other diseases. Furthermore, it is evident that subclinical or borderline inadequacies may affect the individual's performance and well-being. Thus, various biochemical procedures have been developed to detect preclinical thiamin deficiencies. Urinary thiamin excretion and blood pyruvate and lactate levels have been used in the past, but they have many limitations. Baker et al. (1964) developed a microbiological assay as a diagnostic tool for use with any body fluids or tissues. This assay has been shown to be highly sensitive, accurate, and reproducible. However, erythrocyte transketolase activity is considered the most reliable index of the functional state of thiamin. Brin and co-workers (1960) demonstrated that this method is a reliable index of the availability of the coenzyme, thiamin diphosphate, and its activity is well correlated with the degree of deficiency.

G. Sources

Most of the cereal grains used in swine diets are rich in thiamin and, therefore, thiamin is not normally included in vitamin premixes (National Research Council, 1998). However, thiamin is very heat sensitive and is easily destroyed during feed processing, especially in the presence of reducing sugars (National Research Council, 1998). Meat, milk, and egg products can also contain significant amounts of thiamin.

IX. VITAMIN B_6

A. History

Rats fed a diet deficient in what was considered to be the rat pellagra-preventative factor developed what was referred to as "rat pellagra." (It was suggested that this factor be called vitamin B_6.) It was then demonstrated that vitamin B_6 did not cure human pellagra, but it did cure "rat pellagra" (Snell, 1986).

B. Structure and Nomenclature

"The term vitamin B_6 should be used as a generic descriptor for all 2-methyl-3-hydroxy-5-hydroxy methyl pyridine derivatives exhibiting qualitatively the biological activity of pyridoxine in rats" (Anonymous, 1987). "The compound, 3-hydroxy-4,5-bis(hydroxymethyl)2-methylpyridine, formerly known as vitamin B_6, adermin, or pyridoxal, should be designated *pyridoxine*. It should be noted that the term pyridoxine is not synonymous with the generic term *vitamin B_6*. The compound, also known as pyridoxaldehyde, should be designated pyridoxal. The compound, 3-hydroxy-4-methylamino-5-hydroxymethyl-2-methylpyridine, should be designated pyridoxamine" (Anonymous, 1987). For a more complete discussion of the structures of the isomers see Leklem (1996).

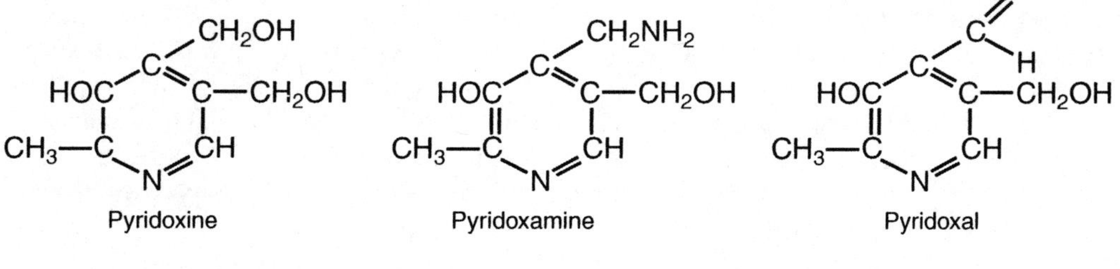

FIGURE 15.8 Isomers of vitamin B_6: pyridoxine, pyridoxamine, and pyridoxal.

C. Metabolism

1. Digestion and Absorption

Research in rats indicates that vitamin B_6 is absorbed from the intestinal tract by a nonsaturable, passive process (Henderson, 1985). Absorption takes place mostly in the jejunum, and absorption is accompanied by the hydrolysis of the 5'-phosphates by nonspecific phosphatases in the gastrointestinal tract (Mehansho et al., 1979; Leklem, 1996). After absorption, the vitamin is phosphorylated back to the original structure (Leklem, 1996).

2. Function

The main active form of vitamin B_6 is pyridoxal phosphate (PLP), which serves as a coenzyme in many metabolic reactions. Pyridoxal phosphate has a functional role, particularly in amino acid metabolism, but also in carbohydrate and lipid metabolism. Pyridoxal phosphate is involved in transaminations, nonoxidative deamination, decarboxylation, and desulfhydration of amino acids. It also seems to affect the conformation of glycogen phosphorylase because the active form (phosphorylase a) contains 4 mol of PLP, whereas the inactive form (phosphorylase b) contains only 2 mol (Yunis et al., 1960). The role of PLP in lipid metabolism is as yet unclear, but it has been shown that carcasses of animals fed deficient levels of B_6 contain less lipid than those of controls (Sauberlich, 1968). A more detailed discussion of the metabolic functions of vitamin B_6 is offered by Driskell (1984) and Leklem (1996).

D. NUTRITIONAL REQUIREMENTS

The vitamin B_6 content of a grain–soybean meal diet for swine is generally adequate to meet the animal's requirement, and thus it is considered unnecessary to supplement the diet (National Research Council, 1998). Easter et al. (1983) demonstrated no benefit from the addition of supplemental vitamin B_6 in nursery, grower, or finisher diets composed of corn and soybean meal. Yen et al. (1976) has reported availability values of vitamin B_6 for the chick to be approximately 40% in corn and 60% in soybean meal. Estimates of the absolute requirement for vitamin B_6 range from 1.0 to 2.0 mg/kg of diet in the baby pig (2 to 10 kg) (Miller et al., 1957a; Kösters and Kirchgessner, 1976a,b) and from 1.2 to 1.8 mg/kg of diet for the nursery pig (10 to 20 kg) (Sewell et al., 1964; Kösters and Kirchgessner, 1976a,b). However, Woodworth et al. (1998) found that the addition of 2.2 to 3.3 mg pyridoxine/kg of diet improved weanling pig performance when fed 0 to 14 days postweaning. No estimates for the growing-finishing pig are available.

Studies conducted with gestating–lactating females have met with mixed results. Draper and co-workers (1958) found no benefit from the addition of pyridoxine to a corn–soybean meal diet for gestating females as measured by the excretion of xanthurenic acid. Ritchie et al. (1960) reported no improvement in reproductive or lactation performance when the diet was supplemented with 10 mg vitamin B_6/kg of diet. However, Easter and co-workers (1983) reported an improvement in litter size at birth and weaning when a corn–soybean meal diet was supplemented with 1 ppm of vitamin B_6. Russell and co-workers (1985a) fed purified diets providing 0.45, 1.5, 2.1, or 83 mg vitamin B_6/day to postpubertal gilts. They used the erythrocyte glutamic-oxaloacetic transaminase coefficient as an indicator of the vitamin B_6 status of the gilts. These researchers demonstrated that the minimum requirement for vitamin B_6 was >2.1 mg/day. This finding was further supported by examining whole-muscle glutamic-oxaloacetic transaminase activity, which was greatly reduced in deficient gilts (Russell et al., 1985b). Knights et al. (1996) have shown a decrease in the days to first postweaning estrus and numerical improvements in litter size in the second parity when high lean genotype sows were fed 15 mg vitamin B_6/kg of diet compared with controls receiving 1 mg/kg of vitamin B_6.

E. DEFICIENCY AND TOXICITY SIGNS

As with many other vitamins, a deficiency of vitamin B_6 results in a reduction in feed intake and growth rate. Other deficiency signs include the development of a brown exudate around the eyes, impaired vision, vomiting, ataxia, epileptiform seizures, coma, and death (Hughes and Squibb, 1942; Wintrobe et al., 1942; 1943c; Lehrer et al., 1951; Miller et al., 1957a). Examination of blood samples taken from deficient animals has revealed microcytic hypochromic anemia, a reduction in albumin, hematocrit, hemoglobin, red blood cells, and lymphocytes, and an increase in gamma globulin (Hughes and Squibb, 1942; Miller et al., 1957a; Harmon et al., 1963). Other signs characteristic of vitamin B_6 deficiency determined at necropsy include degeneration of sensory neurons and fat infiltration of the liver (Wintrobe et al., 1942). A reduction in antibody production as a result of vitamin B_6 deficiency also has been reported (Harmon et al., 1963).

Levels of vitamin B_6 as high as 9.2 mg/kg of diet have been fed to early-weaned pigs with no detrimental effects (Adams et al., 1967). However, toxicity signs, such as ataxia, muscle weakness, and loss of balance, have been reported in other animals (Phillips et al., 1978). It is suggested that dietary levels of at least 50 times the requirement are safe for most species (National Research Council, 1987).

F. Determination of Status

Clinical signs of a vitamin B_6 deficiency in young growing animals appear within 2 to 3 weeks following the removal of the vitamin from the diet (Miller et al., 1957a). Thus, a more sensitive measurement of vitamin B_6 status is required. One of the earliest methods utilized was the tryptophan-loading test (Greenburg et al., 1949), which measures the excretion of xanthurenic acid following a test dose of tryptophan. Other methods include measurement of urinary 4-pyridoxic acid (Baysal et al., 1966), plasma pyridoxal phosphate (Lumeng et al., 1978), and serum transaminases (Linkswiler, 1967). However, due to its simplicity and ease of measurement, the assay for erythrocyte glutamic-oxaloacetic transaminase activity has been suggested as the method of choice in assessing vitamin B_6 status (Russell et al., 1985a).

G. Sources

Vitamin B_6 occurs in feedstuffs as pyridoxine, pyridoxal, pyridoxamine, and pyridoxal phosphate (NRC, 1998). In the chick, vitamin B_6 is about 40% bioavialable in corn and about 60% bioavailable in soybean meal (Yen et al., 1976). Vitamin B_6 concentrations are fairly high in most cereal grains and other common feed ingredients. Vitamin B_6 is normally present in adequate amounts in swine diets and does not require supplementation. However, feed processing and storage can result in the destruction of 10 to 50% of the naturally occurring vitamin B_6 (Woodring and Storvick, 1960; Richardson et al., 1961; Gregory, 1980; Ang, 1981).

X. VITAMIN B_{12}

A. History

Vitamin B_{12}, cyanocobalamin, was the last vitamin to be discovered. Vitamin B_{12} is best known for its association with Addisonian pernicious anemia. Addison (1855) gave a detailed description of the symptoms associated with pernicious anemia. However, it was not until the early 1900s that the feeding of liver as a successful treatment was demonstrated (Minot and Murphy, 1926). Shortly thereafter, Castle (1929) demonstrated that the antipernicious anemia principle in liver required prior binding to an "intrinsic factor" secreted by the stomach for proper intestinal absorption. West (1948), using the vitamin isolated by Rickes and co-workers, definitively demonstrated the association between vitamin B_{12} and pernicious anemia. Hydroxyocobalamin was shown to have the same biological activity as cyanocobalamin (Lichtman et al., 1949), and it was thus determined that the cyanide was apparently an artifact of the original isolation procedure.

B. Structure and Nomenclature

"The term vitamin B_{12} should be used as a generic descriptor for all corrinoids exhibiting qualitatively the biological activity of cyanocobalamin" (Anonymous, 1987). The compound formerly referred to as vitamin B_{12}, or cyanocobalamine, should be designated cyanocobalamin. The compound formerly referred to as vitamin B_{12b} should be designated hydroxocobalamin. Related compounds with vitamin B_{12} activity should be named in accordance with the IUPAC-IUB-CBN, The Nomenclature of Corrinoids, 1973 Recommendations (IUPAC-IUB Commission on Biochemical Nomenclature, 1974).

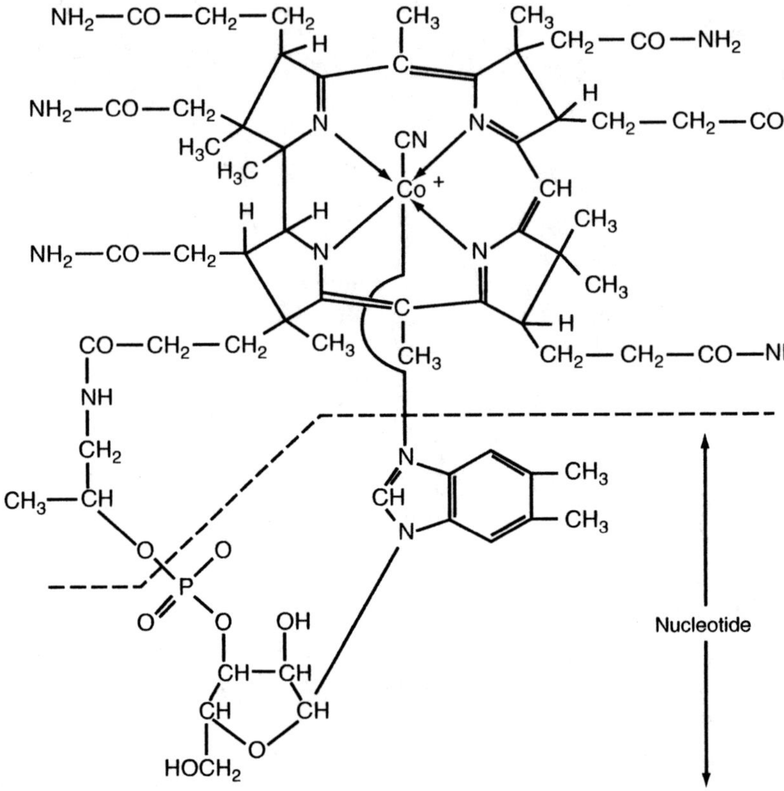

FIGURE 15.9 Vitamin B_{12}.

C. Metabolism

1. Digestion and Absorption

Digestion of vitamin B_{12} begins in the stomach where gastric acids and enzymes free the vitamin B_{12} from its peptide bonds in food by proteolysis. The vitamin B_{12} then binds to salivary protein. As the salivary protein is digested, the B_{12} is freed and then bound to unidentified intrinsic factor secreted by the gastric parietal cells. The intrinsic factor-bound vitamin B_{12} is then absorbed by the ileum (Herzlich and Herbert, 1986; Herbert, 1996).

2. Functions

Two coenzyme forms of vitamin B_{12} are known to exist in animals. These include methylcobalamin, which functions as a methyl carrier, and adenosylcobalamin, which serves as a hydrogen carrier (Stadtman, 1971). The function of methylcobalamin as a methyl carrier is the basis for the interrelationship between vitamin B_{12} and folate. In one such reaction, an enzyme-bound methylcobalamin is formed as an intermediate in the transfer of the methyl moiety of N^5-methyltetrahydrofolate to homocysteine in the resynthesis of methionine (Ellenbogen, 1984). In another reaction, a cobalamin-dependent enzyme removes the methyl group from methylfolate, thereby generating tetrahydrofolate, from which the 5,10-methylenetetrahydrofolate required for thymidylate synthesis is made (Herbert, 1984). In the form of adenosylcobalamin, vitamin B_{12} is a coenzyme for methylmalonyl-CoA mutase, which catalyzes the conversion of methyl-malonyl-CoA to succinyl-CoA (Ellenbogen, 1984). This reaction is a step in the catabolism of propionyl-CoA, which is derived from the breakdown of valine and isoleucine.

D. NUTRITIONAL REQUIREMENTS

In early work with newborn pigs, a synthetic milk ration was found to be deficient in an unknown growth factor contained in purified casein (Neumann et al., 1948). It was subsequently discovered that this deficiency in baby pigs could be alleviated by adding the antipernicious anemia liver extract (Johnson and Neumann, 1948). The factor contained in this extract was shortly thereafter identified as vitamin B_{12}. Thus, it is obvious that the baby pig requires a source of vitamin B_{12} in the diet. However, studies investigating the response to supplemental vitamin B_{12} have met with variable results. This may be partially explained by the fact that ingredients from plant sources are devoid of vitamin B_{12}, whereas animal by-products contain vitamin B_{12} (National Research Council, 1998). However, it has been suggested that microbial synthesis of vitamin B_{12} in the intestinal tract, as well as that supplied via coprophagy, may satisfy the pig's requirement for vitamin B_{12} (Bauriedel et al., 1954; Hendrickx et al., 1964). However, De Passille et al. (1989) found that coprophagy was an insignificant source of vitamin B_{12} in young pigs. Nonetheless, due to the commercial availability of vitamin B_{12} supplements, it is routinely added to grain–soybean meal diets.

Estimates of the vitamin B_{12} requirement of young pigs (1.5 to 20 kg) have ranged from 15 to 20 µg/kg of dry matter in the diet (Anderson and Hogan, 1950a; Nesheim et al., 1950; Frederick and Brisson, 1961). However, Neumann and co-workers (1950) reported suboptimal performance over a similar weight range in pigs receiving 34 µg vitamin B_{12}/kg of diet dry matter. This diet, however, contained sulfasuxidine to inhibit intestinal synthesis of vitamin B_{12}. These studies utilized a synthetic milk diet, and the pigs were housed in wire-floored cages to avoid coprophagy. For pigs ranging in weight from 10 to 45 kg and housed in wire-floored cages, the requirement ranges from 8.8 to 11.0 µg/kg of diet (Richardson et al., 1951; Catron et al., 1952).

The addition of 11 to 1100 µg vitamin B_{12}/kg of diet has been shown to improve reproductive performance of sows (Anderson and Hogan, 1950b; Frederick and Brisson, 1961; Teague and Grifo, 1966; Reinisch et al., 1990). However, Teague and Grifo (1966) observed no improvement in the number of pigs farrowed and weaned or in their weights at birth or weaning in sows supplemented with 110 to 1100 µg vitamin B_{12}/kg of a corn–soybean meal diet for three to four parities. However, increased litter weight was observed in B_{12}-supplemented sows only in the third and fourth parities. Because of the limited information available and wide range of levels of supplementation used, it is difficult to determine an exact requirement of vitamin B_{12} for gestation and lactation, but a level of 15 µg/kg of diet has been suggested (National Research Council, 1998).

E. DEFICIENCY AND TOXICITY SIGNS

A vitamin B_{12} deficiency in pigs is evidenced by a reduction in growth rate and feed intake, rough hair coat, dermatitis, enlarged liver, extreme irritability and sensitivity to touch, posterior incoordination, and unsteadiness of gait (Anderson and Hogan, 1950a; Neumann and Johnson, 1950; Neumann et al., 1950; Richardson et al., 1951; Catron et al., 1952). Deficient pigs exhibited normocytic anemia and high neutrophils with concomitantly low lymphocyte counts (Neumann and Johnson, 1950; Cartwright et al., 1951). Similar to pernicious anemia in humans, a double deficiency of vitamin B_{12} and folic acid has been reported to result in the development of macrocytic anemia and bone marrow hyperplasia (Johnson et al., 1950; Cartwright et al., 1952).

No data are available to suggest an upper safe level of vitamin B_{12} for pigs. Data with chicks suggest an upper safe level at three times the requirement, whereas data in mice indicate that dietary levels of at least several hundred times the requirement are safe (National Research Council, 1987).

F. DETERMINATION OF STATUS

Early studies utilized gross observations and performance are red and white blood cell counts as indicators of status. However, a number of diagnostic tests have been investigated in the area of human nutrition. One of the most commonly used tests is that of serum vitamin B_{12} levels (Herbert,

1979). Newer tests for vitamin B_{12} status include the peripheral blood lymphocyte vitamin B_{12} level (Herbert, 1984) and the whole-blood dU suppression test (Das et al., 1980).

G. Sources

Plants and grain materials are completely devoid of naturally occurring vitamin B_{12}. Vitamin B_{12} found in nature is made exclusively by microorganisms. Fecal material contains high levels of vitamin B_{12}, but vitamin B_{12} is not absorbed from the colon. Meat and meat products are high in vitamin B_{12} (Herbert, 1996).

XI. ASCORBIC ACID

A. History

Ascorbic acid may have influenced the course of history by spontaneously ending many military campaigns and long ocean voyages because of fatal outbreaks of scurvy when rations became depleted of ascorbic acid (Jaffe, 1984). Ascorbic acid, or vitamin C, was recognized as the antiscorbutic factor in fresh fruits and vegetables as early as 1734 (Chick, 1953). However, it was not until 1932 that two different research groups isolated and identified this compound (Svirbely and Szent-Györgyi, 1932; King and Waugh, 1932).

B. Structure and Nomenclature

"The term vitamin C should be used as a generic descriptor for all compounds exhibiting qualitatively the biological activity of ascorbic acid" (Anonymous, 1987). L-Ascorbic acid or simply ascorbic acid, formerly known as vitamin C, cevitamic acid, or hexuronic acid, should be used to designate the compound 2,3-didehydro-L-threohexano-1,4-lactone. "The compound L-threo-hexano-1,4-lactone should be designated L-dehydroascorbic acid or dehydroascorbic acid" (Anonymous, 1987).

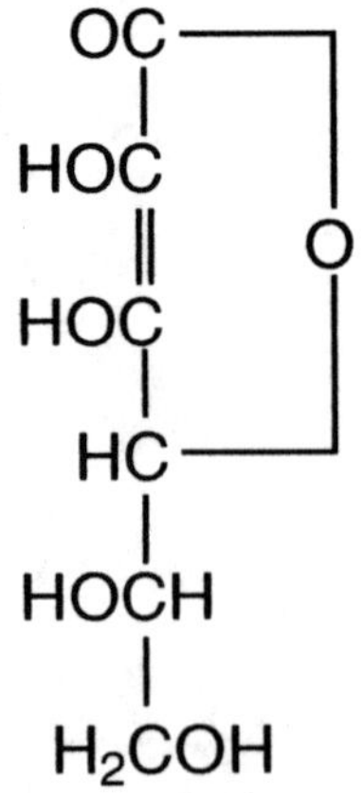

FIGURE 15.10 L-Ascorbic acid.

C. Metabolism

1. Digestion and Absorption

Ascorbate absorption seems to be a protein-mediated active transport in the small intestine (Stevenson and Brush, 1969; Rose et al., 1986). Intestinal absorption of dehydroascorbic acid has not been well characterized (Rose et al., 1988; Levine et al., 1996). There seems to be a different active transport system for dehydroascorbic acid than there is for ascorbate, but the system has not been identified (Levine et al., 1996).

2. Function

Although ascorbic acid has long been known to prevent the occurrence of scurvy, the biochemical function of ascorbic acid is uncertain. An ascorbic acid deficiency may induce various liver lysosomal enzyme activities (Hoehn and Kanfer, 1978) and impair the biosynthesis of collagen (Barnes and Kodicek, 1972). The impairment in collagen synthesis seems to be due to decreased ability to hydroxylate lysine and proline. The hydroxylation of these amino acid residues is required for formation of cross-links in the collagen matrix, which gives strength to the collagen. Collagen is essential for normal growth of bone and cartilage. Ascorbic acid also enhances the formation of intracellular material, the formation of bone matrix, and the formation of tooth dentin (National Research Council, 1998). Ascorbic acid is also involved in the hydroxylation of trimethyllysine and γ-butyrobetaine in carnitine biosynthesis (Broquist, 1982). Ascorbic acid, because of its reducing and chelating properties, also enhances the absorption of Fe from the diet and may be involved in the absorption, mobilization, and distribution of other metal ions throughout the body (Levine et al., 1996). The vitamin has also been implicated in the metabolism of cholesterol (Turley et al., 1976), the synthesis of epinephrine and anti-inflammatory steroids (Broquist, 1982), wound healing (Irwin and Hutchins, 1976), and leukocyte functions (Shilotri, 1977).

D. NUTRITIONAL REQUIREMENTS

It is generally accepted that the pig does not require a dietary source of ascorbic acid (National Research Council, 1998). Some research has suggested that under certain environmental conditions the pig may not be able to synthesize enough ascorbic acid for maximum growth. Riker et al. (1967) reported that plasma ascorbic acid levels were lower for pigs in a hot environment. Kornegay et al. (1986) found no benefit to supplemental ascorbic acid for weaning pigs exposed to cold. There is also a high correlation between energy intake and serum ascorbic acid concentrations (Brown et al., 1970). Ascorbic acid supplementation has been shown to improve growth rate of 3-week-old pigs significantly, especially at a low energy intake (Brown et al., 1975). Dvorak (1974) reported a reduction in liver ascorbic acid levels in 1- and 40-day-old pigs in response to fasting. Studies investigating the effect of ascorbic acid supplementation when no specific stress has been imposed have met with mixed results. Jewell et al. (1981) reported an increase in weight gain in pigs weaned at 1 day of age in one trial, but they were unable to show a response to supplemental ascorbic acid in a second trial. In pigs weaned at 3 to 4 weeks of age, supplemental ascorbic acid significantly increased weight gain (Brown et al., 1975; Yen and Pond, 1981). Parenteral dosing and feed supplementation with ascorbic acid has been reported to improve weight gain in pigs initially weighing 24 kg (Mahan et al., 1966). Cromwell and co-workers (1970) were only able to show an improvement in growth rate in two of three trials when supplemental ascorbic acid was added to the diet of growing pigs. No response to supplemental ascorbic acid has been reported in suckling pigs (Leibbrandt, 1977), pigs weaned at 3 to 4 weeks of age (Mahan and Saif, 1983; Nakano et al., 1983; Yen and Pond, 1983; 1984; 1987; Chiang et al., 1985; Yen et al., 1985), or growing-finishing pigs (Hutagalung et al., 1969; Strittmatter et al., 1978). Housing system (Mahan and Saif, 1983), crowding (Brown and Partridge, 1971; Yen and Pond, 1983; 1987), space allowance (NCR-89 Committee on Confinement Management of Swine, 1989), carbadox (Mahan and Saif, 1983; Yen and Pond, 1984), and Cu (Mahan and Saif, 1983) have also been reported to have no interactive effect with supplemental ascorbic acid.

It also has been postulated that ascorbic acid supplementation may be effective in the prevention or alleviation of osteochondrosis in swine. It was thought that osteochondrosis might be related to insufficient collagen cross-linking due to a reduction in hydroxylation of lysine and proline. However, dietary supplementation with ascorbic acid has been shown to be ineffective in preventing this condition (Strittmatter et al., 1978; Cleveland et al., 1983; Nakano et al., 1983).

Navel bleeding in pigs was reported to be prevented by the addition of 1.0 g ascorbic acid/day to the feed of pregnant sows beginning 6 days before farrowing (Sandholm et al., 1979). In addition, it was noted that the administration of water-soluble vitamin K in the drinking water failed to prevent navel bleeding in newborn pigs. The investigators postulated that the defect in coagulation was due to immature collagen, which did not efficiently induce platelet plug formation, and that the piglets depend on their dam for their supply of ascorbic acid. However, in subsequent studies where navel bleeding was not considered to be a problem, there was no improvement in pig survival or growth rate when 1.0 to 10.0 g ascorbic acid/day was added to sows' diets beginning in late pregnancy (Lynch and O'Grady, 1981; Chavez, 1983; Yen and Pond, 1983).

E. Deficiency and Toxicity Signs

Ascorbic acid is not a dietary essential for the pig because it can be synthesized from carbohydrates such as glucose and galactose. Other species, such as primates and the guinea pig, lack the enzyme L-gulonolactone oxidase that is required for ascorbic acid biosynthesis (Nishikimi and Udenfriend, 1976). Thus, no deficiency signs have been observed in the pig. However, under certain environmental conditions, a reduction in plasma, serum, and liver ascorbic acid concentrations has been reported (Riker et al., 1967; Brown et al., 1970; 1975; Dvorak, 1974).

No signs of ascorbic acid toxicity have been reported in swine. Levels as high as 10 g/kg of diet have been fed to young pigs with no adverse effects (Chavez, 1983). However, excess ascorbic acid results in development of toxicity signs in humans and laboratory animals. These signs include allergic responses, oxaluria, uricosuria, and interference with mixed function oxidase systems (National Research Council, 1987).

F. Determination of Status

Due to the limited knowledge concerning the metabolic functions of ascorbic acid, no completely satisfactory or reliable biochemical procedures to identify a deficiency state or to assess nutritional status have been developed (Jaffe, 1984). However, measurements of ascorbic acid content in serum, plasma, whole blood, leukocytes, and urine have been used to determine inadequacies (Sauberlich et al., 1974). Various fluorometric and colorimetric procedures are available for the measurement of ascorbic acid levels in biological samples (Sauberlich et al., 1974).

G. Sources

Significant concentrations of ascorbate can be found in fruits and vegetables (Haytowitz, 1995). Data concerning the ascorbate content of cereal grains is not readily available. Estimates of the vitamin C content of foods are affected by season, storage, transport methods, and cooking practices (Levine et al., 1996).

REFERENCES

Achuta Murthy, P. N., and S. P. Mistry. 1977. Biotin, *Prog. Food Nutr. Sci.*, 2:405.

Adams, C. R., C. E. Richardson, and T. J. Cunha. 1967. Supplemental biotin and vitamin B_6 for swine, *J. Anim. Sci.*, 26:903 (Abstr.).

Addison, T. 1855. *On the Constitutional and Local Effects of Disease of the Suprarenal Capsules*, Samuel Highely, London.

Anderson, G. C., and A. G. Hogan. 1950a. Adequacy of synthetic diets for reproduction of swine, *Proc. Soc. Exp. Biol. Med.*, 75:288.

Anderson, G. C., and A. G. Hogan. 1950b. Requirements of the pig for vitamin B_{12}, *J. Nutr.*, 40:243.

Anderson, P. A., D. H. Baker, P. A. Sherry, and J. E. Corbin. 1979. Choline-methionine interrelationship in feline nutrition, *J. Anim. Sci.*, 49:552.

Ang, C. Y. N. 1981. Comparison of sample storage methods of vitamin B-6 assay in broiler meats, *J. Food Sci.*, 47:336

Anonymous. 1987. Nomenclature policy: generic descriptors and trivial names for vitamins and related compounds, *J. Nutr.*, 117:7.

Arienti, G., M. S. Simonetti, and F. Fidanza. 1982. The effect of niacin deprivation on nicotinic acid mononucleotide pyrophosphorylase of pig erythrocytes, *Int. J. Vitam. Nutr. Res.*, 52:142.

Baker, H., O. Frank, J. J. Fennelly, and C. M. Leevy. 1964. A method for assaying thiamin status in man and animals, *Am. J. Clin. Nutr.*, 14:197.

Bamji, M. S., and D. Sharada. 1972. Hepatic glutathione reductase and riboflavin concentrations in experimental deficiency of thiamin and riboflavin in rats, *J. Nutr.*, 102:443.

Bane, D. P., R. J. Meade, H. D. Hilley, and A. D. Leman. 1980. Influence of d-biotin and housing on hoof lesions, *Proc. Int. Pig. Vet. Soc.*, 6:334.

Barnes, M. J., and E. Kodicek. 1972. Biological hydroxylations and ascorbic acid with special regard to collagen metabolism, *Vitam. Horm.*, 30:1.

Barnhart, C. E., D. V. Catron, G. C. Ashton, and L. Y. Quinn. 1957. Effects of dietary pantothenic acid levels on the weanling pig, *J. Anim. Sci.*, 16:396.

Bauriedel, W. R., A. B. Hoerlein, J. C. Picken, Jr., and L. A. Underkofler. 1954. Selection of diet for studies of vitamin B_{12} depletion using unsuckled baby pigs, *J. Agric. Food Chem.*, 2:468.

Baysal, A., B. A. Johnson, and H. Linkswiler. 1966. Vitamin B-6 depletion in man: blood vitamin B-6, plasma pyridoxalphosphate, serum cholesterol, serum transaminases and urinary vitamin B-6 and 4-pyridoxic acid, *J. Nutr.*, 89:19.

Bazer, F. W., and T. T. Zavy. 1988. Supplemental riboflavin and reproduction performance of gilts, *J. Anim. Sci.*, 66(Suppl. 1):324 (Abstr.).

Bechgaard, H., and S. Jespersen. 1977. GI absorption of niacin in humans, *J. Pharm. Sci.*, 66:871.

Best, C. H., and M. E. Huntsman. 1932. The effects of the components of lecithin upon deposition of fat in the liver, *J. Physiol.* (London), 75:405.

Blair, J. A., I. T. Johnson, and A. J. Matty. 1976. Aspects of intestinal folate transport in the rat, *J. Physiol.*, 256:197.

Bonjour, J. P. 1984. Biotin. In *Handbook of Vitamins, Nutritional, Biochemical, and Clinical Aspects*, Machlin, L.J., Ed., Marcel Dekker, New York, 403–435.

Bowland, J. P., and B. D. Owen. 1952. Supplemental pantothenic acid in small grain rations for swine, *J. Anim. Sci.*, 11:757 (Abstr.).

Bowman, B. B., and I. H. Rosenberg. 1987. Biotin absorption by distal rat intestine, *J. Nutr.*, 117:2121.

Bowman, B. B., D. B. McCormick, and I. H. Rosenberg. 1989. Epithelial transport of water soluble vitamins, *Annu. Rev. Nutr.*, 9:187.

Boyd, R. D., B. D. Moser, E. R. Peo, Jr., A. J. Lewis, and R. K. Johnson. 1982. Effect of tallow and choline chloride addition to the diet of sows on mik composition, milk yield, and preweaning pig performance, *J. Anim. Sci.*, 54:1.

Braude, R., S. K. Kon, and E. G. White. 1946. Observations on the nicotinic acid requirements of pigs, *Biochem. J.*, 40:843.

Brin, M., M. Tai, A. S. Ostashever, and H. Kalinsky. 1960. The effect of thiamine deficiency on the activity of erythrocyte hemolysate transketolase, *J. Nutr.*, 71:273.

Brooks, P. H., D. A. Smith, and V. C. R. Irwin. 1977. Biotin-supplementation of diets: the incidence of foot lesions and the reproductive performance of sows, *Vet. Rec.*, 101:46.

Broquist, H. P. 1982. Carnitine biosynthesis and function. Introductory remarks, *Fed. Proc.*, 41:2840.

Brown, R. G., and I. G. Partridge. 1971. Influence of supplementary ascorbic acid on performance of crowded swine, *Can. J. Anim. Sci.*, 51:824.

Brown, R. G., V. D. Sharma, and L. G. Young. 1970. Ascorbic acid metabolism in swine. Interrelationships between the level of energy intake and serum ascorbate levels, *Can. J. Anim. Sci.*, 50:605.

Brown, R. G., J. G. Buchanan-Smith, and V. D. Sharma. 1975. Ascorbic acid metabolism in swine. The effects of feeding and level of supplementary ascorbic acid on swine fed various energy levels, *Can. J. Anim. Sci.*, 55:353.

Bryant, K. L., G. E. Combs, and H. D. Wallace. 1977. Supplemental choline for young and growing-finishing swine, Florida Agricultural Experiment Station Twenty-second Annual Swine Field Day. Research Report AL-1977-1, Florida Agricultural Experiment Station, Gainesville, FL.

Bryant, K. L., E. T. Kornegay, J. W. Knight, H. P. Veit, and D. R. Notter. 1985a. Supplemental biotin for swine. III. Influence of supplementation to corn- and wheat-based diets on the incidence and severity of toe lesions, hair, and skin characteristics and structural soundness of sows housed in confinement during four parities, *J. Anim. Sci.*, 60:154.

Bryant, K. L., E. T. Kornegay, J. W. Knight, K. E. Webb, Jr., and D. R. Notter. 1985b. Supplemental biotin for swine. I. Influence on feedlot performance, plasma biotin, and toe lesions in developing gilts, *J. Anim. Sci.*, 60:136.

Bryant, K. L., E. T. Kornegay, J. W. Knight, K. E. Webb, Jr., and D. R. Notter. 1985c. Supplemental biotin for swine. II. Influence of supplementation of corn- and wheat-based diets on reproductive performance and various biochemical criteria of sows during four parities, *J. Anim. Sci.*, 60:145.

Cartwright, G. E., B. Tatting, and M. M. Wintrobe. 1948. Niacin deficiency anemia in swine, *Arch. Biochem.*, 19:109.

Cartwright, G. E., J. G. Palmer, B. Tatting, H. Ashenbrucker, and M. M. Wintrobe. 1949. Experimental production of nutritional macrocytic anemia in swine. III. Futher studies of pteroylglutamic acid deficiency, *Blood*, 4:301.

Cartwright, G. E., B. Tatting, J. Robinson, N. M. Fellows, F. D. Gunn, and M. M. Wintrobe. 1951. Hematological manifestations of vitamin B_{12} deficiency in swine, *Blood*, 6:867.

Cartwright, G. E., B. Tatting, D. Kurth, and M. M. Wintrobe. 1952. Experimental production of nutritional macrocytic anemia in swine. V. Hematologic manifestations of a combined deficiency of vitamin B_{12} and pteroylglutamic acid, *Blood*, 7:992.

Castle, W. B. 1929. Observations on the etiologic relationship of achylia gastriica to pernicious anemia, *Am. J. Med. Sci.*, 178:748.

Catron, D.V., D. Richardson, L. A. Underkofler, H. M. Maddock, and W. C. Friedland. 1952. Vitamin B_{12} requirement of weanling pigs. II. Performance on low level of vitamin B_{12} and requirements for optimum growth, *J. Nutr.*, 47:461.

Catron, D. V., R. W. Binnison, H. M. Maddock, G. C. Ashton, and P. G. Homeyer. 1953. Effects of certain antibiotics and vitamin B_{12} on pantothenic acid requirements of growing-fattening swine, *J. Anim. Sci.*, 12:51.

Chavez, E. R. 1983. Supplemental value of ascorbic acid during late gestation on piglet survival and early growth, *Can. J. Anim. Sci.*, 63:683.

Chiang, S. H., J. E. Pettigrew, R. L. Moser, S. G. Cornelius, K. P. Miller, and T. R. Heeg. 1985. Supplemental vitamin C in swine diets, *Nutr. Rep. Int.*, 31:573.

Chick, H. 1953. Early investigations of scurvy and the antiscorbutic vitamin, *Proc. Nutr. Soc.*, 12:210.

Chung, T. K., and D. H. Baker. 1990. Riboflavin requirement of chicks fed purified amino acid and conventional corn–soybean meal diets, *Poult. Sci.*, 69:1357.

Cleveland, E. R., G. L. Newton, B. G. Mullinix, O. M. Hale, and T. M. Frye. 1983. Foot-leg and performance traits of boars fed two levels of ascorbic acid, *J. Anim. Sci.*, 57(Suppl. 1):387 (Abstr.).

Cooperman, J. M., and R. Lopez. 1984. Riboflavin. In *Handbook of Vitamins: Nutritional, Biochemical, and Clinical Aspects*, Machlin, L. J., Ed., Marcel Dekker, New York, 299–327.

Copelin, J. L., H. Monegue, and G. E. Combs. 1980. Niacin levels in growing-finishing swine diets, *J. Anim. Sci.*, 51(Suppl. 1):190 (Abstr.).

Cromwell, G. L., V. W. Hays, and J. R. Overfield. 1970. Effect of dietary ascorbic acid on performance and plasma cholesterol levels of growing swine, *J. Anim. Sci.*, 31:63.

Cunha, T. J., D. C. Lindley, and M. E. Ensminger. 1946. Biotin deficiency syndrome in pigs fed desiccated egg white, *J. Anim. Sci.*, 5:219.

Cunha, T. J., L. K. Bustad, W. E. Ham, D. R. Cordy, E. C. McCullock, I. F. Woods, G. H. Corner, and M. A. McGregor. 1947. Folic acid, para-aminobenzoic acid and anti-pernicious anemia liver extract in swine nutrition, *J. Nutr.*, 34:173.

Cunha, T. J., R. W. Colby, L. K. Bustad, and J. F. Bone. 1948. The need for and interrelationship of folic acid, anti-pernicious anemia liver extract, and biotin in the pig, *J. Nutr.*, 36:215.

Das, K. C., C. Manusselis, and V. Herbert. 1980. Simplifying lymphocyte culture and the deoxyuridine suppression test by using whole blood (0.1 ml) instead of separated lymphocytes, *Clin. Chem.*, 26:72.

Davey, R. J., and J. W. Stevenson. 1963. Pantothenic acid requirement of swine for reproduction, *J. Anim. Sci.*, 22:9.

Day, P. L., V. Mims, J. R. Totter, E. L. R. Stokstad, B. L. Hutchings, and N. H. Sloane. 1945. The successful treatment of vitamin M deficiency in the monkey with highly purified lactobacilus casei factor, *J. Biol. Chem.*, 157:423.

De Passille, A. M. B., R. R. Bilodeau, C. L. Girard, and J. J. Matte. 1989. A study on the occurrence of coprophagy behavior and its relationship to B-vitamin status in growing-finishing pigs, *Can. J. Anim. Sci.*, 69:299.

Draper, H. H., R. Hironaka, and A. H. Jensen. 1958. A study of xanthurenic acid excretion by swine, *J. Anim. Sci.*, 17:68.

Driessen, A. P. C., W. W. de Jong, G. I. Tesser, and H. Bloemendal. 1985. The mechanism of N-terminal acetylation of proteins, *CRC Crit. Rev. Biochem.*, 18:281.

Driskell, J. A. 1984. Vitamin B-6. In *Handbook of Vitamins, Nutritional, Biochemical, and Clinical Aspects*, Machlin, L. J., Ed., Marcel Dekker, New York, 379–401.

Duquette J., J. J. Matte, C. Farmer, C. L. Girard, and J. P. Laforest. 1997. Pre- and post-mating dietary supplements of folic acid and uterine secretory activity in gilts, *Can. J. Anim. Sci.*, 77:415.

du Vigneaud, V., K. Hofmann, and D. B. Melville. 1942. On the structure of biotin, *J. Am. Chem. Soc.*, 64:188.

Dvorak, M. 1974. Effects of corticotrophin, starvation and glucose on ascorbic acid levels in the blood plasma and liver of piglets, *Nutr. Metab.*, 16:215.

Easter, R. A., P. A. Anderson, E. J. Michel, and J. R. Corley. 1983. Response of gestating gilts and starter, grower and finisher swine to biotin, pyridoxine, folacin, and thiamine additions to a corn–soybean meal diet, *Nutr. Rep. Int.*, 28:945.

Ellenbogen, L. 1984. Vitamin B_{12}. In *Handbook of Vitamins, Nutritional, Biochemical, and Clinical Aspects*, Machlin, L. J., Ed., Marcel Dekker, New York, 497–547.

Ellestad, J. J., R. A. Nelson, M. A. Adson, and W. M. Palmer. 1970. Pantothenic acid and coenzyme A activity in blood and colonic mucosa from patients with chronic ulcerative colitis, *Fed. Proc.*, 29:820.

Ellis, N. R., and L. L. Madsen. 1944. The thiamine requirements of pigs as related to the fat content of the diet, *J. Nutr.*, 27:253.

Elvehjem, C. A., R. J. Madden, F. M. Strong, and D. W. Woolley. 1938. The isolation and identification of the anit-black tongue factor, *J. Biol. Chem.*, 123:137.

Emmert, J. L. 1997. Methyl group metabolism in poultry. In *Proc. Degussa Tech. Symp.*, Degussa Chemical, Indianapolis, IN, 19–40.

Emmert, J. L., and D. H. Baker. 1997. A chick bioassay approach for determining the bioavailable choline concentration in normal and over-heated soybean meal, canola meal, and peanut meal, *J. Nutr.*, 127:745.

Emmert, J. L., T. A. Garrow, and D. H. Baker. 1996. Development of an experimental diet for determining bioavailable choline concentration and its application in studies with soybean lecithin, *J. Anim. Sci.*, 74:2738.

Ensminger, M. E., J. P. Bowland, and T. J. Cunha. 1947. Observations on the thiamine, riboflavin, and choline needs of sows for reproduction, *J. Anim. Sci.*, 6:409.

Esch, N. W., R. A. Easter, and J. M. Bahr. 1981. Effect of riboflavin deficiency on estrous cyclicity in pigs, *Biol. Reprod.*, 25:659.

Evans, I. A., D. J. Humphreys, L. Goulden, A. J. Thomas, and W. C. Evans. 1963. Effects of bracken rhizomes on the pig, *J. Comp. Pathol.*, 73:229.

Fenstermacher, D. K., and R. C. Rose. 1986. Absorption of pantothenic acid in rat and chick intestine, *Am. J. Physiol.*, 250:G155.

Firth, J., and B. C. Johnson. 1956. Quantitative relationships of tryptophan and nicotinic acid in the baby pig, *J. Nutr.*, 59:223.

Forbes, R. M., and W. T. Haines. 1952. The riboflavin requirement of the baby pig, *J. Nutr.*, 47:411.

Fouts, P. J., O. M. Helmer, S. Lepkovsky, and T. H. Jukes. 1937. Treatment of human pellagra with nicotinic acid, *Proc. Soc. Exp. Biol. Med.*, 37:405.

Fox, H. M. 1984. Pantothenic acid. In *Handbook of Vitamins, Nutritional, Biochemical, and Clinical Aspects*, Machlin, L. J., Ed., Marcel Dekker, New York, 437–457.

Frank, G. R., J. M. Bahr, and R. A. Easter. 1984. Riboflavin requirement of gestating swine, *J. Anim. Sci.*, 59:1567.

Frank, G. R., J. M. Bahr, and R. A. Easter. 1988. Riboflavin requirement of lactating swine, *J. Anim. Sci.*, 66:47.

Frederick, G. L., and G. J. Brisson. 1961. Some observations on the relationship between vitamin B_{12} and reproduction in swine, *Can. J. Anim. Sci.*, 41:212.

Freeman, J. J., and D. J. Jenden. 1976. Minireview: the source of choline for acetylcholine synthesis in brain, *Life Sci.*, 19:949.

Funk, C. 1911. On the chemical nature of the substance which cures polyneuritis in birds induced by a diet of polished rice, *J. Physiol.* (London), 43:395.

Gannon, N. J. 1991. The Folic Acid Requirements of the Pig. Ph.D. dissertation, University of Sydney, Camden, NSW, Australia.

Gastaldi, G., U. Laforenza, and G. Ferrari. 1992. Age-related thiamin transport by small intestinal microvillous vesicles of rat, *Biochim. Biophys. Acta*, 1105:271.

Gibson, D. M., J. J. Kennelly, and F. X. Aherne. 1987. The performance and thiamin status of pigs fed sulfur dioxide treated high-moisture barley, *Can. J. Anim. Sci.*, 67:841.

Grandhi, R. R., and J. H. Strain. 1980. Effect of biotin supplementation on reproductive performance and foot lesions in swine, *Can. J. Anim. Sci.*, 60:961.

Gray, T. J. B. 1980. Toxicology. In *Developments in Food Preservation*, Tilbury, R. H., Ed., Applied Science Publishers, London, 53–74.

Green, R. G., W. E. Carlson, and C. A. Evans. 1941. A deficiency disease of foxes produced by feeding fish, *J. Nutr.*, 21:243.

Greenberg, D. M. 1963. Biological methylation, *Adv. Enzymol.*, 25:395.

Greenburg, L. D., D. F. Bohr, H. McGrath, and J. F. Rinehart. 1949. Xanthurenic acid excretion in the human subject on a pyridoxine-deficient diet, *Arch. Biochem.*, 21:237.

Gregory, J. F. 1980. Effects of ε-pyridoxyllysine bound to dietary protein on the vitamin B-6 status of rats, *J. Nutr.*, 110:995.

Gregory, J. F., S. L. Ink, and J. J. Cedra. 1989. Comparison of pteroylpolyglutamate hydrolase (folate conjugase) from porcine and human intestinal brush border membrane, *Comp. Biochem. Physiol.*, 90B:1135.

Gubler, C. J. 1976. Biochemical changes in thiamine deficiencies. In *Thiamine*, Gubler, C. J., M. Fujiwara, and P. M. Dreyfus, Eds., John Wiley & Sons, New York, 121–142.

Gubler, C. J. 1984. Thiamin. In *Handbook of Vitamins, Nutritional, Biochemical, and Clinical Aspects*, Machlin, L. J., Ed. Marcel Dekker, New York, 245–297.

György, P., M. Sullivan, and H. T. Karsner. 1937. Nutritional dermatoses in rats, *Proc. Soc. Exp. Biol. Med.*, 37:313.

György, P., D. B. Melville, D. Burk, and V. du Vingeaud. 1940. The possible identity of vitamin H with biotin and coenzyme R, *Science*, 91:243.

Halama, A. K. 1979. Biotinreaktive Gesundheits- und Leistungsstörungen bei Zuchtschweinen, *Wien. Tierärztl. Mschr.*, 66:370.

Halstead, C. H. 1980. Intestinal absorption and malabsorption of folates, *Annu. Rev. Med.*, 31:79.

Halstead, C. H. 1990. Intestinal absorption of dietary folates. In *Folic Acid Metabolism in Health and Disease*, Picciano, M. F., E. L. R. Sokstad, and J. S. Gregory III, Eds., Wiley-Liss, New York, 23–45.

Hamilton, C. R., and T. L. Veum. 1984. Response of sows and litters to added dietary biotin in environmentally regulated facilities, *J. Anim. Sci.*, 59:151.

Hamilton, C. R., and T. L. Veum. 1986. Effect of biotin and/or lysine additions to corn–soybean meal diets on the performance and nutrient balance of growing pigs, *J. Anim. Sci.*, 62:155.

Hamilton, C. R., T. L. Veum, D. E. Jewell, and J. A. Siwecki. 1983. The biotin status of weanling pigs fed semipurified diets as evaluated by plasma and hepatic parameters, *Int. J. Vitam. Nutr. Res.*, 53:44.

Hanke, H. G., and R. J. Meade. 1971. Biotin and pyridoxine additions to diets for pigs weaned at an early age. 1970–71 Minnesota Swine Research Report H-120, University of Minnesota Press, St. Paul, MN.

Harmon, B. G., E. R. Miller, J. A. Hoefer, D. E. Ullrey, and R. W. Luecke. 1963. Relationship of specific nutrient deficiencies to antibody production in swine. II. Pantothenic acid, pyridoxine or riboflavin, *J. Nutr.*, 79:269.

Harmon, B. G., D. E. Becker, A. H. Jensen, and D. H. Baker. 1969. Nicotinic acid-tryptophan relationship in the nutrition of the weanling pig, *J. Anim. Sci.*, 28:848.

Harmon, B. G., D. E. Becker, A. H. Jensen, and D. H. Baker. 1970. Nicotinic acid-tryptophan nutrition and immunologic implications in young swine, *J. Anim. Sci.*, 31:339.

Harper, A. F., M. D. Lindemann, L. I. Chiba, G. E. Combs, D. L. Handlin, E. T. Kornegay, and L. L. Southern, S-145 Committee on Nutritional Systems for Swine to Increase Reproductive Efficiency. 1994. An assessment of dietary folic acid levels during gestation and lactation on reproductive and lactational performance of sows: a cooperative study, *J. Anim. Sci.*, 72:2338.

Harris, S. A., D. E. Wolf, R. Mozingo, G. E. Arth, R. Christian, C. Anderson, N. R. Easton, and K. Folkers. 1945. Biotin. V. Synthesis of *dl*-biotin, *dl*-allobiotin and *dl-epi*-allobiotin, *J. Am. Chem. Soc.*, 67:2096.

Haytowitz, D. 1995. Information from USDA's nutrient data book, *J. Nutr.*, 125:1952.

Heinemann, W. W., M. E. Ensminger, T. J. Cunha, and E. C. McCulloch. 1946. The relation of the amount of thiamine in the ration of the hog to the thiamine and riboflavin content of the tissue, *J. Nutr.*, 31:107.

Heinle, R. W., A. D. Welch, and J. A. Pritchard. 1948. Essentiality of both the antipernicious anemia factor of liver and pteroylglutamic acid for hematopoiesis in swine, *J. Lab. Clin. Med.*, 33:1647.

Henderickx, H. K., H. S. Teague, D. R. Redman, and A. P. Grifo, Jr. 1964. Absorption of vitamin B_{12} from the colon of the pig, *J. Anim. Sci.*, 23:1036.

Henderson, L. M. 1985. Intestinal absorption of B-6 vitamers. In *Vitamin B-6: Its Role in Health and Disease, Proceeding of a Conference on Vitamin B-6 Nutrition and Metabolism*, Banff Conference Center, Banff, Alberta, Canada, October 8–10, 1985, Reynolds, L. D. and J. E. Leklem, Eds., Liss, New York, 22–33.

Herbert, V. 1979. Vitamin B_{12}. In *Textbook of Medicine*, 15th ed., Beeson, P. B., W. McDermott, and J. B. Wyngaarden, Eds., W. B. Saunders, Philadelphia, 1709.

Herbert, V. 1984. Vitamin B_{12}. In *Nutrition Reviews' Present Knowledge in Nutrition*, 5th ed., The Nutrition Foundation, Washington, D.C., 347–364.

Herbert, V. 1996. Vitamin B_{12}. In *Present Knowledge in Nutrition*, 7th ed., Ziegler, E. E., and L. J. Filer, Jr., Eds., International Life Sciences Institute Press, Washington, D.C., 191–205.

Hershey, J. M. 1930. Substitution of lecithin for raw pancreas in the diet of the depancreatized dog, *Am. J. Physiol.*, 93:657.

Herzlich, B., and V. Herbert. 1986. Rapid collection of human intrinsic factor uncontaminated with cobalophilin (R binder), *Am. J. Gastroenterol.*, 81:678.

Hirsch, M. J., J. H. Growdon, and R. J. Wurtman. 1978. Relations between dietary choline or lecithin intake, serum choline levels, and various metabolic indices, *Metabolism*, 27:953.

Hoehn, S. K., and J. N. Kanfer. 1978. L-Ascorbic acid and lysosomal acid hydrolase activities of guinea pig liver and brain, *Can. J. Biochem.*, 56:353.

Hogan, A. G., and E. M. Parrot. 1940. Anemia in chicks caused by a vitamin deficiency, *J. Biol. Chem.*, 132:507.

Honjo, T., Y. Nishizuka, I. Kato, and O. Hayaishi. 1971. Adenosine diphosphate ribosylation of aminoacyl transferase II and inhibition of protein synthesis by diphtheria toxin, *J. Biol. Chem.*, 246:4251.

Hughes, E. H. 1939. The role of riboflavin and other factors of the vitamin-B complex in the nutrition of the pig, *J. Nutr.*, 17:527.

Hughes, E. H. 1940a. The minimum requirement of riboflavin for the growing pig, *J. Nutr.*, 20:233.

Hughes, E. H. 1940b. The minimum requirement of thiamine for the growing pig, *J. Nutr.*, 20:239.

Hughes, E. H., and N. R. Ittner. 1942. The minimum requirement of pantothenic acid for the growing pig, *J. Anim. Sci.*, 1:116.

Hughes, E. H., and R. L. Squibb. 1942. Vitamin B_6 (pyridoxine) in the nutrition for the growing pig, *J. Anim. Sci.*, 1:320.

Huguenin, M. E., A. Birbaumer, F. P. Brunner, J. Thorhorst, U. Schmidt, U. C. Dubach, and G. Thiel. 1978. An evaluation of the role of tubular obstruction in folic acid-induced acute renal failure in the rat, *Nephron*, 22:41.

Hutagalung, R. I., G. L. Cromwell, V. W. Hays, and C. H. Chaney. 1969. Effect of dietary fat, protein, cholesterol and ascorbic acid on performance, serum, and tissue cholesterol levels and serum lipid levels of swine, *J. Anim. Sci.*, 29:700.

Ijichi, H., A. Ichiyama, and O. Hayaishi. 1966. Studies on the biosynthesis of nicotinamide adenine dinucleotide, *J. Biol. Chem.*, 241:3701.

Irwin, M. I., and B. K. Hutchins. 1976. A conspectus of research on vitamin C requirements of man, *J. Nutr.*, 106:823.

IUPAC-IUB Commission on Biochemical Nomenclature. 1966. Tentative rules: nomenclature and symbols for folic acid and related compounds, *J. Biol. Chem.*, 241:2991.
IUPAC-IUB Commission on Biochemical Nomenclature. 1974. The nomenclature of corrinoids (1973 recommendations), *Biochemistry*, 13:1555.
Ivers, D. J., S. L. Rodhouse, T. L. Veum, and M. R. Ellersieck. 1989. Effects of added niacin on sow and litter performance, *J. Anim. Sci.*, 67(Suppl. 2):120 (Abstr.).
Jacob, R. A., and M. E. Swendseid. 1996. Niacin. In *Present Knowledge in Nutrition*, 7th ed., Zeigler, E. E., and L. J. Filer, Eds., International Life Sciences Institute, Washington, D.C., 184–190.
Jaffe, G. M. 1984. Vitamin C. In *Handbook of Vitamins, Nutritional, Biochemical, and Clinical Aspects*, Machlin, L. J., Ed., Marcel Dekker, New York, 199–244.
Jansen, B. C. P., and W. F. Donath. 1926. On the isolation of the anti-beri-beri vitamin, *Proc. K. Ned. Akad. Wet. (Amsterdam)*, 29:1390.
Jewell, D. E., J. A. Siwecki, and T. L. Veum. 1981. The effect of dietary vitamin C on performance and tissue vitamin C levels in neonatal pigs, *J. Anim. Sci.*, 53(Suppl. 1):98 (Abstr.).
Johnson, B. C., and M. F. James. 1948. Choline deficiency in the baby pig, *J. Nutr.*, 36:339.
Johnson, B. C., and A. L. Neumann. 1948. New factor(s) present in antipernicious anemia liver extract stimulates growth in baby pigs, *J. Anim. Sci.*, 7:528.
Johnson, B. C., M. F. James, and J. L. Krider. 1948. Raising newborn pigs to weaning age on a synthetic diet with attempts to produce a pteroylglutamic acid deficiency, *J. Anim. Sci.*, 7:486.
Johnson, B. C., A. L. Neuman, R. O. Nesheim, M. F. James, J. L. Krider, A. S. Dana, and J. B. Thiersch. 1950. The interrelationship of vitamin B_{12} and folic acid in the baby pig, *J. Lab. Clin. Med.*, 36:537.
Jusko, W. J., and G. Levy. 1967. Absorption, metabolism and excretion of riboflavin-5' phosphate in man, *J. Pharm. Sci.*, 56:58.
Kennedy, E. P., and S. B. Weiss. 1956. The function of cytidine coenzymes in the biosynthesis of phospholipids, *J. Biol. Chem.*, 222:193.
King, C. G., and W. A. Waugh. 1932. The chemical nature of vitamin C, *Science*, 75:357.
Knights, T. E. N., R. R. Grandhi, and S. K. Baidoo. 1996. Effect of feeding supplemental vitamin B_6 on the reproductive performance and the nutrient metabolism in lean genotype sows, *J. Anim. Sci.*, 74(Suppl. 1):190 (Abstr.).
Kodicek, E., R. Braude, S. K. Kon, and K. G. Mitchell. 1956. The effect of alkaline hydrolysis of maize on the availability of its nicotinic acid to the pig, *Br. J. Nutr.*, 10:51.
Kodicek, E., R. Braude, S. K. Kon, and K. G. Mitchell. 1959. The availability to pigs of nicotinic acid in tortilla baked from maize treated with limewater, *Br. J. Nutr.*, 13:363.
Kögl, F. 1935. Über Wuchsstoffe der Auxin- und der Bios-gruppe, *Chem. Ber.*, 68:16.
Kögl, F., and B. Tonnis. 1936. Über das Bios-Problem. Darstellung von krystallisiertem Biotin aus Eigelb, *Hoppe Seylers Z. Physiol. Chem.*, 242:43.
Kornegay, E. T. 1986. Biotin in swine production: a review, *Livest. Prod. Sci.*, 14:65.
Kornegay, E. T., and T. N. Meacham. 1973. Evaluation of supplemental choline for reproducing sows housed in total confinement on concrete or dirt lots, *J. Anim. Sci.*, 37:506.
Kornegay, E. T., J. B. Meldrum, G. Schurig, M. D. Lindemann, and F. C. Gwazdauskas. 1986. Lack of influence of nursery temperature on the response of weanling pigs to supplemental vitamins C and E, *J. Anim. Sci.*, 63:484.
Kösters, W. W., and M. Kirchgessner. 1976a. Gewichtsentwicklung und Futterverwertung frühentwöhnter Ferkel bei unterschiedlicher Vitamin B_6-Versorgung [Growth rate and feed efficiency of early-weaned piglets with varying vitamin B_6 supply], *Z. Tierphysiol. Tierernähr. Futtermittelkd.*, 37:235.
Kösters, W. W., and M. Kirchgessner. 1976b. Zur Veränderung des Futterverzehrs frühentwöhnter Ferkel bei unterschiedlicher Vitamin B_6-Versorgung [Change in feed intake of early-weaned piglets in response to different vitamin B_6 supply], *Z. Tierphysiol. Tierernähr. Futtermittelkd.*, 37:247.
Krampitz, L. O., and D. W. Wooley. 1944. The manner of inactivation of thiamine in fish tissue, *J. Biol. Chem.*, 152:9.
Krider, J. L., S. W. Terrill, and R. F. VanPoucke. 1949. Response of weanling pigs to various levels of riboflavin, *J. Anim. Sci.*, 8:121.
Kroenig, G. H., and W. G. Pond. 1967. Methionine, choline and threonine interrelationships for growth and lipotropic actions in the baby pig and rat, *J. Anim. Sci.*, 26:352.

Kuksis, A., and S. Mookerjea. 1984. Choline. In *Nutrition Reviews' Present Knowledge in Nutrition*, 5th ed., The Nutrition Foundation, Washington, D.C., 383–399.

Lash Miller, W. 1924. Wildiers' bios, *Science*, 59:197.

Lehrer, W. P., Jr., A. C. Wiese, and P. R. Moore. 1952. Biotin deficiency in suckling pigs, *J. Nutr.*, 47:203.

Lehrer, W. P., Jr., A. C. Wiese, P. R. Moore, and M. E. Ensminger. 1951. Pyridoxine deficiency in baby pigs, *J. Anim. Sci.*, 10:65.

Leibbrandt, V. D. 1977. Influence of ascorbic acid on suckling pig performance, *J. Anim. Sci.*, 45(Suppl. 1):98 (Abstr.).

Leklem, J. E. 1996. Vitamin B-6. In *Present Knowledge in Nutrition*, 7th ed., Ziegler, E. E., and L. J. Filer, Jr., Eds., International Life Sciences Institute Press, Washington, D.C., 174–183.

Levine, M., S. Rumsey, Y. Wang, J. Park, O. Kwon, W. Xu, and N. Amano. 1996. Vitamin C. In *Present Knowledge in Nutrition*, 7th ed., Ziegler, E. E., and L. J. Filer, Jr., Eds., International Life Sciences Press, Washington, D.C., 146–159.

Lewis, A. J., G. L. Cromwell, and J. E. Pettigrew. 1991. Effects of supplemental biotin during gestation and lactation on reproductive performance of sows: a cooperative study, *J. Anim. Sci.*, 69:207.

Lichtman, H., J. Watson, V. Ginsberg, J. V. Pierce, E. L. R. Stokstad, and T. H. Jukes. 1949. Vitamin B_{12b}: some properties and its therapeutic use, *Proc. Soc. Exp. Biol. Med.*, 72:643.

Lindemann, M. D. 1993. Supplemental folic acid: a requirement for optimizing swine reproduction, *J. Anim. Sci.*, 71:239.

Lindemann, M. D., and E. T. Kornegay. 1986. Folic acid additions to weanling pig diets, *J. Anim. Sci.*, 63(Suppl. 1):35 (Abstr.).

Lindemann, M. D., and E. T. Kornegay. 1989. Folic acid supplementation to diets of gestating-lactating swine over multiple parities, *J. Anim. Sci.*, 67:459.

Lindley, O. C., and T. J. Cunha. 1946. Nutritional significance of inositol and biotin for the pig, *J. Nutr.*, 32:47.

Linkswiler, H. 1967. Biochemical and physiological changes in vitamin B_6 deficiency, *Am. J. Clin. Nutr.*, 20:547.

Longo, D. L., and V. Herbert. 1976. Radioassay for serum and red cell folate, *J. Lab. Clin. Med.*, 87:138.

Lucas, C. C., and J. H. Ridout. 1967. Fatty livers and lipotropic phenomena, *Proc. Chem. Fats Other Lipids*, 10:1.

Lucas, G. H. W. 1924. The fractionation of bios, and the comparison of bios with vitamins B and C, *J. Phys. Chem.*, 28:1180.

Luce, W. G., E. R. Peo, Jr., and D. B. Hudman. 1966. Availability of niacin in wheat for swine, *J. Nutr.*, 88:39.

Luce, W. G., E. R. Peo, Jr., and D. B. Hudman. 1967. Availability of niacin in corn and milo for swine, *J. Anim. Sci.*, 26:76.

Luce, W. G., D. S. Buchanan, C. V. Maxwell, H. E. Jordan, and R. O. Bates. 1985. Effect of supplemental choline and dichlorvos on reproductive performance of gilts, *Nutr. Rep. Int.*, 32:245.

Luce, W. G., R. D. Geisert, M. T. Zavy, A. C. Clutter, F. W. Bazer, C. V. Maxwell, and M. D. Woltmann. 1990. Effect of riboflavin supplementation on litter parameters of bred sows, *J. Anim. Sci.*, 68(Suppl. 1):42 (Abstr.).

Luecke, R. W., W. N. McMillen, F. Thorpe, Jr., and C. Tull. 1948. Further studies on the relationship of nicotinic acid, tryptophone and protein in the nutrition of the pig, *J. Nutr.*, 36:417.

Luecke, R. W., W. N. McMillen, and F. Thorpe, Jr. 1950. Further studies of pantothenic acid deficiency in weanling pigs, *J. Anim. Sci.*, 9:78.

Luecke, R. W., J. A. Hoefer, and F. Thorpe. 1952. The relationship of protein to pantothenic acid and vitamin B_{12} in the growing pig, *J. Anim. Sci.*, 11:238.

Luecke, R. W., J. A. Hoefer, and F. Thorpe, Jr. 1953. The supplementary effect of calcium pantothenate and aureomycin in a low-protein ration for weanling pigs, *J. Anim. Sci.*, 12:605.

Lumeng, L., M. P. Ryan, and T. K. Li. 1978. Validation of the diagnostic value of plasma pyridoxal 5′-phosphate measurements in vitamin B_6 nutrition of the rat, *J. Nutr.*, 108:545.

Lynch, P. B., and J. F. O'Grady. 1981. Effect of vitamin C (ascorbic acid) supplementation on sows in late pregnancy on piglet mortality, *Irish J. Agric. Res.*, 20:217.

Mahan, D. C., and L. J. Saif. 1983. Efficacy of vitamin C supplementation for weanling pigs, *J. Anim. Sci.*, 56:631.

Mahan, D. C., R. A. Pickett, T. W. Perry, T. M. Curtin, W. R. Featherston, and W. M. Beeson. 1966. Influence of various nutritional factors and physical form of feed on esophagogastric ulcers in swine, *J. Anim. Sci.*, 25:1019.

Mason, J. B. 1992. Intestinal transport of monoglutomyl folates in mammalian systems. In *Folic Acid Metabolism in Health and Disease*, Picciano, M. F., E. L. R. Stohstod, and J. F. Gregory III, Eds., Wiley-Liss, New York, 47–63.

Matte, J. J., and C. L. Girard. 1989. Effects of intramuscular injection of folic acid during lactation on folates in serum and milk and performance of sows and piglets, *J. Anim. Sci.*, 67:426.

Matte, J. J., and C. L. Girard. 1994. Pteroylglutamic (folic) acid in different feedstuffs: the pteroylglutamate content and an attempt to measure the bioavailability in pigs, *Br. J. Nutr.*, 72:911.

Matte, J. J., C. L. Girard, and G. J. Brisson. 1984a. Folic acid and reproductive performance of sows, *J. Anim. Sci.*, 59:1020.

Matte, J. J., C. L. Girard, and G. J. Brisson. 1984b. Serum folates during the reproductive cycle of sows, *J. Anim. Sci.*, 59:158.

Matte, J. J., C. L. Girard, G. A. Tremblay, and G. J. Brisson. 1989. Importance of folic acid in the nutrition of the gestating sow, *Pig News Info.*, 10:331.

Matte, J. J., C. Farmer, C. L. Girard, and J. P. Laforest. 1996. Dietary folic acid, uterine function and early embryonic development in sows, *Can. J. Anim. Sci.*, 76:427.

Maxwell, C. V., R. K. Johnson, and W. G. Luce. 1987. Effect of level of protein and supplemental choline on reproductive performance of gilts fed sorghum diets, *J. Anim. Sci.*, 64:1044.

McCormick, D. B. 1986. Riboflavin. In *Textbook of Clinical Chemistry*, Tietz, N. W., Ed., W. B. Saunders, Philadelphia, PA, 927–964.

McCormick, D. B. 1994. Riboflavin. In *Modern Nutrition in Health and Disease*, 8th ed., Skils, M. E., J. A. Olson, and M. Shike, Eds., Lea and Febiger, Philadelphia, PA, 366–375.

Meade, R. J. 1971. Biotin and pyridoxine supplementation of diets for growing pigs, 1970–71 Minnesota Swine Research Report H-218, University of Minnesota Press, St. Paul, MN.

Meade, R. J., L. E. Hanson, H. E. Hanke, K. P. Miller, J. W. Rust, R. S. Grant, and M. E. Tumbleson. 1969. B-vitamin supplementation of conventional diets for growing swine, Minnesota Agricultural Experiment Station Technical Bulletin 263, University of Minnesota Press, St. Paul, MN.

Mehansho, H., M. W. Hamm, and L. M. Henderson. 1979. Transport and metabolism of pyridoxal and pyridoxal phosphate in the small intestine of the rat, *J. Nutr.*, 109:1542.

Mertz, W. 1975. Effects and metabolism of glucose tolerance factor, *Nutr. Rev.*, 33:129.

Miller, C. O., and N. R. Ellis. 1951. The riboflavin requirement of growing swine, *J. Anim. Sci.*, 10:807.

Miller, C. O., N. R. Ellis, J. W. Stevenson, and R. Davey. 1953. The riboflavin requirement of swine for reproduction, *J. Nutr.*, 51:163.

Miller, E. R., R. L. Johnson, J. A. Hoefer, and R. W. Luecke. 1954. The riboflavin requirement for the baby pig, *J. Nutr.*, 52:405.

Miller, E. R., D. A. Schmidt, J. A. Hoefer, and R. W. Luecke. 1955. The pyridoxine requirement of the baby pig, *J. Nutr.*, 56:423.

Miller, E. R., D. A. Schmidt, J. A. Hoefer, and R. W. Luecke. 1957a. The pyridoxine requirement of the baby pig, *J. Nutr.*, 62:407.

Miller, E. R., D. A. Schmidt, J. A. Hoefer, R. W. Luecke, and W. D. Collings. 1957b. Electrocardiographic patterns of normal and thiamine-deficient baby pigs, *Proc. Soc. Exp. Bio. Med.*, 94:209.

Minot, G. R., and W. P. Murphy. 1926. Treatment of pernicious anemia by special diet, *J. Am. Med. Assoc.*, 91:923.

Misir, R., and R. Blair. 1984. Effect of biotin supplementation on the performance of biotin deficient sows, *J. Anim. Sci.*, 59(Suppl. 1):254 (Abstr.).

Misir, R., and R. Blair. 1986. Effect of biotin supplementation of a barley-wheat diet on restoration of healthy feet, legs, and skin of biotin deficient sows, *J. Res. Vet. Sci.*, 40:212.

Mitchell, H. H., B. C. Johnson, T. S. Hamilton, and W. T. Haines. 1950. The riboflavin requirement of the growing pig at two environmental temperatures, *J. Nutr.*, 41:317.

Mitchell, H. K., E. E. Snell, and R. J. Williams. 1941. The concentration of "folic acid," *J. Am. Chem. Soc.*, 63:2284.

Mock, D. M. 1990. Biotin. In *Present Knowledge in Nutrition*, 6th ed., Brown, M., Ed., International Life Sciences Institute, Washington, D.C., 189–207.

Mock, D. M. 1996. Biotin. In *Present Knowledge in Nutrition*, 7th ed., Ziegler, E. E., and L. J. Filer, Jr., Eds., International Life Sciences Institute, Washington, D.C., 220–235.

Molitoris, B. A., and D. H. Baker. 1976. Assessment of the quantity of biologically available choline in soybean meal, *J. Anim. Sci.*, 42:481.

Mosenthin, R., W. C. Sauer, L. Völker, and M. Frigg. 1990. Synthesis and absorption of biotin in the large intestine of pigs, *Livest. Prod. Sci.*, 25:95.

Mowatt, J. H., J. H. Boothe, B. L. Hutchings, E. L. R. Stokstad, C. W. Waller, R. B. Angier, J. Semb, D. B. Cosulich, and Y. SubbaRow. 1948. The structure of the liver *L. casei* factor, *J. Am. Chem. Soc.*, 70:14.

Nakano, T., F. X. Aherne, and J. R. Thompson. 1983. Effect of dietary supplementation of vitamin C on pig performance and the incidence of osteochondrosis in the elbow and stifle joints in young growing swine, *Can. J. Anim. Sci.*, 63:421.

National Research Council. 1987. *Vitamin Tolerance of Animals*, National Academy Press, Washington, D.C.

National Research Council. 1998. *Nutrient Requirements of Swine*, 10th ed., National Academy Press, Washington, D.C.

Nesheim, R. O., and B. C. Johnson. 1950. Effect of a high level of methionine on the dietary choline requirement of the baby pig, *J. Nutr.*, 41:149.

Nesheim, R. O., J. L. Krider, and B. C. Johnson. 1950. The quantitative crystalline B_{12} requirement of the baby pig, *Arch. Biochem.*, 27:240.

Neumann, A. L., and B. C. Johnson. 1950. Crystalline vitamin B_{12} in the nutrition of the baby pig, *J. Nutr.*, 40:403.

Neumann, A. L., J. L. Krider, and B. C. Johnson. 1948. Unidentified growth factor(s) needed for optimum growth of newborn pigs, *Proc. Soc. Exp. Biol. Med.*, 69:513.

Neumann, A. L., J. L. Krider, M. R. James, and B. C. Johnson. 1949. The choline requirement of the baby pig, *J. Nutr.*, 38:195.

Neumann, A. L., J. B. Thiersch, J. L. Krider, M. F. James, and B. C. Johnson. 1950. Requirement of the baby pig for vitamin B_{12} fed as a concentrate, *J. Anim. Sci.*, 9:83.

Newcomb, M. D., and G. L. Allee. 1986. Water-soluble vitamins for weanling pigs, *J. Anim. Sci.*, 63 (Suppl. 1):108 (Abstr.).

Newport, M. J. 1981. A note on the effect of low levels of biotin in milk substitutes for neonatal pigs, *Anim. Prod.*, 33:333.

Nichoalds, G. E. 1974. Assessment of status of riboflavin nutriture by assay of erythrocyte glutathione reductase activity, *Clin. Chem.*, 20:624.

Nishikimi, N., and S. Udenfriend. 1976. Immunologic evidence that the gene for L-gulono-γ-lactone oxidase is not expressed in animals subject to scurvy, *Proc. Natl. Acad. Sci. U.S.A.*, 73:2066.

Norris, L. C., and A. T. Ringrose. 1930. The occurrence of a pellagrous-like syndrome in chicks, *Science*, 71:643.

North Central Region–42 Committee on Swine Nutrition. 1976. Effects of supplemental choline on reproductive performance of sows: a cooperative regional study, *J. Anim. Sci.*, 42:1211.

North Central Region–42 Committee on Swine Nutrition. 1980. Effect of supplemental choline on performance of starting, growing, and finishing pigs: a cooperative regional study, *J. Anim. Sci.*, 50:99.

North Central Region–89 Committee on Confinement Management of Swine. 1989. Effect of vitamin C and space allowance on performance of weanling pigs, *J. Anim. Sci.*, 67:624.

O'Conner, D. L., M. F. Picciano, T. Tamura, and B. Shane. 1989. Impaired milk folate secretion is not corrected by supplemental folate during iron deficiency in rats, *J. Nutr.*, 120:499.

Olson, R. E. 1984. Pantothenic acid. In *Nutrition Reviews' Present Knowledge in Nutrition*, 5th ed., Nutrition Foundation, Washington, D.C., 377–382.

Omaye, S. T. 1984. Safety of megavitamin therapy, *Adv. Exp. Med. Biol.*, 177:169.

Owen, B. D., and J. P. Bowland. 1952. The pantothenic acid content of the blood and mik of swine fed supplemental levels of the vitamin, *J. Nutr.*, 48:317.

Palm, B. W., R. J. Meade, and A. L. Melliere. 1968. Pantothenic acid requirement of young swine, *J. Anim. Sci.*, 27:1596.

Peng, C. L., and H. Heitman, Jr. 1973. Erythrocyte transketolase activity and the percentage stimulation by thiamin pyrophosphate as criteria of thiamin status in the pig, *Br. J. Nutr.*, 30:391.

Peng, C. L., and H. Heitman, Jr. 1974. The effect of ambient temperature on the thiamin requirement of growing-finishing pigs, *Br. J. Nutr.*, 32:1.

Penny, R. H. C., R. H. A. Cameron, S. Johnson, P. J. Kenyan, H. A. Smith, A. W. P. Bell, J. P. L. Cole, and J. Taylor. 1981. The influence of biotin supplementation on sow reproductive efficiency, *Vet. Rec.*, 109:80.

Peo, E. R., Jr., G. F. Wehrebein, B. Moser, P. J. Cunningham, and P. E. Vipperman, Jr. 1970. Biotin supplementation of baby pig diets, *J. Anim. Sci.*, 31:209 (Abstr.).

Pettigrew, J. E., S. M. El-Kandelgy, L. J. Johnston, and G. C. Shurson. 1996. Riboflavin nutrition of sows, *J. Anim. Sci.*, 74:2226.

Pharazyn, A., and F. X. Aherne. 1987. Folacin requirements of the lactating sow, 66th Annual Feeder's Day Report, University of Alberta, Edmonton, Alberta, 16–17.

Phillips, W. E. J., J. H. L. Mills, S. M. Charbonneau, L. Tryphonas, G. V. Hatina, Z. Zawidzka, F. R. Bryce, and I. C. Munro. 1978. Subacute toxicity of pyrdoxine hydrochloride in the beagle dog, *Toxicol. Appl. Pharmacol.*, 44:323.

Plesofsky-Vig, N. 1996. Pantothenic acid. In *Present Knowledge in Nutrition*, 7th ed., Ziegler, E. E., and L. J. Filer, Jr., Eds., International Life Sciences Institute Press, Washington, D.C., 236–244.

Pond, W. G., E. Kwong, and J. K. Loosli. 1960. Effect of level of dietary fat, pantothenic acid, and protein on performance of growing-fattening swine, *J. Anim. Sci.*, 19:1115.

Powick, W. C., N. R. Ellis, and C. N. Dale. 1948. Relationship of tryptophane to nicotinic acid in the feeding of growing pigs, *J. Anim. Sci.*, 7:228.

Prentice, A. M., and C. J. Bates. 1981. A biochemical evaluation of the erythrocyte glutathione reductase test for riboflavin status, *Br. J. Nutr.*, 45:53.

Rao, B. S. N., and C. Gopalan. 1984. Niacin. In *Nutrition Reviews' Present Knowledge in Nutrition*, 5th ed., Nutrition Foundation, Washington, D.C., 318–331.

Reinisch, F., H. Jerod, and G. Gelbhardt. 1990. Improvement of fertility in sows by means of vitamin B_{12}, *Tierzucht*, 44:76.

Reisenauer, A. M., C. L. Krumdieck, and C. H. Halsted. 1979. Folate conjugase: two separate activities in human jejunum, *Science*, 198:196.

Richardson, D., D. V. Catron, L. A. Underkofler, H. M. Maddock, and W. C. Friedland. 1951. Vitamin B_{12} requirement of male weanling pigs, *J. Nutr.*, 44:371.

Richardson, L. R., S. Wilkes, and S. J. Ritchey. 1961. Comparative vitamin B-6 activity of frozen, irradiated, and heat processed foods, *J. Nutr.*, 73:363.

Riker, J. T., III, T. W. Perry, R. A. Pickett, and C. J. Heidenreich. 1967. Influence of controlled temperatures on growth rate and plasm ascorbic acid values in swine, *J. Nutr.*, 92:99.

Rindi, G. 1996. Thiamin. In *Present Knowledge in Nutrition*, 7th ed., Ziegler, E. E., and L. J. Filer, Jr., Eds., International Life Sciences Institute Press, Washington, D.C., 160–166.

Rindi, G., and G. Ferrari. 1977. Thiamine transport by human intestine *in vitro*, *Experimentia*, 32:211.

Rindi, G., and U. Ventura. 1972. Thiamine intestinal transport, *Physiol. Rev.*, 52:821.

Ringrose, A. T., L. C. Norris, and G. F. Heuser. 1931. The occurrence of a pellegra-like syndrome in chicks, *Poult. Sci.*, 10:166.

Ritchie, H. D., E. R. Miller, D. E. Ullrey, J. A. Hoefer, and R. W. Luecke. 1960. Supplementation of the swine gestation diet with pyridoxine, *J. Nutr.*, 70:491.

Rivlin, R. S. 1996. Riboflavin. In *Present Knowledge in Nutrition*, 7th ed., Ziegler, E. E., and L. J. Filer, Jr., Eds., International Life Sciences Institute Press, Washington, D.C., 167–173.

Robie, T. R. 1967. Cyproheptadine: an excellent antidote for niacin-induced hyperthermia. *J. Schizophr.*, 1:133.

Roe, D. A. 1988. Fiber and riboflavin absorption [letter], *J. Am. Diet. Assoc.*, 88:783.

Rose, R. C. 1980. Water-soluble vitamin absorption in intestine, *Annu. Rev. Physiol.*, 42:157.

Rose, R. C., D. B. McCormick, and T. K. Li. 1986. Transport and metabolism of vitamins, *Fed. Proc.*, 45:30.

Rose, R. C., J. L. Choi, and M. J. Koch. 1988. Intestinal transport and metabolism of oxidized ascorbic acid (dehydroascorbic acid), *Am. J. Physiol.*, 254:G824.

Rosenburg, I. H., J. Zimmerman, and J. Selhub. 1987. Folate transport, *Chimioterapia*, 4:354.

Roth-Maier, D. A., and M. Kirchgessner. 1977. Untersuchungen zum optimalen Pantothensaurebedarf von Mastschweinen [Studies on the optimal pantothenic acid requirement of market pigs], *Z. Tierphysiol. Tierernähr. Futtermittelkd.*, 38:121.

Russell, L. E., P. J. Bechtel, and R. A. Easter. 1985a. Effect of deficient and excess dietary vitamin B_6 on amino transaminase and glycogen phosphorylase activity and pyridoxal phosphate content in two muscles from postpubertal gilts, *J. Nutr.*, 115:1124.

Russell, L. E., R. A. Easter, and P. J. Bechtel. 1985b. Evaluation of the erythrocyte aspartate aminotransferase activity coefficient as an indicator of the vitamin B_6 status of postpubertal gilts, *J. Nutr.*, 115:1117.

Russet, J. C., J. L. Krider, T. R. Cline, H. L. Thacker, and L. B. Underwood. 1979a. Choline-methionine interactions in young swine, *J. Anim. Sci.*, 49:708.

Russet, J. C., J. L. Krider, T. R. Cline, and L. B. Underwood. 1979b. Choline requirement of young swine, *J. Anim. Sci.*, 48:1366.

Said, H. M., D. M. Mock, and J. C. Collins. 1989. Regulation of biotin intestinal transport in the rat: effect of biotin deficiency and supplementation, *Am. J. Physiol.*, 259:G306.

Sandholm, M., T. Honkanen-Buzalski, and V. Rasi. 1979. Prevention of navel bleeding in piglets by preparturient administration of ascorbic acid, *Vet. Rec.*, 104:337.

Sauberlich, H. E. 1967. Biochemical alterations in thiamine deficiency — their interpretation, *Am. J. Clin. Nutr.*, 20:528.

Sauberlich, H. E. 1968. Biochemical systems and biochemical detection of deficiency. In *The Vitamins: Chemistry, Physiology, Pathology, Assay*, Vol. 2, 2nd ed., Sebrell, W. H., Jr., and R. S. Harris, Eds., Academic Press, New York, 44–80.

Sauberlich, H. E., J. H. Skala, and R. P. Dowdy. 1974. *Laboratory Tests for the Assessment of Nutritional Status*, CRC Press, Boca Raton, FL.

Sauer, W. C., R. Mosenthin, and L. Ozimek. 1988. The digestibility of biotin in protein supplements and cereal grains for growing pigs, *J. Anim. Sci.*, 66:2583.

Said, H. M., and I. Derweesh. 1991. Carrier-mediated mechanism for biotin transport in rabbit intestine — studies with brush-border membrane vesicles, *Am. J. Physiol.*, 261:R94.

Schroeter, L. C. 1966. *Sulfur Dioxide*, Pergamon Press, Toronto.

Seerley, R. W., R. A. Snyder, and H. C. McCampbell. 1981. The influence of sow dietary lipids and choline on piglet survival, milk, and carcass composition, *J. Anim. Sci.*, 52:542.

Selhub, J., and I. H. Rosenberg. 1996. Folic Acid. In *Present Knowledge of Nutrition*, 7th ed., Ziegler, E. E., and L. J. Filer, Jr., Eds., International Life Sciences Institute, Washington, D.C., 206–219.

Sewell, R. F., D. G. Price, and M. C. Thomas. 1962. Pantothenic acid requirement of the pig as influenced by dietary fat, *Fed. Proc.*, 21:468.

Sewell, R. F., D. Nugara, R. L. Hill, and W. A. Knapp. 1964. Vitamin B-6 requirement of early-weaned pigs, *J. Anim. Sci.*, 23:694.

Seymour, E. W., V. C. Speer, and V. W. Hays. 1968. Effect of environmental temperature on the riboflavin requirement of young pigs, *J. Anim. Sci.*, 27:389.

Shibata, K., C. J. Gross, and L. M. Henderson. 1983. Hydrolysis and absorption of pantothenate and its coenzymes in the rat small intestine, *J. Nutr.*, 113:2107.

Shilotri, P. G. 1977. Phagocytosis and leukocyte enzymes in ascorbic acid deficient guinea pigs, *J. Nutr.*, 107:1513.

Simmins, P. H., and P. H. Brooks. 1980. The effect of dietary biotin level on the physical characteristics of pig hoof tissue, *Anim. Prod.*, 30:469 (Abstr.).

Simmins, P. H., and P. H. Brooks. 1983. Supplementary biotin for sows: effect on reproductive characteristics, *Vet. Rec.*, 112:425.

Simmins, P. H., and P. H. Brooks. 1985. Effect of different levels of dietary biotin intake on the hoof horn hardness of the gilt, *Anim. Prod.*, 40:544 (Abstr.).

Smith, D. T., J. M. Ruffin, and S. G. Smith. 1937. Pellagra successfully treated with nicotinic acid: a case report, *J. Am. Med. Assoc.*, 109:2054.

Snell, E. E. 1986. Pyridoxal phosphate: history, and nomenclature. In *Pyridoxal Phosphate: Chemical, Biochemical, and Medical Aspects*, Part 1A, Vol. 1A, Dolphin, D., R. Poulson, and O. Avramovic, Eds., John Wiley & Sons, New York, 1–12.

Southern, L. L., and D. H. Baker. 1981. Bioavailable pantothenic acid in cereal grains and soybean meal, *J. Anim. Sci.*, 53:403.

Southern, L. L., D. R. Brown, D. D. Werner, and M. C. Fox. 1986. Excess supplemental choline for swine, *J. Anim. Sci.*, 62:992.

Spies, T. D., C. Cooper, and M. A. Blankenhorn. 1938. The use of nicotinic acid in the treatment of pellagra, *J. Am. Med. Assoc.*, 110:622.

Stadtman, T. C. 1971. Vitamin B_{12}. Biochemical studies elucidate the role of this complex molecule in diverse metabolic processes, *Science*, 171:859.

Stevenson, N. R., and M. K. Brush. 1969. Existence and characteristics of Na positive-dependent active transport of ascorbic acid in guinea pig, *Am. J. Clin. Nutr.*, 22:318.

Stockland, W. L., and L. G. Blaylock. 1974. Choline requirement of pregnant sows and gilts under restricted feeding conditions, *J. Anim. Sci.*, 39:1113.

Stoffel, W., and I. Melzner. 1980. Studies *in vitro* on the biosynthesis of ceramide and sphingomyelin: a reevaluation of proposed pathways, *Hoppe-Seyler's Z. Physiol. Chem.*, 361:755.

Stokstad, E. L., R., B. L. Hutchings, and Y. SubbaRow. 1948. The isolation of the *Lactobacillus casei* factor from liver, *J. Am. Chem. Soc.*, 70:3.

Stothers, S. C., D. A. Schmidy, R. L. Johnson, J. A. Hoefer, and R. W. Luecke. 1955. The pantothenic acid requirement of the baby pig, *J. Nutr.*, 57:47.

Strecker, A. 1862. Über einige neue Bestandtheile der Schweinegalle, *Ann. Chem. Pharm.*, 123:353.

Strecker, A. 1868. Über das Lecithin, *Ann. Chem. Pharm.*, 148:77.

Strittmatter, J. E., D. J. Ellis, M. G. Hogberg, A. L. Trapp, M. J. Parsons, and E. R. Miller. 1978. Effects of vitamin C on swine growth and osteochondrosis, *J. Anim. Sci.*, 47(Suppl. 1):16 (Abstr.).

Svirbely, J. L., and A. Szent-Györgyi. 1932. The chemical nature of vitamin C, *Biochem. J.*, 26:865.

Tahiliani, A. G., and C. J. Beinlich. 1991. Pantothenic acid in health and disease, *Vitam. Horm.*, 46:165.

Tanphaichitr, V., and B. Wood. 1984. Thiamin. In *Present Knowledge in Nutrition*, 5th ed., Nutrition Foundation, Washington, D.C., 273–284.

Teague, H. S., and A. P. Grifo, Jr. 1966. Vitamin B_{12} supplementation of sow rations, *J. Anim. Sci.*, 25:895 (Abstr.).

Teague, H. S., W. M. Palmer, and A. P. Grifo, Jr. 1970. Pantothenic acid efficiency in the reproducing sow, Ohio Agricultural Research Development Center Animal Science Mimeograph 200, Ohio State University Press, Wooster, OH.

Terrill, S. W., C. B. Ammerman, D. E. Walker, R. M. Edwards, H. W. Norton, and D. E. Becker. 1955. Riboflavin studies with pigs, *J. Anim. Sci.*, 14:593.

Thaler, R. C., J. L. Nelssen, R. D. Goodband, and G. L. Allee. 1989. Effect of dietary folic acid supplementation on sow performance through two parities, *J. Anim. Sci.*, 67:3360.

Tilton, S. L., R. O. Bates, and R. J. Moffatt. 1991. Effect of riboflavin supplementation during gestation on reproductive performance of sows, *J. Anim. Sci.*, 69(Suppl. 1):482 (Abstr.).

Tremblay, G. F., J. J. Matte, L. Lemieux, and G. J. Brisson. 1986. Serum folates in gestating swine after folic acid addition to diet, *J. Anim. Sci.*, 63:1173.

Tremblay, G. F., J. J. Matte, J. J. Dufour, and G. J. Brisson. 1989a. Survival rate and development of fetuses during the first 30 days of gestation after folic acid addition to a swine diet, *J. Anim. Sci.*, 67:724.

Tremblay, G. F., J. J. Matte, C. L. Girard, and G. J. Brisson. 1989b. Serum zinc, iron, and copper status during early gestation in sows fed a folic acid-supplemented diet, *J. Anim. Sci.*, 67:733.

Tribble, L. R., J. D. Hancock, and D. E. Orr, Jr. 1984. Value of supplemental biotin on reproductive performance of sows in confinement, *J. Anim. Sci.*, 59(Suppl. 1):245 (Abstr.).

Turley, S. D., C. E. West, and B. J. Horton. 1976. The role of ascorbic acid in the regulation of cholesterol metabolism and in the pathogenesis of atherosclerosis, *Atherosclerosis*, 24:1.

Ullrey, D. E., D. E. Becker, S. W. Terrill, and R. A. Notzold. 1955. Dietary levels of pantothenic acid and reproductive performance of female swine, *J. Nutr.*, 57:401.

Van Etten, C., N. R. Ellis, and L. L. Madsen. 1940. Studies on the thiamine requirement of young swine, *J. Nutr.*, 20:607.

Van Eys, J. 1991. Nicotinic acid. In *Handbook of Vitamins*, 2nd ed. rev. exp., Macklin, L.H., Ed., Marcel Dekker, New York, 311–340.

Warburg, O., and W. Christian. 1936. Pyridin, der wasserstoffdbertragejde Bestandteil von Garungsfermenten (Pyridin-Nudleotide), *Biochem. Z. Band.*, 287:291.

Washam, R. D., J. E. Sowers, and L. W. DeGoey. 1975. Effect of zinc-proteinate or biotin in swine starter rations, *J. Anim. Sci.*, 40:179.

Watkins, K. L., L. L. Southern, and J. E. Miller. 1991. Effect of dietary biotin supplementation on sow reproductive performance and soundness and pig growth and mortality, *J. Anim. Sci.*, 69:201.

Webb, N. G., R. H. C. Penny, and A. M. Johnston. 1984. The effect of a dietary supplement of biotin on pig hoof horn strength and hardness, *Vet. Rec.*, 114:185.

West, R. 1948. Activity of vitamin B_{12} in Addisonian pernicious anemia, *Science*, 107:398.

Whitehead, C. C., D. W. Banister, and J. P. F. D'Mello. 1980. Blood pyruvate carboxylase activity as a criterion of biotin status in young pigs, *Res. Vet. Sci.*, 29:126.

Wiese, A. C., W. P. Lehrer, Jr., P. R. Moore, O. F. Pahnish, and W. V. Hartwell. 1951. Pantothenic acid deficiency in baby pigs, *J. Anim. Sci.*, 10:80.

Wintrobe, M. M., M. H. Miller, R. H. Follis, Jr., H. J. Stein, C. Mushatt, and S. Humphreys. 1942. Sensory neuron degeneration in pigs. IV. Protection afforded by calcium pantothenate and pyridoxine, *J. Nutr.*, 24:345.

Wintrobe, M. M., R. Alcayaga, S. Humphreys, and R. H. Follis, Jr. 1943a. Electrocardiographic changes associated with thiamine deficiency in pigs, *Bull. Johns Hopkins Hosp.*, 73:169.

Wintrobe, M. M., R. H. Follis, Jr., R. Alcayaga, M. Paulson, and S. Humphreys. 1943b. Pantothenic acid deficiency in swine with a particular reference to the effects on growth and on the alimentary tract, *Bull. Johns Hopkins Hosp.*, 73:313.

Wintrobe, M. M., R. H. Follis, Jr., M. H. Miller, H. J. Stein, R. Alcayaga, S. Humphreys, A. Suksta, and G. E. Cartwright. 1943c. Pyridoxine deficiency in swine with particular reference to anemia, epileptiform convulsions and fatty liver, *Bull. Johns Hopkins Hosp.*, 72:1.

Wiseman, S. L., J. R. Wenninghoff, R. D. Saner, and D. M. Danielson. 1991. The effect of supplementary riboflavin fed during the breeding and implantation period on reproductive performance of gilts, *J. Anim. Sci.*, 69(Suppl. 1):359 (Abstr.).

Wolf, B., G. Heard, J. R. S. McVoy, and H. M. Raetz. 1984. Biotinidase deficiency: the possible role of biotinidase in the processing of dietary protein-bound biotin, *J. Inherit. Metab. Dis.*, 7:121.

Wood, H. G., and R. E. Barden. 1977. Biotin enzymes, *Annu. Rev. Biochem.*, 46:385.

Woodring, M. J., and C. A. Storvich. 1960. Vitamin B-6 in milk: review of literature, *J. Assoc. Off. Agric. Chem.*, 43:63.

Woodworth, J. C., R. D. Goodband, J. L. Nelssen, M. D. Tokach, and R. E. Musser. 1998. Pyridoxine, but not thiamin improves weanling pig growth performance, *J. Anim. Sci.*, 76(Suppl. 2):46 (Abstr.).

Yen, J. T., and W. G. Pond. 1981. Effect of dietary vitamin C addition on performance, plasma vitamin C and hematic iron status in weanling pigs, *J. Anim. Sci.*, 53:1292.

Yen, J. T., and W. G. Pond. 1983. Response of swine to periparturient vitamin C supplementation, *J. Anim. Sci.*, 56:621.

Yen, J. T., and W. G. Pond. 1984. Responses of weanling pigs to dietary supplementation with vitamin C or carbadox, *J. Anim. Sci.*, 58:132.

Yen, J. T., and W. G. Pond. 1987. Effect of dietary supplementation with vitamin C or carbadox on weanling pigs subjected to crowding stress, *J. Anim. Sci.*, 64:1672.

Yen, J. T., A. H. Jensen, and D. H. Baker. 1976. Assessment of the concentration of biologically available vitamin B_6 in corn and soybean meal, *J. Anim. Sci.*, 42:866.

Yen, J. T., R. Lauxen, and T. L. Veum. 1978. Effect of supplemental niacin on finishing pigs fed soybean meal supplemented diets, *J. Anim. Sci.*, 47(Suppl. 1):325 (Abstr.).

Yen, J. T., P. K. Ku, W. G. Pond, and E. R. Miller. 1985. Response to dietary supplementation of vitamins C and E in weanling pigs fed low vitamin E-selenium diets, *Nutr. Rep. Int.*, 31:877.

Yunis, A. A., E. H. Fischer, and E. G. Krebs. 1960. Crystallization and properties of human muscle phosphorylases *a* and *b*, *J. Biol. Chem.*, 235:3163.

16 Bioavailability of Minerals and Vitamins

David H. Baker

CONTENTS

I. Introduction 357
II. Mineral Bioavailability 358
    A. Calcium 358
    B. Phosphorus 359
        1. Phytate 359
    C. Sodium and Chloride 360
    D. Magnesium 360
    E. Potassium 360
    F. Copper 361
    G. Iodine 361
    H. Iron 361
    I. Manganese 363
    J. Selenium 363
    K. Zinc 364
III. Vitamin Bioavailability 365
    A. Vitamin A 365
    B. Vitamin D 366
    C. Vitamin E 367
    D. Vitamin K 367
    E. Biotin 367
    F. Choline 368
    G. Folacin 369
    H. Niacin 370
    I. Pantothenic Acid 370
    J. Riboflavin 370
    K. Thiamin 371
    L. Vitamin B6 371
    M. Vitamin B12 372
    N. Vitamin C 372
References 372

I. INTRODUCTION

Minerals and vitamins present in feed ingredients, and even from crystalline sources, are generally not fully available when compared with a common and well-utilized source of the mineral or vitamin in question. Mineral elements may be bound in phytate complexes or attached to fiber, and vitamins often exist as either precursor compounds or as coenzymes that may also be bound or complexed in some manner. Hence, gut processes are required to release or convert both minerals and vitamins to absorbable chemical entities.

The literature on mineral and vitamin bioavailability is much more extensive for chicks and rats than for swine. Indeed, in several instances no data whatsoever exist for bioavailability estimates in swine. This chapter will cover pertinent aspects of mineral and vitamin bioavailability, with an emphasis on swine. Laboratory-animal, poultry, and human data will be used in those cases where limited pig data are available.

II. MINERAL BIOAVAILABILITY

Several excellent reviews are available that deal with comparative mineral bioavailability (Nelson and Walker, 1964; Ammerman and Miller, 1972; Peeler, 1972; Cantor et al., 1975a,b; Hays, 1976; Peo, 1976; Miller, 1978; O'Dell et al., 1979; Harmon, 1979; Miller, 1980; Cromwell, 1992; Ammerman et al., 1995). Most of these have dealt with relative bioavailability of inorganic rather than organic (i.e., feed) sources of mineral elements. Best estimates of true absorption efficiencies of mineral elements will be given, and these will be based primarily on human data. It is deemed important to have some perspective of true absorption efficiency so that relative (to a standard) absorption efficiency can be properly evaluated. Also, to assess the effects of supplemental mineral salts on acid–base balance properly, one needs to have knowledge of true absorption efficiencies. For example, $CaCl_2$ would seem to be equally balanced with regard to its cation:anion ratio, but it is, in fact, very acidic. This occurs because the calcium (alkaline) from this compound is absorbed poorly (less than 50%) relative to the chloride (acidic), which is probably 100% absorbed.

A. Calcium

The true absorption efficiency of Ca for humans consuming a mixed animal- and plant-source diet has been estimated at 30% (Groff et al., 1995). Other than the data from Cromwell's laboratory (Cromwell et al., 1983; Ross et al., 1984; Cromwell et al., 1989a), no definitive information is available on relative Ca bioavailability for swine. The Kentucky work showed that limestone, oyster shell, gypsum, marble dust, and aragonite were essentially 100% available as sources of Ca, relative to a $CaCO_3$ precipitate used as a standard. Calcium bioavailability in dolomitic limestone, however, was lower, ranging from 51 to 78%. Ross et al. (1984) also established that particle size of the Ca sources evaluated had no effect on the bioavailability of Ca. Only one feed ingredient, alfalfa meal, was evaluated by Cromwell et al. (1983). Using slope-ratio analysis (bone-breaking strength regressed on Ca intake), Ca in dehydrated alfalfa meal was only 21% available relative to Ca in the $CaCO_3$ precipitate standard.

Based on poultry data reviewed by Peeler (1972), the relative bioavailability of Ca is 100% in dicalcium phosphate, tricalcium phosphate, defluorinated rock phosphate, Ca gluconate, Ca citrate, Ca lactate, Ca sulfate, and bone meal. Little work has been done on Ca bioavailability in protein- and energy-furnishing feed ingredients in any species. It is nonetheless generally assumed that Ca availability in meat and fish meals is equivalent to that in feed-grade limestone. Plant-source Ca is probably not fully available, although except for the Kentucky work on alfalfa meal (Cromwell et al., 1983), quantitative estimates are not available.

Calcium is a mineral element whose absorption efficiency can be markedly influenced by other dietary factors (Groff et al., 1995). Factors known to increase absorption efficiency are as follows: (1) low (deficient) intakes, (2) presence of lactose in the diet, (3) pregnancy and lactation, and (4) young age. In contrast, several factors are also known to decrease the efficiency of Ca absorption: (1) consumption without food, (2) presence of phytates or oxalates in the diet, (3) excesses of dietary Mg or P, and (4) fat malabsorption problems that cause steatorrhea.

B. Phosphorus

The true absorption efficiency of P from a mixed diet for humans has been estimated at between 70 and 90% (Groff et al., 1995). A summary of P bioavailability estimates in various inorganic and organic feed ingredients for swine and poultry is contained in reviews by Miller (1980) and Soares (1995). Phosphorus bioavailability estimates for swine per se have been published by Cromwell (1992). Current thinking regarding turkey nutrition is that relative to commercial mono-dicalcium phosphate, i.e., $Ca(H_2PO_4)_2$ set at 100%, P availability in commercial dicalcium phosphate is about 90%, and that in defluorinated rock phosphate is about 80% (Waibel et al., 1984). Those familiar with the commercial feed-grade phosphate industry generally assume that all feed-grade dicalcium phosphates are actually mixtures of $Ca(H_2PO_4)_2$ and $CaHPO_4$, and both compounds are variable in water of hydration (e.g., $CaHPO_4 \cdot H_2O$ or $CaHPO_4 \cdot 2H_2O$, Baker, 1989). Thus, Ca or P analysis is perhaps the only accurate means of establishing the ratio of $CaHPO_4$ (23% Ca, 18.5% P) to $Ca(H_2PO_4)_2$ (16% Ca and 21% P). A rule of thumb for swine formulation would consist of setting the P bioavailability in the purchased feed-grade phosphate source at 100% (regardless of whether labeled dicalcium or mono-dicalcium phosphate), and then assuming that P bioavailability in commercial defluorinated phosphate is 90% (Cromwell, 1992). Coffey et al. (1994), however, suggested that P bioavailability (relative to NaH_2PO_4) in defluorinated P sources for chicks and pigs averaged 85%.

Plant-source P is relatively unavailable (Nelson, 1967), although some feed ingredients (e.g., wheat and barley) contain phytase, which may increase P bioavailability somewhat. Most swine nutritionists consider the P contained in corn–soybean meal combinations used in commercial diets to be about 25% bioavailable, primarily because 60 to 70% of the P in corn–soybean combinations is present as phytate-P (Erdman, 1979; Cromwell, 1992). Cromwell (1992) estimated the bioavailability of P in corn to be only 14% and that in soybean meal to be 23 to 31%, relative to $CaHPO_4$. He further estimated that the P in wheat and wheat by-products was 29 to 49% bioavailable; that in rice bran, 25%; cottonseed meal, 1%; and peanut meal, 12%. He considered the P contributed by dried whey, blood meal, fish meal, and alfalfa meal to be close to 100% bioavailable, but his P bioavailability estimate for meat and bone meal was only 67%. High-moisture corn has been estimated to contain up to four times more bioavailable P than dry number-2 yellow corn (Cromwell, 1992).

Fermentation-derived P is highly bioavailable because much of the P in yeast, distillers' solubles, etc., is in the form of nucleic acid-P, most of which is RNA. Research using chicks has established that the P in RNA is close to 100% bioavailable relative to KH_2PO_4 used as a standard (Burns and Baker, 1976). The same is true for P existing in ingredients as phospholipids (D. H. Baker, unpublished data).

1. Phytate

There is much confusion regarding effects of phytates on not only P bioavailability but on the Ca and trace mineral status of animals. Phytates added to various research diets are generally provided as phytic acid or as the Na or Ca salt of phytic acid. These compounds are not the same as the mixed Ca-Mg-K salt of phytic acid generally found in plant-source feed ingredients (Nelson, 1967; Erdman, 1979). Moreover, the negative effects of added phytates on trace mineral utilization are affected significantly by dietary Ca level (O'Dell et al., 1964; Hendricks et al., 1969; Bafundo et al., 1984b). Research in the author's laboratory using chicks, for example, has shown that the Zn-antagonizing effect of 1.2% supplemental Na phytate when added to a typical corn–soybean meal broiler diet is evident only when Ca is provided in the diet in a quantity at least twice the National Research Council (NRC) recommended level (NRC, 1994; Bafundo et al., 1984b).

Knowledge of where phytate occurs in plant-source feedstuffs is important for proper interpretation of effects of such ingredients on mineral bioavailability (Erdman, 1979). Corn is unique among the cereal grains because 90% of the phytate present is located in the germ portion of the kernel. Wheat and rice germ also contain considerable phytate, but the hull portion is also rich. Thus, wheat and rice bran are extremely rich in phytate (Halpin and Baker, 1987). Soybeans, too, are different from most other oilseeds in that phytic acid is contained in protein bodies distributed throughout the seed. Hence, protein isolates are richer in phytate than soybean meal (Erdman, 1979). Phytic acid in peanuts, cottonseed, and sunflower seeds is concentrated only in crystalloid and globoid substructures. Diekert et al. (1962) isolated two protein-rich fractions from peanuts and found one to contain 0.5% phytic acid and the other to contain 5.7% phytic acid.

Clearly, dietary addition of microbial or feed-derived phytase markedly improves the utilization of phytate P by nonruminant animals. Phytase also markedly improves the utilization of Ca, Zn, Mn, and Fe, but it does not improve the utilization of either Cu (Aoyagi and Baker, 1995) or Se (G. F. Combs, Jr., 1999, personal communication). Certain organic acids (citrate, lactate, and formate) also increase phytate P utilization, and they may also function additively with phytase. Low-phytate corn varieties are close to commercialization, and preliminary evidence suggests that the bioavailable P in these varieties is up to three times higher than that in conventional corn varieties. For more detail on the current state of knowledge regarding the beneficial effects of phytase, organic acids, and hydroxylated vitamin D_3 products on P bioavailability, the reader is referred to the recent book by Coelho and Kornegay (1996).

C. Sodium and Chloride

True absorption efficiency of Na and Cl is thought to be very high, approaching 100% (Groff et al., 1995). There appears to be no good evidence on the relative utilization of Na and Cl from various sources. Using information from requirement studies, one can generalize that NaCl, Na_2SO_4, $NaHCO_3$, Na acetate, and Na citrate are equal in bioavailable Na and that NaCl, KCl, NH_4Cl, and $CaCl_2 \cdot 2H_2O$ are equivalent in bioavailable Cl. Because Na and Cl (also K) are so intimately involved in acid–base balance and in urinary excretion of cations and anions, suitable bioassays of availability are difficult to develop. Defluorinated phosphates are generally rich in Na, and this ingredient is common in swine diets. Miller (1980) estimated that Na in defluorinated P is 83% available relative to the Na in NaCl. The Na in aluminosilicate (e.g., zeolite) products is thought to be absorbed as efficiently as the Na in NaCl (Fethiere et al., 1988).

D. Magnesium

Judging from Peeler's review (1972) and from field observation of Mg deficiency, Mg bioavailability is probably more of a problem in ruminant nutrition than in nonruminant nutrition. Miller (1980) estimated that the Mg supplied by feed-grade sources of MgO, $MgSO_4$, and $MgCO_3$ was 100% bioavailable for swine relative to the Mg in reagent-grade MgO. He also estimated that grains and concentrates would have Mg bioavailabilities of 50 to 60% as compared with MgO. Cook's (1973) research using rats appears to be the only nonruminant study in which bioavailability of Mg salts was determined directly, rather than estimated. He found oxide, chloride, carbonate, phosphate, sulfate, and silicate salts of Mg to be equally bioavailable. A report by Guenter and Sell (1974) suggested that the true absorption efficiency of Mg from soybean meal was 60%, about the same as that estimated for $MgSO_4 \cdot 7H_2O$. Thus, it is open to debate whether nonruminant animals utilize Mg as efficiently from plant-based feed ingredients as from inorganic salts of Mg.

E. Potassium

Definitive information on K bioavailability from various K sources is lacking. Corn–soybean meal diets for swine are rich in K, making K bioavailability a subject of primarily academic interest. Peeler (1972) predicted that K_2CO_3, $KHCO_3$, K_2HPO_4, K acetate, and K citrate would be 100%

available, relative to the K in KCl. Groff et al. (1995) have suggested that over 90% of ingested K is absorbed by humans.

E. R. Miller and co-workers addressed the subject of K bioavailability in various K sources for young pigs (Combs et al., 1985; Combs and Miller, 1985). Among response criteria examined, that is, blood K, urinary K, and K retention, only K retention (balance trials) responded linearly to K intake for all K sources examined. Based on slope-ratio methodology and within the realm of experimental error, K from K_2CO_3, $KHCO_3$, corn, and soybean meal was judged essentially 100% bioavailable relative to K acetate, which was used as the standard.

F. COPPER

The true absorption efficiency of Cu from a mixed diet consumed by humans (Groff et al., 1995) has been estimated to range from 25 (high intakes) to 50% (low intakes). Copper bioavailability, like that of Zn, is difficult to quantify accurately. Hence, Cu accumulation in tissues (primarily liver) increases only slightly (and curvilinearly) between deficient levels and a dietary level of about 250 mg Cu/kg diet. Beyond this level, Cu accumulates rapidly, and generally in a linear fashion. Relative to $CuSO_4 \cdot 5H_2O$, Miller (1980) suggested good utilization of the Cu in CuO, $CuCl_2$, and $CuCO_3$, and poor utilization in CuS. More recent pig work by Cromwell et al. (1989b), confirmed in the author's laboratory with chicks (Baker et al., 1991; Aoyagi and Baker, 1993a; Baker and Ammerman, 1995a), has shown that the Cu in CuO is almost totally unavailable for absorption from the gut. Aoyagi and Baker (1993a,b; 1994) and Aoyagi et al. (1995) established a bioavailability assay for Cu in chicks fed Cu either above its requirement (liver Cu accumulation) or below its requirement (gall bladder Cu accumulation). Relative bioavailability (RBV) of Cu for various inorganic and feed-ingredient sources of Cu were in good agreement between the two methods. Relative to analytical-grade $CuSO_4 \cdot 5H_2O$, RBV values for Cu were 145% for analytical-grade CuCl and 95 to 115% for feed-grade $CuSO_4 \cdot 5H_2O$, Cu-lysine, $Cu_2(OH)_3Cl$, and Cu-methionine. Other RBV values were 0% for both analytical-grade and feed-grade CuO, 115% for analytical-grade $Cu(OAc) \cdot H_2O$, 100% for analytical-grade Cu_2O and 100% for analytical-grade $CuCO_3 \cdot Cu(OH)_2$. Among animal- and plant-source proteins, RBV values ranged from 0% for pork liver to 115% for chicken liver. Intermediate values were obtained for poultry by-product meal (90%), beef liver (80%), corn gluten meal (50%), peanut hulls and soy mill run (45%), cottonseed meal and dehulled soybean meal (40%), and rat liver (20%); see Aoyagi et al. (1993).

Copper ingested from fecal material is utilized no better than 30% relative to that provided as $CuSO_4 \cdot 5H_2O$ (Izquierdo and Baker, 1986). Copper absorption from the gut is reduced substantially if Na_2S (Barber et al., 1961; Cromwell et al., 1978), roxarsone (Czarnecki and Baker, 1985; Edmonds and Baker, 1986), or reducing agents such as cysteine or ascorbic acid (Baker and Czarnecki-Maulden, 1987; Aoyagi and Baker, 1994) are included in the diet.

G. IODINE

Little definitive work on I availability has been carried out in any species. What does exist is primarily rat research in which bioavailability assessment was not the primary objective. Nonetheless, Miller (1980) estimated that (relative to NaI) the I in KI, $Ca(IO_3)_2 \cdot 2H_2O$, KIO_3, and CuI was 100% bioavailable. The I in ethylenediamine dihydriodide ($C_2H_8N_2 \cdot 2HI$) is also considered to have an RBV of at least 100% (Miller and Ammerman, 1995). It seems reasonable to assume, also, that the I present in iodized salt is 100% available relative to NaI.

H. IRON

Baby pigs are uniquely susceptible to Fe deficiency anemia because of their rapid growth rate, confinement rearing (little access to soil), and lack of placental or mammary Fe transfer from dam to offspring. Thus, it has become standard practice to give newborn pigs Fe injections during the first few days of life. Braude et al. (1962) and Miller (1980) demonstrated that over 90% of the Fe from Fe-dextran (100- or 200-mg injections) is incorporated into hemoglobin over the ensuing 4 weeks. Later, Harmon et al. (1974), Thoren-Tolling (1975), and Cornelius and Harmon (1976) observed that similar Fe-dextran doses administered orally during the first 12 h after birth (prior to gut closure) likewise promoted efficient Fe incorporation into hemoglobin.

There is no effective means of increasing placental or mammary transfer of Fe from the sow to her offspring. Work at Cornell University showed conclusively that whether Fe sources are administered to dams orally or via injection, neither pig Fe stores at birth nor Fe concentration in milk is increased sufficiently to prevent anemia in the offspring (Pond et al., 1961). Iron sources fed to lactating sows at high levels will elicit hemoglobin responses in the nursing pigs, but this has been shown to be more due to Fe consumption from the Fe in the dam's feces than to an increased concentration of Fe in the dam's milk.

Pig studies on Fe bioavailability have revealed essentially 100% relative bioavailability of Fe in $FeSO_4 \cdot 2H_2O$, $FeSO_4 \cdot 7H_2O$, Fe citrate, and Fe choline citrate, relative to Fe in $FeSO_4 \cdot H_2O$. The chick and rat data of Fritz et al. (1970) have largely confirmed these findings (Harmon et al., 1967; Ullrey et al., 1973; Furugouri and Kawabata, 1975; Miller, 1978). Chick and rat data indicate that Fe ammonium citrate, $FeCl_2$, Fe fumarate, and Fe gluconate are also 100% bioavailable, whereas $FeCl_3$, $Fe_2(SO_4)_3$, and Fe carbonate are less available. Oxides of Fe are almost totally unavailable, whereas carbonates are variable in bioavailability, depending on where they are mined (Harmon et al., 1969; Ammerman et al., 1974; Henry and Miller, 1995).

Commercial dicalcium and defluorinated phosphates are rich in Fe, containing from 2.5 to 3.0% $FePO_4 \cdot 2H_2O$ (Baker, 1989). Bioavailability of Fe in these products generally ranges from 35 to 85% (Ammerman and Miller, 1972; Kornegay, 1972; Miller, 1978; Deming and Czarnecki-Maulden, 1989).

It is conventional in human nutrition to categorize Fe sources as heme or nonheme in nature. However, this categorization often leads to misinterpretation, because many nutritionists unwittingly conclude that all animal sources of Fe are heme Fe, when in fact they are generally a mixture of heme (highly available), ferritin (less available), and hemosiderin (poorly available); see Layrisse et al. (1975) and Bogunjoko et al. (1983). To illustrate the confusion, liver (fresh or dried) is rich in Fe but the Fe present therein is about 10% heme Fe and 90% nonheme Fe. Thus, liver Fe is lower in bioavailability than the Fe in poultry by-product meal or meat meal (Chausow, 1987). While Fe in commercial blood meal would be expected to be highly available, values ranging from 40 to 50% (relative to $FeSO_4 \cdot 7H_2O$) were provided by Miller (1980) for flash-dried blood meal and only 22% was reported by Chausow and Czarnecki-Maulden (1988a). It is probable, therefore, that the drying process influences the bioavailability of Fe in dried blood meals.

The Fe in grains and oilseed meals may be largely bound to or complexed with phytate, fiber, or protein. As such, its bioavailability would be expected to be lower than that of $FeSO_4 \cdot H_2O$. Data on availability of Fe in these sources are limited. Without definitive data, one should probably assume that cereal grain and oilseed Fe sources are no more than 50% available relative to $FeSO_4 \cdot H_2O$.

Chausow (1987) and Chausow and Czarnecki-Maulden (1988a,b) evaluated the utilization of several Fe sources (relative to $FeSO_4 \cdot 7H_2O$) in chicks, cats, and dogs. Based on their chick bioavailability results where hemoglobin repletion of Fe-depleted chicks was regressed on Fe intake, Fe bioavailability was 22% in dried blood meal, 48% in meat and bone meal, 68% in poultry by-product meal, 39% in feather meal, and 32% in fish meal. Among plant-source feed ingredients evaluated, Fe relative bioavailabilities were 96% for sesame meal, 77% for rice bran, 65% for alfalfa meal, 45% for dehulled soybean meal, and 20% for yellow corn (Chausow and Czarnecki-Maulden, 1988a,b).

Boling et al. (1998) used a hemoglobin depletion–repletion assay in chicks to estimate the bioavailability of several Fe sources, relative to either analytical-grade $FeSO_4 \cdot 7H_2O$ or feed-grade $FeSO_4 \cdot H_2O$. The Fe in analytical-grade ferric sulfate, $Fe_2(SO_4)_3 \cdot 7H_2O$, was only 37% bioavailable and that in cottonseed meal was 56% available. Two by-products of the galvanizing industry, mixtures of $FeSO_4 \cdot H_2O$ and $ZnSO_4 \cdot H_2O$, were also evaluated, and the Fe in these products was found to be as bioavailable as that in the ferrous sulfate standard.

The true absorption efficiency of Fe by humans consuming a mixed animal- and plant-based diet is assumed to be about 15% (Groff et al., 1995), but many factors can markedly affect the efficiency of Fe absorption. It is well established that dietary ascorbic acid, cysteine, and organic acids such as citrate or lactate can almost double the efficiency of Fe absorption. On the other hand, dietary phytate, oxalates, and excess dietary Zn (in the presence of phytate) have been shown to decrease the absorption of Fe to less than half that occurring without these antagonizing factors. Also, absorption efficiency is much greater when consumed by Fe deficient than by Fe-adequate animals.

I. Manganese

Manganese is a species mineral problem (i.e., poultry) and is therefore of only minor interest to swine nutritionists. Avian studies from Ammerman's laboratory (Black et al., 1984; 1985; Henry, 1995) and from the author's laboratory (Southern and Baker, 1983a,b; Baker et al., 1986; Halpin and Baker, 1986a,b; Halpin et al., 1986; Halpin and Baker, 1987) have provided considerable information on Mn bioavailability. Tissues (primarily bone) accumulate Mn in a linear fashion, and this fact can be used as a basis for assessing Mn bioavailability. Relative to $MnSO_4 \cdot H_2O$, Mn bioavailability is approximately 100% in $MnCl_2$, 75% in MnO, 55% in $MnCO_3$, and 30% in MnO_2 (Henry, 1995). Availability of Mn in a protein–Mn or a methionine–Mn complex has been observed in the author's laboratory to be at least as high as that in $MnSO_4 \cdot H_2O$ (Baker et al., 1986; Fly et al., 1989). The Mn in corn, soybean meal, wheat bran, and fish meal should probably be considered totally unavailable for poultry and swine (Baker et al., 1986), whereas the considerable Mn present in rice bran should be considered only minimally bioavailable. In practice, excesses of either Fe or cobalt in corn–soybean meal diets have minimal effects on Mn utilization, although considerable excesses of Mn reduce Fe absorption from the gut. Excess dietary P (inorganic or phytate) reduces Mn utilization substantially (Baker and Wedekind, 1988; Wedekind and Baker, 1990a,b; Wedekind et al., 1991a,b; Baker and Oduho, 1994).

Even with a highly available source of Mn such as $MnSO_4 \cdot H_2O$, gut absorption of Mn by chicks is only about 2 to 3% of the ingested dose (Wedekind et al., 1991a,b). Elimination of all fiber and phytate from the diet nearly doubles the absorption efficiency of Mn (Halpin et al., 1986).

J. Selenium

Based on studies by Mathias et al. (1967), Cantor et al. (1975a,b), and Mahan and Moxon (1978), as reviewed by Miller (1980), Se in Na_2SeO_3 and Na_2SeO_4 is well utilized, whereas that existing as selenomethionine is probably utilized somewhat less efficiently. However, based on Se accumulation in tissues, selenomethionine would be judged over 100% bioavailable relative to Na_2SeO_3. Selenium seems to be well utilized from cereal grains (60 to 80%) and extremely well utilized from alfalfa meal (>100%), but utilization is poor from fish and poultry by-product meals (10 to 40%). Poultry data have provided Se bioavailability estimates in soybean meal of only 18% for restoration of glutathione peroxidase activity but 60% for prevention of exudative diathesis (Cantor et al., 1975b). Wedekind et al. (1998) used multiple indices of Se bioavailability in chicks and reported (relative to Na_2SeO_3) that animal-derived feed ingredients had average Se bioavailabilities of 28% whereas plant-derived feed ingredients had Se bioavailabilities of 47%. Selenium-enriched yeast had an Se RBV of 159%.

Mahan and Parrett (1996) compared Se-enriched yeast to Na_2SeO_3 as Se sources for growing-finishing pigs. Based on Se retention in the body, the Se in Se-enriched yeast was more bioavailable than the Se in Na_2SeO_3, but the reverse was true when serum GSH was used as the RBV criterion.

Selenium absorption from the gut is relatively efficient; that is, 63% of an administered dose was found to be absorbed by pigs (Wright and Bell, 1966). A variety of arsenic compounds as well as cysteine, methionine, Cu, tungsten, mercury, cadmium, and silver have been reported to decrease the efficiency of inorganic Se absorption from the gut (Baker and Czarnecki-Maulden, 1987; Lowry and Baker, 1989a).

K. ZINC

True absorption of Zn from a mixed diet consumed by humans is considered to be about 20% (Groff et al., 1995). This estimate presumes an absorption efficiency of less than 10% for the Zn in plant-based foods, but an absorption efficiency of 30% in animal-based food products. It is well known that the Zn in edible meat products such as pork loin and hamburger is efficiently absorbed (Hortin et al., 1991; 1993), and it is thought that cysteine (and cysteine present as glutathione) present in meat products is responsible for the efficient absorption of Zn.

Little swine data exist on RBV of Zn in Zn-containing supplements. Miller et al. (1981) reported that RBV of Zn in Zn dust (99.3% Zn) was high for pigs, relative to analytical-grade ZnO. Feed-grade ZnO for pigs, however, has been reported to have an RBV of only 56% (Hahn and Baker, 1993) to 68% (Wedekind et al., 1994), relative to a feed-grade $ZnSO_4 \cdot H_2O$ standard.

Many of the same factors that affect the efficiency of Fe utilization also apply to Zn. Thus, low intakes of Zn, and dietary reducing agents such as ascorbic acid and cysteine, increase Zn absorption, whereas high Zn intakes and presence of phytate or oxalate in the diet decrease Zn absorption. Stress and/or trauma (e.g., surgery, burns) are also known to decrease the efficiency of Zn absorption in humans (Groff et al., 1995).

Because high levels (2000 to 3000 mg Zn/kg) of feed-grade ZnO are now routinely used in the United States for growth promotion in weanling pigs (Hahn and Baker, 1993), the issue of RBV of Zn in ZnO products has become more important. Early chick work on Zn bioavailability in ZnO had suggested that the Zn in reagent-grade ZnO was as bioavailable as a reagent-grade $ZnSO_4 \cdot 7H_2O$ standard (Edwards, 1959). The author's chick work with feed-grade ZnO, the principal Zn source used in the feed industry, indicated that the RBV of Zn in this product (Waelz process, 72% Zn) was about 50% relative to feed-grade $ZnSO_4 \cdot H_2O$ (Wedekind and Baker, 1990c; Wedekind et al., 1992). The RBV of Zn in feed-grade sources of ZnO and $ZnSO_4$ has been recently reevaluated (Edwards and Baker, 1999). Both weight gain and tibia Zn content were used as dependent variables in chicks fed a Zn-deficient soy concentrate diet. Three sources of feed-grade ZnO were evaluated: source A (78.1% Zn, U.S.), source B (Waelz process, 74.1% Zn, Mexican), and source C (78.0% Zn, Mexican). Also, two sources of feed-grade $ZnSO_4 \cdot H_2O$ were evaluated: source A (36.5% Zn, Mexican) and source B (35.3% Zn, U.S.). The RBV of Zn in both feed-grade sulfate products was not different from the analytical-grade $ZnSO_4 \cdot 7H_2O$ standard. By using an average of the weight gain and tibia Zn RBV values, and setting RBV of feed-grade $ZnSO_4 \cdot H_2O$ at 100%, RBV values for the three ZnO products were 100% for source A, 36% for source B, and 65% for source C. It is apparent from these results that feed-grade ZnO products can vary widely in Zn bioavailability. Clearly, however, the ZnO product produced by the Waelz process has been the product used most extensively in the commercial feed industry, and this product in five separate trials in the author's laboratory has produced low RBV values. Analytical-grade ZnO and at least one feed-grade ZnO product, however, produced Zn RBV values that were not different from the $ZnSO_4 \cdot H_2O$ standard.

Based on the review by Baker and Ammerman (1995b), the Zn in $ZnSO_4 \cdot H_2O$, $ZnCO_3$, $ZnCl_2$, analytical-grade ZnO, Zn methionine, and Zn acetate are all highly available sources of Zn relative to analytical-grade $ZnSO_4 \cdot 7H_2O$. Weight gain and bone Zn accumulation of animals fed Zn-deficient diets are the best measures of RBV of Zn (Fordyce et al., 1987; Wedekind et al., 1992). Soft-tissue Zn, plasma Zn, and plasma alkaline phosphatase activity generally do not respond linearly to Zn supplementation.

Zinc, like many other trace elements, is poorly utilized by nonruminant animals fed conventional corn–soybean meal diets. Indeed, the dietary requirement for Zn is often three- to fourfold higher in animals fed these diets than in those fed phytate-free (e.g., egg white) diets. Also, in the presence of phytate and fiber, excess Ca decreases Zn utilization. Work in the author's laboratory has established that, whereas excess Zn can exacerbate Cu and Fe deficiency states, excesses of either Cu or Fe have minimal effects on Zn utilization (Southern and Baker, 1983c; Bafundo et al., 1984a).

The Zn in soy products is poorly utilized, based on chick bioassays using a Zn-deficient egg white basal diet (Edwards and Baker, 1999). Soybean meal, soy protein concentrate, and soy protein isolate were found to have Zn bioavailabilities (relative to $ZnSO_4 \cdot 7H_2O$) of 34, 18, and 25%, respectively. However, Zn bioavailability in soybean meal in chicks fed a Zn-deficient soy concentrate diet was 77%. Clearly, utilization of Zn is low in plant-source ingredients and higher in animal-source ingredients. The observation of Baker and Halpin (1988) that addition of 10% fish meal to a casein-dextrose diet containing either 68 or 318 mg Zn/kg diet would depress Zn levels in bone, liver, and pancreas of chicks provides evidence that even some animal-source products may contain factors that antagonize Zn utilization. Whether this would have occurred had fish meal been added to a corn–soybean meal diet is problematic.

III. VITAMIN BIOAVAILABILITY

There are two primary concerns regarding vitamin bioavailability in modern swine diets and premixes: (1) stability in vitamin and vitamin–mineral premixes as well as in diets and supplements, and (2) utilization efficiency from plant- and animal-source feed ingredients. Readers are referred to the reviews of Schneider (1986), McGinnis (1986), Wornick (1968), Coelho (1991), Baker (1995), and Zhuge and Klopfenstein (1986) for details of factors affecting the stability of crystalline vitamins in diets and premixes. Regarding vitamin bioavailability in feed ingredients, a paucity of pig research data exists, and even considering chick and rat data, few feed ingredients have been evaluated.

There are many pitfalls in vitamin (and mineral) bioavailability assessment. Body stores often preclude developing a distinct deficiency during the course of a conventional growth trial. Even if a frank deficiency can be produced within the framework of available funding, one must deal with the vexing question of whether the responding criterion (usually weight gain) increased because of the vitamin being supplied or perhaps because of increased diet intake that results from adding the unknown ingredient to an often less than voraciously palatable purified diet. Because water-soluble B vitamins respond better insofar as growth is concerned, they are, in many respects, easier to evaluate than fat-soluble vitamins.

Chick work in the area of vitamin bioavailability has caused the author to come to certain conclusions concerning the proper bioassay methodology for maximum efficacy and extrapolative value of results:

1. Pretest periods to obtain desired deficiency states are generally necessary.
2. Activity of a key enzyme of which the vitamin is a component or cofactor is generally a less desirable dependent variable than weight gain.
3. Precursor materials (e.g., methionine for choline; tryptophan for niacin) must be carefully considered.
4. Use of specific vitamin inhibitors may assist in establishing veracity of assessed bioavailability values.

A. Vitamin A

Vitamin nomenclature policy (Anonymous, 1979) dictates that the term *vitamin A* be used for all B-ionone derivatives, other than provitamin A carotenoids, exhibiting the biological activity of all-*trans* retinol (i.e., vitamin A alcohol or vitamin A_1). Esters of all-*trans* retinol should be referred to as retinyl esters.

Vitamin A is present in animal tissues, whereas most plant materials contain only provitamin A carotenoids, which must be split in the intestinal tract to form vitamin A. In blood, vitamin A is transported as retinol, but it is stored, primarily in the liver, as retinyl palmitate. Absorption efficiency of vitamin A is relatively constant over a wide range of doses (Olson, 1984), but higher doses of carotenoids are absorbed much less efficiently than are lower doses (Erdman et al., 1988).

Vitamin A esters are more stable in feeds and premixes than retinol. The hydroxyl group as well as the four double bonds on the retinol side chain are subject to oxidative losses. Thus, esterification of vitamin A alcohol does not totally protect this vitamin from oxidative losses. Current commercial sources of vitamin A are generally "coated" esters (e.g., acetate or palmitate) that contain an added antioxidant such as ethoxyquin or butylated hyroxytoluene (BHT).

The water content of premixes and feedstuffs has a negative effect on vitamin A stability. Moisture causes vitamin A beadlets to soften and become more permeable to oxygen (Schneider, 1986). Thus, both high humidity and presence of free choline chloride (hygroscopic) enhance vitamin A destruction. Trace minerals also exacerbate vitamin A losses in premixes exposed to moisture. For maximum retention of vitamin A activity, premixes should be as moisture-free as possible and should be made to have a pH above 5. Low pH causes isomerization of all-*trans* vitamin A to less potent *cis* forms and also results in deesterification of vitamin A esters to retinol (DeRitter, 1976). Likewise, heat processing, especially extrusion, can reduce vitamin A bioavailability (Harper, 1988).

Crystalline β-carotene is absorbed from the gut more efficiently than β-carotene existing in foods and feeds (Rao and Rao, 1970). Some of the β-carotene in foods is complexed with protein. Fiber components of feeds, especially pectins, have been shown to reduce β-carotene absorption from the gut in chicks (Erdman et al., 1986).

Ullrey (1972) reviewed the bioavailability aspects of vitamin A precursor materials for swine and reported that pigs were far less efficient than rats in converting carotenoid precursors to active vitamin A. Thus, bioefficacies (wt/wt) ranging from 7 to 14% were observed for corn carotenes in pigs relative to all-*trans* retinyl palmitate. Thus, at best, carotenoid precursors in corn (also corn gluten meal) have no more than 261 IU/mg vitamin A activity when consumed by swine. This is decidedly less than the theoretical potency of 1667 IU/mg (assuming all the carotenoids are all-*trans*-β carotene), which is assumed for the rat. Corn carotenoids consist of about 50% cryptoxanthin, 25% β-zeacarotene, and 25% β-carotene (Ullrey, 1972).

Quantification of vitamin A bioavailability is difficult. Accumulation of vitamin A in the liver may be the most acceptable method (Erdman et al., 1988; Chung et al., 1990).

B. VITAMIN D

The term *vitamin D* is appropriate for all steroids having cholecalciferol biological activity. Cholecalciferol, itself, is synonymous with vitamin D_3, as distinguished from ergocalciferol, which is also called vitamin D_2. Commercially, vitamin D_3 is available as a spray-dried product or (frequently in combination with vitamin A) as gelatin-coated beadlets; one international unit is equal to 0.025 μg of cholecalciferol (Anonymous, 1979). These products are quite stable if stored as the vitamin itself at room temperature. In complete feeds and mineral–vitamin premixes, Schneider (1986) observed activity losses up to 10 and 30%, respectively, after either 4 or 6 months of storage at 22°C.

Vitamin D precursors are present in plant (ergosterol) and animal (7-dehydrocholesterol) feedstuffs, but they require ultraviolet irradiation for conversion into active D_2 and D_3, respectively. Although D_2 and D_3 have long been considered equal in biological activity for pigs, the recent findings of Horst et al. (1982) suggest that D_3 may be more bioactive than D_2. Hydroxylated forms of cholecalciferol [25-OH D_3, 1α-OH D_3, 1,25(OH)$_2$ D_3] contain more D_3 bioactivity than D_3 itself.

C. Vitamin E

Vitamin E is the generic term for all tocol and tocotrienol derivatives having α-tocopherol biological activity. There are eight naturally occurring forms of vitamin E: α-, β-, γ-, and δ- tocopherols and α-, β-, γ-, and δ-tocotrienols. Among these, D-α-tocopherol possesses the greatest biological activity (Bieri and McKenna, 1981). An international unit of vitamin E is the activity of 1 mg of DL-α-tocopheryl acetate. All racemic (i.e., DL-α-tocopherol) has about 70% of the activity of pure D-α-tocopherol. Bieri and McKenna (1981) consider β-tocopherol and γ-tocopherol to have only 40 and 10% of the activity, respectively, of α-tocopherol (set at 100%). The only other natural form to possess activity is α-tocotrienol, which on the rating scale used above was listed by Bieri and McKenna (1981) as containing a biopotency of 25%.

Plant-source ingredients are richer in vitamin E bioactivity than animal-source feed ingredients. Plant oils are particularly rich in bioactive vitamin E, although corn and corn oil contain about six times more γ-tocol than α-tocol (Ullrey, 1981). Fat-extracted soybean meal has very little vitamin E activity.

Vitamin E is subject to destruction by oxidation, and this process is accelerated by heat, moisture, unsaturated fat, and trace minerals. Losses of 50 to 70% have been observed to occur in alfalfa hay stored at 32°C for 12 weeks; losses up to 30% have been known to occur during dehydration of alfalfa (Livingston et al., 1968). Treatment of high-moisture grains with organic acids also greatly enhances vitamin E destruction (Young et al., 1975; 1977; 1978). However, even mildly alkaline conditions of vitamin E storage are also very detrimental to vitamin E stability (Schneider, 1986). Thus, finely ground limestone or MgO coming in direct contact with vitamin E can markedly reduce its bioavailability.

D. Vitamin K

This fat-soluble vitamin exists in three series: phylloquinones (K_1) in plants, menaquinones (K_2) formed by microbial fermentation, and menadiones (K_3), which are synthetic. All three forms of vitamin K are biologically active. Only water-soluble forms of menadione are used to supplement swine diets. The commercially available forms of K_3 supplements are menadione sodium bisulfite (MSB), menadione sodium bisulfate complex (MSBC), and menadione dimethyl pyrimidinol bisulfite (MPB). These contain 52, 33, and 45.5% menadione, respectively. Stability of these K_3 supplements in premixes and diets is impaired by moisture, choline chloride, trace elements, and alkaline conditions. Coelho (1991) suggested that MSBC or MPB may lose almost 80% of bioactivity if stored for 3 months in a vitamin–trace mineral premix containing choline, but losses were suggested as being far less if stored in a similar premix containing no choline. Coated K_3 supplements are generally more stable than uncoated supplements. Bioactivity of MPB is greater than either MSB or MSBC for chicks (Griminger, 1965; Charles and Huston, 1972). Seerley et al. (1976) also found MPB to be effective for swine. Oduho et al. (1993) compared menadione nicotinamide bisulfite (MNB; 45.7% menadione, 32% nicotinamide) to MPB as a source of vitamin K activity for young chicks. Based on prothrombin time, MNB was reported to be equal to MPB in vitamin K activity. Although certain feed ingredients are known to be rich in vitamin K activity for swine (e.g., alfalfa meal; Fritschen et al., 1971), little quantitative information exists on the bioavailability of vitamin K in swine feedstuffs.

E. Biotin

Commercial D-biotin has no specific unit of activity. Thus, 1 g of D-biotin equals 1 g of activity. Pelleting or heat have little effect on biotin activity in feeds, but oxidative rancidity severely reduces biotin bioavailability. Much of the biotin in feed ingredients exists in a bound form, ε-N-biotinyl-L-lysine (biocytin), which is a component of protein. Crystalline biotin is absorbed well from the small intestine, but the bioavailability of biotin in biocytin varies widely and is dependent on the digestibility of the proteins in which it is found (Baker, 1995). Avidin, a glycoprotein found in egg albumen, binds biotin and makes it totally unavailable. Proper heat treatment of egg white will denature avidin and prevent it from binding biotin. Based on bioassay results using biotin-depleted chicks, it is apparent that among the cereal grains, bioavailability of biotin in corn is high ($\geq 100\%$) while that in wheat, barley, and sorghum is about 50% (Anderson and Warnick, 1970; Frigg, 1976; Anderson et al., 1978). Bioavailable biotin concentrations of 0.11 mg/kg in corn, 0.08 mg/kg in barley, 0.09 mg/kg in sorghum, and 0.04 mg/kg in wheat were estimated by Anderson et al. (1978). Feedstuff ingredient tables generally list the biotin concentration in soybean meal as 0.30 mg/kg. Buenrostro and Kratzer (1984) reported that biotin is 100% available in soybean meal and 86% available in meat and bone meal for laying hens. Hence, with considerable bioavailable biotin present in corn–soybean meal diets, growing-finishing pigs fed such diets have generally not responded to supplemental biotin. With sows, Bryant et al. (1985) provided evidence that under some conditions supplemental biotin may increase conception rate, decrease the weaning-to-estrus interval, and improve both foot health and hair coat, particularly in advanced parities. Lewis et al. (1991) reported that addition of 0.33 mg biotin/kg to a corn–soybean meal diet throughout both gestation and lactation increased the number of pigs weaned but did not improve foot health. In a similar study, however, Watkins et al. (1991) observed no benefit from adding 0.44 mg biotin/kg to a corn–soybean meal diet.

Biotin may be the only vitamin where a good test exists to assess the veracity of the bioavailability assay. Thus, growth responses to ingredients added to a biotin-free purified diet can be measured in the presence and absence of crystalline avidin. When the author's laboratory did this, growth rate of biotin-depleted chicks was doubled by supplementation with 20% corn, but it was not significantly increased when the same quantity of corn was fed in the presence of 3.81 mg avidin/kg diet (Anderson et al., 1978). Similar results occurred when barley was evaluated (Anderson et al., 1978). These results, therefore, provide rather convincing evidence that the growth responses observed from cereal-grain supplementation of the biotin-free purified diet resulted from the available biotin per se furnished by the grains.

F. Choline

In animal nutrition, choline remains in the B-vitamin category, even though the quantity required far exceeds the "trace organic nutrient" definition of a vitamin. Choline is absorbed primarily in the small intestine and is required by the body for (1) phospholipid synthesis, (2) acetyl choline formation, and (3) transmethylation of homocysteine to methionine. When a choline deficit is produced experimentally by feeding a choline-free diet to chicks, functions 1 and/or 2 seem to have priority over function 3 in that betaine (the methylated product of choline oxidation) does not elicit a growth response, whereas choline does. When about two thirds of the dietary choline needed for maximal growth is supplied as choline, as in practical diets, then synthetic choline and betaine are equally efficacious (Lowry et al., 1987).

In mammalian but not avian species, the dietary need for choline can be replaced by excess methionine. In crystalline form, choline chloride (74.6% choline) is hygroscopic, and therefore it is considered a stress agent to other vitamins in a vitamin–mineral premix. Crystalline choline is considered quite stable in animal feeds and premixes. Crude plant oils (e.g., corn and soybean oil) contain choline as phospholipid-bound phosphatidyl choline. The bioavailability of choline in this form is at least 100% (Emmert et al., 1996). Refined plant oils generally have been subjected to alkaline treatment and "bleaching," and these processes almost totally remove phospholipids, including phospholipid-bound choline.

Choline bioavailability (relative to crystalline choline chloride) in oilseed meals for chicks has been estimated at 83% in soybean meal (Molitoris and Baker, 1976a; Emmert and Baker, 1997), 76% in peanut meal, and only 24% in canola meal (Emmert and Baker, 1997). Also in chicks, excess dietary protein has been observed to increase the dietary requirement for choline

(Molitoris and Baker, 1976b). Minimizing liver lipid content may require a higher level of dietary choline than that required to maximize rate and efficiency of weight gain (Anderson et al., 1979).

As with niacin, for which tryptophan serves as a precursor, choline bioavailability assessment would be difficult, if not impossible, in pigs, because all common feed ingredients would supply both choline and methionine. Therefore, it would be difficult to separate responses from one or the other, although use of the transmethylation inhibitor ethionine or the inhibitor of methionine methylation of aminoethanol in choline biosynthesis (i.e., 2-amino-2-methyl-1-propanol) might prove useful in this endeavor (Molitoris and Baker, 1976a; Anderson et al., 1979; Lowry et al., 1987).

Corn–soybean meal diets for growing and finishing pigs often do not respond to choline supplementation, probably because soybean meal is so rich in choline content (NCR-42, 1980). Swine pregnancy, however, has been shown to benefit from choline addition to corn–soybean meal diets (Kornegay and Meacham, 1973; Stockland and Blaylock, 1974; NCR-42, 1976). Failure of corn–soybean meal swine and poultry grower diets to respond to vitamin supplementation is not unique to choline (among those generally supplemented). Unpublished work in the author's laboratory has shown that these diets also fail to respond consistently to either nicotinic acid or pantothenic acid. Choline, nicotinic acid, and pantothenic acid should nonetheless be included in swine vitamin mixtures to provide a margin of safety against environmental and stress conditions that might manifest in a swine production operation.

G. Folacin

The term *folacin* is the accepted generic term for folic acid and related compounds exhibiting "folacin" activity. Over 150 forms of folacin are known to exist in foods (McGinnis, 1986). Chemically, folic acid consists of a pteridine ring, *para*-aminobenzoic acid (PABA), and glutamic acid. Animal cells cannot synthesize PABA, nor can they attach glutamic acid to pteroic acid (i.e., pteridine attached to PABA). Thus, folic acid must be supplied in the diet of nonruminant animals. The folacin present in feeds and foods exists largely as polyglutamates. In plants, folacin exists as a polyglutamate conjugate containing a γ-linked polypeptide chain of (primarily) seven glutamic acid residues. The normal gut proteases do not cleave the glutamate residues from this compound. Instead, a group of intestinal enzymes known as conjugases (folyl polyglutamate hydrolases) removes all but the last glutamate residue. Only the monoglutamyl form is thought to be absorbed into the enterocyte. Most of the folic acid taken up by the brush border is reduced to tetrahydrofolate (FH_4) and then methylated to N^5-methyl-FH_4, the predominant form of folate in blood plasma. The majority of the N^5-methyl-FH_4 in plasma is bound to protein.

Like thiamin, folic acid has a free amino group (on the pteridine ring), and this makes it very sensitive to losses in activity due to heat treatment, particularly if heat is applied to foods or feeds containing reducing sugars such as lactose or glucose. Whether the free amino group of folacin (or thiamin) can bind to the free aldehyde moiety of pyridoxal or pyridoxalphosphate is not known. Intestinal conjugase inhibitors may be present in certain beans and pulses, and these may impede folacin absorption (Krumdieck et al., 1973; Bailey, 1988). Adams (1982) reported only 38% retention of folacin activity when folic acid was stored for 3 weeks at 45°C in a mineral-free premix. At room temperature, 57% of original activity was present after 3 months of storage. Verbeeck (1975) observed even greater losses when minerals were included in the premix.

Growing pigs fed conventional corn–soybean meal diets generally do not respond to folacin supplementation. Hence, it is not generally provided at supplemental levels in such diets (Easter et al., 1983). For gestating–lactating sows, however, some workers have observed improvements in reproductive performance as a result of folacin supplementation (Lindemann and Kornegay, 1989; Matte et al., 1992), whereas others have observed no response (Pharazyn and Aherne, 1987; Easter et al., 1983; Harper et al., 1994).

H. Niacin

The term *niacin* is the generic descriptive term for pyridine 3-carboxylic acid and derivatives delivering nicotinamide activity. Thus, pyridine 3-carboxylic acid per se is properly referred to as nicotinic acid (Anonymous, 1979). Niacin is a very stable vitamin when added to feed or premixes, being little affected by heat, oxygen, moisture, or light. In plant-source feed ingredients, much of the niacin activity, mostly nicotinamide nucleotides, is bound and therefore unavailable (Yen et al., 1977). Ghosh et al. (1963) estimated that 85 to 90% of the niacin activity in cereal grains and 40% in oilseeds is in a bound unavailable form. Alkaline hydrolysis is the only means by which niacin can be efficiently released from its bound state in these ingredients. Meat and milk products, on the other hand, contain no bound niacin, but instead contain free nicotinic acid and nicotinamide.

Because excess tryptophan is converted to nicotinic acid and because all common feed ingredients contain tryptophan as well as nicotinic acid, there is no good way to assess the bioavailability of niacin per se. Thus, 50 mg of tryptophan yields 1 mg of nicotinic acid (Baker et al., 1973; Czarnecki et al., 1983). Does excess leucine in corn–soybean meal swine diets antagonize tryptophan or nicotinic acid or does it impair the metabolic conversion of tryptophan to nicotinic acid? This subject is controversial (Anonymous, 1986) and data exist to support both points of view. Recent chick studies suggest that excess leucine has no effect on either tryptophan conversion to niacin or niacin bioavailability (Lowry and Baker, 1989b). Iron, on the other hand, is required in two metabolic reactions in the pathway of tryptophan to nicotinate mononucleotide. Oduho et al. (1994) established that Fe deficiency in chicks will reduce the conversion efficiency of tryptophan to niacin (i.e., from 42:1 to 56:1, wt:wt).

Niacin activity can be purchased as either free nicotinic acid or free nicotinamide. Relative to nicotinic acid, nicotinamide has been observed to be roughly 120% bioavailable in delivering niacin bioactivity (Baker et al., 1976; Oduho and Baker, 1993). Other work, however, has suggested niacin and nicotinamide to be equal in biopotency for chicks (Bao-Ji and Combs, 1986; Ruiz and Harms, 1988).

I. Pantothenic Acid

This B vitamin is generally sold as either D- or DL-Ca pantothenate, and only the D-isomer has bioactivity (Staten et al., 1980). Thus, 1 g of D-Ca pantothenate equals 0.92 g pantothenic acid (PA) activity, and 1 g DL-Ca pantothenate equals 0.46 g of PA activity. Crystalline PA is relatively stable to heat, oxygen, and light, but it can lose activity rapidly when exposed to moisture. Gadient (1986) concluded that PA should retain at least 80% of its activity after 3 months when present in pelleted feed or vitamin–mineral premixes.

Feed ingredients contain PA in the form of coenzyme A, and in this form it may not be fully available for gut absorption. Chick bioassay work suggested that the PA in corn and soybean meal is 100% bioavailable, whereas that in barley, wheat, and sorghum is about 60% bioavailable (Southern and Baker, 1981). Processed feed ingredients may exhibit losses in PA bioavailability, although definitive animal data are lacking on this subject. Sauberlich (1985) estimated that PA in the typical adult American diet was only 50% bioavailable. He further suggested that processing (freezing, canning, refining, etc.) may decrease bioavailability further.

J. Riboflavin

This vitamin is relatively labile, being reduced in bioactivity by light, alkali, and oxygen. In feedstuffs, it exists primarily as nucleotide coenzymes, in which form the bioavailability is probably less than 100%. Chung and Baker (1990) estimated that riboflavin bioavailability in a corn–soybean meal diet is 60% for chicks relative to crystalline riboflavin. Zhuge and Klopenstein (1986) reported that crystalline riboflavin loses activity in vitamin–mineral premixes over time and that high-temperature storage enhances the loss. Gadient (1986), however, suggested that riboflavin activity in feeds is little affected by heat and oxygen and only slightly affected by moisture and light. He observed 95 to 100% retention of riboflavin bioactivity in pelleted feeds stored for 3 months at room temperature.

Jusko and Levy (1975) and Sauberlich (1985) suggested that several factors may reduce the bioavailability of riboflavin in foods. Among the suggested factors antagonizing riboflavin were excess dietary levels of tetracycline, Fe, Zn, Cu, ascorbate, and caffeine. Patel and Baker (1996) used chick growth bioassays to evaluate dietary excesses of Fe (420 mg/kg), Zn (448 mg/kg), Cu (245 mg/kg), ascorbic acid (1000 mg/kg), caffeine (200 mg/kg), or chortetracycline (500 mg/kg), which were added to riboflavin-deficient soy-isolate semipurified diets. None of these supplements was found to decrease the utilization of crystalline riboflavin.

K. Thiamin

Thiamin is available to the food and feed industries as thiamin·HCl (89% thiamin) or thiamin·NO_3 (92% thiamin). These compounds are stable up to 100°C and are readily soluble in water (NRC, 1987). An international unit of thiamin activity is equivalent to 3 µg of crystalline thiamin·HCl. Because it contains a free amino group, heat processing can rapidly destroy thiamin bioactivity via the Maillard reaction. Similarly, any processing procedure that involves alkaline treatment leads to loss of thiamin activity. The thiamin contained in swine feed ingredients is present largely in phosphorylated forms, either as protein–phosphate complexes or as thiamin mono-, di-, or triphosphates. Some raw ingredients (e.g., fish) contain thiaminase, which can destroy thiamin in diets to which it may be added. While thiaminase is of particular concern in the nutrition of cats and fur-bearing animals, it is of little consequence in modern swine feeding. Thiamin in fish meal is lost to the fish solubles fraction when fish meal is made. Thus, fish meal has essentially no bioavailable thiamin. Similarly, as a result of the high-temperature processing, meat meals contain very little bioavailable thiamin activity.

Pelleting results in some loss of thiamin activity, as does premix storage in the presence of minerals (Gadient, 1986). Adams (1982) found 48 and 95% retention of thiamin activity when stored in the form of the HCl and NO_3, respectively, in a premix for 21 days at 40°C and 85% relative humidity. In a complete feed stored under similar conditions, thiamin·HCl retained only 21% of its activity, whereas thiamin·NO_3 retained 97% of its activity. Thus, the mononitrate form of thiamin would seem to be the more stable form when storage in hot environments is anticipated.

Grains and soybean meal are sufficiently rich in thiamin that, even with considerable losses of bioactivity due to heat or lengthy storage, seldom would there be a case where practical-type diets for swine would respond to supplementation with thiamin.

L. Vitamin B_6

Vitamin B_6 is not generally added in supplemental crystalline form to practical-type diets for swine because both corn and soybean meal are plentiful in this B vitamin. Work at the author's laboratory suggests that vitamin B_6 is about 40% bioavailable in corn and about 60% bioavailable in soybean meal (Yen et al., 1976). Moderate heat treatment (80 to 120°C) of corn seems to enhance B_6 bioavailability, whereas greater heat treatment (160°C) decreases availability. Most of the vitamin B_6 activity in corn exists as pyridoxal and pyridoxamine, forms that are more heat-labile than is pyridoxine (Schroeder, 1971). Plant-source feedstuffs may contain B_6 as either pyridoxine glucoside or pyridoxallysine, and both of these compounds have minimal B_6 bioactivity (Gregory and Kirk, 1981; Trumbo et al., 1988). Even with the reduced bioavailability of vitamin B_6 in corn and soybean meal relative to crystalline pyridoxine·HCl, a surfeit of available B_6 would still be present in practical-type diets for swine, thus precluding a response to supplemental vitamin B_6 if added to these diets.

In premixes, vitamin B_6 can lose bioactivity, particularly when minerals in the form of carbonates or oxides are present (Verbeeck, 1975). High temperatures enhance loss of activity. Adams

(1982) found 76% retention of B_6 activity after 3 months of storage at room temperature, but only 45% retention after 3 months of storage at 37°C. Loss of B_6 activity in stored, pelleted complete feeds averages about 20% during 3 months of storage at room temperature (Gadient, 1986).

M. VITAMIN B_{12}

Cyanocobalamin, or B_{12}, is available in crystalline form, where 1 U.S. Pharmacopoeia (USP) unit is considered equivalent to 1 µg of the vitamin. Vitamin B_{12} is essentially devoid in plant-source feed ingredients, existing instead in animal-source proteins and fermentation products, where it is considered (but not proved) to be 100% available.

Both animal and fermentation-based feedstuffs contain B_{12} as methylcobalamin or adenosylcobalamin, which are bound to protein. As in humans, but unlike in sheep and in horses, an "intrinsic" factor is required for gut absorption of B_{12} in swine. Gadient (1986) considers crystalline vitamin B_{12} to be quite stable in feeds and premixes.

N. VITAMIN C

There is little concern about the bioavailability of vitamin C (ascorbic acid) because swine are capable of synthesizing this vitamin. Nonetheless, vitamin C is often included in vitamin premixes for use in purified swine diets because of its antioxidant and putative antistress properties. Adams (1982) observed considerable losses of vitamin C activity in stored layer diets. Coating ascorbate with ethylcellulose minimized the loss of potency. Gadient (1986) noted that both pelleting and extruding can markedly reduce the bioactivity of supplemental ascorbate added to feeds or premixes. Losses due to oxidation are well known, as ascorbic acid (reduced form) can be reversibly oxidized to dehydroascorbic acid, which in turn can be further irreversibly oxidized to diketogulonic acid. Both reduced and oxidized forms of ascorbate retain scurvy-preventing ascorbate activity, but diketogulonic acid has no activity. Both ascorbate and dehydroascorbate are heat labile, particularly when heat is applied in the presence of trace minerals such as Cu, Fe, or Zn.

REFERENCES

Adams, C. R. 1982. Vitamins — the life essentials. In *Proc. of the NFIA Nutr. Institute*, 1.
Ammerman, C. B., and S. M. Miller. 1972. Biological availability of minor mineral ions: a review, *J. Anim. Sci.*, 35:681.
Ammerman, C. B., J. F. Standish, C. E. Holt, R. H. Houser, S. M. Miller, and G. E. Combs. 1974. Ferrous carbonates as sources of iron for weanling pigs and rats, *J. Anim. Sci.*, 38:52.
Ammerman, C. B., D. H. Baker, and A. J. Lewis. 1995. *Bioavailability of Nutrients for Animals: Amino Acids, Minerals, and Vitamins*, Academic Press, San Diego, CA.
Anderson, J. O., and R. E. Warnick. 1970. Studies of the need for supplemental biotin in chick rations, *Poult. Sci.*, 49:569.
Anderson, P. A., D. H. Baker, and S. P. Mistry. 1978. Bioassay determination of the biotin content of corn, barley, sorghum and wheat, *J. Anim. Sci.*, 47:654.
Anderson, P. A., D. H. Baker, P. A. Sherry, and J. E. Corbin. 1979. Choline-methionine interrelationship in feline nutrition, *J. Anim. Sci.*, 49:522.
Anonymous. 1979. Nomenclature policy: generic descriptors and trivial names for vitamins and related compounds, *J. Nutr.*, 109:8.
Anonymous. 1986. Pellagragenic effect of excess leucine, *Nutr. Rev.*, 44:26.
Aoyagi, S., and D. H. Baker. 1993a. Bioavailability of copper in analytical-grade and feed-grade inorganic copper sources when fed to provide copper at levels below the chick's requirement, *Poult. Sci.*, 72:1075.
Aoyagi, S., and D. H. Baker. 1993b. Nutritional evaluation of copper-lysine and zinc-lysine complexes for chicks, *Poult. Sci.*, 72:165.

Aoyagi, S., and D. H. Baker. 1994. Copper-amino acid complexes are partially protected against inhibitory effects of L-cysteine and L-ascorbate, *J. Nutr.*, 124:388.

Aoyagi, S., and D. H. Baker. 1995. Effect of microbial phytase and 1,25-dihydroxycholecalciferol on dietary copper utilization in chicks, *Poult. Sci.*, 74:121.

Aoyagi, S., D. H. Baker, and K. J. Wedekind. 1993. Estimates of copper bioavailability from liver of different animal species and from feed ingredients derived from plants and animals, *Poult. Sci.*, 72:1746.

Aoyagi, S., K. M. Hiney, and D. H. Baker. 1995. Copper bioavailability in pork liver and in various animal by-products as determined by chick bioassay, *J. Anim. Sci.*, 73:799.

Bafundo, K. W., D. H. Baker, and P. R. Fitzgerald. 1984a. The iron-zinc interrelationship in the chick as influenced by *Eimeria acervulina* infection, *J. Nutr.*, 114:1306.

Bafundo, K. W., D. H. Baker, and P. R. Fitzgerald. 1984b. Zinc utilization in the chick as influenced by dietary concentration of calcium and phytate and by *Eimeria acervulina* infection, *Poult. Sci.*, 63:2430.

Bailey, L. B. 1988. Factors affecting folate bioavailability, *Food Technol.*, 42:206.

Baker, D. H. 1989. Phosphorus supplements for poultry, *Multistate Newsl. Poult. Ext. Res.*, 1(5):5.

Baker, D. H. 1995. Vitamin bioavailability. In *Bioavailability of Nutrients for Animals: Amino Acids, Minerals, and Vitamins*, Ammerman, C. B., D. H. Baker, and A. J. Lewis, Eds., Academic Press, San Diego, CA, 399.

Baker, D. H., and C. B. Ammerman. 1995a. Copper bioavailability. In *Bioavailability of Nutrients for Animals: Amino Acids, Minerals, and Vitamins*, Ammerman, C. B., D. H. Baker, and A. J. Lewis, Eds., Academic Press, San Diego, CA, 127.

Baker, D. H., and C. B. Ammerman. 1995b. Zinc bioavailability. In *Bioavailability of Nutrients for Animals: Amino Acids, Mineals, and Vitamins*, Ammerman, C. B., D. H. Baker, and A. J. Lewis, Eds., Academic Press, San Diego, CA, 367.

Baker, D. H., and G. L. Czarnecki-Maulden. 1987. Pharmacologic role of cysteine in ameliorating or exacerbating mineral toxicities, *J. Nutr.*, 117:1003.

Baker, D. H., and K. M. Halpin. 1988. Zinc antagonizing effects of fish meal, wheat bran and a corn–soybean meal mixture when added to a phytate- and fiber-free casein-dextrose diet, *Nutr. Res.*, 8:213.

Baker, D. H., and G. W. Oduho. 1994. Manganese utilization in the chick: effects of excess phosphorus on chicks fed manganese-deficient diets, *Poult. Sci.*, 73:1162.

Baker, D. H., and K. J. Wedekind. 1988. Manganese utilization in chicks as affected by excess calcium and phosphorus ingestion. In *Proc. of the Maryland Nutr. Conf.*, 29.

Baker, D. H., N. K. Allen, and A. J. Kleiss. 1973. Efficiency of tryptophan as a niacin precursor in the chick, *J. Anim. Sci.*, 36:299.

Baker, D. H., J. T. Yen, A. H. Jensen, R. G. Teeter, E. N. Michel, and J. H. Burns. 1976. Niacin activity in niacinamide and coffee, *Nutr. Rep. Int.*, 14:115.

Baker, D. H., K. M. Halpin, G. L. Czarnecki, and C. M. Parsons. 1983. The choline-methionine interrelationship for growth of the chick, *Poult. Sci.*, 62:133.

Baker, D. H., K. M. Halpin, D. E. Laurin, and L. L. Southern. 1986. Manganese for poultry — a review, In *Proc. of the Arkansas Nutr. Conf.*, 1.

Baker, D. H., J. Odle, M. A. Funk, and T. M. Wieland. 1991. Bioavailability of copper in cupric oxide, cuprous oxide and in a copper-lysine complex, *Poult. Sci.*, 70:177.

Bao-Ji, C., and G. F. Combs. 1986. Evaluation of biopotencies of nicotinamide and nicotinic acid for broiler chickens, *Poult. Sci.*, 65(Suppl. 1):24 (Abstr.).

Barber, R. S., J. D. Bowland, R. Braude, K. G. Mitchell, and J. W. G. Porter. 1961. Copper sulphate and copper sulphide (CuS) as supplements for growing pigs, *Br. J. Nutr.*, 15:189.

Bieri, J. G., and M. C. McKenna. 1981. Expressing dietary values for fat-soluble vitamins: changes in concepts and terminology, *Am. J. Clin. Nutr.*, 34:289.

Black, J. R., C. B. Ammerman, P. R. Henry, and R. D. Miles. 1984. Biological availability of manganese sources and effects of high dietary manganese on tissue mineral composition of broiler-type chicks, *Poult. Sci.*, 63:1999.

Black, J. R., C. B. Ammerman, P. R. Henry, and R. D. Miles. 1985. Effect of dietary manganese and age on tissue trace mineral composition of broiler-type chicks as a bioassay of manganese sources, *Poult. Sci.*, 64:688.

Bogunjoko, F. E., R. J. Neale, and D. A. Ledward. 1983. Availability of iron from chicken meat and liver given to rats, *Br. J. Nutr.*, 50:511.

Boling, S. D., H. M. Edwards III, J. L. Emmert, R. R. Biehl, and D. H. Baker. 1998. Bioavailability of iron in cottonseed meal, ferric sulfate and two ferrous sulfate by-products of the galvanizing industry, *Poult. Sci.*, 77:1388.

Braude, R., A. G. Chamberlain, M. Kotarbinska, and K. G. Mitchell. 1962. The metabolism of iron in piglets given labeled iron either orally or by injection, *Br. J. Nutr.*, 16:427.

Bryant, K. L., E. T. Kornegay, J. W. Knight, H. P. Veit, and D. R. Natter. 1985. Supplemental biotin for swine III. Influence of supplementation to corn- and wheat-based diets on the incidence and severity of toe lesions, hair and skin characteristics and structural soundness of sows housed in confinement during four parities, *J. Anim. Sci.*, 60:154.

Buenostro, J. L., and F. H. Kratzer. 1984. Use of plasma and egg yolk biotin of white leghorn hens to assess biotin availability from feedstuffs, *Poult. Sci.*, 63:1563.

Burns, J. M., and D. H. Baker. 1976. Assessment of the quantity of biologically available phosphorus in yeast RNA and single-cell protein, *Poult. Sci.*, 55:2447.

Cantor, A. H., M. L. Langevin, T. Noguchi, and M. L. Scott. 1975a. Efficacy of selenium compounds and feedstuffs for prevention of pancreatic fibrosis in chicks, *J. Nutr.*, 105:106.

Cantor, A. H., M. L. Scott, and T. Noguchi. 1975b. Biological availability of selenium in feedstuffs and selenium compounds for prevention of exudative diathesis in chicks, *J. Nutr.*, 105:96.

Charles, O. W., and T. M. Huston. 1972. The biological activity of vitamin K materials following storage and pelleting, *Poult. Sci.*, 51:1421.

Chausow, D. G. 1987. Selected Aspects of Mineral Nutrition of the Cat and Dog with Special Emphasis on Magnesium and Iron, Ph.D. thesis, University of Illinois, Urbana.

Chausow, D. G., and G. L. Czarnecki-Maulden. 1988a. The relative bioavailability of iron from feedstuffs of plant and animal origin to the chick, *Nutr. Res.*, 8:175.

Chausow, D. G., and G. L. Czarnecki-Maulden. 1988b. The relative bioavailability of plant and animal sources of iron to the cat and chick, *Nutr. Res.*, 8:1041.

Chung, T. K., and D. H. Baker. 1990. Riboflavin requirement of chicks fed purified amino acid and conventional corn–soybean meal diets, *Poult. Sci.*, 69:1357.

Chung, T. K., J. W. Erdman, and D. H. Baker. 1990. Hydrated sodium calcium aluminosilicate: effects on zinc, manganese, vitamin A and riboflavin utilization, *Poult. Sci.*, 69:1364.

Coelho, M. B. 1991. Vitamin stability, *Feed Manag.*, 42(10):24.

Coelho, M. B., and E. T. Kornegay. 1996. *Phytase in Animal Nutrition and Waste Management*, BASF Corp., Mount Olive, NJ, 728 pp.

Coffey, R. D., K. W. Mooney, G. L. Cromwell, and D. K. Aaron. 1994. Biological availability of phosphorus in defluorinated phosphates with different phosphorus solubilities in neutral ammonium citrate for chicks and pigs, *J. Anim. Sci.*, 72:2653.

Combs, N. R., and E. R. Miller. 1985. Determination of potassium availability in K_2CO_3, $KHCO_3$, corn and soybean meal for the young pig, *J. Anim. Sci.*, 60:715.

Combs, N. R., E. R. Miller, and P. K. Ku. 1985. Development of an assay to determine the bioavailability of potassium in feedstuffs for the young pig, *J. Anim. Sci.*, 60:709.

Cook, D. A. 1973. Availability of magnesium: balance studies in rats with various inorganic magnesium salts, *J. Nutr.*, 103:1365.

Cornelius, S. G., and B. G. Harmon. 1976. Sources of oral iron for neonatal piglets, *J. Anim. Sci.*, 42:1351 (Abstr.).

Cromwell, G. L. 1992. The biological availability of phosphorus in feedstuffs for pigs, *Pig News Info.*, 13:75N.

Cromwell, G. L., V. W. Hays, and T. L. Clark. 1978. Effects of copper sulfate, copper sulfide and sodium sulfide on performance and copper stores of pigs, *J. Anim. Sci.*, 46:692.

Cromwell, G. L., T. S. Stahly, and H. J. Monegue. 1983. Bioavailability of the calcium and phosphorus in dehydrated alfalfa meal for growing pigs, *J. Anim. Sci.*, 57(Suppl. 1):242 (Abstr.).

Cromwell, G. L., R. D. Ross, and T. S. Stahly. 1989a. An evaluation of the requirements and biological availability of calcium and phosphorus for swine, *Proc. of the Texas Gulf Nutr. Symp.*, Raleigh, NC, 88.

Cromwell, G. L., T. S. Stahly, and H. J. Monegue. 1989b. Effects of source and level of copper on performance and liver copper stores in weanling pigs, *J. Anim. Sci.*, 67:2996.

Czarnecki, G. L., and D. H. Baker. 1985. Reduction of liver copper concentration by the organic arsenical, 3-nitro-4-hydroxyphenylarsonic acid, *J. Anim. Sci.*, 60:440.

Czarnecki, G. L., K. M. Halpin, and D. H. Baker. 1983. Precursor (amino acid):product (vitamin) interrelationship for growing chicks as illustrated by tryptophan-niacin and methionine-choline, *Poult. Sci.*, 62:371.
Deming, J. G., and G. L. Czarnecki-Maulden. 1989. Iron bioavailability in calcium and phosphorus sources, *J. Anim. Sci.*, 67(Suppl. 1):253 (Abstr.).
DeRitter, E. 1976. Stability characteristics of vitamins in processed foods, *Food Technol.*, 30:48.
Diekert, J. W., J. E. Snowden, Jr., A. T. Moore, D. C. Heinzelman, and A. M. Altschul. 1962. Composition of some subcellular fractions from seeds of *Arachis hypogaea*, *J. Food Sci.*, 27:321.
Easter, R. A., P. A. Anderson, E. J. Michel, and J. R. Corley. 1983. Response of gestating gilts and starter, grower and finisher swine to biotin, pyridoxine, folacin and thiamine additions to corn–soybean meal diets, *Nutr. Rep. Int.*, 28:945.
Edmonds, M. S., and D. H. Baker. 1986. Toxic effects of supplemental copper and roxarsone when fed alone or in combination to young pigs, *J. Anim. Sci.*, 63:533.
Edwards, H. M., Jr. 1959. The availability to chicks of zinc in various compounds and ores, *J. Nutr.*, 69:306.
Edwards, H. M., III, and D. H. Baker. 1999. Bioavailability of zinc in several sources of zinc oxide, zinc sulfate and zinc metal, *J. Anim. Sci.*, 77:2730.
Emmert, J. L., and D. H. Baker. 1997. A chick bioassay approach for determining the bioavailable choline concentration of normal and overheated soybean meal, canola meal and peanut meal, *J. Nutr.*, 127:745.
Emmert, J. L., T. A. Garrow, and D. H. Baker. 1996. Development of an experimental diet for determining bioavailable choline concentration, and its application in studies with soybean lecithin, *J. Anim. Sci.*, 74:2738.
Erdman, J. W., Jr. 1979. Oilseed phytates: nutritional implications, *J. Am. Oil Chem. Soc.*, 56:736.
Erdman, J. W., Jr., G. C. Fahey, and C. B. White. 1986. Effects of purified dietary fiber sources on β-carotene utilization by the chick, *J. Nutr.*, 116:2415.
Erdman, J. W., Jr., C. L. Poor, and J. M. Dietz. 1988. Processing and dietary effects on the bioavailability of vitamin A, carotenoids and vitamin E, *Food Technol.*, 42:214.
Fethiere, R., R. D. Miles, R. H. Harms, and S. M. Laurent. 1988. Bioavailability of sodium in Ethacal® feed component, *Poult. Sci.*, 67(Suppl. 1):15 (Abstr.).
Fly, A. D., O. A. Izquierdo, K. R. Lowry, and D. H. Baker. 1989. Manganese bioavailability in a Mn-methionine chelate, *Nutr. Res.*, 9:901.
Fordyce, E. J., R. M. Forbes, K. R. Robbins, and J. W. Erdman, Jr. 1987. Phytate X calcium/zinc molar ratios: are they predictive of zinc bioavailability, *J. Food Sci.*, 52:440.
Frigg, M. 1976. Bioavailability of biotin in cereals, *Poult. Sci.*, 55:2310.
Fritschen, R. D., O. D. Grace, and E. R. Peo. 1971. Bleeding pig disease, Nebraska Swine Report EC71, 219:22.
Fritz, J. C., G. W. Pla, T. Roberts, J. W. Boehne, and E. L. Hove. 1970. Biological availability in animals of iron from common dietary sources, *J. Agric. Food Chem.*, 18:647.
Furugouri, K., and A. Kawabata. 1975. Iron absorption in nursing piglets, *J. Anim. Sci.*, 41:1348.
Gadient, M. 1986. Effect of pelleting on nutritional quality of feed. In *Proc. of the Maryland Nutr. Conf.*, 73.
Ghosh, H. P., P. K. Sarkar, and B. C. Guha. 1963. Distribution of the bound form of nicotinic acid in natural materials, *J. Nutr.*, 79:451.
Gregory, J. F., III, and J. R. Kirk. 1981. The bioavailability of vitamin B_6 in foods, *Nutr. Rev.*, 39:1.
Griminger, P. 1965. Relative vitamin K potency of two water-soluble menadione analogues, *Poult. Sci.*, 44:210.
Groff, J. L., S. S. Gropper, and S. M. Hunt. 1995. *Advanced Nutrition and Human Metabolism*. West Publishing, St. Paul, MN, 575 pp.
Guenter, W., and J. L. Sell. 1974. A method for determining Atrue@ availability of magnesium from foodstuffs using chickens, *J. Nutr.*, 104:1446.
Hahn, J. D., and D. H. Baker. 1993. Growth and plasma zinc responses of young pigs fed pharmacologic levels of zinc, *J. Anim. Sci.*, 71:3020.
Halpin, K. M., and D. H. Baker. 1986a. Long-term effects of corn, soybean meal, wheat bran and fish meal on manganese utilization in the chick, *Poult. Sci.*, 65:1371.
Halpin, K. M., and D. H. Baker. 1986b. Manganese utilization in the chick: effects of corn, soybean meal, fish meal, wheat bran and rice bran on tissue uptake of manganese, *Poult. Sci.*, 65:995.
Halpin, K. M., and D. H. Baker. 1987. Mechanism of the tissue manganese-lowering effect of corn, soybean meal, fish meal, wheat bran and rice bran, *Poult. Sci.*, 66:332.
Halpin, K. M., D. G. Chausow, and D. H. Baker. 1986. Efficiency of manganese absorption in chicks fed corn-soy and casein diets, *J. Nutr.*, 116:1747.

Harmon, B. G. 1979. Bioavailability of minerals in ingredients for swine, In *Proc. of the Georgia Nutr. Conf.*, 98.

Harmon, B. G., D. E. Becker, and A. H. Jensen. 1967. Efficacy of ferric ammonium citrate in preventing anemia in young swine, *J. Anim. Sci.*, 26:1051.

Harmon, B. G., D. E. Hoge, A. H. Jensen, and D. H. Baker. 1969. Efficacy of ferrous carbonate as a hematinic for young swine, *J. Anim. Sci.*, 29:706.

Harmon, B. G., S. G. Cornelius, J. Totsch, D. H. Baker, and A. H. Jensen. 1974. Oral iron dextran and iron from steel slats as hematinics for swine, *J. Anim. Sci.*, 39:699.

Harper, A. F., M. D. Lindemann, L. I. Chiba, G. E. Combs, D. L. Handlin, E. T. Kornegay, and L. L. Southern. 1994. An assessment of dietary folic acid levels during gestation and lactation on reproductive and lactational performance of sows: a cooperative study, *J. Anim. Sci.*, 72:2338.

Harper, J. M. 1988. Effect of extrusion processing on nutrients. In *Nutritional Evaluation of Food Processing*, 3rd ed., Karmas, E., and R. S. Harris, Eds., Van Nostrand Reinhold, New York.

Hays, V. W. 1976. *Phosphorus in Swine Nutrition*, National Feed Ingredients Association, West Des Moines, IA.

Hendricks, D. G., E. R. Miller, D. E. Ullrey, J. A. Hoefer, and R. W. Luecke. 1969. Effect of level of soybean protein and ergocalciferol on mineral utilization by the baby pig, *J. Anim. Sci.*, 28:342.

Henry, P. R. 1995. Manganese bioavailability. In *Bioavailability of Nutrients for Animals: Amino Acids, Minerals, and Vitamins*, Ammerman, C. B., D. H. Baker, and A. J. Lewis, Eds., Academic Press, San Diego, CA, 239.

Henry, P. R., and E. R. Miller. 1995. Iron bioavailability. In *Bioavailability of Nutrients for Animals: Amino Acids, Minerals, and Vitamins*, Ammerman, C. B., D. H. Baker, and A. J. Lewis, Eds., Academic Press, San Diego, CA, 169.

Horst, R. L., J. L. Napoli, and E. T. Littledike. 1982. Discrimination in the metabolism of orally dosed ergocalciferol and cholecalciferol by the pig, rat, and chick, *Biochem. J.*, 204:185.

Hortin, A. E., P. J. Bechtel, and D. H. Baker. 1991. Efficacy of pork loin as a source of zinc, and effect of added cysteine on zinc bioavailability, *J. Food Sci.*, 56:1505.

Hortin, A. E., G. Oduho, Y. Han, P. J. Bechtel, and D. H. Baker. 1993. Bioavailability of zinc in ground beef, *J. Anim. Sci.*, 71:119.

Izquierdo, O. A., and D. H. Baker. 1986. Bioavailability of copper in pig feces, *Can. J. Anim. Sci.*, 66:1145.

Jusko, W. J., and G. Levy. 1975. Absorption, protein binding and elimination of riboflavin. In *Riboflavin*, Rivlin, R. S., Ed., Plenum Press, New York, 99.

Kornegay, E. T. 1972. Availability of iron contained in defluorinated phosphate, *J. Anim. Sci.*, 34:569.

Kornegay, E. T., and T. N. Meacham. 1973. Evaluation of supplemental choline for reproducing sows housed in total confinement on concrete or in dirt lots, *J. Anim. Sci.*, 37:506.

Krumdieck, C. L., A. J. Newman, and C. E. Butterworth, Jr. 1973. A naturally occurring inhibitor of folic acid conjugase (petroylopolyglutamyl hydrolase) in beans and other pulses, *Am. J. Clin. Nutr.*, 24:460 (Abstr.).

Layrisse, M., C. Martinez-Torres, M. Renzy, and I. Leets. 1975. Ferritin iron absorption in man, *Blood*, 45:689.

Lewis, A. J., G. L. Cromwell, and J. E. Pettigrew. 1991. Effects of supplemental biotin during gestation and lactation on reproductive performance of sows: a cooperative study, *J. Anim. Sci.*, 69:207.

Lindemann, M. D., and E. T. Kornegay. 1989. Folic acid supplementation to diets of gestating-lactating swine over multiple parities, *J. Anim. Sci.*, 67:459.

Livington, A. L., J. W. Nelson, and G. O. Kohler. 1968. Stability of alpha-tocopherol during alfalfa dehydration and storage, *J. Agric. Food Chem.*, 16:492.

Lowry, K. R., and D. H. Baker. 1989a. Amelioration of selenium toxicity by arsenicals and cysteine, *J. Anim. Sci.*, 67:959.

Lowry, K. R., and D. H. Baker. 1989b. Effect of excess leucine on niacin provided by either tryptophan or niacin, *FASEB J.*, 3:A666 (Abstr.).

Lowry, K. R., O. A. Izquierdo, and D. H. Baker. 1987. Efficacy of betaine relative to choline as a dietary methyl donor, *Poult. Sci.*, 66(Suppl. 1):135 (Abstr.).

Mahan, D. C., and A. L. Moxon. 1978. Effect of adding inorganic or organic selenium sources to the diets of young swine, *J. Anim. Sci.*, 47:456.

Mahan, D.C., and N. A. Parrett. 1996. Evaluating the efficacy of selenium-enriched yeast and sodium selenite on tissue selenium retention and serum glutathionine peroxidase activity in grower and finisher swine, *J. Anim. Sci.*, 74:2967.

Mathias, M. M., D. E. Hogue, and J. K. Loosli. 1967. The biological value of selenium in bovine milk for the rat and chick, *J. Nutr.*, 93:14.

Matte, J. J., C. L. Girard, and G. J. Brisson. 1992. The role of folic acid in the nutrition of gestating and lactating primaparous sows, *Livest. Prod. Sci.*, 32:131.

McGinnis, C. H. 1986. Vitamin stability, and activity of water-soluble vitamins as influenced by manufacturing processes and recommendations for the water-soluble vitamins. In *Proc. of the NFIA Nutr. Institute*, 1.

Miller, E. R. 1978. Biological availability of iron in iron supplements, *Feedstuffs*, 50:20.

Miller, E. R. 1980. Bioavailability of minerals. In *Proc. of the Minnesota Nutr. Conf.*, 144.

Miller, E. R., and C. B. Ammerman. 1995. Iodine bioavailability. In *Bioavailability of Nutrients for Animals: Amino Acids, Minerals and Vitamins*, Ammerman, C. B., D. H. Baker, and A. J. Lewis, Eds., Academic Press, San Diego, CA, 157.

Miller, E. R., P. K. Ku, J. P. Hitchcock, and W. T. Magee. 1981. Availability of zinc from metallic zinc dust for young swine, *J. Anim. Sci.*, 52:312.

Molitoris, B. A., and D. H. Baker. 1976a. Assessment of the quantity of biologically available choline in soybean meal, *J. Anim. Sci.*, 42:481.

Molitoris, B. A., and D. H. Baker. 1976b. Choline utilization in the chick as influenced by levels of dietary protein and methionine, *J. Nutr.*, 106:412.

NCR-42 Committee on Swine Nutrition. 1976. Effect of supplemental choline on reproductive performance of sows: a cooperative regional study, *J. Anim. Sci.*, 42:1211.

NCR-42 Committee on Swine Nutrition. 1980. Effect of supplemental choline on performance of starting, growing and finishing pigs: a cooperative regional study, *J. Anim. Sci.*, 50:99.

Nelson, T. S. 1967. The utilization of phytate phosphorus by poultry, *Poult. Sci.*, 46:862.

Nelson, T. S., and A. C. Walker. 1964. The biological evaluation of phosphorus compounds, *Poult. Sci.*, 43:94.

NRC. 1987. *Vitamin Tolerance of Animals*, National Academy Press, Washington, D.C.

NRC. 1994. *Nutrient Requirements of Poultry*, 9th ed., National Academy Press, Washington, D.C.

NRC. 1998. *Nutrient Requirements of Swine*, 10th ed., National Academy Press, Washington, D.C.

O'Dell, B. L., J. M. Yohe, and J. E. Savage. 1964. Zinc availability in the chick as affected by phytate, calcium and ethylenediaminetetracetate, *Poult. Sci.*, 43:415.

O'Dell, B. L., E. R. Miller, and W. J. Miller. 1979. *Copper and Zinc in Poultry, Swine and Ruminant Nutrition*, National Feed Ingredients Association, West Des Moines, IA.

Oduho, G., and D. H. Baker. 1993. Quantitative efficacy of niacin sources for the chick: nicotinic acid, nicotinamide, NAD and tryptophan, *J. Nutr.*, 123:2201.

Oduho, G. W., T. K. Chung, and D. H. Baker. 1993. Menadione nicotinamide bisulfite is a bioactive source of vitamin K and niacin activity for chicks, *J. Nutr.*, 123:737.

Oduho, G., Y. Han, and D. H. Baker. 1994. Iron deficiency reduces the efficacy of tryptophan as a niacin precursor for chicks, *J. Nutr.*, 124:444.

Olson, J. A. 1984. Vitamin A. In *Handbook of Vitamins*, Machlin, L. J., Ed., Marcel Dekker, New York, 1.

Patel, K., and D. H. Baker. 1996. Supplemental iron, copper, zinc, ascorbate caffeine and chlortetracycline do not affect riboflavin utilization in the chick, *Nutr. Res.*, 16:1943.

Peeler, H. T. 1972. Biological availability of nutrients in feeds: availability of major mineral ions, *J. Anim. Sci.*, 35:695.

Peo, E. R. 1976. *Calcium in Swine Nutrition*, National Feed Ingredients Association, West Des Moines, IA.

Pharazyn, A., and F. X. Aherne. 1987. Folacin requirement of the lactating sow. In 66th Annual Feeders Day Report, University of Alberta, 16.

Pond, W. G., R. S. Lowrey, J. H. Maner, and J. K. Loosli. 1961. Parenteral iron administration to sows during gestation or lactation, *J. Anim. Sci.*, 20:747.

Rao, N., and B. S. N. Rao. 1970. Absorption of dietary carotenes in human subjects, *Am. J. Clin. Nutr.*, 23:105.

Ross, R. D., G. L. Cromwell, and T. S. Stahly. 1984. Effects of source and particle size on the biological availability of calicum in calcium supplements for growing pigs, *J. Anim. Sci.*, 59:125.

Ruiz, N., and R. H. Harms. 1988. Comparison of biopotencies of nicotinic acid and nicotinamide for broiler chickens, *Br. Poult. Sci.*, 29:491.

Sauberlich, H. 1985. Bioavailability of vitamins, *Prog. Food Nutr. Sci.*, 9:1.

Schneider, J. 1986. Vitamin stability and activity of fat-soluble vitamins as influenced by manufacturing processes. In *Proc. of the NFIA Nutr. Institute*, 1.

Schroeder, H. A. 1971. Losses of vitamins and trace minerals resulting from processing and preservation of foods, *Am. J. Clin. Nutr.*, 24:562.

Seerley, R. W., O. W. Charles, H. C. McCampbell, and S. P. Bertsch. 1976. Efficacy of menadione dimethylpyrimidinol bisulfite as a source of vitamin K in swine diets, *J. Anim. Sci.*, 42:599.

Soares, J. H. 1995. Phosphorus bioavailability. In *Bioavailability of Nutrients for Animals: Amino Acids, Minerals, and Vitamins*, Ammerman, C. B., D. H. Baker, and A. J. Lewis, Eds., Academic Press, Inc., San Diego, CA, 257.

Southern, L. L., and D. H. Baker. 1981. Bioavailable pantothenic acid in cereal grains and soybean meal, *J. Anim. Sci.*, 53:403.

Southern, L. L., and D. H. Baker. 1983a. *Eimeria acervulina* infection in chicks fed deficient or excess levels of manganese, *J. Nutr.*, 113:172.

Southern, L. L., and D. H. Baker. 1983b. Excess manganese ingestion in the chick, *Poult. Sci.*, 62:642.

Southern, L. L., and D. H. Baker. 1983c. Zinc toxicity, zinc deficiency and zinc-copper interrelationship in *Eimeria acervulina*-infected chicks, *J. Nutr.*, 113:688.

Staten, F. E., P. A. Anderson, D. H. Baker, and P. C. Harrison. 1980. The efficacy of DL-pantothenic acid relative to D-pantothenic acid in chicks, *Poult. Sci.*, 59:1664 (Abstr.).

Stockland, W. L., and L. G. Blaylock. 1974. Choline requirement of pregnant sows and gilts under restricted feeding conditions, *J. Anim. Sci.*, 39:1113.

Thoren-Tolling, K. 1975. Studies on the absorption of iron after oral administration in piglets, *Acta Vet. Scand. Suppl.*, 54:1.

Trumbo, P. R., J. F. Gregory, and D. B. Sartain. 1988. Incomplete utilization of pyridoxine-beta-glucoside as vitamin B_6 in the rat, *J. Nutr.*, 118:170.

Ullrey, D. E. 1972. Biological availability of fat-soluble vitamins: vitamin A and carotene, *J. Anim. Sci.*, 35:648.

Ullrey, D. E. 1981. Vitamin E for swine, *J. Anim. Sci.*, 53:1039.

Ullrey, D. E., E. R. Miller, J. P. Hitchcock, P. K. Ku, R. L. Covert, J. Hegenauer, and P. Saltman. 1973. Oral ferric citrate vs. ferrous sulfate for prevention of baby pig anemia, *Mich. Agric. Exp. Sta. Rep.*, 232:34.

Verbeeck, J. 1975. Vitamin behavior in premixes, *Feedstuffs*, 47(36):45.

Waibel, P. E., N. A. Nahorniak, H. E. Dziuk, M. M. Walser, and W. G. Olson. 1984. Bioavailability of phosphorus in commercial phosphate supplements for turkeys, *Poult. Sci.*, 63:730.

Watkins, K. L., L. L. Southern, and J. E. Miller. 1991. Effect of dietary biotin supplementation on sow reproductive performance and soundness and pig growth and mortality, *J. Anim. Sci.*, 69:201.

Wedekind, K. J., and D. H. Baker. 1990a. Effect of varying calcium and phosphorus level on manganese utilization, *Poult. Sci.*, 69:1156.

Wedekind, K. J., and D. H. Baker. 1990b. Manganese utilization in chicks as affected by excess calcium and phosphorus ingestion, *Poult. Sci.*, 69:977.

Wedekind, K. J., and D. H. Baker. 1990c. Zinc bioavailability in feed-grade sources of zinc, *J. Anim. Sci.*, 68:684.

Wedekind, K. J., M. R. Murphy, and D. H. Baker. 1991a. Manganese turnover as affected by excess phosphorus consumption, *J. Nutr.*, 121:1035.

Wedekind, K. J., E. C. Titgemeyer, A. R. Twardock, and D. H. Baker. 1991b. Phosphorus, but not calcium, affects manganese absorption and turnover in chicks, *J. Nutr.*, 121:1776.

Wedekind, K. J., A. E. Hortin, and D. H. Baker. 1992. Methodology for assessing zinc bioavailability: efficacy estimates for zinc-methionine, zinc sulfate and zinc oxide, *J. Anim. Sci.*, 70:178.

Wedekind, K. J., A. J. Lewis, M. A. Giesemann, and P. S. Miller. 1994. Bioavailability of zinc from inorganic and organic sources for pigs fed corn–soybean meal diets, *J. Anim. Sci.*, 72:2681.

Wedekind, K. J., R. S. Beyer, and G. F. Combs, Jr. 1998. Is selenium addition necessary in pet foods? *FASEB J.*, A823 (Abstr.).

Wornick, R. C. 1968. The stability of microingredients in animal feed products, *Feedstuffs*, 40:25.

Wright, P. L., and M. C. Bell. 1966. Comparative metabolism of selenium and tellurium in sheep and swine, *Am. J. Physiol.*, 211:6.

Yen, J. T., A. H. Jensen, and D. H. Baker. 1976. Assessment of the concentration of biologically available vitamin B_6 in corn and soybean meal, *J. Anim. Sci.*, 42:866.

Yen, J. T., A. H. Jensen, and D. H. Baker. 1977. Assessment of the availability of niacin in corn, soybeans and soybean meal, *J. Anim. Sci.*, 46:269.

Young, L. G., A. Lun, J. Pos, R. P. Forshaw, and D. E. Edmeades. 1975. Vitamin E stability in corn and mixed feed, *J. Anim. Sci.*, 40:495.

Young, L. G., R. B. Miller, D. E. Edmeades, A. Lun, G. C. Smith, and G. J. King. 1977. Selenium and vitamin E supplementation of high moisture corn diets for swine reproduction, *J. Anim. Sci.*, 45:1051.

Young, L. G., R. B. Miller, D. E. Edmeades, A. Lun, G. C. Smith, and G. J. King. 1978. Influence of method of corn storage and vitamin E and selenium supplementation on pig survival and reproduction, *J. Anim. Sci.*, 47:639.

Zhuge, Q., and C. F. Klopfenstein. 1986. Factors affecting storage stability of vitamin A, riboflavin and niacin in a broiler diet premix, *Poult. Sci.*, 65:987.

17 Water in Swine Nutrition

Philip A. Thacker

CONTENTS

I. Functions of Water 381
II. Sources of Water for Swine 382
III. Routes of Water Excretion by Swine 382
IV. Water Balance in Swine 383
V. Water Use by Various Classes of Swine 383
    A. Suckling Pigs 383
    B. Weanling Pigs 385
    C. Growing-Finishing Pigs 385
    D. Gestating Sows 385
    E. Lactating Sows 386
    F. Boars 386
    G. Summary of Water Requirements of Swine 386
VI. Water Delivery Systems for Pigs 387
VII. Consequences of an Inadequate Water Intake 389
VIII. Reducing Water Wastage in Swine Operations 390
IX. Water Quality for Swine 391
    A. Total Dissolved Solids 391
    B. pH 392
    C. Hardness 392
    D. Sulfates 393
    E. Nitrates 393
    F. Other Contaminants 393
    G. Dealing with Poor-Quality Water 393
References 395

I. FUNCTIONS OF WATER

Water is the nutrient that is required in the largest quantity by swine, and it fulfills a number of physiological functions necessary for life (Roubicek, 1969). It is a major structural element giving form to the body through cell turgidity, and it also plays a crucial role in temperature regulation. Water is important in the movement of nutrients to the cells of the body tissues and for the removal of waste products from these cells. In addition, water plays a role in virtually every chemical reaction that takes place in the body (i.e., hydration and hydrolysis). Finally, water is important in the lubrication of joints (i.e., synovial fluid) and in providing protective cushioning for the nervous system (i.e., cerebrospinal fluid).

    The water content of a pig varies with its age. Water accounts for as much as 82% of the empty body weight (whole-body weight less gastrointestinal tract contents) in the 1.5-kg, neonatal pig and declines to 53% in the 90-kg, market hog (Shields et al., 1983). This change with age occurs

TABLE 17.1
Water Content of the Whole Body of Pigs in Relation to Age and Body Weight

Age (days)	Body Weight (kg)	Water Content (%)
1	1.2	81.5
6	2.2	80.6
28	6.9	65.7
70	22.7	64.6
110	56.0	56.4
155	103.2	48.9

Source: Georgievskii, *Mineral Nutrition of Animals*, 1982, 79–89.

principally because the fat content of the pig increases with age and adipose tissue is considerably lower in water content than is muscle (Georgievskii, 1982). The relationship between age and water content of swine is demonstrated in Table 17.1.

II. SOURCES OF WATER FOR SWINE

Swine obtain water from three main sources: (1) water that is consumed (i.e., drinking water); (2) water that is a natural component of feedstuffs; and (3) metabolic water produced from the breakdown of the carbohydrates, fats, and proteins contained in feed ingredients. The ingredients most commonly used in swine diets contain about 10 to 12% water (NRC, 1998), and so the amount of water supplied from this source can be determined by multiplying the expected feed consumption of a pig by the moisture content of its feed. The amount of metabolic water produced can be calculated based on a chemical analysis of the diet assuming the oxidation of 1 kg of fat, carbohydrate, or protein produces 1190, 560, or 450 g of water, respectively (NRC, 1981). According to Yang et al. (1984), every 1 kg of air-dry feed consumed will produce between 0.38 and 0.48 l of metabolic water. Although metabolic water and the water contained in feed reduce the amount of water that the pig must drink to meet its daily requirements, drinking water is by far the most important source of water for swine.

III. ROUTES OF WATER EXCRETION BY SWINE

Water is lost from the body of pigs by four routes: (1) the kidneys (urination); (2) the intestines (defecation); (3) the lungs (respiration); and (4) the skin (evaporation). Urination is the major route of water excretion in swine although the amount of water excreted is highly variable. The kidneys regulate the volume and composition of body fluids by excreting more or less water, depending on water intake and excretion via other routes. Water excretion is increased when pigs are fed diets that contain large amounts of minerals and protein. The greater the amount of protein in the diet, the greater the water loss, and thus the greater the water requirement (Wahlstrom et al., 1970). Similarly, increased intake of salt results in increases in water intake and a concomitant increase in urinary excretion (Sinclair, 1939).

Significant quantities of water are also lost in the feces. The amount of manure a pig produces per day in confinement ranges from 6.5 to 9% of its body weight, with a water content that varies from 62 to 79% (Brooks and Carpenter, 1993). Water loss through the gut will vary with the nature of the diet. In general, the greater the proportion of undigested material, the greater the water loss (Maynard et al., 1979). Water loss increases with the level of fiber intake (Cooper and Tyler, 1959) and with intake of feeds that have laxative properties (e.g., linseed meal). Water excretion via the feces is increased during diarrhea (Thulin and Brumm, 1991).

Moisture is continually lost from the respiratory tract during the normal process of breathing. Incoming air is both warmed and wetted as it passes over the moist lining of the respiratory tract and is expired at approximately 90% saturation (Roubicek, 1969). For pigs in a thermoneutral environment (20°C), daily respiratory water loss has been estimated to be 0.29 and 0.58 l for pigs of 20 and 60 kg (Holmes and Mount, 1967). The amount of loss is affected by both temperature and relative humidity, with water loss increasing with increased temperature and decreasing with increased humidity.

Sweating and insensible water loss from the skin are not major sources of water loss in swine because the sweat glands are largely dormant. Within the thermoneutral zone, the daily rate of moisture loss has been estimated to be between 12 and 16 g/m^2 (Morrison et al., 1967). Increasing the environmental temperature from −5 to 30°C increased daily water loss from 7 to 32 g/m^2 (Ingram, 1964). However, increased relative humidity had no effect on this loss (Morrison et al., 1967). A summary of factors affecting water consumption and excretion by swine is presented in Table 17.2.

TABLE 17.2
Summary of Factors Affecting Water Consumption and Excretion by Swine

Environmental temperature
Relative humidity
Health of pig (i.e., diarrhea)
Amount of feed consumed
Protein content of diet
Salt content of diet
Fiber content of diet
Water content of diet
Water salinity

IV. WATER BALANCE IN SWINE

The body water status of swine is under tight physiological control (Mroz et al., 1995). At a given body weight and body fat content, the water content of a pig's body is remarkably constant. In certain pathological conditions, excess water may be retained in the tissues (i.e., edema), whereas at other times the body tissues may become depleted of water (dehydration). However, these are unusual circumstances and normally there is very little variation in the water content of a pig's body from day to day. The amount of water excreted from the body is essentially matched by water consumption. An example of water balance in swine is presented in Table 17.3.

V. WATER USE BY VARIOUS CLASSES OF SWINE

A. SUCKLING PIGS

It is a common assumption that suckling pigs do not drink water and can completely satisfy their water requirements by drinking milk because milk contains 80% water. However, suckling pigs, in fact, drink water within 1 or 2 days of birth (Aumaitre, 1964). In addition, because milk is a high-protein, high-mineral food, its consumption can cause increased urinary excretion, which might actually lead to a water deficit (Lloyd et al., 1978). As a consequence, research interest in the water requirements of suckling pigs has increased.

TABLE 17.3
Daily Water Balance for Three Categories of Swine

	Growing Pig (60 kg BW)[a]	Pregnant Sow (140 kg BW)[b]	Lactating Sow (160 kg BW)[c]
Water Input (l/day)			
Drinking water	6.50	11.50	17.50
Water contained in feed[d]	0.31	0.24	0.84
Metabolic water[e]	1.07	0.82	2.89
Total water consumption	7.88	12.56	21.23
Water Output (l/day)			
Growth[f]	0.70	0.17	—
Urine	5.22	9.39	9.09
Feces[g]	0.96	0.74	2.60
Milk[h]	—	—	7.20
Skin[i]	0.42	0.72	0.78
Lungs[j]	0.58	1.40	1.56
Other[k]	—	0.14	—
Total water excretion	7.88	12.56	21.23

[a] Water balance for a 60-kg growing pig gaining 1.0 kg/day and consuming 2.6 kg of feed.
[b] Water balance for a 140-kg gestating sow gaining 50 kg in gestation (27.2 kg of maternal gain and 22.8 kg of conceptus) with an expected litter size of ten pigs.
[c] Water balance for a 160-kg sow in lactation, losing 10 kg in a 21-day lactation suckling a litter of ten pigs which are gaining 225 g/day.
[d] Assumes a feed with 12% moisture content and 80% digestibility.
[e] Metabolic water calculated assuming all feeds had 5% fat, 15% crude protein, and 60% carbohydrate, and that the oxidation of 1 kg of fat, carbohydrate or protein produces 1190, 560, or 450 g of water (NRC, 1981).
[f] Assumes body tissue is 70% water.
[g] Assumes feces contain 65% water and all feeds are 80% digestible.
[h] Assumes milk is 80% water.
[i] Equal to 13.2 ml/m^2/h (Mroz et al., 1995).
[j] Equal to 0.01 kg^{-1} BW daily (Mroz et al., 1995).
[k] Fetus, fluids, and membranes that contain 70% water.

Fraser et al. (1988) suggested that providing a supplemental water supply may help to reduce preweaning mortality. They speculated that undernourished pigs, especially those housed in warm environments, may be prone to dehydration during the first few days after farrowing and that at least some pigs have the developmental maturity to compensate by drinking water. Exposed water surfaces (i.e., bowls or cups) are superior to nipple drinkers for this purpose (Phillips and Fraser, 1990; 1991).

Fraser et al. (1988) measured water use by 51 suckling litters during the first 4 days after farrowing. The use varied greatly among litters, ranging from 0 to 200 g/day with an average consumption of 46 g/pig/day. This level of intake is considerably higher than that reported in earlier work in which average water intakes were closer to 10 ml/pig/day. Fraser et al. (1993) speculated that the more recently recorded consumption levels may be a reflection of an increased emphasis on temperature control in farrowing rooms and that the higher temperatures currently used in swine barns may lead to an increase in moisture loss from the pig. Their data showed almost a fourfold increase in water consumption when pigs were housed at 28°C than when housed at 20°C. Pig health is another factor that affects water intake because it has been shown that suckling pigs with diarrhea consumed 15% less water than healthy pigs (Baranyiova and Holub, 1993).

After the first week of life, the principal concern regarding the water consumption of suckling pigs is the role it plays in stimulating creep feed consumption. Although the consumption of creep feed by pigs is usually low during the first 3 weeks, subsequent feed intake is lower if water is not provided (Friend and Cunningham, 1966).

B. Weanling Pigs

Gill et al. (1986) measured the water intake of weaned pigs from 3 to 6 weeks of age. Daily water intake during the first, second, and third week after weaning averaged 0.49, 0.89, and 1.46 l per pig. The relationship between feed intake and water consumption was described by Brooks et al. (1984) using the following equation:

$$\text{Water intake (l/day)} = 0.149 + (3.053 \times \text{kg daily dry feed intake})$$

McLeese et al. (1992) observed two distinct patterns of water intake. During the first phase, lasting about 5 days after weaning, water intake fluctuated independently of apparent physiological need and did not seem to be related to growth, feed intake, or the severity of diarrhea. In the second period, water intake followed a consistent pattern that paralleled growth and feed intake. The authors speculated that during the first few days after weaning, water consumption might be high, as a consequence of a need for gut fill to obtain a sense of satiety in the absense of feed intake. Brooks et al. (1984) reported a diurnal pattern to water intake for weaned pigs housed under conditions of constant light, with a higher consumption from 0830 to 1700 hours than from 1700 to 0830 hours.

The importance of water intake as a factor affecting the performance of weaned pigs cannot be overstated. Restricted water flow reduced feed intake of pigs aged 3 to 6 weeks by approximately 15% and had a similar effect on growth (Barber et al., 1989).

C. Growing-Finishing Pigs

Water consumption by growing-finishing pigs generally has a positive relationship with feed intake and body weight (Evvard, 1929). The minimum requirement for pigs between 20 and 90 kg body weight is approximately 2 kg of water for each 1 kg of feed (Cumby, 1986). The voluntary water intake of growing pigs allowed to consume feed *ad libitum* is approximately 2.5 kg of water for each 1 kg of feed (Braude et al., 1957). Pigs receiving restricted amounts of feed have been reported to consume 3.7 kg of water per 1 kg of feed (Cumby, 1986). The difference between *ad libitum* and restricted-fed pigs might be due to the tendency of pigs to fill themselves with water if their appetite is not satisfied by their feed allowance (Yang et al., 1984).

Olsson and Andersson (1985), using nose-operated drinking devices, concluded that water consumption at feeding for growing-finishing pigs has a distinct periodicity, with a peak at the beginning and end of the feeding period. Water consumption between feeding periods peaked 2 h after the morning feeding and 1 h after the afternoon feeding.

Mount et al. (1971) reported little difference in water consumption by growing pigs kept at temperatures of 7, 9, 12, 20, or 22°C, although there was considerable variation among pigs at any one temperature. However, at 30 and 33°C, the intake of water increased considerably. At 30°C and above, Close et al. (1971) observed behavioral responses to increased temperature. Urine and feces were voided over the whole pen area, and water was spilled from the water bowl presumably in an attempt to cool the pig's body surface.

D. Gestating Sows

The water intake of pregnant gilts increases in correspondence with dry matter intake (Friend, 1971). For unbred gilts, feed and water intake diminished during estrus (Friend, 1973; Friend and Wolynetz, 1981). Nonpregnant gilts consumed 11.5 kg of water daily, whereas gilts in advanced pregnancy consumed 20 kg (Bauer, 1982). These quantities are similar to the values of 13.5 kg reported by Riley (1978), 10.0 kg reported by Lightfoot and Armsby (1984), and 11 to 15 kg reported by Klopfenstein et al. (1994).

The practice of feed or water deprivation before or after weaning as a means of reducing the weaning-to-breeding interval in sows is not well supported by research evidence (Knabe et al., 1986). According to Madec (1984), urinary disorders are quite common in sows, and low water intake is strongly implicated. Pregnant sows given restricted levels of feed intake may show a desire to compensate for inadequate gut fill by an enhanced water intake. Current interest in increasing the fiber content of gestation diets is also likely to increase the required ratio of water to feed.

E. Lactating Sows

Lactating sows need considerable amounts of water, not only to replace the 8 to 12 kg of milk secreted but also to void large amounts of metabolic end products in the urine. Daily water consumption for lactating sows was shown to vary from 12 to 40 l/day, with a mean of 18 l/day (Lightfoot, 1978). These quantities are similar to other recorded values for the daily water intake of lactating sows of 20 kg (Bauer, 1982), 25.1 kg (Riley, 1978), 17.7 kg (Lightfoot and Armsby, 1984), and 20 kg (Klopfenstein et al., 1994).

Fraser and Phillips (1989) reported that suckling pig weight gains were correlated with the sow's water intake during lactation and that water intake was in turn correlated with the sow's degree of physical activity. They suggested that some sows are extremely lethargic during the first days after farrowing and fail to consume adequate amounts of water and that this could contribute to low milk production in early lactation and to reduced pig weight gain and survival.

F. Boars

There are few data on the water requirements of boars, but free access to water is advisable. Straub et al. (1976) observed water intakes in boars (70 to 110 kg) of up to 15 l/day at 25°C compared with about 10 l/day at 15°C.

G. Summary of Water Requirements of Swine

In determining water requirements, care must be taken to distinquish between water consumption and water disappearance. True water usage by pigs is usually overestimated because wastage is generally not taken into account. In addition, as previously noted, factors such as feed intake, ingredients contained in the diet, ambient temperature and humidity, state of health, and stress level will all affect water requirements. It is therefore difficult to provide universal estimates of requirements. Table 17.4 provides a summary of requirement estimates for the various classes of swine.

TABLE 17.4
Estimates of Water Requirements for Various Classes of Swine (l/day)

Class of Swine	Pederson (1994)	Lumb (1998)	Cleary (1983)	Anderson et al. (1984)
Suckling pigs	1–2	0.27	—	—
Weanling pigs	1–5	1.20	—	1.3–2.5
Growing pigs	5–10	2.25	3–7	2.5–3.8
Finishing pigs	5–10	6.00	7–12	3.8–7.5
Gestating sows	12–20	5–8	12–15	13–17
Lactating sows	25–35	15–30	18–23	18–23
Boars	8–10	—	12–15	13–17

VI. WATER DELIVERY SYSTEMS FOR PIGS

The most commonly used drinking devices for providing water to swine can be grouped into three simple categories: bite drinkers, nipple drinkers, and bowls (Gill and Barber, 1990). Bite drinkers release water when a spring-loaded valve is opened by a biting action. In nipple drinkers, the valve is opened when a small teat is pushed in or displaced sideways. Bowl drinkers can be further subdivided into two additional subgroups: the self-refill and the pig-operated types (Gill and Barber, 1990). Self-refill bowls provide a drinking reservoir or a given volume that is held constant by a protected floating valve assemby. This operates like a ball valve in a header tank, thus ensuring that any water removed from the bowl dispenser is immediately replenished. Pig-operated bowl drinkers have a rigid flap or lever that must be pushed against a spring-loaded valve to allow the release of water into a collecting basin. A sampling of the types of drinkers currently available was published in *International Pig Topics* (Vol. 12, No. 7, pp. 35–37).

There has been little research conducted to access accurately what type of drinker is best for each phase of production. For very young pigs, a water bowl is recommended because nipple drinkers are not readily used by suckling pigs (Phillips and Fraser, 1990), and the provision of an obvious source of water seems to result in the pigs finding the water faster (Phillips and Fraser, 1991). A University of Nebraska study reported 70% higher water use by suckling pigs provided water from a cup vs. a bowl although much of the increase was attributed to increased wastage (Carlson and Peo, 1979). The bowl should be set quite low with a fairly deep water level so the pig can immerse its mouth (Upjohn Limited, 1985). A hood is recommended to prevent fecal contamination of the bowl (Gadd, 1988b). Phillips and Fraser (1989) describe a water dispenser that bubbled to attract the pig's attention and thereby increased water use by pigs during the first few days of life.

For weanling pigs, nipple waterers work well, although some producers prefer small bowl waterers for young pigs unaccustomed to nipple waterers. Some producers attempt to attract weanling pigs to the water source by leaving the nipple dripping, but controlled experiments showed there was no advantage in using drip vs. nondrip waterers (Ogunbameru et al., 1991). Several commercial operations have recently adopted the use of turkey drinkers as a means of stimulating water intake of early weaned pigs and have observed an increase in growth (Dunn, 1997; Gadd, 1997; Table 17.5).

Gill and Barber (1990) showed that the performance of growing pigs was not affected by the type of drinker (three bite and one nipple drinker were tested) when tested under *ad libitum* feeding conditions, but daily gain and feed intake increased when water was supplied through one of the bite drinkers used under restricted-feeding conditions. The nipple drinker seemed to result in increased water wastage, and therefore bite drinkers are recommended.

TABLE 17.5
Effect of Type of Drinker on Weanling Pig Performance

	Control Drinker	Turkey Drinker
Starting weight (kg)	6.2	6.2
Finishing weight (kg)	22.1	23.7
Daily gain (g)	388	427
Daily feed intake (g)	686	738
Feed efficiency	1.77	1.73

Source: Gadd, *Pigs*, 13(2):19, 1997.

TABLE 17.6
Comparison of Water Consumption by Lactating Sows Provided Water via a Trough or Drinker

	Water Source	
	Trough	Drinker
Water used (l/d)	23	18
Water spillage (l/d)	ND[a]	3.6
Feed consumption (kg/d)	6.61	6.04
Pig weaning weight (kg)	6.03	5.81

[a] No detectable wastage

Source: Gadd, *West. Hog J.*, 18(2):11–13, 1996.

For sows, particularly during lactation, high water intakes are required to support the demands for milk production. Although nipple and bite drinkers will eventually provide adequate water, some sows become frustrated and stop drinking before sufficient water has been obtained. A recent study suggested that lactating sows receiving water via a trough located next to the feed bowl drank more water and wasted less, resulting in higher feed intakes and therefore weaning heavier pigs (Gadd, 1996; Table 17.6). Many producers find that filling the sow's feed trough with water after feeding is a useful way of stimulating water intake. The depth of water in the trough is very important as pigs are not designed to lick up water. For example, for sows, a depth of 3.8 cm has been recommended (Carr, 1993).

Most animal welfare codes recommend at least one waterer for every 10 to 15 pigs (Ministry of Agriculture, Fisheries and Food, 1983; Agriculture and Agri-Food Canada, 1993). For practical purposes, it is wise to have a minimum of two drinkers per pen, regardless of how few animals are in the pen, in case one drinker ceases to function. In addition, it has been suggested that when only one drinker is present, competition at the drinker results in increased water wastage (Barber et al., 1988).

There would seem to be little benefit from providing additional waterers over the two waterer minimum. Gadd (1988a) showed no difference in performance when growing pigs were given two, three, or four drinkers per pen (40 pigs/pen) and researchers at the Scottish Agricultural College found no detrimental effect on performance from having 20 growing pigs per nipple compared with the 10 recommended by animal welfare codes (Anonymous, 1999a). Where more than one drinker is placed in a pen, the drinkers should be placed far enough apart so that they are outside the attack radius of a pig (i.e., for weanling pigs the nozzles should be >38 cm apart and be >76 cm apart for larger pigs; Gadd, 1988b).

There are few published guidelines on the appropriate height for drinkers for different classes of swine. As a rough guide, it is suggested that positioning the drinker 10 to 15 cm above the pig's backline wastes the least water by getting the pigs head up (Gadd, 1988a). Nozzles should be set at 15 to 25° from the horizontal. Published recommendations for drinker heights are compared in Table 17.7.

Angles of presentation for bite and nipple drinkers have been tested where the direction has been changed from downward to upward (Carlson and Peo, 1982). In this mode of presentation, extra savings in water use has been reported, but there have been problems of blockage by waterborne particles settling in the delivery bend. Therefore, this practice should be avoided because unnoticed restriction can result in considerable animal losses from dehydration.

TABLE 17.7
Recommended Heights (cm) of Nipple Drinkers for Swine[a]

	Agriculture and Agri-Food Canada (1993)	Carr (1993)	Pederson (1994)	Gadd (1988b)
Suckling pigs	15	10–13	10	8–10
Weanling pigs	20	10–13	25–30	35–45
Growing pigs	20–30	13–30	25–30	35–45
Finishing pigs	30–40	30–61	35–45	50–60
Gestating sows	50–61	76–91	75	80–90
Lactating sows	50–61	76–91	75	80–90
Boars	50–61	76–91	—	—

[a] Height of nipple from the floor is based on the nipple being placed at a 90° angle to the wall. Height would be higher for a 45° angle sloping down or lower for a 45° angle sloping up.

VII. CONSEQUENCES OF AN INADEQUATE WATER INTAKE

As stated previously, water is the most essential nutrient for life. Unlike some other nutrients, where failure to meet nutrient requirements may only result in slight reductions in performance, failure to provide an adequate water supply can have devastating consequences and in extreme cases can result in death (Maynard et al., 1979). One of the first symptoms of an inadequate water supply is a reduction in feed intake. Any unexplained drop in feed intake should automatically trigger an immediate check of the water supply. Additional symptoms of water deprivation are summarized in Table 17.8.

There are many situations in which the water supply to pigs may be inadvertently affected (Table 17.9). These can be partitioned into acute and chronic shortages. A sudden reduction in water supply can result if the water is mistakenly turned off. To minimize the possibility of this occurring, barn staff should be made aware of the serious consequences that may follow if such an error is made. More easily prevented are water shortages that occur when the water lines become blocked or frozen. Blockages can occur from hard water scale accumulation, rust, or microbial contamination. Frozen water lines are unlikely to occur in modern confinement operations but have occurred in situations where water lines are placed under ventilation fan openings without proper insulation. Filters should be considered to prevent dirt and debris from entering the watering system.

Acute water shortages are usually obvious and, provided immediate steps are taken to rectify the problem, generally do not result in serious economic loss. Of greater concern are chronic restrictions that may go unnoticed for years. Chronic restriction may be caused by having an

TABLE 17.8
Symptoms of Water Deprivation in Swine

Reduced feed intake
Crowding around drinker
Dehydration
Diarrhea in piglets
Increased heart rate
Increased body temperature
Increased respiration
Death

TABLE 17.9
Possible Reasons for Reduced Water Consumption by Swine

Water supply turned off
Rusted or blocked pipes
Frozen water lines
Low water pressure
Too many pigs in pen
Poor drinker design
Inappropriate drinker height
Poor water quality

inappropriate ratio of pigs to waterers (i.e., too many pigs in a pen), poor drinker design, low water pressure, or poor-quality water. Excessive water pressure may also reduce intakes by preventing drinkers from functioning properly. The force that it takes to open the valve should not be higher than 1000 g for nipple drinkers and 500 g for bite drinkers (Pedersen, 1994).

The appropriate flow rate for swine watering systems has been the subject of some controversy. On the one hand, inadequate flow rate depresses water intake, which may lead to a depression in pig performance. On the other hand, excessive flow rates have been reported to lead to water wastage. For nursery pigs, Barber et al. (1989) reported better performance with increased flow of water. In contrast, Nienaber and Hahn (1984) studied the effects of water flow restriction on the performance of weanling pigs and showed little effect on growth when flow rates were varied between 0.1 and 1.1 l/min. However, water use was significantly higher with a more rapid flow rate, which was attributed to increased wastage of water.

Barber et al. (1988) studied the effect of water delivery rate on the water use of growing pigs. A high (900 ml^3/min) delivery rate increased water use (3.8 l/day) compared with a low (300 ml^3/min) delivery rate (1.9 l/day). However, pig performance was not affected.

Philips et al. (1990) observed no difference in water consumption between sows housed in crates with high (2 l/min) vs. low (0.6 l/min) flow rates of nipple drinkers. However, Hoppe et al. (1987) reported higher lactation feed intakes and lower weight loss for sows provided with a water flow rate of 700 vs. 70 ml/min. Phillips et al. (1995) suggested that a flow rate of 1.8 l/min was adequate for sows, whereas Swedish researchers have recently recommended flow rates as high as 3 to 4 l/min (Anonymous, 1999b).

It should be clear from the discussion above that there is no single recommendation for flow rates that will suit all situations. How much one pays for slurry disposal and whether there is a charge for water usage will both weigh heavily on any decision regarding the establishment of flow rates. The flow rates in Table 17.10 are a compromise and seem adequate for most situations.

VIII. REDUCING WATER WASTAGE IN SWINE OPERATIONS

Although provision of adequate amounts of water is essential, increased water costs plus legislative moves to reduce farm effluent output and limit pollution from intensive units has led to the investigation of methods to minimize water wastage without compromising animal performance. Some potential causes of water wastage were reviewed by Thacker (1998) and are listed in Table 17.11.

The type of drinker will affect water wastage. Gill and Barber (1990) compared four types of drinkers and observed a 40% difference in water usage, with nipple drinkers wasting more water than a bite drinker. One particular feature that seems useful in reducing waste is to mount a metal flange (wing) on both sides of the drinker so that a sideways approach cannot be made (Gill and Barber, 1990). Gadd (1992) reported a 55% reduction in wastage using drinker wings.

TABLE 17.10
Recommended Flow Rates of Water for Different Classes of Swine (l/min)

	Agriculture and Agri-Food Canada (1993)	Carr (1993)	Pederson (1994)	Gadd (1988)	Lumb (1998)
Suckling pigs	0.3	0.3	0.5	0.25	—
Weanling pigs	0.5–1.0	0.7	0.5–0.8	0.50	0.5
Growing pigs	1–1.5	1.0	0.8–1.2	0.66	0.7
Finishing pigs	1–1.5	1.5	0.8–1.2	0.75	0.7
Gestating sows	2	1.5–2.0	1.5–2.0	1.00	1.0
Lactating sows	2	1.5–2.0	4.0	1.00	1.5

TABLE 17.11
Factors Leading to Increased Water Wastage in Swine Operations

Inappropriate flow rates
Inappropriate drinker height
Poor drinker design
Failure to use drinker wings
Poor location of drinker
Improper drinker angle
Inadequate maintenace
Leaking water nipples

The position of the drinker also affects waste. Positioning a drinker 10 to 15 cm above the pig's backline wastes the least amount of water by getting the pigs head up (Gadd, 1988a). Sometimes, drinkers are set too low. As a result, the pig turns sideways to drink and up to 60% of the water flows out of the other side of its mouth (Gadd, 1988b). Therefore, the appropriate heights listed above should be followed. Wastage was reduced by 40% when drinkers were placed on the back of a deliberate division between sleeping and dunging areas so that the drinker faced the dunging area (Olsson, 1983). The flow rate is also important. An excessive flow rate of 900 ml/min compared with a more conventional rate of 300 ml/min with pigs 30 to 60 kg produces an extra 78 l of slurry per pig over 40 days (Gadd, 1988a). In addition, leaking or poorly maintained drinkers will increase water usage.

The way in which pigs use a drinker also has a marked effect on the extent of water wastage from it (Brooks, 1994). A considerable amount of wastage occurs as a result of pigs using the drinker in a manner which the designer had not intended.

Poor diet formulation can also increase water usage unnecessarily. Hagsten and Perry (1976) showed how the water consumption of growing pigs increased in response to salt additions to the diet. Similar findings were reported by Friend and Wolynetz (1981) for gestating and lactating sows. Protein-rich diets are also likely to increase water use and increase the volume of urine (Wahlstrom et al., 1970). Care should be taken to provide adequate but not excessive dietary salt and protein.

IX. WATER QUALITY FOR SWINE

Elements and other substances can occur in water at levels that are harmful to pigs (NRC, 1974). Water may contain a variety of microorganisms, including both bacteria and viruses. Of the former, *Salmonella*, *Leptospira*, and *Escherichia coli* are the most commonly encountered (Fraser et al., 1993). Water can also carry pathogenic protozoa as well as eggs or cysts of intestinal worms. Whether the presence of these microorganisms will be detrimental is largely dependent on the specific types found and their concentration. The Bureau of National Affairs (1973) proposed that water used for livestock should not contain more than 5000 coliforms/100 ml. However, this can only be considered as a guide because some pathogens may be harmful below this level, whereas other, more benign microorganisms can be tolerated at much higher levels. Bacterial contamination is usually more common in surface waters than in underground supplies such as deep wells and artesian water.

A. TOTAL DISSOLVED SOLIDS

Total dissolved solids (TDS) is a measure of the total inorganic matter dissolved in a sample of water. Calcium, magnesium, and sodium in the bicarbonate, chloride, or sulfate form are the most common salts found in water with a high TDS (Thulin and Brumm, 1991). Water containing >6000 ppm TDS may cause temporary diarrhea and increased daily water intake, although health and performance are not usually affected. Paterson et al. (1979), offered water containing 5060 ppm TDS to gilts and sows and reported no significant effects on reproduction. The addition of up to 6000 ppm TDS to water offered to weaned pigs resulted in no effect on growth or feed efficiency. However, increases in water intake were reported along with temporary mild diarrhea and less firm feces for pigs offered the higher TDS levels in their water (Anderson and Stothers, 1978; Paterson et al., 1979).

Total dissolved solids is an inexact measure of water quality. As a general rule, water containing <1000 ppm TDS should be safe, whereas water containing >7000 ppm TDS may present a health risk for pregnant or lactating sows or stressed pigs and should not be offered to swine for consumption (NRC, 1974). Between 1000 and 7000 ppm is a gray area with some producers reporting economical loss at levels well below 7000 ppm, whereas others experience transient or minor inconvenience at worst. Since so many different elements can contribute to a high TDS, further chemical analysis should be conducted on such water to determine whether the soluble minerals present represent a health risk. However, the values in Table 17.12 can be used as a guide.

TABLE 17.12
Evaluation of Water Quality for Pigs Based on Total Dissolved Solids (TDS ppm)

TDS	Rating	Comment
<1000	Safe	No risk to pigs
1000–2999	Satisfactory	Mild diarrhea in pigs not adapted to it
3000–4999	Satisfactory	Temporary diarrhea and water refusal initially when pigs not accustomed to them; may cause increased water consumption
5000–7999	Reasonable	May be used with reasonable safety for growing-finishing pigs; should avoid the use of water approaching the higher levels for breeding stock
>7000	Unfit	Considerable risk may exist with pregnant or lactating sows, or with pigs subjected to heat stress, water loss, or disease conditions

Source: Adapted from NRC (1974).

B. pH

The pH of water has little direct relevance to water quality because almost all samples fall within the acceptable range of 6.5 to 8.5 (Fraser et al., 1993). However, alterations in pH can have a major impact on chemical reactions involved in the treatment of water. High water pH impairs the efficiency of chlorination, and low water pH may cause precipitation of some antibacterial agents delivered via the water system. Sulfonamides are particularly at risk (Russell, 1985) and could lead to potential problems with carcass sulfa residues, because precipitated medication in the water lines may leach back into the water after medication has been terminated.

C. Hardness

Water hardness is caused by multivalent metal cations, principally calcium and magnesium. Water is considered soft if hardness is <60 ppm, hard between 120 and 180 ppm, and very hard when >180 ppm (Durfor and Becker, 1964). Even very hard water rarely causes problems for swine (NRC, 1980), although it does result in the accumulation of scale in water-delivery systems. If this impairs water availabilty, problems can arise. In one survey, water was found to supply as much as 28% of a sow's daily requirement for calcium (Filipot and Ouellet, 1988).

D. SULFATES

Sulfates are the primary cause of water quality problems in well water in many regions of North America. A survey conducted on the Canadian prairies indicated that 25% of wells contained excessive (>1000 ppm) quantities of sulfates (McLeese et al., 1991). Sulfates are not well tolerated in the gut of the pig, resulting in diarrhea and reduced performance when levels are >7000 ppm (Anderson et al., 1994). However, lower levels (2650 ppm) have no detrimental effect on pig performance (Maenz et al., 1994). It would seem that pigs can adapt to elevated sulfate levels within a few weeks of exposure. This explains why weanling pigs are most susceptible to sulfates because they consume little water before weaning and, as a consequence, are not adapted. In addition, water odor is not necessarily an indication of poor quality water. Despite a distinct "rotten egg" smell, water containing 1900 ppm sulfates did not affect pig performance (DeWit et al., 1987).

E. NITRATES

Heavy applications of nitrogenous fertilizers to land and contamination of runoff water by animal wastes can raise nitrate concentrations in water supplies to exceedingly high levels. Factors associated with the nitrate concentration of water wells on farms in the United States were reviewed by Bruning-Fann et al. (1994).

Nitrites impair the oxygen-carrying capacity of the blood by reducing hemoglobin to methemoglobin. Winks et al. (1950) found that conversion of nitrate to nitrite in the water was necessary for toxicity to occur. They reported mortality in swine with access to well water containing 290 to 490 ppm of nitrate nitrogen. However, Seerley et al. (1965) considered it unlikely that sufficient nitrite would be formed and consumed in water alone to cause toxicity in swine unless the initial level of nitrate exceeds 300 ppm of nitrate nitrogen. Nitrite levels greater than 10 ppm are cause for concern (Task Force on Water Quality Guidelines, 1987). Nitrates and nitrites in water also may impair the use of vitamin A by the pig (Wood et al., 1967).

F. OTHER CONTAMINANTS

Additional ions may be found from time to time in water samples. Examples of these are iron, aluminum, beryllium, boron, chromium, cobalt, copper, iodine, manganese, molybdenum and zinc. Safety guidelines for these and other elements are provided in Table 17.13. However, it should be noted that it would be exceedingly rare for these elements to cause any problems for swine either because they do not normally occur at high levels or because they are toxic only at very high concentrations. A survey of 135 wells used to provide water for swine operations in Western Canada showed that the vast majority of water wells produced samples that were significantly below the recommended maximum limit for all of these elements, and many had mineral concentrations below the detectable limits of the chemical analysis used (Table 17.14).

A second group of elements that can be toxic at lower levels includes arsenic, cadmium, fluorine, lead, mercury, and selenium. While these may harm animals that drink these waters, the major concern is that they do not accumulate in pork products used for human consumption. Analyses for these elements are only done when there is good reason to suspect their presence since most water supplies would contain only trace levels of these elements (see Table 17.14).

G. DEALING WITH POOR-QUALITY WATER

In situations where poor-quality water exists, it is essential to determine the impact of the poor-quality water on animal performance. Often, producers are overly concerned about diarrhea in situations where animal performance is not impaired. However, when poor water quality reduces performance, there are a number of things that can be done to alleviate the problem.

TABLE 17.13
Water Quality Guidelines for Swine

	Recommended Maximum (ppm)	
	TFWQG[a]	NRC[b]
Major Ions		
Calcium	1000	—
Nitrate-N + Nitrite-N	100	440
Nitrite-N	10	33
Sulfate	1000	—
Heavy Metals and Trace Ions		
Aluminum	5.0	—
Arsenic	0.5	0.2
Beryllium	0.1	—
Boron	5.0	—
Cadmium	0.02	0.05
Chromium	1.0	1.0
Cobalt	1.0	1.0
Copper	5.0	0.5
Fluoride	2.0	2.0
Lead	0.1	0.1
Mercury	0.003	0.01
Molybenum	0.5	—
Nickel	1.0	1.0
Selenium	0.05	—
Uranium	0.2	—
Vanadium	0.1	0.1
Zinc	50.0	25.0

[a] Task Force on Water Quality Guidelines, 1987. Canadian Water Quality Guidelines, Inland Waters Directorate, Ottawa, Ontario.
[b] Adapted from NRC (1974).

Chlorination disinfects and destroys disease-causing microrganisms. Protozoa and enteroviruses are much more resistant to chlorination than are bacteria (Fraser et al., 1993). The effectiveness of disinfection and the quantity of chlorine required in the water depends on the quantity of nitrites, iron, hydrogen sulfide, ammonia, and organic matter in the water. The presence of organic matter in the water converts the free chlorine to chloramines, which have less disinfecting action. Sodium hypochlorite or laundry bleach (5.25% chlorine solution) is commonly used for chlorination. The higher the pH, the more chlorine that is needed to achieve the same degree of disinfection.

Some changes in the diet may be warranted in response to water quality problems. A reduction in the salt (NaCl) level in the diet is common on farms that use water containing a high mineral (TDS) load. Some salt can usually be removed without causing a problem because most diets contain a reasonable safety margin. However, care must be taken to ensure that adequate chloride levels are maintained in the diet because chloride is not usually found in high concentration in poor-quality water.

Hard water may be improved with a water softener. The most common type is an ion-exchange unit in which sodium replaces calcium and magnesium in the water. This reduces the hardness of the water but has no effect on the overall mineral load (TDS) because the water then has a higher sodium content. Reverse osmosis units are available to remove sulfates, but both the capital and operating costs of the equipment are prohibitive for a livestock unit.

TABLE 17.14
Chemical Analysis of Well Waters (n = 135) Used for Swine Production (mg/l)

	Mean	Minimum	Maximum	% Below Detectable Limits
Aluminum	0.06	0.005	0.48	58.8
Beryllium	0.002	0.001	0.005	79.4
Boron	0.71	0.02	5.70	8.1
Cadmium	0.001	0.001	0.002	96.3
Chromium	0.006	0.001	0.150	44.9
Cobalt	0.002	0.001	0.007	82.4
Copper	0.019	0.001	0.570	41.9
Fluoride	0.35	0.05	4.10	0.0
Lead	0.012	0.010	0.070	20.6
Molybenum	0.014	0.005	0.039	29.4
Nickel	0.006	0.001	0.076	33.8
Silicon	4.58	1.10	9.90	0.0
Silver	0.0	0.0	0.0	99.9
Titanium	0.012	0.001	0.042	90.4
Tungsten	0.0	0.0	0.0	99.9
Vanadium	0.025	0.010	0.070	20.6
Zinc	0.165	0.001	4.20	8.8

Source: Adapted from McLeese et al. (1991).

REFERENCES

Agriculture and Agri-Food Canada. 1993. Recommended code of practice for the care and handling of farm animals: Pigs, Agriculture and Agri-Food Canada Publication 1898/E, Ottawa, Canada.

Anderson, D. M., and S. C. Stothers. 1978. Effects of saline water high in sulfates, chlorides and nitrates on the performance of young weanling pigs, *J. Anim. Sci.*, 47:900.

Anderson, D. M., S. Jaikaran, and S. C. Stothers. 1984. Water for swine, Manitoba Swine Facts, Agdex 440–68.

Anderson, J. S., D. M. Anderson, and J. M. Murphy. 1994. The effect of water quality on nutrient availability for grower/finisher pigs, *Can. J. Anim. Sci.*, 74:141.

Anonymous. 1999a. Water intake in growing pigs, *Pig Int.*, 29(1):35.

Anonymous. 1999b. Water for the nursing sow, *Pig Int.*, 29(1):33.

Aumaitre, A. 1964. Le besoin en eau du porcelet: Étude de la consommation d'eau avant le sevrage. [Water requirements of suckling piglets], *Ann. Zootechnol.*, 13:183.

Baranyiova, E., and A. Holub. 1993. Effect of diarrhaea on water consumption of piglets weaned on the first day after birth, *Acta Vet. Brno*, 62:27.

Barber, J., P. H. Brooks, and J. L. Carpenter. 1988. The effect of water delivery rate and drinker number on the water use of growing pigs, *Anim. Prod.*, 46:521 (Abstr.).

Barber, J., P. H. Brooks, and J. L. Carpenter. 1989. The effects of water delivery rate on the voluntary feed intake, water use and performance of early weaned pigs from 3–6 weeks of age. In *The Voluntary Feed Intake of Pigs*, Forbes, J. M., M. A. Varley, and T. L. J. Lawrence, Eds., British Society of Animal Production, Edinburgh, 103–104.

Bauer, W. 1982. Der Tränkwasserverbrauch güster, hochtragender und laktierender Jungsauen [Consumption of drinking water by nonpregnant, pregnant and lactating gilts], *Arch. Exp. Vet. Med.*, 36:823.

Braude, R., P. M. Clarke, K. G. Mitchell, A. S. Cray, A. Franke, and P. H. Sedgwick. 1957. Unrestricted whey for fattening pigs, *J. Agric. Sci.* (Cambridge), 49:347.

Brooks, P. H. 1994. Water: forgotten nutrient and novel delivery system. In *Biotechnology in the Feed Industry, Proceedings of Alltech's Tenth Annual Symposium*, Lyons, P., and K. A. Jacques, Eds., Nottingham University Press, Loughborough, U.K., 211–234.

Brooks, P. H., and J. L. Carpenter. 1993. The water requirement of growing-finishing pigs: Theoretical and practical considerations. In *Recent Developments in Pig Nutrition*, 2, Coles, D. J., W. Haresign, and P. C. Garnsworthy, Eds., Nottingham University Press, Loughborough, U.K., 179–200.

Brooks, P. H., S. J. Russel, and J. L. Carpenter. 1984. Water intake of weaned piglets from three to seven weeks old, *Vet. Rec.*, 115:513.

Bruning-Fann, C., J. B. Kaneene, R. A. Miller, I. Gardner, R. Johnson, and F. Ross. 1994. The use of epidemiological concepts and techniques to discern factors associated with the nitrate concentration of well water on swine farms in the USA, *Sci. Total Environ.*, 153:85.

Bureau of National Affairs. 1973. EPA drafts water quality criteria as required under federal order law, *Environ. Rep.*, 4:663.

Carlson, R. L., and E. R. Peo. 1979. H_2O — critical swine nutrient, Nebraska Swine Report, Lincoln, NE, 20–21.

Carlson, R. L., and E. R. Peo. 1982. Nipple waterer position: up or down? Nebraska Swine Report, Lincoln, NE, 8–9.

Carr, J. 1993. Are your stockmanship skills a match for your pig's water requirements, *Pig Farm.*, July:26–40.

Cleary, G. 1983. Water requirements of piggeries, Government of Victoria's Department of Agriculture AgNote 2136/83.

Close, W. H., L. E. Mount, and I. B. Start. 1971. The influence of environmental temperature and plane of nutrition on heat losses from groups of growing pigs, *Anim. Prod.*, 13:285.

Cooper, P. H., and C. Tyler. 1959. Some effects of bran and cellulose on the water relationships in the digesta and faeces of pigs. Part 1. The effect of including bran and two forms of cellulose in otherwise normal rations, *J. Agric. Sci.* (Cambridge), 52:332.

Cumby, T. R. 1986. Design requirements of liquid feeding systems for pigs: a review, *J. Agric. Eng. Res.*, 34:332.

DeWit, P., L. G. Young, R. Wenzell, R. Friendship, and D. Peer. 1987. Water quality and pig performance, *Can. J. Anim. Sci.*, 67:1196 (Abstr.).

Dunn, N. 1997. Performance gains from easy access, *Pigs*, 13(6):32.

Durfor, C. M., and E. Becker. 1964. USGS Water-Supply Paper 1812, U.S. Government Printing Office, Washington, D.C.

Evvard, J. M. 1929. A new feeding method and standards for fattening young swine, *Iowa Agric. Exp. Sta. Res. Bull. 118*, Iowa State University Press, Ames.

Filpot, P. M., and G. Ouellet. 1988. Mineral and nitrate content of swine drinking-water in four Quebec regions, *Can. J. Anim. Sci.*, 68:997.

Fraser, D., and P. A. Phillips. 1989. Lethargy and low water intake by sows during early lactation: a cause of low piglet weight gains and survival, *Appl. Anim. Behav. Sci.*, 24:13.

Fraser, D., P. A. Phillips, B. K. Thompson, and W. B. Peeters Weem. 1988. Use of water by piglets in the first days after birth, *Can. J. Anim. Sci.*, 68:603.

Fraser, D., J. F. Patience, P. A. Phillips, and J. M. McLeese. 1993. Water for piglets and lactating sows: Quantity, quality and quandaries. In *Recent Developments in Pig Nutrition*, 2, Cole, D. J., W. Haresign, and P. C. Garnsworthy, Eds., Nottingham University Press, Loughborough, U.K., 200–224.

Friend, D. W. 1971. Self-selection of feeds and water by swine during pregnancy and lactation, *J. Anim. Sci.*, 32:658.

Friend, D. W. 1973. Self-selection of feeds and water by unbred gilts, *J. Anim. Sci.*, 37:1137.

Friend, D. W., and H. M. Cunningham. 1966. The effect of water consumption on the growth, feed intake, and carcass composition of suckling piglets, *Can. J. Anim. Sci.*, 46:203.

Friend, D. W., and M. S. Wolynetz. 1981. Self-selection of salt by gilts during pregnancy and lactation, *Can. J. Anim. Sci.*, 61:429.

Gadd, J. 1988a. Water: the facts and the myths, *West. Hog J.*, 10(1):26.

Gadd, J. 1988b. How much water do pigs really need, *Pigs*, 4(6):14.

Gadd, J. 1992. War on waste, *West. Hog J.*, 13(3):14.

Gadd, J. 1996. Watering that sow in lactation, *West. Hog J.*, 18(2):11.

Gadd, J. 1997. What the textbooks don't tell you about new style weaner drinkers, *Pigs*, 13(2):19.

Georgievskii, V. I. 1982. Water metabolism and the animal's water requirements. In *Mineral Nutrition of Animals*, Georgievskii, V. I., B. N. Annenkov, and V. I. Samokkhin, Eds., Butterworths, London, 79–89.

Gill, B. P., and J. Barber, 1990. Water delivery systems for growing pigs, *Farm Building Progr.*, 102:19.

Gill, B. P., P. H. Brooks, and J. L. Carpenter. 1986. The water intake of weaned pigs from 3 to 6 weeks of age, *Anim. Prod.*, 42:470 (Abstr.).

Hagsten, I., and T. W. Perry. 1976. Evaluation of dietary salt levels for swine. 1. Effect on gain, water consumption and efficiency of feed conversion, *J. Anim. Sci.*, 42:1187.

Holmes, C. W., and L. E. Mount. 1967. Heat loss from groups of growing pigs under various conditions of environmental temperature and air movement, *Anim. Prod.*, 9:435.

Hoppe, M. K., G. W. Libal, and R. C. Wahlstrom. 1987. Effect of water flow rate from nipple drinkers on sow performance during lactation, South Dakota State University Swine Day, 43–45.

Ingram, D. L. 1964. The effect of environmental temperature on heat loss and thermal insulation in the young pig, *Res. Vet. Sci.*, 5:357.

Klopfenstein, C., S. D'Allaire, and G. Martineau. 1994. What sows have to say about water intake, *Proceedings of the 1994 Allen D. Leman Swine Conference*, 71–77.

Knabe, D. A., T. J. Prince, and D. E. Orr, Jr. 1986. Effect of feed and (or) water deprivation prior to weaning on reproductive performance of sows: a cooperative study, *J. Anim. Sci.*, 62:1.

Lightfoot, A. L. 1978. Water consumption of lactating sows, *Anim. Prod.*, 26:386 (Abstr.).

Lightfoot, A. L., and A. W. Armsby. 1984. Water consumption and slurry production of dry and lactating sows, *Anim. Prod.*, 38:541 (Abstr.).

Lloyd, L. E., B. E. McDonald, and E. W. Crampton. 1978. Water and its metabolism. In *Fundamentals of Nutrition*, 2nd ed., W. H. Freeman, San Francisco, 22–34.

Lumb, S. 1998. Water management, *Int. Pig Top.*, 13(1):33.

Madec, F. 1984. Urinary disorders in intensive pig herds, *Pig News Info.*, 5:89.

Maenz, D. D., J. F. Patience, and M. S. Wolynetz. 1994. The influence of the mineral level in drinking water and thermal environment on the performance and intestinal fluid flux of newly-weaned pigs, *J. Anim. Sci.*, 72:300.

Maynard, L. A., J. K. Loosli, H. F. Hintz, and R. G. Warner. 1979, *Animal Nutrition*, 7th ed., McGraw-Hill, New York.

McLeese, J. M., J. F. Patience, M. S. Wolynetz, and G. I. Christison. 1991. Evaluation of the quality of ground water supplies used on Saskatchewan swine farms, *Can. J. Anim. Sci.*, 71:191.

McLeese, J. M., M. L. Tremblay, J. F. Patience, and G. I. Christison. 1992. Water intake patterns in the weanling pig: effect of water quality, antibiotics and probiotics, *Anim. Prod.*, 54:135.

Ministry of Agriculture, Fisheries and Food, 1983. Codes of Recommendations for the Welfare of Livestock: Pigs, Ministry of Agriculture, Fisheries and Food Leaflet 702.

Morrison, S. R., T. E. Bond, and H. Heitman, 1967. Skin and lung moisture loss from swine, *Trans. Am. Soc. Agric. Eng.*, 10:691.

Mount, L. E., C. W. Holmes, W. H. Close, S. R. Morrison, and I. B. Start. 1971. A note on the consumption of water by the growing pig at several environmental temperatures and levels of feeding, *Anim. Prod.*, 13:561.

Mroz, Z., A. W. Jongblod, N. P. Lenis, and K. Vreman. 1995. Water in pig nutrition. physiology, allowance and environmental implications, *Nutr. Res. Rev.*, 8:137.

Nienaber, J. A., and G. L. Hahn. 1984. Effects of water flow restriction and environmental factors on performance of nursery-age pigs, *J. Anim. Sci.*, 59:1423.

NRC. 1974. *Nutrient and Toxic Substances in Water for Livestock and Poultry*, National Academy Press, Washington, D.C., 93 pp.

NRC. 1980. *Mineral Tolerance of Domestic Animals*, National Academy Press, Washington, D.C.

NRC. 1981. Water-environment interactions. In *Effect of Environment on Nutrient Requirements of Domestic Animals*, National Academy Press, Washington, D.C., 39–50.

NRC. 1998. *Nutrient Requirements of Swine*, 10th ed. National Academy Press, Washington, D.C., 189 pp.

Ogunbarmeru, B. O., E. T. Kornegay, and C. M. Wood. 1991. A comparison of drip and non-drip nipple waters used by weanling pigs, *Can. J. Anim. Sci.*, 71:581.

Olsson, O. 1983. Valve drinking systems for growing-finishing pigs. Effects on pig performance and behaviour and biometric considerations for technical design, Swedish University of Agricultural Sciences Report 111, 81 pp.

Olsson, O., and T. Andersson. 1985. Biometric considerations when designing value drinking systems for growing-finishing pigs, *Acta Agric. Scand.*, 35:55.

Paterson, D. W., R. C. Wahlstrom, G. W. Libal, and O. E. Olson. 1979. Effects of sulfate in water on swine reproduction and young pig performance, *J. Anim. Sci.*, 49:664.

Pedersen, B. K. 1994. Water intake and pig performance, *Proceedings Teagasc Pig Conference*, 50–54.

Phillips, P. A., and D. Fraser. 1989. A water dispenser modified to promote water use by piglets in the first days after birth, *Can. Agric. Eng.*, 31:175.

Phillips, P. A., and D. Fraser. 1990. Water bowl size for newborn pigs, *Appl. Eng. Agric.*, 6:79.

Phillips, P. A., and D. Fraser. 1991. Discovery of selected water dispensers by newborn pigs, *Can. J. Anim. Sci.*, 71:233.

Phillips, P. A., D. Fraser, and B. K. Thompson. 1990. The influence of water nipple flow rate and position and room temperature on sow water intake and spillage, *Appl. Eng. Agric.*, 6:75.

Phillips, P. A., D. Fraser, and B. K. Thompson. 1995. A method to evaluate appropriate nipple drinker flow rates for pigs, *Appl. Eng. Agric.*, 11:587.

Riley, J. E. 1978. Drinking "straws": a method of watering housed sows during pregnancy and lactation, *Anim. Prod.*, 26:386 (Abstr.).

Roubicek, C. B. 1969. Water metabolism. In *Animal Growth and Nutrition*, Hafez, E. S., and I. A. Dyer, Eds., Lea and Febiger, Philadelphia, 353–373.

Russell, I. D., 1985. Some fundamentals of water medications, *Poult. Dig.*, 44:422.

Seerley, R. W., R. J. Emerick, L. B. Emery, and O. E. Olson. 1965. Effect of nitrate or nitrite administered continuously in drinking water for swine and sheep, *J. Anim. Sci.*, 24:1014.

Shields, R. G., Jr., D. C. Mahan, and P. L. Graham. 1983. Changes in swine body composition from birth to 145 kg, *J. Anim. Sci.*, 57:43.

Sinclair, R. D. 1939. The salt requirements of growing pigs, *Sci. Agric.*, 20:109.

Straub, G., J. H. Weniger, E. S. Tawfik, and D. Steinhauf. 1976. The effects of high environmental temperatures on fattening performance and growth of boars, *Livest. Prod. Sci.*, 3:65.

Task Force on Water Quality Guidelines. 1987. Canadian Water Quality Guidelines, Inland Waters Directorate, Ottawa, Ontario.

Thacker, P. A. 1998. Water requirements, presented at International Symposium on the Nutrient Requirements of Swine, April 14, Iowa State University, Ames.

Thulin, A. J., and M. C. Brumm. 1991. Water: the forgotten nutrient. In *Swine Nutrition*, Miller, E. R., D. E. Ulrey, and A. J. Lewis, Eds., Butterworth-Heinemann, Stoneham, MA, 315–324.

Upjohn Limited. 1985. Water and Water Medication of Pigs, Upjohn Veterinary Division, West Sussex, England.

Wahlstrom, R. C., A. R. Taylor, and R. W. Seerley. 1970. Effects of lysine in the drinking water of growing swine, *J. Anim. Sci.*, 30:368.

Winks, W. R., A. K. Sutherland, and R. M. Salisbury. 1950. Nitrite poisoning of pigs, *Queensl. J. Agric. Sci.*, 7:1.

Wood, R. D., C. H. Chaney, D. G. Waddill, and G. W. Garrison. 1967. Effect of adding nitrate or nitrite to drinking water on the utilization of carotene by growing swine, *J. Anim. Sci.*, 26:510.

Yang, T. S., M. A. Price, and F. X. Aherne. 1984. The effect of level of feeding on water turnover in growing pigs, *Appl. Anim. Behav. Sci.*, 12:103.

Part III

Factors That Influence Swine Nutrition

18 Antimicrobial and Promicrobial Agents

Gary L. Cromwell

CONTENTS

I. Introduction 401
   A. Definition of Antimicrobial and Promicrobial Agents 401
   B. Background on Use of Antimicrobials 402
   C. Background on Use of Promicrobials 404
II. Antimicrobial Agents 405
   A. Efficacy of Antimicrobials as Growth Promoters 405
   B. Efficacy of Antimicrobials on Reproductive Efficiency 409
   C. Mode of Action of Antimicrobials 409
      1. Metabolic Effect 409
      2. Nutritional Effect 411
      3. Disease Control Effect 412
   D. Proper Usage — Residue Avoidance 413
   E. Safety of Antimicrobials 414
   F. Economic Benefits of Antimicrobials 417
III. Promicrobial Agents 417
   A. Efficacy of Promicrobials 417
   B. Mode of Action of Promicrobials 418
IV. Miscellaneous Agents 419
References 421

I. INTRODUCTION

A. DEFINITION OF ANTIMICROBIAL AND PROMICROBIAL AGENTS

Antimicrobial agents are compounds that, at low concentrations, suppress or inhibit the growth of microorganisms. This class of compounds includes the antibiotics (naturally occurring substances produced by yeasts, molds, and other microorganisms) and the chemotherapeutics (chemically synthesized substances). In addition, the mineral elements copper and zinc have antimicrobial properties when present in high concentrations in diets for young pigs.

Promicrobial agents are live (viable), naturally occurring microorganisms that are fed directly to animals. They include a number of microbials, but the more common ones are species of *Lactobacillus* and *Enterococcus* (formerly called *Streptococcus*) and yeasts. Direct-fed microorganisms, commonly referred to as "probiotics," are thought to affect the host animal beneficially by improving its intestinal microbial balance. Also, some serve as sources of enzymes.

B. Background on Use of Antimicrobials

Antimicrobial agents have been used widely as feed additives for swine since the early 1950s. They are used at low (subtherapeutic) levels in feed for growth promotion, improvement of feed utilization, reduction of mortality, and improvement of reproductive efficiency. Approximately 88% of the total antibiotics used for animals is subtherapeutic usage (IOM, 1988). Antibacterial agents also are used at moderate-to-high (prophylaxis) levels for the prevention of disease in exposed animals and at high (therapeutic) levels for the treatment of certain swine diseases.

The discovery of the growth-stimulating effects associated with the feeding of antibiotics was made in the late 1940s as a result of research involving vitamin B_{12}. Stokstad et al. (1949) fed the fermentation products of the microorganism *Streptomyces aureofaciens* to chicks to assay the amount of vitamin B_{12} and found that the growth rate of the chicks was more than could be accounted for on the basis of the vitamin content. Similar growth responses from fermentation media were subsequently demonstrated in studies with pigs (Cunha et al., 1949; 1950; Jukes et al., 1950; Lepley et al., 1950; Luecke et al., 1950). Stokstad and Jukes identified the agent in the original fermentation media as the antibiotic chlortetracycline.

Soon after the benefits of antibiotics were discovered, swine producers readily accepted them as an integral part of their feeding programs. By 1963, approximately 1 million kg of antibiotics was being used annually in animal feeds (Figure 18.1). In 1988, approximately 13 million kg of antibiotics and chemotherapeutics was produced and 4.65 million kg was sold in the United States, and about one half of these amounts was for feed additive use (U.S. International Trade Commission, 1989). At present, approximately 80 to 90% of pig starting feeds, 70 to 80% of growing feeds, 50 to 60% of finishing feeds, and 40 to 50% of sow feeds contain antimicrobial agents.

In the early years following the discovery of antibiotics, the average cost of feed-grade antibiotics was $200 to $220/kg (Figure 18.2). By the mid-1960s, the average cost of antibiotics decreased to one tenth of the initial cost, and their cost has remained between $20 and $40/kg.

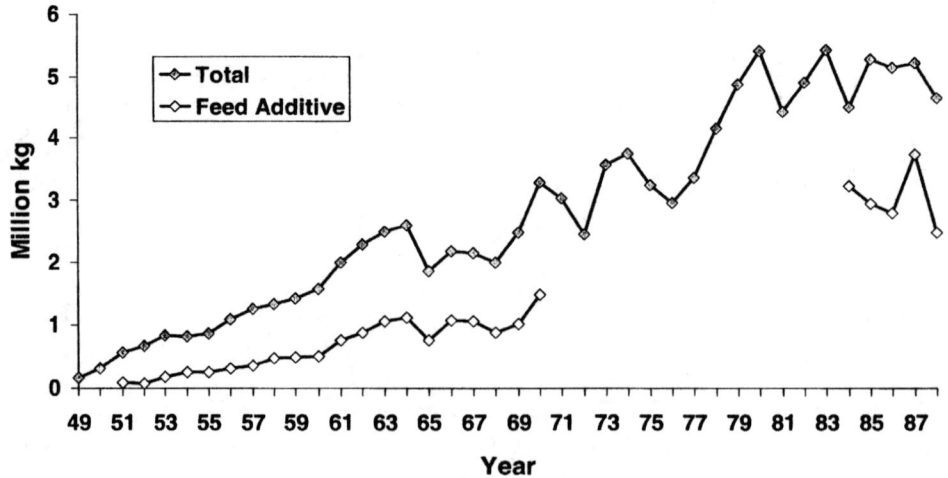

FIGURE 18.1 Sales of total antibiotics for medicinal and nonmedicinal (feed additive) purposes in the United States from 1949 to 1988. (Data are from U.S. Tariff Commission Reports, 1950–1957 and U.S. International Trade Commission Reports, 1958–1989. Reliable data were not obtainable after 1989.)

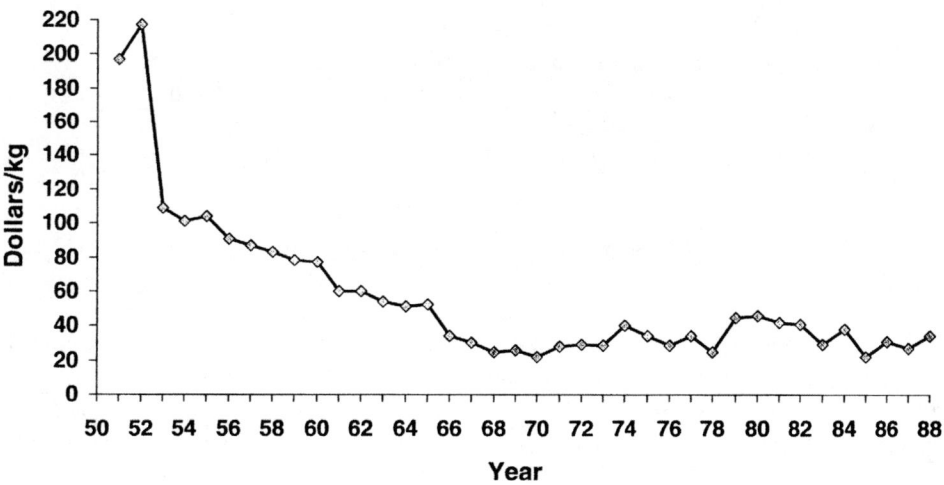

FIGURE 18.2 Average price of antibiotics for nonmedicinal (feed additive) usage in the United States from 1951 to 1988. (Data are from U.S. Tariff Commission Reports, 1950–1957 and U.S. International Trade Commission Reports, 1958–1989. Reliable data were not obtainable after 1989.)

Currently, 17 antimicrobial agents (12 antibiotics, 5 chemotherapeutics) are approved by the Food and Drug Administration (FDA) for use in swine feeds, and these are listed in Table 18.1 (Feed Additive Compendium, 2000). Certain of these antimicrobial agents are approved for combination usage (e.g., chlortetracycline–sulfamethazine–penicillin, neomycin–oxytetracycline), whereas others cannot be used in combination with other drugs. Several other antibiotics (avilamycin, efrotomycin, salinomycin, nosiheptide, and thiopeptin) have potential as growth promoters (Cromwell, 1987) but they have not been approved by the FDA for use in swine feeds.

TABLE 18.1
Antimicrobial Agents Approved for Swine

Antibiotics	Chemotherapeutics
Apramycin	Arsanilic acid
Bacitracin methylene disalicylate	Carbadox
Bacitracin zinc	Roxarsone
Bambermycins	Sulfamethazine
Chlortetracycline	Sulfathiazole
Lincomycin	
Neomycin	
Oxytetracycline	
Penicillin	
Tiamulin	
Tylosin	
Virginiamycin	

Source: Feed Additive Compendium, Miller Publishing Co., Minnetonka, MN, 2000. With permission.

The antimicrobials that are effective in improving performance in pigs have one thing in common: their ability to suppress or inhibit the growth of certain microorganisms. The chemical composition and bacterial spectrum of the antimicrobials vary widely. Some are readily absorbed (e.g., tetracyclines, sulfonamides), whereas others are largely nonabsorbed (e.g., bacitracin, bambermycins). Some are excreted more rapidly than others (e.g., sulfathiazole vs. sulfamethazine). While chemical composition, bacterial spectrum, and absorption–excretion patterns influence the bactericidal and bacteriostatic properties and effectiveness against specific systemic pathogens, these characteristics are less readily associated with the ability of a given antimicrobial agent to stimulate growth.

C. Background on Use of Promicrobials

The philosophy of promicrobial agents goes back to the early 1900s with the studies of Metchnikoff (1903; 1908), who ascribed beneficial effects to the use of lactobacilli by men. He attributed the longevity of Bulgarians to daily consumption of yogurt. Metchnikoff believed that the lactobacilli in yogurt could "balance the intestinal environment," prevent the growth of pathogenic bacteria, and, as a consequence, improve health and prolong life. *Lactobacillus acidophilus* was widely used during the first half of this century, before the introduction of sulfanilamides, to control outbreaks of diarrhea in children (Winkelstein, 1956) and it was subsequently found to have antibacterial activity (Vincent et al., 1959).

The administration of promicrobial agents to animals started in the 1920s. The term, *probiotics* was introduced by Parker (1974) when the production of bacterial feed supplements began on a commercial scale (Fuller, 1992a). Parker used this term to describe organisms and substances that contribute to intestinal microbial balance. This term was used to describe any living or dead microorganisms or fermentation by-products administered to animals (Fox, 1988). Fuller (1989), however, proposed to limit the definition of this class of compounds only to live microorganisms. This revised definition emphasizes the importance of live organisms as an essential component of an effective probiotic and removes the confusion created by the use of the word *substances*.

The FDA now requires manufacturers to use the term *direct-fed microbials* instead of probiotics. The FDA defines direct-fed microbials as "a source of live (viable), naturally occurring microorganisms" (Pendelton, 1992). At present, direct-fed microbials fall into the category classified by FDA and the Association of American Feed Control Officials (AAFCO, 2000) as ingredients that are generally recognized as safe (GRAS). The GRAS status is defined as food and feed additives that have been designated as safe for consumption having been judged by a panel of expert pharmacologists and toxicologists who considered the available data, including technical experience of their common usage in human food (Pollmann, 1986).

At present, 42 different microorganisms are considered GRAS and can be used as direct-fed microbials (Anon, 1992; AAFCO, 2000). A list of these is shown in Table 18.2. They include molds (species of *Asperigillus*) and yeast (*Saccharomyces cerevisiae*), both of which are classified as fungi; Gram-positive bacteria (*Leuconostoc mesenteroide* and species of *Bacillus*, *Bifidobacterium*, *Lactobacillus*, *Pediococcus*, *Propionibacterium*, and *Enterococcus*); and Gram-negative bacteria (species of *Bacteroides*) (Risley, 1992). The species of *Bifidobacterium*, *Lactobacillus*, *Enterococcus*, and *S. cerevisiae*, are usually direct-fed microorganisms, while the species of *Asperigillus* and *Bacillus* are also used as sources of enzymes. *Leuconostoc mesenteroides* and species of *Pediococcus* and *Propionibacterium* are used primarily as silage additives. All of the approved organisms are intestinal strains except for *Lactobacillus bulgaricus* and *E. thermophilus*, which are yogurt starter organisms.

TABLE 18.2
Direct-Fed Microorganisms Approved for Swine and Other Livestock[a]

Asperigillus niger	*B. infantis*	*L. enterii*
A. oryzae	*B. longum*	*Leuconostoc mesenteroides*
Bacillus coagulans	*B. thermophilum*	*Pediococcus acidilacticii*
B. lentus	*Lactobacillus acidolphilus*	*P. cerevisiae*
B. licheniformis	*L. brevis*	*P. pentosaceus*
B. pumilus	*L. bulgaricus*	*Propionibacterium freudenreichii*
B. subtilis	*L. casei*	*P. shermanii*
Bacteroides amphophilus	*L. cellobiosus*	*Saccharomyces cerevisiae*
B. capillosus	*L. curvatus*	*Enterococcus cremoris*
B. ruminocola	*L. delbruekii*	*E. diacetylactis*
B. suis	*L. fermentum*	*E. faecium*
Bifidobacterium adolescentis	*L. helveticus*	*E. intermedius*
B. animalis	*L. lactis*	*E. lactis*
B. bifidum	*L. plantarum*	*E. thermophilus*

[a] Anonymous (1992) and AAFCO (2000). The *Enterococcus* species were formerly cataloged as *Streptococcus* species.

II. ANTIMICROBIAL AGENTS

A. EFFICACY OF ANTIMICROBIALS AS GROWTH PROMOTERS

The efficacy of antibiotics in improving the rate and efficiency of growth in pigs is well documented in numerous research studies (Hays, 1977; CAST, 1981; Zimmerman, 1986; Cromwell and Dawson, 1992). Table 18.3 summarizes data from 1194 experiments conducted in the United States from 1950 to 1985. In studies involving young, weanling pigs from 7 to 25 kg, antibiotics improved growth rate by an average of 16.4% and reduced the amount of feed required per unit of gain by 6.9%. In studies with slightly heavier, growing pigs (from 17 to 49 kg), antibiotics improved growth rate by 10.6% and feed efficiency by 4.5%. Over the entire growing-finishing period (from 24 to 89 kg), growth rate was improved by 4.2% and feed efficiency by 2.2% when antibiotics were fed.

TABLE 18.3
Efficacy of Antibiotics as Growth Promoters for Pigs[a]

Stage	Control	Antibiotic	Improvement (%)
Starting phase (7–25 kg)			
Daily gain (kg)	0.39	0.45	16.4
Feed/gain	2.28	2.13	6.9
Growing phase (17–49 kg)			
Daily gain (kg)	0.59	0.66	10.6
Feed/gain	2.91	2.78	4.5
Growing-finishing phase (24–89 kg)			
Daily gain (kg)	0.69	0.72	4.2
Feed/gain	3.30	3.23	2.2

[a] Data from 453, 298, and 443 experiments, involving 13,632, 5,783, and 13,140 pigs for the three phases, respectively.

Source: Adapted from Hays (1977) and Zimmerman (1986).

TABLE 18.4
Efficacy of Antibiotics from 1950 to 1977 and from 1978 to 1985

	Improvement from Antibiotics (%)	
Stage	1950–1977[a]	1978–1985[b]
Starting phase		
Daily gain	16.1	15.0
Feed/gain	6.9	6.5
Growing-finishing phase		
Daily gain	4.0	3.6
Feed/gain	2.1	2.4

[a] Data from 378 and 279 experiments, involving 10,023 and 5,666 pigs for the two phases, respectively; Hays (1977).
[b] Data from 75 and 164 experiments, involving 3,609 and 7,474 pigs for the two phases, respectively; Zimmerman (1986).

Even though some antibiotics have now been used for nearly five decades, they still are as effective as they were in the early years following their discovery. A comparison of data from the first 28 years of antibiotic usage (1950 to 1977) and for the subsequent 8 years (1978 to 1985) indicates that the overall effectiveness of antibiotics did not diminish (Table 18.4).

The benefits from antibiotics, such as those listed in Tables 18.3 and 18.4, are derived mostly from controlled experiments conducted at universities and other research stations. Antibiotics are likely even more beneficial when used at the farm level. The data shown in Table 18.5 indicate that responses to antibiotics under farm conditions may be twice as great as those occurring in a research station environment, where the facilities are generally cleaner, the disease load is less, and the environment is less stressful.

Since most of the data in Tables 18.3 and 18.4 are based primarily on experiment station studies, the relative benefits from subtherapeutic usage of antibiotics are probably underestimated. In actuality, antibiotics may improve growth rate at the farm level by as much as 25 to 30% and feed efficiency by 12 to 15% in weanling pigs. In growing-finishing pigs, improvements in rate and efficiency of gain may be improved by as much as 8 and 10% and 4 and 5%, respectively, when antibiotics are included in the feed.

TABLE 18.5
Efficacy of Antibiotics in Research Station (University) Tests vs. Farm Tests

		Improvement from Antibiotics (%)	
Location	No. of Trials	Daily Gain	Feed/Gain
Summary 1[a]			
Research station tests	128	16.9	7.0
Farm tests	32	28.4	14.5
Summary 2[b]			
Research station tests	9	13.2	4.7
Farm tests	67	25.5	10.0

[a] Data on 12,000 pigs from 7 to 26 kg. Chlortetracycline–sulfamethazine–penicillin, tylosin–sulfamethazine, tetracycline, and carbadox. Adapted from Hays (1977).
[b] Data on 3321 pigs from 8 to 20 kg. Chlortetracycline–sulfamethazine–penicillin. Adapted from NCR-89 (1984) and Maddock (1985).

TABLE 18.6
Effects of Antibiotics on Performance and Mortality of Young Pigs in Commercial Field Tests[a]

Item	Control	Antibiotics	Improvement (%)
Summary 1[b]			
Daily gain (kg)	0.31	0.40	26
Feed/gain	2.48	2.23	10
Mortality (%)	4.3	2.0	
Summary 2 (high disease level)[c]			
Daily gain (kg)	0.30	0.38	26
Feed/gain	3.07	2.50	19
Mortality	15.6	3.1	

[a] Antimicrobials were chlortetracylcine–sulfamethazine–penicillin or tylosin–sulfamethazine.
[b] 67 field trials from 1960 to 1982, 1597 pigs.
[c] Five field trials under high disease level, 638 pigs, 8 to 31 kg.

Source: Adapted from Maddock (1985).

In addition to growth enhancement, the use of antibiotics in swine feeds has been found to reduce mortality and morbidity, particularly in young pigs. A summary of 67 field trials conducted over a 22-year period indicates that antibiotics reduced mortality by one half (from 4.3 to 2.0%) in young pigs (Table 18.6). The reduction in mortality was even greater under high-disease conditions and environmental stress (15.6 vs. 3.1%; Table 18.6).

Although not generally classified as an antimicrobial, the mineral element copper has antibacterial properties when present at high concentrations. The initial reports on improved pig performance resulting from high dietary copper were by Evvard et al. (1928) at Iowa State University and by Braude (1945) in the United Kingdom. Table 18.7 illustrates that the responses in growth rate and efficiency of feed utilization to high dietary copper (200 to 250 ppm) are similar in magnitude to those resulting from antibiotic feeding. Also, the responses to copper and antibiotics

TABLE 18.7
Effects of Copper Sulfate on Performance of Weanling and Growing-Finishing Pigs

	Added Copper (ppm)[a]		
Stage	0	200–250	Improvement (%)
Starting period (8 to 20 kg)[b]			
Daily gain (kg)	0.34	0.38	11.9
Feed/gain	1.87	1.78	4.5
Growing period (18 to 56 kg)[c]			
Daily gain (kg)	0.67	0.71	6.9
Feed/gain	2.80	2.70	3.6
Growing-finishing period (18 to 93 kg)[c]			
Daily gain (kg)	0.71	0.74	3.1
Feed/gain	3.18	3.10	2.5

[a] The 250 ppm level is in addition to the copper (6–12 ppm) in the trace mineral mix. Copper added as $CuSO_4 \cdot 5H_2O$.
[b] Summary of 23 experiments with 1376 pigs weaned at 3 to 4 weeks of age conducted at the University of Kentucky from 1978 to 1997. The test periods were 4 to 5 weeks in length.
[c] Summary of 18 experiments with 672 pigs conducted at the University of Kentucky from 1970 to 1980.

TABLE 18.8
Effects of Single and Combined Additions of Antibiotics and Copper Sulfate on Performance of Weanling Pigs[a]

Item	Control	Antibiotics	Copper (250 ppm)	Both
Daily gain (kg)	0.26	0.30	0.31	0.34
Daily feed (kg)	0.54	0.58	0.59	0.63
Feed/gain	2.10	1.95	1.91	1.84

[a] Summary of 14 experiments involving 1700 pigs (7 to 18 kg) conducted at six stations.

Source: Adapted from Beames and Lloyd (1965), Mahan (1980), Stahly et al. (1980), Edmonds et al. (1985), Hagen et al. (1987), and Burnell et al. (1988).

are additive in young pigs (Table 18.8); that is, copper is efficacious in both the presence and absence of antibiotics.

Responses to copper are influenced by feeding level of the mineral and by its chemical form. In weanling pigs, 200 to 250 ppm copper seems to be the most efficacious level; 100 to 125 ppm copper results in about 75 to 80% of the maximum response (Cromwell et al., 1989). The sulfate, carbonate, and chloride salts are efficacious forms of copper (Wallace, 1967; Cromwell et al., 1998), but the oxide and sulfide salts are not (Cromwell et al., 1989; Cromwell, 1997). Copper–lysine complex (Coffey et al., 1994; Apgar et al., 1995) and other organic complexes of copper (Bunch et al., 1965; Stansbury et al., 1990) are effective growth promoters in young pigs. High levels of copper (≥500 ppm) should be avoided because of the chances of copper toxicity in pigs, resulting from the marked accumulation of copper in the liver (Cromwell, 1997).

High levels of dietary zinc (2000 to 3000 ppm) as zinc oxide have been found to reduce preweaning diarrhea (Kulwich et al., 1953) and to enhance growth in young pigs (Hahn and Baker, 1993; LeMieux et al., 1995; Hill et al., 2000; Table 18.9). Other forms of zinc have not consistently produced a growth response similar to that obtained from high levels of zinc oxide. High zinc and high copper are not additive in terms of growth promotion when added in combination to diets for young pigs (Hill et al., 2000).

TABLE 18.9
High Dietary Zinc and Copper for Weanling Pigs[a]

Item	Control	Zinc[b]	Copper[c]	Both[b,c]
Daily gain (kg)	0.37	0.42	0.41	0.41
Daily feed (kg)	0.64	0.69	0.67	0.68
Feed/gain	1.71	1.64	1.64	1.63
Fecal color[d]	3.17	3.24	4.32	3.57
Fecal firmness[e]	2.39	2.14	2.14	2.13

[a] Summary of 12, 4-week experiments conducted at 12 universities and involving 1356 pigs initially averaging 6.55 kg and 22.2 days of age. All diets contained 200 g/ton of chlortetracycline.
[b] 3000 ppm added zinc as zinc oxide.
[c] 250 ppm added copper as copper sulfate.
[d] Scored 1 to 5, 1 = yellow, 5 = black.
[e] Scored 1 to 5, 1 = very firm, 5 = very watery.

Source: Hill, G. M. et al., *J. Anim. Sci.*, 28:1010, 2000. With permission.

B. Efficacy of Antimicrobials on Reproductive Efficiency

Antibiotics are not as commonly used in diets for breeding animals as for growing pigs; however, they are quite effective when fed during certain stages of the reproductive cycle, such as at the time of breeding. A summary of nine studies involving 1931 sows shows that feeding a high level (0.5 to 1 g/sow daily) of an absorbable antibiotic at the time of breeding improves conception rate by about 7 percentage points and improves litter size by nearly one half of a pig at the subsequent farrowing (Table 18.10).

TABLE 18.10
Effects of Antimicrobial Agents in the Feed at Breeding on Reproductive Performance of Sows[a,b]

Researcher	Agent	No. of Sows	Farrowing Rate (%)[c] −[d]	Farrowing Rate (%)[c] +[d]	Live Pigs Born/Litter −[d]	Live Pigs Born/Litter +[d]
Dean and Tribble (1962)	OTC, CTC	59	—	—	7.1	9.7
Mayrose et al. (1964)	Ty	192	93.8	91.7	11.0	11.3
Messersmith et al. (1966)	CTC	377	68.5	82.9	9.8	10.0
Ruiz et al. (1968)	ASP	96	87.5	95.8	9.0	10.3
Myers and Speer (1973)	CTC	249	66.9	75.4	9.9	10.3
Soma and Speer (1975)	CTC	239	70.8	72.3	10.2	10.5
Hays et al. (1978)	ASP	182	60.9	70.0	9.8	10.0
Johnson et al. (1985)	CTC	112	77.0	96.0	10.7	11.0
Maxwell et al. (1994)	CTC	425	83.0	85.0	9.5	9.8
Total and weighted averages		1931	75.2	82.1	9.9	10.3

[a] Abbreviations: OTC, oxytetracycline; CTC, chlortetracycline; Ty, tylosin; ASP, combination of chlortetracycline, sulfamethazine, and penicillin.
[b] In most instances, the antimicrobial agent was fed at 0.5 to 1.0 g/day for 1 week before and 2 to 3 weeks after breeding.
[c] 100 × (no. of sows that farrowed/no. of sows exposed to boar).
[d] Without (−) or with (+) antimicrobial agents in the feed at breeding.

Antibiotics also have been shown in some experiments to be beneficial at farrowing and during early lactation. In some instances, high levels of antibiotics in the sow feed have reduced the incidence of agalactia and uterine infections that occasionally occur shortly after farrowing (Langlois et al., 1978a). The data in Table 18.11, based on 13 studies and 2338 litters, indicate a slight improvement in survival and weaning weights of nursing pigs when antibiotics are included in the prefarrowing and lactation diet. Long-term withdrawal of antibiotics from a swine herd has been shown to be associated with a reduction in reproductive performance (Table 18.12).

C. Mode of Action of Antimicrobials

The mechanisms by which antibiotics and other antimicrobial agents stimulate growth in animals are not well understood. Possible modes of action can be grouped into three categories, according to Hays (1978): (1) metabolic effect; (2) nutritional effect; and (3) disease control effect.

1. Metabolic Effect

This mode of action implies that antibiotics may directly influence certain metabolic processes in the animal. Braude and Johnson (1953) demonstrated that chlortetracycline affected water and nitrogen excretion in pigs. Brody et al. (1954) reported that fatty acid oxidation in liver mitochondria

TABLE 18.11
Effects of Antimicrobial Agents in the Prefarrowing and Lactation Diet on Reproductive Performance of Sows[a,b]

Researchers	Agent	No. of Sows	Live Pigs Born/Litter −[d]	Live Pigs Born/Litter +[d]	No. of Pigs Weaned/Litter[c] −[d]	No. of Pigs Weaned/Litter[c] +[d]	Survival to Weaning (%)[c] −[d]	Survival to Weaning (%)[c] +[d]	Weaning Weight (kg)[c] −[d]	Weaning Weight (kg)[c] +[d]
Sewell and Carmon (1958)	CTC	136	8.0	8.6	5.8	7.0	72.1	80.8	4.80	4.90
Wallace and Combs (1962)	Ty	88	10.1	10.4	8.8	9.0	87.1	86.7	3.41	3.53
Jordan and Waitt (1963)	Ty	291	—	—	—	—	93.6	98.0	5.03	4.92
Wallace and Combs (1964)	OTC,CTC	143	11.2	11.8	9.8	10.3	87.8	87.5	3.26	3.34
Mayrose et al. (1964)	Ty	178	11.0	11.3	8.1	8.8	73.1	77.3	3.99	3.99
Wallace et al. (1966)	Cu	50	12.0	12.1	10.0	10.3	83.7	85.4	3.28	3.39
Combs and Wallace (1969)	Bac	91	9.4	9.8	7.8	8.4	83.0	85.7	3.63	3.47
Wallace et al. (1974)	ASP	149	10.6	11.0	9.3	9.4	88.0	85.3	3.80	3.75
Lillie and Frobish (1978)	Cu	32	8.6	8.5	6.7	7.0	78.4	82.2	4.61	4.94
Johnson et al. (1985)	CTC, ASP	97	9.8	9.8	8.5	8.8	86.7	89.2	5.13	5.48
Cromwell et al. (1993)	Cu	167	9.2	9.5	8.0	8.1	84.8	84.8	6.81	7.08
Maxwell et al. (1994)	CTC	850	9.7	9.9	8.2	8.4	85.6	86.4	5.31	5.36
Monegue and Cromwell (1996)	Cu	66	8.9	9.5	8.2	8.3	91.8	87.7	6.17	5.68
Total or average (weighted)		2338	9.9	10.2	8.2	8.6	85.1	86.8	4.86	4.90

[a] *Abbreviations:* CTC, chlortetracycline; Ty, tylosin; OTC, oxytetracycline; Cu, copper sulfate; Bac, bacitracin zinc; ASP, combination of chlortetracycline, sulfamethazine, and penicillin.

[b] In most instances an antimicrobial agent was added at a high dietary level (110 to 275 mg/kg) from 3 to 7 days before farrowing and during a 14- to 21-day lactation period. Copper sulfate was added at 250 ppm copper. Copper sulfate was also included in the gestation diet in the studies of Cromwell et al. (1993) and Monegue and Cromwell (1996).

[c] Weaning age was 21 days in the Sewell and Carmon (1958), Jordan and Waitt (1963), Lillie and Frobish (1978), Johnson et al. (1985), Maxwell et al. (1994) and Monegue and Cromwell (1996) studies, 28 days in the Cromwell et al. (1993) study, and 14 days in all others.

[d] Without (−) or with (+) antimicrobial agents in the prefarrowing and lactation diet.

TABLE 18.12
Effects of Long-Term Antibiotic Withdrawal in a Swine Herd on Reproductive Performance[a,b]

Item	Antibiotics (1963–1972)	No Antibiotics (1972–1985)
No. of litters	398	688
Conception rate (%)	91.4	82.6
No. of pigs born/litter	10.8	10.2
Live pigs born/litter	9.8	9.3
Avg. birth weight (kg)	1.29	1.38
No. of pigs weaned (21 days)	8.8	7.5
Avg weaning weight (kg)	5.67	5.37
Survival of live born (%)	89.7	80.9
Incidence of MMA	<10	66[c]

[a] *Abbreviations:* MMA, mastitis, metritis, agalactia.
[b] Closed, specific-pathogen-free herd at the University of Kentucky. Antibiotics were used in breeding, lactation, starting, growing, and finishing diets from 1963 to 1972. Antibiotics were not used in the feed or for treatment purposes from 1972 to 1985.
[c] For the period 1972 to 1975 only.

was inhibited by tetracyclines. Weinberg (1957) likewise showed, in bacteria, that phosphorylation and oxidation reactions requiring magnesium ions were inhibited by tetracyclines. Hash et al. (1964) demonstrated that protein synthesis was affected by tetracyclines. Similarly, results of studies by Moser et al. (1980) indicate that carbadox increased protein synthesis in pig muscle cells.

Although numerous studies have shown that antibiotics may have metabolic effects, the tissue levels of antibiotics that result from feeding subtherapeutic levels of antibiotics to pigs probably are not high enough to account for the growth-enhancing effects that occur when antibiotics are fed. Furthermore, a metabolic effect certainly does not explain the action of those antibiotics that are not absorbed from the gut.

2. Nutritional Effect

This proposed mechanism has a considerable amount of support. Certain microbes that inhabit the intestinal tract synthesize vitamins and amino acids that are essential to animals, while other microbes compete with the host animal for vitamins, amino acids, and other essential nutrients. Shifts in bacteria populations that are associated with the feeding of antibiotics could account for a greater availability of nutrients to the host animal.

Moore et al. (1946) found that streptomycin stimulated the growth of yeasts, and Anderson et al. (1952) found that penicillin increased the numbers of certain intestinal coliforms. Such organisms synthesize nutrients that are essential for the animal. If a diet is inadequate in certain vitamins, the deficiency could be partially corrected by microbial synthesis.

A depression in growth of certain organisms that could be considered as competitors with the host animal for nutrients has been shown when antibiotics are fed. In early studies, tetracycline was found to inhibit the growth of lactobacilli, microorganisms that require amino acids in about the same proportions as does the pig (March and Biely, 1952; Kellogg et al., 1964) Studies have shown that levels and sources of protein that support maximum growth in pigs are near optimum for the multiplication of lactobacilli in the tract. A reduction in the numbers of these competing microorganisms could be beneficial when diets that are marginally deficient in amino acids or vitamins are fed to pigs.

Studies by Henderickx et al. (1981) have shown that the feeding of virginiamycin results in a shift in the bacterial populations of the intestinal tract, which, in turn, leads to (1) a reduction in ammonia and amine production and (2) a reduction in volatile fatty acid (VFA) and lactic acid production. Hedde (1981) also reported a reduction in lactate and VFA production in the small intestine when virginiamycin was fed to pigs. Since these metabolites represent potential losses of protein and energy, the results of these studies suggest that virginiamycin spares both energy and amino acids for the host animal. Results of studies by Yen et al. (1976) and Moser et al. (1980) also indicate improved utilization of dietary protein when carbadox was fed to pigs.

Another significant change that occurs when antibiotics are fed to animals is a reduction in the thickness of the intestinal wall and an overall decrease in the total gut mass (Braude et al., 1955; Taylor and Harrington, 1955; Yen et al., 1985). Increased gut wall thickness is thought to be caused by the inhabitant bacteria, which either damage intestinal tissue or produce toxins that, in turn, damage the tissues. Greater ammonia production occurs in the gut when antibiotic-free diets are fed and the ammonia (an irritant) may also contribute to increased gut wall thickness and overall mass of the gut (Visek, 1978).

A thinner gut wall could result in greater nutrient absorption, as suggested in studies by Catron et al. (1953) and Henderickx et al. (1981). Additionally, the gut has a high rate of metabolic activity and has been suggested to contribute significantly to total body heat production (Webster, 1981; Koong et al., 1982). The reduced mass of the gut in animals fed antibiotics could mean a greater diversion of energy and other nutrients away from heat production and toward body growth.

If one accepts the concept that certain antibiotics spare energy and protein, it would seem that the dietary requirement for amino acids might be less in pigs fed antibiotics. Early studies by Catron et al. (1952) with chlortetracycline and later studies by Yen et al. (1979) and Moser et al. (1980) with carbadox provide evidence that the pig's dietary protein requirement may be reduced slightly when antibiotics are fed.

3. Disease Control Effect

This mode of action is probably the most commonly accepted theory on how antibiotics function to improve growth in animals. Pigs and other animals are continually exposed to an unfriendly environment of microorganisms that cause varying degrees of nonspecific, subclinical disease. This, in turn, reduces the animal's overall growth performance. The feeding of antibiotics suppresses the hostile microbes and this allows the host animal to perform more closely to its maximum genetic potential.

There are several pieces of evidence to support this proposed mechanism of action. The response to antibiotics is greater in young animals than in older animals, as illustrated in Table 18.3. Young pigs are more susceptible to disease organisms, in that their immunological protection is quite low. The immunoglobulins acquired from the sow's colostrum reach minimal levels in the pig's serum by the time they reach 3 to 5 weeks of age (Miller et al., 1961). This corresponds approximately to the same time as weaning, which adds further stress to pigs. The pig's ability to synthesize antibodies is poor, so immune protection remains low until 6 to 8 weeks of age. As pigs grow older, they develop higher levels of blood immunoglobulins (Miller et al., 1961), which better equip them to cope with the pathogenic organisms in their environment.

Additional evidence to support the disease control mode of action is that the degree of response is strongly influenced by cleanliness of the environment and the disease load of the animals involved. As previously discussed, and as illustrated in Tables 18.5 and 18.6, responses to antibiotics generally are minimal when tested in a clean and less stressful environment. Table 18.13 shows that antibiotics were more effective in a "dirty" nursery building than in a "clean" one (Hays and Speer, 1960). Table 18.14 summarizes experiments in which antibiotics were tested with slow-growing and fast-growing pigs (Braude et al., 1953). Improvements were considerably greater when antibiotics were fed to slow-growing pigs. Again, the greater response to antibiotics in the poor environment and/or

TABLE 18.13
Effects of Cleanliness of Environment on Responses of Young Pigs to Antibiotics[a]

Item	Control	Antibiotics[b]	Improvement (%)
Gain (kg)			
Clean building	8.1	10.4	28
Dirty building	4.8	7.5	55
Feed/gain			
Clean building	1.90	1.74	8
Dirty building	2.89	2.05	29

[a] Data on 615 pigs initially averaging 5.7 kg; 4- to 5-week trials.
[b] Spiramycin, chlortetracycline, or oxytetracycline.

Source: Hays, V. W., and V. C. Speer, *J. Anim. Sci.*, 19:938, 1960. With permission.

TABLE 18.14
Effects of Overall Thriftiness in Pigs on Response to Antibiotics[a]

	Daily Gain (kg)		
No. of Trials	Control	Antibiotics	Improvement (%)
4 slowest growers	0.09	0.25	161
12	0.18	0.34	85
16	0.27	0.45	65
12	0.36	0.50	38
16	0.45	0.57	26
32	0.55	0.63	15
48	0.64	0.71	12
22 fastest growers	0.73	0.79	9

Source: Adapted from Braude et al. (1953).

in unthrifty pigs is attributed to the fact that antibiotics suppress the bacteria that are responsible for reduced animal performance because of subclinical disease.

D. PROPER USAGE — RESIDUE AVOIDANCE

Antimicrobial drugs may be used only in approved combinations and at approved levels, as outlined in the Feed Additive Compendium (2000). Certain drugs require withdrawal from the feed for a prescribed period prior to slaughter so that residues do not occur in edible tissue. Those requiring withdrawal include apramycin, the arsenicals (arsanilic acid, roxarsone), carbadox, neomycin, and the sulfonamides (sulfamethazine, sulfathiazole). Proper use levels and withdrawal times are imperative for the production of residue-free pork.

The most common residue found in pork carcasses is sulfamethazine. Several years ago, sulfa residues were a major problem in the pork industry. The problem stemmed from the fact that only trace amounts of sulfamethazine (2 ppm) in the feed caused a high incidence of residues in liver tissue (Cromwell et al., 1981). Using improper mixing procedures or failure to prevent contamination of "clean" feed with sulfa-containing feed can result in finishing feed having sufficient levels of sulfa to cause a violative residue (0.1 ppm) in liver or muscle tissue. The sulfonamides have electrostatic properties, and they tend to accumulate in feed dust, which can contaminate other batches of feed. Granulated forms of sulfamethazine are now used, and they are less apt to contribute to cross-contamination than powdered sulfamethazine (Cromwell et al., 1982).

E. SAFETY OF ANTIMICROBIALS

Not long after the antibiotics were discovered and accepted into feeding programs for livestock and poultry, questions were raised about their safety. Many of those concerns continue today. The greatest concern is whether the widespread usage of antibiotics in animal feeds contributes to a reservoir of drug-resistant enteric bacteria that are capable of transferring their resistance to pathogenic bacteria (such as the salmonella), thereby causing a potential public health hazard (Smith, 1962; Falkow, 1975; Linton, 1977). The greatest concern is in regard to penicillin and the tetracyclines, because they also are used in human medicine.

Although transfer of antibiotic-resistant plasmids (R-plasmids) occurs rapidly *in vitro*, the extent to which it occurs in the animal, and between animal bacteria and human bacteria, is not well documented. Animal bacteria do not colonize very effectively in humans unless extremely large doses are consumed, and, even then, they are transient (Smith, 1969).

Steps were taken in the early 1970s in Great Britain to restrict the use of certain drugs (those used in human medicine and those capable of cross-resisting with drugs used in human medicine) to a prescription basis (Swann, 1969). A similar plan was proposed by the FDA in the mid-1970s (Kennedy, 1977) but it was never implemented. Shortly after a report by Holmberg et al. (1984), which attempted to link several cases of salmonellosis in humans with the consumption of beef from cattle that had been exposed to antibiotics, a petition was filed by the National Resources Defense Council to declare an immediate ban on penicillin and tetracyclines, claiming that they constitute an imminent hazard to public health. After extensive hearings, however, it was concluded that a ban was not justified, and the petition was denied.

In 1987, the FDA asked the Institute of Medicine of the National Academy of Science to conduct an independent review of the human health consequences and to make a quantitative risk assessment associated with the use of penicillin and the tetracyclines at subtherapeutic levels in animal feeds. The committee was unable to find a substantive body of direct evidence that established the existence of a definite health hazard in humans that could be associated with the use of subtherapeutic concentrations of these antibiotics in animal feeds (IOM, 1988). Other groups of scientists have extensively reviewed the published data and concluded that there is no evidence of human health being compromised by subtherapeutic antimicrobial usage in animals (NRC, 1980; 1999; CAST, 1981).

Whether restricting or even banning the use of certain antibiotics would have a significant influence on the pool of drug-resistant microorganisms is questionable. Action taken by the British government to limit the use of certain drugs to a prescription basis did not reduce the overall usage of tetracyclines, nor did it influence the resistance patterns in enteric bacteria of pigs in Britain (Smith, 1975; 1977; Braude, 1978).

The studies by Langlois et al. (1978a,b; 1986) lend further evidence that even a complete ban on subtherapeutic use of all antibiotics would have only minor influences on antimicrobial resistance levels and patterns. Figure 18.3 illustrates that a rather large percentage of enteric microbes in pigs were resistant to tetracycline, even after 13 years of no antibacterial exposure in a closed swine herd. Multiple resistance also was relatively high in pigs having no exposure to antibacterials for 13 years (Figure 18.4; Table 18.15). Factors such as animal age, type of housing, and transportation stress were found to have as much (or more) of an impact on fecal shedding of resistant organisms as the presence of antibiotics in the feed (Table 18.16).

The question of whether antimicrobial resistance constitutes a significant threat to human health likely will continue to be debated in the scientific community as well as in the political arena. Monitoring and surveillance of microbial resistance in animals and humans has continued with no animal-to-human infection path being clearly delineated. While the incidence of antimicrobial

Antimicrobial and Promicrobial Agents 415

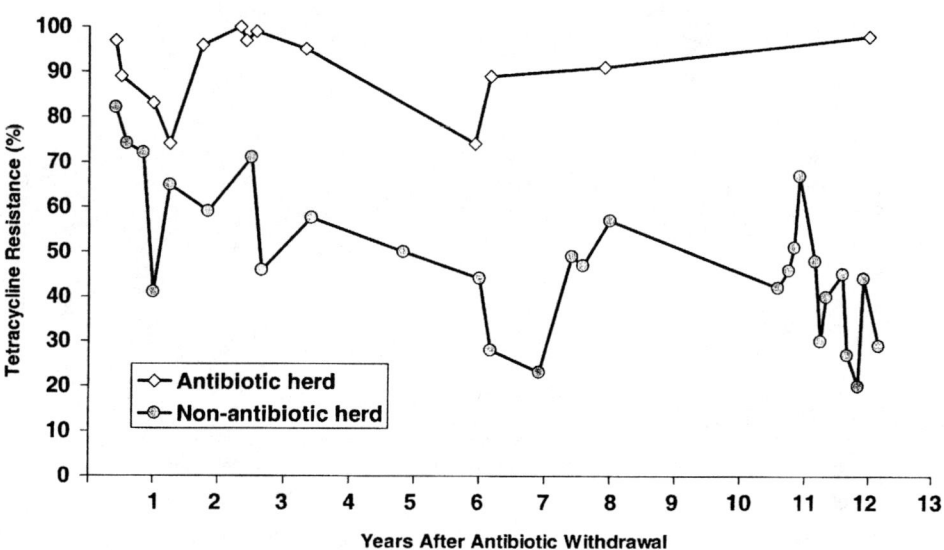

FIGURE 18.3 Tetracycline resistance of fecal coliforms isolated from pigs in a herd not exposed to antibiotics since 1972 (nonantibiotic herd) and in a herd fed chlortetracycline continuously since 1972 (antibiotic herd). (Adapted from Langlois et al., 1986.)

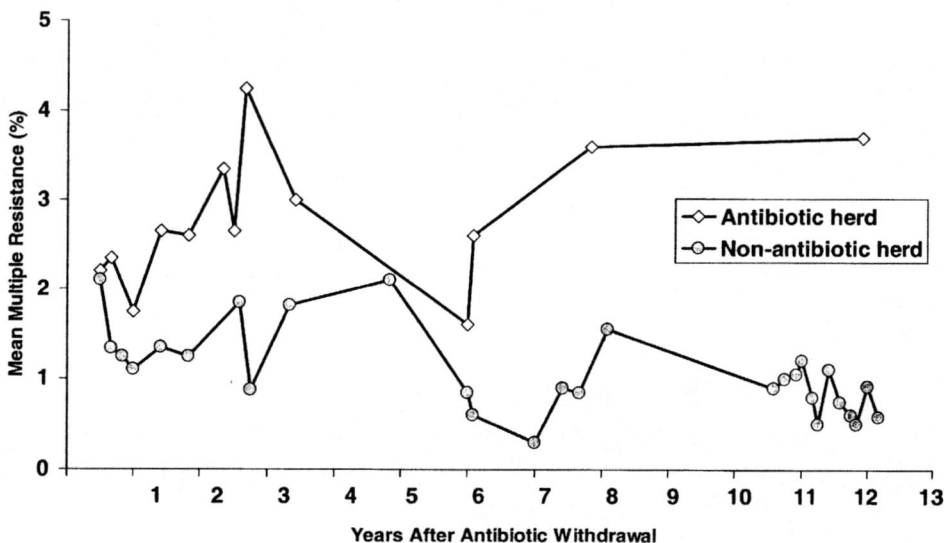

FIGURE 18.4 Mean multiple resistance to ten antimicrobial agents of fecal coliforms isolated from pigs in a herd not exposed to antibiotics since 1972 (nonantibiotic herd) and in a herd fed chlortetracycline continuously since 1972 (antibiotic herd). (Adapted from Langlois et al., 1986.)

TABLE 18.15
Resistance of Fecal Coliform Isolates from Herds Having No Exposure or Continuous Exposure to Antibiotics for 13 Years

Item	Antibiotic Exposure	
	Continuous[a]	None
No. of isolates	1761	4886
Percent of isolates resistant to:		
Ampicillin	25	7
Kanamycin	39	<1
Neomycin	30	<1
Streptomycin	62	20
Sulfisoxazole	32	23
Tetracycline	92	46
Average number of agents to which coliforms were resistant	2.87	1.00

[a] Less than 3% of the isolates from the pigs having antibiotic exposure were resistant to cephalothin, chloramphenicol, gentamicin, and nalidixic acid.

Source: Langlois, B. E. et al., *J. Anim. Sci.,* 62(Suppl. 3):18, 1986. With permission.

TABLE 18.16
Effects of Age, Housing System, and Moving Stress on Tetracycline Resistance of Fecal Coliforms from Pigs Not Exposed to Antibiotics for 13 Years

Item	No. of Isolates	Coliforms Resistant to Tetracycline (% of total)	Multiple Resistance[a]
Age of pigs (months)			
< 2	1069	70	1.52
2 to 6	1110	64	1.38
7 to 11	719	24	0.50
12 to 23	1648	33	0.69
>24	340	29	0.61
Housing			
Farrowing house	464	50	1.11
Feeding floor	1326	69	1.47
Pasture	2421	29	0.62
Moving stress			
Unmoved	4886	46	1.00
After moving 300 km	696	82	2.21

[a] Average number of antimicrobials (of 10 tested) to which fecal coliforms were resistant.

Source: Langlois, B. E. et al., *J. Anim. Sci.,* 62(Suppl. 3):18, 1986. With permission.

resistance in the human population is quite high, there is no evidence that the levels or patterns are changing to any great extent (Lorian, 1986). The high incidence of antimicrobial resistance in humans is likely due to the use of antibiotics prescribed directly for humans, because well over half of the antibiotics produced in the United States is used in human medicine (NRC, 1999).

Although antimicrobial agents have been fed for nearly 50 years to literally billions of animals, there is still no convincing evidence of any unfavorable health effects in humans that can be directly linked to the feeding of subtherapeutic levels of antibiotics to swine or other food-producing animals.

F. Economic Benefits of Antimicrobials

The economic returns to the swine producer using antibiotics in the feeding program are influenced by a number of factors, including the degree of response to the particular antibiotic (i.e., improvement in rate and efficiency of growth, improvement in the reproductive performance, reduction in mortality and morbidity, the cost of the antibiotic, the cost of feed and other production variables, and the market price of hogs). Based on average figures, the total benefit from antimicrobial usage was calculated by Zimmerman (1986) to be $2.64 per marketed pig. More recent calculations indicate that the benefits could be as much as $3.93 per marketed pig (Cromwell, 1999).

The ultimate beneficiary from increased production efficiency is the consumer. In 1981 it was estimated that the use of antimicrobial agents in animal production resulted in a $3.5 billion annual savings in meat costs to the consumer in the United States (CAST, 1981). Likely, this savings is considerably greater today.

III. PROMICROBIAL AGENTS

Promicrobials (formerly called probiotics; now called direct-fed microbials), are live, viable microorganisms that are added to animal feed with the intent of modifying the gut to a more desirable balance of microflora to improve the health and performance of the host animal. A number of reviews have been written on the use of promicrobials for swine (Pollmann, 1986; 1992; Fuller, 1989; 1992a; Vanbelle et al., 1990; Jonsson and Conway, 1992; Stavric and Kornegay, 1995).

The sterile digestive tract of newborn pigs rapidly becomes naturally colonized by a variety of microorganisms as the pigs are exposed to a traditional environment. Under healthy and nonstress conditions, "beneficial" microflora colonize gut surfaces in a symbiotic relationship with the host, and undesirable microbes, which may be pathogenic, are suppressed. The development of a stable, protective microflora is important for the animal's health and well-being. Pigs raised in a sterile environment are more susceptible to bacterial infections apparently because of the establishment of pathogenic organisms that have no competition from normal microflora. When animals are stressed, the balance between beneficial and harmful organisms may be upset, resulting in diarrhea, gastroenteritis, and reduced growth performance. The original concept of administering direct-fed microbials was that the large amounts of beneficial microbes would combat the negative effects of stress by preventing pathogenic organisms from colonizing in the gut (Kung, 1992).

A. Efficacy of Promicrobials

The responses to promicrobials in pigs is considerable less consistent than is the case with antimicrobial agents. In the past, many of the claims of improved growth rate and efficiency of feed utilization, improved health, reduced diarrhea, and improvements in reproductive efficiency were not supported by data from controlled experiments (Pollmann, 1992). This was largely because promicrobials could be added to feed without having claims substantiated by controlled experiments, as was the case with antimicrobials. As a result, many of the microbials and similar products were promoted, sold, and used in the swine industry based on their perceived beneficial value with little or no supporting data demonstrating their efficacy.

Pollmann (1986) conducted an extensive review of the literature in which *Lactobacillus* species were evaluated in young, weanling pigs. A summary of 18 experiments showed that pig performance was numerically improved in 13 of the trials. A review by this author of seven studies with growing-finishing pigs indicated that the addition of either mixed *Lactobacillus* or *E. faecium* failed to consistently improve growth performance. Other studies involving *Bacillus subtilis* additions to pig or sow diets failed to consistently improve growth or reproductive performance (Pollmann, 1986).

A summary of 26 experiments by Nousiainen and Setala (1993) showed positive growth responses to promicrobials in 16 trials (two were significant at $P < 0.05$) and negative growth responses in nine trials (two were significant at $P < 0.05$). Feed:gain responses were positively affected by promicrobials in eight trials and negatively affected in nine trials. Summaries by other authors and reviewed by Stavric and Kornegay (1995) showed similar inconsistent responses to promicrobials in young and growing-finishing pigs.

An extensive study by Cromwell et al. (1991) assessed various combinations of *Saccharomyces cerevisiae*, *L. acidophilus*, and *Streptococcus faecium* added to pig starter diets alone and in combination with antimicrobial agents (a commercial mixture of chlortetracycline, penicillin, and sulfamethazine). The study involved five experiments with 29 pen-replications of six pigs per treatment. The microbial supplements produced no responses in growth rate or efficiency of feed utilization in any of the experiments, while the antimicrobial agents gave positive growth and feed:gain responses in every experiment in which they were tested (Table 18.17).

TABLE 18.17
Effects of Promicrobial and Antimicrobial Agents in Starting Diets for Weanling Pigs[a]

	None	Promicrobials[b]	Antimicrobials[b]	Both
Daily gain (g)[c]	247	237	306	310
Daily feed (g)[c]	467	460	540	550
Feed:gain[c]	1.92	1.96	1.77	1.75

[a] A summary of five experiments involving 764 pigs weaned at 4 weeks of age (7.4 kg body weight); 4-week test period.

[b] Promicrobials were various combinations of *Saccharomyces cerevisiae*, *Lactobacillus acidophilus*, and *Streptococcus faecium*. Antimicrobials were a mixture of chlortetracycline, penicillin, and sulfamethazine.

[c] Effect of antimicrobials ($P < 0.001$).

Source: Adapted from Cromwell et al. (1991).

Despite the lack of consistent responses to promicrobials in controlled experiments, there are claims that the responses are more consistent under field conditions, particularly when disease or stress is high. In controlled studies, promicrobials were found to reduce diarrhea in young pigs in some studies (Hale and Newton, 1979; Maeng et al., 1989; Eigel, 1989), but not in others (Wu et al., 1987; McLeese et al., 1992; De Cupere et al., 1992; Havenaar and Huis in't Veld; 1993; Apgar et al., 1993).

B. Mode of Action of Promicrobials

Numerous authors have speculated on the mode of action of promicrobial agents, but there is little definitive evidence to support any of the proposed mechanisms (Stavric and Kornegay, 1995). Fuller (1992b) suggested four possible mechanisms: (1) competition for adhesion receptors on the gut epithelium, (2) competition for nutrients, (3) production of antibacterial substances, and (4) stimulation of immunity.

Evidence that the indigenous gut microflora have the ability to inhibit colonization of invading microorganisms comes primarily from studies with poultry and germ-free animals (Hentges, 1992). Introduction of gut microflora from healthy birds into newly hatched chicks made them resistant to infection when challenged with salmonella (Nurmi and Rantala, 1973). This process of adhesion of desirable microbes and resulting inhibition or displacement of undesirable microbes on the gut epithelium is called "competitive exclusion." Although lactic acid bacteria are associated with the gut wall of pigs (Barrow et al., 1980), the process of competitive exclusion is not as well documented in pigs as it is in chicks. In one study, homogenates of intestinal mucosa from pigs treated with *L. lactis* were found to have more attached lactobacilli and fewer *Escherichia coli* counts than scouring or nontreated control pigs (Muralidhara et al., 1977).

Competition for nutrients between resident and invading bacteria occurs *in vivo*, but evidence for such competition in the intestine is lacking (Freter, 1992; Hentges, 1992). Colonized lactic acid bacteria may utilize nutrients that would otherwise be available for pathogens or they may produce metabolites that inhibit the growth of pathogens.

Inhibitory compounds produced by lactobacilli are active *in vitro* against a broad spectrum of bacterial species (Juven et al., 1991; Havenaar et al., 1992). These compounds include bacteriocins and bacteriocin-like substances, hydrogen peroxide, and certain organic acids (Juven et al., 1991). However, the role of most of these antagonistic compounds in the intestine is unknown. An exception is the organic acids, which are known to decrease intestinal pH. A lower gut pH seems to be associated with a reduction in the colonization of pathogenic microbes (Stavric and Kornegay, 1995).

Finally, although supporting data are scarce, some have proposed that promicrobials may improve the animal's immune status. This proposed mechanism is based on the fact that conventional animals with complete microflora have higher immunoglobulin levels and phagocytic activity than their germ-free counterparts (Nousiainen and Setala, 1993).

IV. MISCELLANEOUS AGENTS

A few other organic compounds have been found to alter the resident microorganisms in the gut. One such group of compounds is the oligosaccharides. The mannan-oligosaccharides (MOS) are short chains of mannose found in relatively high concentrations in yeast cell walls. These compounds have a high affinity for specific sites on certain pathogenic bacteria, which prevents their attachment to the intestinal epithelium. As a result, the potential pathogens flow out of the intestine, and beneficial microorganisms (e.g., lactobacilli) are given opportunity to attach and colonize. This process is commonly referred to as "competitive exclusion." Although this process has been shown to work effectively with poultry (Newman, 1996), it is less well documented in swine. In one study, oligosaccharides from yeast were found to improve growth rate in young pigs (Schoenherr et al., 1994). In a more recent study, Davis et al. (1999) found that dietary inclusion of MOS was about half as effective in stimulating growth of weanling pigs as inclusion of a high level of copper sulfate, a well-known antimicrobial agent (Table 18.18). In another study (Davis et al., 2000), these same researchers found that MOS was ineffective in stimulating growth of weanling pigs (Table 18.18).

Fructo-oligosaccharides (FOS) are short and medium chains of fructose linked with β-(2-1) osidic bonds and with a terminal glucose unit (Roberfroid et al, 1993). FOS is resistant to acidic and enzymatic hydrolysis in the tract, but is fermented by specific microbes. FOS differs from MOS in that is serves as a substrate for the *Bifidobacterium* species and certain other beneficial microflora in the gut (Russell et al., 1996), and their rapid growth inhibits colonization of pathogenic microbes. When challenged with pathogenic *E. coli*, pigs given FOS had reduced numbers of *E. coli* after several days and there was a reduced incidence of diarrhea and death compared with untreated controls (Bunce et al., 1995). In healthy pigs, inclusion of FOS in the diet increased weight gains in weanling pigs to the same magnitude as supplementing the diet with carbadox (Table 18.19) or tylosin (Russell et al., 1996; Howard et al, 1999). Improvements in intestinal morphology including an increase in villus height and villus:crypt ratio also have been observed in pigs given FOS (Spencer et al., 1997).

TABLE 18.18
Effects of MOS and Antimicrobial Agents in Starting Diets for Weanling Pigs

Item	Control	MOS[a]	Antimicrobial[b]	Both
Experiment 1[c]				
Daily gain (g)	364	402	439	452
Daily feed (g)	564	596	659	638
Feed:gain	1.56	1.45	1.42	1.37
Experiment 2[d]				
Daily gain (g)	413	406	427	437
Daily feed (g)	559	571	587	594
Feed:gain	1.32	1.37	1.33	1.31

[a] Mannan-oligosaccharides (MOS) included at 0.2% of the diet in Exp. 1 and at 0.2 or 0.3% of the diet in Exp. 2.
[b] Antimicrobial in Exp. 1 was copper sulfate at 185 ppm copper, and in Exp. 2 was zinc oxide at 2300 ppm zinc.
[c] Davis et al. (1999). Adapted from summary of a 38-day experiment involving nine replications of six pigs per pen. Pigs weaned at 21 days of age and initially averaged 5.8 kg body weight.
[d] Davis et al. (2000). Adapted from summary of a 38-day experiment involving six replications of six pigs per pen. Pigs weaned at 15 to 21 days of age and initially averaged 4.6 kg body weight.

TABLE 18.19
Effects of FOS and an Antimicrobial Agent in Starting Diets for Weanling Pigs[a]

Item	Control	FOS[b]	Antimicrobial[b]	Both
Daily gain (g)	338	379	380	420
Daily feed (g)	534	594	560	622
Feed:gain	1.58	1.57	1.47	1.48

[a] Russell et al. (1996). Adapted from a summary of two 28-day experiments involving eight replications of four pigs per pen. Pigs weaned at 15 days of age and initially averaged 5.5 kg body weight.
[b] Fructo-oligosaccharides (FOS) provided at 383 mg/day and carbadox included in diet at 55 mg/kg.

TABLE 18.20
Effects of Organic Acids in Starting Diets for Weanling Pigs

Item	Control	Organic Acid	Improvement (%)
Experiments with citric acid[a]			
Daily gain (g)	295	313	5.2
Feed:gain	1.88	1.75	7.2
Experiments with fumaric acid[b]			
Daily gain (g)	309	322	4.1
Feed:gain	1.86	1.73	6.9

[a] Summary of five experiments, 311 pigs, 8.6 to 15.9 kg, 24-day test.
[b] Summary of five experiments, 386 pigs, 9.1 to 17.3 kg, 27-day test.

Source: Adapted from Kirchgessner and Roth (1982), Falkowski and Aherne (1984), Giesting and Easter (1985), Edmonds et al. (1985), and Burnell et al. (1988).

Inclusion of organic acids in diets for early-weaned pigs have been shown to improve postweaning performance (Kirchgessner and Roth, 1982; Falkowski and Aherne, 1984; Edmonds et al., 1985; Giesting and Easter, 1985; Burnell et al., 1988) as shown in Table 18.20. Benefits have been reported for citric acid, fumaric acid, and formic acid. The reduced pH in the upper gastrointestinal tract and its impact on microbial populations in the gut has been suggested as one of the possible modes of action of organic acids in young pigs.

REFERENCES

AAFCO (Association of American Feed Control Officials). 2000. AAFCO Official Publication. P. O. Box 478, Oxford, IN 47971.

Anderson, G. W., J. D. Cunningham, and S. J. Slinger. 1952. Effect of protein level and penicillin on growth and intestinal flora of chickens, *J. Nutr.*, 47:175.

Anonymous. 1992. *1993 Direct-Fed Microbial, Enzyme, and Forage Additive Compendium*, Miller Publishing Co., Minnetonka, MN.

Apgar, G. A., E. T. Kornegay, M. D. Lindemann, and C. M. Wood. 1993. The effect of feeding various levels of *Bifidobacterium globosum* A on the performance, gastrointestinal measurements, and immunity of weanling pigs and on the performance and carcass measurements of growing-finishing pigs, *J. Anim. Sci.*, 71:2173.

Apgar, G. A., E. T. Kornegay, M. D. Lindemann, and D. R. Notter. 1995. Evaluation of copper sulfate and a copper lysine complex as growth promotants for weanling swine, *J. Anim. Sci.*, 73:2640.

Barrow, P. A., B. E. Brooker, R. Fuller, and M. J. Newport. 1980. The attachment of bacteria to the gastric epithelium of the pig and its importance in the microecology of the intestine, *J. Appl. Bacteriol.*, 48:147.

Beames, R. M., and L. E. Lloyd. 1965. Response of pigs and rats to rations supplemented with tylosin and high levels of copper, *J. Anim. Sci.*, 24:1020.

Braude, R. 1945. Some observations on the need for copper in the diet of fattening pigs, *J. Agric. Sci.*, 35:163.

Braude, R. 1978. Antibiotics in animal feeds in Great Britain, *J. Anim. Sci.*, 46:1425.

Braude, R., and B. C. Johnson. 1953. Effect of aureomycin on nitrogen and water metabolism in growing pigs, *J. Nutr.*, 49:505.

Braude, R., H. D. Wallace, and T. J. Cunha. 1953. The value of antibiotics in the nutrition of swine: a review, *Antibiot. Chemother.*, 3:271.

Braude, R., M. F. Coates, M. K. Davies, G. F. Harrison, and K. G. Mitchell. 1955. The effect of aureomycin on the gut of a pig, *Br. J. Nutr.*, 9:363.

Brody, T. M., M. R. Hurwitz, and J. A. Bain. 1954. Magnesium and the effect of the tetracycline antibiotics on oxidative processes in mitochondria, *Antibiot. Chemother.*, 4:864.

Bunce, T. J., M. D. Howard, M. S. Kerley, G. L. Allee, and L. W. Pace. 1995. Protective effect of fructooligosaccharide (FOS) in prevention of mortality and morbidity from infectious *E. coli* K:88 challenge, *J. Anim. Sci.*, 63(Suppl. 1):69 (Abstr.).

Bunch, R. J., J. T. McCall, V. C. Speer, and V. W. Hays. 1965. Copper supplementation for weanling pigs, *J. Anim. Sci.*, 24:995.

Burnell, T. W., G. L. Cromwell, and T. S. Stahly. 1988. Effects of dried whey and copper sulfate on the growth responses to organic acid in diets for weanling pigs, *J. Anim. Sci.*, 66:1100.

CAST. 1981. Antibiotics in Animal Feeds, Report 88, Council for Agricultural Science and Technology, Ames, IA.

Catron, D. V., A. H. Jensen, P. G. Homeyer, H. M. Maddock, and G. C. Ashton. 1952. Re-evaluation of protein requirements of growing-fattening swine as influenced by feeding an antibiotic, *J. Anim. Sci.*, 11:221.

Catron, D. V., M. D. Lane, L. Y. Quinn, G. C. Ashton, and H. M. Maddock. 1953. Mode of action of antibiotics in swine nutrition, *Antibiot. Chemother.*, 3:571.

Coffey, R. D., G. L. Cromwell, and H. J. Monegue. 1994. Efficacy of a copper-lysine complex as a growth promotant for weanling pigs, *J. Anim. Sci.*, 72:2880.

Combs, G. E., and H. D. Wallace. 1969. Recent research on the use of feed additives for swine, Florida Animal Science Mimeograph Series No. 69-11, University of Florida, Gainesville.

Cromwell, G. L. 1987. Recent research on the use of feed additives for swine, *Proc. Georgia Nutr. Conf.*, University of Georgia, Athens, 24–35.

Cromwell, G. L. 1997. Copper as a nutrient for animals. In *Handbook of Copper Compounds and Applications*, H. W. Richardson, Ed., Marcel Dekker, New York, 177–202.

Cromwell, G. L. 1999. Subtherapeutic use of antibiotics for swine: Performance, reproductive efficiency and safety issues, *Proc. 40th Annual George A. Young Swine Health and Management Conf.*, University of Nebraska, Lincoln, 70–87.

Cromwell, G. L., and K. A. Dawson. 1992. Antibiotic growth promotants. In Emerging Agricultural Technology: Issues for the 1990's, Office of Technology Assessment, U.S. Congress, Washington, D.C.

Cromwell, G. L., T. S. Stahly, H. J. Monegue, E. R. Peo, B. D. Moser, and A. J. Lewis. 1981. Effects of sulfamethazine vs. sulfathiazole in finishing feed on sulfa residues in swine, *J. Anim. Sci.*, 53(Suppl. 1):95 (Abstr.).

Cromwell, G. L., R. I. Hutagalung, and T. S. Stahly. 1982. Effects of form of sulfamethazine (powder vs. granular) on sulfa carry-over in swine feed, *J. Anim. Sci.*, 55(Suppl. 1):267 (Abstr.).

Cromwell, G. L., T. S. Stahly, and H. J. Monegue. 1989. Effects of source and level of copper on performance and liver copper stores in weanling pigs, *J. Anim. Sci.*, 67:2996.

Cromwell, G. L., T. S. Stahly, K. A. Dawson, J. J. Monegue, and K. Newman. 1991. Probiotics and antibacterial agents for weanling pigs, *J. Anim. Sci.*, 69(Suppl. 1):114 (Abstr.).

Cromwell, G. L., H. J. Monegue, and T. S. Stahly. 1993. Long-term effects of feeding a high copper diet to sows during gestation and lactation, *J. Anim. Sci.*, 71:2996.

Cromwell, G. L., M. D. Lindemann, H. J. Monegue, D. D. Hall, and D. E. Orr, Jr. 1998. Tribasic copper chloride and copper sulfate as copper sources for weanling pigs, *J. Anim. Sci.*, 76:118.

Cunha, T. J., J. E. Burnside, D. M. Buschman, R. S. Glasscock, A. M. Pearson, and A. L. Shealy. 1949. Effect of vitamin B_{12}, animal protein factor and soil for pig growth, *Arch. Biochem.*, 23:324.

Cunha, T. J., G. B. Meadows, H. M. Edwards, R. F. Sewell, C. B. Shaver, A. M. Person, and R. S. Glasscock. 1950. Effect of aureomycin and other antibiotics on the pig, *J. Anim. Sci.*, 9:653.

Davis, M. E., C. V. Maxwell, E. B. Kegley, B. Z. de Rodas, K. G. Friesen, D. H. Hellwig, and R. A. Dvorak. 1999. Efficacy of mannan oligosaccharide (Bio-Mos) addition at two levels of supplemental copper on performance and immunocompetence of early weaned pigs, *J. Anim. Sci.*, 77(Suppl. 1):63 (Abstr.).

Davis, M. E., C. V. Maxwell, E. B. Kegley, B. Z. de Rodas, K. G. Friesen, D. H. Hellwig, D. C. Brown, and R. A. Dvorak. 2000. Efficacy of mannan oligosaccharide (Bio-Mos) supplementation with and without zinc oxide on performance and immunocompetence of weanling pigs. Abstr. 166 of the Midwestern Section Meeting of the American Society of Animal Science, Des Moines, IA, March 13–15, 2000.

Dean, B. T., and L. F. Tribble. 1962. Effect of feeding therapeutic levels of antibiotics at breeding on reproductive performance of swine, *J. Anim. Sci.*, 21:207.

De Cupere, F., P. Deprez, D. Demeulenaere, and E. Muylle. 1992. Evaluation of the effect of 3 probiotics on experimental *Escherichia coli* enterotoxaemia in weaned piglets, *J. Vet. Med.*, B 39:277.

Edmonds, M. S., O. A. Izquierdo, and D. H. Baker. 1985. Feed additive studies with newly weaned pigs: efficacy of supplemental copper, antibiotics and organic acids, *J. Anim. Sci.*, 60:462.

Eigel, W. N. 1989. Ability of probiotics to protect weanling pigs against challenge with enterotoxigenic *E. coli*. In Proceedings Chr. Hansen Biosystems Technical Conf., San Antonio, TX, 10–19.

Evvard, J. M., V. E. Nelson, and W. E. Sewell. 1928. Copper salts in nutrition, *Proc. Iowa Acad. Sci.*, 35:211.

Falkow, S. 1975. *Infectious Multiple Drug Resistance*, Pion Ltd., London.

Falkowski, J. F., and F. X. Aherne. 1984. Fumaric and citric acid as feed additives in starter pig nutrition, *J. Anim. Sci.*, 58:935.

Feed Additive Compendium, 2000. Miller Publishing Co., Minnetonka, MN.

Fox, S. M. 1988. Probiotics: intestinal inoculants for production animals, *Vet. Med.*, 83:806.

Freter, R. 1992. Factors affecting the microecology of the gut. In *Probiotics: The Scientific Basis*, R. Fuller, Ed., Chapman & Hall, London, 111–144.

Fuller, R. 1989. Probiotics in man and animals, *J. Appl. Bacteriol.*, 66:365.

Fuller, R. 1992a. History and development of probiotics. In *Probiotics: The Scientific Basis*, R. Fuller, Ed., Chapman & Hall, London, 1–8.

Fuller, R. 1992b. Problems and prospects. In *Probiotics: The Scientific Basis*, R. Fuller, Ed., Chapman & Hall, London, 337–386.

Giesting, D. W., and R. A. Easter. 1985. Response of starter pigs to supplementation of corn–soybean meal diets with organic acids, *J. Anim. Sci.*, 60:1288.

Hagen, C. D., S. G. Cornelius, R. L. Moser, J. E. Pettigrew, and K. P. Miller. 1987. High levels of copper alone or in combination with antibacterials in weanling pig diets, *Nutr. Rep. Int.*, 35:1083.

Hahn, J. D., and D. H. Baker. 1993. Growth and plasma zinc responses of young pigs fed pharmacologic levels of zinc, *J. Anim. Sci.*, 71:3030.

Hale, O. M., and G. L. Newton. 1979. Effects of a nonviable lactobacillus species fermentation product on performance of pigs, *J. Anim. Sci.*, 48:770.

Hash, J. H., M. Wishnick, and P. A. Miller. 1964. On the mode of action of the tetracycline antibiotics in *Staphylococcus aureus*, *J. Biol. Chem.*, 239:2070.

Havanaar, R., and J. H. J. Huis in't Veld. 1993. *In vitro* and *in vivo* experiments with two commercial probiotic products containing *Enterococcus faecium* and *Bacillus toyoi*. In *Prevention and Control of Potentially Pathogenic Microorganisms in Poultry and Poultry Meat Processing. Probiotics and Pathogenicity,* Jensen, J. F., M. H. Hinton, and R. W. A. W. Mulder, Eds., COVP-DLO Het Spelderholt, D. A. Bbeekbergen, The Netherlands, 53–62.

Havanaar, R., B. T. Brink, and J. H. J. Huis in't Veld. 1992. Selection of strains for probiotic use. In *Probiotics. The Scientific Basis*, R. Fuller, Ed., Chapman & Hall, London, 209–224.

Hays, V. W. 1977. Effectiveness of Feed Additive Usage of Antibacterial Agents in Swine and Poultry Production, Office of Technology Assessment, U.S. Congress, Washington, D.C. (Edited version: Hays, V. W. 1981. *The Hays Report*, Rachelle Laboratories, Inc., Long Beach, CA).

Hays, V. W. 1978. The role of antibiotics in efficient livestock production. In *Nutrition and Drug Interrelations*, Academic Press, New York.

Hays, V. W., and V. C. Speer. 1960. Effect of spiramycin on growth and feed utilization of young pigs, *J. Anim. Sci.*, 19:938.

Hays, V. W., J. L. Krug, G. L. Cromwell, R. H. Dutt, and D. D. Kratzer. 1978. Effect of lactation length and dietary antibiotics on reproductive performance of sows, *J. Anim. Sci.*, 46:884.

Hedde, R. D. 1981. Intestinal fermentation in the pig and how it is influenced by age and virginiamycin. In *Proceedings of the Growth Promotion Mode-of-Action Symposium*, SmithKline Corp., Philadelphia, 10–20.

Henderickx, H. K., I. J. Vervaecke, J. A. Decuypere, and N. A. Dierick. 1981. Mode of action of growth promotion drugs. In *Proceedings of the Growth Promotion Mode-of-Action Symposium*, SmithKline Corp., Philadelphia, 3–9.

Hentges, D. J. 1992. Gut flora in disease resistance. In *Probiotics: The Scientific Basis*, R. Fuller, Ed., Chapman & Hall, London, 87–110.

Hill, G. M., G. L. Cromwell, T. D. Crenshaw, C. R. Dove, R. C. Ewan, D. A. Knabe, A. J. Lewis, G. W. Libal, D. C. Mahan, G. C. Shurson, L. L. Southern, and T. L. Veum. 2000. Growth promotion effects and plasma changes from feeding high dietary concentrations of zinc and copper to weanling pigs (regional study), *J. Anim. Sci.*, 78:1010.

Holmberg, M. D., M. T. Osterholm, K. A. Senger, and M. L. Cohen. 1984. Drug-resistant salmonella from animals fed antimicrobials, *N. Engl. J. Med.*, 311:617.

Howard, M. D., H. Liu, J. D. Spencer, M. S. Kerley, and G. L. Allee. 1999. Incorporation of short-chain fructooligosaccharides and Tylan into diets of early weaned pigs, *J. Anim. Sci.*, 77(Suppl. 1):63.

IOM. 1988. *Human Health Risks with the Subtherapeutic Use of Penicillin or Tetracycline in Animal Feed*, Institute of Medicine, National Academy of Sciences, National Academy Press, Washington, D.C.

Johnson, D. D., R. G. Eggert, H. M. Maddock, and K. L. Simkins. 1985. Effect of an antibiotic feed medication program in swine herds with a history of respiratory disease on sow reproduction, pig performance, and lung lesions, *J. Anim. Sci.*, 61(Suppl. 1):437 (Abstr.).

Jonsson, E., and P. Conway 1992. Probiotics for pigs. In *Probiotics: The Scientific Basis*, R. Fuller, Ed., Chapman & Hall, London, 260–316.

Jordan, C. E., and W. P. Waitt. 1963. The effect of tylosin when fed to sows during farrowing and early lactation on pig survival and gains, *J. Anim. Sci.*, 22:838.

Jukes, T. H., E. L. R. Stokstad, R. R. Taylor, T. J. Cunha, H. M. Edwards, and G. B. Meadows. 1950. Growth promoting effect of aureomycin on pigs, *Arch. Biochem.*, 26:324.

Juven, B. J., R. J. Meinersmann, and N. J. Stern. 1991. A review. Antagonistic effects of lactobacilli and pediococci to control intestinal colonization by human enterophatogens in live poultry, *J. Appl. Bacteriol.*, 70:95.

Kellogg, T. F., V. W. Hays, D. V. Catron, L. Y. Quinn, and V. C. Speer. 1964. Effect of level and source of dietary protein on performance and fecal flora of baby pigs, *J. Anim. Sci.*, 23:1089.

Kennedy, D. F. 1977. Antibiotics used in animal feeds. In HEW News, April 15, U.S. Department of Health, Education and Welfare, Rockville, MD.

Kirchgessner, M., and F. X. Roth. 1982. Fumaric acid as a feed additive in pig nutrition, *Pig News Info.*, 3:259.

Koong, L. J., J. A. Neinaber, J. C. Pekas, and J. T. Yen. 1982. Effects of plane of nutrition on organ size and fasting heat production in pigs, *J. Nutr.*, 112:1638.

Kulwich, R., S. L. Hansard, C. L. Comar, and G. K. Davis. 1953. Copper, molydenum, and zinc interrelationships in rats and swine, *Proc. Soc. Exp. Biol. Med.*, 84:487.

Kung, L., Jr. 1992. Direct-fed microbial and enzyme feed additives. In *1993 Direct-Fed Microbial, Enzyme, and Forage Additive Compendium*, Miller Publishing Co., Minnetonka, MN, 17–21.

Langlois, B. E., G. L. Cromwell, and V. W. Hays. 1978a. Influence of chlortetracycline in swine feed on reproductive performance and on incidence and persistence of antibiotic resistant enteric bacteria, *J. Anim. Sci.*, 46:1369.

Langlois, B. E., G. L. Cromwell, and V. W. Hays. 1978b. Influence of type of antibiotic and length of antibiotic feeding period on performance and persistence of antibiotic resistant enteric bacteria in growing-finishing swine, *J. Anim. Sci.*, 46:1383.

Langlois, B. E., K. A. Dawson, G. L. Cromwell, and T. S. Stahly. 1986. Antibiotic resistance in pigs following a 13 year ban, *J. Anim. Sci.*, 62 (Suppl. 3):18.

LeMieux, F. M., L. V. Ellison, T. L. Ward, L. L. Southern, and T. D. Bidner. 1995. Excess dietary zinc for pigs weaned at 28 days, *J. Anim. Sci.*, 73(Suppl. 1):72 (Abstr.).

Lepley, K. C., D. V. Catron, and C. C. Culbertson. 1950. Dried whole aureomycin mash and meat and bone scraps for growing-fattening swine, *J. Anim. Sci.*, 9:608.

Lillie, R. J. and L. T. Frobish. 1978. Effect of copper and iron supplements on performance and hematology of confined sows and their progeny through four reproductive cycles, *J. Anim. Sci.*, 46:678.

Linton, A. H. 1977. Antibiotics, animals, and man — an appraisal of a contentious subject. In *Antibiotics and Antibiosis in Agriculture*, M. Woodbine, Ed., Butterworths, Woburn, MA, 315–343.

Lorian, V. 1986. Antibiotic sensitivity patterns of human pathogens in American hospitals, *J. Anim. Sci.*, 62 (Suppl. 3):49.

Luecke, R. W., W. N. McMillan, and F. Thorp, Jr. 1950. The effect of vitamin B_{12} animal protein factor and streptomycin on the growth of young pigs, *Arch. Biochem.*, 26:326.

Maddock, H. M. 1985. Unpublished data.

Maeng, W. J., C. M. Kim, and H. T. Shin. 1989. Effect of feeding lactic acid bacteria concentrate (LBC, *Streptococcus faecium*, Cernelle 68) on the growth rate and prevention of scouring in piglet, *Korean J. Anim. Sci.*, 31:318.

Mahan, D. C. 1980. Effectiveness of antibacterial compounds and copper for weanling pigs, Ohio Swine Research and Industry Report 80-2. Ohio State University, Columbus.

March, B., and J. Biely. 1952. The effect of feeding aureomycin on the bacterial content of chick feces, *Poult. Sci.*, 31:177.

Maxwell, C. V., G. E. Combs, D. A. Knabe, E. T. Kornegay, P. R. Noland, and the S-145 Committee on Nutritional Systems for Swine to Increase Reproductive Efficiency. 1994. Effect of dietary chlortetracycline during breeding and(or) farrowing and lactation on reproductive performance of sows: a cooperative study, *J. Anim Sci.*, 72:3169.

Mayrose, V. B., V. C. Speer, V. W. Hays, and J. T. McCall. 1964. Effect of an antibiotic (tylosin) and protein source on swine reproduction, *J. Anim. Sci.*, 23:737.

McLeese, J. M., M. L. Tremblay, J. F. Patience, and G. I. Christison. 1992. Water intake patterns in the weanling pig: effect of water quality, antibiotics and probiotics, *Anim. Prod.*, 54:135.

Messersmith, R. E., D. D. Johnson, R. F. Elliot, and J. J. Drain. 1966. Value of chlortetracycline in breeding rations for sows, *J. Anim. Sci.*, 25:752.

Metchnikoff, E. 1903. *The Nature of Man. Studies of Optimistic Philosophy*, Heinemann, London.

Metchnikoff, E. 1908. *Prolongation of Life*, G. P. Putnam and Sons, New York.

Miller, E. R., D. E. Ullrey, I. Ackerman, D. A. Schmidt, J. A. Hoefer, and R. W. Luecke. 1961. Swine hematology from birth to maturity. I. Serum proteins, *J. Anim. Sci.*, 20:31.

Monegue, H. J., and G. L. Cromwell. 1996. Effects of high dietary copper for sows on reproductive performance, milk copper, and liver copper in sows and nursing pigs, *J. Anim. Sci.*, 74(Suppl. 1):55 (Abstr.).

Moore, P. R., A. Evenson, T. D. Luckey, E. McCoy, and C. A. Elvehjem. 1946. Use of sulfasuxidine, streptothricin and streptomycin in nutritional studies with the chick, *J. Biol. Chem.*, 165:437.

Moser, B. D., E. R. Peo, Jr., and A. J. Lewis. 1980. Effect of carbadox on protein utilization in the baby pig, *Nutr. Rep. Int.*, 22:949.

Muralidhara, K. S., G. G. Sheggeby, P. R. Elliker, D. C. England, and W. E. Sandine. 1977. Effect of feeding lactobacilli on the coliform and lactobacillus flora of intestinal tissue and feces from piglets, *J. Food Prot.*, 40:288.

Myers, D. J., and V. C. Speer. 1973. Effect of an antibiotic and flushing on performance of sows with short farrowing intervals, *J. Anim. Sci.*, 36:1125.

NCR-89 Committee on Confinement Management of Swine. 1984. Effect of space allowance and antibiotic feeding on performance of nursery pigs, *J. Anim. Sci.*, 58:801.

Newman, K. E. 1996. Nutritional manipulation of the gastrointestinal tract to eliminate salmonella and other pathogens. In *Biotechnology in the Feed Industry*, Lyons, T. P., and K. A. Jacques, Eds., Nottingham University Press, Nottingham, U.K., 37–45.

Nousiainen, J., and J. Setala. 1993. Lactic acid bacteria as animal probiotics. In *Lactic Acid Bacteria*, Salminen, S., and A. von Wright, Eds., Marcel Dekker, New York, 315–356.

NRC (National Research Council). 1980. *Effects on Human Health of Subtherapeutic Use of Antimicrobials in Animal Feed*, National Academy Press, Washington, D.C.

NRC (National Research Council). 1999. *The Use of Drugs in Food Animals: Benefits and Risks*, National Academy Press, Washington, D.C.

Nurmi, E., and M. Rantala. 1973. New aspects of *Salmonella* infection in broiler production, *Nature*, 241:210.

Parker, R. B. 1974. Probiotics, the other half of the antibiotics story, *Anim. Nutr. Health*, 29:4.

Pendelton, B. 1992. Challenges of regulation: United States industry perspective. In *Proceedings of the International Roundtable on Animal Feed Biotechnology — Research and Scientific Regulation*, Leger, D. A., and S. K. Ho, Eds., Agriculture Canada, Ottawa, Canada, 185–189.

Pollmann, D. S. 1986. Probiotics in pig diets. In *Recent Advances in Animal Nutrition*, Haresign, W., and D.J.A. Cole, Eds., Butterworths, London, 193–205.

Pollmann, D. S. 1992. Probiotics in swine diets. In *Proceedings of the International Roundtable on Animal Feed Biotechnology — Research and Scientific Regulation*, Leger, D. A., and S. K. Ho, Eds., Agriculture Canada, Ottawa, Canada, 65–74.

Risley, C. R. 1992. An overview of basic microbiology. In *1993 Direct-Fed Microbial, Enzyme, and Forage Additive Compendium*, Miller Publishing Co., Minnetonka, MN, 11–13.

Roberfroid, M., G. R. Gibson, and N. Delzenne. 1993. The biochemistry of oligofructose, a nondigestible fiber: an approach to calculate its caloric value, *Nutr. Rev.*, 51(5):137.

Ruiz, M. E., V. C. Speer, V. W. Hays, and W. P. Switzer. 1968. Effect of feed intake and antibiotic on reproduction in gilts, *J. Anim. Sci.*, 27:1602.

Russell, R. J., M. S. Kerley, and G. L. Allee. 1996. Effect of fructooligosaccharides on growth performance of the weaned pig, *J. Anim. Sci.*, 74(Suppl. 1):61 (Abstr.).

Sasaki, T., Y. Meade, and S. Namioka. 1987. Immunopotentiation of the mucosa of the small intestine of weaning piglets by peptidoglycans, *Jpn. J. Vet. Sci.*, 49:235.

Schoenherr, W. D., D. S. Pollmann, and J. A. Coalson. 1994. Titration of MacroGard™-S on growth performance of nursery pigs, *J. Anim. Sci.*, 72(Suppl. 2):57 (Abstr.).

Sewell, R. F., and J. L. Carmon. 1958. Reproductive performance of swine fed chlortetracycline over several generations, *J. Anim. Sci.*, 17:752.

Smith, H. W. 1962. The effects of the use of antibiotics on the emergency of antibiotic-resistant disease-producing organisms in animals. In *Proceedings of the University of Nottingham Ninth Easter School in Agricultural Science*, Butterworths, London, 374.

Smith, H. W. 1969. Transfer of antibiotic resistance from animal and human strains of *Escherichia coli* to resistant *E. coli* in the alimentary tract of man, *Lancet*, 1:1174.

Smith, H. W. 1975. Persistence of tetracycline resistance in pig *E. coli*, *Nature*, 258:628.

Smith, H. W. 1977. Antibiotic resistance in bacteria and associated problems in farm animals before and after the 1969 Swann Report. In *Antibiotics and Antibiosis in Agriculture*, Woodbine, M., Ed., Butterworths, Woburn, MA, 344–357.

Soma, J. A., and V. C. Speer. 1975. Effects of pregnant mare serum and chlortetracycline on the reproductive efficiency of sows, *J. Anim. Sci.*, 41:100.

Spencer, J. D., K. J. Touchett, H. Liu, G. L. Allee, M. D. Newcomb, M. S. Kerley, and L. W. Pace. 1997. Effect of spray-dried plasma and fructooligosaccharide on nursery performance and small intestinal morphology of weaned pigs, *J. Anim. Sci.*, 75(Suppl. 1):199 (Abstr.).

Stahly, T. S., G. L. Cromwell, and H. J. Monegue. 1980. Effect of single additions and combinations of copper and antibiotics on the performance of weanling pigs, *J. Anim. Sci.*, 51:1347.

Stansbury, W. F., L. F. Tribble, and D. E. Orr, Jr. 1990. Effect of chelated copper sources on performance of nursery and growing pigs, *J. Anim. Sci.*, 68:1317.

Stavric, S., and E. T. Kornegay. 1995. Microbial probiotics for pigs and poultry. In *Biotechnology in Animal Feeds and Feeding*, Wallace, R. J., and A. Chesson, Eds., VCH Verlagsgesellschaft, Weinheim, Germany, 205–231.

Stokstad, E. L. R., T. H. Jukes, J. Pierce, A. C. Page, Jr., and A. L. Franklin. 1949. The multiple nature of the animal protein factor, *J. Biol. Chem.*, 180:647.

Swann, M. M. 1969. Report of the Joint Committee on the Use of Antibiotics in Animal Husbandry and Veterinary Medicine, Her Majesty's Stationery Office, London.

Taylor, J. H., and G. Harrington. 1955. Influence of dietary antibiotic supplements on the visceral weights of pigs, *Nature*, 175:643.

U.S. International Trade Commission. 1989. Synthetic organic chemicals. In USITC Publication 2219, Washington, D.C.

Vanbelle, M., E. Teller, and M. Focant. 1990. Probiotics in animal nutrition: a review, *Arch. Anim. Nutr. Berlin*, 40(7):543–567.

Vincent, J. G., R. C. Veomett, and R. F. Riley. 1959. Antibacterial activity associated with *Lactobacillus acidophilus*, *J. Bacteriol.*, 78:477.

Visek, W. J. 1978. The mode of growth promotion by antibiotics, *J. Anim. Sci.*, 46:1447.

Wallace, H. D. 1967. *High Level Copper in Swine Feeding*, International Copper Research Association. New York.

Wallace, H. D., and G. E. Combs. 1962. High level antibiotic supplementation of the sow during the farrowing period, Florida Animal Science Mimeograph Series 63-3, University of Florida, Gainesville.

Wallace, H. D., and G. E. Combs. 1964. High level antibiotic supplementation of the sow during the farrowing period, Florida Animal Science Mimeograph Series 64-14, University of Florida, Gainesville.

Wallace, H. D., R. H. Hauser, and G. E. Combs. 1966. High level copper supplementation of the sow during the farrowing and early lactation period, Florida Animal Science Mimeograph Series 66-12, University of Florida, Gainesville.

Wallace, H. D., D. D. Thieu, and G. E. Combs. 1974. Sow farrowing and lactation performance as influenced by diet fortification with aureomycin, penicillin and sulfamethazine. Florida Animal Science Mimeograph Series. No. 74–6. University of Florida, Gainesville.

Webster, A. J. F. 1981. The energetic efficiency of metabolism, *Proc. Nutr. Soc.*, 40:121.

Weinberg, E. D. 1957. The mutual effects of antimicrobial compounds and metallic cations, *Bacteriol. Rev.*, 21:46.

Winkelstein, A. 1956. L. acidophilus tables in the therapy of functional intestinal disorders, *Am. Pract. Dig. Treat.*, 7:1637.

Wu, M. C., L. C. Wung, S. Y. Chen, and C. C. Kuo. 1987. Study on the feeding value of *Streptococcus faecium* M-74 for pigs; I. Large scale of feeding trial of *Streptococcus faecium* M-74 on the performance of weaning pigs, Animal Industry Research Institute, Taiwan Sugar Corp., Chunan Miaoli, Taiwan, 11–12.

Yen, J. T., A. H. Jensen, N. H. Bajjalieh, and V. D. Ladwig. 1976. Effects of methyl-3-(2-quinoxalinylmethylene) carbazate-N^1, N^4-dioxide on nitrogen and energy digestibility in and performance of young pigs, *J. Anim. Sci.*, 42:375.

Yen, J. T., T. L. Veum, and R. Lauxen. 1979. Lysine-sparing effect of carbadox in low protein diet for young pigs, *J. Anim. Sci.*, 49(Suppl. 1):257 (Abstr.).

Yen, J. T., J. A. Neinaber, W. G. Pond, and V. H. Varel. 1985. Effect of carbadox on growth, fasting metabolism, thyroid function, and gastrointestinal tract in young pigs, *J. Nutr.*, 115:970.

Zimmerman, D. R. 1986. Role of subtherapeutic antimicrobials in animal production, *J. Anim. Sci.*, 62 (Suppl. 3):6.

19 Performance-Enhancing Substances*

Diane Wray-Cahen

CONTENTS

I. Introduction 427
II. Nutrient Partitioning 428
III. Porcine Somatotropin 429
   A. Growth 429
   B. Lactation 432
IV. β-Adrenergic Agonists 433
V. Other Potential Performance Enhancers 435
   A. Nutraceuticals 435
   B. Other Hormones 436
VI. Interactions with Immune Function 436
VII. Impact of Performance Enhancement on Nutrient Requirements 438
   A. Amino Acid Requirements 439
   B. Energy Requirements 441
   C. Mineral and Vitamin Requirements 441
VIII. Summary 442
References 442

I. INTRODUCTION

Today's pig reaches market weight more quickly and with a leaner body composition than even a decade ago, reflecting the producer's response to consumer concerns about dietary animal fat. New technologies and strategies have generated greater and more rapid progress toward the objective of a leaner, more healthful pork product. Genetic manipulation through selective breeding practice in swine production has shifted the phenotypic potential from the obesity of the pre–World War II pig to a much leaner modern-day animal. However, a new arsenal of tools is becoming available called metabolic modifiers (or repartitioning agents); these can be partnered with the new genetics (Wray-Cahen et al., 1998). The result is the production of leaner pigs with improved rates and efficiencies of gain. Of the potential metabolic modifiers studied so far, the most dramatic effects on growth performance have been seen with porcine somatotropin (pST) and β-adrenergic agonists. Metabolic modifiers permit an animal to achieve its genetic potential. Some new performance-enhancing strategies such as continuing developments in genetic engineering, transgenics, and even cloning promise to raise the bar higher by actually increasing the animal's genetic potential for

---

* The contents of this publication do not necessarily reflect the views or policies of the U.S. Food and Drug Administration or the U.S. Department of Agriculture, nor does mention of trade names, commercial products, or organizations imply endorsement from the U.S. Government.

lean growth. This chapter focuses on how an animal's nutrient requirements are affected by these performance-enhancers. Stahly and Bark (1991) addressed this subject in the first edition of this book. Since the publication of the first edition, more data are available and new concepts have been developed regarding performance enhancing substances and nutrient requirements for lean tissue growth. This chapter emphasizes research published since the first edition and how current nutritional concepts apply to these performance-enhancing strategies.

Enhancing the performance of meat animals poses a twofold challenge for nutritionists. Not only must the nutritional requirement of the animal be satisfied, but awareness that nutrition influences the effectiveness of metabolism modifiers must also be maintained. This said, the fundamental principles of nutrition discussed in earlier chapters remain the same. As is always the case, one should ideally feed the animal to meet the requirement for the sum of its individual tissue needs. Nutrient requirements of pigs receiving metabolic modifiers are affected because their metabolism has been modified and their rates of lean and fat accretion have been altered. When determining the nutrient requirements of pigs receiving metabolic modifiers (or of pigs that have been genetically engineered), one must consider the impact that the substances have on (1) feed intake, (2) lean and fat accretion rates, and (3) physiological and biochemical processes that consume energy. Therefore, it is essential to understand how metabolic modifiers or other performance-enhancing technologies might work. Some (e.g., pST) alter the animal's response to homeostatic signals such as insulin, which is released in response to nutrient intake and feeding. Some nutrients (e.g., copper, zinc), sometimes referred to as nutraceuticals, may enhance animal performance when fed at higher-than-normal levels by acting as antimicrobial agents (as discussed in Chapter 18) or by improving the immune status of the animal to reduce the energy costs of immune system activation.

Different metabolic modifiers affect tissues and systems (directly or indirectly) via sometimes profoundly different mechanisms, yet may produce a similar net effect. For example, adipose deposition rates can be reduced by decreasing synthesis, by increasing mobilization, or both. It is the balance between these two processes (synthesis vs. degradation/mobilization) that determines the end result, but the energy required to accomplish these differs greatly. The response of the animal to a performance enhancer is the sum of many processes in different tissues. The nutrient requirements of the animal will depend on which processes are affected and how they are affected. The better the mechanisms of action of performance-enhancing substances are understood the better the requirements of the animals can be met and the more feeding of excess nutrients can be reduced.

II. NUTRIENT PARTITIONING

The concept of partitioning or dividing nutrients among tissues with some hierarchy of need is not new. Hammond (1944; 1952) elegantly described this concept over 50 years ago. Hammond based his priority of partition of nutrients in the bloodstream on the metabolic rate of different tissues. He developed his nutrient partitioning model (Figure 19.1) from studies on animals fed at different levels of nutrition. Certain functions and tissues are protected even when nutrition is severely limited. Those that are most essential for survival of the individual (brain and central nervous system) are most protected (with the most arrows in the model diagram; Figure 19.1), followed by those necessary for the production and survival of the animal's offspring (pregnancy and lactation). The tissue that has the lowest priority for nutrient use is adipose tissue. This helps explain the relative ease with which the lipid accretion rates can be nutritionally manipulated. As shown in Figure 19.1, reducing the nutrients available in the bloodstream (e.g., by feeding less) reduces the nutrients available for adipose accretion without severely compromising the nutrients available for muscle accretion and vital bodily functions. Thus, limit feeding is the easiest and cheapest method of altering an animal's body composition and its efficiency of feed utilization. However, limit-feeding, unlike the use of some of the substances discussed below, will not increase the animal's rate of whole body or protein gain. Nutrient repartitioning agents, such as those discussed

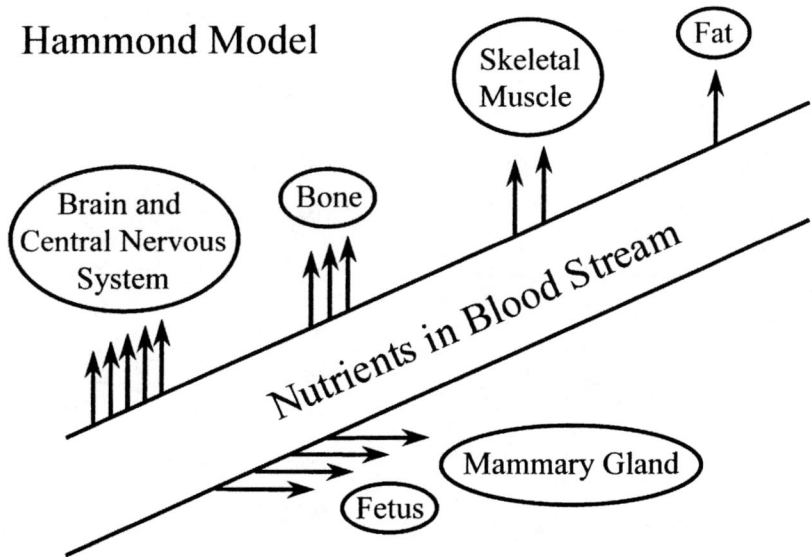

FIGURE 19.1 Priority of partitioning of nutrients according to metabolic rate. The larger the number of arrows leading to a tissue, the higher priority it has. (Adapted from Hammond, 1944; 1952.)

below, shift the tissue accretion priorities, thereby producing a leaner composition of gain while simultaneously increasing the efficiency of growth.

III. PORCINE SOMATOTROPIN

Somatotropin (ST), or growth hormone, is a naturally occurring peptide hormone (containing 191 amino acids), which is secreted by the anterior pituitary gland (Etherton and Bauman, 1998). The growth-promoting effects of somatotropin have been known since Evans and Simpson (1931) first demonstrated that a crude pituitary extract from cows could stimulate growth in rats and then, with Li (Li et al., 1945), isolated ST from the pituitary in the 1940s. Porcine ST was first used in pigs in the 1950s (Turman and Andrews, 1955) and its nutrient repartitioning effects in swine were confirmed by Machlin (1972). However, the usefulness of pST for production purposes was limited by the small supply and the expense of extracting it from the pituitaries of slaughtered pigs. Breakthroughs in biotechnology in the early 1980s allowed for the production of large quantities of ST via recombinant DNA technology. At that time, understanding of the effects of pST on growing pigs (and the mechanisms involved) began an exponential advance. Some of the recombinantly derived pST differ slightly from natural pituitary pST in amino acid composition and/or protein structure, and, consequently, their bioactivity and potency vary (Etherton and Bauman, 1998). However, the growth performance and metabolic effects of variants of pST are similar in most respects to those of the natural pituitary hormone. Unlike steroid hormones, ST is not orally active, and, therefore, it must be administered as an injection or implant. Since the mid-1980s, many studies have been conducted on pigs receiving exogenous pST. The results of these studies have been dramatic. Treatment animals could be identified visually from control animals and the metabolic differences were even more clear-cut. Would that research results were always so clear!

A. Growth

In the growing pig, pST increases muscle accretion rate and decreases adipose accretion rate (e.g., protein and lipid accretion rates in Figure 19.2). The degree to which pST affects these two processes

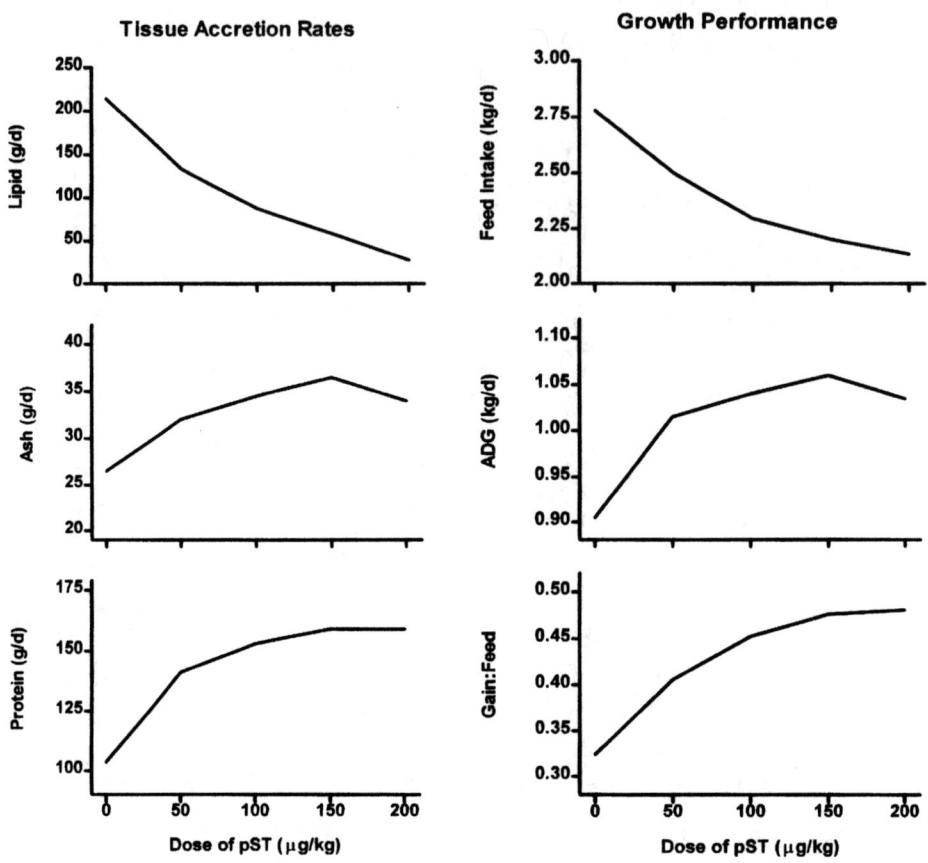

FIGURE 19.2 Effect of dose of somatotropin on body tissue accretion rates and growth performance parameters. (Adapted from Krick et al., 1992.)

varies with the dose of pST, the animal's stage of development, and the composition of the diet. Somatotropin acts both directly on target tissues (e.g., adipose) and indirectly via its stimulation of insulin-like growth factor-I (IGF-I), which in turn elicits responses from other target tissues (e.g., muscle) (Etherton and Bauman, 1998). A proportion of the response to pST is due to direct and indirect alterations in the animal's response to homeostatic signals such as insulin. Insulin stimulates tissue uptake of glucose and amino acids. Altering the response of a tissue to insulin can regulate the postabsorptive use of nutrients, which in turn affects the utilization of nutrients of the tissue (Etherton and Bauman, 1998; Wray-Cahen et al., 1998).

The primary effect of pST on adipose tissue in the growing pig is to decrease both the uptake of glucose into the fat cell and the synthesis of lipid from glucose, rather than to stimulate lipid mobilization (Dunshea et al., 1992a,b; Dunshea, 1993; Harris et al., 1993; Etherton and Bauman, 1998). Therefore, as one might expect, the largest effect of pST on adipose accretion is observed during the finishing phase of growth when pigs normally would have higher rates of lipid deposition. Despite the marked pST-induced reduction in glucose utilization by adipose tissue, glucose uptake and utilization by muscle and other non-adipose tissues seems to be unaffected by pST administration (Dunshea et al., 1992a; Wray-Cahen et al., 1995).

Less is known about the direct or indirect effects of pST on muscle metabolism. Systemically, treatment with pST is associated with lower blood urea nitrogen concentrations, reduced urinary nitrogen output (resulting in a higher nitrogen retention; Table 19.1), and an overall improvement in

TABLE 19.1
Summary of Response of Nutrient Digestibility and Retention to pST Treatment

Treatment	Dose of pST (µg/kg)[a]	Digestibility (%)[b]			Retained Nitrogen		Metabolized Energy	
		N	E	DM	(g/d)	(%)	(Mcal/d)	(%)
Control	0	84.3	85.2		23.0	26.1	9.6	81.8
pST	120	87.5	88.0		38.4	55.5	7.7	85.1
Control	0	84.3		85.4	25.9	30.4		
pST	60	86.2		86.9	34.5	37.9		

[a] Approximate dose of porcine somatotropin based on average weight and amount per day.
[b] N = nitrogen; E = energy; DM = dry matter.

Source: Adapted from Wray-Cahen et al. (1991) and Hansen et al. (1994).

the efficiency of amino acid utilization. The increase in protein deposition rates seems to be primarily due to enhanced rates of protein synthesis with protein degradation remaining unchanged (Etherton and Bauman, 1998). IGF-I is a potent mitogen that stimulates cell proliferation and protein synthesis. Evidence suggests that elevated levels of IGF-I are responsible for the effects of pST on protein accretion and that the protein accretion rates are proportional to stimulation of IGF-I levels (Pursel et al., 1998).

In addition to ST-stimulated synthesis of IGF-I in the liver (and release into the circulation), IGF-I is produced by other tissues in response to pST administration, including muscle. Because it is produced at the target tissue, as well as elevated in the circulating blood, IGF-I may have both endocrine and paracrine functions. Most IGF-I studies have been conducted *in vitro* and/or in rodents, therefore, relatively little is known about the direct effects of IGF-I on growing swine *in vivo*. One recent study examined the endocrine effects of IGF-I in growing pigs (Klindt et al., 1998). Administration of exogenous IGF-I to growing pigs produced only some of the effects usually observed with pST administration. For example IGF-I, unlike pST, did not suppress feed intake. It did improve average daily gain, but not to the same extent as pST. Unlike pST, IGF-I had little effect on organ weights. Although carcass composition was unaffected by IGF-I administration, IGF-I administration did tend to increase protein and ash accretion rates — but less dramatically than pST. The paracrine effects of IGF-I have been recently examined in transgenic gilts expressing IGF-I solely in skeletal muscle, but in an insufficient amount to elevate blood levels of the growth factor (Pursel et al., 1998). In these animals, average daily gain was unaffected, but body fat was reduced 30% and body lean was increased by 9.4%. Therefore, locally produced IGF-I (paracrine function), rather than circulating IGF-I (endocrine function), may be more important in the regulation of muscle growth and body composition (Pursel et al., 1998).

The pig's response to pST varies with the animal's stage of development, but in all ages studied pST consistently raises protein accretion rates and decreases lipid accumulation rates — although not necessarily to the same degree (Table 19.2). Even the newborn pig responds with an increase in average daily gain and feed efficiency over the first week of life, although it is much less sensitive to exogenous pST administration (i.e., a larger dose is required to elicit a response). pST administration in neonatal pigs also increases the weight, protein content, and protein synthesis rate of certain tissues (Wester et al., 1998). In the somewhat older young, growing pigs (10 to 25 kg), pST increases protein accretion rates and decreases adipose accretion rates, without affecting average daily gain or feed efficiency at the dose given (Harrell et al., 1997). The improvements in the composition of gain and growth performance are considerable for both the growing and finishing phases of growth, but the impact of pST on pig performance is greater in the finishing (50 to 100 kg) phase as compared with the growing (20 to 50 kg) phase (Boyd et al., 1991). This may be due to the higher potential for adipose gain in the finishing pig. An example of tissue accretion rates and growth performance responses to pST in finishing pigs is shown in Figure 19.2. In these pigs,

TABLE 19.2
Summary of Effects of Porcine Somatotropin at Different Phases of Growth and β-Adrenergic Agonists in the Finishing Phase on Growth and Performance Parameters (presented as a percentage change from control) from Selected Studies[a]

Treatment	Pig wt (kg)	Feed Intake (kg/day)	ADG (kg/day)	F:G	Body Composition (%)		Accretion Rate (g/day)	
					Fat	Protein	Lipid	Protein
pST	1–3[b]	*	25	–16	ND	ND	ND	ND
	10–25[c]	NC	NC	NC	–26	5	–31	17
	20–60[d]	–10	12	–20	–27	11	–46	32
	60–100[e]	–20	17	–30	–60	28	–82	74
Ractopamine	60–100[f]	–7	12	–14	–7	5	–18	42
Salbutamol	60–90[g]	NR	NC	–20	–11	8	–18	48

Note: * = pigs were fed equal amounts; NR= not reported, NC= no significant change, ND = not determined.

[a] Data used were selected from studies with conditions that the author judged were sufficiently similar to allow averaging within treatment groups. Some studies have been excluded because the diets fed or the feed regime would potentially limit the treatment effect and prejudice the means.
[b] 1000 μg/kg; Wester et al. (1998).
[c] 120 μg/kg; Harrell et al. (1997).
[d] 100 and 150 μg/kg; data combined from Campbell et al. (1988) and Krick et al. (1992).
[e] 100–150 μg/kg; data combined from Campbell et al. (1991), Johnston et al. (1993), Evock et al. (1988), Boyd et al. (1991).
[f] 20 ppm; data combined from Dunshea et al. (1993b), Mitchell et al. (1991), Bark et al. (1992), and Crome et al. (1996).
[g] 2.75 ppm; Hansen et al. (1997b).

lipid accretion rates decrease almost linearly with dose, and this is paralleled by a decrease in feed intake, with no maximal effect achieved over a wide dose range. The response of protein and ash accretion rates to pST in the finishing pig is quadratic rather than linear. The increase in average daily gain in response to pST administration is also quadratic, with a maximum response achieved at approximately 100 μg/kg body weight (BW)/day for these pigs. Although the effect of pST appears to be greatest in the finishing phase of growth, pigs in all phases of growth appear to be responsive to pST to some extent, and therefore pST may affect their nutritional requirements. This is discussed later in this chapter (see Section VII).

B. Lactation

Although somatotropin administration has been extensively studied in lactating dairy cows, fewer studies have been conducted in lactating swine. Somatotropin has been shown to stimulate milk production in sows (Harkins et al., 1989); growth hormone–releasing factor (GRF), a hormone that stimulates endogenous pST release, has also shown potential to stimulate milk production and increase piglet weight through pST-directed increases in milk production (Farmer et al., 1996). However, the results in lactating sows are far from consistent. Some studies have seen no effect of pST (Cromwell et al., 1992; Toner et al., 1996) or GRF (Farmer et al., 1992) on milk production or piglet weight gain.

Too few studies have been conducted, with too-variable results, to allow one to predict accurately how pST or GRF will affect nutritional requirements of lactating or gestating sows. However, most studies have found that pST administration in the lactating sow, as in the growing pig, reduces feed intake and backfat depth. It also tends to result in greater body weight losses for sows during lactation. Table 19.3 illustrates the potential of pST in lactating sows, along with the potential nutrient strain on the sow. Large losses in body mass during lactation have been associated with

TABLE 19.3
Response of Sow Lactation Performance and Composition to pST Administration

Treatment	Feed Intake (kg/day)	Weight Loss (kg)	BF Loss (cm)	Milk Yield (kg/day)	Fat Yield (kg)	Protein Yield (kg)	Piglet ADG (g/day)	Energy Balance (Mcal ME/day)
Control	5.99	−7.0	−0.12	9.0	0.49	0.52	188	−5.43
pST	4.66	−13.6	−0.37	11.0	0.68	0.60	207	−9.99
% change	−28	−94	−208	+22	+39	+15	+10	−84

Source: Adapted from Harkins et al. (1989).

reduced reproductive performance in the sow (Reese et al., 1982; 1984; Nelssen et al., 1985; Brendemuhl et al., 1987); when GRF administration did increase milk yield, sows were delayed in their return to estrus (Farmer et al., 1996). The estimated energy balance for sows shown in Table 19.3 (Harkins et al., 1989) was reduced by 84% with pST administration. This, combined with the consistent further reduction in backfat and reduced feed intake, represents a great nutritional challenge. How does one get enough feed into the pST-treated sow to support increases in milk production and prevent large losses of body reserves? This problem is compounded by the suppression of feed intake with pST administration. In the lactating sow, the primary limiting nutrient is not amino acids, but energy. Therefore, what works for the growing pig will not work for the sow; increasing the nutrient density of the sow's diet is an insufficient method of meeting the sow's requirements. The 2-kg/day increase in milk production would increase the ME requirement by 3.49 Mcal metabolizable (ME)/day, assuming 1.256 Mcal ME/kg milk (ARC, 1981) and a marginal efficiency of use of ME for milk production to be 72% (NRC, 1998). This would require the sow to eat each day an additional 1.1 kg of feed to avoid further losses of body weight; a difficult task given the 1.3 kg decrease in feed intake observed. The amino acid density of the feed can be readily increased to meet the additional amino acid requirement, but increasing the energy density of the feed is unlikely to meet the energy requirement of these animals because of the suppression of feed intake. In growing pigs (Azain et al., 1992), increasing the energy density of the diet by adding fat to the diet does not increase the energy intake of *ad libitum* fed pigs. One could speculate that the feed intake response is associated with leptin, a hormone involved with the regulation of feed intake and linked to somatotropin levels (discussed in Section V), but at this time, there is no known mechanism for increasing feed intake in pST-treated sows.

IV. β-ADRENERGIC AGONISTS

Epinephrine (adrenaline) and norepinephrine (noradrenaline) are naturally occurring adrenergic agonists or catecholamines. They are released by the adrenal medulla (hence, the term *adrenergic*) in small quantities; norepinephrine is also produced and secreted by sympathetic nerve endings (Martin, 1985). Although work with exogenous adrenergic agonists in growing pigs in the 1960s demonstrated that epinephrine could increase average daily gain and nitrogen retention in swine (Cunningham et al., 1963), interest waned and did not resume until the 1980s after several synthetic β-adrenergic agonists were developed. Their structure (Figure 19.3) is similar to the natural catecholamines, as are their pharmacological properties. There are at least six β-adrenergic agonists that have been shown to increase protein deposition in meat animals: ractopamine, cimaterol, L-644,969, isoproterenol, salbutamol, and clenbuterol. Their protein deposition effects are not consistent among species. One advantage of β-adrenergic agonists over pST is their relative ease of administration — unlike pST, they are orally active compounds and can therefore be added to the diet. However, the effects of β-adrenergic agonists in swine are neither as predictable as the effects of pST nor as dramatic as some effects observed with β-adrenergic agonists in ruminants. For

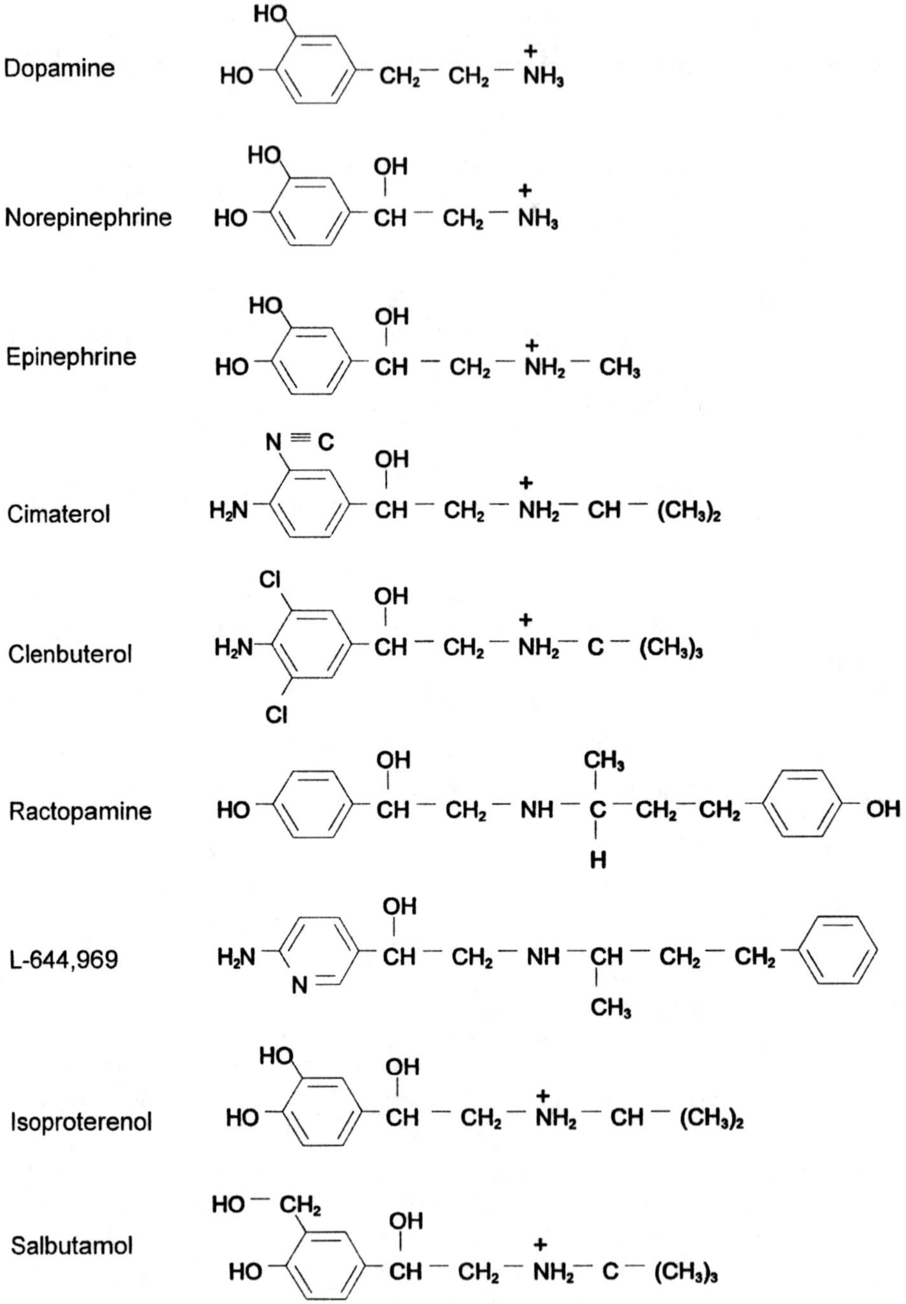

FIGURE 19.3 Chemical structures of some endogenous catecholamines and selected synthetic β-adrenergic agonists.

example, swine seem to be less responsive to cimaterol and clenbuterol than growing ruminants, which have enhanced muscle deposition rates in response to these β-agonists. In some instances, an initial positive effect may wane with time on the treatment (Williams et al., 1994). To add to the confusion, the effect of β-adrenergic agonists on fat metabolism appears to vary not only between species, but also among the different β-adrenergic agonists within a given species (Reeds and Mersmann, 1991). Therefore, one must be cautious when making generalizations about β-adrenergic agonist use and mode of action.

As shown in Table 19.2, both ractopamine and salbutamol can alter body composition and tissue accretion rates in swine. Ractopamine was recently approved (by FDA in December 1999) for use in diets fed to finishing swine to enhance rate of weight gain, feed efficiency, and carcass leanness. The β-agonists can also affect individual tissue weights. For example, salbutamol can increase the loin eye area and individual muscle weights in swine (Hansen et al., 1997a; 1997b). In contrast with pST-treatment, the administration of salbutamol is accompanied by a decrease in the weight of the liver and portal-drained viscera organs. Less is known about the mechanisms by which β-agonists influence protein and lipid deposition than is known for pST administration. Ractopamine stimulates protein synthesis of skeletal muscle myofibrillar proteins, but not connective tissue proteins (Adeola et al., 1992). The protein synthesis stimulation occurs only when high levels of dietary protein were fed. Ractopamine, unlike pST, appears to have little effect on glucose metabolism and does not appear to alter rate of lipid synthesis (Liu et al., 1994; Dunshea and King, 1995). It may alter lipid mobilization rates.

It appears that the effects of β-adrenergic agonists may be greater in older rather than younger pigs (Crome et al., 1996); this is possibly because lipid accretion rates are naturally higher in older pigs. The response to ractopamine, and possibly other β-adrenergic agonists, appears to become refractory (at least for parameters such as average daily gain), meaning that the response is greatest shortly after initiation of treatment and then decreases over time (Williams et al., 1994).

V. OTHER POTENTIAL PERFORMANCE ENHANCERS

A. NUTRACEUTICALS

Somatotropin, IGF-I, and β-adrenergic agonists are not the only substances that have the potential to enhance pig performance. It is also possible that certain nutrients may have pharmacological effects. Termed *nutraceuticals*, these nutrients may stimulate growth or other biological functions when given in doses higher than considered necessary to meet the nutritional requirement for trace or macronutrients. Putative nutraceuticals include chromium, iron, copper, and zinc (see Chapters 12 and 18). Chromium particularly has received a lot of attention over the years and the NRC has published a book on this nutrient (NRC, 1997). Chromium elicits metabolic responses associated with glucose metabolism and chromium increases insulin sensitivity in pigs (Steele et al., 1977; Amoikon et al., 1995). Some investigators have reported that chromium picolinate may decrease backfat and increase lean (Page et al., 1993; Lindemann et al., 1995; Ward et al., 1997), but the results have been mixed, even in trials conducted by a single laboratory. Some studies have reported no response to chromium (Evock-Clover et al., 1993; Ward et al., 1997) and others suggest that responses to chromium may depend upon the stress level in the animal's environment (NRC, 1997). The conditions under which chromium can elicit a growth performance response are unclear and results are too variable to support its use as a growth promoter.

Betaine (trimethyl glycine), a by-product of beet sugar production, is another nutrient with potential as a performance enhancer. Betaine, a metabolite of choline, aids in osmotic regulation. It serves as a methyl donor in the animal and is involved in methionine metabolism. Its use has proved beneficial in poultry production and aquaculture, but no affirmation is yet available in swine. Some studies have seen a decrease in backfat, but this response has not been consistent across farms. Fernandez-Figares and colleagues (2000) observed enhanced protein deposition rates and decreases in carcass fat when betaine was fed to energy-restricted pigs. Feeding betaine may also lower plasma levels of urea nitrogen and possibly improve nitrogen retention (Matthews et al., 1998). Although it is too early to tell at this point, betaine may improve both nitrogen and energy utilization, but its effectiveness may depend on energy status.

Carnitine, another tri-methylated compound, is similar in structure to betaine and may have performance-enhancing potential. And like betaine, carnitine is a naturally produced metabolite that plays a role in methyl group metabolism. Although not thought to be an essential nutrient for adult mammals, it may be conditionally essential for the neonate (Odle, 1995). Owen and co-workers (1996) reported that L-carnitine improved feed efficiency and reduced carcass lipid accretion in early-weaned pigs. L-Carnitine supplementation in piglets has also been shown to increase both fatty acid oxidation rate (van Kempen and Odle, 1993) and nitrogen retention (Bohles et al., 1984). However, some studies have seen no effects of L-carnitine on lipid or nitrogen metabolism (Hoffman et al., 1993). Data on older pigs, especially in the finishing phase, are limited, but there have been some positive results reported (see Odle, 1995). As with betaine, it is too early to tell whether carnitine is an effective growth promoter in swine.

Conjugated linoleic acids (CLA) are a recent arrival to the performance-enhancing scene. There are different chemical forms of CLA and each may elicit different responses. Some reports have suggested that feeding certain forms of CLA may result in leaner animals; other forms may prevent cancer. Possibly due to the differences in chemical forms, the early trials in pigs are inconclusive. However, some studies have reported a decrease in backfat and an increase in percent lean. Most have noted an improvement in fat quality and firmness (Eggert and Belury, 1998). At this writing it is too early to evaluate their potential use in animal agriculture.

B. OTHER HORMONES

Protein hormones other than pST may improve milk production or the efficiency and/or composition of animal growth. Prolactin is a protein hormone that, like pST, is produced in the anterior pituitary. It is in the same family of hormones as pST. Recombinant prolactin is less readily available to researchers than pST; therefore, very few studies have been conducted in swine. In growing pigs, prolactin does not appear to affect feed intake, feed efficiency, average daily gain, or carcass composition, despite elevating IGF-I concentrations (McLaughlin et al., 1997). Prolactin does appear to simulate mammary development in these growing pigs; this may have implications for increasing milk production, but further work needs to be done.

Another protein hormone arrived on the scene in the 1990s: leptin. Leptin is a protein hormone produced by adipose tissue. It is thought to be the link between adipose tissue and its role in the regulation of food intake and the control of body fat stores. Its mechanism(s) of action are not yet well understood, but initial studies in swine suggest that leptin administration can reduce feed intake in a dose-responsive manner (Barb et al., 1998; Ramsay, 1999). At this writing, no one has enough leptin to conduct a growth performance trial in pigs; however, leptin affects the pST/IGF axis and the existing evidence suggests that it has nutrient partitioning properties. Because feed intake limits protein deposition in the linear (growing) phase of growth (Figures 19.4 and 19.5), transitory immunization against leptin could increase average daily gain and protein deposition rates in growing pigs.

VI. INTERACTIONS WITH IMMUNE FUNCTION

Hormones, including pST, and nutrients can interact extensively with the immune system; immune status can affect tissue accretion rates and turnover. Some performance-enhancing substances may interact with the immune system as illustrated in Figure 19.6; their ability to enhance growth may be associated with this effect, rather than a direct effect on lipid or protein accretion rates. Increased growth may be a beneficial consequence of improved health as nutrients spared from immune responses are more available for growth. For further discussion of this, see Chapter 24.

Performance-Enhancing Substances

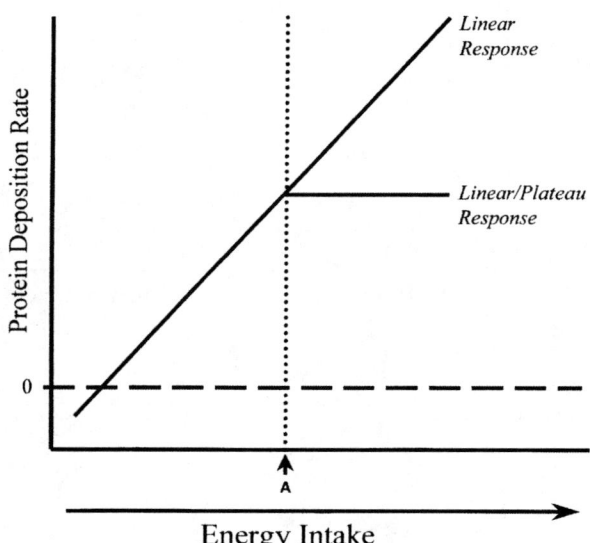

FIGURE 19.4 This diagram shows the relationship between dietary energy intake and protein deposition rates during the growing (linear) stage and finishing (linear/plateau) stage of growth. Point A on the x-axis represents the energy intake required to achieve the maximal protein deposition response in finishing pigs. (Adapted from Steele et al., 1994; NRC, 1994; and SCA, 1987.)

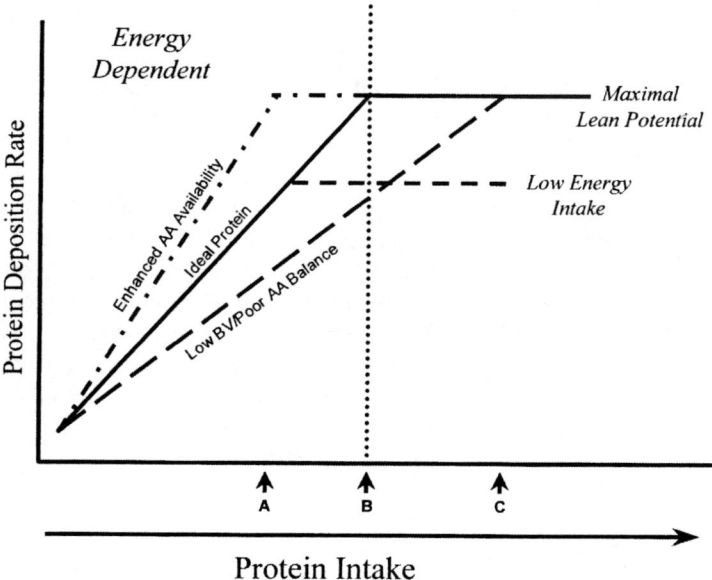

FIGURE 19.5 This diagram demonstrates the relationship between dietary protein intake and whole body tissue deposition rates. Point B represents the dietary protein intake required to achieve the maximal potential for protein deposition when energy is not limiting and an ideal protein is fed. Point A represents the dietary protein requirement when amino acid availability is enhanced or a growth modifier is administered. Point C represents the dietary protein requirement when pigs are fed a poor-quality feed. This figure also illustrates the effect on protein deposition rate when energy intake is limited. (Adapted from Steele et al., 1994; NRC, 1994; and SCA, 1987.)

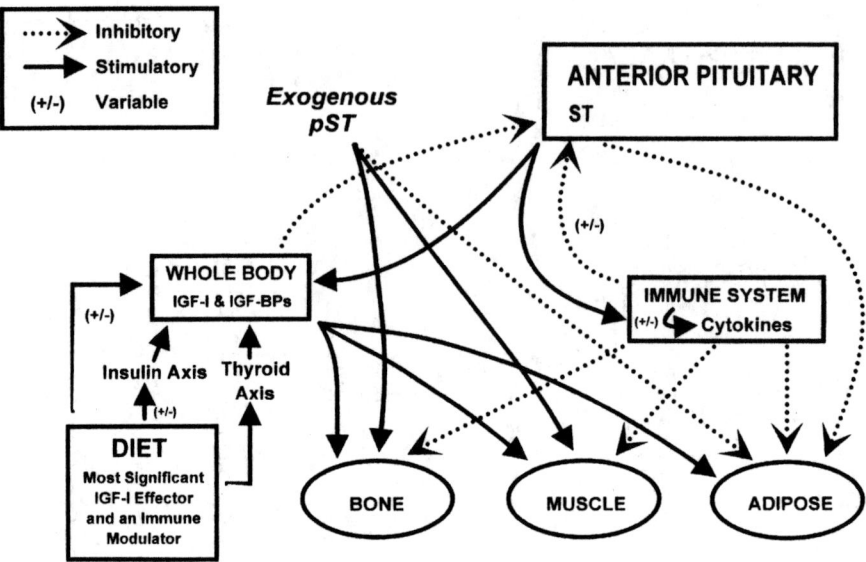

FIGURE 19.6 Diagram illustrating some of the interactions between the endocrine signals that stimulate growth and maintain tissue stability (somatotropic axis: ST and IGF-I) and the endocrine and cytokine systems that mobilize stored tissue products and divert nutrients from growth. The balance between these systems determines to what extent nutrients partitioned toward growth processes or diverted from them to address an imposed stress. ST, somatotropin; IGF-I, insulin-like growth factor-I; IGF-BPs, IGF binding proteins. (Adapted from Wray-Cahen et al., 1998 and Elsasser et al., 1995.)

VII. IMPACT OF PERFORMANCE ENHANCEMENT ON NUTRIENT REQUIREMENTS

Although the maximal growth potential of an animal is determined by its genotype, sex, and stage of development, the animal's environment — including nutrition — can limit the animal's ability to achieve its maximal potential. The same holds true for the animal's response to metabolic modifiers; without the appropriate conditions and nutrition their full effect cannot be realized. Diet and nutritional status are significant regulators of insulin and the ST/IGF axis (see Figure 19.6). Fasted pigs do not elicit an IGF-I response to ST and pigs fed at maintenance levels have a much reduced response compared with pigs fed four times maintenance (Ozawa et al., 1996). Nutritional stress can even trigger the immune system (see Figure 19.6), negatively influencing growth and metabolism (Elsasser et al., 1995; Wray-Cahen et al., 1998). Inadequate levels of either amino acids or energy can limit or seriously interfere with (or even block) the effects of metabolic modifiers.

As illustrated earlier with the Hammond model (see Figure 19.1), if muscle growth is to be maximized there must be sufficient nutrients provided to meet the requirements of the muscle tissue plus the requirements of more "metabolically essential," higher priority tissues. The primary nutritional limits on protein deposition are protein and energy. The relationship among protein deposition, protein intake, and energy intake is illustrated in Figures 19.4 and 19.5. This relationship varies with stage of development (Figure 19.4). Young (growing) pigs appear to have a linear response to energy for protein deposition, while older (finishing) pigs have an initial linear response to energy intake, after which protein deposition reaches a plateau. When energy intake is higher than that required for maximal protein deposition in older pigs, the animals become fatter, as would be predicted by the Hammond model. Young pigs may also have a theoretical plateau, but voluntary feed intake becomes a limiting factor before a plateau is reached. As shown in Figure 19.5, protein deposition is unaffected by additional dietary protein if energy is limiting (i.e., low energy intake line). When a low level of energy is fed, maximal protein deposition cannot be achieved. During the energy-dependent phase, protein deposition increases with increasing protein intake, unless an energy limit is reached. In addition, the slope of the protein deposition curve is affected by the quality and balance of the protein source. The solid line in Figure 19.5 represents an ideal protein. If amino acid availability is enhanced (dotted line), then the slope of the protein deposition line increases, resulting in the maximal protein deposition being achieved at a lower protein intake. If the biological value or amino acid balance of the protein is poor (dashed line), then the slope of the line decreases and a higher protein intake is required to achieve maximal protein deposition.

Three factors must be considered regarding the effect of a substance on nutrient requirements: (1) feed intake, (2) digestive processes, and (3) postabsorptive use of nutrients (Boyd et al., 1991). The third category includes any changes in the following: the animal's maintenance requirements, its efficiency of nutrient utilization, and its pattern of nutrient deposition (rate and composition of body growth).

Except in the very young pig, pST administration reduces feed intake. This appears to be true with β-adrenergic agonists as well. The impact of these metabolic modifiers on feed intake (as well as some other parameters) is greater in the finishing phase than in the growing phase of production (see Table 19.2). This may be associated with the difference in the relative protein and lipid deposition rates in the growing vs. the finishing animal, but the basis for the difference in feed intake suppression is not known.

One likely effect of the reduction in feed intake is a reduction in the treated pig's rate of digesta passage through the gastrointestinal tract; a slower rate of passage may improve feed digestibility. As shown in Table 19.1, pST administration results in a dose-dependent improvement in digestibility of nitrogen, energy, and dry matter. The observed improvements in digestibility are exactly what would be predicted by the percentage reduction in voluntary feed intake observed in these studies (Haydon et al., 1984; Verstegen et al., 1990). Therefore, little to no improvement in digestibility would be expected in pigs already restrictively fed. When feed intake is suppressed, even if the absolute nutrient requirements (other than energy) are unaffected, adjustments must be made to the diet similar to dietary adjustments required with limit feeding. If performance-enhancing substances have no impact on nonenergy nutrient requirements on a gram per day basis, the diet should be adjusted so that it contains a higher (nonenergy) nutrient density to compensate for the reduction in feed consumption. (See Chapter 32 for more on the related topic of limit feeding.)

A greater percentage of the nitrogen and energy absorbed (i.e., digestible nitrogen and energy) is retained by the animal when pST is administered; it is upon this postabsorptive use of nutrients that metabolic modifiers or repartitioning agents have the greatest impact. In pST-treated pigs, total nitrogen retained (g/day) is also increased, reflecting the increase in whole body protein deposition (Wray-Cahen et al., 1991; Hansen et al., 1994). This increase in nitrogen retention is also associated with an increase in protein turnover in growing pigs which in turn is likely reflected in an increased metabolic rate (Tomas et al., 1992). Although a greater percentage of digestible energy is retained or metabolized, metabolized energy in Mcal/day is reduced by pST treatment, reflecting the reduced feed intake.

A. AMINO ACID REQUIREMENTS

As discussed in Chapter 8, the amino acid requirements of a pig are defined by the potential for the animal to accrue protein. Performance-enhancing substances such as pST and β-adrenergic agonists increase the protein accretion potential of the pig. Although the capacity of protein accretion is determined by genotype (including genetically engineered genotypes), gender, and stage of growth, inadequate intake of either energy or protein can limit the protein accretion potential of an animal (Black et al., 1986; SCA, 1987). As mentioned earlier (see Figure 19.5), failure to provide adequate protein or energy to the animal will limit the ability of an animal to achieve its potential biological response to a performance-enhancing substance. The American (NRC, 1998), British (ARC, 1981), and Australian (SCA, 1987) nutrient recommendations all base the protein/amino acid requirement on the expected protein accretion potential of the pig.

In an elegant study conducted by Krick and co-workers (Krick et al., 1993) on pigs in the growing phase of production (20 to 60 kg, 150 µg pST/kg BW) using diets based on the ideal protein concept, the maximum protein accretion rates achieved by control and pST-treated pigs were 118 and 150 g/day, respectively. In this study, the amount of lysine required to maximize protein accretion rates for pigs receiving pST (with *ad libitum* access to feed) was increased from 22 g/day for control pigs to only 24 g/day. This means that a mere 9% increase in protein intake was required to achieve a 27% increase in protein accretion rate. A similar finding with restrictively fed growing pigs (30 to 60 kg, 90 µg pST/kg BW) was made by Campbell et al. (1990); they found that a 4% increase in the level of ideal protein allowed an 18 to 24% increase in protein deposition rate. This strongly suggests that pST improves the efficiency of amino acid utilization and shifts the response curve to the left as shown in Figure 19.5 by the dotted line. Studies conducted during the finishing phase indicate that the increase in lysine requirement with pST treatment is more dramatic than in the growing phase. In a study where pigs were able to regulate their own protein intake, pigs receiving pST chose a higher-protein diet (Roberts and Azain, 1997). In some studies care was not taken to ensure that the amino acid profile approached that of an ideal protein (see Chapter 8 for discussion of ideal protein). However, studies on pST-treated finishing pigs fed diets based on the ideal protein profile also found a different relationship between protein intake and protein deposition than observed during the growing phase (Boyd et al., 1991; Campbell et al., 1991). In most cases, when protein intake is limiting protein accretion rate, any additional energy is partitioned into fat. Therefore, another reason to meet the amino acid requirement of the growing pig is to reduce the amount of energy partitioned into adipose tissue.

Although metabolic modifiers, such as pST, alter the rate of whole body protein accretion, they do not appear to alter the amino acid composition of that gain. Although the amino acid concentration is higher in the tissues and carcass of pST-treated pigs, the amino acid composition of the pigs, including the ratio of essential amino acid to total amino acid, is not affected by treatment (Caperna et al., 1995). Although Krick et al. (1993) observed a slight increase in whole-body lysine and a decrease in glycine, a different dietary amino acid balance is likely not required for pST-treated pigs.

Unlike pST, β-adrenergic agonists are very tissue specific with regard to protein deposition. β-Adrenergic agonists appear to increase protein deposition only in muscle (Reeds and Mersmann, 1991). Because only one tissue is affected, it is possible that, in contrast to pST, which increases protein deposition throughout the body, the amino acid composition of gain may be affected by β-adrenergic agonist administration. Although the ideal protein composition may differ slightly for β-adrenergic agonist–treated animals, the difference is probably of little consequence in practical diets.

The protein deposition response of ractopamine is highly dependent on the level of amino acids or protein in the diet. Dunshea et al. (1993a) found that ractopamine was unable to stimulate protein deposition at dietary protein concentrations of less than 14% in finishing pigs, a level that allowed maximal protein deposition for control animals. A 20% increase in dietary protein was required to achieve maximal protein deposition in pigs receiving ractopamine, with maximal stimulation being 23% greater than controls. In contrast, Mitchell et al. (1991) was able to elicit a response at lower protein levels. They found that the impact of ractopamine on protein and lipid accretion rates and on body composition was actually greater at lower CP intake (12 vs. 18%) in finishing pigs. Both the absolute protein accretion rate and the percent change from the control were higher in the lower-protein diet. As expected, the high-protein diet had the lower lipid accretion rate, but ractopamine reduced the lipid accretion rates more in the lower-protein diet, both in absolute value and as a percentage of the control.

B. ENERGY REQUIREMENTS

The pST-induced reduction in voluntary feed intake is associated with reduced lipid accretion rates and the response is dose dependent (see Figure 19.2). It is likely closely linked to the animal's reduced energy requirement. The degree of the reduction in feed intake depends on the energy composition of the gain allowed by the performance enhancer. Including fat in the diet does not increase the energy consumption of finishing pigs receiving pST, but results in the same reduction of feed intake seen in control animals (Azain et al., 1991).

Administration of pST increases the maintenance energy expenditure in pigs. Noblet et al. (1992) reported an increase in the ME requirement for maintenance in finishing pigs treated with pST and suggested that the greater mass of the liver, kidneys, and heart may account for the higher maintenance with pST treatment. The basal metabolic rate of pigs (80 kg) treated with pST is higher than control animals (Verstegen et al., 1991). Metabolic rate is 14.5 kcal/kg$^{0.75}$/day (7%) higher in pST- treated pigs. This was also associated with a slightly higher body temperature. This increase in metabolic rate may be associated with the increased protein turnover (Tomas et al., 1992). In growing animals, it is estimated that protein turnover accounts for approximately 18% of energy expenditure and Na/K pumping and the triacylglycerol cycle account for 23 and 6%, respectively (Reeds and Mersmann, 1991). Although protein turnover could, in theory, account for the increase, all of these processes may in fact contribute to the increase observed. The increase in maintenance does not equate to an increase in the animal's total energy requirement. The large reduction in adipose accretion, even when combined with higher energy requirements for maintenance, results in a lower ME requirement for the pST-treated growing pig. Increasing energy intake also improves feed efficiency in pST-treated finishing swine (Nossaman et al., 1991).

In finishing pigs fed ractopamine, increasing dietary energy intake resulted in a linear increase in average daily gain. Fat gain was stimulated with increasing energy intake in control and ractopamine pigs. Lean gain increased with energy intake, but this response was muted with ractopamine. The efficiency of lean gain (gain per kilogram of feed) decreased with increasing energy intake when pigs were fed ractopamine (Williams et al., 1994). In contrast to pST-treated pigs, the response to ractopamine was essentially eliminated even at high protein levels when energy intake was restricted (Mitchell et al., 1991).

C. MINERAL AND VITAMIN REQUIREMENTS

Information on the mineral and vitamin requirements of animals receiving performance-enhancing substances is limited primarily to alterations in calcium, phosphorus, and vitamin D metabolism in pST-treated pigs. Ash deposition increases with pST administration in a dose-dependent manner (Figure 19.2) and bone accretion rate is also increased (Caperna et al., 1989; Denis et al., 1994b). However, the mineral composition of the animal is little altered (Caperna et al., 1989). Therefore, while additional minerals may be required, it is likely that the relative proportions will remain the same. Finishing pigs treated with pST do require higher phosphorus levels (Carter and Cromwell, 1998b) and higher daily intakes of P are required to maximize protein deposition rates and to minimize lipid accretion rates (Carter and Cromwell, 1998a). Increased P is especially important to ensure optimum bone traits, such as strength, weight, and wall thickness (Carter and Cromwell, 1998b). Calcium and phosphorus absorption and retention appears to be increased by pST administration (Denis et al., 1994a). This may contribute to the increase in bone growth, especially when combined with the stimulation of vitamin D metabolism with an increase in 1,25-dihydroxy-vitamin D levels (Goff et al., 1990; Denis et al., 1994b). There have been no reported symptoms of vitamin deficiencies with pST or β-adrenergic agonists administration; but possible effects may have been masked because many researchers have increased the vitamin and mineral mix along the same lines as protein concentrations.

VIII. SUMMARY

β-Adrenergic agonists and pST can have a profound effect on the rate and composition of body growth. Other substances and technologies also hold promise as performance enhancers and nutrient-partitioning agents. When determining the nutrient requirements for pigs receiving any given performance enhancer, one must evaluate the impact of the substances on feed intake, tissue accretion and turnover, and the efficiency of nutrient utilization. There is little evidence that performance-enhancing substances sufficiently alter the relative composition of whole-body protein or minerals to require a change in the concept of an ideal protein or to alter the micronutrient proportions relative to the rate of tissue gain. Reductions in feed intake call for an increase in the nutrient density of the diet, but the amino acid requirements of a "performance-enhanced" pig will depend both on the degree of change of tissue accretion rates (dependent dose of enhancer administered) and the stage of growth of the animal. Pigs in the linear growing phase of production require a different strategy than those in the finishing phase. While feeding performance-enhanced pigs may pose some challenges, enhancing animal performance with metabolism modifiers does not change the fundamental concepts of nutrition.

REFERENCES

Adeola, O., R. O. Ball, and L. G. Young. 1992. Porcine skeletal muscle myofibrillar protein synthesis is stimulated by ractopamine, *J. Nutr.*, 122:488.

ARC (Agricultural Research Council). 1981. *The Nutrient Requirements of Pigs*, Commonwealth Agricultural Bureaux, Page Bros Ltd., Norwich, England.

Amoikon, E. K., J. M. Fernandez, L. L. Southern, D. L. Thompson, Jr., T. L. Ward, and B. M. Olcott. 1995. Effect of chromium tripicolinate on growth, glucose tolerance, insulin sensitivity, plasma metabolites, and growth hormone in pigs, *J. Anim. Sci.*, 73:1123.

Azain, M. J., R. W. Seerley, J. O. Reagan, and M. K. Anderson. 1991. Effect of a high-fat diet on the performance response to porcine somatotropin (pST) in finishing pigs, *J. Anim. Sci.*, 69:153.

Azain, M. J., K. D. Bullock, T. R. Kasser, and J. J. Veenhuizen. 1992. Relationship of mode of porcine somatotropin administration and dietary fat to the growth performance and carcass characteristics of finishing pigs, *J. Anim. Sci.*, 70:3086.

Barb, C. R., X. Yan, M. J. Azain, R. R. Kraeling, G. B. Rampacek, and T. G. Ramsay. 1998. Recombinant porcine leptin reduces feed intake and stimulates growth hormone secretion in swine, *Domest. Anim. Endocrinol.*, 15:77.

Bark, L. J., T. S. Stahly, G. L. Cromwell, and J. Miyat. 1992. Influence of genetic capacity for lean tissue growth on rate and efficiency of tissue accretion in pigs fed ractopamine, *J. Anim. Sci.*, 70:3391.

Black, J. L., R. G. Campbell, I. H. Williams, K. J. James, and G. I. Davis. 1986. Simulation of energy and amino acid utilization in the pig, *Res. Dev. Agric.*, 3:121.

Bohles, H., H. Segerer, and W. Fekl. 1984. Improved N-retention during L-carnitine-supplemented total parenteral nutrition, *J. Parenter. Enteral Nutr.*, 8:9.

Boyd, R. D., D. E. Bauman, D. G. Fox, and C. G. Scanes. 1991. Impact of metabolism modifiers on protein accretion and protein and energy requirements of livestock, *J. Anim. Sci.*, 69:56.

Brendemuhl, J. H., A. J. Lewis, and E. R. Peo, Jr. 1987. Effect of protein and energy intake by primiparous sows during lactation on sow and litter performance and sow serum thyroxine and urea concentrations, *J. Anim. Sci.*, 64:1060.

Campbell, R. G., N. C. Steele, T. J. Caperna, J. P. McMurtry, M. B. Solomon, and A. D. Mitchell. 1988. Interrelationships between energy intake and endogenous porcine growth hormone administration on the performance, body composition and protein and energy metabolism of growing pigs weighing 25 to 55 kilograms live weight, *J. Anim. Sci.*, 66:1643.

Campbell, R. G., R. J. Johnson, R. H. King, M. R. Taverner, and D. J. Meisinger. 1990. Interaction of dietary protein content and exogenous porcine growth hormone administration on protein and lipid accretion rates in growing pigs, *J. Anim. Sci.*, 68:3217.

Campbell, R. G., R. J. Johnson, M. R. Taverner, and R. H. King. 1991. Interrelationships between exogenous porcine somatotropin (PST) administration and dietary protein and energy intake on protein deposition capacity and energy metabolism of pigs, *J. Anim. Sci.*, 69:1522.

Caperna, T. J., R. G. Campbell, and N. C. Steele. 1989. Interrelationships of exogenous porcine growth hormone administration and feed intake level affecting various tissue levels of iron, copper, zinc and bone calcium of growing pigs, *J. Anim. Sci.*, 67:654.

Caperna, T. J., R. G. Campbell, M. R. Ballard, and N. C. Steele. 1995. Somatotropin enhances the rate of amino acid deposition but has minimal impact on amino acid balance in growing pigs, *J. Nutr.*, 125:2104.

Carter, S. D., and G. L. Cromwell. 1998a. Influence of porcine somatotropin on the phosphorus requirement of finishing pigs: II. Carcass characteristics, tissue accretion rates, and chemical composition of the ham, *J. Anim. Sci.*, 76:596.

Carter, S. D., and G. L. Cromwell. 1998b. Influence of porcine somatotropin on the phosphorus requirement of finishing pigs: I. Performance and bone characteristics, *J. Anim. Sci.*, 76:584.

Crome, P. K., F. K. McKeith, T. R. Carr, D. J. Jones, D. H. Mowrey, and J. E. Cannon. 1996. Effect of ractopamine on growth performance, carcass composition, and cutting yields of pigs slaughtered at 107 and 125 kilograms, *J. Anim. Sci.*, 74:709.

Cromwell, G. L., T. S. Stahly, L. A. Edgerton, H. J. Monegue, T. W. Burnell, B. C. Schenck, and B. R. Schricker. 1992. Recombinant porcine somatotropin for sows during late gestation and throughout lactation, *J. Anim. Sci.*, 70:1404.

Cunningham, H. M., D. W. Friend, and J. W. G. Nicholson. 1963. Effect of epinephrine on nitrogen and fat deposition of pigs, *J. Anim. Sci.*, 22:632.

Denis, I., M. Thomasset, and A. Pointillart. 1994a. Influence of exogenous porcine growth hormone on vitamin D metabolism and calcium and phosphorus absorption in intact pigs, *Calcif. Tissue Int.*, 54:489.

Denis, I., E. Zerath, and A. Pointillart. 1994b. Effects of exogenous growth hormone on bone mineralization and remodeling and on plasma calcitriol in intact pigs, *Bone*, 15:419.

Dunshea, F. R. 1993. Effect of metabolism modifiers on lipid metabolism in the pig, *J. Anim. Sci.*, 71:1966.

Dunshea, F. R., and R. H. King. 1995. Responses to homeostatic signals in ractopamine-treated pigs, *Br. J. Nutr.*, 73:809.

Dunshea, F. R., D. M. Harris, D. E. Bauman, R. D. Boyd, and A. W. Bell. 1992a. Effect of porcine somatotropin on *in vivo* glucose kinetics and lipogenesis in growing pigs, *J. Anim. Sci.*, 70:141.

Dunshea, F. R., D. M. Harris, D. E. Bauman, R. D. Boyd, and A. W. Bell. 1992b. Effect of somatotropin on nonesterified fatty acid and glycerol metabolism in growing pigs, *J. Anim. Sci.*, 70:132.

Dunshea, F. R., R. H. King, and R. G. Campbell. 1993a. Interrelationships between dietary protein and ractopamine on protein and lipid deposition in finishing gilts, *J. Anim. Sci.*, 71:2931.

Dunshea, F. R., R. H. King, R. G. Campbell, R. D. Sainz, and Y. S. Kim. 1993b. Interrelationships between sex and ractopamine on protein and lipid deposition in rapidly growing pigs, *J. Anim. Sci.*, 71:2919.

Eggert, J. M., and M. A. Belury. 1998. Conjugated linoleic acid effects studied, *Nat. Hog Farm.*, (Dec. 15):52.

Elsasser, T. H., N. C. Steele, and R. Fayer. 1995. Cytokines, stress, and growth modulation. In *Cytokines in Animal Health and Disease*, Myers M. J. and M. P. Murtaugh, Ed., Marcel Dekker, New York, 261.

Etherton, T. D., and D. E. Bauman. 1998. Biology of somatotropin in growth and lactation of domestic animals, *Physiol. Rev.*, 78:745.

Evans, H. M., and M. E. Simpson. 1931. Hormones of the anterior hypophysis, *Am. J. Physiol.*, 98:511.

Evock, C. M., T. D. Etherton, C. S. Chung, and R. E. Ivy. 1988. Pituitary porcine growth hormone (pGH) and a recombinant pGH analog stimulate pig growth performance in a similar manner, *J. Anim. Sci.*, 66:1928.

Evock-Clover, C. M., M. M. Polansky, R. A. Anderson, and N. C. Steele. 1993. Dietary chromium supplementation with or without somatotropin treatment alters serum hormones and metabolites in growing pigs without affecting growth performance, *J. Nutr.*, 123:1504.

Farmer, C., D. Petitclerc, G. Pelletier, and P. Brazeau. 1992. Lactation performance of sows injected with growth hormone-releasing factor during gestation and/or lactation, *J. Anim. Sci.*, 70:2636.

Farmer, C., S. Robert, and J. J. Matte. 1996. Lactation performance of sows fed a bulky diet during gestation and receiving growth hormone-releasing factor during lactation, *J. Anim. Sci.*, 74:1298.

Fernandez-Figares, I., D. Wray-Cahen, N. C. Steele, R. G. Campbell, D. D. Hall, E. Virtanen, and T. J. Caperna. 2000. Effects of betaine on nutrient partitioning in feed-restricted pigs, *J. Anim. Sci.*, 78 (Suppl. 1):146 (Abstr.).

Goff, J. P., T. J. Caperna, and N. C. Steele. 1990. Effects of growth hormone administration on vitamin D metabolism and vitamin D receptors in the pig, *Domest. Anim. Endocrinol.*, 7:425.
Hammond, J. 1944. Physiological factors affecting birth weight, *Proc. Nutr. Soc.*, 1:8.
Hammond, J. 1952. Physiological limits to intensive production in animals, *Br. Agric. Bull.*, 4:222.
Hansen, J. A., J. L. Nelssen, R. D. Goodband, and J. L. Laurin. 1994. Interactive effects among porcine somatotropin, the beta-adrenergic agonist salbutamol, and dietary lysine on growth performance and nitrogen balance of finshing swine, *J. Anim. Sci.*, 72:1547.
Hansen, J. A., J. T. Yen, J. Klindt, J. L. Nelssen, and R. D. Goodband. 1997a. Effects of somatotropin and salbutamol in three genotypes of finishing barrows: blood hormones an metabolites and muscle characteristics, *J. Anim. Sci.*, 75:1810.
Hansen, J. A., J. T. Yen, J. L. Nelssen, J. A. Nienaber, R. D. Goodband, and T. L. Wheeler. 1997b. Effects of somatotropin and salbutamol in three genotypes of finishing barrows: growth, carcass, and calorimeter criteria, *J. Anim. Sci.*, 75:1798.
Harkins, R. D., R. D. Boyd, and D. E. Bauman. 1989. Effect of recombinant porcine somatotropin on lactational performance and metabolite patterns in sows and growth of nursing pigs, *J. Anim. Sci.*, 67:1997.
Harrell, R. J., M. J. Thomas, R. D. Boyd, S. M. Czerwinski, N. C. Steele, and D. E. Bauman. 1997. Effect of porcine somatotropin administration in young pigs during the growth phase from 10 to 25 kilograms, *J. Anim. Sci.*, 75:3152.
Harris, D. M., F. R. Dunshea, D. E. Bauman, R. D. Boyd, S. Y. Wang, P. A. Johnson, and S. D. Clarke. 1993. Effect of *in vivo* somatotropin treatment of growing pigs on adipose tissue lipogenesis, *J. Anim. Sci.*, 71:3293.
Haydon, K. D., D. A. Knabe, and T. D. J. Tanksley. 1984. Effects of level of feed intake on nitrogen, amino acid and energy digestibilities measured at the end of the small intestine and over the total digestive tract of growing pigs, *J. Anim. Sci.*, 59:717.
Hoffman, L. A., D. J. Ivers, M. R. Ellersieck, and T. L. Veum. 1993. The effect of L-carnitine and soybean oil on performance and nitrogen and energy utilization by neonatal and young pigs, *J. Anim. Sci.*, 71:132.
Johnston, M. E., J. L. Nelssen, R. D. Goodband, D. H. Kropf, R. H. Hines, and B. R. Schricker. 1993. The effects of porcine somatotropin and dietary lysine on growth performance and carcass characteristics of finishing swine fed to 105 or 127 kilograms, *J. Anim. Sci.*, 71:2986.
Klindt, J., J. T. Yen, F. C. Buonomo, A. J. Roberts, and T. Wise. 1998. Growth, body composition, and endocrine responses to chronic administration of insulin-like growth factor I and/or porcine growth hormone in pigs, *J. Anim. Sci.*, 76:2368.
Krick, B. J., K. R. Roneker, R. D. Boyd, D. H. Beermann, P. J. David, and D. J. Meisinger. 1992. Influence of genotype and sex on the response of growing pigs to recombinant porcine somatotropin, *J. Anim. Sci.*, 70:3024.
Krick, B. J., R. D. Boyd, K. R. Roneker, D. H. Beermann, D. E. Bauman, D. A. Ross, and D. J. Meisinger. 1993. Porcine somatotropin affects the dietary lysine requirement and net lysine utilization for growing pigs, *J. Nutr.*, 123:1913.
Li, C. H., M. E. Simpson, and H. M. Evans. 1945. Isolation and properties of the anterior hypophysial growth hormones, *J. Biol. Chem.*, 353.
Lindemann, M. D., C. M. Wood, A. F. Harper, E. T. Kornegay, and R. A. Anderson. 1995. Dietary chromium picolinate additions improve gain:feed and carcass characteristics in growing-finishing pigs and increase litter size in reproducing sows, *J. Anim. Sci.*, 73:457.
Liu, C. Y., A. L. Grant, K. H. Kim, S. Q. Ji, D. L. Hancock, D. B. Anderson, and S. E. Mills. 1994. Limitations of ractopamine to affect adipose tissue metabolism in swine, *J. Anim. Sci.*, 72:62.
Machlin, L. J. 1972. Effect of porcine growth hormone on growth and carcass composition of the pig, *J. Anim. Sci.*, 35:794.
Martin, C. R. 1985. *Endocrine Physiology*, Oxford University Press, New York.
Matthews, J. O., L. L. Southern, J. E. Pontif, A. D. Higbie, and T. D. Bidner. 1998. Interactive effects of betaine, crude protein, and net energy in finishing pigs, *J. Anim. Sci.*, 76:2444.
McLaughlin, C. L., J. C. Byatt, D. F. Curran, E. L. Veenhuizen, M. F. McGrath, F. C. Buonomo, R. L. Hintz, and C. A. Baile. 1997. Growth performance, endocrine, and metabolite responses of finishing hogs to porcine prolactin, *J. Anim. Sci.*, 75:959.
Mitchell, A. D., M. B. Solomon, and N. C. Steele. 1991. Influence of level of dietary protein or energy on effects of ractopamine in finishing swine, *J. Anim. Sci.*, 69:4487.

Nelssen, J. L., A. J. Lewis, E. R. Peo, Jr., and J. D. Crenshaw. 1985. Effect of dietary energy intake during lactation on performance of primiparous sows and their litters, *J. Anim. Sci.*, 61:1164.

Noblet, J., P. Herpin, and S. Dubois. 1992. Effect of recombinant porcine somatotropin on energy and protein utilization by growing pigs: interaction with capacity for lean tissue growth, *J. Anim. Sci.*, 70:2471.

Nossaman, D. A., A. P. Schinckel, L. F. Miller, and S. E. Mills. 1991. Interaction of somatotropin and genotype on the requirement for energy in two lines of finishing pigs, *J. Nutr.*, 121:223.

NRC (National Research Council). 1994. *Metabolic Modifiers: Effects on the Nutrient Requirements of Food-producing Animals*, National Academy Press, Washington, D.C.

NRC (National Research Council). 1997. *The Role of Chromium in Animal Nutrition*, National Academy Press, Washington, D.C.

NRC (National Research Council). 1998. *Nutrient Requirements of Swine*, National Academy Press, Washington, D.C.

Odle, J. 1995. Betaine and carnitine — evaluation of performance and carcass effects, *Proc. Carolina Nutr. Conf.*, 11:1.

Owen, K. Q., J. L. Nelssen, R. D. Goodband, T. L. Weeden, and S. A. Blum. 1996. Effect of L-carnitine and soybean oil on growth performance and body composition of early-weaned pigs, *J. Anim. Sci.*, 74:1612.

Ozawa, A., K. Hodate, and T. Johke. 1996. Plasma concentrations of hormones and metabolic substrates in growing pigs after bovine growth hormone injections under various nutritional conditions, *Endocr. J.*, 43:357.

Page, T. G., L. L. Southern, T. L. Ward, and D. L. Thompson, Jr. 1993. Effect of chromium picolinate on growth and serum and carcass traits of growing-finishing pigs, *J. Anim. Sci.*, 71:656.

Pursel, V. G., R. J. Wall, A. D. Mitchell, T. H. Elsasser, M. B. Solomon, M. E. Coleman, F. DeMayo, and R. J. Schwartz. 1998. Expression of insulin-like growth factor-I in skeletal muscle of transgenic swine. In *Transgenic Animals in Agriculture*, Murray, J. D., G. B. Anderson, A. M. Oberbauer, and M. M. McGloughlin, Ed., CAB International, Oxford, 131.

Ramsay, T. G. 1999. Leptin: a regulator of feed intake and physiology in swine, *Proc. Maryland Nutr. Conf.*, 46:195.

Reeds, P. J., and H. J. Mersmann. 1991. Protein and energy requirements of animals treated with β-adrenergic agonists: a discussion, *J. Anim. Sci.*, 69:1532.

Reese, D. E., B. D. Moser, E. R. Peo, Jr., A. J. Lewis, D. R. Zimmerman, J. E. Kinder, and W. W. Stroup. 1982. Influence of energy intake during lactation on the interval from weaning to first estrus in sows, *J. Anim. Sci.*, 55:590.

Reese, D. E., E. R. Peo, Jr., and A. J. Lewis. 1984. Relationship of lactation energy intake and occurrence of postweaning estrus to body and backfat composition in sows, *J. Anim. Sci.*, 58:1236.

Roberts, T. J., and M. J. Azain. 1997. Somatotropin treatment reduces energy intake without altering protein intake in pigs selecting between high and low protein diets, *J. Nutr.*, 127:2047.

Stahly, T. S., and L. J. Bark. 1991. Impact of porcine somatotropin and beta-adrenergic agonists in swine. In *Swine Nutrition*, Miller, E. R., D. E. Ullrey, and A. J. Lewis., Ed., Butterworth-Heinemann, Boston, MA, 103.

SCA (Standing Committee on Agriculture). 1987. *Feeding Standards for Australian Livestock: Pigs*, CSIRO, East Melbourne, Australia.

Steele, N. C., R. D. Boyd, and R. G. Campbell. 1994. Growth, metabolic modifiers, and nutrient considerations. In *Low-Fat Meats: Design Strategies and Human Implications*, Hafs, H. D., and R. G. Zimbelman, Ed., Academic Press, San Diego, CA, 167.

Steele, N. C., T. G. Althen, and L. T. Frobish. 1977. Biological activity of glucose tolerance factor in swine, *J. Anim. Sci.*, 45:1341.

Tomas, F. M., R. G. Campbell, R. H. King, R. J. Johnson, C. S. Chandler, and M. R. Taverner. 1992. Growth hormone increases whole-body protein turnover in growing pigs, *J. Anim. Sci.*, 70:3138.

Toner, M. S., R. H. King, F. R. Dunshea, H. Dove, and C. S. Atwood. 1996. The effect of exogenous somatotropin on lactation performance of first-litter sows, *J. Anim. Sci.*, 74:167.

Turman, E. J., and F. N. Andrews. 1955. Some effects of purified anterior pituitary growth hormone on swine, *J. Anim. Sci.*, 14:7.

van Kempen, T. A., and J. Odle. 1993. Medium-chain fatty acid oxidation in colostrum-deprived newborn piglets: stimulative effect of L-carnitine supplementation, *J. Nutr.*, 123:1531.

Verstegen, M. W., W. van der Hel, A. M. Henken, J. Huisman, E. Kanis, P. van der Wal, and E. J. van Weerden. 1990. Effect of exogenous porcine somatotropin administration on nitrogen and energy metabolism in three genotypes of pigs, *J. Anim. Sci.*, 68:1008.

Verstegen, M. W., W. van der Hel, H. A. Brandsma, A. M. Henken, E. Kanis, and P. van der Wal. 1991. Effects of recombinant porcine somatotropin on metabolic rate in growing pigs, *J. Anim. Sci.*, 69:2961.

Ward, T. L., L. L. Southern, and T. D. Bidner. 1997. Interactive effects of dietary chromium tripicolinate and crude protein level in growing-finishing pigs provided inadequate and adequate pen space, *J. Anim. Sci.*, 75:1001.

Wester, T. J., T. A. Davis, M. L. Fiorotto, and D. G. Burrin. 1998. Exogenous growth hormone stimulates somatotropic axis function and growth in neonatal pigs, *Am. J. Physiol.*, 274:E29-E37.

Williams, N. H., T. R. Cline, A. P. Schinckel, and D. J. Jones. 1994. The impact of ractopamine, energy intake, and dietary fat on finisher pig growth performance and carcass merit, *J. Anim. Sci.*, 72:3152.

Wray-Cahen, D., D. A. Ross, D. E. Bauman, and R. D. Boyd. 1991. Metabolic effects of porcine somatotropin: nitrogen and energy balance and characterization of the temporal pattern of blood metabolites and hormones, *J. Anim. Sci.*, 69:1503.

Wray-Cahen, D., A. W. Bell, R. D. Boyd, D. A. Ross, D. E. Bauman, B. J. Krick, and R. J. Harrell. 1995. Nutrient uptake by the hindlimb of growing pigs treated with porcine somatotropin and insulin, *J. Nutr.*, 125:125.

Wray-Cahen, D., D. E. Kerr, C. M. Evock-Clover, and N. C. Steele. 1998. Redefining body composition: nutrients, hormones, and genes in meat production, *Annu. Rev. Nutr.*, 18:63.

20 Feed Intake in Growing-Finishing Pigs

Michael Ellis and Nathan Augspurger

CONTENTS

I. Introduction 447
II. Physiological Control of Feed Intake 447
III. Nutritional Factors Influencing Voluntary Feed Intake 448
IV. Animal Factors Influencing Voluntary Feed Intake 451
V. Environmental Factors Influencing Voluntary Feed Intake 454
VI. Feeding Behavior 458
VII. Measuring and Predicting Feed Intake 462
References 463

I. INTRODUCTION

Growing-finishing pigs are provided feed on an *ad libitum* basis for most, if not all, of the production period under normal conditions in the United States and many other countries. Consequently, the amount of feed consumed is central to determining their growth performance in terms of both live weight and tissue accretion rates. In addition, knowledge of the feed intake of pigs on commercial units is essential to formulating diets to meet the animal's requirements within its intake limit.

Curtis (1996), after Forbes (1995), defined *voluntary feed intake* as the total weight of feed ingested in a given period of free access to feed (usually a day), and the *potential feed intake* as the weight of feed required to fulfill all of the animal's nutrient requirements. In practice, voluntary feed intake is usually significantly lower than potential intake because of a range of internal animal constraints, environmental limitations, and/or nutritional factors. The range of factors that interact to determine the voluntary feed intake of growing-finishing pigs under commercial conditions is discussed in this chapter.

II. PHYSIOLOGICAL CONTROL OF FEED INTAKE

The regulation of feed intake is complex, involving the central nervous system and many other systems and nutrients or metabolites in the body. The hypothalamus has been shown to be a center of control of feed intake, with numerous studies illustrating its involvement in feed intake regulation in the pig (Martin et al., 1989). Theories have been developed to explain the overall control of feed intake incorporating the hypothalamus and other body systems and components into a central theme of feed intake regulation. These theories are briefly summarized in this chapter. A more comprehensive review of the physiological mechanisms involved in the regulation of feed and energy intake has been published by Martin et al. (1989).

There are a number of theories that have been proposed to explain the short-term control of feed intake. These include the glucostatic theory of feed intake control that was presented by Mayer (1953) and is based upon the premise that feeding is stimulated in response to a decrease in glucose utilization by neurons in the ventromedial hypothalamus, due to a reduction in circulating glucose levels (Martin et al., 1989). In studies in the pig, depriving the central nervous system and, thus, the hypothalamus of glucose via insulin administration had mixed effects on feed intake, but administration of 2-deoxy-D-glucose, a nonmetabolizable glucose analog, did increase feed intake (Houpt, 1984). Regulation of feed intake due to plasma amino acid balance has been established, but this mechanism is not apparent when diets are balanced and nonlimiting (Martin et al., 1989). It has also been hypothesized that total energy intake also regulates feed intake. This theory suggests that the animal will match its energy intake to its immediate or past energy needs, which in turn influences meal size and time between meals to affect feed intake. In addition, gastric distension and gastric emptying have been shown to exert a regulatory influence on feed intake (Martin et al., 1989).

Theories relating to the longer-term control of feed intake include the set-point theory, which suggests that feed intake is regulated by the ability of blood metabolites to be incorporated into adipose tissue. The proposed set point is that at which an adipocyte reaches a certain size and releases more fatty acids into circulation. These fatty acids are then detected by the brain, and subsequent feed intake is decreased (Martin et al., 1989). It has also been shown that leptin, a protein produced in adipocytes, is also released into the circulation at this point and this compound has also been implicated in feed intake regulation. One hypothesis is that leptin acts on the brain via leptin receptors in different nuclei of the hypothalamus to reduce feed intake and increase energy expenditure to regulate body weight (Carro et al., 1997). The roles of leptin in feed intake regulation, energy expenditure, and energy balance have been reviewed by Houseknecht et al. (1998).

A number of other peripheral mechanisms have been implicated in feed intake regulation including various hormones and neurotransmitters. Cholecystokinin is a hormone released from the small intestine during feed ingestion that is thought to be a humoral satiety signal (Scharrer, 1991). Exogenous cholecystokinin has been shown to reduce feed intake in the pig (Scharrer, 1991); however, although cholecystokinin may have a satiety effect, this hormone may also cause general sedation (Houpt, 1985). A number of other hormones and neurotransmitters have been investigated regarding their potential role in feed intake control; these include norepinephrine, γ-amino butyric acid, neuropeptide Y, peptide YY, opioids, growth hormone–releasing factor, insulin, thyrotropin-releasing hormone, corticotropin-releasing factor, and calcitonin gene-related peptide (Martin et al., 1989).

III. NUTRITIONAL FACTORS INFLUENCING VOLUNTARY FEED INTAKE

There is a substantial volume of literature relating to the relationship between nutritional factors and feed intake in the pig, with the bulk of this literature addressing the impact of dietary energy density on intake. The statement that "pigs eat for calories" is borne out by a large number of studies with growing-finishing pigs that supports the concept that energy balance mechanisms are probably operating in young, rapidly growing animals (Martin et al., 1989).

A graphical model illustrating the potential relationship between energy density of the diet and feed and energy intake levels is represented schematically in Figure 20.1, which was derived from Cole et al. (1971). Conceptually, there are a wide range of dietary energy levels within which the pig can adjust its feed intake to maintain a constant energy intake. However, according to this model (Figure 20.1), at relatively high or low dietary energy concentrations this ability is compromised. At the extremes, the physiological control of feed intake probably involves mechanisms other than those associated with maintenance of energy balance. Cole et al. (1971) suggested that these mechanisms could involve physical limitations to gut capacity with diets of low nutrient density and a lack of gut fill with diets of high nutrient density.

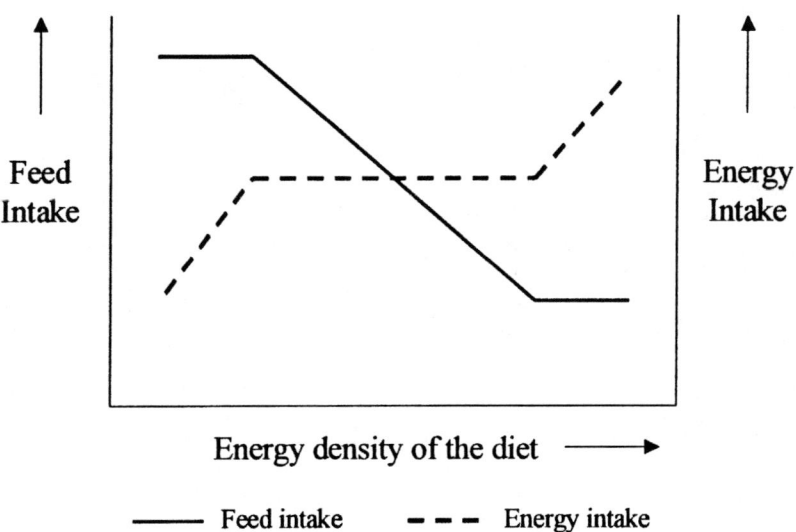

FIGURE 20.1 Schematic representation of the relationship between feed and energy intakes and the energy density of the diet. (Adapted from Cole et al., 1971.)

There are few studies that have titrated the relationship between dietary energy concentration and feed and energy intake across a wide-enough range of dietary energy concentrations to test the validity of the concepts represented in Figure 20.1. However, a number of factors of practical significance will impact these relationships and determine the feed intake of pigs fed a particular diet. These factors include the size, genotype, and sex of the pig, the previous nutrition of the animal, the dietary concentration of protein, amino acids, and other nutrients, and the source(s) of energy in the diet, particularly in relation to the type of fat or fiber used.

Giles et al. (1998) suggested that pigs weighing less than 20 kg seem unable to increase feed intake to adjust for reductions in dietary energy density below a digestible energy concentration of approximately 16 MJ/kg. In contrast, these authors suggested that pigs weighing from 20 to 50 kg or above 70 kg live weight could increase feed intake down to dietary digestible energy concentrations of 14 and 10 MJ/kg, respectively. In addition, there are substantial differences between genotypes and sexes for the level of feed intake and, presumably, also for the relationship between dietary energy concentration and feeding level, although there has been little research conducted in this area.

Madsen (1985) reviewed published relationships between dietary energy density and feed intake, including studies where relatively high levels of fiber or fat had been used to produce diets with relatively low and high energy concentrations, respectively. This author concluded that the impact of these ingredients on feed and energy intake varied with the type of fiber or fat used. One practical situation where diets with elevated fat and energy concentrations have been used is under hot conditions. The relationship between high dietary fat levels and the performance of pigs under hot conditions has been reviewed by Cisneros (1997). Generally speaking, growing-finishing pigs fed fat-supplemented diets compared with standard corn–soybean meal diets under hot conditions had similar feed intakes; however, energy intake and, consequently, growth rates were increased for the fat-supplemented diets. Interestingly, carcass fat levels were also increased for pigs fed the high-fat diets, suggesting that under hot conditions a major portion of the increased energy intake achieved with high-fat diets went into fat rather than protein synthesis.

A potential practical application of diets with reduced energy density is to reduce energy intakes and, subsequently, carcass fat levels in pigs given *ad libitum* access to feed. This concept has been investigated in a number of studies including that of Stein and Easter (1996), which was conducted

TABLE 20.1
Influence of Dietary Energy Concentration on Growth and Carcass Traits[a,b]

Diet	1	2	3	4	5
Energy concentration (kcal ME/kg)	3,500	3,300	3,100	2,900	2,700
Feed intake (kg/d)	2.91[c]	3.28[d]	3.36[d]	3.23[d]	3.31[d]
Energy intake (Mcal/day)	10.17[cd]	10.83[c]	10.41[c]	9.36[de]	8.93[e]
Daily gain (g)	1017[c]	1038[c]	1006[cd]	931[de]	872[e]
Gain:feed (kg/kg)	0.35[c]	0.32[d]	0.30[de]	0.29[e]	0.26[f]
Gain:feed (g/Mcal)	100	96	97	100	98
Carcass lean (%)	50.78[cd]	50.42[d]	51.72[cd]	52.32[c]	52.0[cd]
Daily lean gain (g)	392[c]	382[cd]	386[cd]	358[de]	330[e]

[a] Growth period was from 54 to 112 kg live weight.
[b] Means in the same row followed by different superscripts differ ($P < 0.05$).

Source: Adapted from Stein and Easter (1996).

at the University of Illinois. Finishing pigs (55 to 112 kg live weight) were given *ad libitum* access to diets with a range of energy concentrations, 2700 to 3500 kcal metabolizable energy (ME)/kg, achieved using a combination of fat, wheat bran, corn gluten feed, and alfalfa meal. The results of this study are summarized in Table 20.1. Feed intake increased as dietary energy decreased from 3500 to 3300 kcal ME/kg, but no further change was noted at lower energy concentrations (Table 20.1). Consequently, energy intake, growth rate, and gain:feed ratio (on a weight for weight basis) were generally reduced, and carcass lean content was increased with reduced dietary energy concentrations below 3300 kcal ME/kg. Energy conversion efficiency (i.e., gain:feed ratio expressed as grams of gain per megacalorie ME) was unaffected by dietary energy concentration (Table 20.1). Thus, feeding diets with reduced dietary energy concentration is a potential tool to increase carcass lean content. However, there are a number of potential problems with such an approach, including an increased output of fecal matter, and an increase in the bulk of feedstuffs, which can increase handling and transportation costs. In addition, high-fiber ingredients are not necessarily low cost and the economics of such an approach will be dictated by the increased costs in terms of diets, feed and manure handling, and reduced growth rate set against the increased value of improved carcass lean content.

As well as the energy concentration of the diet, the voluntary feed intake of pigs in a given situation will also be influenced by the level of other essential nutrients in the diet, particularly in terms of any deficiencies or imbalances. In relation to dietary protein and amino acid levels, a number of studies have shown that feed intake can be reduced in growing-finishing pigs fed diets that are deficient in protein or essential amino acids (Rogerson and Campbell, 1982; Hahn et al., 1995) or have an amino acid balance that is not ideal (Henry et al., 1992a,b; Henry, 1995; Hahn and Baker, 1995). However, other studies have shown an increase in feed intake in response to dietary protein deficiency (Friesen et al., 1994).

Deficiencies in dietary minerals and vitamins also have been shown to reduce feed intake. Combs et al. (1991) fed pigs diets containing phosphorus and calcium at 70, 85, 100, 115, and 130% of NRC (1988) requirements from 10 to 110 kg live weight. Feed intake was decreased with decreasing levels of phosphorus and calcium. Deficiencies of vitamins are often associated with reduced feed intake and poor growth, along with a myriad of other physiological symptoms (NRC, 1998).

In addition, there are a wide range of compounds that are found in certain dietary ingredients under certain conditions, such as antinutritive factors and toxins, that can dramatically reduce feed intake levels. Van Heugten discusses some of these factors in Chapter 25 of this book.

IV. ANIMAL FACTORS INFLUENCING VOLUNTARY FEED INTAKE

The genotype of an animal influences both its feed intake and lean growth potential. These two factors in combination will determine the diet that must be fed to meet the animal's requirements within its intake capacity. Breed differences in feed intake have been reported in a number of studies. For example, the results of a recent comparison of a number of sire breeds and lines used in the United States (NPPC, 1995) are summarized in Table 20.2. The sire lines were all mated to a common dam line and the differences among the progeny presented in Table 20.2 represent half the difference between the sire lines themselves. The between-line range in feed intake was 0.16 kg/day or approximately 6% of the mean with the Berkshire, Duroc, and Spot progeny having the highest intake and the lines originating from Europe (Danbred HD and Newsham Hybrid) having the lowest (Table 20.2). A breed that is relatively widely used in Europe and North America is the Pietrain; however, there is little current information on the relative performance of this breed. Historically, comparisons involving the Pietrain have generally shown a lower feed intake and relatively slow growth compared with Yorkshire, Duroc, or Hampshire pigs (Miller, 1998). Thus, the increased carcass lean content generally associated with the Pietrain results largely from this lower feed intake rather than from any increase in the rate of lean deposition.

The variation in feed intake and growth performance within a breed and between lines of similar genetic composition from different breeding stock suppliers is probably greater than that across breeds. This is illustrated by historical data from a U.K. study that compared lines with similar breed composition from four breeding companies (MLC, 1988; Table 20.3). The range in growth performance was substantial, with the difference between the highest and lowest lines being 0.22 kg/day or 10.2% of the mean for daily feed intake, 115 g/day or 13.7% of the mean for daily live weight gain, 0.42 kg or 16.2% of the mean for feed:gain ratio, and 85 g/day or 23.3% of the mean for lean growth rate. This highlights the importance to the producer of choice of breeding stock supplier and of an understanding of the performance level of the breeding stock being used.

Gu et al. (1991a,b) compared a range of crossbreds typical of the U.S. industry and also showed substantial variation between genotypes for feed intake and growth (Table 20.4). Generally speaking, the genotypes with the highest lean growth rates tended to have the lowest feed intakes. This has obvious implications for the nutrient concentrations in the diet that would be required to meet the nutrient requirements of each genotype, which is illustrated by comparing genotypes 4 and 5 from this study (Table 20.4). Genotype 5 had a higher lean growth rate (61 g/day) but consumed

TABLE 20.2
Breed and Genetic Line Differences in Growth Performance Traits[a,b]

	Average Daily Feed Intake (kg)	Average Daily Gain (g)	Feed:Gain Ratio	Lean Growth Rate (g/day)
Berkshire	2.66[cf]	840[e]	3.07[e]	286[e]
Danbred HD	2.47[c]	831[e]	2.88[cd]	327[c]
Duroc	2.61[e]	885[c]	2.91[d]	318[cd]
Hampshire	2.57[de]	849[cd]	2.92[d]	322[c]
NGT Large White	2.53[cd]	849[de]	2.94[d]	295[e]
NE SPF Duroc	2.62[e]	894[c]	2.89[cd]	331[c]
Newsham Hybrid	2.51[cd]	863[cd]	2.83[c]	331[c]
Spot	2.68[f]	835[e]	3.14[f]	285[e]
Yorkshire	2.53[d]	835[e]	2.93[d]	309[d]

[a] Growth period was from 29.5 to 113.5 kg live weight.
[b] Means in the same column followed by different letters differ ($P < 0.05$).

Source: Adapted from National Pork Producers Council (1995).

TABLE 20.3
Range in Performance for Four Breeding Companies

	Overall Mean	Company Range
Number of piglets born alive	10.2	9.8–10.8
Daily feed intake (kg)	2.16	2.07–2.29
Daily gain (g)	842	775–890
Feed conversion ratio	2.59	2.45–2.87
Dressing percentage	75.7	74.7–76.5
Carcass lean (%)	55.2	51.6–58.2
Lean growth rate (g/day)	365	315–400

Source: Adapted from Meat and Livestock Commission (1988).

TABLE 20.4
Genotype Effects on Feed Intake and Growth

Genotype	Feed Intake (kg/day)	Daily Gain (g)	Lean Growth Rate (g/day)
1	3.145	916	329
2	3.019	924	361
3	3.055	1010	390
4	3.238	1001	332
5	3.028	1017	393

Source: Adapted from Gu et al. (1991a,b).

210 g/day less feed compared with genotype 4 (Table 20.4). Obviously, the dietary concentrations of essential amino acids and other nutrients to meet the requirements of these two genotypes within their feed intake capacity would be markedly different.

A number of genotype comparisons, including the study of Gu et al. (1991a,b), have suggested a negative association between feed intake and lean growth rate, and there is evidence that selection for genetic improvement of carcass lean content has resulted in reduced feed intake in some selection programs (Smith et al., 1991). However, the relationship between the genetic change in lean growth and feed intake is not fixed and will depend on the combination of testing environment and selection objectives under which particular lines have been developed (Fowler et al., 1976). For example, when pigs are tested under *ad libitum* feeding conditions and the selection criteria emphasizes increased carcass leanness and improved feed efficiency, then reductions in feed intake have occurred (Smith et al., 1991), whereas, when increasing lean growth rate was the selection objective, genetic increases in feed intake have been found. This is illustrated by the results of a four-generation selection experiment carried out in the United Kingdom that compared three different selection objectives, namely, lean growth rate, lean feed efficiency, or daily feed intake, under *ad libitum* feeding (Cameron and Curran, 1994). The responses are summarized in Table 20.5, where they are expressed as the difference between selected and control populations. Selection for lean feed efficiency, which emphasized increased carcass lean content and feed conversion efficiency (measured as backfat thickness and feed:gain ratio) resulted in an improvement in carcass lean and feed efficiency, but a reduction in daily live weight gain and feed intake. In contrast, selection for lean growth rate, which emphasized live weight gain and carcass lean content, actually increased growth rates and feed intakes (Table 20.5). As anticipated, selection for daily feed intake produced increases in feed intake, growth rate, and carcass fatness, and also led to an increase in feed:gain ratio. This illustrates the potential variation that could exist in feed intake and lean growth rate in lines of pigs

TABLE 20.5
Response to Four Generations of Selection for Different Selection Objectives in a Large White Population

Selection Objective	Deviation of Selected and Control Populations		
	Lean Growth Rate	Lean Feed Efficiency	Daily Feed Intake
Live weight gain (g/day)	+55	−24	+96
Backfat thickness (mm)	−0.40	−1.35	+2.79
Feed:gain	−0.034	−0.028	+0.030
Daily feed intake (g/day)	+105	−68	+242

Source: Derived from Cameron and Curran (1994).

that have been subjected to different selection strategies, and also highlights the importance of quantifying these traits for specific genotypes.

A large number of studies have been conducted worldwide where differences between the sexes for feed intake and growth performance have been estimated. A summary of selected recent studies that have compared castrates and gilts is presented in Table 20.6. The difference in daily feed intake between these two sexes, expressed as castrate minus gilt, varied considerably among studies with a range from −0.01 (Van Lunen and Cole, 1996) to +0.44 kg/day (Henry et al., 1992b; Table 20.6). To a certain extent, this may reflect the weight ranges over which the sexes were

TABLE 20.6
Selected Studies Reporting on the Differences in Feed Intake and Growth Performance Between Castrates and Gilts

Reference	Genotype[a]	Weight Range (kg)	Difference (Castrate-Gilt)[b]		
			ADFI (kg)	ADG (g)	G:F
Cisneros et al., 1996	Hybrid, HYD	60–130	+0.14	+56	+0.008
Cromwell et al., 1993	Crossbred	35–99	+0.32	+98	+0.002
		50–105	+0.35	+61	−0.015
		50–105	+0.34	+95	−0.004
Friesen et al., 1994	HL, ML	44–127	+0.27	+50	−0.008
Fuller et al., 1995	Hybrid	37–85	+0.04	+40	+0.009
Haydon et al., 1989	Crossbred	18–105	+0.16	+57	+0.002
Henry et al., 1992a	LW	42–100	+0.23	+55	−0.005
Henry et al., 1992b	LW	44–100	+0.44	+128	−0.003
		50–70	+0.14	+79	+0.015
Henry, 1995	LW	53–88	+0.15	+62	+0.011
			+0.25	+87	+0.014
Hyun et al., 1997	PIC	27–83	+0.10	+52	+0.01
Knight et al., 1991	Crossbred	67–100	+0.22	+50	−0.005
		72–100	+0.39	+90	−0.009
Langlois and Minvielle, 1989	Crossbred	33–95	+0.19	+98	+0.018
Lopez et al., 1991a	HYD	90–110	+0.17	+30	−0.004
Lopez et al., 1991b	HYD	85–105	+0.32	+90	+0.004
Van Lunen and Cole, 1996	PIC	25–90	−0.01	−10	−0.003
Weatherup et al., 1998	LD x LW	50–125	+0.42	+87	−0.026

[a] HYD = Hampshire, Yorkshire, Duroc crossbred; HL = high lean; ML = medium lean; LW = Large White; PIC = PIC hybrid offspring; LD = Landrace.
[b] ADFI = Average daily feed intake; ADG = Average daily gain; G:F = Gain to feed ratio.

TABLE 20.7
Relative Performance of Entire Males and Castrates (castrate performance level = 100)

	Relative Performance	Range Within Which Most Trial Results Fall
Daily feed intake	91	±5
Daily live weight gain	103	±2
Dressing percentage	99	±1
Gain:feed ratio	113	±5
P2 fat thickness	80	±5
Carcass lean percentage	106	±3
Carcass fat percentage (separable)	89	±4
Daily lean growth rate	116	±5
Lean gain:feed	125	±5

Source: Adapted from Kempster and Lowe (1993).

compared in the various studies; there is evidence that sex differences for feed intake and growth increase with live weight (Hamilton, 1999; Wolter, 1999). However, variation in the relative differences between castrates and gilts cannot be discounted. Kempster and Lowe (1993) reviewed the literature comparing growth and carcass characteristics of entire males and castrates. This review is summarized in Table 20.7 and shows that, on average, boars consumed 9% less feed than castrates, and that most of the results from studies fell within the range of 4 to 14% lower feed intake for the entire male.

Feed intake obviously changes as pigs grow. In a review focusing on the prediction of feed intake, NRC (1987) described feed intake (digestible energy intake) as an asymptotic function of live weight between 4.5 and 117 kg, with the maximum energy intake attained between 100 and 120 kg live weight. Bigelow and Houpt (1988) reported increases in feed intake of 188% from 10 kg live weight to a maximum at 110 kg live weight, with feed intake then slightly decreasing as pigs grew to 130 kg live weight. Hyun et al. (1997) reported that feed intake for pigs 25 to 85 kg live weight increased linearly with increasing body weight. These authors also showed a correlation of +0.58 between body weight and daily feed intake. In the most recent edition of *Nutrient Requirements of Swine* (NRC, 1998), feed intake in growing-finishing pigs is described as a cubic function of body weight between 20 and 120 kg live weight. According to this relationship, feed intake increases the fastest between live weights of 20 and 70 kg while beyond 70 kg, feed intake increases at a slower rate.

V. ENVIRONMENTAL FACTORS INFLUENCING VOLUNTARY FEED INTAKE

Most aspects of the pig's environment can influence its voluntary feed intake if the environmental conditions fall outside the animal's capacity to adapt. In practice, most commercial environments within which pigs are kept are limiting in some or many respects, and feed intake levels achieved on the farm are generally significantly below the pig's potential feed intake. The major environmental factors that can compromise the feed intake of the animal include climatic, physical, social, and disease aspects.

The major climatic factor that directly influences feed intake is the environmental temperature or, more precisely, the effective environmental temperature to which the animal is exposed. Curtis (1983) defined effective environmental temperature as the "total effect of a particular environment on an animal's heat balance, which the animal has some control over through changing its body orientation to the surroundings." The effective environmental temperature is the result of the interaction between

Feed Intake in Growing-Finishing Pigs

ambient temperature and other environmental factors such as air speed, humidity, number of pigs in the pen, flooring type, and availability of cooling systems such as water drips and sprays.

Conceptually, pigs attempt to maintain a stable body temperature in the face of widely varying environmental temperatures and one of the major mechanisms to achieve this is variation in feed intake. The literature relating to changes in feed intake under hot and cold climatic conditions has been reviewed by Giles et al. (1998). In general, animals will increase intake in response to cold conditions and reduce intake in response to hot conditions. In fact, feed intake generally declines with increases in ambient temperature across the range likely to be encountered in most housed situations (0 to 40°C); however, the rate of the decline varies with the absolute temperature and also with the size of the pig. Close (1989) showed that heavier pigs (≥90 kg) when kept at temperatures below the pigs' lower critical temperature generally show a greater increase in feed intake than lighter animals (≤60 kg). In addition, pigs weighing less than 18 kg showed no increase in feed intake at low ambient temperatures, presumably because of some limitation in gut capacity (Close, 1989).

A summary of a number of studies that have investigated the influence of environmental temperature on feed intake in growing and finishing pigs is presented in Figures 20.2 and 20.3, respectively, which have been adapted from Cisneros (1997). Giles et al. (1998) suggested that decreases in feed intake above the evaporative critical temperature (i.e., the temperature at which animals must start to increase evaporative heat loss to maintain body temperature) were associated with a rise in body temperature. These authors looked at the relationship between body temperature and "relative" voluntary feed intake (i.e., the ratio of feed intake at high temperature relative to that under thermoneutral conditions) in growing pigs. They showed a negative linear regression with "relative" feed intake declining by 40% per degree Celsius rise in body temperature above 39.2°C, and that animals stopped eating when body temperature approached 41.3°C.

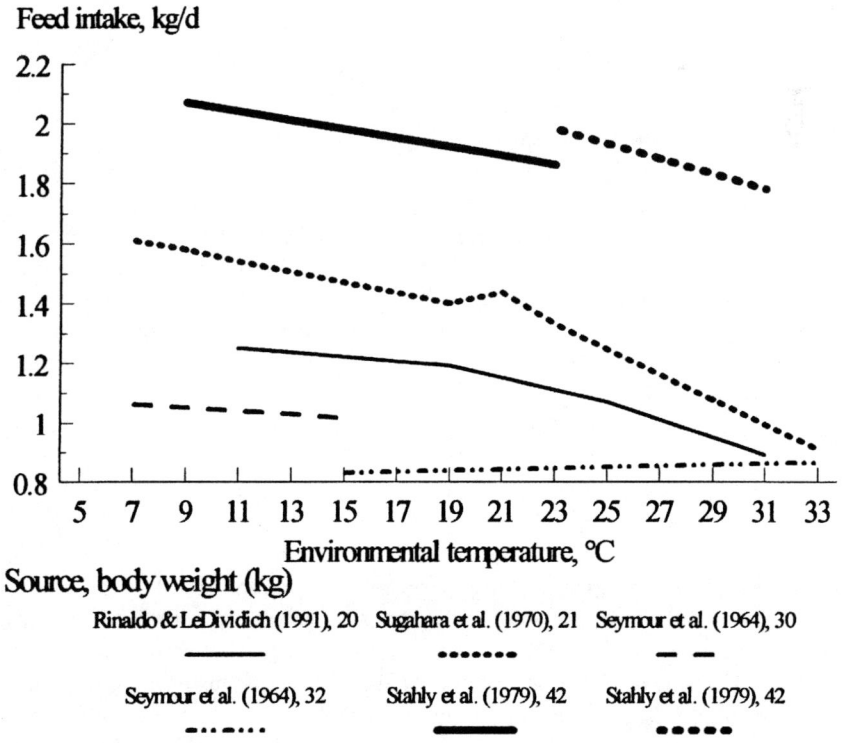

FIGURE 20.2 Effect of environmental temperature on the voluntary feed intake of growing swine. (Adapted from Cisneros, 1997.)

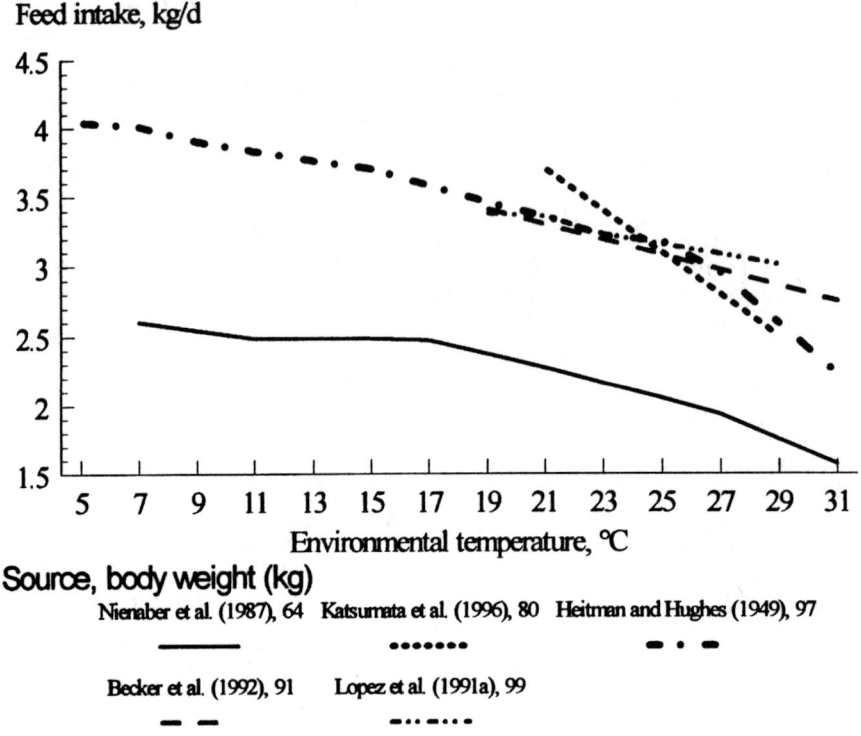

FIGURE 20.3 Effect of environmental temperature on the voluntary feed intake of finishing swine. (Adapted from Cisneros, 1997.)

Two factors that will influence the impact of environmental temperature on feed intake of pigs under practical conditions are diurnal fluctuations in temperature and the degree of adaptation of the animal to the temperature conditions. In hot weather conditions, such as those experienced in the summer in many parts of the world where pigs are produced, ambient temperatures are lower during the evening, nighttime, and early morning. Pigs will generally respond to such conditions by decreasing intake during the hot periods and increasing intake during the cooler periods of the day (Xin and De Shazer, 1992). The study of Feddes et al. (1989) suggested that the impact of cyclic temperatures on feed intake was similar to the effect observed with a constant temperature that was the average temperature of the cyclic regime. Conceptually, pigs will show adaptative changes to prolonged exposure to high environmental temperatures, which could impact the rate of reduction in feed intake with increasing environmental temperatures. However, published data in support of this concept are scarce; Giles and Black (1991) showed no increase in feed intake in pigs (90 kg live weight) maintained at 31°C ambient temperature for a 12-day period even though body temperature had declined during the test period. Similarly, Morrison and Mount (1971) found that feed intake of growing pigs was unchanged when they were exposed to high temperatures for 30 days.

The impact of photoperiod on feed intake and growth has not been widely researched in the pig. McGlone et al. (1988) compared photoperiod regimes of 1 h light:23 h dark and 16 h light:8 h dark in nursery pigs and found no effect on feed intake, growth rate, or feed efficiency ratio over a 28-day period following weaning. In addition, Ntunde et al. (1979) compared three photoperiods (24 h complete darkness, except for 1 to 1.5 h of dim red light during experimental procedures; 18 h artificial light:6 h dark; and natural winter photoperiod, 9 to 10.8 h light daily) in gilts from 100 days of age to approximately 105 kg live weight and also found no effect on daily gain and feed efficiency. These limited results would suggest that feed intake and growth of swine are not influenced by photoperiod.

There are a wide range of aspects of the pig's social, physical, and disease environment that affect feed intake, and under practical conditions they are a major cause of reduced voluntary feed intake and growth performance. The impact of the social and physical environment on feed intake has been reviewed by Curtis (1996); important aspects include group size, floor space, regrouping, feeder design, pen layout (size, shape, and location of resources), waterer design and operation, water quality, waste handling and removal, pen cleanliness, ventilation system, air movement and air quality (in terms of dust and gas levels). Many of these aspects are covered in detail by Brumm and Gonyou in Chapter 22 of this book.

Although disease is probably the biggest single factor reducing feed intake and growth of pigs under commercial conditions, there is surprisingly little data quantifying the impact of specific diseases on pig performance. The role of disease and immune system stimulation on energy expenditure and growth has been reviewed by Johnson (1996), and the feed intake response to infection has been quantified in some studies (e.g., Bray, 1996). Research at Iowa State University (Williams et al., 1997b) has shown that pigs kept under a management scheme designed to minimize immunological challenges had higher feed intake and growth rate, and retained more nitrogen compared with those that were immunologically challenged (Williams et al., 1997a). Johnson (1996) suggested that sickness in pigs, which is manifest as reduced feed intake and lowered lean growth, results from the increased synthesis by the animal of certain cytokines. This area is being extensively researched in a number of laboratories and is reviewed in Chapter 24 of this book by Johnson. This research offers the potential to clarify understanding of the association among disease challenge, immunological changes, and voluntary feed intake.

Most research investigating the impact of the animal's environment on growth performance has generally studied individual factors in isolation. However, under commercial conditions, pigs are generally exposed to multiple stressors concurrently. A recent study conducted at the University of Illinois (Hyun et al., 1998a) looked at the effect of three stressors (high ambient temperatures, reduced floor space, and regrouping) singly and in combination, on growth performance of growing pigs. The effects of the three stressors were generally additive for feed intake, growth rate, and feed efficiency (Figure 20.4). In addition, Drummond et al. (1981) showed that the effects of high atmospheric ammonia and ascarid infection were additive in terms of depressing feed intake and growth rate. These results were very similar to those obtained by McFarlane et al. (1989) who studied six different stressors in poultry and showed that their effects on feed intake and growth were also largely additive.

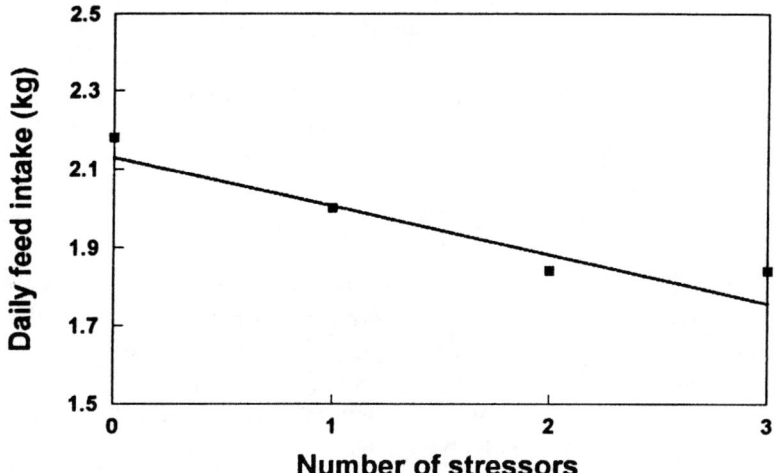

FIGURE 20.4 The effect of multiple stressors on average daily feed intake. (Adapted from Hyun et al., 1998a.)

VI. FEEDING BEHAVIOR

Although there is a large volume of empirical research relating to the effects of genetic and environmental factors on feed intake, these data have largely been measured for groups of animals over the entire growing-finishing period or a large part of it. Consequently, there is relatively little information on feeding behavior, which, to a large extent, reflects the practical problems associated with collecting detailed data on feeding behavior for individual animals within a group. Studies that have attempted to determine detailed feeding behavior have used observations of feeder-related activity and/or have attempted to monitor feed disappearance using weighing devices such as load cells fitted to feeders. A number of studies have investigated feed intake and feeding behavior for individually penned animals (e.g., De Haer and Merks, 1992) and these have generally shown higher intake levels and much different feeding patterns compared with group-housed animals.

The development of computerized feed intake recording equipment, which was primarily designed for performance testing pigs in genetic selection programs, has provided the opportunity to collect detailed information on feed intake and feeding behavior for individual pigs when housed in groups. The results of a number of studies that have used such equipment to study feeding patterns in growing-finishing pigs are summarized in Table 20.8. There is considerable variability between studies in the mean values for the feeding pattern traits; for example, the number of daily feeder visits ranged from approximately 10 to approaching 45, feed intake per visit ranged from around 95 g to in excess of 285 g, feeder occupation time per visit was between 3.1 and 11.3 min, feeder occupation time per pig per day ranged from 53.8 to 115.5 min, and feed consumption rate (i.e., feed consumed per visit divided by feeder occupation time per visit) ranged from approximately 15 to greater than 40 g/min. To a certain extent, this variation results from inclusion of individually housed pigs in the studies of De Haer and Merks (1992) and De Haer and De Vries (1993a). However, as well as differences in group size, the studies reported in Table 20.8 differed in many other respects that could influence feeding behavior, including the form of the feed used (pellets or meal), the live weight, genotype and sex of the pigs, and floor space allowance.

Only one study used more than one genotype (De Haer and De Vries, 1993b) and this suggested similar feed intakes but substantial differences in feeding behavior between Dutch Landrace and Yorkshire pigs (see Table 20.8). A number of studies have compared the sexes for feeding patterns and although there are reports of differences between boars, barrows, and gilts, these seem to be modest (see Table 20.8).

Using the number of visits to the feeder as a measure of feeding behavior may actually overestimate the number of discrete meals consumed by the pig. Forbes (1995) defined a meal as distinct eating periods that may include short breaks but that are separated by longer intervals. In feeding behavior studies, meal frequency can be determined by calculating a minimum intermeal interval from the frequency plot of intervals between consecutive feeder visits (Petrie and Gonyou 1988; Curtis, 1996). When a behavior occurs in bouts, such as visits to a feeder, the plot of intervals between visits can generally be divided into two sections. The first part of the distribution consists of a high frequency of short intervals within a meal (intrameal intervals), and the remainder of the distribution consists of longer, between-meal intervals (Clifton, 1987). Hyun et al. (1997) calculated an intrameal interval of 28 min for mixed-sex groups (boars, barrows, and gilts) of 15 pigs (27 to 87 kg live weight) fed from a computerized feed intake recording system. On this basis, the number of meals consumed per day was around seven compared to the number of feeder visits per day which averaged approximately 12. However, it has not always been possible to define an intrameal interval using the above approach in certain studies (e.g., Hyun et al., 1998b).

Research at the University of Illinois has suggested that feeding behavior is affected by pig weight (Hyun et al., 1997). In this study, boars, barrows, and gilts were grown from 27 to 82 kg live weight in groups of 15 pigs, and fed via a computerized feed intake recording system. The regression equations relating feeding pattern traits to live weight were relatively weak with R^2 values ranging between 0.05 and 0.43 for the equations for number of meals per day and feed

TABLE 20.8
Summary of Published Literature of Feed Intake Behavior in Growing-Finishing Pigs Using Computerized Feed Intake Recording Systems

Reference	Feed System[b]	Genotype[c]	Sex[d]	Weight Range (kg)	Group Size	Diet Form[e]	Feed Intake Traits[a]							Treatment
							ADFI (g)	ADG (g)	NFV	FIV (g)	FOV (min)	FOD (min)	FCR (g/min)	
De Haer and Merks, 1992	IVOG	DL	B, G	25–100	1, 8	—	2123	—	36.5	98.3	3.1	73.8	29.6	
De Haer and De Vries, 1993a	IVOG	DL	B, G	25–100	1, 8	—	2005	692	44.5	95.4	3.07	72.9	29.7	
De Haer and De Vries, 1993b	IVOG	DL, GY	B, G	25–100	8		1866	659	18.0	137.1	3.93	56.9	34.9	
Hall et al., 1999	FIRE	LW	B, G	45–95	12	P	2060	990	10.1	198	6.01	58.3	42.0	
Hyun, 1997	FIRE	PIC	C, G	25–50	2–12	M	1699	769	20.2	95.3	—	115.5	15.5	
	FIRE	PIC	C, G	85–115	2–12	M	3038	989	11.8	287	9.2	99.0	32.0	
Hyun et al., 1997	FIRE	PIC	B,C,G	25–80	15	M	1727	778	12.0	152	6.6	75.8	23.7	
Hyun et al., 1998b	FIRE	Y, H, D	C, G	35–55	8	M	1983	719	13.5	170.9	10.7	124.7	16.8	0.56/0.25 m²/pig
Labroue et al., 1994	ACEMA	FL, FLW	B, C	35–100	9–14	P	2234	866	14.5	420	11.3	59.3	40.8	
Morgan et al., 1998	FIRE	LW × LD	B	40–70	10	P	1786	772	11.2	178.0	5.26	53.8	34.0	Straw provision
Morgan et al., 1999	FIRE	LW × LD	B	41	10	P	2074	916	10.1	223.6	5.85	54.7	39.3	Straw provision
Nielsen et al., 1995a	FIRE	LW × LD	B	38	5–20	P	1494	723	12.5	142.9	5.21	56.6	27.3	
Nielsen et al., 1995b	FIRE	LW × LD	B	30–60	10	P	1962	792	12.6	177	5.3	59.0	34.3	Feeding protection
Young and Lawrence, 1994	FIRE	LW × LD	B, G	32–69	10	P	—	922	12.0	—	—	—	—	

[a] ADFI = average daily feed intake; ADG = average daily gain; NFV = number of feeder visits; FIV = feed intake per visit; FOV = feeder occupation time per visit; FOD = feeder occupation time per day; FCR = feed consumption rate.
[b] IVOG = individual voluntary food intake recording in group housing; FIRE = feed intake recording equipment; ACEMA = ACEMA-48 feeder.
[c] DL = Dutch Landrace; GY = Great Yorkshire; LW = Large White; Y = Yorkshire; H = Hampshire; D = Duroc; FL = French Landrace; FLW = French Large White; LD = Landrace.
[d] B = Boar; C = Castrate; G = Gilt.
[e] P = pellets, M = meal.

consumption rate, respectively. Number of meals per day showed a modest decline from approximately 7.5 to 6.0 over the weight range studied. In contrast, there were substantial increases in feed intake per meal (from around 220 to over 300 g/day) and feed consumption rate (from approximately 15 to above 35 g/min) resulting in a substantial decline in feeder occupation time per visit (from approximately 14 to a low of above 8 min) and per day (from approximately 105 to 60 min) as live weight increased from 27 to 82 kg. These data suggest that the feeder occupation time required for pigs to achieve their daily voluntary intake decreases with live weight. In addition, Hyun (1997) evaluated the impact of increasing group size from 2 to 12 pigs in both growing and finishing pigs. In finishing pigs (85 to 113 kg live weight), the number of feeder visits generally decreased and feed intake per visit and feed consumption rate generally increased with group size, resulting in little change in daily feed intake. In contrast, with growing pigs (26 to 48 kg live weight), the number of feeder visits and feed consumption rate were relatively unaffected by group size; however, feeder occupation time per pig per day was significantly reduced by increasing group size, resulting in a reduced daily feed intake and average daily gain for pigs in the larger groups. Kornegay and Notter (1984) also found that the reduction in daily feed intake with increasing group size was less in growing compared with finishing pigs on conventional feeders (–0.30 and +0.13% per pig, respectively).

A characteristic diurnal feeding pattern also has been shown in a number of studies and this is illustrated in Figure 20.5, which is taken from the study of Hyun et al. (1997), which used computerized feed intake recording equipment. A similar pattern has generally been found for pigs on conventional feeders (Montgomery et al., 1978). Pigs made relatively few visits to the feeder between 2000 and 0500 hours (Figure 20.5); feeder visits peaked between 0700 to 1100 hours and then declined steadily throughout the remainder of the day. Some studies (Montgomery et al., 1978; De Haer and Merks, 1992) have shown a second peak in feeder activity in the afternoon, which Feddes et al. (1989) suggested was primarily a response to light:dark patterns. However, this relationship between feeding pattern and photoperiod has not been substantiated. During peak feeder activity, the feeding behavior of pigs also changes with decreases in feeder occupancy time and feed intake per visit and increases in feed consumption rate. Apparently, the pig is attempting to compensate for increased competition at the feeder by increasing eating speeds.

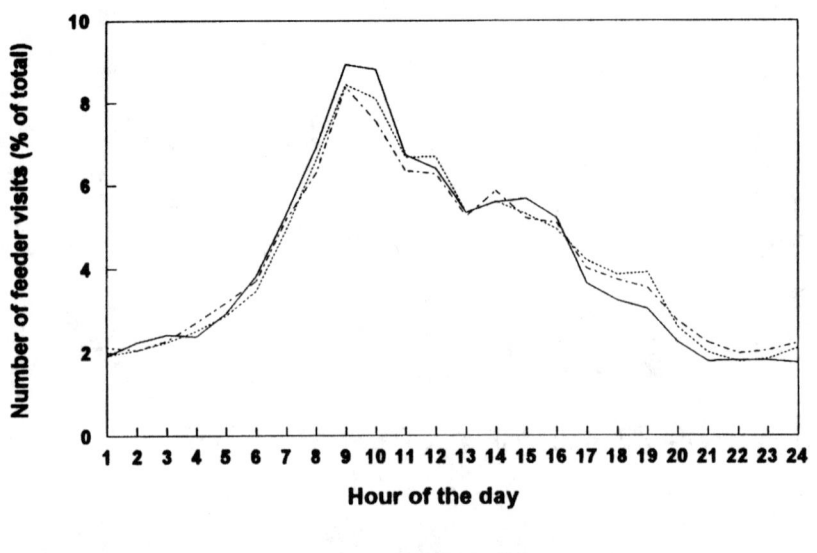

FIGURE 20.5 Diurnal pattern of feeder visits by growing-finishing pigs. (Adapted from Hyun et al., 1997.)

This characteristic diurnal feeding pattern can be altered by a number of factors including group size, floor space allowance, and environmental temperature. Generally speaking, any factor that increases competition for feeder access, such as increased group size or reduced floor space allowance, will tend to reduce the extent of the diurnal variation in feeder related activity (Hyun et al., 1998b). In addition, high environmental temperatures, as well as reducing the absolute feed intake of the animal, are also likely to shift feeding away from the hotter parts of the day into the evening, nighttime, and early morning (Xin and De Shazer, 1992).

Another extremely interesting finding that has emerged from the analysis of feeding patterns for pigs on computerized feed intake recording equipment is the enormous variation in feeder-related activity and feed intake level between individual pigs within a group, and for the same pig between consecutive days. For example, in the study of Hyun et al. (1997), the range in the number of feeder visits per day for individual pigs of the same genotype, sex, and weight was from 8 to 33. Young and Lawrence (1994) found an even greater range of 3 to 69 visits per day for individual pigs housed in groups. Day-to-day variation in feed intake for two pigs that were selected from the data set of Hyun et al. (1997) to have either relatively high or relatively low variation in daily feed intake is illustrated in Figure 20.6. There was considerable day-to-day variation in feed intake for the pig showing low variability; however, the daily variation in the pig exhibiting high variability was huge. The significance of this striking daily variability in feeding behavior and feed intake level in terms of animal performance and nutritional programs is not obvious but requires further investigation.

Phenotypic correlations between feeding pattern traits and growth performance have generally been low (De Haer and Merks, 1992; Young and Lawrence, 1994; Hyun et al., 1997) suggesting that the variation between pigs in feeder-related activity has limited impact on growth performance. The exception to this is feed consumption rate, which has been shown in a number of studies to be moderately correlated (approximately 0.3) with average daily gain and daily feed intake. This suggests that pigs that eat faster may have production advantages in terms of intake level and growth rate, and further study aimed at understanding the basis for variation in consumption rates is warranted.

Computerized feed intake recording equipment such as that used in the studies described above has a protective race in front of the feed trough that prevents more than one pig from accessing the feeder simultaneously, but also protects the animal during feeding. There are a number of different race designs, ranging from short versions that protect only the head and shoulders of the pig, to longer versions that protect all of the pig's body. However, this protection reduces the competition for feeder access and results in different feeding behavior compared with conventional

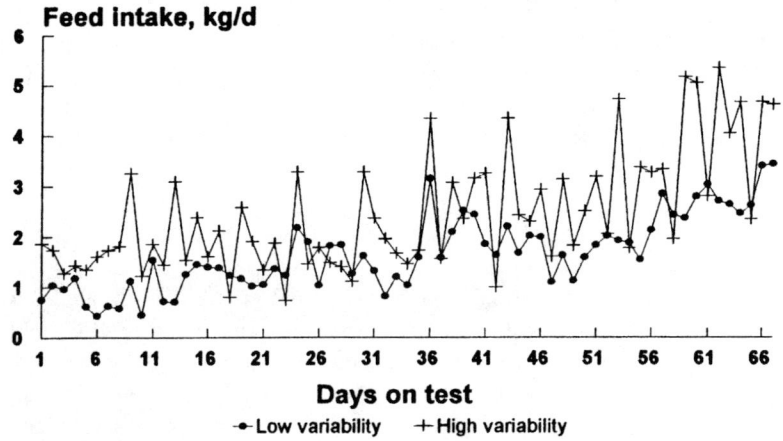

FIGURE 20.6 Daily feed intake variation in two growing pigs. (Adapted from Hyun, unpublished data.)

feeders that give limited protection for the feeding animal. This is illustrated by the data of Nielsen et al. (1995b), which showed that feeder occupation time per visit and feed intake per visit increased, and feed consumption rate decreased for feeder races that provided a high compared with a low degree of protection for the feeding pig. Interestingly, growth rates for pigs on computerized compared with conventional feeders seem to be very similar (Hyun et al., 1998b).

Curtis (1996) described the daily behavior of growing-finishing pigs housed in groups of 16 on a conventional feeder in a naturally ventilated, intensive growing-finishing house with partially slatted concrete floors as follows: lying or sitting 19.9 h (83%); eating 2.2 h (9%); walking or running 1.4 h (6%); other activities 0.5 h (2%). Pigs averaged 26 meals daily and a total of 132 min/day eating, with a meal duration of approximately 5 min (Curtis, 1996). These results were very similar to those found in a study carried out 30 years earlier (Haugse et al., 1965). However, other studies carried out with conventional feeders have shown a lower number of feeder visits (Xin and DeShazer, 1992; Nienaber et al., 1996) than suggested by Haugse et al. (1965) and Curtis (1996). As previously discussed, feeding behavior can be influenced by a number of animal, nutritional, and environmental factors.

VII. MEASURING AND PREDICTING FEED INTAKE

Obtaining an accurate estimate of feed intake of pigs on a particular production unit is an essential prerequisite to formulating diets accurately that meet the pig's nutritional requirements. There are two obvious approaches to this, namely, prediction or direct measurement. The major factors involved in determining the feed intake of growing pigs and, therefore, those that conceptually should be considered in the development of prediction equations have been reviewed by Giles et al. (1998).

These authors used the concept of the potential voluntary feed intake of an animal that is assumed to be a function of the voluntary energy demand, which is the sum of the energy required for maintenance and tissue deposition. Maintenance activities include the energy costs associated with fasting, activity, maintenance of body temperature, and disease. The energy costs associated with tissue deposition are directly related to the composition of the gain in terms of the amount of lean and fat, which will be a function of the genotype, sex, and weight of the animal. In addition, feed intake will be influenced by the range of factors discussed above, including nutrient deficiencies and imbalances, gut capacity, environmental conditions (such as climatic factors and air quality), social factors (such as floor space allowance and number of pigs per pen), and disease (Giles et al., 1998). Ideally, equations to predict feed intake should take into account all these factors. Published equations for predicting energy or feed intake are presented in Table 20.9.

The concept of predicting feed intake from equations that take account of the major factors that influence voluntary feed intake in practice has been incorporated into the model developed as part of the most recent *Nutrient Requirements of Swine* (NRC, 1998). Digestible energy intake is predicted using a cubic regression equation based on body weight (BW in kilograms) as follows (NRC, 1998):

Digestible energy intake (kcal/day) = $1250 + (188 \times BW) - (1.4 \times BW^2) + (0.0044 \times BW^3)$

The above equation is for a combination of barrows and gilts, but there are adjustment factors for sex and for variation in ambient temperature and in floor space per pig (NRC, 1998). Obviously, this ignores a number of factors that influence feed intake that have been discussed above, particularly disease. In addition, there are no data available that compare the accuracy of predicted compared with actual feed intake using the NRC (1998) or other equations under practical conditions from which to assess the robustness of these equations.

TABLE 20.9
Published Equations for Prediction of Energy and Feed Intake in Growing-Finishing Pigs[a]

Reference	Equation	Units of Intake
Kyriazakis and Emmans, 1999	$DEI = 1.93W - 0.0407W^2 - 6.40$	MJ/day
	$dF/dt = (1/FEC) * (MH + k_1 dP/dt + k_2 dL/dt)$	g/day
	$DEI = 0.44W^{0.75} + 52 dP/dt + 53 dL/dt$	MJ/day
NRC, 1987	$DEI = 575 BW^{0.675}$	kcal/day
	$DEI = 13{,}162(1 - e^{-0.0176 BW})$	kcal/day
NRC, 1998	$DEI = 1250 + 188 BW - 1.4 BW^2 + 0.0044 BW^3$	kcal/day

[a] DEI = digestible energy intake; W = body weight, kg; dF/dt = feed intake per unit time; FEC = energy content of the feed, kJ/g; MH = maintenance heat production, kJ/day; k_1, k_2 = energy constants; dP/dt = estimation of the potential rate of protein accretion; dL/dt = estimation of the potential rate of lipid accretion; BW = body weight, kg.

Direct measurement of feed intake under the conditions in which the information is to be applied would, on the face of it, seem to be the most accurate approach to obtaining feed intake data for use in developing diet formulations. However, measuring feed intake accurately and in a timely manner on commercial operations can also be problematic. Although there are a number of potential approaches for measuring feed intake in commercial barns, including volumetric and gravimetric methods, there has been little if any research comparing the different methods. One of the major challenges to improving the precision of nutritional programs for growing-finishing pigs will be to develop accurate, practically robust approaches to measure accurately and/or predict feed intake levels under commercial conditions.

REFERENCES

Becker, B. A., C. D. Knight, F. C. Buonomo, G. W. Jesse, H. B. Hedrick, and C. A. Baile. 1992. Effect of a hot environment on performance, carcass characteristics and blood metabolites of pigs treated with porcine somatotropin, *J. Anim. Sci.*, 70:2732.

Bigelow, J. A., and T. A. Houpt. 1988. Feeding and drinking patterns in young pigs, *Physiol. Behav.*, 43:99.

Bray, H. J. 1996. The Physiological Response of Growing Pigs to Pleuropneumonia, Ph.D. dissertation, University of Sydney, Australia.

Cameron, N. D., and M. K. Curran. 1994. Selection for components of efficient lean growth rate in pigs. 4. Genetic and phenotypic parameter estimates and correlated responses in performance test traits with *ad libitum* feeding, *Anim. Prod.*, 59:281.

Carro, E., R. Senaris, R. V. Considine, F. F. Casanueva, and C. Dieguez. 1997. Regulation of *in vivo* growth hormone secretion by leptin, *Endocrinology*, 138:2203.

Cisneros, F. 1997. Performance and Body Composition in Swine as Affected by Environmental Temperature, Ph.D. dissertation, University of Illinois, Urbana-Champaign.

Cisneros, F., M. Ellis, F. K. McKeith, J. McCaw, and R. L. Fernando. 1996. Influence of slaughter weight on growth and carcass characteristics, commercial cutting and curing yields, and meat quality of barrows and gilts from two genotypes, *J. Anim. Sci.*, 74:925.

Clifton, P. G. 1987. Analysis of feeding and drinking patterns. In *Techniques in Behavioral and Neural Sciences*, Toates, F. M., and N. E. Rowland, Eds., Elsevier Science, New York, 19.

Close, W. H. 1989. The influence of the thermal environment on the voluntary food intake of pigs. In *The Voluntary Food Intake of Pigs*, Forbes, J. M., M. A. Varley, and T. L. J. Lawrence, Eds., British Society of Animal Production, Edinburgh, 88.

Cole, D. J. A., B. Hardy, and D. Lewis. 1971. Nutrient density of pig diets. In *Pig Production, Proceedings of the Eighteenth Easter School in Agricultural Science*, University of Nottingham, Butterworths, London, 243.

Combs, N. R., E. T. Kornegay, M. D. Lindemann, and D. R. Notter. 1991. Calcium and phosphorus requirement of swine from weaning to market weight: I. Development of response curves for performance, *J. Anim. Sci.*, 69:673.

Cromwell, G. L., T. R. Cline, J. D. Crenshaw, T. D. Crenshaw, R. C. Ewan, C. R. Hamilton, A. J. Lewis, D. C. Mahan, E. R. Miller, J. E. Pettigrew, L. F. Tribble, and T. L. Veum. 1993. The dietary protein and/or lysine requirements of barrows and gilts, *J. Anim. Sci.*, 71:1510.

Curtis, S. E. 1983. *Environmental Management in Animal Agriculture*, Iowa State University Press, Ames.

Curtis, S. E. 1996. Effects of environmental design on the pig's voluntary feed intake, presented at Pork Industry Conference, University of Illinois, 60.

De Haer, L. C. M., and A. G. De Vries. 1993a. Feed intake patterns of and feed digestibility in growing pigs housed individually or in groups, *Livest. Prod. Sci.*, 33:277.

De Haer, L. C. M., and A. G. De Vries. 1993b. Effects of genotype and sex on the feed intake pattern of group housed growing pigs, *Livest. Prod. Sci.*, 36:223.

De Haer, L. C. M., and J. W. M. Merks. 1992. Patterns of daily food intake in growing pigs, *Anim. Prod.*, 54:95.

Drummond, J. G., S. E. Curtis, J. Simon, and H. W. Norton. 1981. Effects of atmospheric ammonia on young pigs experimentally infected with *Ascaris suum*, *Am. J. Vet. Res.*, 42:969.

Feddes, J. J. R., B. A. Young, and J. A. De Shazer. 1989. Influence of temperature and light on feeding behaviour of pigs, *Appl. Anim. Behav. Sci.*, 23:215.

Forbes, J. M. 1995. *Voluntary Food Intake and Diet Selection in Farm Animals*, CAB International, Wallingford, U.K.

Fowler, V. R., M. Bichard, and A. Pease. 1976. Objectives in pig breeding, *Anim. Prod.*, 23:365.

Friesen, K. G., J. L. Nelssen, J. A. Unruh, R. D. Goodband, and M. D. Tokach. 1994. Effects of the interrelationship between genotype, sex, and dietary lysine on growth performance and carcass composition in finishing pigs fed to either 104 or 127 kilograms, *J. Anim. Sci.*, 72:946.

Fuller, M. F., M. F. Franklin, R. McWilliam, and K. Pennie. 1995. The responses of growing pigs, of different sex and genotype, to dietary energy and protein, *Anim. Sci.*, 60:291.

Giles, L. R., and J. L. Black. 1991. Voluntary food intake in growing pigs at ambient temperatures above the zone of thermal comfort. In *Manipulation Pig Production III*, Batterham, E. S., Ed., Australasian Pig Science Association, Attwood, Victoria, 162.

Giles, L. R., M. L. Lorschy, H. J. Bray, and J. L. Black. 1998. Predicting feed intake in growing pigs. In *Progress in Pig Science*, Wiseman, J., M. A. Varley, and J. P. Chadwick, Eds., Nottingham University Press, Nottingham, 209.

Gu, Y., A. P. Schinckel, J. C. Forrest, C. H. Kuei, and L. E. Watkins. 1991a. Effects of ractopamine, genotype, and growth phase on finishing performance and carcass value in swine. I. Growth performance and carcass merit, *J. Anim. Sci.*, 69:2685.

Gu, Y., A. P. Schinckel, J. C. Forrest, C. H. Kuei, and L. E. Watkins. 1991b. Effects of ractopamine, genotype, and growth phase on finishing performance and carcass value in swine. II. Estimation of lean growth rate and lean feed efficiency, *J. Anim. Sci.*, 69:2694.

Hahn, J. D., and D. H. Baker. 1995. Optimum ratio to lysine of threonine, tryptophan, and sulfur amino acids for finishing swine, *J. Anim. Sci.*, 73:482.

Hahn, J. D., R. R. Biehl, and D. H. Baker. 1995. Ideal digestible lysine level for early- and late-finishing swine, *J. Anim. Sci.*, 73:773.

Hall, A. D., W. G. Hill, P. R. Bampton, and A. J. Webb. 1999. Genetic and phenotypic parameter estimates for feeding pattern and performance test traits in pigs, *Anim. Sci.*, 68:43.

Hamilton, D. N. 1999. Genetic and Environmental Effects on Growth Performance, Carcass Characteristics and Meat Quality in Pigs, M.S. dissertation, University of Illinois, Urbana-Champaign.

Haugse, C. N., W. E. Dinusson, D. O. Erickson, J. N. Johnson, and M. L. Buchanan. 1965. A day in the life of a pig, Bimonthly Bulletin, North Dakota Agric. Exp. Sta., Fargo, 18.

Haydon, K. D., M. D. Harrison, and C. R. Dove. 1989. Effect of varying ideal protein level on the performance of growing-finishing swine, *Nutr. Rep. Int.*, 40:939.

Heitman, H., and E. H. Hughes. 1949. The effects of air temperature and relative humidity on the physiological well-being of swine, *J. Anim. Sci.*, 8:171.

Henry, Y. 1995. Effects of dietary tryptophan deficiency in finishing pigs, according to age or weight at slaughter or live weight gain, *Livest. Prod. Sci.*, 41:63.

Henry, Y., Y. Colleaux, and B. Seve. 1992a. Effects of dietary level of lysine and of level and source of protein on feed intake, growth performance, and plasma amino acid pattern in the finishing pig, *J. Anim. Sci.*, 70:188.

Henry, Y., B. Seve, Y. Colleaux, P. Ganier, C. Saligaut, and P. Jego. 1992b. Interactive effects of dietary levels of tryptophan and protein on voluntary feed intake and growth performance in pigs, in relation to plasma free amino acids and hypothalamic serotonin, *J. Anim. Sci.*, 70:1873.

Houpt, T. R. 1984. Controls of feeding in pigs, *J. Anim. Sci.*, 59:1345.

Houpt, T. R. 1985. The physiological determination of meal size in pigs, *Proc. Nutr. Soc.*, 44:323.

Houseknecht, K. L., C. A. Baile, R. L. Matteri, and M. E. Spurlock. 1998. The biology of leptin: a review, *J. Anim. Sci.*, 76:1405.

Hyun, Y. 1997. Nutritional and Environmental Factors Affecting Feed Intake Level and Pattern in Growing and Finishing Pigs, Ph.D. dissertation, University of Illinois, Urbana-Champaign.

Hyun, Y., M. Ellis, F. K. McKeith, and E. R. Wilson. 1997. Feed intake pattern of group-housed growing-finishing pigs monitored using a computerized feed intake recording system, *J. Anim. Sci.*, 75:1443.

Hyun, Y., M. Ellis, G. Riskowski, and R. W. Johnson. 1998a. Growth performance of pigs subjected to multiple concurrent environmental stressors, *J. Anim. Sci.*, 76:721.

Hyun, Y., M. Ellis, and R. W. Johnson. 1998b. Effects of feeder type, space allowance, and mixing on the growth performance and feed intake pattern of growing pigs, *J. Anim. Sci.*, 76: 2771.1.

Johnson, R. W. 1996. The energy cost of illness in swine, presented to Swine Energetics, University of Illinois Pork Industry Conference, Urbana-Champaign, 10.

Katsumata, M., Y. Kaji, and M. Saitoh. 1996. Growth and carcass fatness responses of finishing pigs to dietary fat supplementation at high ambient temperature, *Anim. Sci.*, 62:591.

Kempster, A. J., and D. B. Lowe. 1993. Meat production with entire males. In *44th Annual Meeting of the European Association for Animal Production*, Arhus, Denmark, 2.1.

Knight, C. D., T. R. Kasser, G. H. Swenson, R. L. Hintz, M. J. Azain, R. O. Bates, T. R. Cline, J. D. Crenshaw, G. L. Cromwell, H. B. Hedrick, S. J. Jones, D. H. Kropf, A. J. Lewis, D. C. Mahan, F. K. McKeith, C. L. McLaughlin, J. L. Nelssen, J. E. Novakofski, M. W. Orcutt, and N. A. Parrett. 1991. The performance and carcass composition responses of finishing swine to a range of porcine somatotropin doses in a 1-week delivery system, *J. Anim. Sci.*, 69:4678.

Kornegay, E. T., and D. R. Notter. 1984. Effects of floor space and number of pigs per pen on performance, *Pigs News Info.*, 5:23.

Kyriazakis, I., and G. C. Emmans. 1999. Voluntary food intake and diet selection. In *A Quantitative Biology of the Pig*, Kyriazakis, I., Ed., CABI Publishing, Wallingford, 229.

Labroue, F., R. Gueblez, P. Sellier, and M. C. Meunier-Salaun. 1994. Feeding behaviour of group-housed Large White and Landrace pigs in French central test stations, *Livest. Prod. Sci.*, 40:303.

Langlois, A., and F. Minvielle. 1989. Comparisons of three-way and backcross swine: I. Growth performance and commercial assessment of the carcass, *J. Anim. Sci.*, 67:2018.

Lopez, J., G. W. Jesse, B. A. Becker, and M. R. Ellersieck. 1991a. Effects of temperature on the performance of finishing swine: I. Effects of a hot, diurnal temperature on average daily gain, feed intake, and feed efficiency, *J. Anim. Sci.*, 69:1843.

Lopez, J., G. W. Jesse, B. A. Becker, and M. R. Ellersieck. 1991b. Effects of temperature on the performance of finishing swine: II. Effects of a cold, diurnal temperature on average daily gain, feed intake, and feed efficiency, *J. Anim. Sci.*, 69:1850.

Madsen, A. 1985. Energy density in pig diets: a review, presented at 36th Annual Meeting of the European Association for Animal Production, Halkidiki, Greece, 1.

Martin, R. J., J. L. Beverly, and G. E. Truett. 1989. Energy balance regulation. In *Animal Growth Regulation*, Campion, D. R., G. J. Hausman, and R. J. Martin, Eds., Plenum Press, New York, 211.

Mayer, J. 1953. Glucostatic mechanism of regulation of food intake, *N. Engl. J. Med.*, 249:13.

McFarlane, J. M., S. E. Curtis, R. D. Shanks, and S. G. Carmer. 1989. Multiple concurrent stressors in chicks. 1. Effect on weight gain, feed intake, and behavior, *Poult. Sci.*, 68:501.

McGlone, J. J., W. F. Stansbury, L. F. Tribble, and J. L. Morrow. 1988. Photoperiod and heat stress influence on lactating sow performance and photoperiod effects on nursery pig performance, *J. Anim. Sci.*, 66:1915.

Miller, K. D. 1998. The Detection and Characterization of Pigs with Differing Glycolytic Potential Levels within United States Swine Populations, Ph.D. dissertation, University of Illinois, Urbana-Champaign.

MLC. 1988. Stotfold Pig Development Unit, First Trial Results; Meat and Livestock Commission, Milton Keynes, England.

Montgomery, G. W., D. S. Flux, and J. R. Carr. 1978. Feeding patterns in pigs: the effects of amino acid deficiency, *Physiol. Behav.*, 20:693.

Morgan, C. A., L. A. Deans, A. B. Lawrence, and B. L. Nielsen. 1998. The effects of straw bedding on the feeding and social behaviour of growing pigs fed by means of single-space feeders, *Appl. Anim. Behav. Sci.*, 58:23.

Morgan, C. A., L. A. Deans, A. B. Lawrence, and B. L. Nielsen. 1999. The effects of changing straw provision on the feeding behaviour and activity of growing pigs given food through single-space feeders, *Anim. Sci.*, 68:19.

Morrison, S. R., and L. E. Mount. 1971. Adaptation of growing pigs to changes in environmental temperature, *Anim. Prod.*, 13:51.

Nielsen, B. L., A. B. Lawrence, and C. T. Whittemore. 1995a. Effect of group size on feeding behaviour, social behaviour, and performance of growing pigs using single-space feeders, *Livest. Prod. Sci.*, 44:73.

Nielsen, B. L., A. B. Lawrence, and C. T. Whittemore. 1995b. Effects of single-space feeder design on feeding behaviour and performance of growing pigs, *Anim. Sci.*, 61:575.

Nienaber, J. A., G. L. Hahn, and J. T. Yen. 1987. Thermal environment effect on growing-finishing swine. Part I — Growth, feed intake and heat production, *Trans. Am. Soc. Agric. Eng.*, 30:1772.

Nienaber, J. A., G. L. Hahn, T. P. McDonald, and R. L. Korthals. 1996. Feeding patterns and swine performance in hot environments, *Trans. Am. Soc. Agric. Eng.*, 39:195.

NPPC. 1995. *Genetic Evaluation: Terminal Line Program Results*, National Pork Producers Council, Des Moines, IA.

NRC. 1987. *Predicting Feed Intake of Food-Producing Animals*, National Academy Press, Washington, D.C.

NRC. 1998. *Nutrient Requirements of Swine*, 10th ed., National Academy Press, Washington, D.C.

Ntunde, B. N., R. R. Hacker, and G. J. King. 1979. Influence of photoperiod on growth, puberty and plasma LH levels in gilts, *J. Anim. Sci.*, 48:1401.

Petrie, C. L., and H. W. Gonyou. 1988. Effects of auditory, visual and chemical stimuli on the ingestive behavior of newly weaned piglets, *J. Anim. Sci.*, 66:661.

Rinaldo, D., and J. Le Dividich. 1991. Assessment of optimal temperature for performance and chemical body composition of growing pigs, *Livest. Prod. Sci.*, 29:61.

Rogerson, J. C., and R. G. Campbell. 1982. The response of early-weaned piglets to various levels of lysine in diets of moderate energy content, *Anim. Prod.*, 35:335.

Scharrer, E. 1991. Peripheral mechanisms controlling voluntary food intake in the pig, *Pig News Info.*, 12:377.

Seymour, E. W., V. C. Speer, V. W. Hays, D. W. Mangold, and T. E. Hazen. 1964. Effects of dietary protein level and environmental temperature on performance and carcass quality of growing-finishing swine, *J. Anim. Sci.*, 23:375.

Smith, W. C., M. Ellis, J. P. Chadwick, and R. Laird. 1991. The influence of index selection for improved growth and carcass characteristics on appetite in a population of Large White pigs, *Anim. Prod.*, 52:193.

Stahly, T. S., G. L. Cromwell, and M. P. Aviotti. 1979. The effect of environmental temperature and dietary lysine source and level on the performance and carcass characteristics of growing swine, *J. Anim. Sci.*, 49:1242.

Stein, H. H., and R. A. Easter. 1996. Dietary energy concentration affects carcass leanness in finishing hogs, University of Illinois Swine Research Reports, Urbana-Champaign, 41.

Sugahara, M., D. H. Baker, B. G. Harmon, and A. H. Jenson. 1970. Effect of ambient temperature on performance and carcass development in young swine, *J. Anim. Sci.*, 31:59.

Van Lunen, T. A., and D. J. A. Cole. 1996. The effect of lysine/digestible energy ratio on growth performance and nitrogen deposition of hybrid boars, gilts and castrated male pigs, *Anim. Sci.*, 63:465.

Weatherup, R. N., V. E. Beattie, B. W. Moss, D. J. Kilpatrick, and N. Walker. 1998. The effect of increasing slaughter weight on the production performance and meat quality of finishing pigs, *Anim. Sci.*, 67:591.

Williams, N. H., T. S. Stahly, and D. R. Zimmerman. 1997a. Effect of chronic immune system activation on body nitrogen retention, partial efficiency of lysine utilization, and lysine needs of pigs, *J. Anim. Sci.*, 75:2472.

Williams, N. H., T. S. Stahly, and D. R. Zimmerman. 1997b. Effect of chronic immune system activation on the rate, efficiency, and composition of growth and lysine needs in pigs fed from 6 to 27 kg, *J. Anim. Sci.*, 75:2463.

Wolter, B. F. 1999. The Effects of Nutritional Management, Group Size and Floor Space Allowance on the Growth Performance of Weanling Pigs, M.S. dissertation, University of Illinois, Urbana-Champaign.

Xin, H., and J. A. De Shazer. 1992. Feeding patterns of growing pigs at warm constant and cyclic temperatures, *Trans. Am. Soc. Agric. Eng.*, 35:319.

Young, R. J., and A. B. Lawrence. 1994. Feeding behaviour of pigs in groups monitored by a computerized feeding system, *Anim. Prod.*, 58:145.

21 Use of Ingredient and Diet Processing Technologies (Grinding, Mixing, Pelleting, and Extruding) to Produce Quality Feeds for Pigs

Joe D. Hancock and Keith C. Behnke

CONTENTS

I. Introduction 469
II. Quality Control in Procurement of Feed Ingredients..470
III. Grinding Feedstuffs...470
IV. Mill Type...474
V. Mixing Diets 476
VI. Pelleting...480
VII. Pellet Size..481
VIII. Pellet Quality...483
IX. Pellet Mill Conditioners..483
X. Pellet Binders..485
XI. Extrusion of Cereals and Complete Diets..486
XII. Extruded Soybeans..488
XIII. Stomach Morphology..490
XIV. Conclusions...492
References..492

I. INTRODUCTION

In today's swine industry, few producers or nutritionists would consider feeding pigs without giving great attention to energy and amino acid concentrations and ratios, and to optimum vitamin and mineral supplementation. Selection of reasonably priced, good-quality ingredients and proper processing of those ingredients into complete diets is equally important to the overall profitability of a swine farm, yet good feed manufacturing practices often are given little emphasis. This chapter is a review of basic considerations for feed manufacturing that can be used to maximize nutritional value of ingredients and complete diets for pigs.

II. QUALITY CONTROL IN PROCUREMENT OF FEED INGREDIENTS

The effects of antinutritional factors and toxicants that can contaminate feeds and feedstuffs used in diets for pigs are discussed in detail in Chapter 25. However, in a chapter designed to discuss the preparation of high-quality diets for pigs, one would be remiss not to reiterate that swine producers should constantly be aware of the potential problems caused by such antinutrients as molds and mycotoxins, protease inhibitors, β-glucans, arabinoxylans, and tannins.

Unfortunately, many of the reasons for the presence and/or development of antinutrients are not under the control of a swine producer. Unusual weather patterns such as drought (aflatoxin) and cool and wet weather during silking (vomitoxin) are thought to trigger development of mycotoxins. Similarly, the organisms that yield problematic concentrations of zearalenone, fumonisin, ochratoxin, and a host of other mycotoxins (there are thought to be more than 200) also are opportunistic in their proliferation. Thus, safeguards during the purchase and delivery of corn and other cereal grains should not be limited only to monitoring moisture and foreign material, but also should include occasional screening for mycotoxins.

Recent refinements in analytical procedures (e.g., immunoassays) have made screening for mycotoxins possible. However, cost of these assays will most likely limit screening to those toxins that are most common (e.g., aflatoxin, vomitoxin, and zearalenone). If mycotoxins are discovered, there are ways to avoid mycotoxicosis in pigs (e.g., blending contaminated grain with clean grain to achieve acceptably low concentrations of toxins, use of clays to bind aflatoxin, ammoniation of the grain, or simply rejecting the load of grain). Thus, not knowing is perhaps the greatest concern when dealing with mycotoxins.

Other prudent measures to ensure the absence of antinutritional factors include an occasional analysis for residual urease activity (an indicator of protease inhibitors) in soybean products. This analysis can be particularly useful when purchasing roasted, extruded, or expelled soybeans from a local feed manufacturer. Also, unless the origin of sorghum grain is known, it is advisable to screen deliveries for the presence of tannins. Tannins are not common in the U.S. sorghum supply (in contrast to their prevalence in sorghums grown in Southeast Asia, China, Africa, and Central/South America), but, nonetheless, there are small quantities of bird-resistant (high-tannin) sorghum produced domestically each year. Finally, there are feed-grade enzyme products that effectively eliminate the "antidigestive" effects of β-glucans in certain varieties of barley and arabinoxylans in certain varieties of wheat. Thus, once again, the primary concern is not that these antinutritional factors occur naturally in feedstuffs but, rather, not knowing that they are present.

Once suitable feedstuffs have been secured, proper storage is required to prevent loss of intrinsic nutritional value. The most difficult and frustrating aspect of grain storage is moisture management. To avoid problems with bridging and mold growth, it is important to set strict standards for moisture content of delivered grain. Also, aeration and turning (i.e., emptying and refilling bins on occasion) are practices often used to minimize opportunity for mold growth.

In conclusion, the first step in producing high-quality feed is to purchase high-quality ingredients and to store them properly. Although the importance of these aspects of feed manufacturing seem intuitive, quality control programs are never easy to establish and/or maintain. Due diligence is required on the part of the swine producer/feed manufacturer to ensure satisfactory ingredients are used in preparation of diets.

III. GRINDING FEEDSTUFFS

The first steps toward the grain processing techniques that are prevalent today were taken when Fraps (1932) reported improved nutrient digestibility of ground sorghum grain compared with whole sorghum grain. Aubel (1945; 1955) also reported improved efficiency of feed utilization when milled sorghum was fed rather than whole grain. Woodsman et al. (1932) reported increased digestibility of oat-based diets with smaller particle size of the cereal. However, these reports did not address the extent of grinding needed to maximize pig performance.

Wondra et al. (1995b) milled corn with a hammermill to geometric mean particle sizes (ASAE, 1983) of 1000, 800, 600, and 400 µm and reported that milling energy increased slightly (from 2.7 to 3.8 kWh/t) as particle size was decreased from 1000 to 600 µm (Figure 21.1). However, the energy required to reduce particle size another 200 µm (to a geometric mean particle size of 400 µm) was more than twice (i.e., 8.1 kWh/t) the energy required to mill the corn to 600 microns. Production rate also decreased only slightly as mean particle size was decreased from 1000 to 600 µm, compared to the marked decrease when the corn was milled to 400 µm. The data clearly demonstrated that energy requirements increased and production rates decreased when corn was milled to smaller particle sizes. Healy et al. (1994) collected milling data when corn and two varieties of sorghum (a hard endosperm sorghum and a soft endosperm sorghum) were ground to mean particle sizes of 900, 700, and 500 µm. The different grains varied in milling characteristics with more energy required to grind the corn than either of the sorghums (Table 21.1). There was little difference between the energy required to grind the soft- and hard-endosperm sorghums. Baker (1960) also found that sorghum grain was easier to grind than corn, and that corn was easier to grind than oats. Silver (1932) reported that the energy required for milling corn was less than that for milling barley, which was less than that for milling oats.

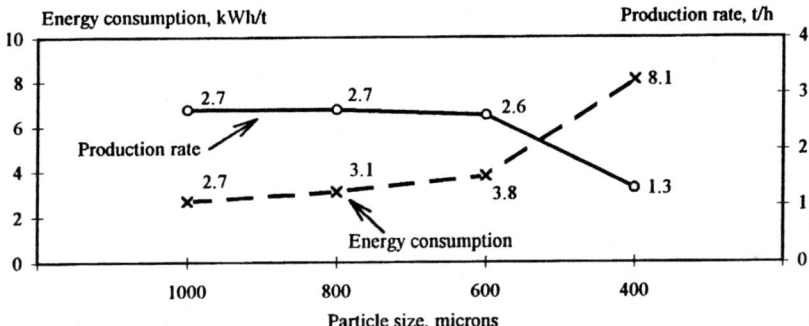

FIGURE 21.1 Energy consumption and production rates when hammermilling corn. (Data from Wondra et al., *J. Anim. Sci.*, 73:757, 1995.)

Hedde et al. (1985) reported an 8% increase in rate of gain for finishing pigs fed corn-based diets when the particle size was reduced from a coarse grind (<20% of the ground grain passing through a 1.2-mm screen) to a fine grind (>80% of the ground grain passing through a 1.2-mm screen). Lawrence (1983) reported 12% greater gain/feed when the particle size of oats was reduced from coarse (>1000 µm) to fine (<600 µm). Goodband and Hines (1988) fed nursery pigs a barley-whey-based diet with the barley ground to mean particle sizes of 768 and 635 µm. They reported a 5% increase in rate of gain for pigs fed barley ground to the smaller particle size. Mavromichalis et al. (1998) reported 10 and 9% improvements in rate and efficiency of gain in nursery pigs as the particle size of wheat was reduced from 1300 to 600 µm. The authors also reported improved efficiency of growth in finishing pigs as particle size of the wheat was reduced from 1300 to 600 to 400 µm.

Giesemann et al. (1990) reported improved efficiency of gain for finishing pigs fed corn and a bronze sorghum variety as particle size was reduced from 1500 to 640 µm. These data are in general agreement with those of Cabrera et al. (1994), who reported that efficiency of gain was increased by 7 and 6% in soft- and hard-endosperm sorghum when particle size was reduced from 800 to 400 µm. Wondra et al. (1995b) ground corn to particle sizes ranging from 1000 to 400 µm and reported a 1.3% improvement in gain:feed for every 100 µm decrease in particle size of the

TABLE 21.1
Processing Characteristics of Corn and Hard and Soft Sorghums and Economic Evaluation of Particle Size Reduction[a]

	Corn			Hard Sorghum			Soft Sorghum		
Item	**900**	**700**	**500**	**900**	**700**	**500**	**900**	**700**	**500**
d_{gw} (μm)[b]	919	702	487	902	741	512	888	715	497
s_{gw} (μm)[c]	1.9	1.9	1.7	2.1	2.0	1.9	2.0	1.8	1.8
Surface area (cm^2/g)[d]	61	79	106	65	77	107	64	75	107
Grinding energy (kWh/t)	5.3	9.2	15.7	1.7	2.4	3.8	1.9	2.5	4.3
Production rate (t/h)	1.76	0.97	0.63	5.95	4.12	2.37	4.48	3.43	1.89
Milling costs ($/t)[e]									
Fixed	1.59	2.89	4.41	0.47	0.68	1.18	0.62	0.81	1.48
Variable	0.53	0.92	1.57	0.17	0.24	0.38	0.19	0.25	0.43
Total	2.12	3.81	5.98	0.64	0.92	1.56	0.81	1.06	1.91
Cost of gain ($/100 kg)[f]	36.18	35.33	35.63	39.49	38.63	37.09	39.51	37.48	36.82

[a] Grains were milled using a roller mill. Bolded numbers represent particle size in μm.
[b] Geometric mean particle size (ASAE, 1983).
[c] Log normal standard deviation (ASAE, 1983).
[d] ASAE (1983).
[e] Estimates derived from McEllhiney (1983). The costs (other than electrical energy) suggested by McEllhiney were inflated by 10%. Electrical energy cost was $0.06/kW.
[f] Calculated from performance of nursery pigs (36 to 57 day of age) fed diets with the milled grains substituted on a weight/weight basis.

Source: Healy, B. J. et al., *J. Anim. Sci.*, 72:2227, 1994. With permission.

corn. Indeed, a thorough review of the literature suggests that a 1.2 to 1.4% improvement in gain:feed for each 100-μm reduction in mean particle size of corn as an appropriate "rule of thumb" for growing pigs. Table 21.2 is a summary of several experiments in which grain was ground to different particle sizes and fed to growing pigs.

Unfortunately, experiments designed to determine the effects of feed processing on performance of lactating sows are very few in number. It is generally recognized that high-producing sows have nutrient requirements that may not be met by traditional dietary regimens. Increased nutrient intake of sows has been shown to improve performance (Brooks and Cole, 1972; Reese et al., 1982; King and Williams, 1984; Brendemuhl et al., 1987). The method most often used to increase nutrient intake of sows is to increase nutrient density of the diet by adding more protein and/or fat (both of which increase diet costs). Surprisingly little attention has been given to the possibility of increasing digestibility of the nutrients already in the diet.

Wondra et al. (1995e) fed 100 primiparous sows diets with corn milled to four particle sizes (1200, 900, 600, and 400 μm). Feed intake increased as particle size of corn was reduced from 1200 to 400 μm, as did digestibility of nutrients (Figure 21.2). This increased feed intake and marked increases in nutrient digestibility resulted in a 14% greater intake of digestible energy (DE) and an 11% increase in litter weight gain. Also, because of the improved digestibility of nutrients with reduction of particle size, a 21% decrease in fecal excretion of dry matter (DM) and a 31% decrease in fecal excretion of N occurred. These reductions in fecal excretion of nutrients have obvious and immediate implications in reducing the burden of waste management for swine operations.

As mentioned in the previous section, the improved performance of growing pigs and lactating sows in response to grinding ingredients results largely from greater nutrient digestibility. Owsley et al. (1981) reported that reduction of particle size in sorghum (from 1262 to 471 μm) improved

TABLE 21.2
Effects of Particle Size Reduction on Growth Performance of Pigs

	Particle Size						
Item	Coarse (>1,000 μm)	Med. (700 to 900 μm)	Fine (<600 μm)	Initial and Final Pig wt (kg)	No. Pigs	Grain	Ref.
ADG (kg)	0.71	0.79	0.74	19–55	36	Corn	Mahan et al. (1966)
Gain:feed	0.337	0.329	0.341				
ADG (kg)	0.62	0.74	0.73	25–70	72	Oats	Lawrence (1983)
Gain:feed	0.322	0.366	0.362				
ADG (kg)	0.68	—	0.73	35–97	160	Corn	Hedde et al. (1985)
Gain:feed	0.266	—	0.288				
ADG (kg)	0.686	—	0.719	32–91	192	Corn	Giesemann et al. (1990)
Gain:feed	0.257	—	0.279				
ADG (kg)	0.696	—	0.699	32–91	192	Sorghum	Giesemann et al. (1990)
Gain:feed	0.259	—	0.272				
ADG (kg)	—	1.00	0.99	54–120	70	Sorghum	Cabrera et al. (1994)
Gain:feed	—	0.295	0.316				
ADG (kg)	—	1.02	1.04	54–120	70	Sorghum	Cabrera et al. (1994)
Gain:feed	—	0.290	0.307				
ADG (kg)	0.98	0.98	0.99	55–115	160	Corn	Wondra et al. (1995b)
Gain:feed	0.298	0.305	0.321				
ADG (kg)	0.88	—	0.91	67–115	160	Wheat	Mavromichalis et al. (1998)
Gain:feed	0.285	—	0.322				

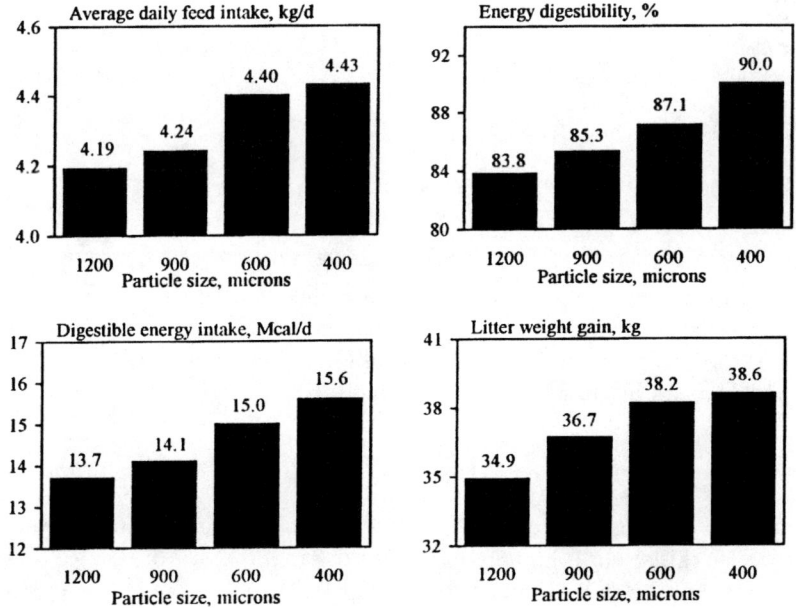

FIGURE 21.2 Effects of corn particle size on lactation performance of primiparous sows and apparent digestibility and intake of energy. (Data from Wondra et al., *J. Anim. Sci.*, 73:421, 1995.)

the apparent digestibilities of DM, starch, N, and gross energy measured at the terminal ileum and for the total digestive tract of growing pigs. Giesemann et al. (1990) reported greater digestibilities of DM, N, and gross energy of corn-based diets fed to growing-finishing pigs as particle size was reduced from 1500 to 640 μm. Sauer et al. (1977) determined that apparent ileal recoveries of amino acids were significantly less for finely ground wheat than for cracked wheat. Lawrence (1967; 1970) reported greater digestibilities of nutrients as particle size was decreased in corn-, sorghum-, and barley-based diets. Ohh et al. (1983) suggested that increased surface area of finely ground feedstuffs and increased fluidity of the digesta (thus, more potential for mixing with digestive enzymes) might be involved in improved digestibility of diets for swine.

Wondra et al. (1995d) fed 38 second-parity sows corn–soybean meal-based diets during lactation with the corn ground to 1200, 900, 600, and 400 μm. The results indicated greater digestibilities of DM, N, and gross energy as corn particle size was reduced from 1200 to 400 μm (Table 21.3). Digestible energy and ME values were maximized with the diet having 400-μm corn. Indeed, the ME concentration of the diet was increased from 3399 to 3745 kcal/kg as particle size of corn was reduced from 1200 to 400 μm. To achieve the same increase in energy density with diet formulation methods, a 9% addition of soybean oil would be needed.

TABLE 21.3
Effects of Corn Particle Size on Nutrient Metabolism in Second-Parity Sows during Lactation[a]

	Particle Size (μm)			
Item	1200	900	600	400
DM digestibility (%)[b]	82.2	85.2	85.6	88.1
N digestibility (%)[c]	80.7	85.6	86.9	88.5
Biological value (%)	55.0	62.7	62.0	57.0
N retention (g/day)[c]	50.9	63.0	63.3	56.7
GE digestibility (%)[b]	81.9	85.5	86.3	89.9
GE retention (Mcal/d)[b]	13.2	14.1	14.4	14.3
DE (kcal/kg of diet)[b]	3513	3668	3705	3857
ME (kcal/kg of diet)[b]	3399	3572	3601	3745

[a] All values are apparent.
[b] Linear effect of particle size reduction ($P < 0.02$).
[c] Quadratic effect of particle size reduction ($P < 0.03$).

Source: Modified from Wondra et al., J. Anim. Sci., 73:427, 1995.

Thus, in experiments with nursery pigs, finishing pigs, and lactating sows, data indicate significant improvements in performance with fine grinding of feedstuffs. Furthermore, the marked improvements in nutrient digestibility associated with fine grinding undoubtedly contribute greatly to the observed responses in growth and lactation performance.

IV. MILL TYPE

Of the various mill designs that can be used to grind feedstuffs (attrition mills, pin mills, hammermills, roller mills, etc.), hammermills and roller mills are by far the most commonly used in production of pig feeds. Hammermills (Figure 21.3) are simpler to operate than roller mills and require little oversight, even when grinding a wide variety of feedstuffs. Roller mills (Figure 21.4) generate less heat than hammermills while grinding and, thus, are more efficient (Heimann, 1983). McEllhiney (1983) suggested several advantages for roller mills compared to hammermills that included lower-energy requirements when grinding, quieter operation, more

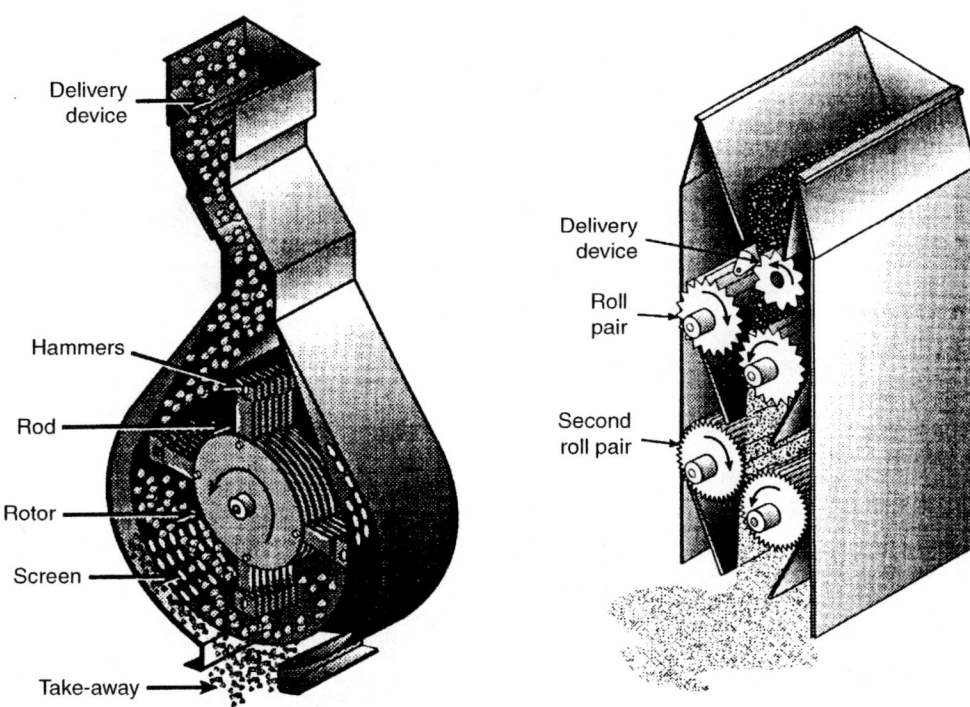

FIGURE 21.3 A basic hammermill design. As a kernel enters the mill, it is struck by a hammer and shattered. Once the kernel is shattered into small enough pieces, it can escape from the mill by passing through the screen. Particle size is controlled primarily by size of the holes in the screen. (From Koch, K., Kansas State University Coop. Ext. Serv. Bull. MS-496, 1996.)

FIGURE 21.4 A basic roller mill design. The rolls have different configurations of groves and corrugations and the roll pairs turn at different speeds. Grinding results from crushing, cutting, and shearing as the kernels are pulled between the rolls. Particle size is controlled by adjusting the gap between the rolls. (From Koch, K., Kansas State University Coop. Ext. Serv. Bull. MS-496, 1996.)

exact control of particle size, reduced moisture loss from the grain (i.e., shrink), and lower maintenance costs. Vermeer (1993) compared the economics of grinding with roller mills vs. hammermills and found that the cost of the grinders and related equipment for hammermill systems was half that of roller mill systems; however, the larger motors of hammermill systems cost twice as much to wire for electricity. Thus, initial setup costs were only slightly lower for the hammermill systems.

As for effects of roller mills and hammermills on growth performance of pigs, some suggest that the more uniform particle size (i.e., lower standard deviation, or s_{gw}, of the mean particle size) achieved with roller mill grinding has nutritional significance. Wondra et al. (1995c) reported data from an experiment with the treatments: (1) a blend of coarsely rolled and finely ground corn with a large s_{gw} of 2.7; (2) hammermilled corn with an s_{gw} of 2.3; and (3) roller-milled corn with an s_{gw} of 2.0. Mean particle size of the corn was similar for all three treatments. Digestibilities of DM, N, and GE were greater when the s_{gw} was smaller but no differences in growth performance were noted (Figure 21.5). In the same paper, the authors reported data from a second experiment where pigs were fed corn ground in a hammermill or roller mill to 800 or 400 μm. Corn ground in the hammermill had s_{gw} of 2.5 and 1.7, and corn ground in the roller mill had s_{gw} of 2.0 and 1.9 at 800 and 400 μm, respectively. Pigs fed corn ground to 800 μm in the roller mill had greater digestibility of nutrients than pigs fed corn ground to

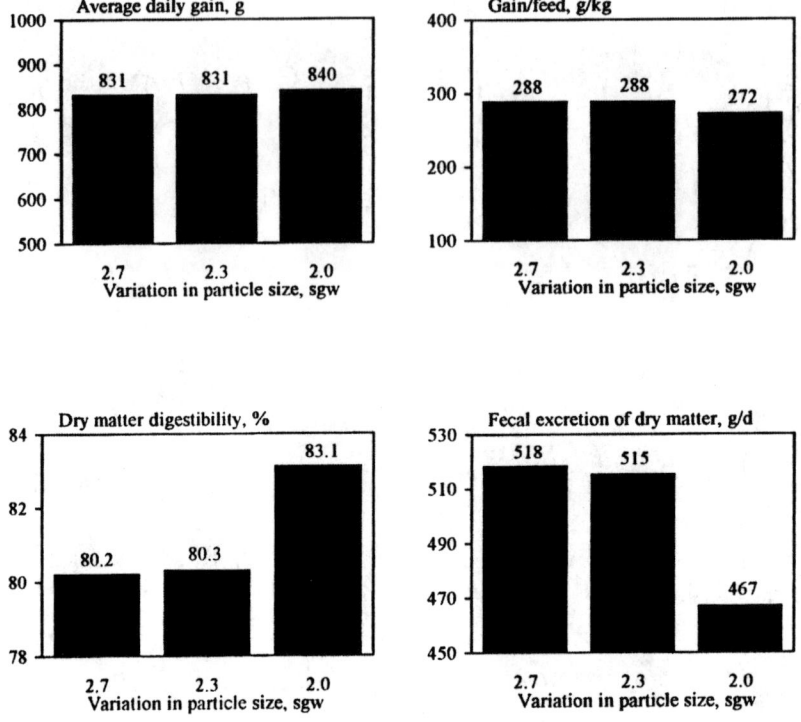

FIGURE 21.5 Particle size uniformity did not affect rate or efficiency of gain. But, as uniformity was increased, digestibility of dry matter increased and excretion of dry matter in feces decreased. (Data from Wondra et al., *J. Anim. Sci.*, 73:2564, 1995.)

800 μm in the hammermill (Table 21.4). Also, digestibilities were greater when corn was milled to 400 μm in the roller mill even though the hammermilled corn had a slightly lower s_{gw}. This suggested an effect of mill type separate from any s_{gw} effect. Reece et al. (1985) described particles of hammermilled corn as more spherical in shape with more uniform edges than particles of roller milled corn. The spherical shape would reduce susceptibility to attack by digestive enzymes, thus decreasing digestibility of nutrients in hammermilled corn. This explanation is difficult to verify, but the possibility of particle shape affecting nutritional value of cereals is intriguing. Equally interesting observations involve the anecdotal reports of greater flowability and improved handling characteristics for the uniform and granular particles resulting from roller mills compared with the less uniform particles resulting from hammermill grinding.

Thus, increased particle size uniformity (i.e., using a roller mill) may improve digestibility of nutrients, but this effect does not seem to be accompanied by predictable improvements in growth performance. Therefore, the industry has focused attention on the consistent improvements in performance that accompany decreased mean particle size rather than the subtle changes associated with greater uniformity of particle size. Because of the focus on reducing mean particle size with as much ease as possible, the hammermill continues to be the favorite grinding system used for manufacture of pig feeds.

V. MIXING DIETS

There are numerous mixer designs, with the most common being vertical screw, horizontal paddle, and horizontal ribbon (Figure 21.6). Suggested mix times are generally near 15 min for a vertical

TABLE 21.4
Effects of Mill Type and Particle Size (μm) on Grain Characteristics and Utilization of Nutrients in Pigs[a]

Item	Hammermill 800	Hammermill 400	Roller Mill 800	Roller Mill 400
Grain characteristics				
Mean particle size (μm)	826	419	793	415
Variation of particle size (s_{gw})	2.5	1.7	2.0	1.9
Growth performance				
ADG (kg)	0.93	0.96	0.96	0.92
Gain:feed[c]	0.284	0.308	0.291	0.305
Apparent digestibility (%)				
DM[b,c,d]	82.5	86.0	86.6	87.3
N[b,c]	72.1	80.1	76.0	82.6
GE[b,c,d]	81.2	86.7	85.9	87.7
Fecal excretion (g/d)				
DM[b,c,d]	517	396	397	347
N[b,c]	18.4	12.6	16.3	10.9

[a] A total of 128 pigs with an average initial weight of 55 kg and an average final weight of 112 kg.
[b] Hammermill vs. roller mill ($P < 0.03$).
[c] 800 vs. 400 μm ($P < 0.004$).
[d] Hammermill vs. roller mill × 800 vs. 400 μm ($P < 0.04$).

Source: Modified from Wondra et al., J. Anim. Sci., 73:2564, 1995.

screw mixer, 6 to 7 min for a horizontal paddle mixer, and 3 to 4 min for a horizontal ribbon mixer. Experience suggests that any of these mixer designs will provide satisfactory mix uniformity if given enough mix time. Thus, feed manufactures and nutritionists should focus on mix uniformity and not mix time as a desired end point.

From a feed manufacturing viewpoint, the optimum mixing procedure would require minimal inputs of time, electricity, and labor. Thus, a standard is needed to indicate adequate (but minimal) mix uniformity. That standard typically is a coefficient of variation (CV) for the distribution of some nutrient or marker within the feed, and a CV of ≤10% has been suggested by Beumer (1991), Lindley (1991), and Wicker and Poole (1991). In reality, however, there is no official testing procedure to describe mix uniformity. Chemical assays for drugs, vitamins, and crystalline amino acids have been used but are time-consuming, expensive, and/or noted for variability. Mineral element analyses are accurate and the distribution of Cr after adding a bolus of chromic oxide to a batch of feed has been used for many years by researchers as a measurement of mix uniformity. However, Cr determination (like that of most other minerals) is complicated and time-consuming and tends to require expensive equipment. One notable assay that has gained much favor in the feed industry is the Quantab® assay for salt (actually, Cl ions). This procedure is used to indicate mix uniformity with generally good success, but it is not satisfactory for diets with salt from several sources (e.g., whey, fishmeal, blood products, and salt) that would confound interpretation of the results. For such problem applications, colored iron filings (the Microtracer™ procedure) often are used. The iron filings (colored with a water-soluble dye) are added to the mixer and then counted in samples of the finished feed. The question still remains, however, of just how well any of these assays predict differences in nutritional value of a finished feed.

Holden (1988) stated that improper mixing of one batch of feed rarely would cause serious problems in growing pigs because a single batch will be consumed in such a short period of time. Traylor et al. (1994) conducted a 21-day growth assay with weanling pigs with mix time treatments

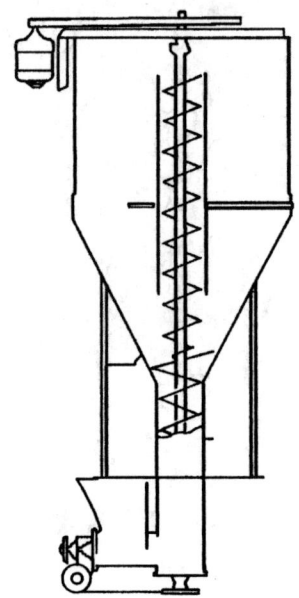

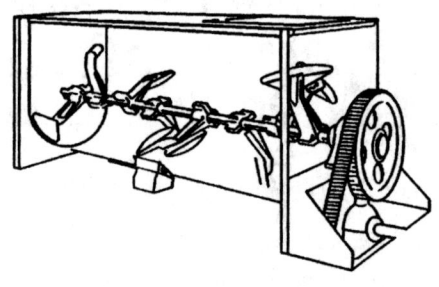

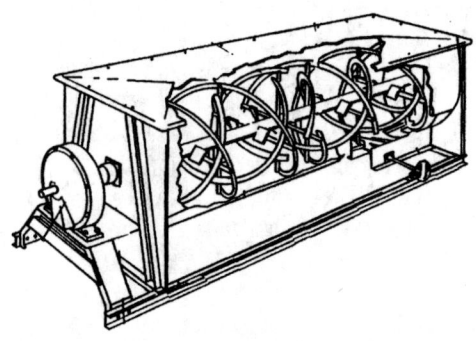

FIGURE 21.6 Basic design of vertical screw, horizontal paddle, and horizontal ribbon mixers. Mixer design affects the aggressiveness (ribbon > paddle > screw) of the mixing process and, thus, the time needed to achieve the desired mix uniformity. (From Wilcox, R. A. and Unruh, D. L., Kansas State University Coop. Ext. Serv. Bull. MF-829, 1986.)

of 0, 0.5, 2, and 4 min in a double-ribbon mixer. Increasing mix time from 0 to 0.5 min decreased the CV for Cr (chromic oxide was the marker used in this experiment) concentration from 107 to 28% (Table 21.5). Diet uniformity was improved further as mix time was increased to 4 min (i.e., a CV of 12%). Rate and efficiency of gain increased markedly as mixing time was increased from 0 to 0.5 min, with little response to increasing mixing time further to 4 min. The authors used the same mix time treatments to prepare diets for finishing pigs. Growth performance was not affected (Table 21.6) by reducing the CVs of the diet from nearly 54% (0 min mixing time) to <10% (4 min mixing time). Bone strength did not differ among pigs fed the various treatments, suggesting that minimal mixing of the diets did not create problems with Ca or P status of the pigs. Numerically at least, the lowest ADG and gain:feed and fattest carcasses were for pigs fed the diet with 0 min mix time (i.e., the CV of 54%). Nonetheless, these two experiments suggest that growing pigs are probably less sensitive to diet nonuniformity than once thought and that a CV of something more than 10% (perhaps 15 to 20%) is quite adequate.

TABLE 21.5
Effects of Mix Time on Diet Uniformity and Growth Performance of Nursery Pigs[a]

Item	Mix Time (min)				SE	Probability Value (P <)		
	0	0.5	2	4		Linear	Quad	Cubic
CV for Cr (%)[b]	106.5	28.4	16.1	12.3	N/A[c]	N/A	N/A	N/A
ADG (g)	267	379	383	402	18	0.01	0.02	0.01
ADFI (g)	598	711	701	720	22	0.01	0.08	0.02
Gain:feed	0.446	0.533	0.546	0.558	0.017	0.01	0.03	0.02

[a] A total of 120 weanling pigs (average initial body weight of 5.5 kg) with five pigs/pen and six pens/treatment.
[b] Coefficient of variation for Cr was determined from ten samples for each batch of feed.
[c] Statistical prcedures were not applicable for mix analyses.

Source: Modified from Traylor et al., *J. Anim. Sci.*, 72(Suppl. 2):59, 1994.

TABLE 21.6
Effects of Mix Time on Diet Uniformity and Growth Performance of Finishing Pigs[a]

Item	Mix Time (min)				SE	Probability Value (P <)		
	0	0.5	2	4		Linear	Quad	Cubic
CV for salt (%)[b]	53.8	14.8	12.5	9.6	N/A[c]	N/A	N/A	N/A
ADG (g)	777	807	793	787	15	—[d]	—	—
ADFI (kg)	2.95	2.90	2.89	2.88	0.05	—	—	—
Gain/feed	0.263	0.278	0.274	0.273	0.005	—	—	0.13
Dressing percentage (%)	73.7	73.3	73.1	73.0	0.2	0.04	—	—
Fat thickness (mm)	30.5	27.6	28.9	29.9	0.5	—	0.04	0.01
Bone strength (kg of force)	230	236	239	218	10	—	—	—

[a] A total of 128 pigs (average initial body weight of 56.3 kg) with eight pigs/pen and four pens/treatment.
[b] Coefficient of variation for salt was determined from ten samples for each batch of feed.
[c] Statistical procedures were not applicable for mix analyses.
[d] Dashes indicate $P > 0.15$.

Source: Modified from Traylor et al., *J. Anim. Sci.*, 72(Suppl. 2):59, 1994.

VI. PELLETING

Once ingredients have been ground and mixed, they can either be fed as a mash or subjected to further processing that usually involves heat or heat and pressure in combination. The most common forms of this "thermal processing" encountered in the feed industry are pelleting, roasting, steam flaking, and extrusion/expansion. Roasting often is used to prepare full-fat soy products (e.g., roasted soybeans) but is not used extensively for processing cereal grains. Steam flaking is used routinely to prepare sorghum grain for feedlot cattle but not to prepare diets for swine. Extrusion is a preferred means to process whole soybeans but generally is considered cost-prohibitive as a way to prepare cereals for pig diets (except, perhaps, for weanling pigs and lactating sows). This leaves pelleting, and, indeed, pelleted swine diets have become extremely popular during the last four decades.

From a feed manufacturer's perspective, benefits of pelleting include decreased segregation of mixed feedstuffs, increased bulk density, reduced dustiness, and improved handling characteristics. Additionally, swine producers often complain about poor flowability of feed through storage bins and feeders when diets are made with finely ground (i.e., particle size of <600 µm) cereals. Pelleting is a process that eliminates bridging problems, making it less problematic to feed diets with finely ground ingredients.

Hanke et al. (1972), Baird (1973), and Wondra et al. (1995b) reported that pelleted diets improved rate of gain. A number of other scientists, however, reported no significant effect of pelleting on growth rate (i.e., NCR-42 Committee on Swine Nutrition, 1969). Nonetheless, when all of the reports in Table 21.7 were considered, they showed an average improvement of 6% in rate of gain and improvements of 6 to 7% in efficiency of gain for growing-finishing pigs fed pelleted diets.

There is little consensus about the reason for increased growth performance of pigs fed pelleted diets. Skoch et al. (1983a) suggested that pelleting increased the bulk density of diets and reduced dustiness, making the diets more palatable. However, improved palatability is inconsistent with the decreased feed intake frequently observed for pigs fed pelleted diets. In experiments reported by Wondra et al. (1995b,c), DM, N, and gross energy digestibilities were increased by pelleting. Jensen and Becker (1965) suggested that pelleting gelatinized starch, thus making it more susceptible to enzymatic digestion. Although some argue that conditions during the pelleting process are not sufficient to gelatinize starch, others contend that the heat, hydration, and shear when pelleting do indeed disrupt the structure of starch and protein molecules, making them more accessible for digestive enzymes. Alternatively, many researchers tend to attribute the improved performance of

TABLE 21.7
Effects of Pelleting on Growth Performance[a]

			Meal			Pellet		
Reference	Pig wt (kg)	No. of Pigs	ADG (kg)	ADFI (kg)	G/F	ADG (kg)	ADFI (kg)	G/F
NCR-42 Committee on Swine Nutrition (1969)	20–91	556	0.77	—	0.31	0.78	—	0.32
Hanke et al. (1972)	58–99	379	0.75	—	0.29	0.80	—	0.31
Baird (1973)	15–100	120	0.69	2.52	0.270	0.72	2.43	0.292
Tribble et al. (1975)	29–100	192	0.66	—	0.265	0.68	—	0.291
Harris et al. (1979)	70–100	98	0.61	2.34	0.261	0.66	2.34	0.282
Tribble et al. (1979)	59–98	144	0.62	2.54	0.244	0.70	2.56	0.273
Skoch et al. (1983a)	49–98	60	0.77	2.39	0.323	0.84	2.44	0.344
Wondra et al. (1995b)	55–115	160	0.96	3.22	0.297	1.00	3.16	0.318

[a] All diets were corn based except the diets used by Tribble et al. (1975; 1979) and Harris et al. (1979), which were sorghum based.

pigs fed pelleted diets to decreased feed wastage. This hypothesis would be valid if only efficiency of gain were improved, but it does not explain the improvements in nutrient digestibility and rate of gain so often observed in pigs fed pelleted diets.

Whether the factors that increase digestibility are changes in feeding behavior, changes in the way digestive tracts react to pelleted vs. meal diets (e.g., altered flow of digesta), or a direct effect of thermal processing (e.g., gelatinization of starch and denaturation of proteins) are yet to be determined. Nonetheless, nutrient excretion from pigs in regions of intensive livestock production is causing environmental concerns, and Wondra et al. (1995b) reported 23 and 22% reductions in excretion of DM and N in feces, respectively, as a result of pelleting. Therefore, grain-processing techniques that increase nutrient digestibility and reduce nutrient excretion have special value to the swine industry. Government regulations are now forcing careful evaluation of every aspect of livestock production in an attempt to minimize waste production, and processing methods that maximize nutrient digestibility have special significance.

VII. PELLET SIZE

From an efficiency-of-milling standpoint, a large-diameter pellet produced with a very thin die would maximize pellet mill output with minimum inputs of time and electricity. Lavorel et al. (1984) conducted a nursery experiment evaluating 2.5-, 3-, and 5-mm-diameter pellets. The authors reported that weanling pigs fed the 2.5-mm pellets had greater growth rate than pigs fed the 5-mm pellets during the first 2 wk postweaning. During the second 2 wk (d 14 to 28), there were no differences in growth performance among pigs fed the different pellet sizes. The few data that address the issue of pellet size in growing finishing pigs are summarized in Table 21.8. Luce et al. (1973) fed pellets with diameters of 4.8, 6.4, and 9.5 mm to finishing pigs. The authors reported that pellet size had little effect on growth performance in pigs fed the sorghum-based diets; however, pigs fed 4.8-mm wheat-based pellets had greater ADG than those fed the 9.5-mm pellets and greater gain:feed than those fed the 6.4- and 9.5-mm pellets. Harris et al. (1979) suggested that finishing pigs fed 4.8-mm pellets were more efficient than pigs fed 6.4-mm pellets. However, concurrent research from that same laboratory (Tribble et al., 1979) indicated no differences in ADG or gain:feed among finishing pigs fed pellets ranging in size from 4.8 to 12.7 mm. Therefore, in the few reports that address pellet size there is little consensus about the actual effects on growth

TABLE 21.8
Effect of Pellet Size on Swine Performance in Growing-Finishing Phase

Reference	No. of Pigs	Pellet Size (mm)	ADG (kg)	ADFI (kg)	G/F
Luce et al. (1973)	208	4.8	0.82	2.49	0.33
		6.4	0.85	2.59	0.33
		9.5	0.82	2.49	0.33
Luce et al. (1973)	144	4.8	0.75	2.14	0.35
		6.4	0.72	2.14	0.34
		9.5	0.71	2.15	0.33
Harris et al. (1979)	66	4.8	0.66	2.17	0.30
		6.4	0.66	2.50	0.26
Tribble et al. (1979)	108	4.8	0.71	2.42	0.29
		6.4	0.71	2.83	0.25
		12.7	0.68	2.44	0.28
Hanrahan (1984)	1360	5.0	0.49	1.94	0.25
		10.0	0.49	1.99	0.25

TABLE 21.9
Effects of Pellet Size on Growth Performance of Nursery Pigs[a]

		Pellet Diameter (mm)				
Item	Meal	2	4	8	12	SE
Day 0 to 5						
ADG (g)[b]	124	151	148	165	158	12
ADFI (g)	153	134	132	162	142	11
Gain/feed[b]	0.810	1.127	1.121	1.019	1.113	0.061
Day 0 to 29						
ADG (g)	358	362	371	362	364	7
ADFI (g)	537	510	516	541	532	11
Gain:feed[b,c,d]	0.667	0.710	0.719	0.669	0.684	0.012

[a] A total of 210 pigs with six pens per treatment.
[b] Meal vs. pellets ($P < 0.04$).
[c] Linear effect of pellet size ($P < 0.05$).
[d] Cubic effect of pellet size ($P < 0.04$).

Source: Modified from Traylor et al., *J. Anim. Sci.*, 74(Suppl. 1):67, 1996.

performance in pigs. Also, there still exists the belief that small pigs prefer small pellets and large pigs prefer large pellets; therefore, many die sizes are needed to process feed.

To address the issue of optimum pellet size for pigs, Traylor et al. (1996) conducted experiments to determine the effects of pellet size on growth performance in nursery and finishing pigs. For the nursery experiment, weanling pigs (average initial body weight of 5.4 kg) were used in a 29-d growth assay. The dietary treatments were a corn-based meal control and 2-, 4-, 8-, and 12-mm pellets. For d 0 to 5, pelleting improved ADG by 25% and gain:feed by 36% (Table 21.9). However, pellet size did not affect growth performance. Overall (d 0 to 29), pelleting improved gain:feed by 4% compared with the meal diets, with maximum gain:feed at a pellet size of 4 mm. In the finishing experiment, 80 barrows (average initial body weight of 58 kg) were fed a corn–soybean meal-based diet with the same pellet size treatments used in the nursery experiment. Rate of gain was not affected by pelleting, but pigs fed pelleted diets tended to have improved gain:feed (Table 21.10). As pellet size was increased, ADG was improved and the 4-mm pellets supporting the greatest gain:feed. Thus, it seems that producing several different pellet sizes for pigs of various sizes is

TABLE 21.10
Effects of Pellet Size on Growth Performance and Carcass Measurements of Finishing Pigs[a]

		Pellet Diameter (mm)				
Item	Meal	2	4	8	12	SE
ADG (kg)[b]	1.03	0.94	1.01	1.02	1.05	0.22
ADFI (kg)[b,c]	3.01	2.62	2.76	2.85	3.05	0.69
Gain/feed[b,c]	0.342	0.361	0.365	0.357	0.343	0.007
Last rib fat depth (mm)	24.6	23.2	23.1	23.6	23.4	1.0
Dressing percentage (%)	72.4	72.4	72.5	72.5	72.1	0.3

[a] A total of 80 pigs with eight pens per treatment.
[b] Linear effect of pellet size ($P < 0.07$).
[c] Meal vs. pellets ($P < 0.08$).

Source: Modified from Traylor et al., *J. Anim. Sci.*, 74(Suppl. 1):67, 1996.

not necessary. Furthermore, a single die with 4- to 5-mm holes seems to be adequate for both nursery and finishing pigs. These findings suggest that significant savings of time and money are possible with use of a single die to prepare diets for pigs from weaning to market.

VIII. PELLET QUALITY

Pellet quality is defined as the ability of a pellet to withstand repeated handling without excessive breakage. For determination of pellet quality, the feed industry generally has adopted the "tumbling box" method suggested by Young (1970) and published as an official ASAE procedure (ASAE, 1987). Reimer (1992) suggested that many factors affect pellet quality, with the largest contributors being diet formulation, particle size, and conditioning (Figure 21.7). The authors' experiences at Kansas State University confirm that diet formulation can have marked beneficial effects, e.g., when wheat enters into formulations (Traylor et al., 1999) or waxy endosperm cereals are used (Froetschner at al., 1998). Also, in the authors' experiments, as particle size of the diet was decreased, pellet durability was improved (Wondra et al., 1995b). In contrast, simple cereal–soybean meal formulations with >1 or 2% fat added in the mixer tend to produce poor-quality pellets (Stark, 1994). Thus, there are several factors recognized to affect pellet quality. However, this still leaves one to wonder just how important pellet quality really is to profitability of a swine operation.

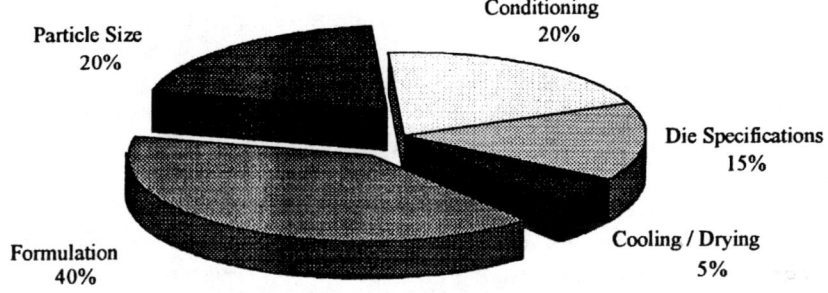

FIGURE 21.7 Factors affecting pellet durability. (Adapted from Reimer, 1992.)

In an attempt to define the effects of pellet quality (e.g., percentage fines in the diet) on growth performance, Stark et al. (1994) conducted a series of experiments with nursery and finishing pigs. In two nursery experiments, a meal control diet was compared with diets with as much as 30% fines. Pelleting improved gain:feed by 12 to 15% compared with the meal control. Compared with scalped pellets (i.e., pellets sieved to remove the fines), concentrations of 25 to 30% pellet fines decreased gain:feed by 3 to 4%. In the finishing experiment, pigs fed the screened pellets had 3% greater ADG and 5% greater gain:feed compared with pigs fed the meal diet (Table 21.11). Pellet fines did not affect ADG, but gain:feed tended to decrease as the amount of fines increased. Perhaps the most troubling observation was that pigs fed diets with high concentrations of fines (between 20 and 40%) were no more efficient than pigs fed the meal control. In a similar experiment with finishing pigs, Amornthewaphat et al. (1999) reported a linear decrease in efficiency of growth as pellet fines was increased from none (7% greater gain:feed than the meal control) to 50% (2% greater gain:feed compared with the meal control). Thus, if the pelleting process is not done properly and results in excessive (perhaps as little as 20 to 40%) fines at the feeder, the benefits of pelleting disappear rapidly.

IX. PELLET MILL CONDITIONERS

To combat the loss of growth performance associated with pellet fines, proper conditioning of the diet becomes a first line of defense. Conditioners usually are purchased as part of the pellet mill,

TABLE 21.11
Effects of Pellet Fines on Growth Performance of Finishing Pigs

		Percentage Fines						
Item	Meal	0%	20%	25%	40%	50%	60%	SE
Stark et al. (1994)[a]								
ADG (kg)	0.93	0.97	0.97	—	0.96	—	0.94	0.02
Gain/feed	0.362	0.379	0.360	—	0.361	—	0.355	0.008
Amornthewaphat et al. (1999)[b]								
ADG (kg)	0.89	0.96	—	0.93	—	0.90	—	0.01
Gain/feed	0.359	0.384	—	0.379	—	0.367	—	0.008

[a] A total of 80 pigs with eight pens per treatment.
[b] A total of 192 pigs with four pens per treatment.

and their purpose is to add heat and moisture (steam) before pelleting. This conditioning of the mash before pelleting softens the particles and makes the proteins and carbohydrates tacky. All this is done with the goal of creating a more durable pellet.

In a standard steam conditioner, the mash is heated to 75 or 85°C (depending on the formulation) with a retention time of only a few seconds. As an alternative, long-term conditioners (also called two-pass or double-pass conditioners) can have retention times of several minutes. This allows greater penetration of the steam into the feed particle and increases starch gelatinization and protein denaturation. This technology is used extensively in the aquaculture industry to make feeds that sink and hold their shape while submerged in water.

Compactors and expanders are used in combination with steam conditioners to enhance pellet quality even further. These machines are placed between the steam conditioners and the pellet mill and use high pressure to enhance the starch gelatinization and protein denaturation that was started in the conditioner. Expanders are more complicated (and expensive) than compactors, and differ little from extruders in their principle of operation, that of high-temperature, short-time processing. Indeed, expanders have been used, like extruders, to produce full-fat soybean meal (Cao et al., 1998a,b). However, expanders initially were designed to condition complete diets and their benefit is thought primarily to be enhanced pellet quality (Peisker, 1994b). Traylor et al. (1999) demonstrated that expanding increased pellet durability indexes of corn-, sorghum-, wheat midds-, and wheat-based diets by 39, 20, 6, and 3%, respectively. Other benefits of expanding are flexibility in formulation (e.g., 5 to 7% fat added at the mixer will not ruin pellet quality), reduced pellet die wear and increased pellet mill throughput (by as much as 25%), feed sterilization, and decreased activity of antinutritional components. However, few published data are available that evaluate the effects of expander technology on growth performance of pigs.

Peisker (1994a) reported improved rates of gain in nursery pigs fed diets with 30% expanded wheat bran and a complete expanded diet compared with an untreated starter diet. In contrast, Hongtrakul et al. (1996) and Johnston et al. (1999b) reported reduced ADG in weanling pigs fed complex nursery diets that were expanded. In work with finishing pigs, Peisker (1996) reported that pigs fed expanded diets had 8% greater ADG and 7% greater gain:feed compared with pigs fed a meal control diet. More recently, Johnston et al. (1999c) reported that finishing pigs fed expanded diets in mash or pelleted form had improved efficiencies of gain compared with pigs fed diets subjected to long- or short-term conditioning. In a comparison of corn- and sorghum-based diets fed to finishing pigs (Johnston et al., 1999a), digestibilities of DM and gross energy were ranked: expander conditioned pellets > standard steam-conditioned pellets > meal control. Also, efficiency of gain tended to be greatest for the expander conditioned pellets. Finally, Park et al.

(1998) reported that conventional steam conditioning and pelleting of a wheat-based diet improved efficiency of gain by 2% and expander processing prior to pelleting improved efficiency of gain by 7% compared with a meal control.

Thus, there does seem to be some benefit from expanding diets for at least growing and finishing pigs. However, the purchase price ($300,000 to $500,000) and maintenance requirements must be considered carefully before installation of such sophisticated processing equipment.

X. PELLET BINDERS

As a seemingly final option in the quest for better pellet quality, some feed manufacturers and pig producers have turned to pellet binders. Pellet binders are, as the name implies, compounds added to diets in hopes of creating more durable pellets. These binders come in various forms, but the more common products are lignosulfonates (co-products of paper manufacturing), sodium and calcium bentonites (mined from clay deposits), hemicellulose extracts (co-product of hardboard manufacturing), and modified starch products (gelatinized cereal starch that enhances "tackiness" during steam conditioning). Surprisingly, there are few published data to indicate the most effective dietary concentrations of these materials for enhanced pellet quality and even fewer data that indicate the effects of these materials on growth performance of pigs.

Lindemann et al. (1993) reported that sodium bentonite and hydrated sodium calcium aluminosilicate improved growth performance of pigs fed corn contaminated with aflatoxin but not of pigs fed "clean" corn. Their experiments were not designed to evaluate the clays as pellet binders so the diets were fed in meal form. Tribble et al. (1980) reported that a modified starch product (Nutri-Binder™) enhanced pellet quality (although pellet durability indexes were not given) without affecting growth performance in finishing pigs. Starkey and Hancock (unpublished data) found that energy required to pellet decreased, and pellet mill production rate and pellet durability index increased as dietary concentration of calcium lignosulfonate was increased from none to 2% (Table 21.12). In a follow-up experiment, the authors found that at the manufacturer's suggested inclusion rate of 0.5% lignosulfonate, pellet durability index of a simple corn–soybean meal finishing diet was increased from 59 to 73%. But, the improvement in pellet quality did not improve growth performance of finishing pigs above that observed for those fed pellets without the added binder (Table 21.13). Note, however, that these diets were pelleted, bagged, and taken directly to the research farm. Thus, there was not a great deal of fines generated among the softer, less durable pellets (without binder) as would be expected to result from the handling in augers, trucks, and bins typical at a commercial feedmill/swine operation.

TABLE 21.12
Effects of a Pellet Binder on Milling Characteristics and Pellet Quality in a Simple, Corn–Soybean Meal Diet for Finishing Pigs

		Ca Lignosulfonate (%)		
Item	Control	0.5	1	2
Production rate (kg/h)	1031	1097	1183	1289
Energy consumption (kWh/t)	9.7	9.3	8.6	7.9
Pellet durability index (%)[a]	53.1	66.8	73.3	80.0
Fines at the scalper (%)	25.7	17.4	13.5	9.5

[a] ASAE (1983).

Source: Unpublished data (Starkey and Hancock).

TABLE 21.13
Effects of a Pellet Binder on Growth Performance and Nutrient Digestibility in Finishing Pigs[a]

Item	Control Mash	Control Pellet	0.5% Lignosulfonate
Pellet durability index (%)	—	59	73
ADG (kg)	1.05	1.09	1.08
ADFI (kg)	2.88	2.77	2.81
Gain/feed	0.365	0.390	0.384
DM digestibility (%)	89.4	89.5	89.9
N digestibility (%)	88.4	88.7	88.3

[a] Two pigs per pen and eight pens per treatment.

Source: Unpublished data (Starkey and Hancock).

Thus, it does appear that pellet binders increase pellet durability and hardness. However, the ability of this binder-induced increase in pellet quality to enhance growth performance of pigs is yet to be demonstrated.

XI. EXTRUSION OF CEREALS AND COMPLETE DIETS

Extrusion of dietary ingredients and finished diets has been limited almost exclusively to pet and aquaculture feeds that allow sufficient markup in price to compensate for the increased processing costs. However, some recent data indicate improved growth performance and/or nutrient digestibility in pigs fed extruded cereal grains and extruded soybeans compared with diets based on ground grain–soybean meal–animal/vegetable fat. Thus, extrusion technology offers numerous specialized applications that make some discussion of this technology appropriate in a text on swine nutrition.

Extrusion processing is not a new concept; it has been used in the preparation of human foodstuffs for more than 50 years (Ferket, 1991) and is used to manufacture everything from cheesepuffs to candy bars to protein-rich meat extenders. The material to be extruded is fed from a holding bin, through a mixing cylinder, and into the extruder barrel (Figure 21.8). The extruder barrel houses a series of locks, dies, and orifices with greater and greater restrictions from inlet to outlet. The material being extruded is subjected to increasing pressure, friction, and attrition as it passes through the extruder barrel, such that the material is heated from room temperature to 135 to 160°C at pressures of 15 to 40 atm in as little as 30 s. As the extruded material exits the extruder barrel, the sudden drop in pressure results in violent expansion as steam escapes from the product. Loss of steam reduces moisture content of the extruded material by as much as one half, depending on initial moisture content. From a nutritional standpoint, desired effects common to extruders are shearing and gelatinization of starch, denaturation and shearing of protein, destruction of microorganisms and some toxicants, and dehydration.

Noland et al. (1976) reported that extrusion improved energy and N digestibility of high-tannin sorghum grain when fed to nursery pigs, but growth performance was not affected. Herkelman et al. (1990) reported that extrusion of corn did not affect utilization of N or lysine in nursery pigs, but extruded corn had greater energy value (i.e., increased DE and ME) compared with ground corn. Fadel et al. (1988) extruded a barley–soybean mixture and digestibilities of DM, GE, starch, and N at the terminal ileum were increased by 12, 12, 16, and 11%, respectively (Table 21.14). Hancock et al. (1991a) reported that substitution of extruded for hammermilled sorghum did not affect ADG but increased efficiency of gain by 5% in finishing pigs. This increased gain:feed was accompanied by increases of 8 and 23% in digestibilities of DM and N, respectively. Replacing

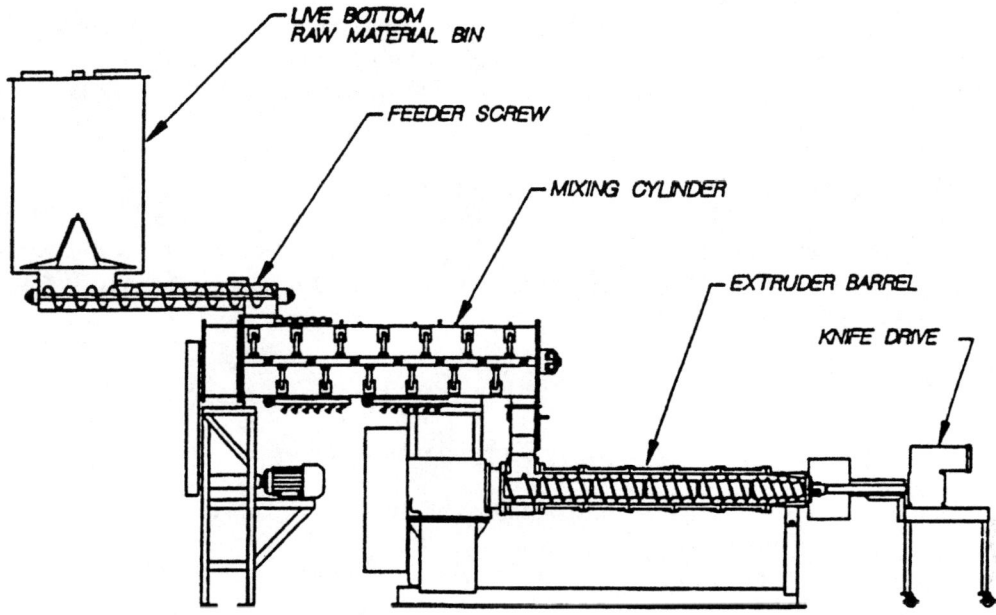

FIGURE 21.8 Typical design for a moist extruder. For moist extrusion, steam is injected into the mixing cylinder. A dry extruder would not have the mixing cylinder. Both extruder designs use a series of screws, locks, dies, and constrictions in the extruder barrel to move the extrudate through the barrel and generate shear and heat (via friction) under extremely high pressure.

TABLE 21.14
Extrusion of Barley Improves Apparent Digestibility of Nutrients in Finishing Pigs

	Apparent Digestibility (%)			
	Ileum[a]		Total Tract	
Item	Ground	Extruded	Ground	Extruded
DM	55.6[b]	62.0[c]	77.4	78.0
Gross energy	57.9[b]	64.9[c]	74.6	79.6
Starch	83.7[b]	96.9[c]	97.0	99.7
N	62.4	69.2	74.1	80.6

[a] Means in the same row with different superscripts differ ($P < 0.05$).

Source: Adapted from Fadel et al. (1988).

---

soybean meal and soy oil with extruded soybeans also improved efficiency of gain by 5%, but the greatest efficiency of gain was in pigs fed diets with extruded sorghum plus extruded soybeans (i.e., a 10% improvement vs. the control). In a second experiment (Hancock et al., 1991b), the authors reported improved gain:feed and DM and N digestibilities when ground sorghum grain, soybean meal, and soybean oil were blended and extruded before use in diets for finishing pigs. A further increase in gain:feed (18% improvement compared with control pigs) was observed when extruded whole soybeans were blended with the ground sorghum grain and then extruded. Finally, Hancock et al. (1992) reported that extrusion improved gain:feed by 4, 9, 6, and 3% in finishing pigs fed corn-, sorghum-, wheat-, and barley-based diets, respectively, compared with simply grinding the cereals in a hammermill. Digestibility of nutrients closely paralleled the differences in gain:feed: corn had greater digestibilities of DM and N than the average of the other grains, sorghum and wheat were more digestible than barley, and extruded grains were more digestible than ground grains. In concluding, the authors stressed that when compared with the ground corn control, the extruded corn- and sorghum-based diets supported greater gain:feed and had greater digestibility of nutrients. Skoch et al. (1983b) compared the effects of pelleting with and without steam conditioning, and extrusion before steam conditioning and pelleting, on the nutritional value of a diet based on corn–wheat middlings in growing-finishing pigs. Pelleting and extruding increased gain/feed and digestibility of GE, but ADG was not affected.

Thus, extrusion processing of fibrous (e.g., wheat middlings) and starchy (e.g., cereal grains) feedstuffs can improve nutrient utilization. But, the added cost of extruding cereals or a complete diet (estimated to be $11 to $15/ton) can make the technology too expensive for routine use in preparation of feed for pigs. This does not, however, preclude the possible use of extrusion to enhance the nutritional value of specialty diets (e.g., baby pig chows) or high-cost ingredients (e.g., protein meals).

XII. EXTRUDED SOYBEANS

Of the nutrient classes (e.g., carbohydrates, proteins, fats, vitamins, and minerals), published reports about extrusion processing of protein sources dominate the literature. Furthermore, a major portion of any discussion of the effects of extrusion processing on protein feedstuffs undoubtedly will concern soybean proteins.

The Chinese have recognized for thousands of years that soybeans are an excellent human foodstuff when cooked, fermented, or otherwise processed. More than 70 years ago, data were published (Osborne and Mendel, 1917) demonstrating that heat-treatment of soybeans greatly improved their nutritional value for growing rats. Thus, early work with extrusion was to use it as a heat treatment process and decisions to feed extruded soybeans were made by comparing costs of soybean meal and feed-grade fat to the cost of extruded soybeans. Briefly, the first decision was whether adding fat was economical. In pigs, fat may or may not improve rate of gain, but a 2% increase in efficiency of gain for every 1% fat added to the diet can be expected. Also, consideration must be given to the physical benefits of adding fat (i.e., decreased dustiness in confinement facilities) and the increased nutrient density of diets that nutritionists desire when feed intake is depressed by hot weather. A simple formula to determine whether feeding extruded soybeans is economical follows:

$$\text{ADVANTAGE} = 0.81 \times \text{SBM} + 0.17 \times \text{FAT} - (\text{BEANS} + \text{PROCESSING}),$$

where:
ADVANTAGE = cost advantage (positive or negative) of feeding 1 ton of extruded soybean seeds
0.81 = adjustment for lower protein in processed soybean seeds vs. soybean meal (i.e., 38% CP/47% CP = 0.81)
SBM = cost of 1 ton of 47% CP soybean meal
0.17 = allowance for 18% fat in soybean seeds minus 1% fat in soybean meal
FAT = value of 1 ton of feed-grade fat
BEANS = value of 1 ton of raw soybean seeds
PROCESSING = cost of extruding 1 ton of soybean seeds.

These calculations assume that full-fat soybean preparations have equal feeding value to soybean meal plus feed-grade fat. This may or may not be correct. Hancock et al. (1990a; 1991c) demonstrated improved soybean protein utilization by nursery pigs when dry-roasting was replaced by extrusion processing. In a protein quality assay, extrusion improved ADG of nursery pigs fed soybeans with and without the Kunitz trypsin inhibitor by 21% compared to pigs fed dry-roasted soybeans (Figure

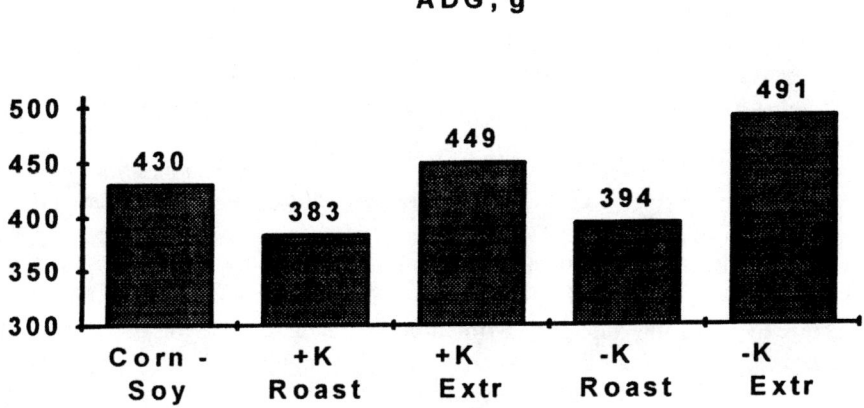

FIGURE 21.9 Extrusion processing improved growth rate of nursery pigs fed soybeans with (+K) or without (–K) gene expression for the Kunitz trypsin inhibitor. Means are for four pigs per pen and five pens per treatment with an average initial weight of 7.5 kg and fed for 5 weeks. (From Hancock, J. D. et al., Kansas State University Swine Day, Agric. Exp. Sta. Prog. No. 610, 52, 1990.)

21.9). Also, ADG for pigs fed low-inhibitor extruded soybeans was 14% greater than that of pigs fed commercially prepared soybean meal plus soybean oil. Digestibilities of N and DM responded in a similar manner, with improvements for pigs fed low-inhibitor and/or extruded soybeans. To investigate the nutritional value of roasted and extruded soybean preparations further, Kim et al. (2000b) fed 90 pigs (5- and 10-kg body weight) in two metabolism experiments. For the experiment with newly weaned (5-kg) pigs, N digestibility, biological value, percentage N retention, gross energy digestibility, percentage ME, and villus height were greater for pigs fed extruded soybeans than for those fed roasted soybeans. Also, N digestibility, biological value, and percentage N retention were greater for pigs fed low-inhibitor soybeans than for those fed the conventional soybeans. For the older (10-kg) pigs, that were allowed to adjust to the nursery environment before being given the soybean treatments, utilization of nutrients was greater for all of the soy sources. However, there still were several advantages in nutrient digestibility and utilization for extruded compared with roasted, and low-inhibitor compared with normal, soybeans. Based on their findings, the authors argued that the 1988 NRC value for ME (3624 kcal/kg) of "heat-processed soybean seeds" overestimated the ME content of roasted soybeans by 368 kcal/kg in 5-kg pigs and by 150 kcal/kg in 10-kg pigs. In contrast, the ME content of extruded soybeans was underestimated by 230 kcal/kg in 5-kg pigs and by 438 kcal/kg in 10-kg pigs. This disparity in nutritional value of heat-processed soy products was evidenced further by Kim et al. (2000a), where the ileal digestibilities for lysine in growing pigs were 83, 67, 86, and 88% for soybean meal, roasted soybeans, extruded soybeans, and soybeans processed with an extrusion aid (sodium sulfite). Unfortunately, the new NRC (1998) still categorizes all full-fat soy products as "heat processed seeds" although it seems a differentiation among the processes used to create full-fat soy products is in order.

Thus, there is general agreement that improved digestibility of nutrients is a major contributor to the high nutritional value of extruded soybeans. However, the actual physical/chemical mechanism that facilitates the improved nutritional value is debatable, especially when biological value and villus measurements are greater in piglets fed extruded vs. roasted soybeans.

Increased energy value of extruded vs. roasted soybeans has been attributed to disruption of the soybean fat globules, which improves accessibility by lipase enzymes. The same disruption also could contribute to improved protein digestibility because limited denaturation of proteins increases their susceptibility to enzymatic attack. However, the denaturation associated with extrusion is far from mild with radical disruption of native proteins by breaking bonds, shearing molecules, and actually stimulating formation of new bonds and configurations. Thus, not only does extrusion leave protein molecules more susceptible to proteases, but biologically active proteins (e.g., trypsin inhibitors and lectins) would also be inactivated. Also, there is a considerable pool of data (Barratt et al., 1978; Kilshaw and Sissons, 1979; Seegraber and Morrill, 1979; Dunsford et al., 1989; Li et al., 1990) that suggests the major storage proteins in soybean seeds (conglycinin and β-conglycinin) have antigenic properties. Soybean preparations with low antigenic potential have been prepared by extraction with hot aqueous ethanol (Sissons et al., 1979; 1982). This reduction in antigenicity was given credit for lower antisoy titers and improved digestive function in preruminant calves. Hancock et al. (1990b,c) reported that extraction with ethanol before heat treatment of soyflakes resulted in improved rates and efficiencies of gain, greater digestibility of nutrients, and larger villi in nursery pigs. These responses were especially apparent if the soy bean flakes were under- or overprocessed by autoclaving. Thus, the denaturation of biologically active proteins, whether by extrusion treatment, extraction with aqueous alcohol, or a combination of the two technologies (as used commercially to prepare soy protein concentrates) undoubtedly contributes to the improved nutritional value of the end product.

In conclusion, extrusion processing is widely used in preparation of expanded pet and fish feeds and, to some extent, to manufacture specialty items used in livestock feeding (e.g., soy preparations for newly weaned calves and pigs). However, when a large number of experiments are considered (Table 21.15), especially those where fat and energy of the diets are equalized, extruded soybeans are at least equal to, if not 3 to 5% better than, soybean meal plus added fat in diets for pigs.

XIII. STOMACH MORPHOLOGY

Stomach lesions were proposed as a concern in commercial production of swine when Bullard (1951) documented esophagogastric ulcers as the cause of death in an adult boar. In the past 5 to 7 years, with the widespread use of European genotypes and modern grain-processing techniques, ulcers have emerged as a major problem in the United States. Studies indicate that, as particle size of cereal grains is reduced, the incidence of ulcers tends to increase in nursery pigs (Healy et al., 1994), growing-finishing pigs (Mahan et al., 1966; Pickett et al., 1969; Cabrera et al., 1994; Eisemann and Argenzio, 1999b), and lactating sows (Wondra et al., 1995d,e). Reimann et al. (1968), Maxwell et al. (1970; 1972), and Regina et al. (1999) reported that smaller particle sizes increased fluidity of stomach contents and/or increased the concentration of pepsin in the stomach. These authors hypothesized that the increased fluidity allowed more mixing of stomach contents; thus, pepsin and digestive acids were continuously in contact with the unprotected mucosa of the esophageal region of the stomach. Pelleting also has been shown to increase ulcers in growing-finishing pigs (Chamberlain et al., 1967; Wondra et al., 1995b,c; Amornthewaphat et al., 1999). Note, however, that incidence of stomach lesions also is probably affected by grain type and stressful housing and shipping conditions (Ricker et al., 1967; Pickett et al., 1969; Lawrence et al., 1998). Perhaps the most significant factor in stomach lesion development was suggested by Berruecos and Robison (1972), where the heritability estimate for gastric lesions in pigs was estimated to be 0.52 (i.e., as highly heritable as many carcass characteristics). Thus, interactions with management and genetic factors may affect the extent to which particle size of cereal grains can be reduced, at least until those problems are corrected.

Despite recognition of several factors that contribute to increased incidence of stomach ulcers, many producers feel they have few viable options for combating this problem. To forfeit the improvements in feed efficiency and decreased fecal excretion of nutrients resulting from fine grinding and pelleting would decrease the competitiveness of a producer's farm. Yet, major changes in genetics and management practices to avoid difficulties with stomach lesions are at the least very expensive and cumbersome. So, it seems producers are constantly seeking alternatives that address the issue.

Ayles et al. (1996) suggested that occasionally to change (e.g., when pigs are moved or sorted) from fine-ground to coarse-ground and back to fine-ground diets could be effective at preventing

TABLE 21.15
Growth Performance of Pigs Fed Extruded Soybeans vs. Soybean Meal

Author(s)	Phase of Production[a]	Percentage Change from Soybean Meal					Treatment Conditions
		ADG	Efficiency of Gain	Carcass Leanness	Apparent N Digestibility	
Carlisle et al. (1973)	N	↓1	↑10	—	—	Fat and energy not equalized
Faber and Zimmerman (1973)	N	↑6	↑12	—	↑2	Soy oil used to equalize energy and CP:energy
Jurgens (1982)	N	↑9	↑1	—	—	Soy oil used to equalize ME and lysine:ME
Myer and Froseth (1983)	N	↑11	↑8	—	—	2% animal fat used to equalize CP:ME
Jurgens (1983)	N	↑4	↑4	—	—	Soy oil used to equalize ME and lysine:ME
Marty and Chavez (1993)	N	—	—	—	↑15	Fat and energy not equalized
Kim et al. (1998b)	N	↓3	↑5	—	—	Nutrient:calorie ratios not equalized
Kim et al. (1998b)	N	Equal	↑9	—	—	Soy oil used to equalize nutrient:calorie ratios
Noland et al. (1969)	G-F	↑1	Equal	—	—	Animal fat used to equalize energy and CP:energy
Koch et al. (1970)	G-F	↑2	↓2	—	—	Fat and energy not equalized
Carlisle et al. (1973)	G-F	↑3	↑12	—	—	Energy and fat not equalized, Exp. 1
Carlisle et al. (1973)	G-F	↓7	↑7	—	—	Energy and fat not equalized, Exp. 2
Bayley and Summers (1975)	G-F	—	—	↑3	↓3	Fat not equalized
Myer and Froseth (1983)	G-F	↑4	↓9	—	—	2% animal fat used to equalize lysine:ME
Rudolph et al. (1983)	G-F	—	—	—	↓15 (ileum)	Fat not equalized
Jurgens (1985)	G-F	↑9	↑9	↓2	—	Fat and ME not equalized
Wahlstrom et al. (1986)	G-F	↑5	↑8	↓4	—	Fat and ME not equalized
Hancock et al. (1991b)	G-F	↑1	↑5	—	↑7	Soy oil used to equalize ME and lysine:ME
Marty and Chavez (1993)	G-F	—	—	—	↑5	Fat and energy not equalized
Kim et al. (1998a)	G-F	↑5	↑14	↓4	—	Nutrient:calorie ratios not equalized

[a] Phase of production: N = nursery; G-F = growing-finishing.

ulcers in pigs while capturing most of the benefits of fine grinding. Also, there has been much interest in identification of a diet supplement that would allow swine producers to capitalize on the growth performance improvements from advanced feed manufacturing practices without compromising health status of their pigs. Patience et al. (1986) indicated that pH of the gastrointestinal tract was altered by adding buffers to the diet. Because Maxwell et al. (1970) observed a correlation between decreased pH in the stomach and increased ulceration, alkaline salts (buffers) could help to neutralize the acidity of the stomach and improve morphology of the gastric mucosa. Wondra et al. (1995a) fed pigs corn–soybean meal diets with 1% $NaHCO_3$ or 1% $KHCO_3$ and reported a mild reduction in scores for stomach lesions. This difference resulted from fewer pigs developing lesions (26 vs. 37% for the buffer vs. control treatments, respectively). Similar results were reported by Sorrell et al. (1996) where 1% $NaHCO_3$ in diets for finishing pigs decreased scores for stomach lesions. More research is needed to verify this response and to evaluate other antiulcer feed additives that might be economically viable for use in the swine industry.

XIV. CONCLUSIONS

Through use of advanced grain-processing technologies such as fine grinding, pelleting, and extrusion/expansion, the swine industry can greatly improve feed utilization. From the literature reviewed for this chapter, "rules of thumb" of 1.3% greater efficiency of gain for every 100-µm decrease in particle size of corn and additional 6 and 7% improvements in rate and efficiency of gain, respectively, with pelleting are proposed.

Because feed costs are easily the greatest economic input into swine production, maximizing nutrient utilization is an area that will continue to receive much attention. Even though improvements have been significant during the past 20 to 30 years, the next two to three decades undoubtedly hold exciting and profound technological advancements in ingredient processing for use in swine diets.

REFERENCES

Amornthewaphat, N., J. D. Hancock, K. C. Behnke, R. H. Hines, G. A. Kennedy, H. Cao, J. S. Park, C. S. Maloney, D. W. Dean, J. M. Derouchey, and D. J. Lee. 1999. Effects of feeder design and pellet quality on growth performance, nutrient digestibility, carcass characteristics, and water usage in finishing pigs, *J. Anim. Sci.*, 77(Suppl. 1):55 (Abstr.).

ASAE. 1983. Method of determining and expressing fineness of feed materials by sieving, American Society for Agricultural Engineers, Standard S319, Yearbook of Standards, 325.

ASAE. 1987. Wafers, pellets, crumbles — definitions and methods for determining density, durability, and moisture content, American Society for Agricultural Engineers, Standard S269, Yearbook of Standards, 318.

Aubel, C. E. 1945. The comparative value of various sorghum grains as swine fattening feeds, *Kans. Agric. Exp. Sta. Circ.*, 258:4.

Aubel, C. E. 1955. The comparative value of corn and whole and ground milo as swine fattening feeds, *Kans. Agric. Exp. Sta. Circ.*, 320:24.

Ayles, H. L., R. M. Friendship, and R. O. Ball. 1996. Effect of dietary particle size on gastric ulcers, assessed by endoscopic examination, and relationship between ulcer severity and growth performance of individually fed pigs, *Swine Health Prod.*, 4:211.

Baird, D. M. 1973. Influence of pelleting swine diets on metabolizable energy, growth, and carcass characteristics, *J. Anim. Sci.*, 36:516.

Baker, R. J. 1960. Factors That Affect the Granulation and Capacity in Grinding of Corn, Oats, and Sorghum Grain with a Hammermill, M.S. thesis, Kansas State University, Manhattan.

Barratt, M. E. J., P. J. Strachan, and P. Porter. 1978. Antibody mechanisms implicated in digestive disturbances following ingestion of soya protein in calves and piglets, *Clin. Exp. Immunol.*, 31:305.

Bayley, H. S., and J. D. Summers. 1975. Nutritional evaluation of extruded full-fat soybeans and rapeseeds using pigs and chickens, *Can. J. Anim. Sci.*, 55:441.

Berruecos, J. M., and O. W. Robison. 1972. Inheritance of gastric ulcers in swine, *J. Anim. Sci.*, 35:20.

Beumer, I. H., 1991. Quality assurance as a tool to reduce losses in animal feed production, *Adv. Feed Technol.*, 6:6.

Brendemuhl, J. H., A. J. Lewis, and E. R. Peo, Jr. 1987. Effect of protein and energy intake by primiparous sows during lactation on sow and litter performance and sow serum thyroxine and urea concentrations, *J. Anim. Sci.*, 64:1060.

Brooks, P. H., and D. J. A. Cole. 1972. Studies in sow reproduction. 1. The effect of nutrition between weaning and remating on the reproductive performance of primiparous sows, *Anim. Prod.*, 15:259.

Bullard, J. J. 1951. Gastric ulcers in a large boar, *J. Am. Vet. Med. Assoc.*, 119:120.

Cabrera, M. R., J. D. Hancock, R. H. Hines, K. C. Behnke, and P. J. Bramel-Cox. 1994. Sorghum genotype and particle size affect milling characteristics, growth performance, nutrient digestibility, and stomach morphology in finishing pigs, *J. Anim. Sci.*, 72(Suppl. 1):55 (Abstr.).

Cao, H., J. D. Hancock, J. M. Jiang, J. R. Froetschner, J. S. Park, K. C. Behnke, and R. H. Hines. 1998a. Effects of expander processing (after steam conditioning) on the nutritional value of whole soybeans in nursery pigs, *J. Anim. Sci.*, 76(Suppl. 1):183 (Abstr.).

Cao, H., J. D. Hancock, J. M. Jiang, J. R. Froetschner, J. S. Park, C. S. Maloney, K. C. Behnke, and R. H. Hines. 1998b. Effects of expander processing on nutritional value of whole soybeans in nursery pigs, *J. Anim. Sci.*, 76(Suppl. 2):49 (Abstr.).

Carlisle, G. R., D. H. Baker, B. G. Harmon, and A. H. Jensen. 1973. Roasted and extruded soybeans in diets for swine, In *Proc. Illinois Pork Industry Day*, December 4, p. 11.

Chamberlain, C. C., G. M. Merriman, E. R. Lidvall, and C. T. Gamble. 1967. Effects of feed processing method and diet form on the incidence of esophagogastric ulcers in swine, *J. Anim. Sci.*, 26:72.

Dunsford, B. R., D. A. Knabe, and W. E. Haensly. 1989. Effect of dietary soybean meal on the microscopic anatomy of the small intestine in the early weaned pig, *J. Anim. Sci.*, 67:1855.

Eisemann, J. H., and R. A. Argenzio. 1999a. Effects of diet and housing density on growth and stomach morphology in pigs, *J. Anim. Sci.*, 77:2709.

Eisemann, J. H., and R. A. Argenzio. 1999b. Effects of diets differing in propensity to promote gastric lesions on defense systems in gastric mucosae, *J. Anim. Sci.*, 77:2715.

Faber, J. L., and D. R. Zimmerman. 1973. Evaluation of infrared-roasted and extruder-processed soybeans in baby pig diets, *J. Anim. Sci.*, 36:902.

Fadel, J. G., C. W. Newman, R. K. Newman, and H. Graham. 1988. Effects of extrusion cooking of barley on ileal and fecal digestibilities of dietary components in pigs, *Can. J. Anim. Sci.*, 68:891.

Ferket, P. R. 1991. Technological advances could make extrusion an economically feasible alternative to pelleting, *Feedstuffs*, 63(9):1.

Fraps, G. S. 1932. Digestibility and production coefficients of pig feeds, *Tex. Agric. Exp. Sta. Bull.*, 454.

Froetschner, J. R., J. D. Hancock, K. C. Behnke, B. W. Senne, and Z. J. Cheng. 1998. Effects of sorghum genotype and processing method on growth performance of nursery pigs, *J. Anim. Sci.*, 76(Suppl. 1):182 (Abstr.).

Giesemann, M. A., A. J. Lewis, J. D. Hancock, and E. R. Peo, Jr. 1990. Effect of particle size of corn and grain sorghum on growth and digestibility of growing pigs, *J. Anim. Sci.*, 68(Suppl. 1):104 (Abstr.).

Goodband, R. D., and R. H. Hines. 1988. An evaluation of barley in starter diets for swine, *J. Anim. Sci.*, 66:3086.

Hancock, J. D., R. H. Hines, G. E. Fitzner, and T. L. Gugle. 1991a. Effect of extrusion processing on the nutritional value of sorghum and soybeans for finishing pigs, In *Proc. 17th Biennial Grain Sorghum Utilization Conference*, February 17–20, Lubbock, TX, p. 113.

Hancock, J. D., R. H. Hines, and T. L. Gugle. 1991b. Extrusion of sorghum, soybean meal, and whole soybeans improves growth performance and nutrient digestibility in finishing pigs, Kansas State University Swine Day, Kansas Agric. Exp. Sta. Rep. Prog. No. 641, p. 92.

Hancock, J. D., R. H. Hines, B. T. Richert, and T. L. Gugle. 1992. Extruded corn, sorghum, wheat, and barley for finishing pig, Kansas State University Swine Day, Agric. Exp. Sta. Rep. Prog. No. 667, p. 130.

Hancock, J. D., A. J. Lewis, D. B. Jones, M. A. Giesemann, and B. J. Healy. 1990a. Processing method affects the nutritional value of low-inhibitor soybeans for nursery pigs, Kansas State University Swine Day, Kansas Agric. Exp. Sta. Rep. Prog. No. 610, p. 52.

Hancock, J. D., A. J. Lewis, P. G. Reddy, D. B. Jones, and M. A. Giesemann. 1991c. Extrusion processing of low-inhibitor soybeans improves growth performance of nursery pigs fed protein-adequate diets, Kansas State University Swine Day, Kansas Agric. Exp. Sta. Rep. Prog. No. 641, p. 40.

Hancock, J. D., E. R. Peo, Jr., A. J. Lewis, and J. D. Crenshaw. 1990b. Effects of ethanol extraction and duration of heat treatment of soybean flakes on the utilization of soybean protein by growing rats and pigs, *J. Anim. Sci.*, 68:3233.

Hancock, J. D., E. R. Peo, Jr., A. J. Lewis, and R. A. Moxley. 1990c. Effects of ethanol extraction and heat treatment of soybean flakes on function and morphology of pig intestine, *J. Anim. Sci.*, 68:3244.

Hanke, H. E., J. W. Rust, R. J. Meade, and L. E. Hanson. 1972. Influence of source of soybean protein and of pelleting on rate of gain and gain/feed of growing swine, *J. Anim. Sci.*, 35:958.

Hanrahan, T. J. 1984. Effect of pellet size and pellet quality on pig performance, *Anim. Feed Sci. Technol.*, 10:277.

Harris, D. D., L. F. Tribble, and D. E. Orr, Jr. 1979. The effects of meal versus different size pellets of sorghum-soybean meal diets for finishing swine, Proc. 27th Annual Swine Short Course, Texas Tech University, Agric. Sci. Tech. Rep. T-5–144, p. 57.

Healy, B. J., J. D. Hancock, G. A. Kennedy, P. J. Bramel-Cox, K. C. Behnke, and R. H. Hines. 1994. Optimum particle size of corn and hard and soft sorghum for nursery pigs, *J. Anim. Sci.*, 72:2227.

Hedde, R. D., T. O. Lindsey, R. C. Parish, H. D. Daniels, E. A. Morgenthien, and H. B. Lewis. 1985. Effect of diet particle size and feeding H_2-receptor antagonists on gastric ulcers in swine, *J. Anim. Sci.*, 61:179.

Heimann, M. A. 1983. Energy consumption and machine efficiency in particle reduction: a roller mill and hammermill comparison. First International Symposium on Particle Size Reduction in the Feed Industry. Kansas State University, Manhattan.

Herkelman, K. L., S. L. Rodhouse, T. L. Veum, and M. R. Ellersieck. 1990. Effect of extrusion on the ileal and fecal digestibilities of lysine in yellow corn in diets for young pigs, *J. Anim. Sci.*, 68:2414.

Holden, P. J. 1988. Diagnosing feed mixing problems is swine herds, *Agri-Practice*, 9(4):3.

Hongtrakul, K., J. R. Bergstrom, R. D. Goodband, K. C. Behnke, I. H. Kim, W. B. Nessmith, M. D. Tokach, and J. L. Nelssen. 1996. The effect of ingredients processing and diet complexity on growth performance of the segregated early-weaned pig, Kansas State University Swine Day, Kansas Agric. Exp. Sta. Rep. Prog. No. 772, p. 43.

Jensen, A. H., and D. E. Becker. 1965. Effect of pelleting diets and dietary components on the performance of young pigs, *J. Anim. Sci.*, 24:392.

Johnston, S. L., J. D. Hancock, R. H. Hines, G. A. Kennedy, S. L. Traylor, B. J. Chae, and I. K. Han. 1999a. Effects of expander conditioning of corn- and sorghum-based diets on pellet quality and performance in finishing pigs and lactating sows, *Asian-Aust. J. Anim. Sci.*, 12:565.

Johnston, S. L., R. H. Hines, J. D. Hancock, K. C. Behnke, S. L. Traylor, B. J. Chae, and I. K. Han. 1999b. Effects of expander conditioning of complex nursery diets on growth performance of weanling pigs, *Asian-Aust. J. Anim. Sci.*, 12:395.

Johnston, S. L., R. H. Hines, J. D. Hancock, K. C. Behnke, S. L. Traylor, B. J. Chae, and I. K. Han. 1999c. Effects of conditioners (standard, long-term, and expander) on pellet quality and growth performance in nursery and finishing pigs, *Asian-Aust. J. Anim. Sci.*, 12:558.

Jurgens, M. H. 1982. Performance of early-weaned pigs fed extruded soybean products, Iowa Agric. Exp. Sta. Rep. Prog. AS-535-E, p. 1.

Jurgens, M. H. 1983. Performance of early weaned pigs fed extruded soybean products, Iowa Agric. Exp. Sta. Rep. Prog. No. AS-539-E, p. 1.

Jurgens, M. H. 1985. Performance and carcass measurements of growing-finishing pigs fed extruded soybean products, Iowa Agric. Exp. Sta. Rep. Prog. No. AS-570-E, p. 1.

Kilshaw, P. J., and J. W. Sissons. 1979. Gastrointestinal allergy to soybean protein in preruminant calves. Antibody production and digestive disturbances in calves fed heated soybean flour, *Res. Vet. Sci.*, 27:361.

Kim, I. H., J. D. Hancock, L. L. Burnham, G. A. Kennedy, R. H. Hines, and C. S. Kim. 1998a. Effects of feeding diets containing dry-extruded whole soybeans on growth, carcass characteristics, and stomach morphology in finishing pigs, *Kor. J. Anim. Nutr. Feed.*, 22:73.

Kim, I. H., J. D. Hancock, M. R. Cabrera, J. H. Kim, and C. S. Kim. 1998b. Effects of alternative soy sources and dry-extruded whole soybeans, with or without adjustment for nutrient:calorie ratios in early-weaned pigs, *Kor. J. Anim. Sci.*, 40:165.

Kim, I. H., J. D. Hancock, and R. H. Hines. 2000a. Influence of processing method on ileal digestibility of nutrients from soybeans in growing and finishing pigs, *Asian-Aust. J. Anim. Sci.*, 13:192.

Kim, I. H., J. D. Hancock, R. H. Hines, and T. L. Gugle. 2000b. Roasting and extruding affect nutrient utilization from soybeans in 5- and 10-kg nursery pigs, *Asian-Aust. J. Anim. Sci.*, 13:200.

King, R. H., and I. H. Williams. 1984. The effect of nutrition on the reproductive performance of first-litter sows. 2. Protein and energy intakes during lactation, *Anim. Prod.*, 38:249.

Koch, B. A., R. H. Hines, and D. T. Lafferty. 1970. Processed whole soybeans in growing-finishing rations, Proc. Kansas State University Swine Day, p. 7.

Koch, K. 1996. Hammer mills and roller mills, Kansas State University Coop. Extension Service Bull. MS-496.

Lavorel, O., J. Fekete, and M. Leuillet. 1984. A comparative study concerning the utilization of pellets of different diameters by the weaned piglet; 14th French Swine Research Day, Institut National de la Recherche Agronomique, Paris, p. 36.

Lawrence, B. V., D. B. Anderson, O. Adeola, and T. R. Cline. 1998. Changes in pars esophageal tissue appearance of the porcine stomach in response to transportation, feed deprivation, and diet composition, *J. Anim. Sci.*, 76:788.

Lawrence, T. L. J. 1967. High level cereal grain diets for the growing-finishing pig. II. The effect of cereal preparation on the performance of pigs fed diets containing high levels of maize, sorghum, and barley, *J. Agric. Sci.* (Cambridge), 69:271.

Lawrence, T. L. J. 1970. Some effects of including differently processed barley in the diet of the growing pig. 1. Growth rate, food conversion efficiency, digestibility, and rate of passage through the gut, *Anim. Prod.*, 12:139.

Lawrence, T. L. J. 1983. The effects of cereal particle size and pelleting on the nutritive value of oat-based diets for the growing pig, *Anim. Feed Sci. Technol.*, 8:91.

Li, D. F., J. L. Nelssen, P. G. Reddy, F. Blecha, J. D. Hancock, G. L. Allee, R. D. Goodband, and R. D. Klemm. 1990. Transient hypersensitivity to soybean meal in the early weaned pig, *J. Anim. Sci.*, 68:1790.

Lindemann, M. D., D. J. Blodgett, E. T. Kornegay, and G. G. Schurig. 1993. Potential amelioration of aflatoxicosis in weanling/growing swine, *J. Anim. Sci.*, 71:171.

Lindley, J. A., 1991. Mixing processes for agricultural and food materials: I. Fundamentals of mixing, *Agric. Eng. Res.*, 48:153.

Luce, W. G., I. T. Omtvedt, and C. V. Maxwell. 1973. Effect of pellet size on pig performance, *J. Anim. Sci.*, 36:204 (Abstr.).

Mahan, D. C., R. A. Pickett, T. W. Perry, T. M. Curtin, W. R. Featherson, and W. M. Beeson. 1966. Influence of various nutritional factors and physical form of feed on esophagogastric ulcers in swine, *J. Anim. Sci.*, 25:1019.

Marty, B. J., and E. R. Chavez. 1993. Effect of heat processing on digestive energy and other nutrient digestibilities of full-fat soybeans fed to weaner, grower, and finishing pigs, *Can. J. Anim. Sci.*, 73:411.

Mavromichalis, I., J. D. Hancock, G. A. Kennedy, R. H. Hines, J. M. Derouchey, B. W. Senne, and S. P. Sorrell. 1998. Effects of enzyme supplementation and particle size of wheat-based diets on nursery and finishing pigs, Kansas State University Swine Day, Kansas Agric. Exp. Sta. Rep. Prog. No. 819, p. 239.

Maxwell, C. V., E. M. Reimann, W. G. Hoekstra, T. Kowalczyk, N. J. Benevenga, and R. H. Grummer. 1970. Effect of dietary particle size on lesion development and on the contents of various regions of the swine stomach, *J. Anim. Sci.*, 30:911.

Maxwell, C. V., E. M. Reimann, W. G. Hoekstra, T. Kowalczyk, N. J. Benevenga, and R. H. Grummer. 1972. Use of tritiated water to assess, *in vivo*, the effect of dietary particle size on the mixing of stomach contents of swine, *J. Anim. Sci.*, 34:212.

McEllhiney, R. R. 1983. Roller mill grinding, *Feed Manag.*, 34:42.

Myer, R. O., and J. A. Froseth. 1983. Extruded mixtures of beans (*Phaseolus vulgaris*) and soybeans as protein sources in barley-based swine diets, *J. Anim. Sci.*, 57:296.

NCR-42 Committee on Swine Nutrition. 1969. Cooperative regional studies with growing swine: effects of source of ingredient, form of diet, and location on rate and efficiency of gain of growing swine, *J. Anim. Sci.*, 29:927.

Noland, P. R., C. A. Baugus, R. O. Lawrence, and Z. Johnson. 1969. Potential role of extruded soybeans in swine rations, Feed Bag Mag., October 18, p. 17.

Noland, P. R., D. R. Campbell, R. K. Gage, Jr., R. N. Sharp, and Z. B. Johnson. 1976. Evaluation of processed soybeans and grains in diets for young pigs, *J. Anim. Sci.*, 43:763.

NRC. 1988. *Nutrient Requirements of Swine*, 9th ed., National Academy Press, Washington, D.C.
NRC. 1998. *Nutrient Requirements of Swine*, 10th ed., National Academy Press, Washington, D.C.
Ohh, S. J., G. L. Allee, K. C. Behnke, and C. W. Deyoe. 1983. Effect of particle size of corn and sorghum grain on performance and digestibility of nutrients for weaned pigs, *J. Anim. Sci.*, 57(Suppl. 1):260 (Abstr.).
Osborne, T. B., and L. B. Mendel. 1917. The use of soybean as food, *J. Biol. Chem.*, 32:369.
Owsley, W. F., D. A. Knabe, and T. D. Tanksley, Jr. 1981. Effect of sorghum particle size on digestibility of nutrients at the terminal ileum and over the total digestive tract of growing-finishing pigs, *J. Anim. Sci.*, 52:557.
Park, J. S., J. D. Hancock, C. A. Maloney, H. Cao, and R. H. Hines. 1998. Effects of expander processing of wheat-based diets for finishing pigs, *J. Anim. Sci.*, 76(Suppl. 1):186 (Abstr.).
Patience, J. F., R. E. Austic, and R. D. Boyd. 1986. The effect of sodium bicarbonate or potassium bicarbonate on acid-base status and protein and energy digestibility in swine, *Nutr. Res.*, 6:263.
Peisker, M. 1994a. An expander's affect on wheat bran in piglet rations, *Extrusion Commun.*, 7(2):18.
Peisker, M. 1994b. Influence of expansion on feed components, *Feed Mix*, 2(3):26.
Peisker, M. 1996. Expanders in the feed industry and economics of using them, presented at American Feed Industry Assoc. Nutrition Symposium, St. Louis, MO.
Pickett, R. A., W. H. Fugate, R. B. Harrington, T. W. Perry, and T. M. Curtin. 1969. Influence of feed preparation and number of pigs per pen on performance and occurrence of esophagogastric ulcers in swine, *J. Anim. Sci.*, 28:837.
Reece, F. N., B. D. Lott, and J. W. Deaton. 1985. The effects of feed form, grinding method, energy level, and gender on broiler performance in a moderate (21°C) environment, *Poult. Sci.*, 64:1834.
Reese, D. E., B. D. Moser, E. R. Peo, Jr., A. J. Lewis, D. R. Zimmerman, J. E. Kinder, and W. W. Stroup. 1982. Influence of energy intake during lactation on the interval from weaning to first estrus in sows, *J. Anim. Sci.*, 55:590.
Regina, D. C., J. H. Eisemann, J. A. Lang, and R. A. Argenzio. 1999. Changes in gastric contents in pigs fed a finely ground and pelleted or coarsely ground meal diet, *J. Anim. Sci.*, 77:2712.
Reimann, E. M., C. V. Maxwell, T. Kowalczyk, N. J. Benevenga, R. H. Grummer, and W. G. Hoekstra. 1968. Effect of fineness of grind of corn on gastric lesions and contents of swine, *J. Anim. Sci.*, 27:992.
Reimer, L. 1992. Conditioning, Proc. Northern Crops Institute Feed Mill Management and Feed Manufacturing Technol. Short Course, California Pellet Mill Co., Crawfordsville, IN, p. 7.
Ricker, J. T., III, T. W. Perry, R. A. Pickett, and T. M. Curtin. 1967. Influence of various grains on the incidence of esophagogastric ulcers in swine, *J. Anim. Sci.*, 26:736.
Rudolph, B. C., L. S. Boggs, D. A. Knabe, T. D. Tanksley, Jr., and S. A. Anderson. 1983. Digestibility of nitrogen and amino acids in soybean products for pigs, *J. Anim. Sci.*, 57:373.
Sauer, W. C., S. C. Stothers, and G. D. Phillips. 1977. Apparent availability of amino acids in corn, wheat, and barley for growing pigs, *Can. J. Anim. Sci.*, 57:585.
Seegraber, F. J., and J. L. Morrill. 1979. Affect of soy protein on intestinal absorptive ability of calves by the xylose absorption test, *J. Dairy Sci.*, 62:972.
Silver, E. R. 1932. Characteristics of feed mill performance, *Agric. Eng.*, 13:31.
Sissons, J. W., R. H. Smith, and D. Hewitt. 1979. The effect of giving feeds containing soya-bean meal treated or extracted with ethanol on digestive processes in the preruminant calf, *Br. J. Nutr.*, 42:477.
Sissons, J. W., R. H. Smith, D. Hewitt, and A. Nyrup. 1982. Prediction of the suitability of soya-bean products for feeding to preruminant calves by an *in vitro* immunochemical method, *Br. J. Nutr.*, 47:311.
Skoch, E. R., S. F. Binder, C. W. Deyoe, G. L. Allee, and K. C. Behnke. 1983a. Effects of pelleting conditions on performance of pigs fed a corn–soybean meal diet, *J. Anim. Sci.*, 57:922.
Skoch, E. R., S. F. Binder, C. W. Deyoe, G. L. Allee, and K. C. Behnke. 1983b. Effects of steam pelleting conditions and extrusion cooking on a swine diet containing wheat middlings, *J. Anim. Sci.*, 57:929.
Sorrell, P., J. D. Hancock, I. H. Kim, R. H. Hines, G. A. Kennedy, and L. L. Burnham. 1996. Effects of fat and sodium bicarbonate on growth performance and stomach morphology in finishing pigs, *J. Anim. Sci.*, 74(Suppl. 1):178 (Abstr.).
Stark, C. R. 1994. Functional characteristics of ingredients in the formation of quality pellets. In Pellet Quality, Ph.D. dissertation, Kansas State University, Manhattan.
Stark, C. R., K. C. Behnke, J. D. Hancock, S. L. Traylor, and R. H. Hines. 1994. Effect of diet form and fines in pelleted diets on growth performance of nursery pigs, *J. Anim. Sci.*, 72(Suppl. 1):214.

Traylor, S. L., J. D. Hancock, K. C. Behnke, C. R. Stark, and R. H. Hines. 1994. Uniformity of mixed diets affects growth performance in nursery and finishing pigs, *J. Anim. Sci.*, 72(Suppl. 2):59.

Traylor, S. L., K. C. Behnke, J. D. Hancock, P. Sorrell, and R. H. Hines. 1996. Effects of pellet size on growth performance in nursery and finishing pigs, *J. Anim. Sci.*, 74(Suppl. 1):67.

Traylor, S. L., K. C. Behnke, J. D. Hancock, R. H. Hines, S. L. Johnston, B. J. Chae, and I. K. Han. 1999. Effects of expander operating conditions on nutrient digestibility in finishing pigs, *Asian-Aust. J. Anim. Sci.*, 12:400.

Tribble, L. F., and A. M. Lennon. 1975. Meal versus pelleted sorghum-soybean meal rations for growing-finishing swine. Proc. 23rd Annual Swine Short Course, Texas Tech University Agric. Sci. Tech. Rep. No. T-5-111, p. 31.

Tribble, L. F., D. D. Harris, and D. E. Orr, Jr. 1979. Effect of pellet size (diameter) on performance of finishing swine. Proc. 27th Swine Short Course, Texas Tech University Agric. Sci. Tech. Rep. T-5-144, p. 59.

Tribble, L. F., D. E. Orr, Jr., C. R. Richardson, and D. Tunmire. 1980. Value of a pellet binder for growing-finishing swine. Proc. 28th Annual Swine Short Course, Texas Tech University Agric. Sci. Tech. Rep. T-5, p. 154.

Vermeer, M. E. 1993. Roller mills versus hammermills: grinding economics, *Feed Manag.*, 44(9):39.

Wahlstrom, R. C., B. S. Borg, and G. W. Libal. 1986. Extruded soybeans for finishing swine, South Dakota State University Swine Day Rep., p. 1.

Wicker, D. L., and D. R. Poole. 1991. How is your mixer performing? *Feed Manag.*, 42(9):40.

Wilcox, R. A., and D. L. Unruh. 1986. Feed mixers and feed mixing times, Kansas State University Coop. Extension Service Bull. MF-829.

Wondra, K. J., J. D. Hancock, K. C. Behnke, and R. H. Hines. 1995a. Effects of dietary buffers on growth performance, nutrient digestibility, and stomach morphology in finishing pigs, *J. Anim. Sci.*, 73:414.

Wondra, K. J., J. D. Hancock, K. C. Behnke, R. H. Hines, and C. R. Stark. 1995b. Effects of particle size and pelleting on growth performance, nutrient digestibility, and stomach morphology in finishing pigs, *J. Anim. Sci.*, 73:757.

Wondra, K. J., J. D. Hancock, K. C. Behnke, and C. R. Stark. 1995c. Effects of mill type and particle size uniformity on growth performance, nutrient digestibility, and stomach morphology in finishing pigs, *J. Anim. Sci.*, 73:2564.

Wondra, K. J., J. D. Hancock, G. A. Kennedy, K. C. Behnke, and K. R. Wondra. 1995d. Effects of reducing particle size of corn in lactation diets on energy and nitrogen metabolism in second-parity sows, *J. Anim. Sci.*, 73:427.

Wondra, K. J., J. D. Hancock, G. A. Kennedy, R. H. Hines, and K. C. Behnke. 1995e. Reducing particle size of corn in lactation diets from 1,200 to 400 micrometers improves sow and litter performance, *J. Anim. Sci.*, 73:421.

Woodsman, H. E., R. E. Evans, and A. W. M. Kitchin. 1932. The value of oats in the nutrition of swine, *J. Agric. Sci.* (Cambridge), 22:657.

Young, L. R. 1970. Mechanical Durability of Feed Pellets, M.S. thesis, Kansas State University, Manhattan.

22 Effects of Facility Design on Behavior and Feed and Water Intake

Michael C. Brumm and Harold W. Gonyou

CONTENTS

I. Introduction 499
II. Characteristics of Pigs' Eating Behavior 500
    A. Meal Frequency 500
    B. Diurnal Patterns and Light:Dark Sequences 500
    C. Eating Speed and Total Duration 501
    D. Feed Restriction 501
    E. Eating Behavior after Weaning 502
III. Effect of Feeder Design on Feed Intake 502
    A. Number of Feeding Spaces 502
    B. Quality of Feeding Spaces 503
    C. Feeder Design and Feed Wastage 504
    D. Wet and Wet/Dry Feeders 505
    E. Social Facilitation 506
IV. Impact of Drinker Design/Location on Feed Intake 508
    A. General 508
    B. Extraneous Voltage 509
V. Impact of Space Allocation and Group Size on Feed Intake 510
    A. General 510
    B. Pigs per Social Group 512
    C. Interaction of Diet and Space 513
VI. Conclusions 514
References 514

I. INTRODUCTION

Management is the means by which producers attempt to maximize the productivity and profitability of a swine enterprise. Good management is based on knowledge of the biological characteristics of the animal and technology available to provide an environment that complements these features. Feed intake is one of the primary determinants of efficient pig production, including the design of nutritional programs. As various feeding technologies available to the swine industry are considered, one should consider the characteristics of the pig that will determine their success or failure. These biological characteristics include eating behavior.

Animals are able to adapt their behavior to their environment, using both an innate ability and their previous experience. This plasticity of behavior is often taken for granted, and it is assumed that animals can adapt to any situation. Although behavioral adaptation is very robust, one must be aware of the potential limitations to this flexibility. This chapter examines aspects of the eating behavior of pigs and how feeding and facility management affects feed intake.

II. CHARACTERISTICS OF PIGS' EATING BEHAVIOR

Pigs have been described as nibblers, implying that they eat small amounts of feed on a frequent basis. This description would seem to be based on casual observations and not on a systematic analysis of data. The key to studying eating behavior is to determine when the motivation of the animal changes from that of eating to another activity. The analysis involves examining the pattern of intervals between periods of eating (Martin and Bateson, 1993). Shorter intervals result from pauses during eating to apprehend food, obtain water, or reposition, but do not represent a change in motivation. Longer intervals separate true bouts of eating behavior or meals. The first such analysis of intermeal intervals in growing pigs resulted in average meal criteria intervals of 20 min; that is, breaks in eating of less than 20 min are considered part of the same meal, while those >20 min are separate meals (Hsia and Wood-Gush, 1984). More recent data, involving more animals, suggests a meal criteria interval of approximately 5 to 6 min for either group or individually penned pigs (Petrie and Gonyou, 1988; de Haer and Merks, 1992).

A. Meal Frequency

Only after a meal criteria interval has been established is it possible to determine the number, length, and size of meals. Individually penned pigs eat 12 meals/day when on an 8.5:15.5 light:dark (L:D) cycle, and 18 meals/day when in continuous light (Hsia and Wood-Gush, 1984). de Haer and Merks (1992) reported 20 and 9 meals/day for individually penned and groups of eight pigs, respectively. Fewer meals occur when pigs are older, in groups, and exposed to normal daylengths. More meals occur in individually penned pigs, if light is continuous, and in young pigs.

B. Diurnal Patterns and Light:Dark Sequences

In general, pigs are diurnal animals. That is, they are most active during the day. However, feral pigs are able to adapt to a night-active, or nocturnal, activity pattern if exposed to even moderate hunting levels (Hanson and Karstad, 1959). The eating pattern observed in domestic pigs seems to be affected by illumination patterns and accessibility to the feeder. A crepuscular (morning and afternoon peaks) eating pattern is most common if lights are programmed for 8 to 12 h of light a day (Walker, 1991; de Haer and Merks, 1992). It is not uncommon for producers with confinement finishing facilities to install lighting with timers in the belief that longer periods of lighting will stimulate activity and hence feed intake, resulting in improved rates of gain. Research results do not support this belief.

Furlan et al. (1986a) reported no difference in daily gain and poorer feed conversion during the growing phase as lighting periods increased from natural day length to 18 to 24 h of light. The intensity of the light provided for the 18- and 24-h treatment was not specified. In a second experiment (Furlan et al., 1986b), they reported the best gain and feed intakes occurred in pigs given no daylight when compared with natural daylight and various L:D cycles.

In 1977, Baldwin and Meese demonstrated that pigs prefer light, but will not perform operant responses to obtain prolonged illumination. Using a light:dark preference method in which the pigs could turn on lighting for as long as desired, pigs spent 72% of their time in light when tests started in darkness and 78% of their time in light when tests started with light.

Feeding behavior and feed consumption of 32-kg growing pigs were reported to exhibit two peaks in response to a 16L:8D regimen (Feddes et al., 1989). The first occurred when the lights were turned on and the second shortly after the lights were turned off. If a cyclic temperature pattern (26 to 40°C) was imposed in addition to lighting pattern, the feed consumption shifted to the coolest part of the thermal cycle.

Petchey (1987), in a review of the literature, concluded there was less social and exploratory behavior in the dark. He concluded that whereas newly weaned pigs probably have a minimum requirement of 6 h of low-intensity light offered in two daily periods, the effect of light on performance of growing-finishing pigs is less conclusive.

Ingram et al. (1985) demonstrated that whether pigs were grown in regimens of 12L:12D or 9L:9D, feed intake per 24-h period and body weights at age-constant times were similar. They concluded that although additional light was found to be associated with longer and leaner carcasses in ruminants (Forbes, 1982), genetic selection of swine has resulted in animals that readily conform with the conditions imposed in husbandry practices. In studies using continuous illumination, a single peak of eating extending from morning to afternoon is common (Gonyou et al., 1992). The crepuscular pattern may also occur as pigs avoid eating during the heat of the day. These results suggest that daytime patterns are very flexible, and that eating activity during the night is usually low.

C. Eating Speed and Total Duration

Eating speed seems to be proportional to live weight (Hsia and Wood-Gush, 1984). The fact that feed intake is proportional to metabolic weight, whereas rate of eating is proportional to body weight, results in greater total duration of eating (minutes per day) for small pigs than for large. Hyun et al. (1997) reported that total duration of eating dropped from over 100 min/day for 25-kg pigs, to <70 min/day for 75-kg pigs. The negative relationship between pig weight and total duration of eating means that the appropriate group size for a single space feeder is less for small pigs than for large.

The form in which a diet is presented will affect eating speed. In a study with sows feeding from a single space feeder (H. Gonyou, personal communication), meal feed took approximately 50% more time to be consumed than pellets. Addition of 30% water to the meal increased eating speed to that of pellets, but adding water to pellets had no effect. Gonyou and Lou (1999), using meal feed, determined that pigs eat as much as three times more quickly if the feed is mixed with water (1:1) before presentation, and that pigs fed from wet/dry feeders spend 17% less time eating but consume 5% more feed than those eating from dry feeders.

As a result of these and other factors, eating speeds derived from published reports differ considerably. Small and large pigs ate at rates of approximately 15 and 28 g/min, respectively, in the study by Hyun et al. (1997). The pigs of de Haer and Merks (1992) consumed feed at the rates of 32 and 27 g/min in group and individual pens, respectively. In the study by Walker (1991), pigs eating from spacious feeders ate at a rate of 37 g/min, whereas those of Gonyou et al. (1992), eating from a more restrictive feeder, consumed feed at a rate of only 22 g/min.

D. Feed Restriction

In some growing-finishing systems, feed is restricted to improve carcass characteristics. The resulting competition among the pigs for feed leads to variation among the animals in eating patterns, intake, and growth, particularly if feed access is limited (Botermans et al., 1997). Feed is also restricted in breeding boars and gestating sows, with the result that the level of hunger in the animals is quite high (Lawrence et al., 1988, Hutson, 1995). Under feed-restricted conditions, behaviors that are adjunctive to eating increase in frequency (Rushen, 1984), and may develop into stereotypies (Lawrence and Terlouw, 1993). Although other environmental conditions may play some role in the development of these activities, feed restriction is the predominant cause (Terlouw et al., 1991). Sows fed at maintenance levels or below spent 19% of their time engaged in repetitive behavior, compared with only 6% for those fed above maintenance (Cronin et al., 1986). Sows showing a high level of stereotypies produced 36% more heat than low stereotypies animals (Cronin et al., 1986).

E. Eating Behavior after Weaning

Pigs must make a transition in their eating behavior following weaning. In most cases this involves a change from suckling to eating solid feed. With weaning increasingly occurring before 3 weeks of age, few pigs have learned to eat solid feed before removal from the sow (Pajor et al., 1991). Pigs weaned at 21 days reach normal levels of eating behavior by approximately 24 h postweaning, compared with 36 h for those weaned at 12 days (Gonyou et al., 1998). A similar delay in feed intake is seen in pigs weaned at 14 vs. 28 days (Metz and Gonyou, 1990). Early weaning (<21 days) results in an increase in belly-nosing, which seems to be similar to the massage phase of suckling behavior (Metz and Gonyou, 1990; Gonyou et al., 1998; Worobec et al., 1999). The motivation for belly-nosing does not seem to be hunger, because it does not begin until 4 days postweaning, by which time pigs are already eating solid feed, and peaks 2 to 3 weeks postweaning, when the possibility of hunger seems remote (Gonyou et al., 1998).

III. EFFECT OF FEEDER DESIGN ON FEED INTAKE

A. Number of Feeding Spaces

Traditionally, advisors to the swine industry have recommended one feeding space per four pigs for the growing pig and one feeding space for four or five pigs for the finishing pig (MWPS, 1991). However, this recommendation makes no mention as to the dimensions of the space, the location of the space within the animal's environment, or other factors that influence the growing pig's interaction with the feed delivery device. Australian guidelines are somewhat more specific by recommending one space for four growing pigs with the space recommended to be 250 mm in length (Farrin, 1990). The European recommendation is one space per four pigs with the space averaging 59 mm/pig for 50-kg pigs and 74 mm/pig for 100-kg pigs (English et al., 1988).

The effect of feeder design was highlighted by the results of Morrow and Walker (1994b). In this study, groups of 20 pigs were provided a single-space feeder that had a nipple drinker in the feeder bowl. The addition of a stall to protect the eating pig from pen mates decreased the number of feeder visits per day, increased the average length of each feeder visit, and decreased aggressive behavior at the feeder. The authors concluded this was a larger change in behavior than that brought about by decreasing the number of pigs per feeder (Walker, 1991), or by doubling the number of feeders (Morrow and Walker, 1994a). Although not reported in this study, reductions in aggressive encounters at the feeder have been reported to reduce feed wastage (Baxter, 1986) and to improve feed conversion (Stoltenberg and Heege, 1984).

However, some competition at the feeder is apparently necessary. Hsia and Wood-Gush (1983) demonstrated that mild competition for feed access in groups with a stable social hierarchy leads to greater intake of feed in a shorter period of time. The competition must be for access to feed, not for delivery of feed. Morrow and Walker (1994a) demonstrated that the amount of effort a pig will expend to obtain feed is limited. If severe enough restrictions are imposed, the pig will restrict feed intake to a level less than that necessary to support maximum daily gain or to satisfy appetite, even if feeder access is available.

Research on feeder space allocations is surprisingly limited. Wahlstrom and Seerley (1960) concluded that one feeder space per six pigs within the weight range for 30 to 91 kg was probably adequate. They went on to add that research with more than six pigs per space must be conducted to establish the maximum number of pigs per feeder space with optimum performance.

Using 12 pigs per pen, Wahlstrom and Libal (1977) concluded there was no difference in performance when three, four, or six pigs were allotted for each available feeder space when wooden feeders were used as the feed delivery device for pigs from 28 to 70 kg. Leibbrandt (1978) provided either one 9.5-cm opening or four openings per pen of ten 6-kg weaned pigs. During the 4-week trial, daily gain and feed conversion were not significantly affected.

Brumm and Carlson (1985) reported on the effect of providing one, three, or five 14 × 14 cm feeder holes per pen of eight weaned pigs. They concluded that the best performance with the least amount of variation in gain for the 5-week nursery trial occurred in the pens with three feeder holes per eight pigs. Pigs in pens with one feed hole (eight pigs per hole) had the greatest weight variation, while pens with five feed holes (1.6 pigs/hole) had problems with messy feeders and wasted feed. Their conclusion was the recommendation of two to three pigs per feed hole for newly weaned pigs in flat deck nurseries.

Lindemann et al. (1987) investigated the interaction of feeder space allowance and floor space allowance on weaned pig performance. They concluded there were no interactions between feeder space allowance and floor space allowance within the range of allowances studied (2 to 12, 15.2-cm feeder sections and 5 to 12 pigs per pen). Unlike the results of Brumm and Carlson (1985), feeder space allowance did not result in any differences of within-pen variation in body weight or daily gain. These authors went on to cite results of McGlone et al. (1983) that evaluated physical and behavioral measures of feeding space for nursery-age swine. McGlone et al. (1983) observed that when pigs were housed four per pen and allowed varying amounts of feeding space over time, that the number of pigs feeding at one time never statistically equaled four, even when the feeding space provided was 50% larger than the total width of the pigs' heads.

More recently, McGlone et al. (1993) provided one, two, or three feeder spaces for 20 pigs/pen from 61 to 104 kg live weight. Using a meal diet, they concluded that the feeder space requirement is one space per ten pigs. Bates et al. (1993) in a study at a commercial swine finishing unit, also concluded that growing-finishing pigs can be stocked at a rate of ten pigs per feeder hole.

Morrow and Walker (1994c) recommended that two, single-space feeders be used in pens of 20 finishing pigs when meal diets are available *ad libitum*. They also recommended that the feeders be sited some distance apart (>2 m), not side by side, when pigs are provided 0.60 m^2 per pig pen space from 37 to 91 kg live weight. Growing pigs in this study showed a clear feeder preference, with a higher proportion of feed consumed from the feeder nearest the service passage.

Nielson et al. (1995) provided one single-space feeder for 5, 10, 15, or 20 pigs. Pigs in the 20 pigs/pen group made fewer but longer visits to the feeder when compared with the mean of the 5, 10, and 15 pigs groups. There was no difference between group sizes in daily feed intake, gain, or feed conversion for the 29-day observation period beginning at 34 kg initial weight with a pen space allocation of 1.05 m^2 per pig. Water was provided by a nipple drinker located in the feeder bowl.

B. QUALITY OF FEEDING SPACES

One of the critical factors limiting feed intake is feeder stocking rate (pigs/feeder space). Acceptable feeder stocking rates are dependent on the number of feeding spaces and the total duration of eating (minutes per pig per day). Although many feeders have some type of feeder space division, they may not accurately reflect the true space requirements. Baxter (1991) suggested that the minimum width of a feeding space should be the shoulder width of the pig, plus 10% to accommodate pig variability and movement. The shoulder width of a pig, in centimeters, is approximately $6.1 \times BW^{0.33}$, with body weight expressed in kilograms (Petherick, 1983). Thus, the width of feeder spaces for 5-, 25-, 50-, and 120-kg pigs would be 11.1, 19.8, 24.8, and 32.8 cm, respectively.

Baxter (1989) assessed the level of aggression among pigs when different amounts of trough space were provided. When no trough divisions were provided, aggression increased as trough length decreased. However, by providing head-sized barriers between standard feeding spaces, as defined above, aggression was reduced to the same level observed when four standard feeding spaces were provided per pig. Unless large amounts of trough space are provided, feeder spaces should be separated by head or head and shoulder barriers to minimize aggression at the feeder. The minimum distance between these dividers is the width of a feeding space for the largest pig intended to use the feeder. Wider feeding spaces not only make inefficient use of feeder space, but allow more than one pig to eat from a feeder space if the pigs are small. For example, a feeder space that is 40 cm wide can accommodate two 25-kg pigs, but a feeder space properly sized to accommodate one 120-kg pig (33 cm), will only accommodate one 25-kg pig.

Multiple spaced feeders must be carefully assessed for true feeding spaces when determining stocking density. A 170-cm feeder, with head divisions at 42 cm, can only accommodate four market-weight pigs. The same feeder with divisions at 33 cm, can accommodate five pigs. However, if nose dividers are provided at 28 cm, only five market weight pigs can be accommodated even though six "spaces" exist because shoulder/head dimensions are larger than facial/nose dimensions..

Baxter (1989) also examined the preference of pigs to eat at different heights. Although pigs prefer to eat from a surface at or slightly above floor level, they can eat from levels as high as their shoulders. Some feeders may have an elevated feeding surface or feed access lever, which could limit feeding if these exceed shoulder height. Elevated feeding surfaces usually require pigs to stand at an angle to the feeder and rotate their heads when eating (Gonyou and Lou, 1998).

The depth of the feeder, from the lip at the front of the feeder to the feed access point at the back, determines the extent to which pigs will step into the feed bowl or trough while eating. When feeder depth was only 20 cm, approximately 50% of 20-kg pigs would step into the feeder while eating. For 95-kg pigs, none would step in at feeder depths of 20 cm, <20% at a depth of 30 cm, and all of the pigs would when the depth was 40 cm (Gonyou and Lou, 1998). However, large pigs (95 kg) have difficulty eating from an area closer than 20 cm from the front of the feeder.

A compromise in feeder depth is needed when feeders are used over a wide range of pig body weights. Gonyou and Lou (1998) suggest that feeder depths for growing-finishing pigs should be 20 to 30 cm.

All the design concepts discussed above assume that the pig is standing at right angles to the feeder. However, when pigs are allowed to eat feed placed on the floor along a wall, they stand at an angle of approximately 30° from the vertical surface (Gonyou and Lou, 1998). Such a position may facilitate apprehension of the feed. It may be advisable to consider designs that provide such an angle to the feed access point.

C. Feeder Design and Feed Wastage

The traditional approach to reduce feed wastage has been to increase the difficulty of accessing the feed. Two ways of achieving this restriction are to reduce the gap at the point of feed access, and to restrict head movement in the feeder bowl or trough. Taylor (1990) and Baxter (1989) both developed feeders that encouraged free movement of the pig's head while eating with the assumption that more natural eating movements do not contribute to feed wastage. The resulting feeders have both been reported to have low wastage rates. Many feeders designed in this manner have a fixed-width feed delivery gap that allows feed to flow relatively freely. In addition, these nonrestrictive feeders may facilitate eating and increase eating speed. The eating speed of 80-kg pigs from a "spacious" feeder was approximately 37 g/min (Walker, 1991), but it was only 22 g/min for similar-sized pigs eating from a more "restrictive" feeder (Gonyou et al., 1992). As feeder stocking rate is dependent on eating rate, a more spacious design should accommodate more pigs.

The movements associated with feed falling onto the floor (feed wastage) were studied by Gonyou and Lou (1998). The most common movements associated with feed wastage were backing away from the feeder, eating while the head was raised, fighting, and stepping into the feeder. Two of these behaviors, fighting and stepping, were more common for smaller pigs that also waste a higher percentage of feed. Fighting was more common among smaller pigs as some of the feeders studied had wider feeder spaces than recommended and two pigs would eat from the same space. As indicated above, when feeders have depths exceeding 20 cm, as required for large pigs, small pigs must step into the feeder while they eat. The compromise required when a wide range of pig sizes are fed from the same feeder results in greater wastage by the smaller pigs.

D. WET AND WET/DRY FEEDERS

Wet feeding (feed combined with water) is used to improve feed efficiency and use liquid feedstuffs such as whey. Wet feeding systems are often designed to limit feed intake, with several meals each day. Because of the limited amount of time that feed is available, the feeder should accommodate all the pigs in the pen simultaneously. This is usually accomplished with a trough providing space sufficient for all pigs to eat at once. Wastage can be extensive from these systems, particularly when the pigs are small. The troughs usually do not have dividers in them, and aggressive pigs can move along the trough displacing other animals. Trough dividers would reduce this problem.

An alternative to wet feeding is to allow pigs to access both water and dry feed from the feeder, with the option to combine them before consumption. This is referred to as a wet/dry feeder. Various methods are used to provide access to feed in these feeders. Some feeders allow access to dry feed on an elevated platform or shelf. The pigs may eat from this shelf or push the feed into the bottom pan of the feeder where it can be combined with water. Another method of accessing dry feed is to press a lever or bar that drops feed into the feeder pan. Water is normally available from a nipple that may be oriented downward or horizontally. A key feature to wet/dry feeders is that there is a separation of the water from the access point of the dry feed. Otherwise the water will "wick" into the feed storage and plug the feeder.

Although the majority of feeders installed in facilities in North America are classified as dry feeders, there is an increasing amount of interest is the idea of locating the watering device (generally a nipple drinker of some type) in the feeder bowl. Part of the recent interest is the adoption of fully slatted finishing facilities as the standard by the North American swine industry. With partially slatted facilities, a concern often expressed by those considering wet/dry feeders was wetness around the feeder location when the feeder was located on the solid portion of a partially slatted pen.

Reese et al. (1990) concluded that a wet/dry feeder that allowed weanling pigs to consume either dry or wet feed or both offered no advantage over a conventional feeding system in which feed and water were offered in separate areas of the pen. In this study, the wet/dry feeder offered two 20-cm feeding spaces and one nipple drinker per ten pigs and the dry feeder had a 55.9-cm trough divided into four feeding spaces.

Walker (1990) reported an increase in daily gain and feed intake when water was available at the feeder vs. located 3 m distant from the feeder. Patterson (1991) reported no benefit to pig performance for wet/dry feeders.

The decision on wet/dry feeders vs. dry feeders and nipple drinkers located at a distance from the feeder is often based on issues not related to pig performance. Gadd (1988) summarized a series of on-farm experiences and concluded that slurry production was reduced as much as 50% with wet/dry feeders vs. dry feeders. Maton and Daelemans (1992) concluded all wet/dry feeders reduce water spillage, resulting in a 20 to 30% reduction in slurry volume. Brumm and Dahlquist (1997), using a two-hole wet/dry feeder for 24 pigs per pen also reported a 30% reduction in slurry volume.

Both Rantanen et al. (1995) at Kansas State University and Brumm and Dahlquist (1997) at the University of Nebraska report a significant reduction in daily water use for pigs on wet/dry feeders vs. dry feeders and nipple drinkers separate from the feeder. The Kansas workers reported total water disappearance of 6.25 l/pig/day for the dry feeders vs. 4.16 l/pig/day for the wet/dry feeder from 48 to 83 kg live weight. The Nebraska workers reported total water disappearance of 6.06 l/pig/day for the dry feeders vs. 4.50 l/pig/day for the wet/dry feeders from 19 to 108 kg live weight.

Pig performance on the wet/dry feeders compared with the dry feeders in the Kansas and Nebraska studies was variable, with instances of improved daily feed intake and rates of gain compared to dry feeders and instances of no difference. In no trial was performance poorer on the wet/dry feeder.

Of concern to producers using wet/dry feeders is the possibility of bacteria and mold buildup in the trough where feed and water mixing occurs. Hansen and Mortensen (1989, as cited in Van Loozen, 1990) reported that wet feeding systems are populated by lactic acid bacteria and yeasts and concluded that these microorganisms may limit the growth of disease-causing bacteria and molds.

Several studies have indicated that one model of wet/dry feeder resulted in increased intake compared with a particular dry feeder (Anderson et al., 1990; Walker, 1990). In a summary of several on-farm tests, Payne (1991) concluded that the wet/dry feature resulted in increased growth but no increase in apparent feed intake. However, he suggested that the level of feed wastage may have been less in wet/dry feeders and that actual intake may have been higher. Gonyou and Lou (2000) compared feed intake and growth from six models of wet/dry feeders with that of six models of dry feeders. The wet/dry feature resulted in a 5% increase in both feed intake and growth rate.

E. Social Facilitation

Social facilitation occurs when one animal increases performance of a behavior due to the presence of another animal performing the same behavior. Synchronized eating has been reported under experimental conditions for growing pigs (Hsia and Wood-Gush, 1984), raising the possibility of using pen and feeder design to increase intake though social facilitation. Gonyou et al. (1992) reported that pigs in adjoining pens (with spindle penning) ate simultaneously more often if the feeders were adjacent to the same pen wall. Feeders that allowed pigs to see pigs in the adjacent pens were reported to promote the pig's feed consumption, in short-term trials (Hutson, 1995). Allowing pigs in adjoining pens to have contact within the feeder resulted in more simultaneous eating, but did not increase total duration of eating or feed intake (Gonyou, 1999). Feeder and pen design can lead to synchronized eating in adjacent pens, but does not seem to increase intake on a long-term basis.

Gonyou and Lou (2000) studied the eating behavior of pigs on 12 models of commercial feeders to determine the effect of feeder design on eating behavior and production. Feeders were classified according to their feed form (dry vs. wet/dry) and space (single vs. multiple space). There were two single-space dry (SS-D), three single-space wet/dry (SS-WD), four multiple-space dry (MS-D), and three multiple-space wet/dry (MS-WD). The average daily gain (ADG) and average daily feed intake (ADFI) were 5% greater with wet/dry feeders than with dry, but the effect of wet/dry feeders on growth was only evident during the final 8 weeks of the trial. Feed intake tended to be higher with wet/dry feeders throughout the trial. Pigs using single and multiple space feeders did not differ in either gain or intake during any of the trial periods, and feed efficiency did not differ among feeder classes. Dry feeders yielded a slightly higher lean percentage of carcass than did wet/dry feeders.

The same 12 models were examined for feed wastage due to spillage on the floor, amount of feed left on and in the feeder, and adherence to the pig that was subsequently wasted. All of the tested feeders were within the range of "good" feeders, with a feed spillage rate of 2 to 5.8% of offered feed. The size of pigs had an effect on feed wastage. Although large and small pigs spilled the same absolute amount of feed, spillage as a percentage of feed disappearance was greater for small (4.4%) compared with large (2.4%) pigs. The amount of feed left within the feeder was greater for large than for small pigs. The differences between feeder categories (dry vs. wet/dry, single vs. multiple space) were not statistically detectable.

The occurrence of feed spillage due to eating, fighting, and stepping into feeder was affected by the size of pigs. Two pigs were often observed eating simultaneously from feeder spaces that were 39 cm wide. The shoulder width of a pig is approximately $6.1 \times BW^{0.33}$, with width in centimeters and body weight in kilograms. Two, 25-kg pigs have a combined shoulder width of approximately 36.5 cm. It is not surprising that fighting, resulting from two pigs attempting to eat at once, is more common among small than large pigs. It is suggested that the width of a feeder space should be approximately 33.5 cm for 115-kg pigs, and that this width should not be exceeded in order to reduce spillage due to fighting.

Gonyou and Lou (2000) constructed an adjustable feeder for an ergonomic study. The width (inside dimension), depth (feeder lip to feed access), and lip height could be adjusted independently. The dimension having the greatest effect on the proportion of pigs stepping into the feeder was depth. Small pigs (22 kg) began stepping into the feeder when depth was set at 20 cm, whereas larger pigs would not step in until the depth reached 30 cm. The authors suggested that a depth of 25 cm may best accommodate both large and small pigs. It is recommended that feeders be appropriately sized for the pigs using them (Hyun et al., 1997).

Electronic stalls (feeding stalls where access is controlled via a unique identification collar or eartag that each pig wears) will affect eating behavior. Because only one pig can eat at a time, social status is likely to affect when pigs eat. Slightly different diurnal eating patterns were reported for boars than for gilts in the same pen with an electronic stall (Nielsen et al., 1996a).

Such is the case in commercial practice when single-space feeders are used. Small, probably subordinate pigs, shift their eating pattern away from the typical crepuscular cycle maintained by larger pigs. Of interest is that if pigs once fed in a group using an electronic stall are then penned individually, their behavior remains similar to that when they were in the group. This suggests that the constraints on feeding behavior result in adaptation, not restriction (Nielsen et al., 1996b). Of particular interest to the applicability of electronic stall data to a single-space commercial feeder system is the effect of protection provided by the stall, which is common in the electronic system. Pigs fed from electronic systems with either a standard stall or a short (head only) stall did not differ in number of visits per day, length of those visits, or total duration of eating (Walker, 1991). However, pigs having only a short stall ate more quickly and therefore consumed slightly more feed during the day.

Increasing the number of pigs eating from a single-space feeder results in changes in eating patterns. Ten pigs are able to maintain a crepuscular pattern, but the pattern is less distinct when 20 pigs eat from the same feeder space, and feeding becomes essentially continuous throughout the 24 h when 30 pigs are fed. As indicated earlier, pigs make the transition from diurnal to nocturnal activity patterns voluntarily in feral and wild conditions. It is not known how stressful the transition from diurnal to continuous eating patterns, which occurs with crowded feeders, is to pigs. The diurnal pattern of eating activity can be used to determine the degree of crowding that occurs at the feeder.

The number of pigs eating from a single-space feeder will also affect eating speed. As indicated earlier, feeder design has changed in recent years to ease access to the feed and facilitate eating. Thus, eating speed differences among reports often reflect the design of the feeder. Other factors such as presence of water or feeder space divisions may affect eating speed. Maximal feeder space stocking density is dependent on total duration of eating, which is dependent upon both ADFI and rate of eating. Recommendations for feeder space stocking density should take into account the design of the feeder, the size of the pig, and the type of feed, all of which affect total duration of eating.

In their study of 12 commercial feeders, Gonyou and Lou (2000) determined the total duration of eating for each model at two different stages in the growing-finishing phase. Based on the total duration of eating, and assuming a maximal utilization level of 80% occupancy, suggested feeder space stocking densities varied from 10 to 15 pigs/space on the different feeders (Gonyou, 1999). However, these suggestions were extrapolated from data obtained with 12 pigs/feeder. Walker (1991) demonstrated that eating rate increases as more pigs are fed from a feeder space, such that finishing pigs stocked at 30 pigs/feeder space ate 62 g/min, while those stocked at 10 pigs/feeder space ate only 36 g/min. It is also not clear what the maximal occupancy rate is (% of time) before feed intake is reduced. The groups of 30 pigs in Walker's study occupied the feeder for 92% of the time without evidencing a reduction in intake. Only when pigs were small, and therefore total duration of eating was increased, was feed intake reduced compared with lower feeder space stocking densities.

IV. IMPACT OF DRINKER DESIGN/LOCATION ON FEED INTAKE

A. General

Nipple drinker devices have traditionally been preferred for all classes of swine. The use of nipple drinking devices ensures that all pigs have access to clean water every time they drink. Barber et al. (1989) reported that when given a choice between drinking from a clean water bowl or a nipple drinker, the bowl was preferred. However, as soon as the bowl became contaminated with feed, pigs preferred the nipple drinker. In most extension specialists' experiences, cup drinking devices are not cleaned frequently enough to ensure cleanliness. In addition, University of Nebraska research (Carlson and Peo, 1979) suggests less total water disappearance with nipple vs. cup drinkers when the nipple drinkers are mounted at a 45° angle pointing up from the floor of the pen. This can be economically important in determining the size and cost of manure storage and if water is purchased from a rural water district.

Although the popular press has given many consultants' opinions as to the minimum flow rate for water from nipple drinkers, research has suggested that pigs compensate for low flow rates by spending more time at the drinking device. Flows as low as 250 ml/min in finishing pens with up to 22 pigs/nipple have not been demonstrated to affect performance, even in summer heat with no sprinkling for cooling (Brumm and Mayrose, 1991). However, pig behavior was altered with more social disruptions reported for the low flow rates.

Barber et al. (1988) demonstrated that weaned pigs compensated for reduced delivery rates by spending more time drinking up to a certain point. They concluded that 3-week-old weaned pigs on the most-restricted water delivery rate were not prepared to extend their drinking time to obtain a greater water intake. The NCR-89 Regional Committee on Swine Management has investigated the effect of nipple drinker flow rates on pig performance. In a study involving five experiment stations (NCR-89, 1991) a reduction in feed intake was associated with reduced nipple drinker flow rates (70 vs. 700 ml/min) and summer conditions for lactating sows.

A recent report from Canada (Philips et al., 1990) suggested that a flow of 600 ml/min (0.19 gal/h) does not impede sow water intake during lactation. Flow rates of 2000 ml/min were associated with greater spillage. In this study, spillage (waste) averaged 23% on the low flow rate vs. 80% on the high flow rate.

The MWPS (1991) recommends one waterer space per 10 weaned pigs and one waterer space per 15 growing pigs. As with feeder recommendations, this recommendation makes no mention of differences in delivery devices, water flow rate, location within the pen, or location with respect to the feeder.

The number of pigs per nipple drinking device is also unclear from the literature. Brumm and Shelton (1986), in comparing one vs. two nipple drinkers for a pen of 16 weaned pigs reported an increase in the variation of weight gain when only one nipple drinker was available. In general, the number of allowable pigs per nipple drinker increases with pig size and ability to adapt to social stress.

Similar to the use of wet/dry feeders, decisions on water delivery devices are now also including consideration of slurry volume in addition to pig performance. Brumm and Dahlquist (1997), in a trial involving nipple drinkers suspended on a chain in the middle of a pen of 24 pigs vs. conventionally mounted nipple drinkers on pen partitions, reported an 11% reduction in total water use and a 16% reduction in manure volume for the suspended nipple device.

More recently, Brumm and Heemstra (1999) reported a 24% reduction in water disappearance (3.79 vs. 5.03 l/day/pig) for bowl drinkers vs. a swinging nipple drinker for the entire growing-finishing period (18 to 115 kg). In addition to a slight improvement in feed conversion efficiency (2.49 vs. 2.55, $P < 0.1$), there was a 22% reduction in manure volume recorded for the bowl drinker. During a period when sulfadimethoxine was administered to all pigs, drug expense/use was twice as high for the swinging nipple drinker as for the bowl drinker.

This raises the issue of appropriate dosage estimates for medications administered via water delivery systems. That is, if a certain intake is desired (as an example, milligrams of drug per pig per day), and water use decreases due to a reduction in wastage, the amount of water consumed per pig does not change. Thus, revising the amount of drug dispensed per liter of water may alter the actual amount of drug consumed by the pig, and the effectiveness of the drug may be compromised or the compound may be administered at rates higher or lower than intended.

The results of Brumm and Dahlquist (1997) and Brumm and Heemstra (1999) suggest that dosages should not be altered if water use is reduced compared with expectations due to equipment selection. That is, the amount of drug per liter of water should remain the same if the total water use is 4 l of water per day or 6 l of water per day because the pig consumes the same amount of water regardless of the delivery device. The only difference is the amount of water wasted during the drinking process.

Thus, if dosages are altered in response to changes in total daily water disappearance, one needs to keep in mind the fact that water wastage as influenced by water delivery devices needs to be considered. The actual daily intake of water per pig is probably not different among delivery devices, just the amount of water wasted. This difference in total water use is different from factors known to influence actual water intake such as dietary ingredients and temperature referred to in Chapter 17.

From the data of Brumm and Dahlquist (1997) and Brumm and Heemstra (1999) it is possible to estimate the water:feed (kg/kg) ratio for these experiments. As shown in Table 22.1, in experiments where pig performance was similar between water delivery devices, water:feed estimates varied considerably.

TABLE 22.1
Effect of Water Delivery Device on Growing-Finishing Pig Water:Feed Ratios (kg water/kg feed)

	Water Delivery Device			
Reference	Wet/Dry	Nipple	Water Swing	Bowl
Brumm and Dahlquist, 1997	1.78	2.79		
		2.64	2.34	
Brumm and Heemstra, 1999			2.41	1.89

B. Extraneous Voltage

Similar to dairy cows, swine have proved to be sensitive to small electrical currents. The problem of extraneous or "stray" voltage has been identified as the cause of poor water consumption on many swine farms. The problem of stray voltage limiting water intake has occurred in all phases of production, but seems to be most evident in farrowing and nursery facilities where pigs are often on metal floors and/or have frequent contact with metal crates/gates while drinking. However, serious problems of extraneous voltage have been reported during the growing-finishing phase also (Gerald Bodman, University of Nebraska, personal communication).

Research at the University of Minnesota (Gustafson et al., 1986) has demonstrated that growing-finishing pigs, given an alternative, showed a preference for a water source with no current compared with those at ≥ 0.25 mA. However, when no alternative source existed, >3.0 mA was needed to affect drinking time and ≥ 4.0 mA to affect consumption.

Pigs forced to drink from water devices that result in electric shock exhibit agitated behavior. Sows in farrowing crates will have reduced feed intake and lower milk output as a result of depressed water intake. Nursery and growing-finishing pigs exhibit nervousness around the drinking devices and feed intake will be reduced.

Producers who suspect stray voltage as a cause of reduced water intake are urged to contact their utility supplier, a qualified electrician, and/or extension agricultural engineer for assistance in diagnosing and alleviating the source of the stray voltage. Any voltage between animal contact points of 0.5 V (AC) is reason for concern. Voltages of 0.2 to 0.3 V AC are fairly common. Proper equipment and techniques are essential to diagnose properly and to correct extraneous voltage problems (Surbrook et al., 1988).

V. IMPACT OF SPACE ALLOCATION AND GROUP SIZE ON FEED INTAKE

A. GENERAL

Stocking density, in terms of floor area, has traditionally been expressed as area per pig, or when a pen of known area is used, as pigs per pen. Under conventional management, pigs remain in the same pen for several weeks and space allowance is based on the maximum space required during that period. For pigs that are removed from the pen as a group, such as when pigs are moved from a nursery to a growing-finishing barn, the maximum space requirement occurs on the day of leaving the pen. For finishing pigs, the maximum space requirement usually occurs the day that the first pig is marketed.

Space allowance can be expressed as an allometric relationship between body weight and body dimensions. Because body weight is proportional to volume, it can be considered a three-dimensional measure. Floor area requirement will be proportional to the surface area of a pig, which is a two-dimensional measure. The relationship between space allowance (A) and body weight (BW) can therefore be expressed as $A = k \times BW^{2/3}$ (Petherick and Baxter, 1981), where k = an empirical coefficient.

Gonyou and Stricklin (1998) adjusted the size of pens for growing-finishing pigs (25 to 105 kg) at 2-week intervals to determine if space allowances based on allometric relationships had consistent effects over a wide range of body weights. Using an equation based on area in square meters and body weight in kilograms, they used coefficients (k) of 0.030, 0.039, and 0.048. Regardless of the weight of the pigs, space allowances based on coefficients of 0.039 and 0.048 yielded similar weight gains, whereas those based on the lower coefficient were depressed by approximately 5%. Edwards et al. (1988) examined a lower range of coefficients and determined that weight gain responds to increasing space allowance up to their highest coefficient of 0.034. Based on these studies, it appears that maximum growth rate will be achieved at a coefficient of between 0.035 and 0.040. Reduction of space allowance to that determined by a coefficient of 0.030 will result in a growth reduction of 5%.

The more conventional means of determining space allowance recommendations has been to use empirical studies that provide a set amount of space per animal throughout the entire study. The general recommendations for floor space have been 0.46 m² for pigs from 27 to 45 kg, 0.56 m² from 45 to 68 kg, and 0.74 m² from 68 kg to market (Fritschen and Muehling, 1986).

In some management systems it is common for pigs to be crowded at more than one stage of production or for various periods of time. While many research centers have examined the effects of space allocation on performance, Kornegay and Notter (1984) compiled a summary of the data on the effects of floor space and number of pigs per pen on pig performance. In their analysis, for the growing pig with a range of space per pig from 0.15 to 0.80 m²/pig, the following equations predicted the effect of decreasing space allocation on pig performance:

Daily gain (kg):

$$0.489 + 0.520(S) - 0.281(S^2) \ (R^2 = 0.93)$$

Daily feed intake (kg):

$$1.542 + 0.856(S) - 0.404(S^2) \ (R^2 = 0.93)$$

Feed per gain:

$$3.3037 - 0.734(S) + 0.406(S^2) \quad (R^2 = 0.94)$$

where S = space per pig in m²/pig.

For the finishing pig with space per pig allocations ranging from 0.4 to 1.0 m/pig, the prediction equations were

Daily gain (kg):

$$0.398 + 0.704(S) - 0.340(S^2) \quad (R^2 = 0.69)$$

Daily feed (kg):

$$1.619 + 1.833(S) - 0.837(S^2) \quad (R^2 = 0.74)$$

Feed per gain:

$$3.840 - 0.927(S) + 0.502(S^2) \quad (R^2 = 0.40)$$

Using this equation, maximum rate of gain is achieved at a k value of 0.048. Recent reports have indicated that maximum gains are achieved when pigs are provided, throughout the growing-finishing period, floor areas equivalent to k values of 0.040 (NCR-89, 1993), 0.029 (McGlone and Newby, 1994), and between 0.032 and 0.038 (Brumm and NCR-89, 1996). It should be noted that the estimate of floor area allowance by McGlone and Newby (1994) may be low, because they reported only the weight at which pigs were marketed, not the average weight for the pen when the first pigs were removed.

Although valuable for predicting performance, a limitation of the data reviewed in the Kornegay and Notter (1984) summary is that the average final weight for the finishing pigs was approximately 93 kg. In an attempt to build on the existing data, the NCR-89 regional research committee dealing with swine management initiated a research effort investigating the effects of space allocation on pigs taken to 114 kg (NCR-89, 1993). New performance curves were developed for the finishing phase using these data (Powell et al, 1993). Data for the new finishing curves were bounded by 0.56 m² (6 ft²)/pig on the low side to 1.11 m² (12 ft²)/pig on the high side. Any effects due to number of pigs per pen were ignored in this analysis because of the smaller group sizes used in the NCR-89 experiment. The new finishing performance curves are predicted by

Daily gain (lb):

$$1.0783 + 0.0444(S) \quad (R^2 = 0.64)$$

Daily feed intake (lb):

$$4.8850 + 0.1004(S) \quad (R^2 = 0.60)$$

Feed per gain:

$$\text{Daily feed/daily gain}$$

where S is space per pig in ft²/pig.

As average U.S. slaughter weights continue to increase in response to packer merit pricing systems, knowledge of appropriate space allocations is limited. Recent results of space studies of barrows taken to 136 kg (Brumm and NCR-89, 1996) suggest little if any improvement in performance beyond 0.83 to 0.93 m²/pig. In both trials reported, there was only a 2 to 3% improvement in daily gain as space allocations increased by 28% (0.65 to 0.83 m²) or by 43% (0.65 to 0.93 m²). In both experiments, the best feed conversion occurred with the 0.65 m²/pig treatment.

Brumm and Dahlquist (1995) reported that pigs raised in crowded nurseries were not as affected by crowded growing-finishing conditions as those that were not crowded in the nursery phase. In other words, the pigs were able to adapt to crowded conditions to some extent. Gonyou (1999) exposed grower-finisher pigs to crowded conditions for 1 to 3 months during the growing-finishing phase and found that growth rate was dependent only on the degree of crowding being experienced, and was not affected by previous conditions. Thus, pigs do not seem to be able to adapt to crowded conditions under all situations, and age may be a factor in this capability.

Based on a coefficient of 0.035, the recommended floor space allowance for pigs at 90, 100, 110, 120, 130, and 140 kg would be 0.704, 0.755, 0.804, 0.853, 0.900, and 0.945 m²/pig, respectively. Thus, producers should adjust space allowance based upon their market weights to achieve maximal growth. However, the level for optimal efficiency of floor area may be considerably lower than that for maximal individual weight gain (Edwards et al., 1988; Powell et al., 1993). The industry is faced with the dilemma of choosing between the most profitable system, and one that maximizes individual growth, which is often cited as evidence of good welfare.

B. Pigs per Social Group

Confounding space considerations is the impact of group size on pig performance for confinement pigs. In general, pigs use their sense of smell to locate their peers within a social group (Ewbank et al., 1974). As long as the social group is <20 to 25 pigs/pen, pigs apparently can rely on these olfactory clues and form stable social hierarchies (Ewbank, 1976).

Kornegay and Notter (1984) also examined the question of social group size (i.e., pigs/pen). For the range of 5 to 30 pigs/pen, they developed the following equations to predict the effect of number of pigs/pen on pig performance:

Daily gain (kg):

    Growing $0.6407 - 0.0019(N)$ $(R^2 = 0.43)$

    Finishing $0.7497 - 0.0012(N)$ $(R^2 = 0.82)$

Daily feed intake (kg):

    Growing $1.5950 - 0.0025(N)$ $(R^2 = 0.87)$

    Finishing $2.3748 + 0.0032(N)$ $(R^2 = 0.92)$

Feed per gain:

    Growing $2.4974 + 0.0037(N)$ $(R^2 = 0.94)$

    Finishing $3.2182 + 0.0060(N)$ $(R^2 = 0.72)$

where N = number of pigs/pen or social grouping.

These equations suggest that for each additional pig within a pen, daily gain decreases 0.0019 kg/day during the growing phase and 0.0012 kg/day during the finishing phase. The reader is cautioned that these equations are only valid for group sizes of <30.

There are studies in the literature that suggest the impact of group size may not be as severe as originally thought. Mortensen (1988) suggested that in groups of 48 vs. 16 pigs there is a tendency for the pigs in large groups to show fewer social interactions than for pigs in smaller groups. McGlone and Newby (1994) investigated group sizes of 10, 20, and 40 pigs/pen. As group size increased, free space per pig increased with limited differences in performance. They concluded that as group size increased, the space needs per pig decreased slightly. Petherick et al. (1989) reported a decrease in gain for groups of 36 pigs/pen, compared with groups of 8 or 16 pigs. However, Randolph et al. (1981) reported no difference between group sizes of 5 and 20, and Walker (1991) reported no differences among 10, 20, and 30 pigs per group, even when feeder space was held constant.

Gonyou and Stricklin (1998) reported a decrease in ADG of 4% when group size was increased from 3 to 5 to 10, and an additional decrease of 5% when group size was further increased to 15 pigs/pen. In an earlier study, Gonyou et al. (1992) reported a substantial reduction in gain when groups of five were compared with individually penned animals. Aggression, expressed on a per pig basis, is maximal when group size is 5 to 7, and reduced when group size is 3, or ≥10 (Moore et al., 1996). These results suggest that the social structure of groups of pigs changes from very stable linear hierarchies for small groups, to less stable hierarchies requiring more aggression, to a social system which requires little aggression to maintain in large groups.

Both space restriction and increased group size affect average daily gain and feed intake. It may be that both conditions have their effect on productivity by making it difficult for the pigs to access feed. If this were the case, increasing the nutrient density of the diet might compensate for the reduction in nutrient intake even though the amount of feed consumed is reduced. However, such is not the case. Space-restricted pigs reduced their nutrient intake when fed either high- or regular-density diets (Brumm and Miller, 1996). It seems more likely that nutrient intake is reduced under crowded conditions or when group size is suboptimal, because of a reduction in growth potential (Chapple, 1993).

C. Interaction of Diet and Space

As the previous discussion has documented, when pigs are given less space, feed intake is decreased, usually resulting in a reduction in daily gain. Feed conversion efficiency may or may not be affected. It would seem logical then that when pigs are given less space and feed intake is reduced, increasing the nutrient density of the diet should maintain daily gain if the cause of the reduced gain is a reduction in lysine or energy intake associated with the reduction in feed intake.

In a series of studies with growing-finishing pigs (Brumm and Miller, 1996), the addition of fat, lysine, or fat and lysine to control diets had no effect on overcoming the reduction in feed intake or daily gain associated with crowding. Although Kornegay et al. (1993b) theorized that the most probable reason for reduced performance of nursery pigs given less space was an absolute decrease in energy intake, the results of Brumm and Miller (1996) do not support this hypothesis. In their experiments, the lysine:energy ratio was constant across the experimental diets. The calculated lysine and energy intakes did not differ between different space allocations, and yet ADG was decreased with less space per pig and more pigs per social group.

Impaired efficiency of feed utilization due to chronic stress has been suggested by Paterson and Pearce (1991) as one mechanism by which crowding reduces growth. Using computer modeling to confirm field observations, Chapple (1993) suggested that the "stress" of being reared in a group reduces the capacity of the pig to deposit protein and that this causes a reduction in feed intake and efficiency of feed use. Chapple went on to hypothesize that when space is limited, stress is mediated through biochemical factors that direct downregulated tissue growth, lower nutrient requirements, and reduced feed intake.

Kornegay et al. (1993a) concluded that the addition of lysine to diets of weanling pigs was not effective in overcoming the reduction in performance caused by a restriction in space allowance. These results are also supported by NCR-42 (1993) results in which the reduction in ADG due to crowding of finishing pigs was not prevented by the addition of 5% added fat and 0.05% added lysine to the control diets.

Zimmerman (1986) in a literature review concluded that there was no interaction between the response to space restrictions and the response to dietary antibiotics. Pigs experiencing space restrictions responded to dietary antibiotics similarly to pigs without space restrictions.

Walker (1989) reported an interaction between the number of pigs per pen (stocking density) and diet form. He concluded that when diets are in meal form, high stocking rates result in reduction in daily gain, while there is no effect of stocking density when diets are pelleted. However, more recently, Brumm (1998) reported no interaction of diet form (pellets vs. meal) and space allocation.

VI. CONCLUSIONS

Nutritional management is becoming more intensive and precise, but to this point the emphasis has been on the nutrient requirements of the pigs. The point at which feeding method and differences in eating behavior should also be considered in formulations may be approaching. Should diets for wet/dry feeders differ from those used in dry feeders because of the expected differences in intake? Does the number and distribution of meals throughout a day affect the uptake and utilization of nutrients? One may need to ask similar questions as feeding programs for gestating sows are considered. Avoiding increasing feed allowance, yet reducing the incidence of stereotypies, may require consideration of alternative feeding methods or nutrient forms that reduce hunger.

Feed intake remains a problem for early weaned pigs, for at least 24 to 36 h after weaning. The incidence of anomalous behaviors that seem to be related to eating behavior in early-weaned pigs is also a concern that may require modifications in management. Although productivity remains the most critical goal of animal management, society will place limitations on certain practices unless some of its concerns can be successfully addressed, and this is already seen with early weaning.

A point at which nutritional management is operating counter to other biological principles may be approaching. There is evidence to suggest that the optimal social environment for productivity may differ from that required for developing nutritional programs. If such is the case, new systems that may retain both sets of advantages need to be devised. Choice feeding is one such system that has potential but may only prove effective if developed using a multidisciplinary approach.

REFERENCES

Anderson, D. M., T. A. VanLunen, and D. Sproule. 1990. Performance of grower finisher pigs obtaining feed from dry feeders or wet/dry feeders with different feeding spaces, *Can. J. Anim. Sci.*, 70:1197 (Abstr.).

Appleby, M. C., and A. B. Lawrence. 1987. Food restriction as a cause of stereotypic behaviour in tethered gilts, *Anim. Prod.*, 45:103.

Baldwin, B. A., and G. B. Meese. 1977. Sensory reinforcement and illumination preference in the domesticated pig, *Anim. Behav.*, 25:497.

Barber, J., P. H. Brooks, and J. L. Carpenter. 1988. *Proc. Br. Soc. Anim. Prod.*, Winter Meeting, Scarborough, Paper 127.

Barber, J., J. L. Carpenter, and P. H. Brooks. 1989. Fresh perspectives on the economic supply of water to housed pigs. In *Land and Water Use*, Dodd, V. A., and P. M. Grace, Eds., Balkema, Rotterdam, 1113.

Bates, R. O., S. L. Tilton, J.C. Rea, and S. Woods. 1993. Performance of pigs stocked at either 5 or 10 per feeder space in grow-finish, University of Missouri, Swine Day Research Report, Columbia.

Baxter, M. R. 1991. The design of the feeding environment for pigs. In *Manipulating Pig Production III, Proceedings of the Third Biennial Conference of the Australian Pig Science Association*, Batterham, E. S., Ed., Australasian Pig Science Association, Attwood, Australia, 150.

Botermans, J. A., J. Svendsen, and B. Westrom. 1997. Competition at feeding of growing-finishing pigs, *Proc. 5th International Livestock Environment Symposium*, American Society of Agricultural Engineers, Minneapolis, MN, 591.

Brumm, M. C. 1998. Pen space allocations and pelleting of swine diets, Nebraska Swine Report EC98-219, University of Nebraska Coop. Ext., Lincoln, 44.

Brumm, M., and D. Carlson. 1985. Nursery feeder space — how much? Nebraska Swine Report EC85-219, University of Nebraska Coop. Ext., Lincoln, 17.

Brumm, M. C., and J. M. Dahlquist. 1995. Nursery and growing-finishing space interactions, Nebraska Swine Report EC95–219, University of Nebraska Coop. Ext., Lincoln, 44.

Brumm, M. C., and J. M. Dahlquist. 1997. Impact of feeder and drinker designs on pig performance, water use, and manure production, Nebraska Swine Report EC97–219, University of Nebraska Coop. Ext., Lincoln, 34.

Brumm, M. C., and J. Heemstra. 1999. Impact of drinker type on pig performance, water use, and manure production, Nebraska Swine Report EC99–219, University of Nebraska Coop. Ext., Lincoln, 49.

Brumm, M. C., and V. B. Mayrose. 1991. Nipple drinkers for finishing pigs, Nebraska Swine Report EC91–219, University of Nebraska Coop. Ext., Lincoln, 41.

Brumm, M. C., and P. S. Miller. 1996. Response of pigs to space allocation and diets varying in nutrient density, *J. Anim. Sci.*, 74:2730.

Brumm, M., and NCR-89 Committee on Management of Swine. 1996. Effect of space allowance on barrow performance to 136 kilograms body weight, *J. Anim. Sci.*, 74:745.

Brumm, M. C., and D. P. Shelton. 1986. Nursery drinkers — how many? Nebraska Swine Report EC86-219, University of Nebraska Coop. Ext., Lincoln, 5.

Carlson, R., and E. R. Peo, Jr. 1979. H_2O — critical swine nutrient, Nebraska Swine Report EC79-219, University of Nebraska Coop. Ext., Lincoln, 20.

Chapple, R. P. 1993. Effect of stocking arrangement on pig performance. In *Manipulating Pig Production IV*, Batterham, E. S., Ed., Australasian Pig Science Association, Attwood, Australia, 87.

Cronin, G. M., J. M. F. M. van Tartwijk, W. van der Hel, and M. W. A. Verstegen. 1986. The influence of degree of adaptation to tether-housing sows in relation to behaviour and energy metabolism, *Anim. Prod.*, 42:257.

de Haer, L. C. M., and J. W. M. Merks. 1992. Patterns of daily food intake in growing pigs, *Anim. Prod.*, 54:95.

Edwards, S. A., A. W. Armsby, and H. H. Spechter. 1988. Effects of floor area allowance on performance of growing pigs kept on fully slatted floors, *Anim. Prod.*, 46:453.

English, P., V. Fowler, S. Baxter, and B. Smith. 1988. *The Growing and Finishing Pig: Improving Efficiency*, Farming Press Limited, Ipswich, England.

Ewbank, R. 1976. Social hierarchy in suckling and fattening pigs: a review, *Livest. Prod. Sci.*, 3:363.

Ewbank, R., G. B. Meese, and J. E. Cox. 1974. Individual recognition and the dominance hierarchy in the domesticated pig: the role of sight, *Anim. Behav.*, 22:473.

Farrin, I. G. 1990. Requirements of effective housing systems. In *Pig Production in Australia*, Gardner, J., A. Dunkin, and L. Lloyd, Eds., Butterworths, Boston.

Feddes, J. J. R., B. A. Young, and J. A. DeShazer. 1989. Influence of temperature and light on feeding behavior of pigs, *Appl. Anim. Behav. Sci.*, 23:215.

Forbes, J. 1982. Effect of lighting pattern on growth, lactation and food intake of sheep, cattle and deer, *Livest. Prod. Sci.*, 9:361.

Fritschen, R., and A. J. Muehling. 1986. Space requirements for swine, *Pork Industry Handbook*, Coop. Ext. Service, Purdue University, West Lafayette, IN, PIH-55.

Furlan, A. C., J. A. Def. Lima, A. I. G. DeOliveira, M. Del Soares, and B. L. DeOliveira. 1986a. Different light regimens for growing-finishing pigs. Experiment 1, *Rev. Soc. Bras. Zootec.*, 15(5):372.

Furlan, A. C., J. A. Def. Lima, A. I. G. DeOliveira, M. Del Soares, and B. L. DeOliveira. 1986b. Different light regimens for growing-finishing pigs. Experiment 2, *Rev. Soc. Bras. Zootec.*, 15(5):378.

Gadd, J. 1988. Mix at trough feeding, a quiet revolution, *Pigs*, Jan./Feb., 26.

Gonyou, H. W. 1999. Four weeks of crowding will reduce overall performances during the grow/finish phase, *Adv. Pork Prod.*, 1:A-16 (Abstr.).

Gonyou, H. W., and Z. Lou. 1998. Grower/Finisher Feeders: Design, Behaviour and Performance. Prairie Swine Centre Monograph 97-01, Saskatoon, SK, 1.

Gonyou, H. W., and Z. Lou. 2000. Effects of eating space and availability of water in feeders on productivity and eating behavior of grower-finisher pigs, *J. Anim. Sci.*, 78:865.

Gonyou, H. W., and W. R. Stricklin. 1981. Eating behavior of beef cattle groups fed from a single stall or trough, *Appl. Anim. Ethol.*, 7:123.

Gonyou, H. W., and W. R. Stricklin. 1998. Effects of floor area allowance and group size on the productivity of growing/finishing pigs, *J. Anim. Sci.*, 76:1326.

Gonyou, H. W., R. P. Chapple, and G.R. Frank. 1992. Productivity, time budgets and social aspects of eating in pigs penned in groups of five or individually, *Appl. Anim. Behav. Sci.*, 34:291.

Gonyou, H. W., E. Beltranena, D. L. Whittington, and J. F. Patience. 1998. The behaviour of pigs weaned at 12 and 21 days of age from weaning to market, *Can. J. Anim. Sci.*, 78:517.

Grandin, T. 1980. Pen size and shape in livestock confinement systems, *Feedstuffs*, Oct. 13, 23.

Gustafson, R. J., R. D. Appleman, and T. M. Brennan. 1986. Electrical current sensitivity of growing/finishing swine for drinking. *Trans. ASAE*, 29:592.

Hansen, I. D., and B. Mortensen. 1989. Pipecleaners beware, *Pig Int.*, 19(11):8.

Hanson, R. P., and L. Karstad. 1959. Feral swine in the southeastern United States, *J. Wildl. Manag.*, 23:64.

Hsia, L.C., and D. G. M. Wood-Gush. 1983. A note on social facilitation and competition in the feeding behavior of pigs, *Anim. Prod.*, 37:149.

Hsia, L. C. and D. G. M. Wood-Gush. 1984. The temporal patterns of food intake and allelomimetic feeding by pigs of different ages, *Appl. Anim. Ethol.*, 11:271.

Hutson, G. D. 1995. Effect of enclosure of the feeding space on feeding behaviour of growing pigs. In *Manipulating Pig Production V*, Batterham, E. S., Ed., Australasian Pig Science Association, Attwood, Australia, 21.

Hyun, Y., M. Ellis, F. K. McKeith, and E. R. Wilson. 1997. Feed intake pattern of group-housed growing-finishing pigs monitored using a computerized feed intake recording system, *J. Anim. Sci.*, 75:1443.

Ingram, D. L., M. J. Dauncey, and K. F. Legge. 1985. Synchronization of motor activity in young pigs to a non-circadian rhythm without affecting food intake or growth, *Comp. Biochem. Physiol.*, 80A(3):363.

Kornegay, E. T., M. D. Lindemann, and V. Ravindran. 1993a. Effects of dietary lysine levels on performance and immune response of weanling pigs housed at two floor space allowances, *J. Anim. Sci.*, 71:552.

Kornegay, E. T., J. B. Meldrum, and W.R. Chickering. 1993b. Influence of floor space allowance and dietary selenium and zinc on growth performance, clinical pathology measurements and liver enzymes, and adrenal weights of weanling pigs, *J. Anim. Sci.*, 71:3185.

Kornegay, E. T., and D. R. Notter. 1984. Effects of floor space and number of pigs per pen on performance, *Pig News Info.*, 5(1):23.

Lawrence, A. B., and E. M. C. Terlouw. 1993. A review of behavioral factors involved in the development and continued performance of stereotypic behaviors in pigs, *J. Anim. Sci.*, 71:2815.

Lawrence, A. B, M. C. Appleby, and H. A. MacLeod. 1988. Measuring hunger in the pig using operant conditioning: the effect of food restriction, *Anim. Prod.*, 47:131.

Leibbrandt, V. D. 1978. Effect of feeder space availability on performance by early weaned pigs, University of Florida 23rd Annual Swine Day, Marianna.

Lindemann, M. D., E. T. Kornegay, J. B. Meldrum, G. Schurig, and F. C. Gwazdauskas. 1987. The effect of feeder space allowance on weaned pig performance, *J. Anim. Sci.*, 64:8.

Martin, P. R., and P. P. G. Bateson. 1993. *Measuring Behaviour: An Introductory Guide*, 2nd ed., Cambridge University Press, Cambridge.

Maton, A., and J. Daelemans. 1992. Third comparative study viz. the circular wet-feeder versus the dry-feed hopper for *ad libitum* feeding and general conclusions concerning wet feeding versus dry feeding of finishing pigs, *Landbouwtijdschr. Rev. l'Agric.*, 45(3):532.

McGlone, J. J., and B. E. Newby. 1994. Space requirements for finishing pigs in confinement: behavior and performance while group size and space vary, *Appl. Anim. Behav. Sci.*, 39:331.

McGlone, J. J., T. E. Heald, and S. L. Hayden. 1983. Physical and behavioral measures of feeding space for nursery-age swine, *J. Anim. Sci.*, 57(Suppl. 1):140 (Abstr.).

McGlone, J. J., T. Hicks, R. Nicholson, and C. Fumuso. 1993. Feeder space requirement for split sex or mixed sex pens. Texas Tech University Agric. Sci. Tech. Rep. T-5–327.

Metz, J. H. M., and H. W. Gonyou. 1990. Effect of age and housing conditions on the behavioural and haemolytic reaction of piglets to weaning, *Appl. Anim. Behav. Sci.*, 27:229.

Moore, C. M., J. Z. Zhou, W. R. Stricklin, and H. W. Gonyou. 1996. The influence of group size and floor area space on social organization of growing-finishing pigs. In *Proc. 30th Cong. Int. Soc. Appl. Ethol.*, I. J. H. Duncan, T.M Widowski, and D.B. Haley, Eds., University of Guelph, 34.

Morrow, A. T. S., and N. Walker. 1994a. The behavioral and production responses of finishing pigs to increasing workload to obtain food *ad libitum* from hopper feeders, *Anim. Prod.*, 59:125.

Morrow, A. T. S., and N. Walker. 1994b. A note on changes to feeding behavior of growing pigs by fitting stalls to single-space feeders, *Anim. Prod.*, 59:262.

Morrow, A.T.S., and N. Walker. 1994c. Effects of number and siting of single-space feeders on performance and feeding behavior of growing pigs, *J. Agric. Sci.* (Cambridge), 122:465.

Mortensen, B. 1988. Type of pens and stocking density for growing-finishing pigs. In *Livestock Environment III, Proceedings of the Third International Livestock Environment Symposium*, ASAE, St. Joseph, MI, 142.

MWPS. 1991. Swine Housing and Equipment Handbook, Midwest Plan Service MWPS-8, 4th ed., 3rd printing, Ames, IA.

NCR-42 Committee on Swine Nutrition. 1993. An attempt to counteract growth depression from overcrowding of finishing pigs with nutrient-dense diet, *J. Anim. Sci.*, 71(Suppl. 1):179 (Abstr.).

NCR-89 Committee on Confinement Management of Swine. 1993. Space requirements of barrows and gilts penned together from 54 to 113 kilograms, *J. Anim. Sci.*, 71:1088.

NCR-89 Committee on Confinement Management of Swine. 1991. Effect of nipple drinker water flow rate and season on swine lactation performance, *J. Anim. Sci.*, 69(Suppl. 1):482 (Abstr.).

Nielsen, B. L., A. B. Lawrence, and C. T. Whittemore. 1996a. Effect of individual housing on the feeding behaviour of previously group housed growing pigs, *Appl. Anim. Behav. Sci.*, 47:149.

Nielsen, B. L., A. B. Lawrence, and C. T. Whittemore. 1996b. Effects of single-space feeder design on feeding behaviour and performance of growing pigs, *Proc. Br. Soc. Anim. Sci.*, Scarborough, paper 204.

Nielsen, B. L., A. B. Lawrence, and C. T. Whittemore. 1995. Effect of group size on feeding behavior, social behavior and performance of growing pigs, *Anim. Sci.*, 61:575.

Pajor, E. A., D. Fraser, and D. L. Kramer. 1991. Consumption of solid food by suckling pigs: individual variation and relation to weight gain, *Appl. Anim. Behav. Sci.*, 32:139.

Paterson, A. M., and G. P. Pearce. 1991. The effect of space restriction during rearing on growth and cortisol levels of male pigs. In *Manipulating Pig Production III*, Batterham, E. S., Ed., Australasian Pig Science Association, Attwood, Australia, 68.

Patterson, D. C. 1991. A comparison of offering meal and pellets to finishing pigs from self-feed hoppers with and without built-in watering, *Anim. Feed. Sci. Tech.*, 34:29.

Payne, H. G. 1991. The evaluation of single-space and wet-and-dry feeders for the Australasian Environment. In *Manipulating Pig Production III*, Batterham, E. S., Ed., Australasian Pig Science Association, Attwood, Australia, 158.

Petchey, A. M. 1987. Supplementary light and pig performance, *Farm Building Progr.*, 63:17.

Petherick, J. C. 1983. A note on allometric relationships in Large White × Landrace pigs, *Anim. Prod.*, 36:497.

Petherick, J. C., and S. H. Baxter. 1981. Modeling the static spatial requirements of livestock, CIGR Section II Seminar, Aberdeen.

Petherick, J. C., A. W. Beattie, and D. A. V. Bodero. 1989. The effect of group size on the performance of growing pigs, *Anim. Prod.*, 49:497.

Petrie, C. L., and H. W. Gonyou. 1988. Effects of auditory, visual and chemical stimuli on the ingestive behavior of newly weaned piglets, *J. Anim. Sci.*, 66:661.

Philips, P. A., D. Fraser, and B. K. Thompson. 1990. The influence of water nipple flow rate and position, and room temperature on sow water intake and spillage, *Appl. Eng. Agric.*, 6(1):75.

Powell, T., M. C. Brumm, and R. E. Massey. 1993. Economics of space allocation for grower-finisher hogs: a simulation approach, *Rev. Agric. Econ.*, 15(1):135.

Randolph, J. H., G. L. Cromwell, T. S. Stahly, and D. D. Kratzer. 1981. Effects of group size and space allowance on performance and behavior of swine, *J. Anim. Sci.*, 53:922.

Rantanen, M., J. Hancock, R. Hines, and I. Kim. 1995. Feeder design and pelleting affect on growth performance and water use in finishing pigs, Kansas State University Swine Day Proceedings, Manhattan.

Reese, D., L. Gama, C. Naber, and T. Radke. 1990. Wet/dry vs. dry feeders for weanling pigs, Nebraska Swine Report EC90–219, University of Nebraska Coop. Ext., Lincoln, 9.

Rushen, J. 1984. Stereotyped behaviour, adjunctive drinking and the feeding periods of tethered sows, *Anim. Behav.*, 32:1059.

Stoltenberg, R. M., and H. J. Heege. 1984. Individual dribble-feeding for fattening pigs, *Landtechnik*, 39:144.

Surbrook, T. C., J. R. Althouse, and N. D. Reese. 1988. Stray voltage diagnostic procedures, Paper 88–3520, American Society of Agricultural Engineers, St. Joseph, MI.

Taylor, I. A.. 1990. Design of The Sow Feeder: A Systems Approach, Ph.D. thesis, University of Illinois, Urbana.

Terlouw, E. M. C., and A. B. Lawrence. 1993. Long-term effects of food allowance and housing on development of stereotypies in pigs, *Appl. Anim. Behav. Sci.*, 38:103

Terlouw, E. M. C., A. B. Lawrence, and A. W. Illius. 1991. Influences of feeding level and physical restriction on development of stereotypies in sows, *Anim. Behav.*, 42:981.

Van Loozen, G. 1990. Wet and dry feeding in combination, *Feed Manag.*, 41(2):19.

Wahlstrom, R., and G. Libal. 1977. Effect of housing type, feeder space and pen space on performance of growing-finishing pigs, South Dakota State University 21st Annual Swine Day, Brookings.

Wahlstrom, R., and R. Seerley. 1960. Feeder space requirements for growing-finishing swine, South Dakota State University 4th Annual Swine Day, Brookings.

Walker, N. 1989. The interactions of stocking density, form of diet and sex group of finishing pigs fed *ad libitum*, *Ir. J. Agric. Res.*, 28:109.

Walker, N. 1990. A comparison of single- and multi-space feeders for growing pigs fed non-pelleted diets *ad libitum*, *Anim. Feed Sci. Technol.*, 30:169.

Walker, N. 1991. The effects on performance and behavior of number of growing pigs per mono-place feeder, *Anim. Feed Sci. Technol.*, 35:3.

Worobec, E. K., I. J. H. Duncan, and T. M. Widowski. 1999. The effects of weaning at 7, 14, and 28 days on piglet behaviour, *Appl. Anim. Behav. Sci.*, 62:173.

Zimmerman, D. 1986. Interrelationship between antibiotic feeding and space allowance of pigs, *Pig News Info.*, 7(2):183.

23 Thermal Environment and Swine Nutrition

Jean Noblet, Jean Le Dividich, and Jaap Van Milgen

CONTENTS

I. Introduction 519
II. General Aspects..520
III. Effects of Environmental Temperature on the Young Pig...522
    A. The Neonatal Period (Birth to 2 Days of Age)..522
        1. Neonatal Mortality 522
        2. Susceptibility of the Newborn to Cold during the Critical Period of 24 to 48 h after Birth 522
        3. Mechanisms of Heat Production in the Cold...523
        4. Provision of Energy 523
        5. Provision of an Adequate Microenvironment..525
        6. The Key Role of Cold Stress in Neonatal Mortality and Poor Growth 526
    B. The Remainder of the Suckling Period...526
    C. Effects of Thermal Environment on the Weaned Pig 527
        1. Ambient Temperature...527
        2. Relative Humidity and Ventilation...529
IV. Effects of Ambient Temperature on Production Traits in the Growing-Finishing Pig and in the Pregnant and Lactating Sow...529
    A. The Growing and Finishing Pig 529
        1. Feed Intake 529
        2. Growth Rate and Feed Efficiency..531
        3. Carcass Composition..532
    B. The Pregnant and Lactating Sow..534
V. Nutritional Interactions with Ambient Temperature 535
    A. Dietary Energy Concentration 535
    B. Amino Acid Supply and Balance 536
VI. Conclusion: Significance of an Optimal Temperature 537
References 538

I. INTRODUCTION

Thermal environment has direct effects on the pigs' energy expenditure and voluntary intake and therefore on its production performance. Hence, interest lies in determining the range of ambient temperatures (Ta) over which heat loss from the animal is minimal with a subsequent maximum energy retention. This range is called the thermoneutral zone with the lower limit called the lower critical temperature (LCT). Variation of Ta on either side of this range results in activation of thermoregulatory mechanisms that consist of behavioral, physiological, and anatomical responses affecting the energy metabolism. Within classes of pigs, the newborn is very sensitive to cold and failure to thermoregulate may be a cause of mortality. In heavier pigs, cold represents a smaller problem compared with heat, especially in animals allowed *ad libitum* access to feed. The effects of thermal environment on the energy metabolism of the pig, including the pathway of heat exchanges and the determination of the thermoneutral zone in relation to animal, nutritional, and environmental factors have been extensively studied (Mount, 1968; Holmes and Close, 1977; Close, 1981; Curtis, 1983; Verstegen and Close, 1994). Data presented in this chapter focus on the following main points: a brief recall of the concept of thermal neutrality and the factors that influence it, the effects of thermal environment on the newborn and suckling pig, on the weaned pig, on production traits in the growing-finishing pig, and in the pregnant and lactating sow, and, finally, the nutritional interaction with Ta. Unless specified otherwise, pigs will be considered as being raised in modern conditions of housing and fed as in practice (close to *ad libitum* intake). More-detailed aspects of thermoregulation of the newborn pig have been described by Le Dividich et al. (1998).

II. GENERAL ASPECTS

In thermoneutral conditions, body heat production (HP) represents heat associated with the utilization of metabolizable energy (ME) for maintenance and productive processes, including a minimal "normal" physical activity. At maintenance, all ingested ME is ultimately converted to heat. Heat associated with productive processes results from the synthesis of new tissues or products (muscle and fat tissues, fetal tissues, milk). The efficiencies of ME utilization for growth and reproduction are in the range of 70 to 75% (Close et al., 1985b; Noblet et al., 1999), the value for milk production being 72% (Noblet and Etienne, 1987). However, HP is also dependent on the nature of energy intake; the ratio of net energy to ME ranges from 0.60 for protein to 0.90 for fat (Noblet et al., 1994). Finally, extra heat is produced as a result of less than optimal thermal environment. The contribution of maintenance HP to total body HP varies with the level of production, averaging 70 to 72% in the growing pig (Noblet et al., 1999), 90 to 92% in the pregnant sow (Noblet et al., 1997), and 65% in the lactating sow (Noblet and Etienne, 1987).

Ambient temperature is a major component of the thermal environment. The relation between Ta and the balance of HP and heat loss is schematically illustrated in Figure 23.1. The thermoneutral zone is defined as "the range of Ta over which, at a fixed level of food intake, HP is minimal and constant" (Mount, 1974). The lower and the upper limits of the thermoneutral zone are called the lower (LCT) and the upper critical temperature (UCT), respectively. Factors that affect HP including animal and environmental factors have been reviewed by Holmes and Close (1977). However, it is of interest to note that Ta affects both total heat loss and its partition into sensible and evaporative heat loss. Below the LCT, sensible heat loss is predominant and affected by Ta, whereas above the LCT the contribution of evaporative heat loss to total heat loss increases with Ta. Because the pig has relatively few functional sweat glands (Ingram, 1965), the major component of the increased heat loss is through an increased respiratory ventilation rate, suggesting that adaptation of pigs to hot conditions is limited.

Very little information exists on the extent of the zone of thermoneutrality and especially on values of the UCT. In contrast, studies on the LCT are well documented. The LCT depends on several factors including animal factors (age/weight, physiological state, size of the group, amount of feed intake) and environmental factors (Ta, air movement, relative humidity, type of floor, radiant heat). These factors have also been discussed by Holmes and Close (1977). Values of the LCT for different classes of pigs reared in modern intensive conditions are given in Table 23.1. Furthermore, the effect of a given Ta on pig response is dependent on other environment factors such as wind speed, radient temperature, or floor conductance. The concept of effective ambient temperature (effective Ta) has then been proposed (review by Mount, 1978) to combine all environmental effects in a single effect of Ta; effective Ta is calculated from Ta, wind speed, and radient temperature.

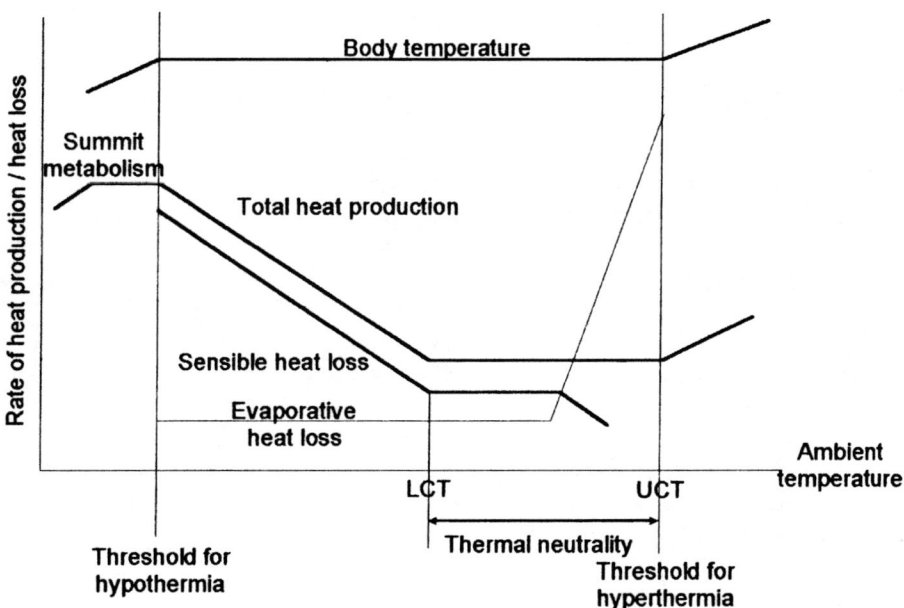

FIGURE 23.1 Diagrammatic representation of the relation between heat production (heat loss) and body temperature as affected by ambient temperature. (Adapted from Mount, 1968.)

Below the LCT, HP increases linearly with a decrease in Ta. The slope of the regression line relating HP to Ta represents the rate of extra heat produced in the cold, and is called the extra thermoregulatory heat production (ETH). Values of ETH for different classes of pigs are presented in Table 23.1. The corresponding feed requirement (as ME) necessary to maintain retained energy at a constant level when Ta is reduced below the LCT can be estimated as ETH divided by the efficiency of ME for energy gain under these climatic conditions.

TABLE 23.1
Values of the Lower Critical Temperature and Extra Thermoregulatory Heat Production in the Cold

Class of Pigs	Housing Conditions	LCT (°C)	ETH (kJ/kg$^{0.75}$/°C)
1-day-old pig	Individually[a]	34	48
2-day-old pig	Individually[b]	30	48
	Group[c]	26	—
3- to 4-kg pig	Group[c]	20	—
Weaned pig	Individually[d]	—	18
	Group[e]	26–28	13
60-kg pig	Individually[f]	—	15
	Group[g]	18–20	7–10
Pregnant sow	Individually[h]	20–23	15–18
	Group[i]	14	8–10
Lactating sow	Individually[j]	12	—

[a] Mount (1968) and Berthon et al. (1994); [b] Berthon et al. (1994); [c] Kovacs and Rafaï (1973); [d] Jordan et al (1985) and Rinaldo and Le Dividich (1991a); [e] Le Dividich et al. (1980); [f] Fuller and Boyne (1972), Noblet et al. (1985), Verstegen and Close (1994); [g] Verstegen et al. (1973), Henken et al. (1991), and Quiniou et al. (1999a); [h] Geuyen et al. (1984) and Noblet et al. (1989); [i] Geuyen et al. (1984); [j] Kemp and Verstegen (1987) and Black et al. (1993).

III. EFFECTS OF ENVIRONMENTAL TEMPERATURE ON THE YOUNG PIG

A. The Neonatal Period (Birth to 2 Days of Age)

1. Neonatal Mortality

It is well established that birth to weaning pig mortality is a source of serious losses to the swine industry, with an average rate of 19% (English and Morrison, 1984; Svendsen, 1992; Holyoake et al., 1995; ITP, 1998). Most (70 to 80%) of this mortality occurs within 72 h of birth, a period when infectious agents play a relatively minor role. The incidence of stillbirth, 70 to 80% of which are intrapartum deaths, usually accounts for 5 to 7% of total pigs born. However, supervision of the farrowings and provision of assistance to disadvantaged pigs could save many pigs (Holyoake et al., 1995). In addition, preweaning mortalities usually average 12 to 13% or more of live born pigs. A survey of the literature indicates that preweaning mortality increases with litter size and, within the litter, pigs of low birth weight are at particular risk. The ultimate cause of preweaning mortality is usually crushing by the sow. However, the primary causes are chilling and starvation. Both weaken the newborn animal and make it prone to be crushed by the sow (English and Edwards, 1996). This indicates that maintenance of a homeothermic balance and establishment of early and regular nutrition are of utmost importance for the survival of the pigs.

2. Susceptibility of the Newborn to Cold during the Critical Period of 24 to 48 h after Birth

The newborn pig has a very low capacity to conserve heat, being virtually hairless and devoid of subcutaneous fat. Its thermal insulation is maximal at Ta of 26°C (Berthon, 1994) and, although a warm microenvironment is usually provided in the farrowing pen, the pig tends to ignore it during the first day. At birth, the typical Ta of 20 to 24°C is 14 to 10°C below the LCT of a single pig and is close to the temperature of 18°C at which the metabolic rate is maximal (Berthon et al., 1993; Table 23.2). In fact, the pig experiences a dramatic period of cold stress until it displays an efficient thermoregulatory response consisting essentially of the ability to locate itself in the heated area and in huddling, and a regular colostrum and milk intake is established. This period is associated with a temporary fall in rectal temperature during which both the extent of the initial drop and the time taken for the subsequent recovery mainly depend on Ta and body weight (BW) (Hata et al., 1985).

Cold resistance is positively related to BW in that the higher the BW is the more resistant to cold the pig is (Curtis et al., 1967; Le Dividich et al., 1991). The impaired ability of small pigs compared with large ones to maintain homeothermic balance during cold exposure is largely

TABLE 23.2
Minimal (mmR) and Maximal (MmR) Metabolic Rate, Lower Critical Temperature (LCT), and Ambient Temperature at Which Maximal Metabolic Rate (TMmR) Is Reached in Pigs (aged from 2 to 48 h)

	Age (h)		
	2	24	48
mmR (kJ/h/kg BW)	12.9	16.9	20.2
MmR (kJ/h/kg BW)	36.6	43.3	>46.8
LCT (°C)	34.2	33.1	30.2
TMmR (°C)	17.8	12.8	ND

ND: not determined.

Source: Adapted from Berthon et al., 1993; 1994.

explained by their greater ratio of surface area to body mass, which results in relatively greater heat loss. Nevertheless, the effects of BW on cold resistance decline rapidly after birth in the fed animals. For example, one can calculate (Le Dividich et al., 1991) that a 200-g difference in BW is associated with a change in rectal temperature of 0.036°C/min during exposure to Ta of 6 to 7°C at 2 h of age, whereas the corresponding change is 0.021°C/min at 24 h. This underlines that newborns of low BW are of particular risk from hypothermia during the very first hours following birth. Genotype is also an important component of cold resistance. This has been demonstrated when comparing Chinese (Meishan breed) to European (Large White breed) pigs (Le Dividich et al., 1991) but reasons for the greater cold resistance of Meishan pigs are not clear. However, cold resistance in fed pigs improves markedly during the early postnatal period. This is shown by the improvement in the ability to maintain rectal temperature during exposure to a cold environment during the first day of life (Curtis et al., 1967; Le Dividich et al., 1991) and by the 4°C decrease in LCT between birth and 48 h of life (Berthon et al., 1993).

3. Mechanisms of Heat Production in the Cold

The inadequacy of protection against heat loss suggests that maintenance of the homeothermic balance and improvement in neonatal thermostability both largely depend on the ability of the newborn to produce heat. This ability is already well developed at birth. For example, metabolic rate is 30% higher at 18 than at 31°C within the first 20 min after birth (Noblet and Le Dividich, 1981), with the difference increasing to 100% in the first 90 min (Herpin et al., 1994). Maximal and minimal metabolic rate (Berthon et al., 1993) are increased by 28 and 56%, respectively, during the first 48 h of life (Table 23.2). However unlike most farm animals, the newborn pig has no dissectable brown adipose tissue as confirmed by the immunoblotting studies of Trayhurn et al. (1989) on the uncoupling protein. Shivering is the predominant mechanism of thermogenesis in the cold. Tremendous amounts of heat can be produced during shivering, but the mechanism is not very efficient because it occurs at the periphery of the body. Heat produced after meal consumption can also contribute to thermoregulation heat produced in the cold. However, this contribution is low because the high efficiency of colostral ME for energy retention (91% according to Le Dividich et al., 1994). Nevertheless, the extra heat produced in the cold amounts to 2 kJ/h/kg BW/°C (Berthon et al., 1994) which is 2.6 times higher than values found in the weaned pig. This suggests that maintenance of a high metabolic rate during this period of cold stress is closely dependent on both the availability of energy substrates and on the ability of the newborn to utilize these as energy sources.

4. Provision of Energy

The requirement for energy is met by body energy reserves and colostrum. Attempts have been made to provide weaker and less competitive newborns with exogenous energy, mainly as medium-chain triglycerides (MCT).

Body energy reserves. Body energy reserves are present as glycogen and fat. Total body glycogen stores range from 30 to 38 g/kg/BW at birth, and liver and skeletal muscle account for 10 and 89% of total body glycogen, respectively. The glycogen reserves decrease rapidly after birth. In conventional environmental conditions, 75% of liver glycogen and 41% of muscle glycogen are utilized by 12 h postpartum (Elliot and Lodge, 1977), and a cold environment hastens the depletion rate in both tissues (McCance and Widdowson, 1959). The total amount of fat in the newborn pig is very low, ranging from 1 to 2%, and most fat is structural fat and therefore not available for mobilization. In addition, selection of growing pigs for reduced carcass fatness results in leaner pigs at birth (Herpin et al., 1993). Overall, available energy derived from glycogen and fat is low (Table 23.3), amounting to about 420 kJ/kg/BW (i.e., 8% of that found in the newborn infant). Although there is some placental transfer of fatty acids during late gestation (Rooke et al., 1998), attempts to improve energy stores do not usually result in

TABLE 23.3
Energy Stores in the Newborn Pig and Human Infant

	Newborn Pig	Human Infant
Glycogen (g/kg)		
Liver	4.5	4.2
Muscle	26.5	10.0
Total	31.0	14.2
Available energy (kJ/kg)	377	167
Fat (g/kg)	15	150
Available energy (kJ/kg)	<80	5440
Total available energy (kJ/kg)	460	5607

Source: Mellor and Cockburn, 1986.

substantial increases in fat and glycogen deposition, which emphasizes the importance of colostrum as an energy source.

Colostrum. The production of colostrum is reported to be continuous during parturition (Hemsworth et al., 1976). The first suckling usually occurs within 20 to 30 min of birth and the rate of intake is very high in the first postnatal hour, representing up to 5 to 7% of BW (Fraser and Rushen, 1992). Consumption is positively related to BW (Fraser and Rushen, 1992), averaging 315 to 340 g/kg/BW in the first day of life (Le Dividich and Noblet, 1981; Milon et al., 1983). However, consumption is highly variable, as suggested by changes in body weight, ranging between −136 and +233 g during the first postnatal day (Thompson and Fraser, 1988). When pigs are supplied with an unlimited availability of colostrum, they consume up to 450 g/kg/BW (Le Dividich et al., 1997), this amount being relatively independent on its fat content, suggesting that the ingestive capacity of the pig is very high at birth and could compensate for its limited energy reserves. Colostrum provides large amounts of lactose and fat, which are readily digested by the newborn pig. Among the nutrients absorbed, lactose is the most quickly metabolized (Holmes et al., 1990). Colostrum is also characterized by a high protein content, but the newborn pig has a very low capacity to oxidize proteins, even in drastic conditions of starvation or/and cold stress. However, the progressive decline in respiratory quotient during the first postnatal day provides evidence for an early involvement of lipids as an energy source (Noblet and Le Dividich, 1981; Berthon et al., 1993). Overall, the thermogenic importance of colostrum is illustrated by the direct linear relationship between heat production (and rectal temperature) and the amount of colostrum consumed by the newborn pig during the first day postpartum, when kept at an environmental temperature of 18°C (Figure 23.2) (Noblet and Le Dividich, 1981).

Exogenous Nutrients. A variety of energy compounds including glucose, lactose, oleic acid, and corn oil (Pettigrew et al., 1986) have been tested as energy supplements for neonatal pigs with little success. Attention is now focused on the utilization of MCT (C8, C10) (Benevenga et al., 1989), which are largely used in colostrum and milk substitutes. MCT are completely digested and readily absorbed (Lee and Chiang, 1994). However, provision of MCT did not increase or may even decrease the survival of neonatal pigs. In fact, *in vitro* studies (Schmidt and Herpin, 1998) indicate that octanoate is poorly oxidized by isolated muscle mitochondria. Similarly, *in vivo* studies in respiration chambers (Léon et al., 1998) provide evidence that, compared with the long-chain triglycerides of colostrum, feeding MCT at physiological doses does not improve the energy status of the newborn, even in cold conditions (Table 23.4). It is suggested the oxidation rate of both long-chain triglycerides and MCT shortly after birth could be limited by the amount of liver and muscle mitochondria (Schmidt and Herpin, 1997).

Thermal Environment and Swine Nutrition

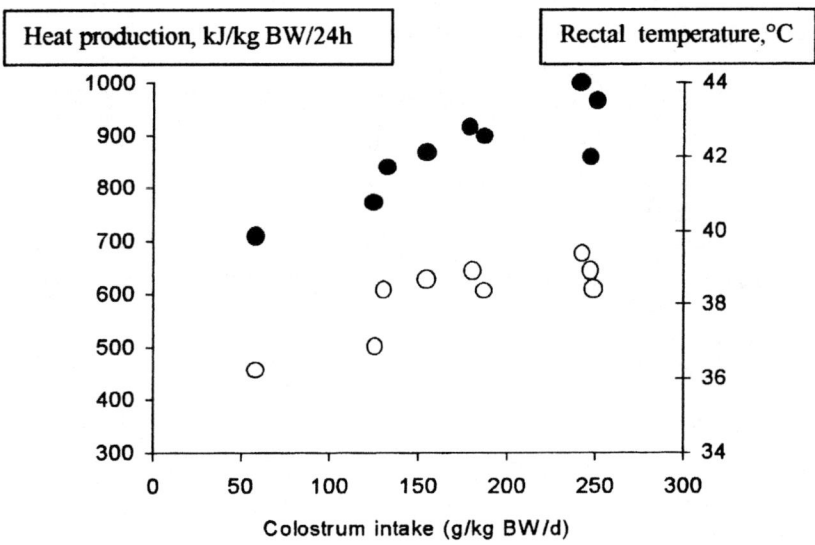

FIGURE 23.2 Heat production (●) and rectal temperature (○) in relation to colostrum intake in pigs kept at 18°C. (Adapted from Noblet and Le Dividich, *Biol. Neonate*, 40:175, 1981.)

TABLE 23.4
Effect of Substitution of Medium- (MCT) for Long- (LCT) Chain Triglycerides in Colostrum on the Energy Metabolism of the Newborn Pig in Relation to Environmental Temperature

Colostrum[a]	LCT		MCT	
Temperature (°C)	34	24	34	24
ME intake (kcal/kg BW/26 h)	230	230	230	230
Heat production (kcal/kg BW/26 h)	107	204	107	191
Respiratory quotient	0.83	0.86	0.84	0.84
Rectal temperature (°C)	38.8	38.2	39.2	38.1

[a] LCT colostrum contained 4.4% LCT and MCT colostrum contained 1.2% LCT and 4.0% MCT.

Source: Adapted from Léon et al., 1998.

5. Provision of an Adequate Microenvironment

Provision of an adequate thermal environment and hence minimizing heat loss from the pig is a major goal during the first postnatal days. However, the high environmental temperature requirement of the newborn pig (32 to 34°C) conflicts with the needs of the lactating sow (12 to 15°C). An infrared (IR) lamp located over the creep area and/or a heated floor are the most common methods used to provide a thermal environment suitable for the neonatal pig. With regard to their effect on the sow's environment, the IR lamp increases Ta, whereas the heated floor with a surface temperature of 35°C does not. In that way, the heated floor would have less detrimental effects on sow appetite during warm conditions. However, provision of an adequate environment must take into account the behavior of the newborn. Indeed, during the first day of life, the newborn pig prefers to lie close to the udder of the sow rather than in the heated area (Hrupka et al., 1998) and this undoubtedly increases the probability of being crushed by the sow. Usually, a movable IR lamp is placed at the rear of the sow during parturition to avoid excessive changes in the pig's temperature. Thereafter, the lamp is used in an attempt to direct the piglets away from the "danger zone" of the sow and to attract them progressively toward the heating device in the creep area.

6. The Key Role of Cold Stress in Neonatal Mortality and Poor Growth

Under severe cold, some pigs may undergo deep hypothermia. This was found to be the direct cause of death of 10 to 31% of the pigs farrowed at Ta of ≤10°C (Hata et al., 1985). Deep hypothermia (rectal temperature of 32 to 33°C) impairs glucose metabolism through a suppression of insulin release, leading to a decrease in glucose utilization rate (Close et al., 1985a). This suppression is largely explained by the increased release of catecholamines and can be reversed by rewarming the hypothermic pig (Lossec et al., 1998). At 18 to 20°C, which is close to the temperature corresponding to the maximum metabolic rate, pigs consume 27% less colostrum than their littermates kept at 30 to 31°C (Le Dividich and Noblet, 1981). It is assumed that an increase in the interval between birth and the first suckling may reduce the ingestion of immunoglobulins (Ig) (Coalson and Lecce, 1973), with the first colostrum the highest in Ig. Pigs of low BW (Hoy et al., 1994) and those suffering from hypoxia during parturition (Herpin et al., 1996) are at greater risk in this respect, since they take longer to achieve the first suckle. Thus, the reduced colostrum intake caused by cold stress has a dual detrimental effect: it decreases ingestion of protective Ig and shortens the supply of dietary energy necessary to sustain a high metabolic rate. Cold stress also increases the susceptibility of the newborn to enterotoxigenic *Escherichia coli*-induced diarrhea (Sarmiento, 1983), which in turn reduces the cold resistance (Balsbaugh et al., 1986). Furthermore, pigs that died before weaning were found to have lower levels of Ig at 14 (Blecka and Kelley, 1981) and 24 h of life (Hendrix et al., 1978) than the surviving littermates. The complex ethiology of pig mortality and the central role of cold stress based on this analysis is illustrated in Figure 23.3.

B. The Remainder of the Suckling Period

During the remainder of suckling (i.e., between 2 days and weaning), the thermal insulation of the pig improves rapidly because of peripheral fat accretion. Furthermore, in the presence of a supple-

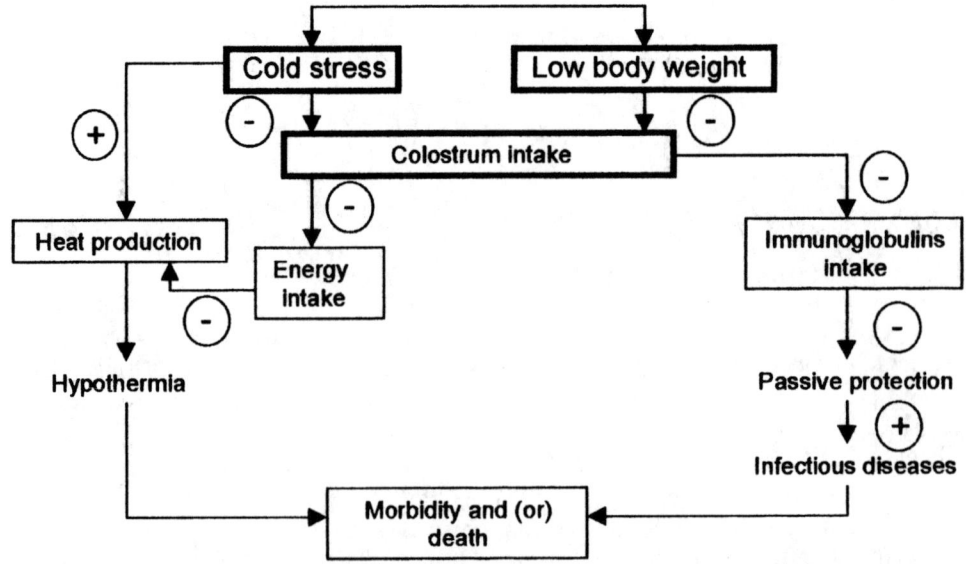

FIGURE 23.3 Schematic representation of the possible effects of cold and low birthweight on colostrum intake and the health of the neonatal pig. (Adapted from Kelley, 1982; Close and Le Dividich, 1982.)

mental source of heat in the farrowing pen, the pig fully expresses its thermoregulatory behavior. These changes result in minimizing heat loss and hence the extra thermoregulatory heat demand. During this period, the preweaning growth rate of pigs is mainly dependent on milk availability, and the thermal environment is usually a secondary issue.

C. Effects of Thermal Environment on the Weaned Pig

1. Ambient Temperature

The requirement for temperature depends on several factors, among which the level of feed intake is the most important. In this respect, it is well established that weaning at 3 to 4 weeks of age is associated with a critical period of underfeeding during which the pig is learning to eat the dry feed (Leibbrandt et al., 1975; Sève, 1982). The duration of this period is very variable, however; usually 2 weeks is required to attain the preweaning level of ME intake (Figure 23.4). Under these conditions, the temperature requirements of the weaning pig may be divided into two periods (Le Dividich and Herpin, 1994): (1) the critical period of about 2 weeks following weaning, representing the period of underfeeding and corresponding to the time required to attain the preweaning level of ME intake and (2) the postcritical period.

The critical period. As a consequence of the low feed intake and a high physical activity associated with the formation of the new social group (McCracken and Caldwell, 1980), pigs are often in negative energy balance during a period of 3 to 6 days following weaning, while the nitrogen balance remains positive (Le Dividich et al., 1980; Close and Stanier, 1984b). This implies that the energy required for maintenance, protein synthesis, and physical activity results in a loss of body fat, which becomes more severe if energy is required for thermoregulation (Whittemore et al., 1978; Le Dividich et al., 1980). This loss of body fat results in a decrease in backfat thickness and body insulation. The combination of lowered insulation and reduced heat associated with the thermic value of feed results in an LCT close to 26 to 28°C during the first postweaning week (McCracken and Caldwell, 1980; Le Dividich et al., 1980; Jordan et al., 1985), which then decreases to 23 to 24°C in the second postweaning week (Close and Stanier, 1984b; McCracken and Gray,

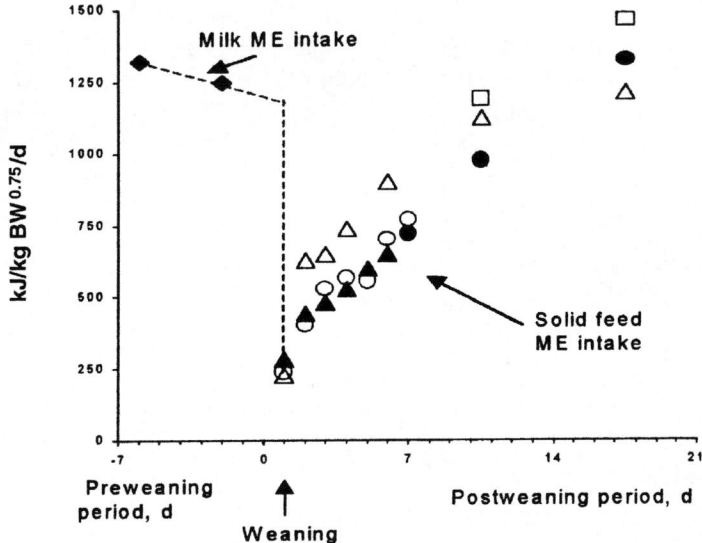

FIGURE 23.4 Effect of weaning between 3 and 4 weeks of age on voluntary ME intake in pigs. (From Leibbrandt et al., 1975 (□); Le Dividich et al., 1980 and Le Dividich, 1981 (▲●); Bark et al., 1986 (○); Noblet and Etienne (1987) (◆); and Le Dividich, unpublished data (△).

1984). Maintaining the ambient temperature at or above the LCT during the critical period of weaning helps to avoid excessive loss of body fat and hence to limit the reduction of thermal insulation and perhaps to attenuate the consequences of the rather frequent disease problems associated to weaning.

The postcritical period. Once regular feed intake is well established and as long as no problem of diarrhea is present, the air temperature of the weaning house can be rapidly reduced. Most studies suggest a 2 to 3°C weekly decrease in ambient temperature until the temperature to be maintained in the finishing house is reached (Le Dividich, 1981; Close and Stanier, 1984a; Feenstra, 1985). In addition, the weaned pig is to some extent able to compensate for a suboptimum environment by increasing its voluntary feed intake. The adjustment in feed intake is rapid and stabilizes within 6 days after exposure to "cold" (Verhagen et al., 1988). Within the 25 to 15°C temperature interval, growth rate remains practically constant (Rinaldo and Le Dividich, 1991c). Because of the relatively high ambient temperature considered essential for optimal performance, the weaning house requires considerable heating. Consequently, several ways of reducing the heating requirement while maintaining pig performance at an acceptable level have been investigated. These include the provision of a microenvironment, reduction in nocturnal air temperature, and, lastly, a reduction in overall temperature in the weaning house while accepting an increase in the feed required per unit of gain.

Provision of a microenvironment. A simple way to save energy is to create a microenvironment for the pig within the weaning house. Use of covers are alternatives that offer the possibility to reduce the heating cost. Pigs provided with hovers or covers at moderate air temperatures (18 to 20°C) had performance similar to those maintained at recommended temperatures (Shelton and Brumm, 1983; Feenstra, 1985). The hovers reduce draughts and, to some extent, trap the heat produced by the pigs.

Reduction of the nocturnal temperature. Another alternative is based on the fact that the pig displays a marked circadian variation in metabolic rate, which is lower during the nighttime than during the daytime. This variation in metabolic rate results in a variation of the LCT, which is lower during the night than during the day (van der Hel et al., 1985). Compared with a constant temperature, a 4 to 9°C reduction in nocturnal temperature (RNT) does not affect the pig's performance, but it decreases heating cost by 30 to 35% (Shelton and Brumm, 1984) with no adverse consequence during the finishing phase (Brumm and Shelton, 1988). However, pigs on an RNT treatment tended to have a greater incidence and severity of scouring. Data obtained by Rinaldo et al. (1989) also reported that within the 12- to 30-kg live weight interval, pigs subjected to a 8°C RNT had similar growth rate as those maintained at a constant temperature of 22°C (Table 23.5). However, the RNT treatment was associated with an overall increase in

TABLE 23.5
Effect of a Reduction of 8°C in Nocturnal Temperature on the Performance of Weaned Pigs Raised in Groups[a]

Temperature	Constant (22°C)	Reduced Nocturnal (22–14°C)
Growth rate (g/day)	626	643
Feed intake (g/day)	1070	1210
Feed conversion ratio	1.71	1.88

[a] Piglets were weaned at 24 days and temperature was progressively decreased from 28 to 22°C over the 3 following weeks; it then remained constant (22°C) or was reduced by 8°C during the nighttime (20 h–8 h). Initial body weight averaged 12.3 kg.

Source: Adapted from Rinaldo et al., 1989.

feed intake with a greater proportion (38 vs. 32%) consumed during the nighttime. Also, pigs on the RNT treatment huddled more during the night. However, repeated fluctuations (3 to 4°C) in temperature (four to six times a day or more) may be detrimental to the health of the pigs (Le Dividich, 1981).

Reduction in overall temperature. The last alternative consists in reducing the overall temperature in the weaning house. Its suitability depends on the amount of extra feed required to compensate for the growth reduction occurring in the cold. From data of Le Dividich and Noblet (1982) and Close and Stanier (1984a), it can be calculated that, at a similar feed intake, growth rate decreases at the rate of 13 g/day/°C coldness, which can be compensated for by an extra feed intake of 13 g/day/°C. In this way, the cost of the extra feed can be compared with the additional cost of heating at optimum.

2. Relative Humidity and Ventilation

Little attention has been paid to the effect of relative humidity and air velocity on the performance of the weaned pig. Relative humidity is not expected to have much influence on the performance of the weaned pig maintained within thermoneutrality. For example, at 24°C, changing the relative humidity from 90 to between 50 and 60% had no effect on performance (Bresk and Stolpe, 1988). Results of Hacker et al. (1979) indicate that below the LCT (18°C), an increase in air velocity from 0 (still air) to 50 cm/s resulted in a 15% decrease in growth rate and a 23% decrease in gain:feed ratio in pigs weaned at 21 to 25 days of age. Similarly, Riskowski et al. (1990) calculated that during the second postweaning week within the temperature range of 24 to 35°C, each 10 cm/s increase in air velocity was associated with a 25 g/day decrease in growth rate. However, because the ventilation rate accounts for most (80 to 90%) of the heat loss in the weaning house, the current recommendation during cold weather is "as low an air velocity as possible." Finally, adverse effects of draughty conditions on performance are noticeable. According to Muehling and Jensen (1961) draught-free weaned pigs grew 6% faster on 25% less feed than did draught-exposed pigs. Moreover, negative effects of draughts are the most detrimental in the immediate postweaning period. During this period, a 106 g/day decrease in growth rate was found by Scheepens et al. (1991) due to draught, the decrease amounting to 155 g/day when draughts were superimposed on fluctuating temperature (25/15°C) (Verhagen, 1987).

IV. EFFECTS OF AMBIENT TEMPERATURE ON PRODUCTION TRAITS IN THE GROWING-FINISHING PIG AND IN THE PREGNANT AND LACTATING SOW

A. THE GROWING AND FINISHING PIG

When supplied nutritionally adequate diets, the level of feed or energy intake is the first factor limiting the pig's performance. In addition, changing the feed intake is an efficient strategy used by the animal to cope with changes in Ta. So, interest lies in determining to what extent feed intake is affected by Ta and examining the effects of Ta on growth rate and carcass composition.

1. Feed Intake

When pigs are allowed *ad libitum* access to feed, they adjust their intake to compensate for changes in Ta. This adjustment is rapid in the cold because feed intake is stabilized within 6 days in response to a decrease in Ta from 20 to 15°C (Verhagen, 1987); the time to adjust feed intake to high Ta is even shorter (<3 days according to Giles, 1992). According to data obtained over a large range of constant Ta by Rinaldo and Le Dividich (1991a) in young growing pigs (10 to 30 kg BW; Ta range 12 to 31.5°C), by Nienaber and Hahn (1983) in finishing pigs (43 to 85 kg BW; Ta range 5 to 30°C), and by Quiniou et al. (2000a) in 30- to 90-kg pigs (Ta range:

12 to 29°C), respectively, voluntary feed intake (VFI) is related to Ta (°C) and BW (kg) according to the following equations:

$$VFI_1 \text{ (g/day)} = 1162 + 16.8Ta - 0.82Ta^2 \ (R^2 = 0.73) \tag{23.1}$$

$$VFI_2 \text{ (g/day)} = 1521 + 10.6BW + 55Ta - 2.6Ta^2 \ (R^2 = 0.67) \tag{23.2}$$

$$VFI_3 \text{ (g/day)} = -1264 + 117Ta - 2.04Ta^2 + 73.6BW - 0.26BW^2 - 0.95Ta \times BW \tag{23.3}$$
$$(R^2 = 0.59)$$

All three equations indicate a curvilinear decrease in feed intake with an increase in Ta. In the early growing period (10 to 30 kg BW; Equation 23.1), intake decreases at the rate of 12 g/day/°C between 15 and 20°C and then at the rate of 24 g/day/°C between 20 and 30°C. In heavier pigs (Equation 23.2), intake changes at the rate of 35 g/day/°C between 15 and 20°C and 75 g/day/°C between 20 and 30°C. Equation 23.3 confirms this higher reduction of VFI at higher temperatures, but it also indicates that the effect of temperature is dependent on BW with, as illustrated in Figure 23.5, larger negative effects of high ambient temperatures in heavier pigs. Finally, it should be mentioned that between 20 and 30°C, the change in VFI in growing–finishing pigs is variable, values ranging from 40 to 50 g/day/°C (Close and Mount, 1978; Vajrabukka et al., 1987; Lopez et al., 1991) to 60 to 80 g/day/°C (Nienaber and Hahn, 1983; Massabie et al., 1997; Quiniou et al., 2000a). In fact, the rate of change in feed intake may depend on several factors including breed, body weight, diet, degree of fatness, and temperature range. Furthermore, it is suggested that there is a temperature threshold above which VFI drops abruptly (see Figure 23.5).

Feed intake is also influenced by other thermal components including relative humidity (RH) and air renewal, but to a much smaller extent than Ta. For example, at a Ta of 24 to 25°C, a 10% increase in RH between 45 and 90% induces a 24 g/day reduction in VFI (Massabie et al., 1997). At a higher Ta (33°C), the corresponding decrease is 32 g/day (Morrison et al., 1969). On the other hand, increasing the air renewal from 0.16 to between 0.40 to 0.50 m³/h/pig at 25°C increases VFI by an average of 160 g/day (Massabie et al., 1997).

Feeding behavior also depends on Ta. A constant-cold Ta does not change the nycthemeral distribution of feed intake in weaned piglets (Herpin et al., 1987), whereas an RNT increases the proportion of feed consumed during the nighttime (Rinaldo et al., 1989). In individually housed

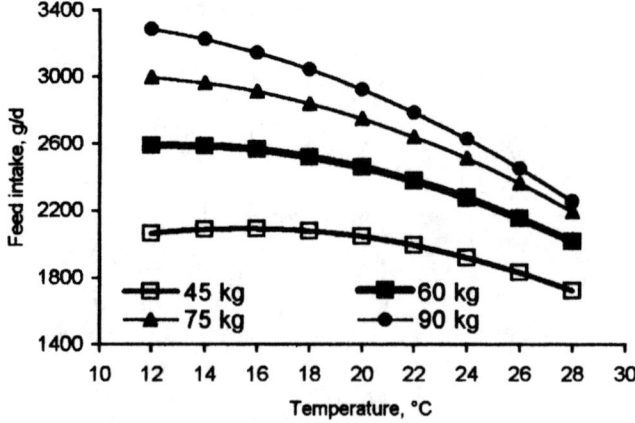

FIGURE 23.5 Effect of ambient temperature and body weight on voluntary feed intake in growing pigs. (Modified from Quiniou et al., *Livest. Prod. Sci.*, 63:245, 2000.)

pigs, the number of meals is increased in the cold and their size is maintained (Nienaber et al., 1990). In contrast, in group-housed pigs, Nienaber et al. (1996) and Quiniou et al. (2000a) failed to detect any change in the number of meals when Ta was decreased, but both their duration and size were increased. At a high Ta, no change was observed in the number of meals, but both their duration and size are reduced (Nienaber et al., 1996; Quiniou et al., 2000a). On a daily basis, when maintained in a hot, cyclic Ta, pigs shift, to some extent, their feeding activity during cooler periods to minimize the detrimental effect of high Ta (Feddes and Deshazer, 1988; Giles, 1992).

2. Growth Rate and Feed Efficiency

The influence of Ta on growth rate or average daily gain (ADG) and feed conversion ratio (FCR) of young pigs and growing-finishing pigs allowed *ad libitum* access to feed is illustrated in Figure 23.6. At both stages, the response of ADG to Ta is curvilinear, the response being maximal between 15 and 25°C and 10 and 20°C in young pigs and growing-finishing pigs, respectively. Corresponding Ta ranges for minimal FCR are 25 to 30°C and 20 to 25°C, respectively. At a lower Ta, FCR increases at the rate of 0.026 and 0.038/°C in young and growing-finishing pigs, respectively (Le Dividich and Rinaldo, 1989). However, studies conducted in equalized feeding conditions indicate that ADG decreases in the cold as a result of an increased heat loss leading to a reduction of energy available for growth. This decrease amounts to 11 to 13 and to 15 to 17 g/day/°C coldness in young and growing-finishing pigs, respectively (Le Dividich, 1991). Alternatively, the additional daily amount of feed required to sustain a similar ADG in the cold as in the optimum Ta is 12 to 14 g/°C coldness in the young pig and 39 to 42 g/°C in the growing-finishing pig. It should be pointed out that the extra feed required in the cold is essentially energy in nature and that protein metabolism and therefore daily protein requirements are only marginally affected in moderate cold conditions (Close et al., 1978; Table 23.6).

At a Ta higher than the optimal range, ADG decreases primarily as a result of the severe decline in feed intake. But, it is of major interest to notice that most studies indicate that a hot environment (27 to 29°C) had no marked effect on FCR (Stahly et al., 1979; Le Dividich et al., 1985; 1987; Giles et al., 1988; Rinaldo and Le Dividich, 1991a; Nienaber et al., 1996; Massabie et al., 1997).

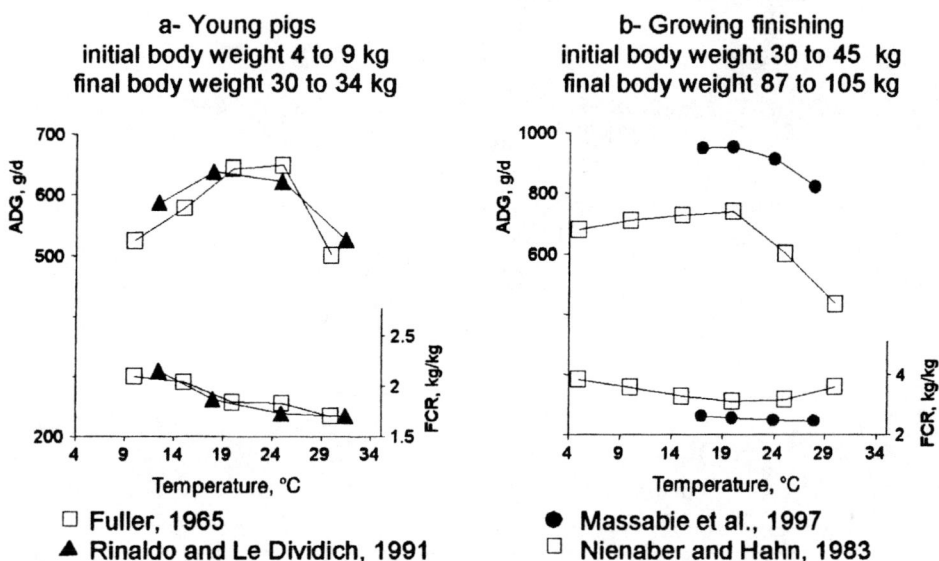

FIGURE 23.6 Effect of environmental temperature on average daily gain (ADG) and feed conservation ratio (FCR) in young pigs (a) and growing-finishing pigs (b).

TABLE 23.6
Performance of Growing-Finishing Pigs Fed Extra Energy to Compensate for the Low Ambient Temperature[a]

	Ambient Temperature (°C)	
	12	20
Feed intake (g/day)		
Basal diet	2234	2234
Corn starch	245	—
Growth rate (g/day)	761	753
Lean tissue gain (g/day)	294	292
Fat tissue gain (g/day)	210	215
Feed conversion ratio	3.26	2.97

[a] There were 18 Large White castrated pigs per treatment. Initial and final BW were 34 and 95 kg, respectively. The basal diet contained (g/kg) 165 g CP and 7.8 g lysine and 12.9 kJ/ME/g during the growing phase (34 to 63 kg), 135 g CP and 6.6 g lysine and 13.1 kJ ME/g during the finishing phase. Extra energy provided per 1°C coldness was calculated according to Le Dividich et al. (1985) and amounted to 28.0 and 19.5 kJ ME/kg $BW^{0.75}$ in the growing and finishing phase, respectively.

Source: Adapted from Rinaldo and Le Dividich (1991a).

In these conditions, the use of techniques that help to alleviate heat stress may be beneficial. For example, wetting of the skin at 32°C results in a similar feed intake and ADG as that at 22°C (Giles et al., 1987).

In practice, conditions may fluctuate and are not constant as in the above-mentioned studies. It is assumed that performance of pigs exposed to diurnal fluctuation in temperature is equivalent to that in a constant temperature of the mean value (Morrison et al., 1975). Bresk and Stolpe (1980) suggested that fluctuations in the range of ±5°C around the mean are acceptable for groups of finishing pigs. On the basis of performance and immune response, larger fluctuations (±12°C) from a mean Ta of 20°C should be avoided (Nienaber et al., 1986).

3. Carcass Composition

Effects of Ta on carcass composition are closely dependent on feeding conditions. Under *ad libitum* intakes, carcass fatness is little affected or unaffected in the cold (Phillips et al., 1982; Le Dividich and Rinaldo, 1989), which is consistent with the recent findings of Quiniou et al. (2000b) that in growing-finishing pigs raised in a group daily energy retention is relatively constant over the temperature range of 12 to 22°C (Figure 23.7). In contrast, at high Ta, carcass fatness is reduced as a result of the decrease in VFI (Nienaber and Hahn, 1983; Giles et al., 1988; Rinaldo and Le Dividich, 1991a). Under constant feeding level, the decrease in energy retained as fat is more pronounced than the energy retained as protein with cold exposure and carcass fatness is subsequently reduced; the effect of cold exposure is then equivalent to the effect of energy restriction (Le Dividich et al., 1985). In pigs fed to achieve similar ADG in the cold as in the warm, little or no effect of Ta is observed (Verstegen et al., 1985; Le Dividich et al., 1987; Giles et al., 1987).

Regardless of feeding conditions, body fat distribution is affected by Ta because, even for similar fatness, percentage of internal fat (viscera, leaf fat) is increased as Ta is increased at the expense of backfat, the opposite being observed in the cold (Le Dividich et al., 1987; Rinaldo and Le Dividich, 1991a; Katsumada et al., 1996). A reduced activity of lipogenic enzymes in backfat and the higher activity of lipoprotein lipase in leaf fat observed at high Ta are consistent with this shift of body fat distribution from external sites toward internal sites (Lefaucheur et al., 1991;

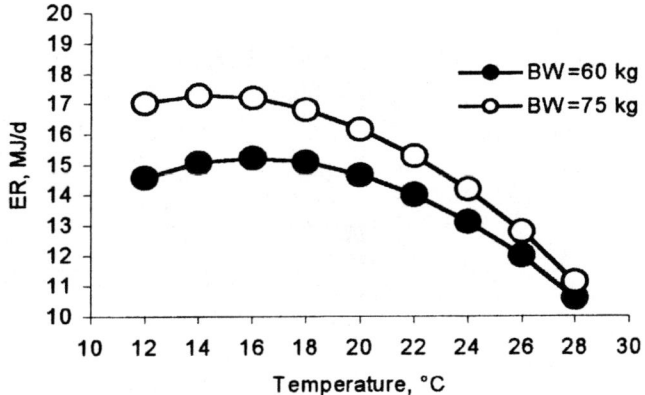

FIGURE 23.7 Effect of ambient temperature on energy retention (ER) in 60- and 75-kg BW growing pigs given *ad libitum* access to feed. (Modified from Quiniou et al., *Br. J. Nutr.*, 2000b.)

Rinaldo and Le Dividich, 1991b). However, further investigations are necessary to elucidate the precise mechanisms by which Ta can alter body fat distribution.

Composition of fat depots is also affected by Ta (Table 23.7). High Ta results in low degree of unsaturation of backfat compared with exposure to cold or thermoneutral temperature (Tonks et al., 1972; Fuller et al., 1974; Le Dividich et al., 1987; Katsumata et al., 1995). Cold exposure induces changes in muscle histology and enzyme activity toward a more oxidative metabolism (Dauncey and Ingram, 1988). This is suggested by the increase in percentage of type I fibers in red muscles (semispinalis, rhomboideus) (Lefaucheur et al., 1991; Herpin and Lefaucheur, 1992) while their mean cross-sectional area is slightly reduced (Table 23.8). Concomitantly, activities of citrate synthase (an indicator of oxidative capacity) and of β-hydroxy-acyl-coenzyme A dehydrogenase (an indicator for lipid oxidation) are also increased. However, whether these changes affect meat quality remains to be elucidated.

Prolonged exposure of the pig to a cold or warm environment is known to affect body conformation and to induce anatomical changes (Dauncey and Ingram, 1986). Pigs living in warm environments have a longer appearance with a longer total body length as well as longer limbs, tail and snout, and longer ears than cold-reared littermates. These, and the changes in body fat distribution, represent adaptation mechanisms that facilitate heat dissipation in the warm through an increased surface exposure and reduced thermal insulation and minimize heat loss in the cold. The mass of internal organs including the liver, kidneys, and the digestive tract (full or empty) is reduced at high Ta, as a result of the decrease in feed intake, and this results in an improvement in dressing percentage (Nienaber and Hahn, 1983; Lefaucheur et al., 1991).

TABLE 23.7
Effect of Environmental Temperature on the Unsaturation Rate of Backfat

	Environmental Temperature			
	Cold (12–13°C)	Thermoneutral (20–23°C)	Warm (28–30°C)	Ref.
Iodine value	—	62.7	60.2	Tonks et al. (1972)
	67.2	64.1	—	Fuller et al. (1974)
Unsaturated fatty acids (% of total fatty acids)	62.8	60.8	58.0	Le Dividich et al. (1987)
	57.4	—	52.0	Lefaucheur et al. (1991)
	—	60.7	58.5	Katsumata et al. (1995)

TABLE 23.8
Effect of Environmental Temperature on Characteristics of Type I Muscle Fibers

	Environmental Temperature (°C)		
	10–12	23	28
Rhomboideus, 20-kg pig[a]			
Percentage	77.4	63.4	—
Area (μm^2)	814	900	—
Relative area (%)	71	58	—
Semispinalis, 90-kg pig[b]			
Percentage	58.4	—	42.6
Area (μm^2)	3,125	—	3,530
Relative area (%)	55	—	39

[a] Herpin and Lefaucheur (1992).
[b] Lefaucheur et al. (1991).

B. THE PREGNANT AND LACTATING SOW

There is no evidence that cold conditions impair the normal course of pregnancy in the sow. However, pregnant sows are often exposed to Ta lower than their LCT (20 to 23°C when single housed or approximately 15°C when group housed), which compromises the building of body energy reserves unless feeding level is increased. To compensate for the effects of cold, 10 to 18 kJ ME/kg$^{0.75}$/°C are required, depending on the degree of coldness and housing conditions (Noblet et al., 1997); this is equivalent to 40 to 70 g feed/°C coldness in 200-kg sows. In contrast to cold stress, severe heat stress may result in a significant embryo and fetal mortality. For example, a brief exposure of 2 h at 40°C between day 2 and 13 can cause embryo mortality to be as high as 63% (Wildt et al., 1975). Similarly, exposure of the sow to 37.8°C for 17 h daily, then 32.2°C for the remaining 7 h between day 102 and 110 is also reported to cause a fetal mortality of 44% (Omtvedt et al., 1971). However, constant moderate heat stress (33°C) during the first month of gestation has no adverse effect on embryo mortality (Liao and Veum, 1994).

During lactation, heat stress is of major importance. Indeed, in relation to high feed intakes during this period, LCT is in the range of 15 to 18°C and Ta of the farrowing house is seldom below 18 and 20°C in winter and often is above the UCT of 22 to 25°C (Kemp and Verstegen, 1987; Black et al., 1993; Quiniou and Noblet, 1999) during summer. The reduction in HP under hot conditions is mainly achieved by a decrease in feed intake, averaging 2.4 MJ DE/1°C rise in Ta between 16 and 32°C (Black et al., 1993). However, recent results of Quiniou and Noblet (1999) indicate a curvilinear decrease of VFI with temperature increase, the decrease being quite pronounced above 25 to 27°C (6.7 MJ DE/1°C rise). The weaning weight of the litter is also 10 to 23% lower at 27 to 30°C compared with 18 to 20°C (Lynch, 1977; Stansbury et al., 1987; Schoenherr et al., 1989; Prunier et al., 1997; Quiniou and Noblet, 1999; Table 23.9) suggesting a negative effect of high Ta on milk yield. Direct measurement of milk production, using the D_2O technique, indicates a 10% decrease in milk yield between 20 and 30°C for the overall period of lactation (Schoenherr et al., 1989). The growth reduction of the litter is also more pronounced with the advancement of lactation (Prunier et al., 1997). There is no evidence that the decrease in milk yield is caused by a lower nursing demand of the piglets because provision of supplemental milk replacer has a more-pronounced effect on the growth of suckling piglets during the warm than during the cold season (Azain et al., 1996). More likely, the reduced milk yield may reflect the inability of the sow to produce more milk at high Ta. In this respect, findings of Prunier et al. (1997) indicate that primiparous sows fed similarly in a thermoneutral (20°C) and a hot (30°C) environment mobilize 27% less body reserves at high Ta, suggesting that the ability to mobilize body reserves

TABLE 23.9
Effect of Ambient Temperature on Performance of Multiparous Lactating Sows

Temperature (°C)	18	22	25	27	29
Daily feed intake (g/day)					
Day 1 to day 21	5666	5419	4947	4520	3079
Day 7 to day 19	7161	6401	6084	5321	3483
Body weight loss (kg)	23	22	25	30	35
Backfat thickness loss (mm)	2.1	1.9	2.7	3.5	3.5
Pig growth rate (g/day/pig) (day 1 to day 21)	244	245	233	212	189

[a] Mean litter size was 10.2 pigs and BW after farrowing averaged 275 kg; sows were given *ad libitum* access to feed after day 6 of lactation.

Source: Adapted from Quiniou and Noblet (1999).

is also limited at high Ta. As a whole, the lowered milk production and the reduced feed intake undoubtedly contribute to reduced HP and milk yield at high Ta.

Attempts have been made to maintain milk yield at high Ta, mainly through the improvement of energy intake by the sow (Black et al., 1993). In brief, the type of floor has little effect upon the appetite, but sows that had access to snout coolers at 30°C consume 1.0 kg more feed per day then did sows without access (Stansbury et al., 1987). McGlone et al. (1988) also demonstrated the benefit of snout coolers, but intermittent water drip on the neck and head of the sow was the most effective in enhancing feed intake in hot environments. Use of underground pipes is also an effective method of air-conditioning farrowing houses (Neukermans et al., 1989) during summer conditions.

From a nutritional point of view, attempts have been made to increase energy intake by increasing the energy density of the diet. In thermoneutral conditions, Dourmad (1988) reported a 7% decrease in food intake but a 9% increase in ME intake when dietary energy content was increased from 12.5 to 14.6 MJ ME/kg. However, in hot conditions, the benefit of increasing the dietary energy density by inclusion of fat is questionable because it results primarily in an increased milk fat content (Schoenherr et al., 1989; Chen et al., 1990) and has little benefit on maintaining body condition of the sow.

V. NUTRITIONAL INTERACTIONS WITH AMBIENT TEMPERATURE

A. DIETARY ENERGY CONCENTRATION

Studies conducted at the Universities of Georgia (Seerley et al., 1978; Coffey et al., 1982) and Kentucky (Stahly and Cromwell, 1979; 1986) suggest an interaction between dietary energy density and Ta on the performance of growing-finishing pigs. When pigs are allowed *ad libitum* feeding, high-energy diets (i.e., high in fat) as compared with low-energy diets (i.e., high in fiber) improve ADG and, to some extent, ME efficiency, under warm environments, whereas in the cold, low- and high-energy diets result in similar performance. This interaction is largely explained by the variations in thermic effect of feed (TEF) between diets and its fate depending on Ta, and by the interaction between dietary energy density and Ta on ME intake. According to Noblet et al. (1994), TEF is higher for high-fiber diets than for high-fat or high-starch diets. In the cold, dietary energy density has little effect on the ME intake (Stahly et al., 1981; Coffey et al., 1982; Le Dividich and Noblet, 1986) and TEF is partly utilized to compensate for some of the extra-thermoregulatory heat production. In the support of this latter view are: (1) the increased efficiency of ME intake utilization for energy retention from an average value of 70 to 75% within the zone

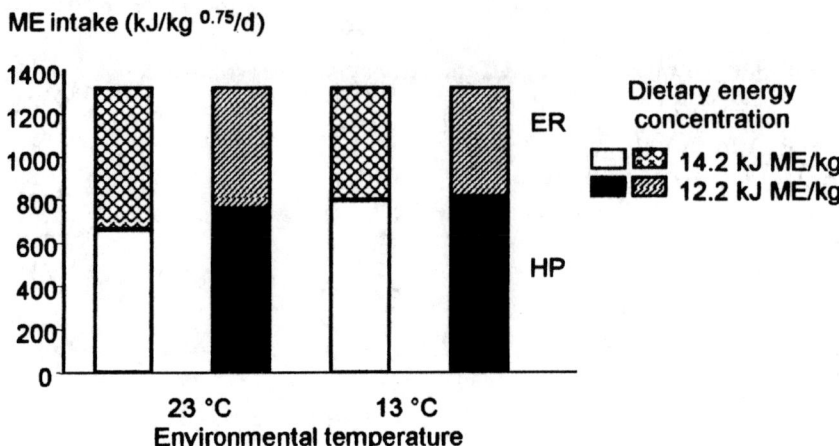

FIGURE 23.8 Effects of dietary energy concentration and ambient temperature on heat production (HP) and energy retention (ER) in pigs (average body weight = 49.5 kg) fed constant ME intake (1324 kJ/kg$^{0.75}$). (Adapted from Noblet et al., 1985.)

of thermoneutrality to 90 to 100% in the cold (Verstegen et al., 1973; Close, 1978; Noblet et al., 1989; Quiniou et al., 2000b) and (2) the findings of Noblet et al. (1985) that in the cold, low- and high-energy diets result in similar HP (Figure 23.8). It follows that the relative nutritional value of diets high in fiber is maximized in the cold. For example, the net energy value of wheat straw for a pregnant sow amounts to 2.5 MJ/kg in thermoneutral conditions and 4.2 MJ/kg in the cold (Noblet et al., 1989). In the warm, high-energy diets are better tolerated because these (1) are associated with a reduced TEF, which must be dissipated to the environment (Figure 23.8), and they (2) result in higher energy intake, which counterbalances to some extent the reduction in VFI occurring in the warm (Stahly and Cromwell, 1979; Le Dividich and Noblet, 1986; Katsumata et al., 1996). These effects undoubtedly contribute for the improved performance of pigs given *ad libitum* access to high-energy diets under warm conditions.

B. Amino Acid Supply and Balance

With regard to the interactive effect between Ta and amino acid supply, two major questions arise: Are the requirements for a given level of performance (lean tissue gain) and is the optimal amino acid balance altered by Ta? There is some evidence that total protein or amino acid requirement or, in other words, maintenance needs and efficiencies of protein supply for protein gain are not affected by Ta. This view is supported by metabolic studies of Verstegen et al. (1973), Close et al. (1978), and Phillips et al. (1982) indicating that protein accretion is largely independent on Ta unless dietary amino acid and/or energy available for protein deposition is becoming limiting (Berschauer et al., 1983; Campbell and Taverner, 1988). Data from growth trials (see Table 23.6) also show that cold-exposed, growing-finishing pigs fed supplemental energy as starch to compensate for the extra-thermoregulatory heat production, perform similarly to those maintained in thermoneutral conditions at equal daily intake of the limiting amino acid. Furthermore, the relationship between ADG (Figure 23.9) or protein gain (Ferguson and Gous, 1997) and the limiting amino acid (lysine) intake clearly suggests that, at equal limiting amino acid intake, ADG is equal in both hot and thermoneutral environments. However, because of changes of feed intake with Ta, the dietary concentration of protein and/or amino acid may need to be altered. For example, Rinaldo and Le Dividich (1991c) calculated that in *ad libitum* conditions, lysine requirement decreases by 0.009 g/MJ ME/°C decrease in Ta between 20 and 12°C and increases by 0.005 g/MJ ME/°C increase in Ta between 20 and 28°C. More generally, exposure of growing pigs to temperatures

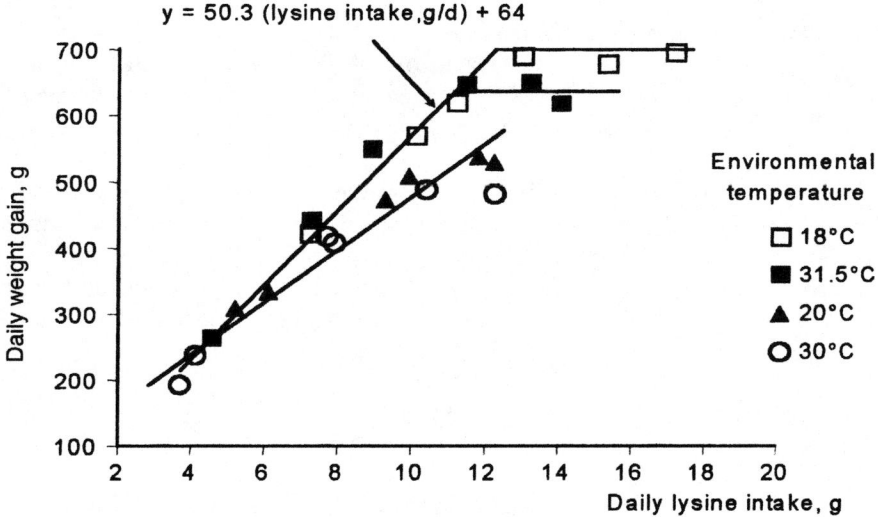

FIGURE 23.9 Effect of environmental temperature on pig growth in relation to lysine intake. (Adapted from Schenk et al., 1992 (▲○) and Rinaldo and Le Dividich, unpublished data (■□).

lower than their LCT is associated with a reduction of protein requirements, expressed as percentage of the diet, while increase of Ta above LCT induces a negligible effect on diet protein content. The effect of high Ta is then comparable with the effect of energy restriction (Quiniou et al., 1996).

As for the interactive effects between Ta and dietary amino acid adequacy, diets containing a deficient amino acid level (Stahly and Cromwell, 1987) have more detrimental effects on performance of pigs exposed to hot environment than to thermoneutral or cold conditions. Indeed, elevation of feed intake due to cold exposure results in an increased intake of the limiting amino acid, thereby minimizing the effect of the inadequacy. In contrast, in hot conditions, the deficient amino acid level may accentuate the reduction in feed intake and hence the intake of the limiting amino acid. Furthermore, in hot conditions, excess levels of protein or amino acids may create problems of heat stress through the relatively high TEF that is due to the metabolism of excess dietary protein or amino acid. This results in a reduction in net energy intake, thereby accentuating the energy deficit. This view is substantiated by the findings of Stahly et al. (1979) that a high-protein diet tended to be utilized less efficiently in a hot environment than an isolysine, low-protein diet supplemented with crystalline L-lysine. However, surprisingly enough, low-protein diets formulated on an ideal protein basis failed to improve the performance of finishing pigs exposed to a hot environment (Lopez et al., 1994).

VI. CONCLUSION: SIGNIFICANCE OF AN OPTIMAL TEMPERATURE

The thermal requirements of the pig are often based on the determination of the LCT. Indeed, the energy retention is maximized at the LCT, and hence satisfactory weight gains are expected. In fact, the LCT corresponds to the optimum temperature of the pig at birth and at weaning, and for the pregnant sow. At the critical periods of birth and weaning, the main goals are (1) to minimize heat loss in the newborn and to maximize the availability of energy intake for retention and fat accretion thus improving the body insulation, and (2) to avoid excessive loss of body fat at weaning and hence minimizing the decrease in thermal insulation. Also, at both periods, resistance to diseases is maximal at the LCT. On the other hand, the pregnant sow is fed restrictively and any change in her maintenance energy requirement in connection with thermoregulation demand will markedly affect the amount of energy available for building her body reserves. In conventional growing-finishing pigs with *ad libitum* access to feed, it is suggested that there is an optimum range of Ta for each production trait. Insofar as decreasing carcass fatness and improving feed efficiency are the main objectives, the range of Ta optimizing overall performance is higher than LCT while remaining within the thermoneutral zone. However, at this range of Ta, the growth rate is somewhat reduced, and hence it is necessary to take into account the increase in time required to reach slaughter weight.

The extent to which performance is affected by the cold is reasonably well established in different classes of pigs. Except at the critical periods of birth and weaning, performance can be maintained by extra feed consumption or by heating the animal house. Choice of either strategy depends largely on the relative costs of feed and heating energy. Under high Ta, it is important to alleviate heat stress, by increased evaporative heat loss or diet manipulation, to maintain performance at an acceptable level, especially in the finishing pig and in the lactating sow.

REFERENCES

Azain, M. J., T. Tomkins, J. S. Sowinski, R. A. Arentson, and D. E. Jewell. 1996. Effect of supplemental pig milk replacer on litter performance: seasonal variation in response, *J. Anim. Sci.*, 74:2195.

Balsbaugh, R. K., S. E. Curtis, R. C. Meyer, and A. W. Norton. 1986. Cold resistance and environmental temperature preference in diarrheic piglets, *J. Anim. Sci.*, 62:315.

Bark, L. J., T. D. Crenshaw, and V. D. Leibbrandt. 1986. The effect of meal intervals and weaning on feed intake of early weaned pigs, *J. Anim. Sci.*, 62:1233.

Benevenga, N. J., J. K. Steinman-Goldsworthy, T. D. Crenshaw, and J. Odle. 1989. Utilization of medium-chain triglycerides by neonatal piglets: I. Effects on milk consumption and body fuel utilization, *J. Anim. Sci.*, 67:3331.

Berschauer, F., W. H. Close, and D. B. Stephens. 1983. The influence of protein: energy value of the ration and level of feed intake on the energy and nitrogen metabolism of the growing pig. 2. N metabolism at two environmental temperature, *Br. J. Nutr.*, 49:271.

Berthon, D. 1994. Thermogénèse néonatale chez le porcelet, Thèse Européenne, Université Claude Bernard, Lyon, 122 pp.

Berthon, D., P. Herpin, C. Duchamp, M. J. Dauncey, and J. Le Dividich. 1993. Modification of thermogenic capacity in neonatal pigs by changes in thyroid status during late gestation, *J. Dev. Physiol.*, 19:253.

Berthon, D., P. Herpin, and J. Le Dividich. 1994. Shivering thermogenesis in the neonatal pig, *J. Therm. Biol.*, 6: 413.

Black, J. L., B. P. Mullan, M. L. Lorschy, and L. R. Giles. 1993. Lactation in the sow during heat stress. In *Biology of Lactation in Farm Animals*, Enright, W. J., D. Peticlerc, and P. Politiek, Eds., Elsevier, Amsterdam, 153–170.

Blecka, F., and K. W. Kelley. 1981. Cold stress reduces the acquisition of colostral immunoglobulins in piglets, *J. Anim. Sci.*, 52:594.

Bresk, B., and J. Stolpe. 1980. On the optimal range of the temperature of the air for breeding fattening pigs, *Arch. Tierernähr.*, 30:759.

Bresk, B., and J. Stolpe. 1988. Effect of high and medium relative humidities on live weight of weaned piglets exposed to different ambient temperature, *Monatsh. Veterinärmed.*, 48:191.

Brumm, M. C., and D. P. Shelton. 1988. A modified reduced nocturnal temperature regimen for early-weaned pigs, *J. Anim. Sci.*, 66:1067.

Campbell, R. G., and M. R. Taverner. 1988. Relationships between energy intake and protein and energy metabolism, growth and body composition of pigs kept at 14 or 32°C from 9 to 29 kg, *Livest. Prod. Sci.*, 18:289.

Chen, S. C., F. S. Chang, T. S. Yang, and S. Y. Chen. 1990. Effect of energy content in lactation diet on lactation and reproductive performance of sows in a hot environment, *Proceedings of the 5th AAAP Animal Science Congress*, Taipei, Vol. 3, AAAP, 13.

Close, W. H. 1978. The effects of plane of nutrition and environmental temperature on the energy metabolism of the growing pig. 3. The efficiency of energy utilization for maintenance and growth, *Br. J. Nutr.*, 40: 433.

Close, W. H. 1981. The climatic environments of the pig. In *Environmental Aspects of Housing for Animal Production*, Clark, J. A., Ed., Butterworths, London, 149–166.

Close, W. H., and J. Le Dividich. 1982. Nutritional and environmental factors influencing the growth and the development of the young piglet, paper presented at the 33rd Annual Meeting of EAAP, Leningrad, U.S.S.R.

Close, W. H., and L. E. Mount. 1978. The effects of plane of nutrition and environmental temperature on the energy metabolism of the growing pig. 1. Heat loss and critical temperature, *Br. J. Nutr.*, 40:413.

Close, W. H., and M. W. Stanier. 1984a. Effects of plane of nutrition and environmental temperature on the growth and development of the early weaned piglet, 1. Growth and body composition, *Anim. Prod.*, 38:211.

Close, W. H., and M. W. Stanier. 1984b. Effects of plane of nutrition and environmental temperature on the growth and development of the early weaned piglet, 2. Energy metabolism, *Anim. Prod.*, 38:221.

Close, W. H., L. E. Mount, and D. Brown. 1978. The effects of plane of nutrition and environmental temperature on the energy metabolism of the growing pig. 2. Growth rate, including protein and fat deposition, *Br. J. Nutr.*, 40:423.

Close, W. H., J. Le Dividich, and P.H. Duée. 1985a. The influence of environmental temperature on glucose tolerance and insulin response in the newborn piglet, *Biol. Neonate*, 47:84.

Close, W. H., J. Noblet, and R. P. Haevens. 1985b. Studies on the energy metabolism in pregnant sow. 2. The partition and utilization of metabolizable energy intake in pregnant and non-pregnant animals, *Br. J. Nutr.*, 53:267.

Coalson, J. A., and J. G. Lecce. 1973. Influence of nursing intervals on changes in serum proteins (immunoglobulins) in neonatal pigs, *J. Anim. Sci.*, 36:381.

Coffey, M. J., R. W. Seerley, D. W. Funderbucke, and H. C. McCampbell. 1982. Heat increment and level of dietary energy and environmental temperature on the performance of growing-finishing swine, *J. Anim. Sci.*, 54:95.

Curtis, S. E.. 1983. *Environmental Management in Animal Agriculture*, Iowa University Press, Ames, 390 pp.

Curtis, S. E., C. J. Heidenreich, and R. B. Harrington. 1967. Age dependent changes of thermostability in neonatal pigs, *Am. J. Vet. Res.*, 28:1887.

Dauncey, M. J., and D. L. Ingram. 1986. Acclimatization to warm and cold temperatures and the role of food intake, *J. Therm Biol.*, 11:89.

Dauncey, M. J., and D. L. Ingram. 1988. Influence of environmental temperature and energy intake on skeletal muscle respiratory enzymes and morphology, *Eur. J. Appl. Physiol.*, 58:239.

Dourmad, J. Y. 1988. Ingestion instantanée d'aliment chez la truie en lactation: de nombreux facteurs de variation, *Prod. Anim.*, 1:141.

Elliot, J. I., and G. A. Lodge. 1977. Body composition and glycogen reserves in the neonatal pig during the first 96 hours post-partum, *Can. J. Anim. Sci.*, 57:141.

English, P. R., and S. A. Edwards. 1996. Management of the nursing sow and her litter, In *Pig Production*, Taverner, M. R., and A. C. Dunkin, Eds., Elsevier, Amsterdam, 113–140.

English, P. R., and V. Morrison. 1984. Causes and prevention of piglet mortality, *Pig News Info.*, 5:369.

Feenstra, A. 1985. Effects of air temperature on weaned piglets, *Pig News Info.*, 6:295.

Feddes, J. J. R., and J. A. Deshazer. 1988. Energetic responses of growing pigs to high cyclic and constant temperatures, *Trans. Am. Soc. Agric. Eng.*, 31:1203.

Ferguson, N. S., and R. M. Gous. 1997. The influence of heat production on voluntary food intake in growing pigs given protein-deficient diets, *Anim. Sci.*, 64:365.

Fraser, D., and J. Rushen. 1992. Colostrum intake by newborn piglets, *Can. J. Anim. Sci.*, 72:1.

Fuller, M. F., and A. W. Boyne. 1972. The effects of environmental temperature on the growth and metabolism of pigs given different amount of food. 2. Energy metabolism, *Br. J. Nutr.*, 28:373.

Fuller, M. F., W. R. H. Duncan, and A. W. Boyne. 1974. Effects of environmental temperature on the degree of insaturation of depot fats of pigs given different amounts of food, *J. Sci. Food Agric.*, 25:205.

Geuyen, T. P. A., J. M. F. Verhagen, and M. W. A. Verstegen. 1984. Effect of housing and temperature on metabolic rate of pregnant sow, *Anim. Prod.*, 38:477.

Giles, L. R. 1992. Energy Expenditure of Growing Pigs at High Ambient Temperatures, Ph.D. thesis, University of Sydney, 162 pp.

Giles, L. R., J. L. Black, and E. B. Dettman. 1987. Influence of high temperature and skin wetness on voluntary intake and performance of pigs from 50 to 80 kg live weight. In *Proceedings of Inaugural Conference of the Australasian Pig Science Association*, Albury, 140.

Giles, L. R., E. B. Dettman, and R. F. Lowe. 1988. Influence of diurnally fluctuating high temperature on growth and energy retention of growing pigs, *Anim. Prod.*, 47:467.

Hacker, P. R., G. S. Wogar, and J. R. Ogilvie. 1979. Environment indices for weaned pig, ASAE paper 79–4017, ASAE, St. Joseph, MI.

Hata, H., H. Abe, N. Sugimoto, H. Miyazaki, E. Deguechi, and K. Tokoro. 1985. Effects of environmental temperature on the rectal temperature and mortality of newborn piglets, *Jpn. J. Swine Sci.*, 22:174.

Hel, W. van der, M. W. A. Verstegen, W. Baltussen, and H. Brandsma. 1985. The effects of ambient temperature on diurnal rythm in heat production and activity in pigs kept in groups, *Int. J. Biometeorol.*, 28:303.

Hemsworth, P. H., C. G. Winfield, and P. D. Mullaney. 1976. A study of the development of teat order in piglets, *Appl. Anim. Ethol.*, 2:225.

Hendrix, W. F., K. W. Kelley, C. T. Gaskins, and D. J. Hinrichs. 1978. Porcine neonatal survival and serum gamma globulins, *J. Anim. Sci.*, 47:1281.

Henken, A. M., H. A. Brandsma, W. Van der Hel, and M. W. A. Verstegen. 1991. Heat balance characteristics of limit-fed growing pigs of several breed kept in groups at and below thermal neutrality, *J. Anim. Sci.*, 69:2434.

Herpin, P., R. Bertin, J. Le Dividich, and R. Portet. 1987. Some regulatory aspects of thermogenesis in cold-exposed piglets, *Comp. Biochem. Physiol.*, 84: 1073.

Herpin, P., and L. Lefaucheur. 1992. Adaptative changes in oxidative metabolism in skeletal muscle of cold-acclimated piglets, *J. Therm. Biol.*, 17:277.

Herpin, P., J. Le Dividich, and N. Amaral. 1993. Effect of selection for lean tissue growth on body composition and physiological state of the pig at birth, *J. Anim. Sci.*, 71:2645.

Herpin, P., J. Le Dividich, D. Berthon, and J. C. Hulin. 1994. Assessment of thermoregulatory and postprandial thermogenesis over the first 24 hours after birth in pigs, *Exp. Physiol.*, 79:1011.

Herpin, P., J. Le Dividich, J. C. Hulin, M. Fillaut, F. de Marco, and R. Bertin. 1996. Effects of level of asphyxia during delivery on viability at birth and postnatal vitality of newborn pigs, *J. Anim. Sci.*, 79:1111.

Holmes, C. W., and W. H. Close. 1977. The influence of climatic variables on energy metabolism and associated aspects of productivity in pigs, In *Nutrition and the Climatic Environment*, Haresign, W., H. Swan, and D. Lewis, Eds., Butterworths, London, 51–74.

Holmes, M. A., P. G. Arthur, and P. E. Hartman. 1990. Changes in the concentration of glucose and galactose in the peripheral blood of suckling piglets, *J. Dairy Res.*, 57:331.

Holyoake, P. K., G. D. Dial, T. Trigg, and V. King. 1995. Reducing pig mortality through supervision during the perinatal period, *J. Anim. Sci.*, 73:3453.

Hoy, S., C. Lutter, M. Wähner, and B. Puppe. 1994. Influence of birth weight on the early postnatal vitality of piglets, *Dtsch. Tierärztl. Wochenschr.*, 101:393.

Hrupka, B. J., V. D. Leibbrant, T. D. Crenshaw, and N. J. Benevenga. 1998. The effect of farrowing crate heat lamp location on sow ands pig patterns of lying and pig survival, *J. Anim. Sci.*, 76:2995.

Ingram, D. L.. 1965. Evaporative cooling in the pig, *Nature* (London), 207:415.

ITP. 1998. *Pig Performance 97*, ITP, Paris, 64 pp.

Jordan, J. W., A. McAllister, and S. T. C. Weatherup. 1985. A note on the critical temperature of the fasted and fed early-weaned pig, *Anim. Prod.*, 41:425.

Katsumata, M., Y. Kaji, and M. Saitoh. 1996. Growth and carcass fatness responses of finishing pigs to dietary fat supplementation at high ambient temperature, *Anim. Sci.*, 62: 591.

Katsumata, M., H. Hirose, Y. Kaji, and M. Saitoh. 1995. Influence of a high ambient temperature and dietary fat supplementation on fatty acid composition of depot fat in finishing pigs, *Anim. Sci. Technol.* (Japan), 66:225.

Kelley, K. W.. 1982. Immunobiology of domestic animals as affected by hot and cold weather, In *Proceedings of the Second International Livestock Environment Symposium*, Ames, IA, 470–482.

Kemp, B., and M. W. A. Verstegen. 1987. The influence of climatic environment on sows, In *Energy Metabolism in Farm Animals*, Verstegen, M. W. A., and A. H. Henken, Eds., Martinus Nijhoff Publishers, Dordrecht, The Netherlands, 115–132.

Kovacs, F., and P. Rafaï. 1973. Investigation on the metabolism of newborn and young piglets, *Magy. Allatorv. Lapja*, 28:182.

Le Dividich, J. 1981. Effects of environmental temperature on the growth rates of early weaned piglets, *Livest. Prod. Sci.*, 8:75.
Le Dividich, J. 1991. Effect of thermal environment on the performance of intensively-reared growing pig, *Sel. Vet.*, 32:191.
Le Dividich, J., and P. Herpin. 1994. Effects of climatic conditions on the performance, metabolism and heath status of weaned piglets: a review, *Livest. Prod. Sci.*, 38:79.
Le Dividich, J., and J. Noblet. 1981. Colostrum intake and thermoregulation in the neonatal pig in relation to environmental temperature, *Biol. Neonate*, 40:167.
Le Dividich, J., and J. Noblet. 1982. Growth rate and protein and fat gain in early weaned piglets housed below thermoneutrality, *Livest. Prod. Sci.*, 9:731.
Le Dividich, J., and J. Noblet. 1986. Effect of dietary energy level on the performance of individually housed early-weaned piglets in relation to environmental temperature, *Livest. Prod. Sci.*, 16:255.
Le Dividich, J., and D. Rinaldo. 1989. Effets de l'environnement thermique sur les performances du porc en croissance, *J. Rech. Porcine Fr.*, 21:219.
Le Dividich, J., M. Vermorel, J. Noblet, J. C. Bouvier, and A. Aumaitre. 1980. Effects of environmental temperature on heat production, energy retention, protein and fat gain in early weaned piglets, *Br. J. Nutr.*, 44:313.
Le Dividich, J., B. Desmoulin, and J. Y. Dourmad. 1985. Influence de la température ambiante sur les performances du porc en croissance-finition en relation avec le même niveau alimentaire, *J. Rech. Porcine Fr.*, 17:275.
Le Dividich, J., J. Noblet, and T. Bikawa. 1987. Effects of environmental temperature and dietary energy concentration on the performance and carcass characteristic of growing-finishing swine fed to equal rate of gain, *Livest. Prod. Sci.*, 17:235.
Le Dividich, J., P. Mormède, M. Catheline, and J. C. Caritez. 1991. Body composition and cold resistance of the neonatal pig from European (Large White) and Chinese (Meishan) breeds, *Biol. Neonate*, 59:268.
Le Dividich, J., P. Herpin, and R. M. Rosario-Ludovino. 1994. Utilization of colostral energy by the newborn pig, *J. Anim. Sci.*, 72:2082.
Le Dividich, J., P. Herpin, C. Cano, and F. Strullu. 1997. Effect of fat content of colostrum on voluntary colostrum intake and fat utilization in newborn pigs, *J. Anim. Sci.*, 75:707.
Le Dividich, J., J. Noblet, P. Herpin, J. van Milgen, and N. Quiniou. 1998. Thermoregulation, In *Progress in Pig Science*, Wiseman, J., M. A. Varley, and J. P. Chadwick, Eds., Nottingham University Press, Nottingham, 229–263
Lee, H. F., and S. H. Chiang. 1994. Energy value of medium-chain triglycerides and their efficacy in improving survival of neonatal pigs, *J. Anim. Sci.*, 72:133.
Lefaucheur, L., J. Le Dividich, J. Mourot, G. Monin, P. Ecolan, and D. Kraus. 1991. Influence of environmental temperature on growth, muscle and adipose tissue metabolism and meat quality in swine, *J. Anim. Sci.*, 69:2844–2854.
Leibbrandt, V. D., R. C. Ewan, V. C. Speer, and D. R. Zimmerman. 1975. Effect of age and calorie: protein ratio on performance and body composition of the baby pig, *J. Anim. Sci.*, 40:1070.
Léon, A. I. Schmidt, F. Strullu, M. Fillaut, J. Gautier, J. C. Hulin, Y. Lebreton, P. Herpin, and J. Le Dividich. 1998. Effects of substitution of medium-for long chain triglycerides in colostrum on the energy metabolism of the newborn pig in relation to environmental temperature, *J. Rech. Porcine Fr.*, 30:275.
Liao, C. W., and T. L. Veum. 1994. Effects of dietary energy intake by gilts and heat stress from days 3 to 24 or 30 after mating on embryo survival and nitrogen and energy balance, *J. Anim. Sci.*, 72:2369.
Lopez, J., G. W. Jesse, B. A. Becker, and M. R. Ellersieck. 1991. Effects of temperature on the performance of finishing swine. 1. Effects of a hot diurnal temperature on average daily gain, feed intake and feed efficiency, *J. Anim. Sci.*, 69:1843.
Lopez, J., R. D. Goodband, G. L. Allee, G. W. Jesse, J. L. Nelssen, M. D. Tokach, D. Spiers, and B. A. Becker. 1994. The effects of diets formulated on an ideal protein basis on growth performance, carcass characteristics, and thermal balance of finishing gilts housed in a hot, diurnal environment, *J. Anim. Sci.*, 72:367.
Lossec, G., P. Herpin, and J. Le Dividich. 1998. Thermoregulatory responses of the newborn pig during experimentally induced hypothermia and rewarming, *Exp. Physiol.*, 83:667.
Lynch, P. B. 1977. Effect of environmental temperature on lactating sows and their litters, *Ir. J. Agric. Sci.*, 16:123.

Massabie, P., R. Granier, and J. Le Dividich. 1997. Effects of environmental conditions on the performance of growing-finishing pigs, In *Proceedings of the 5th International Livestock Environment Symposium*, Bloomington, MN, 1010–1016.

McCance, R. A., and E. M. Widdowson. 1959. Effect of lowering the ambient temperature on the metabolism of the newborn pig, *J. Physiol.* (London), 147:124.

McCracken, K. J., and B. J. Caldwell. 1980. Studies of diurnal variations of heat production and the effective lower critical temperature of early-weaned pigs under commercial conditions of feeding and management, *Br. J. Nutr.*, 43:321.

McCracken, K. J., and R. Gray. 1984. Further studies on the heat production and effective lower critical temperature of early-weaned pigs under commercial conditions of feeding and management, *Anim. Prod.*, 39:283.

McGlone, J. J., W. F. Stansbury, and L. F. Tribble. 1988. Management of lactating sows during heat stress: effects of water drip, snout coolers, floor type and a high energy-density diet, *J. Anim. Sci.*, 66:885.

Mellor, D. J., and C. Cockburn. 1986. A comparison of energy metabolism in the newborn infant, piglet and lamb: a review, *Q. J. Exp. Biol.*, 71:361.

Milon, A., A. Aumaitre, J. Le Dividich, J. Frantz, and J. J. Metzger. 1983. Influence of birth prematurity on colostrum composition and subsequent immunity of piglets, *Ann. Rech. Vet.*, 14:533.

Morrison, S. R., H. Heitman, and T. E. Bond. 1969. Effect of humidity on swine and temperatures above optimum, *Int. J. Biometeorol.*, 13:135.

Morrison, S. R., H. Heitman, and R. L. Givens. 1975. Effect of diurnal air temperature cycles on growth and food conversion in pigs, *Anim. Prod.*, 20:287.

Mount, L. E. 1968. *The Climatic Physiology of the Pig*, Edward Arnold, London.

Mount, L. E. 1974. The concept of thermal neutrality, In *Heat Loss from Animals and Man*, Monteith, J. L., and L. E. Mount, Eds., Butterworths, London, 426–439.

Mount, L. E.. 1979. *Adaptation to Thermal Environment: Man and His Productive Animals*, Edward Arnold, London.

Muehling, A. J., and A. H. Jensen. 1961. Environmental studies with early-weaned pigs, Agriculture Experimental Station, Bull. 670, University of Illinois, Urbana.

Neukermans, G. K., K. De Schrijvere, M. Debruyckere, W. Van Der Biest, and L. Balemans. 1989. Conditionnement de l'air de ventilation des porcheries d'élevage par l'échangeur thermique enterré dans le sol, In *Proceedings of the 11th International Congress on Agricultural Engineering*, Dodd, V. A., and P. M. Grace, Eds., 1385–1392.

Nienaber, J. A., and G. L. Hahn. 1983. Performance of growing-finishing swine in response to thermal environment, ASAE paper 83–137, St. Joseph, MI.

Nienaber, J. A., G. L. Hahn, H. G. Klemcke, B. A. Becker, and F. Blecka. 1986. Cyclic temperature effects on growing-finishing swine, American Society of Agricultural Engineers, paper 86–4026.

Nienaber, J. A., T. P. McDonald, G. L. Hahn, and Y. R. Chen. 1990. Eating dynamics of growing-finishing swine, *Trans. Am. Soc. Agric. Eng.*, 33:2011.

Nienaber, J. A., G. L. Hahn, T. P. McDonald, and R. L. Korthals. 1996. Feeding pattern and swine performance in hot environments, *Trans. Am. Soc. Agric. Eng.*, 39:195.

Noblet, J., and M. Etienne. 1987. Metabolic utilization of energy and maintenance requirements in lactating sows, *J. Anim. Sci.*, 64:774.

Noblet, J., and J. Le Dividich. 1981. Energy metabolism of the newborn pig during the first 24 h after birth, *Biol. Neonate*, 40:175.

Noblet, J., J. Le Dividich, and T. Bikawa. 1985. Interaction between energy level in the diet and environmental temperature on the utilization of energy in growing pigs, *J. Anim. Sci.*, 61:452.

Noblet, J., J. Y. Dourmad, J. Le Dividich, and S. Dubois. 1989. Effect of ambient temperature and addition of straw of alfalfa in the diet on energy metabolism in pregnant sow, *Livest. Prod. Sci.*, 21:309.

Noblet, J., H. Fortune, X. S. Shi, and S. Dubois. 1994. Prediction of net energy value of feed for growing pigs, *J. Anim. Sci.*, 72:344.

Noblet, J., J. Y. Dourmad, M. Etienne, and J. Le Dividich. 1997. Energy metabolism in pregnant sows and newborn pig, *J. Anim. Sci.*, 75:2708.

Noblet, J., C. Karege, S. Dubois, and J. Van Milgen. 1999. Metabolic utilization of energy and maintenance requirements in growing pigs: effect of sex and genotype, *J. Anim. Sci.*, 77:1208.

Omtvedt, I. T., R. E. Nelson, R. L. Edwards, D. F. Stephens, and E. J. Turman. 1971. Influence of heat stress during early, mid and late pregnancy of gilts, *J. Anim. Sci.*, 32:312.

Pettigrew, J. E., S. G. Cornelius, R. L. Moser, T. R. Heeg, K. P. Miller, and C. D. Hagen. 1986. Effects of oral doses of corn oil and other factors on preweaning survival and growth of piglets, *J. Anim. Sci.*, 62:601.

Phillips, P. A., B. A. Young, and J. B. McQuitty. 1982. Liveweight, protein deposition and digestibility responses in growing pig exposed to low temperature, *Can. J. Anim. Sci.*, 62:95.

Prunier, A., M. Messias de Bragança, and J. Le Dividich. 1997. Influence of high ambient temperature on performance of reproductive sows, *Livest. Prod. Sci.*, 52:123.

Quiniou, N., and J. Noblet. 1999. Influence of high ambient temperatures on performance of multiparous lactating sows, *J. Anim. Sci.*, 77:2124.

Quiniou, N., J. Y. Dourmad, and J. Noblet. 1996. Effect of energy intake on the performance of different types of pig from 45 to 100 kg body weight. 1. Protein and lipid deposition, *Anim. Sci.*, 63:277.

Quiniou, N., J. Noblet, and S. Dubois. 2000a. Voluntary feed intake and feeding behaviour of group-housed growing pigs are affected by ambient temperature and body weight, *Livest. Prod. Sci.*, 63:245.

Quiniou, N., J. Noblet, J. van Milgen, and S. Dubois. 2000b. Modelling heat production and energy balance in group-housed growing pigs exposed to cold or hot ambient temperatures, *Br. J. Nutr.* (in press).

Rinaldo, D., M. C. Salaün, and J. Le Dividich. 1989. Influence d'une réduction de la température ambiante ou d'un abaissement nocturne de la température ambiante sur les performances du porcelet sevré, *J. Rech. Porcine Fr.*, 21:239.

Rinaldo, D., and J. Le Dividich. 1991a. Assessement of optimal temperature for performance and chemical body composition of growing pigs, *Livest. Prod. Sci.*, 29:61.

Rinaldo, D., and J. Le Dividich. 1991b. Effect of warm exposure on adipose tissue and muscle metabolism in growing pigs, *Comp. Biochem. Physiol.*, 100A:995.

Rinaldo, D., and J. Le Dividich. 1991c. Influence de la température ambiante sur les performances de croissance du porc, *Prod. Anim.*, 4:57.

Riskowski, G. L., D. S. Bundy, and J. A. Mathews. 1990. Huddling behavior and hematology of weanling pigs as affected by air velocity and temperature, *Trans. Am. Soc. Agric. Eng.*, 33:1677.

Rooke, J. A., I. M. Bland, and S. A. Edwards. 1998. Effect of feeding tuna oil or soyabean oil as supplements to sows in late pregnancy on piglet tissue composition and viability, *Br. J. Nutr.*, 80:273.

Sarmiento, J. I.. 1983. Environmental Temperature: A Predisposing Factor in the Enterotoxigenic *Escherichia coli*-Induced Diarrhea in Newborn Pig, M.Sc. dissertation, University of Guelph, 123 pp.

Scheepens, C. J. M., M. J. M. Tielen, and M. J. C. Hessing. 1991. Influence of daily intermittent draught on the health status of weaned pigs, *Livest. Prod. Sci.*, 29:241.

Schenck, B. C., T. S. Stahly, and G. L. Cromwell. 1992. Interactive effects of thermal environment and dietary lysine and fat levels on rate, efficiency and composition of growth of weaning pigs, *J. Anim. Sci.*, 70:3791.

Schmidt, I., and P. Herpin. 1997. Postnatal changes of mitochondrial protein mass and respiration in skeletal muscle from the newborn pig, *Comp. Biochem. Physiol.*, 118B:639.

Schmidt, I., and P. Herpin. 1998. Carnitine palmitoytransferase and its regulation by malonyl-CoA are modulated by age and cold exposure in skeletal muscle mitochondria from newborn pigs, *J. Nutr.*, 128:886.

Schoenherr, W. D., T. S. Stahly, and G. L. Cromwell. 1989. The effects of dietary fat or fiber addition on yield and composition of milk from sows house in a warm or hot environment, *J. Anim. Sci.*, 67:482.

Seerley, R. W., M. C. McDaniel, and H. C. McCampbell. 1978. Effects of sows' dietary energy on source of sows' milk and piglet carcass composition, *J. Anim. Sci.*, 47:427.

Sève, B. 1982. Age at weaning, development of chemical body components, and energy utilization in piglets from 3–25 kg live weight, *Livest. Prod. Sci.*, 9:603.

Shelton, D. P., and M. C. Brumm. 1983. Hovers in flat-deck swine nursery pens, ASAE paper 83-4010, ASAE, St. Joseph, MI.

Shelton, D. P., and M. C. Brumm. 1984. Response of nursery pigs to reduced nocturnal temperatures, ASAE paper 84-4021, ASAE, St. Joseph, MI.

Stahly, T. S., and G. L. Cromwell. 1979. Effects of environmental temperature and dietary fat supplementation on the performance and carcass characteristics of growing and finishing swine, *J. Anim. Sci.*, 49: 1478.

Stahly, T. S., and G. L. Cromwell. 1987. Optimal dietary lysine levels for pigs as influenced by thermal environment, Swine Research Report 299, Department of Animal Science, University of Kentucky, Lexington, 15–18.

Stahly, T. S., G. L. Cromwell, and M. P. Aviotti. 1979. The effects of environmental temperature and dietary lysine source and level performance and carcass characteristics of growing swine, *J. Anim. Sci.*, 49:1242.

Stahly, T. S., G. L. Cromwell, and J. R. Overfield. 1981. Interactive effects of season and year and dietary fat supplementation, lysine source and lysine levels of the performance of swine, *J. Anim. Sci.*, 53:1269.

Stahly, T. S., and G. L. Cromwell. 1986. Responses to dietary additions of fiber (alfalfa meal) in growing pigs housed in a cold, warm or hot thermal environment, *J. Anim. Sci.*, 63:1870.

Stansbury, W. F., J. L. Mc Glone, and L.F. Tribble. 1987. Effects of season, floor type, air temperature and snout coolers on sow and litter performance, *J. Anim. Sci.*, 65:1507.

Svendsen, J. 1992. Perinatal mortality in pigs, *Anim. Reprod. Sci.*, 28:59.

Thompson, B. K., and D. Fraser. 1988. Variation in piglet weights: weight gain in the first day after birth and their relationship with later performance, *Can. J. Anim. Sci.*, 68:581.

Tonks, H. M., W. C. S. Smith, and J. M. Bruce. 1972. The influence of a high temperature, high humidity indoor environment on the performance of bacon pig, *Vet. Rec.*, 90:531.

Trayhurn, D. R., N. J. Temple, and J. Van Aerde. 1989. Evidence from immunoblotting studies on uncoupling protein that brown adipose tissue is not present in the domestic pig, *Can. J. Physiol. Pharmacol.*, 67:1480.

Vajrabukka, C., C. J. Thwaites, and D. J. Farrell. 1987. The effects of duration of sprinkling and temperature of the drinking water of the feed intake and growth of pigs at high temperature, *J. Agric. Sci.* (Cambridge), 109:409.

Verhagen, J. M. F. 1987. Acclimation of Growing Pigs to Climatic Environment, Ph.D. thesis, Wageningen, The Netherlands, 128 pp.

Verhagen, J. M. F., R. Geers, and M. W. A. Verstegen. 1988. Time taken for growing pigs to acclimate to change in ambient temperature, *Neth. J. Agric. Sci.*, 36:1.

Verstegen, M. W. A., and W. H. Close. 1994. The environment and the growing pig, In *Principles of Pig Science*, Cole, D. J. A., J. Wiseman, and M. A. Varley, Eds., Nottingham University Press, Nottingham, 333–353.

Verstegen, M. W. A., W. H. Close, I. B. Start, and L. E. Mount. 1973. The effects of environmental temperature and plane of nutrition on heat loss, energy retention and deposition of protein and fat in groups of growing pigs, *Br. J. Nutr.*, 30:21.

Verstegen, M. W. A., H. A. Brandsma, and G. Mateman. 1985. Effect of ambient temperature and feeding level on slaughter quality in fattening pigs, *Neth. J. Agric. Sci.*, 33:1.

Whittemore, C. T., A. Aumaitre, and I. H. Williams. 1978. Growth of body components in young weaned pigs, *J. Agric. Sci.* (Cambridge), 91:681.

Wildt, D. E., G. D. Riegle, and W. R. Dukelow. 1975. Physiological temperature response and embryonic mortality in stressed swine, *Am. J. Physiol.*, 229:1471.

24 Nutrition and Immunology of Swine

Rodney W. Johnson, Jeffery Escobar, and Douglas M. Webel

CONTENTS

I. Introduction 545
II. Basic Concepts in Porcine Immunology 546
III. Inflammatory Cytokines Alter Metabolism 547
IV. Impact of Cytokines on Nitrogen Metabolism 548
V. Nutrient Requirements of the Immune System 550
    A. Amino Acids 551
    B. Lipids 553
    C. Zinc 554
    D. Iron and Copper 555
    E. Vitamin E and Selenium 556
    F. Vitamin A 556
VI. Concluding Remarks 557
References 557

I. INTRODUCTION

In modern, high-density production systems, swine live surrounded by pathogenic microorganisms — bacteria, viruses, and parasites that can cause infectious disease or pathology. Nonetheless, pigs become ill relatively infrequently because they are equipped with a highly evolved immune system that affords protection against infectious microorganisms. This protection can be costly, however, as a number of studies have established that animals reared in unsanitary environments that afford a high level of host–pathogen interaction grow more slowly and consume less feed than animals reared in more sanitary environments (Coates et al., 1963; Roura et al., 1992; Williams et al., 1997b). The view is that nutrients that might have otherwise gone to support growth are redirected to support the host's defenses against pathogenic microorganisms.

An important yet unresolved issue is whether animals that are subjected to varying degrees of immunological stress (i.e., stress caused by exposure to pathogens) have different nutrient requirements. The nutrient requirements for swine established by the National Research Council (NRC) are, for the most part, based on experiments conducted in laboratory situations where environmental stresses are minimized. Therefore, the estimated nutrient requirements for pigs have been established to maximize production of healthy animals that in all likelihood are exposed to fewer infectious microorganisms than what is usual. Another important issue is whether the nutrient requirements established by NRC to maximize production also afford "optimum" immunity. At times, it may be preferential to enhance immune responses while at other times it may be better to inhibit them. Importantly, specific nutrients have been identified that can either enhance or inhibit the response of the immune system to pathogenic microorganisms. Therefore, it is possible that animals reared in environments that afford different levels of exposure to pathogens require more or less of a given nutrient to optimize the immune response. However, specific nutrient requirements for optimal immune function have not been determined.

This chapter attempts to shed light on these issues by briefly describing the immune system, what constitutes an immune response, and how the immune system interacts with disparate physiological systems to alter protein accretion. The chapter also briefly discusses the nutrient requirements of the immune system and how certain nutrients can either enhance or inhibit immunity.

II. BASIC CONCEPTS IN PORCINE IMMUNOLOGY

The different types of white blood cells or leukocytes that mediate host defense against infection are derived from hematopoietic stem cells that are found in the bone marrow. The myeloid progenitors differentiate to produce the polymorphonuclear leukocytes, including monocytes that further differentiate into macrophages in the tissues. The immune cells derived from myeloid progenitors are critical for innate immunity — the nonspecific defense against infectious microorganisms that is completely independent of prior exposure to the pathogen. The lymphoid progenitors give rise to T and B lymphocytes, which are responsible for adaptive or acquired immunity — a highly specific response to a specific pathogen that is acquired over time through previous exposure to that same pathogen. The B lymphocyte or B cell differentiates in the bone marrow and, upon activation, differentiates further into an antibody-producing plasma cell. However, T cells differentiate in the thymus and, when activated, differentiate into cells that can kill infected cells (cytotoxic CD8 T cells) or activate other cells (inflammatory and helper CD4 T cells) of the immune system. Therefore, B cells and T cells are responsible for humoral and cell-mediated immunity, respectively, which sum to form acquired immunity (Table 24.1).

Each individual lymphocyte (i.e., mature T and B cells) possesses receptors for just one antigen, but the animal's entire lymphocyte receptor repertoire allows it to recognize all possible antigens except those of self. When a lymphocyte encounters a foreign antigen from a pathogenic microorganism, for example, each activated lymphocyte proliferates to produce a clone of progeny bearing the same receptor. These processes, known as clonal selection and clonal expansion, are

TABLE 24.1
Key Leukocytes That Are Involved in Innate and Acquired Immunity

Leukocyte	Primary Function
	Innate Immunity
Neutrophil	Phagocytosis and destruction of bacteria
	Produce inflammatory response mediators
Macrophage	Phagocytosis and destruction of bacteria
	Produce inflammatory cytokines that activate other leukocytes and that initiate other components of the acute-phase response
	Antigen presentation
Natural killer cell	Provide early defense against viruses and certain intracellular pathogens
	Acquired Immunity
B lymphocyte	Produce antibody
	Antigen presentation
T lymphocyte	Combat intracellular pathogens by activating macrophages (inflammatory CD4 T cells, T_H1)
	Combat extracellular pathogens by stimulating B cells to produce antibody (helper CD4 T cells, T_H2)
	Destroy infected cells (CD8 cytotoxic T cells)

the basic premise of acquired immunity. These cells then differentiate into effector cells, which can do away with the microorganism, thereby causing the response to cease. The initial response to the antigen generates a population of lymphocytes with immunological memory so that if the pathogen is encountered a second time, these so-called memory cells can rapidly proliferate and differentiate into effector cells that eliminate the pathogen before visible symptoms of infection are evident. This, of course, is the biological basis for long-term immunity following infection or successful vaccination.

Host defense systems that are nonspecific to the various pathogenic microorganisms are referred to as innate immunity because they are inherent, and the capacity to respond does not change or adapt from one infection to another. When a pathogen penetrates the epithelial barriers to infection (Table 24.2), the innate immune system is next in line. The nonadaptive or early-induced responses that are part of innate immunity are induced by macrophages and polymorphonuclear neutrophilic leukocytes, which recognize pathogens using relatively invariant receptors. Therefore, the same response is usually made to all pathogens. The purposes of the early-induced nonadaptive response are to ward off invading pathogens or to hold them in check until an adaptive immune response can be mounted. For example, neutrophils engulf and kill extracellular pathogens, whereas natural killer cells are important in innate immunity to viruses and certain intracellular pathogens. Macrophages ingest and degrade pathogenic microorganisms, present antigen to lymphocytes, and are activated to secrete inflammatory cytokines. The cytokine molecules initiate an inflammatory response and activate B and T lymphocytes and therefore promote adaptive immunity. Inflammatory cytokines, however, do more than mediate communication among leukocytes — they also act as hormones that enable the immune system to communicate with other disparate physiological systems. This allows the immune system to reorganize the animal's biological priorities in response to infection. Because several inflammatory cytokines are metabolically active, this aspect of immunophysiology has lately captured the attention of swine nutritionists.

III. INFLAMMATORY CYTOKINES ALTER METABOLISM

It is well established that animals reared in environments where they are exposed to a high number of pathogens neither eat well nor grow well, even when no clinically identifiable disease is present. The early research by Coates et al. (1963) demonstrated that chicks reared in a germ-free environment grew faster and consumed more feed than animals reared in a conventional environment. Until recently, it was thought that a bacterial or viral contaminant was directly responsible for decreasing the performance of the host. However, it has been proposed that an immunological mechanism is at least partly, if not totally, responsible for the decreased performance of immune-challenged animals (Klasing et al., 1987; Kelley et al., 1994; Johnson, 1997).

Several years ago it was proposed that cytokines released during an immune challenge were responsible for the changes observed in intermediary metabolism following an immune challenge (Klasing, 1988). This hypothesis was based on a series of experiments that demonstrated that chicks

TABLE 24.2
Epithelial Barriers to Infection

Mechanical	Epithelial cells joined by tight junctions
	Ciliated epithelial cells and mucin that trap and remove pathogens
Chemical	Bactericidal enzymes in saliva, sweat, tears, and gut
	Low pH in stomach
	Antibacterial peptides
Microbiological	Normal flora in gastrointestinal tract produce antibacterial substances and compete against pathogenic microorganisms

challenged with inflammatory agents had lower rates of weight gain, feed intake, and feed efficiency than chicks not injected with inflammatory agents (Klasing et al., 1987; Klasing, 1988; Klasing and Barnes, 1988). Klasing and co-workers (1987) observed similar changes in performance and metabolism when chicks were treated with a cell-free supernatant derived from stimulated macrophages. This finding strongly supported the hypothesis that a component produced by macrophages was responsible for the anorectic and metabolic effects associated with immune challenge. The work of Klasing's group with birds confirmed previous work in rats and mice, and provided convincing evidence that a group of proteins released from macrophages, called cytokines, were involved in the changes observed in sick or immunologically challenged animals.

Cytokines are hormone-like proteins released by a variety of cell types, including mononuclear myeloid cells (e.g., monocytes and macrophages). As the first line of defense against invading pathogens (i.e., as part of the innate immune response), mononuclear myeloid cells are uniquely suited to identify and respond to pathogens and provide a signal to the rest of the body concerning an impending infection (Klasing and Johnstone, 1991; Johnson, 1997). Recent research has shown that if macrophages do not produce cytokines there is a complete breakdown in communication between immune and nonimmune tissues (Segreti et al., 1997; Finck et al., 1998). Although many cytokines have been identified, the inflammatory cytokines, interleukin-1 (IL-1), interleukin-6 (IL-6), and tumor necrosis factor-α (TNF-α) are thought to be the primary cytokines involved in metabolic regulation. Several important immunological and metabolic effects of these molecules are presented in Table 24.3. The metabolic changes induced by these molecules are homeostatic in nature and thus nutrients that would have gone toward growth and skeletal muscle accretion now go to support host defense systems, which at the time are of higher priority. Because rapid efficient protein accretion is a goal of swine production and inflammatory cytokines have profound effects on protein accretion, this issue is discussed in more detail below.

IV. IMPACT OF CYTOKINES ON NITROGEN METABOLISM

The net effect of cytokine synthesis and release is a decrease in whole-body protein accretion. The alterations in whole-body protein and skeletal muscle metabolism are attributed to a decrease in protein synthesis and an increase in protein degradation, with the combination of these processes leading to a decrease in protein accretion and an increase in nitrogen excretion. This is illustrated

TABLE 24.3
Immunologic and Metabolic Effects of Cytokines Produced by Macrophages

Interleukin-1	Interleukin-6	Tumor Necrosis Factor-α
	Major Immunological Effects	
Activates lymphocytes	Activates lymphocytes	Inflammation
	Antibody production	
	Acute-phase protein synthesis	
	Major Metabolic Effects	
Muscle protein degradation	Muscle protein degradation	Muscle protein degradation
Reduced muscle protein synthesis	Reduced muscle protein synthesis	Reduced muscle protein synthesis
Fever	Fever	Fever
Anorexia	Acute-phase protein synthesis	Anorexia
Hypoferremia		Lipolysis
Hypozincemia		
Hypercuppremia		

by the work of Flores et al. (1989), which demonstrated that exogenous IL-1 and TNF-α elicit a negative nitrogen balance that is accompanied by a decrease in whole-body protein synthesis and an increase in skeletal muscle protein degradation. Consistent with these results, peak plasma concentrations of TNF-α, IL-6, and urea nitrogen were evident, respectively, in pigs that were fasted and then challenged with lipopolysaccharide (LPS; Webel et al., 1997).

The influence of cytokines on protein synthesis and degradation seems to be dependent on the tissue and skeletal-muscle fiber type. In general, protein synthesis is decreased in skeletal muscle and is increased in liver, lung, and heart (Charters and Grimble, 1989; Fong et al., 1989; Ballmer et al., 1991). The effects of cytokines on protein kinetics are vastly different from those induced by fasting, where peripheral proteins are spared and visceral proteins are broken down. In addition to the tissue-specific effects, it is apparent that the fiber type of a muscle can also influence protein turnover. Vary and Kimball (1992) demonstrated that muscles consisting of fast-twitch fibers were subject to breakdown during sepsis whereas protein kinetics were unaffected by sepsis in muscles consisting of slow-twitch fibers.

The distinct differences in muscle protein kinetics during sepsis between muscles composed of fast-twitch and slow-twitch fibers could be of importance. In recent years, pigs and chickens intended for meat production have been selected for maximal lean growth rate and increased breast meat yield, respectively. Because pigs selected for maximal lean growth rate have a greater proportion of muscles containing fast-twitch vs. slow-twitch muscles (Rahelic and Puac, 1981) and chickens selected for maximal breast-meat yield likewise have higher levels of fast-twitch fibers, the effects of cytokines on muscle tissue growth are potentially more deleterious in leaner, more modern genotypes (Williams, 1995).

The increase in protein synthesis in the liver is most likely due to an increase in the synthesis of the acute-phase proteins. Numerous *in vivo* and *in vitro* studies have demonstrated that synthesis of the positive acute-phase proteins is mediated by the direct action of cytokines upon the hepatocyte, and indirectly as the result of hormonal changes brought about by cytokines (Rothwell and Grimble, 1992). The inflammatory cytokines IL-1, IL-6, and TNF-α are known to increase the rate of hepatic amino acid uptake (Argiles et al., 1989; Argiles and Lopez-Soriano, 1990) and protein synthesis (Klasing and Austic, 1984; Geiger et al., 1988; Ballmer et al., 1991). The increase in hepatic protein synthesis results in a net increase in hepatic protein accretion and an increase in protein release into the circulation (Geiger et al., 1988). It is generally accepted that the increase in acute-phase protein production is of fundamental importance and is an adaptive response necessary for survival of the animal (Beisel, 1977). The proteins released by the liver have a wide array of functions, and, for many, the functions have yet to be elucidated. Acute-phase proteins are known to enhance macrophage phagocytosis and lysis ability, inhibit serum protease activity, and alter plasma mineral concentrations, among other functions.

There is a substantial quantity of acute-phase proteins synthesized shortly after an infectious insult in humans. In fact, it has been estimated that up to 850 mg of acute-phase proteins are synthesized per kg body weight in a typical acute-phase response (Reeds et al., 1994). Although acute-phase protein production has not been as well documented in either chickens or pigs, several of the acute-phase proteins have been described in these species. Serum levels of α_1-acid glycoprotein (AGP), haptoglobin, and C-reactive protein (CRP) have been explored as measures of stress in swineherds. Specific-pathogen-free pigs have been shown to possess threefold lower levels of AGP when compared with pigs infected with *Actinobacillus pleuropneumonia* and atrophic rhinitis (Itoh et al., 1992). In addition, Williams et al. (1997a,b) compared AGP levels of pigs reared in environments that presented either a high or low level of immune stimulation. They reported that the level of immune stimulation and the plasma concentration of AGP were positively correlated. Serum levels of CRP and haptoglobin have also been shown to be elevated in infected swine (Burger et al., 1992; Hall et al., 1992). Furthermore, Pfeiffer et al. (1993) demonstrated that growth rate was negatively correlated with serum concentrations of ceruloplasmin, fibrinogen, and haptoglobin in sheep challenged with yeast.

V. NUTRIENT REQUIREMENTS OF THE IMMUNE SYSTEM

Nutrient requirements established by the NRC for swine can be defined as levels adequate to permit the maintenance of normal health and productivity. These estimates are, for the most part, based on experiments conducted in laboratory situations where environmental stresses are minimized. This leads one to question whether animals reared under field conditions require more or less of a given nutrient to maximize performance and maintain normal health. Indeed, it is common practice in commercial animal production to feed levels of nutrients well above those proposed by the NRC. Interactions between nutrition and the immune system can affect animal productivity and nutrient requirements in at least two ways. First, immune responses to pathogenic microorganisms reduce growth and alter metabolism such that nutrient requirements are impacted. Second, nutrition can impact the immunocompetence of animals and thus their resistance to infectious disease (Table 24.4).

The effects of nutrients on immunocompetence have received considerable attention. Chandra (1992) reviewed the effects of protein and energy malnutrition (PEM) on immunocompetence and found that humans with prolonged PEM have reduced lymphocyte numbers, decreased humoral immune responsiveness, and reduced neutrophil bactericidal activity. Furthermore, moderate to severe deficiencies of protein or specific amino acids have been shown to induce changes in immune responses. These changes include depression of antibody titers to specific antigens, reduced lymphocyte populations, reduced complement and acute-phase protein production, and increased susceptibility to infection (Grimble, 1990; Dietert et al., 1994). In addition, several vitamins and trace minerals have been shown to impact immune function. In particular, antioxidants such as α-tocopherol and Se have received considerable attention. Supplementation of domestic animals with vitamin E has been shown to potentiate antibody responses to a variety of killed preparations as well as live organisms (Finch and Turner, 1996). However, recent evidence suggests that vitamin E, as well as other antioxidants, may reduce cytokine production from cultured macrophages and monocytes (Eugui et al., 1994; Bulger et al., 1997) and in pigs challenged with LPS (Webel et al., 1998).

Although, marked deficiencies in trace nutrients, protein, or amino acids are not likely to occur in swine reared in commercial situations, marginal nutrient deficiencies could occur in certain situations. It is possible that these deficiencies may not impact growth or productivity but may influence other physiological variables, such as the immune system (Klasing, 1996). However, specific nutrient requirements for optimal immune function have not been determined. Part of the reason that nutrient requirements have not been determined for immune function is that a specific response criterion has not been established. For example, numerous investigators have measured

TABLE 24.4
Several Items Associated with Immunity and Disease Resistance That Can Be Affected by Nutrients

Epithelial barrier function
Chemotaxis
Phagocytosis
Production of reactive oxygen species and other inflammatory mediators
Cytokine production
Production of acute-phase proteins and complement
Lymphoid tissues
Lymphocyte populations
Lymphocyte proliferation
Antibody synthesis

specific titers to antibodies or levels of immunoglobulins in relation to amino acid intake to determine a requirement. However, the importance of maximizing the response to a specific antigen is questionable because very low levels of IgG are required for an animal to mount a normal immune response and fight off infection (Kelley and Easter, 1987).

A. Amino Acids

Although numerous amino acids have important roles in the proper functioning of the immune system, methionine, arginine, glutamine, and possibly the aromatic amino acids seem to be the ones that are required in the greatest quantities during an immune response. Methionine is the first limiting amino acid in most practical poultry diets, and it is the second or third limiting amino acid in barley and wheat-based swine diets, making it a primary concern for marginal deficiency. Tsiagbe et al. (1987) showed that chicks required a greater quantity of methionine to maximize responses to sheep red blood cells and delayed-type hypersensitivity to phytohemagglutinin, but other investigators have not observed this relationship (Bhargva et al., 1970). The idea that animals may require methionine for immune function at levels above those that support maximal growth is not entirely agreed upon. In fact, Klasing and Barnes (1988) demonstrated that activation of the immune system by LPS decreased the methionine requirement of chicks for maximal growth and feed efficiency.

Arginine is considered a semiessential amino acid for humans and other mammals because it is synthesized from other amino acids via the urea cycle. However, exogenous arginine is required for growth in young animals and in various stress situations (e.g., sepsis, trauma) to optimize growth and minimize nitrogen excretion (Barbul and Dawson, 1994). The recent discovery that arginine is a direct precursor of nitric oxide (NO), a potent cytotoxic agent produced by macrophages and neutrophils, highlights the importance of arginine in immune function.

Nitric oxide production is known to occur in a number of mammalian tissues including endothelial cells, macrophages, neutrophils, T lymphocytes, and Kupffer cells, to name a few (reviewed by Barbul and Dawson, 1994). Production of NO occurs via a deaminase reaction where arginine is the primary substrate and NO and citrulline are the products. The role of NO in immune function is twofold. First, NO increases the influx of immune cells into tissues by increasing vasculature dilation and enhancing leukocyte adhesion to the endothelial cell wall (Barbul and Dawson, 1994). Second, neutrophils and macrophages are known to exert their cytotoxic effect against bacteria and parasites via NO (Stuehr and Marletta, 1985; Denis, 1991).

The possibility of a marginal deficiency of arginine in practice is not usually considered important because diets formulated using common ingredients have adequate arginine to support maximal growth. However, research in mice and chickens has demonstrated that NO production from macrophages cultured *in vitro* is dependent upon the concentration of arginine in the culture medium, and that NO production is maximized at a concentration of approximately 0.40 mM arginine (Granger et al., 1988; Sung et al., 1991). The level of arginine that maximizes NO production from macrophages *in vitro* is considerably higher than the concentration found in plasma from animals receiving a diet with levels of arginine capable of supporting maximal growth (Dietert et al., 1994), indicating that plasma arginine may be limiting NO production *in vivo*.

Although glutamine is not considered to be an indispensable amino acid for growth of animals, recent research has indicated that it may be conditionally essential in times of immune system activation (Newsholme et al., 1988; Lacey and Wilmore, 1990). This hypothesis stemmed from research showing that glutamine is essential for the normal functioning of macrophages and lymphocytes during an immune response (Lacey and Wilmore, 1990; Dudrick et al., 1994). The requirement for glutamine in these cells stems from increased metabolic activity following stimulation by an infectious pathogen. The accelerated metabolism is necessary to facilitate cell division and the secretion of antibodies and cytokines, all processes that require amino acids and energy. The importance of glutamine metabolism in lymphocytes and macrophages is illustrated by the essentiality of glutamine in the media for proliferation of these cells *in vitro* (Eagle et al., 1956).

Glutamine is a primary carrier of nitrogen in the blood, and its concentration is generally maintained within a relatively small range. However, during catabolic states like sepsis, there is an increased demand for glutamine as a substrate for cells of the immune system. A well-documented response to septic insult is a rapid mobilization of amino acids from skeletal muscle, provided by enhanced protein breakdown. This release of amino acids has typically been thought of as a general release of amino acids from skeletal muscle to fuel hepatic acute-phase protein synthesis and gluconeogenesis. Recent evidence would indicate that this might not be the case, as the release of glutamine from skeletal muscle exceeds the release of other amino acids (Dudrick et al., 1994). This has led to the hypothesis that glutamine is necessary for proper immune function and that the release of amino acids from skeletal muscle is a specific response necessary to provide glutamine for the immune system. Support for this hypothesis is provided by studies conducted in rodents and humans where the addition of glutamine to diets of infected individuals decreased muscle protein breakdown and reduced nitrogen excretion (reviewed by Ziegler et al., 1994). That glutamine administration ameliorates muscle protein catabolism and nitrogen excretion in septic animals indicates that glutamine, or the nitrogen from glutamine, may be a limiting factor for the resynthesis of muscle protein from endogenous amino acids.

Reeds et al. (1994) proposed that a significant portion of nitrogen excreted during an inflammatory response was the result of excessive demands for the aromatic amino acids phenylalanine, tyrosine, and tryptophan. Their conclusions were based on a comparison of the amino acid profiles of the major acute-phase proteins produced by humans and the amino acid profile of mixed muscle protein. Analysis of the acute-phase proteins indicated that four of the six proteins contained high levels of phenylalanine, five of the proteins were rich in tryptophan, and three contained high levels of tyrosine. By calculating the quantity of amino acids incorporated into a typical acute-phase protein mixture (850 mg/kg BW) they calculated that 1980 mg of mixed muscle protein per kilogram body weight would need to be liberated to supply an adequate quantity of phenylalanine for the increased hepatic protein synthesis. The amino acids that are released in excess of the need for acute-phase protein production (1980 − 850 = 1130 mg/kg) are catabolized because they cannot be used for protein resynthesis due to the phenylalanine limitation, with the end result being an excessive excretion of nitrogen. Assuming that pigs have a similar pattern and quantity of acute-phase proteins, it is apparent that an infectious insult could result in a substantial amount of protein breakdown and nitrogen excretion. For example, for a 100-kg pig there would be roughly 200 g of protein broken down to supply amino acids for acute-phase protein synthesis, and approximately 13 g nitrogen would be excreted.

As discussed in previous sections, stimulation of an animal's immune system disturbs normal body processes, and immunological, metabolical, and physiologic responses are required so that homeostasis may be achieved. These alterations have the potential to reduce growth and body protein accretion, which in turn will likely have an effect on amino acid requirements. Recent studies in chicks and pigs suggest that activation of the immune system by LPS results in decreased growth rates and feed efficiency (Klasing and Barnes, 1988; van Heughten et al., 1994). Because of the reduction in feed intake associated with immunological stress, it has been suggested that the concentration of amino acids in the diet may need to be increased so that growth can be maintained. However, recent research in chicks demonstrated that the requirements for lysine and methionine for maximal gain and feed efficiency are decreased in LPS-treated chicks (Klasing and Barnes, 1988; Webel et al., 1998). Furthermore, Williams et al. (1997a,b) demonstrated that pigs kept in management schemes that presumably provide fewer immunological challenges ate more, grew faster, and had higher requirements for lysine than their counterparts reared in a less sanitary environment.

Because of the reductions in feed intake and growth caused by immunological stress, it seems reasonable to postulate that the quantity of an amino acid required to support maximal growth in a disease-challenged animal is less than the amount required by a healthy animal. Support for this hypothesis is provided by research on amino acid requirements in other stress situations, such as heat stress or crowding, where a reduction in feed intake is also typical. In these situations it has been shown that animals require a smaller *quantity* of dietary amino acids to maximize performance. However, in many of these studies, it is apparent that animals require a similar *concentration* of dietary amino acids to maximize weight gain and feed efficiency (Han and Baker, 1993; Myer and Bucklin, 1993; Edmonds et al., 1998).

The metabolic changes brought on by immunological stress are different from those seen during either heat stress or crowding. The need for amino acids to support cells of the immune system, hepatic acute-phase protein synthesis, and gluconeogenesis are unique to animals that have an activated immune system. Although the amino acid requirements for these functions have not been determined, it is apparent that the requirements for certain amino acids could be increased (Reeds et al., 1994). Therefore, it seems possible that immunological stress may alter not only amino acid requirements, but also the profile of amino acids relative to lysine that the animal requires. As discussed previously, the needs for the sulfur amino acids, arginine, glutamine, and the aromatic amino acids may be increased relative to lysine to support the metabolic and physiological changes associated with immunological stress. In addition, in immunologically stressed animals where food intake and growth are depressed, maintenance amino acid requirements will comprise a greater portion of the total requirement. In this situation, it can be hypothesized that the requirements for amino acids that have a high maintenance component (i.e., sulfur amino acids and threonine) may be increased relative to lysine.

Williams (1995) proposed a simple factorial model that illustrated how lysine needs for growing pigs can be affected by immunological stress. The primary factors used in the model included: (1) rate of protein accretion; (2) lysine content of whole-body protein; (3) maintenance lysine requirement; (4) lysine required for protein accretion; (5) efficiency of lysine utilization; and (6) digestibility of lysine in the diet. He assumed that protein accretion, feed intake, and the digestibility of lysine were decreased as a result of immunological stress. In addition, the utilization of lysine above maintenance and the maintenance lysine requirement were assumed to be unaffected by immunological stress. Although the assumptions used were the best available, they are inadequate to make accurate predictions. For example, determining a value for the efficiency of lysine utilization is not without problems under ideal conditions, and there is literally no information on what effect immunological stress has on this value. Nevertheless, the model predicted that the immunologically stressed animals required substantially less lysine than animals that are not stressed. The model proposed by Williams (1995) is not adequate to predict amino acid requirements accurately, but it is useful, because it clearly illustrates the gaps in present knowledge of the factors that affect the amino acid requirements of animals.

B. Lipids

Feeding high-fat diets reduces *in vitro* mitogen-stimulated lymphocyte proliferation, when compared with low-fat diets, but the precise effects depend on the amount and type of dietary fat (reviewed by Calder, 1998a,b). As discussed elsewhere in this book, there are two major classes of polyunsaturated fatty acids (PUFAs) — the n-6 and the n-3 families. Linoleic acid is the precursor of the n-6 family, and it is found in plant oils, including corn and soybean oil. In animals, linoleic acid is converted to arachidonic acid, which can account for 25% of the total fatty acids in the plasma membranes of immune cells. The amount of arachidonic acid in the plasma membrane is important immunologically, because it is the precursor of several prostaglandins and leukotrienes that have potent inflammatory effects. The precursor of the n-3 PUFAs is α-linolenic acid, which in animal tissues is converted to eicosapentaenoic and docosahexaenoic acids. As opposed to n-6 PUFAs that are inflammatory, n-3 PUFAs are anti-inflammatory. This may be the reason populations that consume diets rich in n-3 PUFAs (e.g., diets that include large quantities of fish oil) have very low incidence of inflammatory and autoimmune diseases (Calder, 1998a).

Compared with diets rich in n-6 PUFAs, feeding laboratory animals diets rich in fish oil (i.e., diets rich in eicosapentaenoic and docosahexaenoic acids) results in suppressed proliferation of spleen lymphocytes stimulated with T- or B-cell mitogens, decreased IL-2 production by lymphocytes, decreased T-lymphocyte cytotoxicity, decreased natural killer cell activity, and decreased macrophage-mediated cytolysis (Alexander and Smythe, 1988; Meydani et al., 1988; Somers et al., 1989; Fritsche and Johnston, 1990; Fritsche et al., 1991; Lumpkin et al., 1993; Yaqoob and Calder, 1995). Consistent with studies in rodents, in pigs dietary fish oil decreased leukocyte phagocytosis, lymphocyte proliferation, and natural killer cell activity (Thies et al., 1999). The production of IL-1, IL-6, and TNF-α by peripheral blood mononuclear cells is also inhibited by n-3 PUFAs. Because these three cytokines are partly to blame for the cachexia observed in people and animals with chronic autoimmune and neoplastic disease, n-3 PUFAs have been evaluated for the ability to prevent body wasting. In patients with pancreatic cancer who were cachectic, the release of IL-6 was reduced and body weight stabilized by daily oral administration of 6 g of eicosapentaenoic acid (Wigmore et al., 1996; 1997).

Diets rich in n-3 PUFAs decrease inflammation at least two ways. First, consumption of a diet rich in n-3 PUFAs increases membrane levels of eicosapentaenoic and docosahexaenoic acids at the expense of arachidonic acid. Thus, when immune cells are stimulated, there is less arachidonic acid available to generate prostaglandins and leukotrienes, which are inflammatory in nature. In pigs, consumption of fish oil resulted in decreased arachidonic acid and increased n-3 PUFAs in serum, thymus, lymph nodes, spleen cells, and alveolar macrophages (Fritsche et al., 1993; Thies et al., 1999). Second, eicosapentaenoic acid is a substrate for the same enzymes that metabolize arachidonic acid. However, the products of eicosapentaenoic acid metabolism are less potent inflammatory molecules than are those generated by metabolism of arachidonic acid. Accordingly, alveolar macrophages from pigs fed fish oil produced less PGE_2 (a metabolite of arachidonic acid) compared with alveolar macrophages from pigs fed a lard-rich diet (Fritsche et al., 1993). For these reasons, most studies on lipids and immunity have examined the effects of replacing membrane arachidonic acid with n-3 PUFAs.

Although it might be useful to consume high levels of n-3 PUFAs to decrease inflammation associated with autoimmune or neoplastic disease, the immunosuppression may render animals more susceptible to infectious disease. Indeed, several studies have shown that dietary fish oil can increase the susceptibility of animals to some bacterial infections. For example, mice fed fish oil for 4 weeks and then challenged with *Salmonella typhimurium* presented the highest number of bacteria 7 days postinoculation and had a higher mortality rate, when compared with mice fed low-fat diets or diets rich in either corn oil or hydrogenated coconut oil (Chang et al., 1992). Similar results were reported for mice fed fish oil and challenged with *Listeria monocytogenes* (Fritsche et al., 1997). Thus, inclusion of fish or other n-3 PUFA–rich oils in pig diets should be approached with caution to avoid increased incidence of infections. The ideal level of dietary fish oil might be different for pigs kept in a good environment that minimizes host–pathogen interaction, when compared with pigs kept in a less hygienic environment.

C. ZINC

In the late 1940s and early 1950s the disease parakeratosis caused significant economic losses in the swine industry, and it was caused by inadequate intake of bioavailable Zn (Luecke, 1984). Zinc is a component of at least 100 enzymes, and inadequate intake of Zn renders animals severely immunodeficient and highly susceptible to viral, bacterial, and parasitic microorganisms (Shankar and Prasad, 1998). Both innate and acquired immunity is affected. Thymulin is a hormone secreted by thymic epithelial cells to promote T-cell maturation, IL-2 production, and cytotoxicity (Pleau et al., 1980). For activation, thymulin must undergo a conformational change, which is induced by binding Zn. Therefore, in Zn-deficient animals even though thymulin is detectable in serum, it is inactive and the utility of T-cells is severely diminished. For example, mice fed Zn-deficient diets had moderate thymic involution after 2 weeks (Fernandes et al., 1979). After 4 weeks, the thymus was only 25% of its original size and after 6 weeks, only a few thymocytes were found in the thymic capsule. The thymus was restored when mice were fed diets adequate in Zn.

A marginal deficiency in Zn, which is more of a concern for swine production, had little effect on the thymus of adult mice (Luecke et al., 1978), but did decrease the size of the thymus gland of neonatal pups (Beach et al., 1979). Interestingly, pigs nursed by sows exposed to aflatoxins have symptoms suggesting Zn deficiency, including growth retardation, thymic involution, and impaired immunocompetence. Thymulin in pigs exposed to maternal aflatoxins was inactive, but could be activated *in vitro* by addition of physiologically relevant levels of Zn (Mocchegiani et al., 1998).

To the authors' best knowledge, there have been no studies in pigs to determine if the Zn required for optimum immunity is higher than that for optimum growth performance. Several studies in rodents and humans suggest that it might. During the acute-phase response Zn is redistributed from the plasma to the liver and lymphocytes. In humans, daily Zn supplementation reduced the incidence and duration of diarrhea and reduced the incidence of acute and lower respiratory infections (Sazawal et al.,1996; 1998). Strains of mice that were genetically susceptible to infection by C. albicans became resistant when fed a Zn-enriched diet or when injected intraperitoneally with Zn, whereas normally resistant mice became susceptible when fed diets inadequate in Zn (Salvin et al., 1987). These results suggest that the immune system's requirement for Zn might be higher than for other physiological processes.

D. IRON AND COPPER

The effect of Fe on immunocompetence is not as clear as that of Zn; however, generally speaking, an imbalance in Fe intake — either too much or too little — decreases immunity. One of the acute responses induced by inflammatory stimuli is hypoferremia. The inflammatory cytokines released by activated macrophages initiate a cascade of events that cause Fe to be sequestered. Because Fe is a rate-limiting nutrient for the growth of several pathogenic microorganisms, its removal from blood and temporary storage in compartments that are not accessible to pathogens is considered part of the host defense. Iron-binding proteins chelate most Fe; however, supplementation can saturate these proteins, leaving excess Fe available to pathogens. For example, pigs that were given 100 mg Fe dextran and then inoculated with *Escherichia coli* into ligated intestines demonstrated increased total Fe-binding capacity, increased liver Fe content, and decreased plasma Fe concentration (Knight et al., 1984). However, pigs that received 400 mg Fe dextran prior to inoculation with *E. coli* had increased Fe in liver, but they were not able to increase total Fe-binding capacity and thus could not limit the availability of Fe to the pathogenic microorganism (Knight et al., 1984). Serum from 1- to 3-day-old pigs injected with 100 or 200 mg of Fe-dextran enhanced growth of *E. coli* when compared with serum from control pigs (Knight et al., 1983). Similarly, addition of Fe to milk enhanced proliferation of *E. coli* both *in vitro* and in isolated intestinal segments (Klasing et al., 1980). Pigs that were challenged with an enterotoxigenic strain of *E. coli* had more diarrhea and a higher mortality rate when administered excess Fe by the oral route (Kadis et al., 1984). Thus, even though supplemental Fe is needed to prevent anemia in newborn pigs, excess Fe can actually enhance the growth of certain pathogenic microorganisms.

Copper status is determined primarily by the plasma concentration of the acute-phase protein ceruloplasmin. The inflammatory cytokine, IL-1, induces synthesis of ceruloplasmin. Therefore, whereas pathogens decrease circulating Fe, they increase circulating Cu. The increase in plasma Cu may be to enhance lymphocyte responses. Splenocytes isolated from Cu-deficient rats produced less IL-2 *in vitro* when compared with splenocytes from controls (Hopkins and Failla, 1995; Percival, 1998). Interleukin-2 is a cytokine produced by T cells that acts in an autocrine manner to promote proliferation. Accordingly, the proliferation of splenocytes from Cu-deficient rats also decreased when compared with control splenocytes. To the authors' best knowledge, there have been no studies in pigs to determine if the Cu required for optimum immunity is higher than that for optimum growth and performance.

E. VITAMIN E AND SELENIUM

It is apparent from the information available at present that the primary role of vitamin E in nutrition is to protect cellular membranes from peroxidative damage (Sheffy and Shultz, 1979), whereas Se is an integral component of glutathione peroxidase. Numerous studies have suggested that vitamin E and Se also play an active role in the host's response to infection (Meydani and Beharka, 1998). Lessard et al. (1991) fed pigs a diet adequate in vitamin E and Se or a diet deficient in both for 21 days before the pigs were inoculated with *S. typhisuis*. Lymphocytes were isolated from blood collected just before inoculation and 4 days later to examine proliferation in response to several mitogens. Whereas vitamin E and Se deficiency did not influence the proliferation of lymphocytes from unchallenged pigs, it markedly suppressed the proliferation of lymphocytes that were obtained from pigs that had been inoculated with *Salmonella*. The suppression was only evident when cells were cultured in autologous serum, which could have been deficient in vitamin E and Se or possibly contained some suppressive factor.

Vitamin E and Se supplementation in excess of minimal requirements has been shown to increase antibody production and lymphocyte proliferation in pigs (Ellis and Vorhies, 1976; Mahan and Moxon, 1980; Larsen and Tollersrud, 1981; Peplowski et al., 1981). Plasma tocopherols and glutathione peroxidase are very low in newborn piglets, but both are substantially increased after consumption of colostrum (Loudenslager et al., 1986). Therefore, vitamin E and Se in colostrum may be important to enhance development of the pig's immature immune system (Kelley and Easter, 1991). Vitamin E supplementation also enhances the random migration, chemotaxis, and phagocytic activity of mouse peritoneal macrophages (Del Rio et al., 1998). Moreover, recent studies indicate that vitamin E reduces the production of certain cytokines in pigs (Webel et al., 1998). Prior administration of d-α-tocopherol reduced LPS-induced secretion of IL-6 by more than half. Exposure of macrophages to LPS induces the production of reactive oxygen intermediates. In addition to their toxic extracellular effects that can be partially mitigated by vitamin E, it is now known that reactive oxygen species play a role in intracellular signaling pathways by activating a variety of nuclear transcription factors (Eugui et al., 1994). As it would be, reactive oxygen species activate transcription factor NF-κB and AP-1, which are required for the expression of certain inflammatory cytokines, including IL-6 (Hirano et al., 1990). Therefore, one way to regulate metabolically active cytokines might be by use of antioxidants like vitamin E.

F. VITAMIN A

Studies concerning the effects of vitamin A and related retinoids on immunity have recently been reviewed (Semba, 1998). The immunological effects of vitamin A deficiency seem to be mediated by its metabolites, all-*trans* and 9-*cis* retinoic acids, which alter gene expression via two families of nuclear receptors (i.e., retinoic acid receptors and retinoid X receptors). Vitamin A deficiency severely compromises the integrity of mucosal epithelial cells in the respiratory, gastrointestinal, and uterine tracts. In the respiratory tract, ciliated columnar epithelium with mucus and goblet cells trap and remove inhaled microorganisms. In animals deficient in vitamin A, ciliated epithelial cells are replaced by stratified, keratinized epithelium, and there is a decrease in mucin. This might explain why children marginally deficient in vitamin A have an increased risk of respiratory disease (Sommer et al., 1984). Similarly, in the small intestine, vitamin A deficiency results in a loss of microvilli, goblet cells, and mucin (DeLuca et al., 1969; Rojanapo et al., 1980). Other effects of vitamin A deficiency on innate immunity include changes in epidermal keratins that disrupt skin barrier function (Molloy and Laskin, 1985); defects in chemotaxis, adhesion, phagocytosis, and the ability to produce reactive oxygen species in neutrophils (Twining et al., 1997); decreased number of natural killer cells and cytotoxicity (Zhao et al., 1994; Zhao and Ross, 1995); and a decrease in the expression of CD14 (a receptor that recognizes LPS), as well as the secretion of inflammatory cytokines by macrophages and monocytes (Semba, 1998).

An adequate level of vitamin A is also necessary to support acquired immunity. The growth and activation of B cells requires retinol. Experiments at Michigan State University showed that pigs deficient in vitamin A synthesize less than one tenth of the amount of antibody produced by pigs fed vitamin A–fortified diets (Harmon et al., 1963). In animals deficient in vitamin A, infection with *Trichinella spiralisa*, which normally induces strong T-helper type 2–like responses (i.e., high levels of parasite-specific IgG and production of IL-4, IL-5, and IL-10), induced inappropriate strong T-helper type 1–like responses (i.e., production of interferon-γ and IL-12) (Carman et al., 1992; Cantorna et al., 1994; 1995). In T lymphocytes, retinoids increased expression of IL-2 receptors (Sidell et al., 1993) and increased antigen-specific proliferation (Friedman et al., 1993). In chickens infected with Newcastle disease virus, vitamin A deficiency impaired T-lymphocyte cytotoxicity (Sijtsma et al., 1990).

VI. CONCLUDING REMARKS

It is now evident that the immune system influences nutrient requirements and specific nutrients can either enhance or inhibit the immune response. A better understanding of this interaction is required, but several pragmatic applications of nutrient–immune interaction are already in sight. First, that immunological stress (i.e., exposure to pathogens) changes the pig's physiological state and alters nutrient requirements is inevitable. If these alterations in nutrient requirements can be precisely defined, it will be possible to formulate cost-effective diets that maximize growth performance, even if that performance is less than it would have been had the pig been in an environment that reduced exposure to pathogens. Second, it might be possible to develop diets that promote "optimal" immune responses. What is considered optimal may change from one production system to another, or even within a system depending on the disease environment at a given time. The goal need not always be to minimize the immune response, for in certain environments this might result in increased incidence of infection. Similarly, the goal need not always be to maximize the immune response because an overzealous response to nonpathogenic organisms can be counterproductive. Finally, it is important to recognize that the physiological state of a pig is very different prior to disease, during disease, and while recovering from disease. Therefore, the nutrient requirements of the immune system and growth during these three critical stages are likely to be different as well. A useful indicator of immunological stress or disease is needed to facilitate movement of these concepts from the laboratory to the field. Unfortunately, no such indicator is currently available.

REFERENCES

Alexander, N. J., and N. L. Smythe. 1988. Dietary modulation of *in vitro* lymphocyte function, *Ann. Nutr. Metab.*, 32:192.

Argiles, J. P., and F. J. Lopez-Soriano. 1990. The effects of tumor necrosis factor α (cachechtin) and tumor growth on hepatic amino acid utilization in the rat, *Biochem. J.*, 266:123.

Argiles, J. P., F. J. Lopez-Soriano, D. Wiggins, and D. H. Williamson. 1989. Comparative effects of tumour necrosis factor-α (cachechtin), interleukin-1-β and tumour growth on amino acid metabolism in the rat *in vivo*. Absorption and tissue uptake of alpha-amino[1-14C]isobutyrate, *Biochem. J.*, 261:357.

Ballmer, P. E., M. A. McNurlan, B. G. Southorn, I. Grant, and P. J. Garlick. 1991. Effects of human recombinant interleukin-1β on protein synthesis in rat tissues compared with a classical acute-phase reaction induced by turpentine, *Biochem. J.*, 279:683.

Barbul, A., and H. Dawson. 1994. Arginine and immunity. In *Diet, Nutrition and Immunity*, Forse, A., Ed., CRC Press, Boca Raton, FL, 199.

Beach, R. S., M. E. Gershwin, and L. S. Hurley. 1979. Altered thymic structure and mitogen responsiveness in postnatally zinc-deprived mice, *Dev. Comp. Immunol.*, 3:725.

Beisel, W. R. 1977. Metabolic and nutritional consequences of infection. In *Advances in Nutritional Research*, Vol. I, Draper, H. H., Ed., Plenum Press, New York, 125.

Bhargva, K. K., R. P. Hanson, and M. L. Sunde. 1970. Effects of methionine and valine on antibody production in chicks infected with Newcastle disease virus, *J. Nutr.*, 100:241.

Bulger, E. M., W. S. Helton, C. M. Clinton, R. P. Roque, I. Garcia, and R. V. Maijer. 1997. Enteral vitamin E supplementation inhibits the cytokine response to endotoxin, *Arch. Surg.*, 132:1337.

Burger, W., E. M. Fennert, M. Poble, and H. Wesemier. 1992. C-reactive protein — a characteristic feature of health control in swine, *J. Vet. Med. Assoc.*, 39:635.

Calder, C. P. 1998a. Dietary fatty acids and the immune system, *Nutr. Rev.*, 56:S70.

Calder, C. P. 1998b. Fat change of immunomodulation, *Immunol. Today*, 19:244.

Cantorna, M. T., F. E. Nashold, and C. E. Hayes. 1994. In vitamin A deficiency multiple mechanisms establish a regulatory T helper cell imbalance with excess Th1 and insufficient Th2 function, *J. Immunol.*, 152:1515.

Cantorna, M. T., F. E. Nashold, and C. E. Hayes. 1995. Vitamin A deficiency results in a priming environment conducive for Th1 cell development, *Eur. J. Immunol.*, 25:1673.

Carman, J. A., L. Pond, F. Nashold, D. L. Wassom, and C. E. Hayes. 1992. Immunity to *Trichinella spiralis* infection in vitamin A-deficient mice, *J. Exp. Med.*, 175:111.

Chandra, R. K. 1992. Protein-energy malnutrition and immunological responses, *J. Nutr.*, 122:597.

Chang, H. R., A. G. Dulloo, I. R. Vladoianu, P. F. Piguet, D. Arsenijevic, L. Girardier, and J. C. Pechere. 1992. Fish oil decreases natural resistance of mice to infection with *Salmonella typhimurium*, *Metabolism*, 41:1.

Charters, Y., and F. Grimble. 1989. Effect of recombinant human tumour necrosis factor α on protein synthesis in liver, skeletal muscle and skin of rats, *Biochem. J.*, 258:493.

Coates, M. E., R. Fuller, G. F. Harrison, M. Lev, and S. F. Suffolk. 1963. A comparison of the growth of chicks in the Gustafsson germ-free apparatus and in a conventional environment, with and without dietary supplements of penicillin, *Br. J. Nutr.*, 17:141.

De Luca, L., E. P. Little, and G. Wolf. 1969. Vitamin A and protein synthesis by rat intestinal mucosa, *J. Biol. Chem.*, 244:701.

Del Rio, M., G. Ruedas, S. Medina, V. M. Victor, and M. De la Fuente. 1998. Improvements by several antioxidants of macrophage function *in vitro*, *Life Sci.*, 63:871.

Denis, M. 1991. Tumor necrosis factor and granulocyte macrophage-colony stimulating factor stimulate human macrophages to restrict growth of *Mycobacterium avium* and to kill avirulent *M. avium*: killing effector mechanism depends on the generation of reactive oxygen intermediates, *J. Leuk. Biol.*, 49:380.

Dietert, R. R., K. A. Golemboski, and R. E. Austic. 1994. Environment-immune interactions, *Poult. Sci.*, 73:1062.

Dudrick, P. S., J. C. Alverdy, and W. W. Souba. 1994. Glutamine and the immune system. In *Diet, Nutrition and Immunity*, Forse, A., Ed., CRC Press, Boca Raton, FL, 217.

Eagle, H., V. I. Oyama, M. Levy, C. L. Horton, and R. Fleischman. 1956. The growth response of mammalian cells in tissue culture to L-glutamine and L-glutamic acid, *J. Biol. Chem.*, 218:607.

Edmonds, M. S., B. E. Arentson, and G. A. Mente. 1998. Effect of protein levels and space allocation on performance of growing-finishing pigs, *J. Anim. Sci.*, 76:814.

Ellis, R. P., and M. W. Vorhies. 1976. Effect of supplemental dietary vitamin E on the serologic response of swine to an *Escherichia coli* bacterin, *J. Am. Vet. Med. Assoc.*, 168:231.

Eugui, E. M., B. Delustro, S. Rouhafza, M. Linicka, S. W. Lee, R. Wilhelm, and A. C. Allison. 1994. Some antioxidants inhibit, in a co-ordinate fashion, the production of tumor necrosis factor-α, IL-1β, and IL-6 by human peripheral blood mononuclear cells, *Int. Immunol.*, 6:409.

Fernandes, G., M. Nair, K. Onoe, T. Tanaka, R. Floyd, and R. A. Good. 1979. Impairment of cell-mediated immunity functions by dietary zinc deficiency in mice, *Proc. Natl. Acad. Sci., U.S.A.*, 76:457.

Finch, J. M., and R. J. Turner. 1996. Effects of selenium and vitamin E on the immune responses of domestic animals, *Res. Vet. Sci.*, 60:97.

Finck, B. N., K. W. Kelley, R. Dantzer, and R. W. Johnson. 1998. *In vivo* and *in vitro* evidence for the involvement of tumor necrosis factor-α in the induction of leptin by lipopolysaccharide, *Endocrinology*, 139:2278.

Flores, E. A., B. R. Bistrian, J. J. Pomposelli, C. A. Dinarello, G. L. Blackburn, and N. W. Istfan. 1989. Infusion of tumor necrosis factor/cachechtin promotes muscle protein catabolism in the rat, *J. Clin. Invest.*, 83:1614.

Fong, Y., L. L. Moldawer, M. Marano, H. Wei, A. Barber, K. Manogue, K. J. Tracey, G. Kuo, D. A. Fischman, A. Cerami, and S. F. Lowry. 1989. Cachechtin/TNF or IL-1α induces cachexia with redistribution of body proteins, *Am. J. Physiol.*, 256:R659.

Friedman, A., O. Halevy, M. Schrift, Y. Arazi, and D. Sklan. 1993. Retinoic acid promotes proliferation and induces expression of retinoic acid receptor-alpha gene in murine T lymphocytes, *Cell Immunol.*, 152:240.

Fritsche, K. L., and P. V. Johnston. 1990. Effect of dietary omega-3 fatty acids on cell-mediated cytotoxic activity in BALB/c mice, *Nutr. Res.*, 10:577.

Fritsche, K. L., N. A. Cassity, and S. C. Huang. 1991. Effect of dietary fat source on antibody production and lymphocyte proliferation in chickens, *Poult. Sci.*, 70:611.

Fritsche, K. L., D. W. Alexander, N. A. Cassity, and S. C. Huang. 1993. Maternally-supplied fish oil alters piglet immune cell fatty acid profile and eicosanoid production, *Lipids*, 28:677.

Fritsche, K. L., L. M. Shahbazian, C. Feng, and J. N. Berg. 1997. Dietary fish oil reduces survival and impairs bacterial clearance in C3H/Hen mice challenged with *Listeria monocytogenes*, *Clin. Sci.*, 92:95.

Geiger, T., T. Andus, J. Klapproth, T. Hirano, T. Kishimoto, and R. C. Heinrich. 1988. Induction of rat acute phase proteins by interleukin-6 *in vivo*, *Eur. J. Immunol.*, 18:717.

Granger, D. L., J. B. Hibbs, J. R. Perfect, and D. T. Durak. 1988. Specific amino acid (L-arginine) requirement for the microbiostatic activity of murine macrophages, *J. Clin. Invest.*, 81:1129.

Grimble, R. F. 1990. Nutrition and cytokine action, *Nutr. Res. Rev.*, 3:193.

Hall, W. F., T. E. Eurell, R. D. Hansen, and L. G. Herr. 1992. Serum haptoglobin concentration in swine naturally or experimentally infected with *Actinobacillus pleuropneumonia*, *J. Am. Vet. Med. Assoc.*, 20:1730.

Han, Y., and D. H. Baker. 1993. Effects of sex, heat stress, body weight and genetic strain on the lysine requirement of broiler chicks, *Poult. Sci.*, 72:701.

Harmon, B. G., E. R. Miller, J. A. Hoefer, D. E. Ullrey, and R. W. Luecke. 1963. Relationships of specific nutrient deficiencies to antibody production in swine. I, Vitamin A, *J. Nutr.*, 79:263.

Hirano, T., S. Akira, T. Taga, and T. Kishimoto. 1990. Biological and clinical aspects of interleukin-6, *Immunol. Today*, 11:443.

Hopkins, R. G., and M. L. Failla. 1995. Chronic intake of a marginally low copper diet impairs *in vitro* activities of lymphocytes and neutrophils from male rats despite minimal impact on conventional indicators of copper status, *J. Nutr.*, 125:2658.

Itoh, H., K. Tamura, M. Izumi, Y. Motoi, K. Kidoguchi, and Y. Funayama. 1992. The influence of age and health status on serum alpha-1 acid glycoprotein levels of conventional and pathogen-free pigs, *Can. J. Vet. Res.*, 57:74.

Johnson, R. W. 1997. Inhibition of growth by pro-inflammatory cytokines: an integrated view, *J. Anim. Sci.*, 75:1244.

Kadis, S., F. A. Udeze, J. Polanco, and D. W. Dreesen. 1984. Relationship of iron administration to susceptibility of newborn pigs to enterotoxic colibacillosis, *Am. J. Vet. Res.*, 45:255.

Kelley, K. W., and R. A. Easter. 1987. Nutritional factors can influence immune responses of swine, *Feedstuffs*, 59:14.

Kelley, K. W., and R. A. Easter. 1991. Nutritional and environmental influences on immunocompetence. In *Swine Nutrition*, Miller, E. R., D. E. Ullrey, and A. J. Lewis, Eds., Butterworth-Heinemann, Stoneham, MA, 401.

Kelley, K. W., R. W. Johnson, and R. Dantzer. 1994. Immunology discovers physiology, *Vet. Immunol. Immunopathol.*, 43:157.

Klasing, K. C. 1988. Nutritional aspects of leukocytic cytokines, *J. Nutr.*, 118:1436.

Klasing, K. C. 1996. Interactions between nutrition and infectious disease, *Proc. Maryland Nutr. Conf.*, March 21–22, College Park, MD, 137.

Klasing, K. C., and R. E. Austic. 1984. Changes in protein synthesis due to an inflammatory challenge, *Proc. Soc. Exp. Biol. Med.*, 176:285.

Klasing, K. C., and D. M. Barnes. 1988. Decreased amino acid requirements of growing chicks due to immunologic stress, *J. Nutr.*, 118:1158.

Klasing, K. C., and B. J. Johnstone. 1991. Monokines in growth and development, *Poult. Sci.*, 70:1781.

Klasing, K. C., C. D. Knight, and D. M. Forsyth. 1980. Effects of iron on the anti-coli capacity of sow's milk *in vitro* and in ligated intestinal segments, *J. Nutr.*, 110:1914.

Klasing, K. C., D. E. Laurin, R. K. Peng, and D. M. Fry. 1987. Immunologically mediated growth depression in chicks: influence of feed intake, corticosterone and interleukin-1, *J. Nutr.*, 117:1629.

Knight, C. D., K. C. Klasing, and D. M. Forsyth. 1983. *E. coli* growth in serum of iron dextran-supplemented pigs, *J. Anim. Sci.*, 57:387.

Knight, C. D., K. C. Klasing, and D. M. Forsyth. 1984. The effects of intestinal *Escherichia coli* 263, intravenous infusion of *Escherichia coli* 263 culture filtrate and iron dextran supplementation on iron metabolism in the young pig, *J. Anim. Sci.*, 59:1519.

Lacey, J. M., and D. W. Wilmore. 1990. Is glutamine a conditionally essential amino acid? *Nutr. Rev.*, 48:297.

Larsen, H. J., and S. Tollersrud. 1981. Effect of dietary vitamin E and selenium on phytohaemagglutinin response of pig lymphocytes, *Res. Vet. Sci.*, 31:301.

Lessard, M., W. C. Yang, G. S. Elliott, A. H. Rebar, J. F. Van Fleet, N. Deslauriers, G. J. Brisson, and R. D. Schultz. 1991. Cellular immune responses in pigs fed a vitamin E- and selenium-deficient diet, *J. Anim. Sci.*, 69:1575.

Loudenslager, M. J., P. K. Ku, P. A. Whetter, D. E. Ullrey, C. K. Whitehair, H. D. Stowe, and E. R. Miller. 1986. Importance of diet of dam and colostrum to the biological antioxidant status and parenteral iron tolerance of the pig, *J. Anim. Sci.*, 63:1905.

Luecke, R. W. 1984. Domestic animals in the elucidation of zinc's role in nutrition, *Fed. Proc.*, 43:2823.

Luecke, R. W., C. E. Simonel, and P. J. Fraker. 1978. The effect of restricted dietary intake on the antibody mediated response of the zinc deficient A/J mouse, *J. Nutr.*, 108:881.

Lumpkin, E. A., J. J. McGlone, J. L. Sells, and J. M. Hellman. 1993. Modulation of murine natural killer cell cytotoxicity by dietary fish oil, corn oil or beef tallow, *J. Nutr. Immunol.*, 2:43.

Mahan, D. C., and A. L. Moxon. 1980. Effects of dietary selenium and injectable vitamin E-selenium for weaning swine, *Nutr. Rep. Int.*, 21:829.

Meydani, S. N., and A. A. Beharka. 1998. Recent developments in vitamin E and immune response, *Nutr. Rev.*, 56:S49.

Meydani, S. N., G. Yogeeswaran, S. Liu, S. Baskar, and M. Meydani. 1988. Fish oil and tocopherol-induced changes in natural killer cell-mediated cytotoxicity and PGE_2 synthesis in young and old mice, *J. Nutr.*, 118:1245.

Mocchegiani, E., A. Corradi, L. Santarelli, A. Tibaldi, E. DeAngelis, P. Borghetti, A. Bonomi, N. Fabris, and E. Cabassi. 1998. Zinc, thymic endocrine activity and mitogen responsiveness (PHA) in piglets exposed to maternal aflatoxicosis B1 and G1, *Vet. Immunol. Immunopathol.*, 62:245.

Molloy, C. J., and J. D. Laskin. 1985. Alterations in mouse epidermal keratin production induced by dietary vitamin A deficiency, *Ann. N.Y. Acad. Sci.*, 455:739.

Myer, R. O., and R. A. Bucklin. 1993. Effect of increased dietary lysine on performance and carcass characteristics of growing-finishing swine reared in a hot, humid environment, University of Florida Swine Field Day, p. 52.

Newsholme, E. A., P. Newsholme, R. Curi, E. Challoner, M. Salleh, and M. Ardawi. 1988. A role for muscle in the immune system and its importance in surgery, trauma, sepsis and burns, *Nutrition*, 4:261.

Peplowski, M. A., D. C. Mahan, F. A. Murray, A. L. Moxon, A. H. Cantor, and K. E. Ekstrom. 1981. Effect of dietary and injectable vitamin E and selenium in weanling swine antigenically challenged with sheep red blood cells, *J. Anim. Sci.*, 51:344.

Percival, S. S. 1998. Copper and immunity, *Am. J. Clin. Nutr.*, 67:1064S.

Pfeiffer, A., K. M. Rogers, L. O'Keeffe, and P. J. Osborn. 1993. Acute phase protein response, food intake, live weight change and lesions following intrathoracic injection of yeast in sheep, *Res. Vet. Sci.*, 55:360.

Pleau, J. M., V. Fuentes, J. L. Morgat, and J. F. Bach. 1980. Specific receptors for the serum thymic factor (FTS) in lymphoblastoid cultured cell lines, *Proc. Natl. Acad. Sci. U.S.A.*, 77:2861.

Rahelic, S., and S. Puac. 1981. Fiber types in longissimus dorsi from wild and highly selected pig breeds, *Meat Sci.*, 5:439.

Reeds, P. J., C. R. Field, and F. Jahoor. 1994. Do the differences between the amino acid compositions of acute phase and muscle proteins have a bearing on nitrogen loss in traumatic states? *J. Nutr.*, 124:906.

Rojanapo, W., A. J. Lamb, and J. A. Olson. 1980. The prevalence, metabolism and migration of goblet cells in rat intestine following the induction of rapid, synchronous vitamin A deficiency, *J. Nutr.*, 110:178.

Rothwell, N. J., and R. F. Grimble. 1992. Metabolic and nutritional effects of TNF. In *The Molecules and Their Emerging Role in Medicine*, Beutler, B., Ed., Raven Press, New York, 237.

Roura, E., J. Homedes, and K. C. Klasing. 1992. Prevention of immunological stress contributes to the growth-promoting ability of dietary antibiotics in chicks, *J. Nutr.*, 122:2382.

Salvin, S. B., B. L. Horecker, L. X. Pan, and B. S. Rabin. 1987. The effect of dietary zinc and prothymosin alpha on cellular immune responses of RF/J mice, *Clin. Immunol. Immunopathol.*, 43:281.

Sazawal, S., R. E. Black, M. K. Bhan, S. Jalla, N. Bhandari, A. Sinha, and S. Majumdar. 1996. Zinc supplementation reduces the incidence of persistent diarrhea and dysentery among low socio-economic children in India, *J. Nutr.*, 126:443.

Sazawal, S., R. E. Black, S. Jalla, S. Mazumdar, A. Sinha, and M. K. Bhan. 1998. Zinc supplementation reduces the incidence of acute lower respiratory infections in infants and preschool children: a double-blind, controlled trial, *Pediatrics*, 102:1.

Segreti, J., G. Gheusi, R. Dantzer, K. W. Kelley, and R. W. Johnson. 1997. Defect in interleukin-1β secretion prevents sickness behavior in C3H/HeJ mice, *Physiol. Behav.*, 61:873.

Semba, R. D. 1998. The role of vitamin A and related retinoids in immune function, *Nutr. Rev.*, 56:S38.

Shankar, A. H., and A. S. Prasad. 1998. Zinc and immune function: the biological basis of altered resistance to infection, *Am. J. Clin. Nutr.*, 68:447S.

Sheffy, B. E., and R. D. Schultz. 1979. Influence of vitamin E and selenium on immune response mechanisms, *Fed. Proc.*, 38:2139.

Sidell, N., B. Chang, and L. Bhatti. 1993. Upregulation by retinoic acid of interleukin-2-receptor mRNA in human T lymphocytes, *Cell Immunol.*, 146:28.

Sijtsma, S. R., J. H. Rombout, C. E. West, and A. J. van der Zijpp. 1990. Vitamin A deficiency impairs cytotoxic T lymphocyte activity in Newcastle disease virus-infected chickens, *Vet. Immunol. Immunopathol.*, 26:191.

Somers, S. D., R. S. Chapkin, and K. L. Erickson. 1989. Alteration of *in vitro* murine peritoneal macrophage function by dietary enrichment with eicosapentaenoic and docosahexaenoic acids in menhaden fish oil, *Cell Immunol.*, 123:201.

Sommer, A., J. Katz, and I. Tarwotjo. 1984. Increased risk of respiratory disease and diarrhea in children with preexisting mild vitamin A deficiency, *Am. J. Clin. Nutr.*, 40:1090.

Stuehr, D. J., and M. A. Marletta. 1985. Mammalian nitrate biosynthesis: mouse macrophages produce nitrite and nitrate in response to *Escherichia coli* lipopolysaccharide, *Proc. Natl. Acad. Sci. U.S.A.*, 82:7738.

Sung, Y. J., J. H. Hotchkiss, R. E. Austic, and R. R. Dietert. 1991. L-Arginine-dependent production of a reactive nitrogen intermediate by macrophages of a uricoletic species, *J. Leuk. Biol.*, 50:49.

Thies, F., L. D. Peterson, J. R. Powell, G. Nebe-von-Caron, T. L. Hurst, K. R. Matthews, E. A. Newsholme, and P. C. Calder. 1999. Manipulation of the type of fat consumed by growing pigs affects plasma and mononuclear cell fatty acid compositions and lymphocyte and phagocyte functions, *J. Anim. Sci.*, 77:137.

Tsiagbe, V. K., M. E. Cook, A. E. Harper, and M. L. Sunde. 1987. Enhanced immune responses in broiler chicks fed methionine-supplemented diets, *Poult. Sci.*, 66:1147.

Twining, S. S., D. P. Schulte, P. M. Wilson, B. L. Fish, and J. E. Moulder. 1997. Vitamin A deficiency alters rat neutrophil function, *J. Nutr.*, 127:558.

van Heughten, E., J. W. Spears, and M. T. Coffey. 1994. The effect of dietary protein on performance and immune response in weanling pigs subjected to inflammatory challenge, *J. Anim. Sci.*, 72:2661.

Vary, T. C., and S. R. Kimball. 1992. Sepsis-induced changes in protein synthesis: differential effects on fast- and slow-twitch muscles, *Am. J. Physiol.*, 262:C1513.

Webel, D. M., B. N. Finck, D. H. Baker, and R. W. Johnson. 1997. Time course of elevated plasma cytokines, cortisol, and urea-nitrogen in pigs following intraperitoneal injection of lipopolysaccharide, *J. Anim. Sci.*, 75:1514.

Webel, D. M., D. C. Mahan, R. W. Johnson, and D. H. Baker. 1998. Pretreatment of young pigs with vitamin E attenuates the elevation in plasma interleukin-6 and cortisol caused by a challenge dose of lipopolysaccharide, *J. Nutr.*, 128:1657.

Wigmore, S. J., J. A. Ross, J. S. Falconer, C. E. Plester, M. J. Tisdale, D. C. Carter, and K. C. Fearon. 1996. The effect of polyunsaturated fatty acids on the progress of cachexia in patients with pancreatic cancer, *Nutrition*, 12:S27.

Wigmore, S. J., K. C. Fearon, J. P. Maingay, and J. A. Ross. 1997. Down-regulation of the acute-phase response in patients with pancreatic cancer cachexia receiving oral eicosapentaenoic acid is mediated via suppression of interleukin-6, *Clin. Sci.*, 92:215.

Williams, N. H. 1995. Impact of Immune System Activation on the Rate, Efficiency, and Composition of Growth, the Efficiency of Nutrient Utilization and Lysine Needs of Growing Pigs, Ph.D. dissertation, Iowa State University, Ames.

Williams, N. H., T. S. Stahly, and D. R. Zimmerman. 1997a. Effect of chronic immune system activation on body nitrogen retention, partial efficiency of lysine utilization, and lysine needs of pigs, *J. Anim. Sci.*, 75:2472.

Williams, N. H., T. S. Stahly, and D. R. Zimmerman. 1997b. Effect of chronic immune system activation on the rate, efficiency, composition of growth, and lysine needs of pigs fed from 6 to 27 kg, *J. Anim. Sci.*, 75:2463.

Yaqoob, P., and P. C. Calder. 1995. The effects of dietary lipid manipulation on the production of murine T cell-derived cytokines, *Cytokine*, 7:548.

Zhao, Z., and A. C. Ross. 1995. Retinoic acid repletion restores the number of leukocytes and their subsets and stimulates natural cytotoxicity in vitamin A-deficient rats, *J. Nutr.*, 125:2064.

Zhao, Z., D. M. Murasko, and A. C. Ross. 1994. The role of vitamin A in natural killer cell cytotoxicity, number and activation in the rat, *Nat. Immun.*, 13:29.

Ziegler, T. R., C. Gatzen, and D. W. S. Wilmore. 1994. Strategies for attenuating protein-catabolic responses in the critically ill, *Annu. Rev. Med.*, 45:459.

25 Mycotoxins and Other Antinutritional Factors in Swine Feeds

Eric van Heugten

CONTENTS

I. Mycotoxins 563
    A. Introduction 563
    B. Aspergillus and Penicillium Toxins 565
        1. Aflatoxin 565
        2. Ochratoxins 566
        3. Citrinin 567
    C. Fusarium Toxins 567
        1. Trichothecenes 568
            a. Deoxynivalenol or Vomitoxin 568
            b. T-2 Toxin and Diacetoxyscirpenol 569
        2. Zearalenone 569
        3. Fumonisins 570
    D. Mycotoxin Interactions 571
    E. Controlling Mycotoxins 572
II. Other Antinutritional Factors 572
    A. Introduction 572
    B. Protease Inhibitors 573
    C. Lectins 574
    D. Tannins 575
    E. Other Factors 576
    F. Reducing Antinutritional Factors 577
References 578

I. MYCOTOXINS

A. INTRODUCTION

Mycotoxins are products of fungal metabolism that can cause serious problems in the quality of agricultural commodities. More than 300 different mycotoxins have been identified; however, based on their prevalence in feedstuffs and their toxicity, aflatoxin, deoxynivalenol (DON or vomitoxin), zearalenone, fumonisin, and T-2 toxin are generally considered most problematic. The Council for Agricultural Science and Technology estimated that 25% of the world's food crops are affected by mycotoxins annually (CAST, 1989). The economic losses associated with mycotoxins are difficult to estimate, but are likely to be high considering they would include losses in crop yield and value, processing costs, losses associated with animal production, the cost of regulatory control programs, and analytical costs (CAST, 1989).

Contamination of agricultural commodities with mycotoxins will vary yearly, depending on preharvest and postharvest conditions. Temperature and moisture under field conditions and storage, insect damage, drying conditions, harvesting, and processing methods are all factors that can influence the extent of mycotoxin contamination (Nelson, 1993; Bilgrami and Choudhary, 1998; Lopez-Garcia and Park, 1998). Controlling some of these processes can reduce the incidence of mycotoxins, but is unlikely to eliminate them completely. Therefore, monitoring mycotoxin levels in feedstuffs is necessary to ensure the quality of the food supply. Analytical techniques have improved substantially in recent years, allowing for the identification and quantification of mycotoxins in feedstuffs. These techniques have been described in recent reviews (Chu, 1992; Wilson et al., 1998).

The total impact of mycotoxins on swine production should be considered from a feed ingredient, an animal production, and a human perspective. First, mold growth on ingredients can degrade the nutritional content of feedstuffs and reduce their feeding value. Second, direct losses from mycotoxin contamination can be experienced from losses in pig growth rate, reduced feed efficiency, impaired reproduction, and increased incidence of disease. Third, contamination of meat products derived from animals that had consumed feeds containing mycotoxins may reduce human health and subsequently consumer acceptance of meat products. The effects of mycotoxins on swine production are discussed in this chapter, emphasizing the most recent research. Table 25.1 provides a summary of the main mycotoxins and the molds that produce them, the crops commonly affected

TABLE 25.1
Summary of Major Mycotoxins Produced by Fungi in Commonly Used Feedstuffs in Swine, Their Toxic Effects in Swine, and Suggested Cautionary Levels

Mycotoxin	Main Producing Molds	Crops Commonly Affected	Major Symptoms	Cautionary Levels[a] (ppm)
Aflatoxin	Aspergillus flavus; A. parasiticus; A. nominus	Corn; peanuts; cottonseed	Reduced weight gain and feed intake; liver damage; systemic hemorrhages; thymic atrophy; reduced immunity	0.02
Ochratoxin	A. ochraceus; Penicillium verrucosum	Barley; oilseed crops	Reduced weight gain and feed intake; kidney dysfunction; increased water consumption; polyuria; reduced immunity	0.20
Deoxynivalenol (vomitoxin)	Fusarium graminearum; F. culmorum	Corn; wheat; barley; rye; oats	Reduced feed intake; feed refusal; vomiting; reduced body weight gain	1.0
T-2	F. sporotrichoides; F. tricinctum; F. poae	Wheat; barley	Reduced body weight gain and feed intake; dermatitis; necrosis of lymphoid tissue; reduced sow fertility	0.5
Zearalenone	F. graminearum; F. culmorum; F. tricinctum	Corn; wheat; barley; rye	Hyperestrogenism; reduced reproductive performance; infertility	0.5
Fumonisin	Fumonisin moniliforme; F. proliferatum	Corn	Reduced body weight gain and feed intake; liver disease; pulmonary edema	5.0

[a] These levels are guidelines and indicate levels of concern. The impact of mycotoxins on swine production depends on many factors and, therefore, lower levels than those indicated here may result in economic losses.

by these molds, the symptoms associated with mycotoxicosis in swine, and suggested levels that should be considered detrimental to swine production.

B. ASPERGILLUS AND PENICILLIUM TOXINS

1. Aflatoxin

Aflatoxins are mycotoxins primarily produced by *Aspergillus flavus*, *A. parasiticus*, and *A. nominus* (Smith, 1997). These molds preferentially grow under hot and humid conditions with an optimal temperature range of 25 to 33°C, but growth can still occur between 2 and 47°C (Nelson, 1993). Corn, peanuts, and cottonseed are the crops that are most commonly affected by *Aspergillus* spp., and drought, insect infestation, and poor storage conditions can increase their occurrence.

Aflatoxins are the most widely studied mycotoxins because of their widespread distribution, their potent toxicity, and their potential as carcinogens in humans. The aflatoxins consist of four naturally occurring compounds that are characterized by dihydrofuran or tetrahydrofuran moieties linked to a substituted coumarin moiety. The most toxic and carcinogenic form is aflatoxin B_1, followed by aflatoxin G_1, B_2, and G_2. Other forms of aflatoxin may occur as products of microbial, animal, or human metabolism. The hydroxylated metabolite of aflatoxin B_1, aflatoxin M_1, is most significant in this context because of its excretion in milk (Smith, 1997).

Because of the recognized toxicity of aflatoxins, this is the only mycotoxin that is currently regulated in the United States and the European Community (EC). The U.S. FDA regulatory guidelines for total aflatoxin level in commodities is set at 20 ppb. Other guidelines restrict aflatoxin levels in corn and peanut products fed to breeding swine to 100 ppb and those fed to finishing swine >100 lb (45 kg) to 200 ppb. The maximum level for cottonseed meal is 300 ppb (Smith, 1997). Efforts in the EC to provide consistent guidelines have led to the recommendation that complete feeds for pigs may not contain >20 ppb of aflatoxin B_1 (10 ppb for young pigs) and that feed ingredients used in pig feeds may not contain >30 ppb of aflatoxin B_1.

The liver is the primary target organ for aflatoxins, where damage occurs following the metabolic activation of aflatoxin to the aflatoxin-8,9-epoxide by the microsomal mixed-function oxidases (Coulombe, 1993). This highly reactive metabolite can bind to proteins, DNA, and RNA, and this is thought to be the mechanism of toxicity. Detoxification occurs mainly by adduct formation of the epoxide with glutathione or via conjugation with sulfates and glucuronic acid. Acute effects of aflatoxicosis include reduced body weight gain, depression of feed intake, liver damage, and systemic hemorrhages (CAST, 1989). Gross examination of the liver indicates icterus, liver enlargement, hepatic degeneration, and fatty infiltration, while microscopic changes include cytoplasmic vacuolation, portal fibrosis, and bile duct hyperplasia. Changes in biochemical measures, including aspartate transaminase, alkaline phosphatase, γ-glutamyl transferase, cholinesterase, urea nitrogen, and albumin are indicative of liver damage in aflatoxicosis (Harvey et al., 1994a). In general, chronic aflatoxin toxicity will result in similar signs of growth retardation and liver damage, although they may be more subtle than in acute toxicity. In addition to the liver, the thymus is another organ that is targeted by aflatoxins. Thymic atrophy and hypoplasia of the thymic cortex have been reported (Pier, 1987).

Pigs are highly susceptible to aflatoxins. The mean oral lethal dose (LD_{50}) for swine is approximately 0.62 mg/kg, compared with 1.0 to 1.5, 2.0, and 6.5 mg/kg for calves (estimated), sheep, and chickens, respectively (Pier, 1987). Sensitivity to aflatoxins will also vary depending on age, with young pigs being more susceptible than older pigs. Pier (1987) summarized that reduced weight gain generally could be detected in pigs consuming 260 ppb of aflatoxin. Other research reported a linear reduction in growth and feed intake in weanling pigs fed 140 or 280 ppb of aflatoxin (van Heugten et al., 1994). Coffey et al. (1989) observed a reduction in growth rate and feed intake in weanling pigs fed 125 ppb of aflatoxin when the diet contained 18% crude protein, but not in pigs receiving diets containing 20% crude protein. The variation in response to aflatoxin among trials is likely due to differences in age, exposure time, the presence of other mycotoxins, and the level of nutrients in the diet they receive. In pigs, Coffey et al. (1989) reported that methionine supplementation could alleviate some of the toxic effects of aflatoxin, although this result was not observed in a subsequent study (van Heugten et al., 1994). Supplementation of aflatoxin-contaminated diets (840 ppb) with 2 ppm of folic acid improved weight gain of weanling pigs in one trial, but not in another (Lindemann et al., 1993). Addition of selenium in that study had no effect on pig performance. An in-depth review of nutrient interactions with mycotoxins is available (Schaeffer and Hamilton, 1991).

Aflatoxins can also affect susceptibility to disease through their effect on the immune system. Aflatoxins cause thymic atrophy and hypoplasia of the thymic cortex, but do not affect the number of circulating T cells (Pier, 1991). Cellular immunity is most consistently affected by aflatoxin, as measured by peripheral blood lymphocyte proliferation, lymphokine production by T cells, and delayed type hypersensitivity. Additionally, macrophage phagocytosis and reduced complement activity are generally observed as a result of aflatoxin consumption. Depression in antibody responses are observed only at high doses of aflatoxins (Pier, 1991). Studies in pigs have shown variable results on immune response when aflatoxin levels ranging from 140 to 800 ppb were fed (Miller et al., 1978; 1981; Panangala et al., 1986; van Heugten et al., 1994).

Direct effects of aflatoxin on reproductive performance seem to be lacking (Diekman and Green, 1992). However, aflatoxins can be transferred *in utero* from the sow to the fetus, are excreted in the milk, and can exert a negative effect on suckling pig performance. Silvotti et al. (1997) reported that supplementation of sow diets during gestation and lactation with 800 ppb of aflatoxin B_1, G_1, or a combination of the two resulted in impaired lymphocyte and macrophage function in their offspring. The level of aflatoxins in the sow milk was 0.9 ppb, which seemed too low to have a direct effect on pigs during suckling. The authors speculated that aflatoxin exposure *in utero* may have compromised their immune system. These results are in agreement with those of Mocchegiani et al. (1998), who reported growth retardation, thymic involution, and impaired lymphocyte proliferation in pigs from sows that were exposed to aflatoxin.

2. Ochratoxins

Ochratoxins are toxic compounds that are mainly produced by *A. ochraceus* (now referred to as *A. alutaceus*) and *Penicillium verrucosum* (Marquardt and Frohlich, 1992). Ochratoxin-producing molds grow best under high moisture conditions as indicated by the optimal water activity values (defined as the partial pressure of water vapor above a sample divided by the partial pressure of water in the liquid form) ranging from 0.95 to 0.99 (Krogh, 1991). The optimum temperature range for ochratoxin production by *A. ochraceus* is 12 to 37°C and that of *P. verrucosum* is 4 to 31°C. This is in agreement with the observation that *P. verrucosum* is primarily responsible for ochratoxin production in colder climates and *A. ochraceus* has the greatest ochratoxin production potential in warmer climates (Krogh, 1991). Grains, particularly barley, and oilseed crops are susceptible to ochratoxin contamination, primarily under storage conditions (Marquardt and Frolich, 1992).

Ochratoxins are a group of closely related isocoumarin derivatives linked to L-β-phenylalanine. Ochratoxin A is the most common form produced and ochratoxin B can occur sporadically as a natural contaminant. This group of mycotoxins has received considerable attention in recent years because of its impact on animal performance and the potential transmission of ochratoxin into the human food chain. Ochratoxin A contamination has been reported in meat products from nonruminant animals (Marquardt and Frolich, 1992). Surveys by the USDA and the FDA have indicated that ochratoxin contamination was not a major problem in the United States, and therefore regulatory limits for ochratoxins were not established (Wood and Trucksess, 1998).

Ochratoxins exert their toxic effect mainly on the kidney. Following absorption in the upper gastrointestinal tract, ochratoxin binds primarily to the albumin fraction of the blood. Excretion takes place in the urine as α-ochratoxin and to a lesser extent ochratoxin A, with some excretion also occurring in the feces. The half-life of ochratoxin A after intravenous administration has been reported as 150 h in pigs. The levels of ochratoxin in blood remain relatively high due to enterohepatic recycling of ochratoxin and an efficient reabsorption of ochratoxin by the renal tubules of the kidney. Toxic effects are evidenced by reduced performance and feed consumption, renal disturbances (including damage to the proximal tubules and interstitial cortical fibrosis), increased water consumption, and polyuria. Further details on ochratoxin metabolism, mechanisms of action, and their effects on animals and humans can be found in recent reviews (Krogh, 1991; Marquardt and Frohlich, 1992).

The acute toxicity of ochratoxin A in pigs as measured by LD_{50} is 1.0 to 6.0 mg/kg of body weight. The kidney is the principal organ affected by ochratoxins at levels that occur under field conditions (0.20 to 4.0 ppm). At higher levels (5 to 10 ppm), other organ systems such as the liver, intestine, spleen, lymphoid tissue, and leukocytes can be affected (CAST, 1989). Madsen et al. (1982) reported reduced growth performance in pigs fed 1.4 to 2.3 ppm of ochratoxin, but no effect was observed when levels of 0 to 0.2 ppm of ochratoxin were fed. Harvey et al. (1989a; 1992; 1994b) reported consistently reduced growth in growing pigs fed 2.0 or 2.5 ppm of ochratoxin. In contrast, Tapia and Seawright (1984) did not observe a significant reduction in pig growth at 2.0 ppm of ochratoxin, but daily gain was linearly decreased when ochratoxin was included at 4.0, 8.0, and 16.0 ppm. Nephropathy may occur at lower levels of ochratoxin based on the observation that 0.2 to 4.0 ppm of ochratoxin caused kidney lesions in pigs after 4 months of exposure (Krogh et al., 1974).

Ochratoxin can also affect the gut-associated lymphoid tissue (GALT), deplete lymphoid cells in the Peyers patches, and possibly affect the thymus (Pier, 1991). Circulating levels of IgG and IgM are reduced and antibody formation is diminished in ochratoxicosis. In addition, reduced macrophage phagocytosis has been reported (Pier, 1991). Harvey et al. (1992) reported reduced *in vivo* cellular immunity as measured by a phytohemagglutinin (PHA) skin thickness response, reduced delayed-type hypersensitivity to tuberculin, decreased lymphocyte proliferation and interleukin production *in vitro*, and decreased macrophage phagocytic activity when ochratoxin was fed at 2.5 ppm to growing gilts. However, immunoglobulin concentrations and antibody response to chicken red blood cells were not affected. In a subsequent study (Harvey et al., 1994b), ochratoxin inclusion in the diet at 2.5 ppm reduced macrophage phagocytosis, but did not affect lymphocyte proliferation. A summary of the effects of ochratoxin on the immune response in other species was published by Richard (1991).

3. Citrinin

Citrinin is produced by *P. citrinum* and *P. verrucosum* on cereal and oilseed crops. It produces effects similar to those of ochratoxin *in vivo*, most notably nephropathy (Abramson, 1997). Because citrinin and ochratoxin often occur together as contaminants of feedstuffs, the impact of each of these mycotoxins on porcine nephropathy is difficult to distinguish (Krogh, 1991).

C. Fusarium Toxins

There are approximately 20 *Fusarium* species reported in cereal grains capable of producing toxic metabolites. The identification of the *Fusarium* species and the toxins they produce is confusing because of different taxonomic systems and incorrect identification of isolates and mycotoxins (Chelkowski, 1998). Nonetheless, 150 mycotoxins isolated from *Fusarium* molds have been reported (Wood, 1992). Of these, the trichothecenes (most notably T-2 toxin, deoxynivalenol, or DON, which is also called vomitoxin, and nivalenol), zearalenone, and the fumonisins are most important based on their occurrence and toxicity. *Fusarium graminearum* and *F. culmorum* are most frequently encountered in wheat, barley, corn, and rye and are producers of DON and zearalenone. *Fusarium sporotrichioides* and *F. tricinctum* produce T-2 toxin and some other trichothecenes, but they are rarely found in agricultural products. *Fusarium poae* cause contamination of grains with nivalenol and fusarenone. More recently, fumonisin produced by *F. moniliforme* has surfaced as a major contaminant of corn products with significant negative effects on animal performance. *Fusarium* molds thrive best under cool and wet weather conditions (Wood, 1992). Nelson (1993) suggested that the optimal temperature for T-2 production by *Fusarium* was between 5 and 15°C, although production of T-2 toxin still occurred at lower and higher temperatures.

1. Trichothecenes

Trichothecenes are a group of structurally related compounds consisting of a tetracyclic sesquiterpene structure with a six-membered oxygen-containing ring, an epoxide group in the 12, 13 position, and an unsaturated bond in the 9, 10 position (Swanson and Corley, 1989). Diacetoxyscirpenol (DAS), T-2 toxin, DON, and nivalenol are four of the most important trichothecenes. The toxic effects of trichothecenes can be characterized by gastrointestinal disorders, such as vomiting, diarrhea, and hemorrhaging; feed refusal; compromised growth; abortion; anemia; and leukopenia (Smith, 1992; Coulombe, 1993). Several reviews have been written discussing current knowledge of trichothecenes (Smith, 1992), their metabolism (Swanson and Corley, 1989), their immunotoxicity (Taylor et al., 1989), and their reproductive toxicity (Francis, 1989).

a. Deoxynivalenol or vomitoxin

Deoxynivalenol or vomitoxin is considered to be one of the trichothecenes with the lowest toxicity, but it is important because it is widely distributed in foods and feeds throughout the world (Rotter et al., 1996). Based on survey data on the occurrence of DON in wheat and wheat products and toxicological data, the FDA issued advisory levels for DON, recommending that levels >1 ppm in finished wheat products are a concern. In addition, FDA recommended that wheat and wheat milling by-products for animal feeds should preferably contain <4 ppm of DON, and grains and grain products for swine diets should contain <5 ppm of DON and not exceed 20% of the diet (Wood and Trucksess, 1998).

Swine are very sensitive to DON. A reduction in feed consumption and weight gain can generally be observed at 2 to 3 ppm of purified DON, whereas poultry and ruminants can tolerate levels of 20 ppm of DON (Rotter et al., 1996). When naturally contaminated feedstuffs are fed, reduced feed intake and growth performance can occur at levels ≤2 ppm of DON. Pigs seem to be more sensitive to DON when they are fed naturally contaminated diets, which may be related to the presence of other mycotoxins in addition to DON (Diekman and Green, 1992). Trenholm et al. (1994) reported that feed intake and body weight gain were 18 and 23% lower, respectively, when diets naturally contaminated with DON were fed compared with diets containing an equal amount of purified DON. Smith et al. (1997) concluded that fusaric acid may play a role in the greater toxicity of DON in naturally contaminated diets. They reported that the toxicity of DON was enhanced in pigs when fusaric acid was added to the diets at levels of 12 to 16 ppm. Rotter et al. (1996) summarized that a substantial reduction in feed intake in growing pigs could be observed at 1.3 ppm of DON, complete feed refusal was evident at 12 ppm, and vomiting occurred at 20 ppm. The reduction in feed intake accounts for the lower growth rates in pigs fed DON-contaminated diets, although specific changes, not related to feed intake, such as stomach appearance and biochemical measures, due to DON contamination occur (Rotter et al., 1994; 1995). Some adaptation to DON exposure may occur as evidenced by reduced negative effects of DON on intake and growth performance and a normalization of blood parameters over time (Rotter et al., 1995).

Information on the immunotoxicity of DON in swine is limited. Overnes et al. (1997) reported a linear reduction in the secondary antibody response to tetanus toxoid when DON levels were increased from control levels to 1.8 and 4.7 ppm. However, antibody response to four other antigens or *in vitro* lymphocyte proliferation to three different mitogens were not affected by DON. Rotter et al. (1994) noted a delayed response in achieving maximum titers to sheep red blood cells (SRBC) vaccination, only when pigs fed DON-contaminated diets were compared with pair-fed control pigs, but not pigs allowed *ad libitum* access to feed. No differences were detected in *in vitro* lymphocyte blastogenic response. Bergsjo et al. (1992) detected no differences in serum IgA in pigs fed up to 4 ppm of DON, whereas Rotter et al. (1995) reported no differences in natural killer cell activity between control pigs and pigs exposed to 4 ppm of DON. These experiments indicate that the effects of DON on immune function seem to be minimal in pigs fed diets with naturally occurring levels of DON.

Limited research with sows indicates that DON has no specific detrimental effects on reproductive performance (Francis, 1989; Diekman and Green, 1992).

b. T-2 Toxin and diacetoxyscirpenol

Swine have been used extensively as a model to study the toxicology, pharmacokinetics, metabolism, and treatment strategies of T-2 toxin and DAS. The LD_{50} following intravenous administration for T-2 toxin and DAS have been reported as 1.2 and 0.38 mg/kg, respectively, which rates pigs as being sensitive to T-2 toxin and very sensitive to DAS (Wannemacher et al., 1991). The levels of T-2 toxin and DAS in feed that will exert negative effects on pig performance, reproduction, and health are less well documented.

Friend et al. (1992) reported a tendency of reduced daily gain and feed intake when T-2 toxin was included in the diet at 0.4, 0.8, 1.6, and 3.2 ppm. Although some effects of the low levels of T-2 toxin supplementation were observed, they concluded that a reduction in performance may occur at approximately 3 ppm. Rafai et al. (1995) reported that supplementation of 2 ppm of T-2 toxin to 9-kg pigs for 3 weeks reduced daily gain, but that feed intake was negatively affected at 0.5 ppm of T-2 toxin. Pigs fed T-2 toxin reduced their feed intake by 5 to 41% for low T-2 toxin levels (0.5, 1, 2, and 3 ppm) up to 52 to 84% for the higher T-2 toxin levels (4, 5, 10, and 15 ppm) in that study. Previous work (Weaver et al., 1978a) suggested that pigs readily consume diets with up to 10 to 12 ppm of T-2 toxin. The daily intake of toxin by pigs when administered through the diet can be controlled to some extent by lowering feed consumption. This may explain differences between studies in which the toxin was administered by injection or parenterally and feeding studies. Rafai et al. (1995) reported plasma glucose levels well below normal in pigs fed 1, 2, or 3 ppm of T-2 toxin. Levels of 4, 5, 10, and 15 ppm of T-2 toxin caused dermatitis of the skin on the snout, dorsal part of the nose, the buccal commissures, behind the ears, and around the prepuce as well as on the mucous membrane of the oral cavity and the tongue. Similar observations were reported by Harvey et al. (1990) in pigs fed 10 ppm of T-2 toxin. Exposure of pigs to T-2 toxin has been reported to result in necrosis of lymphoid tissues, reduced leukocyte counts, and impaired lymphocyte blastogenic response to mitogens (Sharma, 1993). Sow fertility was compromised in sows consuming diets containing 12 ppm of T-2 toxin for a prolonged period of time (Weaver et al., 1978c).

Feeding of 2 ppm of DAS reduced daily gain in 9-week-old barrows (Harvey et al., 1991). Similarly, Weaver et al. (1978b) reported decreased weight gain in pigs fed 2 ppm of DAS, but not at lower levels. Complete feed refusal and oral, cutaneous, and intestinal lesions were documented in that study at levels >10 ppm.

2. Zearalenone

Zearalenone is a resorcyclic acid lactone compound with estrogenic properties. Although zearalenone differs structurally from the estrogens, it is capable of binding to estrogen receptors. Therefore, toxicity signs for zearalenone are evidenced by hyperestrogenism, which is characterized by reddening and swelling of the vulva, increased size of the uterus, mammary enlargement, and rectal and vaginal prolapse in gilts (Etienne and Dourmad, 1994). In boars, testis atrophy, nipple enlargement, and rectal prolapse may be observed. Prolonged estrus, ovarian atrophy, pseudopregnancy, abortion, increased embryonic mortality, stillbirths, and birth of weak pigs have been reported in sexually mature sows (Etienne and Dourmad, 1994).

Swine are very sensitive to zearalenone, and, within the species, prepubertal gilts seem to be most sensitive (Diekman and Green, 1992). Hyperestrogenism can be observed in immature gilts within 1 week of feeding zearalenone at 1.5 to 2.0 ppm (Rainey et al., 1990). Similarly, Friend et al. (1990) reported reddening and swelling of the vulva and increased uterus weight in pigs fed zearalenone at low concentrations for 9 weeks and concluded that 0.5 ppm of zearalenone was estrogenic. These effects seem to be reversible and usually disappear 1 to 2 weeks after withdrawal of zearalenone-contaminated feed (Etienne and Dourmad, 1994). The impact of the estrogenic effect of zearalenone on attainment of puberty and subsequent reproduction is not clear. Diekman and Green (1992) summarized the results from three studies, in which an increase, no effect, and a decrease in the age of first estrus were observed, and generally there were no effects on ovulation rate, litter size, or length of the estrus cycle. The duration of feeding of zearalenone, the level of contamination, and the age of the gilts when feeding was initiated varied among the studies and may account for the differences in response.

In cycling gilts, an extended interestrous interval has been consistently reported when zearalenone was fed at levels ranging from 3.6 to 20 ppm (Diekman and Green, 1992). Return to estrus after weaning was also delayed for gilts and sows when levels >3 ppm of zearalenone were fed (Etienne and Dourmad, 1994). In studies where zearalenone was fed during pregnancy, increased embryo mortality and decreased litter size were reported, usually at levels >10 ppm. Additionally, reduced weight of fetuses at 80 days of gestation and lowered pig weight at birth have been observed in gilts fed diets containing levels of ≥4 ppm of zearalenone (Etienne and Dourmad, 1994). These negative effects of zearalenone can be observed even at short periods of exposure during critical periods of the reproductive cycle. Zearalenone may further decrease pig survival from birth to weaning when sows are fed zearalenone during gestation and lactation, and there may be estrogenic effects in pigs nursing sows exposed to high levels of zearalenone, possibly via the milk (Etienne and Dourmad, 1994). Diekman and Green (1992) summarized that levels of 40 to 600 ppm of zearalenone reduced testis weight and libido in boars and that sperm motility was reported to be reduced in boars fed 9 ppm of zearalenone.

3. Fumonisins

The fumonisins are a group of compounds most commonly found in corn and corn products. To date, seven fumonisins have been isolated, fumonisin A_1, A_2, B_1, B_2, B_3, B_4, and C_1, of which fumonisin B_1 and B_2 are most abundant (Wood and Trucksess, 1998). The concentration of fumonisin B_1 in field samples is typically three times greater than that of fumonisin B_2 (Ross et al., 1992). The FDA has provided guidelines for fumonisins for livestock feeds, due to the high frequency of fumonisins in corn products and their potential carcinogenecity. The maximum level of fumonisins in complete swine feeds suggested by FDA is 10 ppm (Wood and Trucksess, 1998).

In swine, fumonisins cause porcine pulmonary edema syndrome and hepatic injury (Harrison et al., 1990; Colvin et al., 1993). The liver is a primary target organ in fumonisin toxicosis in most species, but the lung and the pancreas are specific targets in swine (Harrison et al., 1990; Haschek et al., 1992). Additionally, keratosis of the distal esophagus has been reported in swine (Casteel et al., 1993). Greater levels of fumonisins are required to induce pulmonary edema than liver disease. Colvin et al. (1993) concluded that pigs intubated with a minimum of 16 mg FB_1/kg body weight daily developed pulmonary edema and that levels <16 mg FB_1/kg body weight or 200 ppm FB_1 in feed caused icterus and hepatic necrosis. Motelin et al. (1994) fed 175, 101, 39, 23, 5, and 0 ppm of total fumonisins and reported pulmonary edema at 175 ppm of fumonisin only. Liver pathology in that study was evident at levels >23 ppm, whereas changes in serum enzyme concentrations indicative of liver damage (particularly alkaline phosphatase) were estimated to occur at levels >12 ppm. The no-adverse-effect level for weight gain was estimated to be 22 ppm (Motelin et al., 1994). Rotter et al. (1997) observed no negative effects of 0.11, 0.33, or 1 ppm of FB_1 on growing-finishing pig performance or carcass characteristics; however, they noted increased variability in feed consumption and carcass merit in pigs fed 1 ppm of FB_1.

The sphinganine-to-sphingosine ratio may be a sensitive indicator of fumonisin toxicosis, because changes in the ratio occur at low levels of fumonisins (Riley et al., 1993). A linear increase in this ratio was observed with increasing fumonisin concentration, with significant effects at levels >5 ppm. Fumonisin B_1 is an inhibitor of the enzyme sphinganine N-acyltransferase causing a reduction in sphingolipid synthesis and an alteration of the sphinganine-to-sphingosine ratio (Wang et al., 1991). Sphingolipids are components of cell membranes and play an important role in cell signaling and the reduction in these compounds has been implicated as a mechanism in fumonisin toxicosis (Merrill et al., 1997).

The effects of fumonisin on immune responses of swine are not clear. Osweiler et al. (1993) reported a decreased lymphocyte blastogenesis and antibody titer response to pseudorabies virus (PRV) on day 14, but not on day 21 in pigs fed 33 ppm of fumonisin. Harvey et al. (1995; 1996) observed a decrease in lymphocyte blastogenesis in barrows fed 50 or 100 ppm of fumonisin. However, feeding of 100 ppm of fumonisin for 17 days did not affect T-lymphocyte function in sows (Becker et al., 1995). Pulmonary clearance of particulates and bacteria was compromised in pigs fed 20 mg/kg body weight of hydrolyzed fumonisin daily, due to decreased phagocytosis by pulmonary intravascular macrophages (Smith et al., 1996).

Fumonisins did not seem to be transferred into the milk of lactating sows when fed at 100 or 200 ppm for 17 days and were not toxic to suckling pigs (Becker et al., 1995).

D. Mycotoxin Interactions

Interactions among different mycotoxins are likely to occur in practical pig production. Diets for swine typically consist of a mixture of multiple ingredients, each of which could potentially be contaminated with different mycotoxins. Additionally, molds of the same genus can produce more than one mycotoxin, contributing to possible coexistence of several mycotoxins in feeds. Further, numerous mold species can be present in ingredients at the same time and produce different mycotoxins. Interactions among mycotoxins may be an explanation for the common observation that studies using naturally contaminated feeds as the source of mycotoxin often report a larger impact on swine performance compared with studies using purified compounds. Responses to multiple mycotoxin exposure under experimental conditions have been primarily additive in nature, as reported for the combinations of aflatoxin and ochratoxin, aflatoxin and DAS, or T-2 toxin and ochratoxin (Huff et al., 1988; Harvey et al., 1989a; 1991; 1994b). In contrast, Tapia and Seawright (1985) observed that the combination of aflatoxin and ochratoxin was not additive, but that toxicity was mainly due to ochratoxin. No toxic interactions were observed when aflatoxin was fed in combination with DON or when T-2 toxin was fed with DON (Harvey et al., 1989b; Friend et al., 1992). Similarly, Rotter et al. (1992) reported no interactive effects between DON and other F. graminearum metabolites. Synergistic effects were evident when combinations of aflatoxin and fumonisin, DON and fumonisin, or DON and fusaric acid were fed (Harvey et al., 1995; 1996; Smith et al., 1997). Harvey et al. (1990) noted a sparing effect for weight gain, and for serum biochemical and hematological values when aflatoxin and T-2 toxin combinations were fed. In that study, the toxic effects of the combination of aflatoxin and T-2 toxin were less severe than the effects of either of these toxins alone. Coffey et al. (1990) summarized that zearalenone improved growth performance in pigs fed aflatoxin. The interactions between mycotoxins are complex and may be antagonistic, additive, or synergistic in nature, which may vary depending on mycotoxin combination, level, and the type of measurement. Care should be taken in interpreting data from experiments using naturally contaminated ingredients because of the possible presence of other mycotoxins or metabolites unrelated to the one that is being studied. Further information on mechanistic interactions among mycotoxins was reviewed by Riley (1998).

E. CONTROLLING MYCOTOXINS

Numerous reviews have been published on the control of mycotoxin levels postharvest through detoxification strategies (CAST, 1989). These strategies may rely on physical or chemical separation of mycotoxins from products (West and Bullerman, 1991), physical degradation of mycotoxins (Samarajeewa, 1991), chemical degradation (Pemberton and Simpson, 1991), or biological detoxification (Bhatnagar et al., 1991). Although some of these approaches can yield promising results, they do not seem to represent economically feasible solutions.

Alumino silicate compounds have been used with success in ameliorating the effects of aflatoxin in swine and other species. These compounds, describing any mineral containing alumina and silica, can be subdivided into the clays (phyllosilicates) and the zeolites (molecular sieves) (Taylor, 1999). Clays are layered silicate minerals and one particular clay, montmorillonite, which is the mineral contained in bentonite, has been investigated extensively as an aflatoxin-binding agent. The zeolites are highly porous arrays that have also been evaluated. Taylor (1999) pointed out the diversity in compounds within the alumino silicates and reported that their *in vitro* binding capacity for aflatoxin can vary from 16.9 to 99.2%. Although *in vitro* binding capacity does not necessarily correspond to effectiveness *in vivo*, several alumino silicates have been reported to reduce the negative effects of aflatoxin. The presumed mechanism of action is a direct irreversible binding of the clay or zeolite to the toxin, thereby preventing absorption by the animal. Their effectiveness against zearalenone and ochratoxin A seems to be limited and they have not shown a positive effect against trichothecenes (Ramos and Hernandez, 1997). Schell et al. (1993b) reported that the reduction in daily gain associated with feeding diets containing 500 or 800 ppb of aflatoxin could be corrected by as much as 31 to 88% by inclusion of various alumino silicates. Based on their work, the reduction in average daily gain due to aflatoxin could be recovered by an average of 77% for hydrated sodium calcium aluminosilicate (HSCA), 78% for bentonite (sodium or calcium bentonite), 42% for polygorskite, 68% for sepiolite, and 60% for zeolite. Similarly, Lindemann et al. (1993) reported that both HSCA and sodium bentonite were effective in improving growth performance in pigs fed 800 or 840 ppb of aflatoxin (83 and 89% recovery), whereas Harvey et al. (1994a) observed 65 to 69% protection from HSCA in pigs fed 3000 ppb of aflatoxin. The optimal level of inclusion seems to be 0.5% (Lindemann et al., 1993; Schell et al., 1993b). Higher levels of inclusion may reduce feed efficiency because of a dilution effect from adding an inert compound (Schell et al., 1993b). Mineral absorption may be compromised with the inclusion of zeolites and clays because of their high adsorptive capacity (Schell et al., 1993a). These effects were most pronounced in pigs fed aflatoxin. In addition, some clays can bind drugs and should be used with caution in medicated feeds. Although many of these products are "Generally Recognized as Safe (GRAS status)," they have not been approved by the FDA as aflatoxin binders.

II. OTHER ANTINUTRITIONAL FACTORS

A. INTRODUCTION

A number of factors present in agricultural commodities fed to farm animals, collectively termed *antinutritional factors*, have been recognized to have negative effects on digestive and metabolic processes and subsequently meat, milk, and egg production. These compounds include protease inhibitors (trypsin, chymotrypsin, and α-amylase inhibitors), lectins, tannins, antigenic proteins, estrogens, flatulence factors, antivitamins, glucosinolates, and phytate (Liener, 1994; Wareham et al., 1994). They are thought to play a protective role in plant tissues against diseases, insects, and animals. Of these factors, protease inhibitors, lectins, and tannins are most important for swine, because they occur at the greatest level in the most commonly used legume seeds such as soybeans and peas and to a lesser extent in cereal grains (Huisman, 1989). Multiple antinutritional factors are present in feedstuffs and ultimately diets for swine at the same time, and this makes their effects on metabolism and pig performance difficult to predict.

B. PROTEASE INHIBITORS

The most well known protease inhibitors are those that inhibit the serine proteases trypsin and chymotrypsin (Gueguen et al., 1993). Two main categories of protease inhibitors for legume seeds can be distinguished: those belonging to the Bowman–Birk family and those to the Kunitz protease inhibitor family (Liener, 1994). The Bowman–Birk inhibitors are protein molecules that are characterized by a molecular weight of 6 to 10 kDa, and seven disulfide bridges (Liener, 1994). The Bowman–Birk inhibitors have two distinct reactive sites, one that binds trypsin and one that binds chymotrypsin (Gueguen et al., 1993). The Kunitz protease inhibitors are proteins with a molecular weight of approximately 20 kDa that contain two disulfide bridges. They primarily bind with trypsin at a 1:1 ratio (Liener, 1994).

Trypsin and chymotrypsin inhibitors can be found in largest quantities in soybeans, peas, and *Phaseolus* beans (such as navy beans, pinto beans, kidney beans, etc.), but have also been detected at moderate levels in some varieties of triticale and rye. Trypsin inhibitor activity (TIA) is highest in raw soybeans at levels of 20.8 to 32.6 mg pure trypsin inhibited per gram of dry matter (DM), whereas the levels in toasted soybean meal are much lower (2.9 to 4.1 mg/g DM) (Huisman, 1990). The level of TIA in peas ranges from 0.1 to 7.9 mg/g DM, depending on variety, and Phaseolus beans were reported to contain 3.8 to 22.4 mg TIA/g DM (Huisman, 1990). As a proportion of protein, the trypsin inhibitor activity is higher in peas and *Phaseolus* beans than in soybean meal. Care should be taken in interpreting data from the literature because different units have been used to express TIA. For comparison purposes, Rackis et al. (1986) suggested that 1.9 trypsin inhibitor units (TIU) or trypsin units inhibited (TUI) was equivalent to 1 mg pure trypsin inhibited per gram of sample. Detailed information on trypsin inhibitor analysis has been reviewed recently (Gueguen et al., 1993; Trugo and von Baer, 1998).

Trypsin inhibitors reduce the growth performance of pigs and interfere with the digestion and metabolic utilization of protein. The exact impact of trypsin inhibitors on these factors and the assignment of threshold values are difficult to establish because of variation in experimental protocols and possible confounding of results. Le Guen and Birk (1993) pointed out that specific effects of trypsin inhibitors are difficult to distinguish from effects of other antinutritional factors that may be present in supplements tested. Further, experiments may use varieties of feedstuffs with different levels of trypsin inhibitors that may also be different in amino acid, starch, or fiber composition. In addition, processing of feedstuffs (e.g., thermal treatment) to obtain different levels of antinutritional factors may also alter other dietary factors, such as available amino acid composition.

Herkelman et al. (1992) reported that raw soybeans with low TIA (TIA was 9.9 mg/g) fed to 24-kg pigs improved average daily gain (ADG) by 9% compared with conventional raw soybeans (TIA was 20.9 mg/g). In the same study, heated soybeans with low trypsin inhibitor (TIA was 1.2 mg/g) resulted in an 11% improvement in ADG compared with heated conventional soybeans (TIA was 4.8 mg/g). Improvements in ADG were 40% when conventional soybeans were heated and 43% when low trypsin inhibitor soybeans were heated (Herkelman et al., 1992). Other studies in which low trypsin inhibitor peas or pea fractions containing antinutritional factors were used have been reported to reduce ADG (Huisman, 1990; Jondreville et al., 1992). Schultze et al. (1993a) reported a reduction in growth rate in 5-week-old pigs fed 2.4 and 7.2 mg added isolated soy trypsin inhibitor per kilogram of diet of 13 and 32%, respectively. Jansman et al. (1998) studied the N retention in young barrows (8.8 kg) fed eight different levels of trypsin inhibitor, ranging from 0.1 to 3.1 mg/g, added as purified Kunitz trypsin inhibitor from soybeans. They concluded that there seemed to be a breakpoint for N retention at 0.77 mg/g and that above this level N retention was reduced by 0.28 g/day for each milligram of TIA per gram of diet. The authors point out that the use of purified Kunitz trypsin inhibitor may not accurately reflect situations where both Kunitz and Bowman–Birk inhibitors are present or when they are present in a natural matrix.

The negative effects of trypsin inhibitors on pig performance can be largely attributed to the reduced apparent ileal amino acid digestibility that has been reported in pigs fed raw soybeans, high trypsin inhibitor soybeans, or purified trypsin inhibitors (Herkelman et al., 1992; Schultze et al., 1993b; Grala et al., 1998a). Studies using peas or pea protein concentrates as the source of trypsin inhibitors have been less consistent in their effect on apparent ileal N digestibility (Lallès and Jansman, 1998). Protease inhibitors may exert their effect by direct inhibition of trypsin and chymotrypsin in the small intestine, thus lowering the digestion of proteins. In addition, negative feedback of low trypsin levels in the intestine stimulates the pancreas through the release of cholecystokinin to produce more trypsin, chymotrypsin, elastase, and amylase causing pancreatic enlargement in some species (Huisman and Jansman, 1991; Liener, 1994). However, in pigs pancreas weight is not affected by trypsin inhibitors, whereas trypsin activity in the pancreas has been reported to be reduced or to remain constant (Huisman, 1990; Schultze et al., 1993a). The differences in response to trypsin inhibitors between species suggests that careful consideration should be given to extrapolating data from one species to another. Furthermore, the use of bovine trypsin in the analysis of TIA of feedstuffs used in swine may not be the most appropriate choice considering these differences (Huisman, 1989; 1990; Liener, 1994). The reduction in ileal digestibility of amino acids in pigs fed trypsin inhibitors seems to be due to a reduction in the true ileal digestibility (the digestibility of the dietary components) and an increase in the endogenous protein losses (Schultze et al., 1993b; Grala et al., 1998a). The effect of trypsin inhibitor on endogenous losses was more pronounced at low TIA levels, whereas the true ileal N digestibility was reduced at higher (>2.5 mg/g) levels of trypsin inhibitor (Schultze et al., 1993b). Grala et al. (1998b) reported that increased endogenous N losses associated with trypsin inhibitors resulted in increased urinary N excretion, tended to reduce N retention, and lowered the efficiency of N utilization for retention. Summarizing some recent studies, Huisman et al. (1998) suggested that as a rule of thumb the amount of apparent undigested protein at the end of the ileum of pigs was increased by 9 g for every unit increase in TIA.

C. Lectins

Lectins are glycoproteins that have the ability to bind to carbohydrate-containing molecules (Grant and van Driessche, 1993; Liener, 1994). They are also often referred to as hemagglutinins, based on their ability to agglutinate red blood cells. However, not all lectins possess the ability to agglutinate red blood cells, but they can bind to the intestinal wall and cause damage (Grant and van Driessche, 1993). Lectins are present at high levels in *Phaseolus* beans and soybeans and to a lesser extent in peas and field beans (Gatel, 1994). The level of lectins present in feedstuffs has traditionally been expressed as hemagglutinin activity units, defined as the smallest amount of sample needed to agglutinate red blood cells. Huisman (1989) demonstrated that identical samples gave different hemagglutinin activity units depending on the animal source of the red blood cells. Additionally, the fact that not all lectins agglutinate red blood cells and the existence of substantial differences in pathogenicity of lectins indicate that this method of analysis does not seem to be sufficiently specific and sensitive (Huisman, 1989; Guenguen et al., 1993). New methods of analysis (functional lectin immunoassay or FLIA) have been developed that specifically measure the ability of lectins to bind to carbohydrate structures or brush border membranes in microtiter plates (Huisman and Jansman, 1991). These methods should more accurately reflect lectin levels in feedstuffs that affect animals and could be adapted to measure lectin activity specifically in the target species under study. Further discussion on the analysis of lectins has been provided by Huisman and Jansman (1991), Guenguen et al. (1993), Liener (1994), and Trugo and von Baer (1998).

Most of the research with lectins has been conducted using *P. vulgaris* beans, primarily using laboratory animals (Huisman, 1990; van der Poel, 1990). In these studies, levels of lectins evaluated are typically higher than levels commonly encountered in practical swine diets (Huisman, 1990). In general, lectins are resistant to proteolytic degradation in the digestive tract, which is a first requirement to elicit toxic effects *in vivo* (Grant and van Driessche, 1993). The second requirement is their ability to bind to the glycoproteins expressed on the epithelial cells of the intestinal mucosa. The glycosylation pattern of the gut epithelial cells differs with species and age, which may affect the susceptibility to lectins of different species at different ages (Huisman, 1990; Grant and van Driessche, 1993). The extent to which binding occurs determines the toxicity of the lectins (Pusztai, 1991; Grant and van Driessche, 1993). Lectins from *P. vulgaris*, for example, are highly toxic to pigs because of their ability to enter the systemic circulation after attachment to the gut epithelium. This specific uptake of dietary lectins into the circulation results in antibody formation against the lectin; increased catabolism of adipose lipid, liver glycogen, and skeletal muscle protein; and a reduced pancreatic insulin synthesis and secretion (Pusztai, 1991; Grant and van Driessche, 1993). In addition, lectins stimulate growth of the small intestine and the pancreas, either through direct interaction with endocrine cells in the intestine (possibly cholecystokinin is involved in pancreatic enlargement) or through the systemic circulation (Putztai, 1991). Further, metabolism in the small intestine is impaired by lectins, which is also often observed when lectins of lesser toxicity, such as soybean lectins, are included in the diet. Binding of lectins to the epithelial cells of the intestinal mucosa results in damage to the microvilli, increased cell turnover and shedding, increased mucus production, reduced enzyme production, and a reduction in digestive and absorptive capacity (Pusztai, 1991; Grant and van Driessche, 1993). Schultze et al. (1995) demonstrated that total N at the terminal ileum was increased by 8 and 36% with the inclusion of 160 and 960 mg added purified soybean lectins/kg of diet, respectively, compared with control pigs. A considerable portion of these increased N losses were of endogenous origin. The endogenous N flow was increased by 31 and 47% compared with control pigs for the 160 and 960 mg/kg added lectin diets, respectively. The levels of lectins added to the test diets were targeted to represent lectin levels in a normally toasted soybean meal diet and a diet containing approximately 10% raw soybeans, respectively (Schultze et al., 1995). Huisman et al. (1998) estimated that undigested endogenous protein at the end of the ileum is increased on average by 13 g for each gram of functional (measured by the FLIA method) lectins per kilogram. Lectins from peas and faba beans seem to be relatively nontoxic, presumably because of their low binding capacity to gut epithelial cells (Grant and van Driessche, 1993).

D. Tannins

Tannins are polyphenolic compounds of various molecular weights and complexities that can bind to proteins and carbohydrates. These compounds are water soluble, have a molecular weight of between 500 and 3000, and can be roughly divided into hydrolyzable tannins (for example, tannic acid) and condensed tannins (for example, catechin). They occur mostly as condensed tannins in grains and legume seeds. The chemistry of tannins was described by Jansman (1993). Tannins can be found at high concentrations in sorghum grains, with levels ranging from 27 to 102 mg/g catechin equivalents. In faba beans, mean tannin concentrations range from 0.6 to 21.5 mg/g in whole beans, with the largest concentration found mainly in the testa of colored flowering varieties (Jansman, 1993). Tannins are also present at lower levels in barley, millet, peas, *Phaseolus* beans, chickpeas, cowpeas, and lentils (Jansman and Longstaff, 1993). Several different assays are available to analyze the tannin content of feedstuffs. Although not very specific, colorimetric assays based on the vanillin and acid butanol procedures are most widely used. Analytical methods for tannin determination have been reviewed (Butler and Bos, 1993; Jansman, 1993; Trugo and von Baer, 1998).

The effect of tannins on animal performance is variable and is dependent on a variety of factors including animal species and age, stage of production, source of tannin (e.g., feedstuff type, tannin-containing plant fraction, or purified tannins), level of tannin inclusion, length of the experimental period, and diet composition (Jansman, 1993). However, in general, feeding of tannins results in a reduction of the apparent digestibility of N, amino acids, and, to a lesser extent, energy, resulting in reduced weight gain and feed efficiency (Jansman, 1993). Feed intake may be reduced because of the bitter or astringent taste of tannins, especially at high levels. In pigs, however, feeding of 20% faba beans high in tannin content (10 mg/g catechin equivalents) did not adversely affect feed intake (Jansman et al., 1993).

Tannins have the ability to form complexes with proteins. Rats and mice responded to high dietary tannin levels with hypertrophy of the parotid gland and an increase in the secretion of proline-rich proteins. These proteins bind with tannins to form inactive tannin complexes and may be a adaptive defensive response against their toxic effects (Jansman and Longstaff, 1993). This adaptive response has not been observed in pigs (Jansman et al., 1993). The affinity of tannins for proteins can result in binding of tannins to dietary proteins and endogenous proteins, and can interfere with intestinal enzyme activity (Jansman and Longstaff, 1993). Jansman et al. (1995) reported that apparent ileal digestibility of N was reduced from 82.7 to 74.1% and true ileal digestibility of N from 94.4 to 90.5% when high-tannin-containing hulls of faba beans were included in the diet compared with low-tannin hulls (tannin content was 6.9 mg/g and <1 mg/g catechin equivalents, respectively). The reduction in the apparent digestibility of protein was due to an increased secretion of endogenous protein, which accounted for approximately 45% of this reduction. Approximately 55% of the reduction in digestibility was accounted for by an increased amount of extra protein from undigested dietary protein. Based on research in the Netherlands with faba beans, Huisman et al. (1998) estimated that on average an additional 1.5 g of protein was excreted at the end of the ileum for every gram of catechin equivalent. Binding of tannins to key carbohydrate-degrading enzymes may interfere with carbohydrate digestion and absorption, and this needs further study (Lallès and Jansman, 1998).

Systemic toxic effects on the liver and kidneys have been reported for hydrolyzable tannins, but not for condensed tannins (Jansman, 1993). Condensed tannins seem to be resistant to degradation and are believed to be too large to be absorbed intact (Lallès and Jansman, 1998). However, potential effects of tannins on the endocrine system through an interaction with gut proteins cannot be ruled out (Jansman and Longstaff, 1993).

E. OTHER FACTORS

Antigenic proteins such as certain legume proteins have been shown to cause hypersensitivity reactions in the gut of piglets. Negative effects of antigenic factors include changes in gut structure including shortening of intestinal villi and crypt hyperplasia, a reduction in absorptive capacity, decreased intestinal enzyme activity, and ultimately depressed growth. Makkink and Heinz (1991) reported that the true ileal N digestibility of a soybean meal diet did not differ from that of a skim milk diet. However, endogenous N excretion at the end of the ileum in pigs fed soybean meal was nearly double compared with pigs fed skim milk, resulting in a lowered apparent ileal digestibility. These effects may be related to antigenic factors in soybean meal, although this was not confirmed. The responses to antigenic proteins seem to be transient as evidenced by a normalization of gut morphology within 7 to 14 days and a lack of differences in pig weights after 3 to 5 weeks (Lallès et al., 1993). Tolerance to dietary protein acting as allergens appears to be established at 12 weeks of age, which implies that particular attention should be given to the source and antigenicity of dietary protein products in young pigs (Miller et al., 1994). The type of allergens involved and the exact contribution of allergens to the postweaning diarrhea syndrome have not been established (Lallès and Jansman, 1998). Circulating antibodies (IgG and IgM) and intestinal IgG and secretory IgA to soy antigens have been reported in pigs. The involvement of T-cell-mediated immunity in the response of pigs to antigenic proteins is less clear based on both positive and negative reports (Lallès et al., 1993). The specific allergens involved in the hypersensitivity process need to be identified and studied with respect to their effect on intestinal damage and the mechanism by which this damage occurs (Lallès and Jansman, 1998).

Glucosinolates are found primarily in rapeseed, but their levels have been reduced significantly in recent years from approximately 150 mmol/kg to about 10 mmol/kg by plant breeding. Canola is defined as rapeseed with <30 mmol/kg of glucosinolates and <2% of the total fatty acids as erucic acid (Bell, 1993). Hydrolysis products of glucosinolates are most toxic and can interfere with iodine uptake by the thyroid, thyroid hormone production, and growth (Pusztai, 1989). Campbell and Schöne (1998) concluded in their review that a concentration of 2 mmol/kg of glucosinolates could be considered the no-effect level in pigs. This was similar to the suggestion by Etienne and Dourmad (1994) that glucosinolate levels of <2 mmol/kg diet did not affect sow reproductive performance.

Alkaloids represent a group of chemical compounds that contain a heterocyclic ring containing N and possess alkaline properties. More than 200 different alkaloids have been discovered in lupins. Wareham et al. (1994) concluded, based on their review, that 0.20 g/kg seemed to be the threshold level in growing pigs. Hill and Pastuszewska (1993) suggested that the response of pigs to alkaloids may depend in part on their age and indicated that levels > 0.30 g/kg could be considered detrimental. High levels of lupin alkaloids can cause feed rejection due to their bitterness, vomiting, respiratory paralysis, and mortality in pigs (Keeler, 1989).

F. Reducing Antinutritional Factors

Industrial processing techniques can be used to lower the antinutritional factors in feedstuffs and improve their nutritional quality. Heat treatment can denature proteins and subsequently reduce the activity of protease inhibitors and lectins. Additionally, heat treatment can increase the accessibility of proteins to enzymatic degradation (van der Poel, 1990). A number of factors influence the effectiveness of heat treatment on nutritional value, such as processing temperature, heating time, particle size, moisture content of the feedstuff, and the addition of moisture during processing. In a review, van der Poel (1990) summarized the effect of different heat processing methods (autoclaving, steam heating, extrusion, and dry roasting) on the reduction in trypsin inhibitor activity and hemagglutinating activity in Phaseolus vulgaris beans. Depending on process conditions and bean type, reductions in trypsin inhibitor activity ranged from 29 to 100% and reductions in hemagglutinating activity ranged from 74 to 100%. Pelleting of complete diets seemed to have little effect on antinutritional factors as compared to extrusion because of relatively low processing temperature used (Wareham et al., 1994). However, effects of pelleting on antinutritional factors needs to be better quantified, especially with new emerging developments and technologies in pelleting (Melcion and van der Poel, 1993). Liener (1994) concluded that heat treatment for most soybean products for human consumption was sufficient to reduce trypsin inhibitor activity by at least 80%. Excessive heat processing may adversely affect the availability of amino acids, particularly lysine, arginine, methionine, and cystine (van der Poel, 1990). In addition, the effect of residual antinutritional factors not destroyed by heat on pig performance needs to be considered. Thus, according to Melcion and van der Poel (1993), the preferred method to assess the effectiveness of heat processing or other processing methods involves measuring the response of the animal to diets containing the final product. Pelleting and other feed-processing methods are discussed in Chapter 21.

Tannins are heat-stable compounds that can be found in the hull fraction of certain legume species. Mechanical separation of hulls from the kernel fraction seems to be a successful method of reducing the tannin content and increasing the protein value of the final product. Dehulling and air classification (particle separation after grinding based on size, shape, and density) are commonly used industrial processes. Dehulling reduced the tannin content of *Phaseolus* beans by 68 to 95% and improved protein digestibility by 2.3 to 4.3% (van der Poel, 1990). However, trypsin inhibitor activity increased by 2 to 36% by dehulling, whereas lectins and enzyme inhibitors in the protein fraction following air classification was increased by 171 to 225% (van der Poel, 1990). Further processing of this protein fraction is required to reduce the antinutritional factors remaining and requires further study.

Other technologies to reduce antinutritional factors in feed ingredients include the use of enzymes and plant breeding. Enzymes provide an opportunity to improve the nutritional quality of feeds as evidenced by recent developments with phytase. The exact impact of enzyme supplementation on antinutritional factors and subsequently animal performance remains to be elucidated (Classen et al., 1993; Bedford and Schulze, 1998; Campbell and van der Poel, 1998). Recent developments in plant breeding to reduce antinutritional factors have been reviewed by Helsper (1998).

REFERENCES

Abramson, D. 1997. Toxicants of the genus *Penicillium*. In *Handbook of Plant and Fungal Toxicants*, D'Mello, J. P. F., Ed., CRC Press, Boca Raton, FL, chap. 21.

Becker, B. A., L. Pace, G. E. Rottinghaus, R. Shelby, M. Misfeldt, and P. F. Ross. 1995. Effects of feeding fumonisin B_1 in lactating sows and their suckling pigs, *Am. J. Vet. Res.*, 56:1253.

Bedford, M. R., and H. Schulze. 1998. Exogenous enzymes for pigs and poultry, *Nutr. Res. Rev.*, 11:91.

Bell, J. M. 1993. Factors affecting the nutritional value of canola meal: a review, *Can. J. Anim. Sci.*, 73:679.

Bergsjo, B., T. Matre, and I. Nafstad. 1992. Effects of diets with graded levels of deoxynivalenol on performance in growing pigs, *J. Vet. Med. Ser. A*, 39:752.

Bhatnagar, D., E. B. Lillehoj, and J. W. Bennett. 1991. Biological detoxification of mycotoxins. In *Mycotoxins and Animal Foods*, Smith, J. E., and R. S. Henderson, Eds., CRC Press, Boca Raton, FL, chap. 36.

Bilgrami, K. S., and A. K. Choudhary. 1998. Mycotoxins in preharvest contamination of agricultural crops. In *Mycotoxins in Agriculture and Food Safety*, Sinha, K. K., and D. Bhatnagar, Eds., Marcel Dekker, New York, chap. 1.

Butler, L. G., and K. D. Bos. 1993. Analysis and characterization of tannins in faba beans, cereals, and other seeds. A literature review. In *Recent Advances of Research in Antinutritional Factors in Legume Seeds*, van der Poel, A. F. B., J. Huisman, and H. S. Saini, Eds., Wageningen Pers, The Netherlands, 81.

Campbell, G. L., and A. F. B. van der Poel. 1998. Use of enzymes and process technology to inactivate antinutritional factors in legume seeds and rapeseed. In *Recent Advances of Research in Antinutritional Factors in Legume Seeds and Rapeseed*, Jansman, A. J. M., G. D. Hill, J. Huisman, and A. F. B. van der Poel, Eds., Wageningen Pers, The Netherlands, 377.

Campbell, L. D., and F. Schöne. 1998. Effects of antinutritional factors in rapeseed. In *Recent Advances of Research in Antinutritional Factors in Legume Seeds and Rapeseed*, Jansman, A. J. M., G. D. Hill, J. Huisman, and A. F. B. van der Poel, Eds., Wageningen Pers, The Netherlands, 185.

CAST (Council for Agricultural Science and Technology). 1989. Mycotoxins: Economic and Health Risks, Task Force Report 116, Ames, IA.

Casteel, S. W., J. R. Turk, R. P. Cowart, and G. E. Rottinghaus. 1993. Chronic toxicity of fumonisin in weanling pigs, *J. Vet. Diagn. Invest.*, 5:413.

Chelkowski, J. 1998. Distribution of Fusarium species and their mycotoxins in cereal grains. In *Mycotoxins in Agriculture and Food Safety*, Sinha, K. K., and D. Bhatnagar, Eds., Marcel Dekker, New York, chap. 2.

Chu, F. S. 1992. Recent progress on analytical techniques for mycotoxins in feedstuffs, *J. Anim. Sci.*, 70:3950.

Classen, H. L., D. Balnave, and M. R. Bedford. 1993. Reduction of legume antinutritional factors using biotechnological techniques. In *Recent Advances of Research in Antinutritional Factors in Legume Seeds*, van der Poel, A. F. B., J. Huisman, and H. S. Saini, Eds., Wageningen Pers, The Netherlands, 501.

Coffey, M. T., W. M. Hagler, Jr., and J. M. Cullen. 1989. Influence of dietary protein, fat or amino acids on the response of weanling swine to aflatoxin B_1, *J. Anim. Sci.*, 67:465.

Coffey, M. T., W. M. Hagler, Jr., E. E. Jones, and J. M. Cullen. 1990. Interactive effects of multiple mycotoxin contamination of swine diets, *Biodeterioration Res.*, 3:117.

Colvin, B. M., A. J. Cooley, and R. W. Beaver. 1993. Fumonisin toxicosis in swine: clinical and pathologic findings, *J. Vet. Diagn. Invest.*, 5:232.

Coulombe, R. A., Jr. 1993. Symposium: biological action of mycotoxins, *J. Dairy Sci.*, 76:880.

Diekman, M. A., and M. L. Green. 1992. Mycotoxins and reproduction in domestic livestock, *J. Anim. Sci.*, 70:1615.

Etienne, M., and J. Y. Dourmad. 1994. Effects of zearalenone or glucosinolates in the diet on reproduction in sows: a review, *Livest. Prod. Sci.*, 40:99.

Francis, B. M. 1989. Reproductive toxicology of trichothecenes. In *Trichothecene Mycotoxicosis: Pathophysiologic Effects*, Vol. II, Beasley, V. R., Ed., CRC Press, Boca Raton, FL, 143.

Friend, D. W., H. L. Trenholm, B. K. Thompson, K. E. Hartin, P. S. Fiser, E. K. Asem, and B. K. Tsang. 1990. The reproductive efficiency of gilts fed very low levels of zearalenone, *Can. J. Anim. Sci.*, 70:635.

Friend, D. W., B. K. Thompson, H. L. Trenholm, H. J. Boermans, K. E. Hartin, and P.L. Panich. 1992. Toxicity of T-2 toxin and its interaction with deoxynivalenol when fed to young pigs, *Can. J. Anim. Sci.*, 72:703.

Gatel, F. 1994. Protein quality of legume seeds for non-ruminant animals: a literature review, *Anim. Feed Sci. Technol.*, 45:317.

Grala, W., M. W. A. Verstegen, A. J. M. Jansman, J. Huisman, and P. van Leeuwen. 1998a. Ileal apparent protein and amino acid digestibilities and endogenous nitrogen losses in pigs fed soybean and rapeseed products, *J. Anim. Sci.*, 76:557.

Grala, W., M. W. A. Verstegen, A. J. M. Jansman, J. Huisman, and J. Wasilewko. 1998b. Nitrogen utilization in pigs fed diets with soybean and rapeseed products leading to different ileal endogenous nitrogen losses, *J. Anim. Sci.*, 76:569.

Grant, G., and E. van Driessche. 1993. Legume lectins: Physicochemical and nutritional properties. In *Recent Advances of Research in Antinutritional Factors in Legume Seeds*, van der Poel, A. F. B., J. Huisman, and H. S. Saini, Eds., Wageningen Pers, The Netherlands, 219.

Guenguen, J., M. G. van Oort, L. Quillien, and M. van Hessing. 1993. The composition, biochemical characteristics and analysis of proteinaceous antinutritional factors in legume seeds. A review. In *Recent Advances of Research in Antinutritional Factors in Legume Seeds*, van der Poel, A. F. B., J. Huisman, and H. S. Saini, Eds., Wageningen Pers, The Netherlands, 9.

Harrison, L. R., B. M. Colvin, J. T. Greene, L. E. Newman, and J. R. Cole. 1990. Pulmonary edema and hydrothorax in swine produced by fumonisin B_1, a toxic metabolite of Fusarium moniliforme, *J. Vet. Diagn. Invest.*, 2:217.

Harvey, R. B., T. S. Edrington, L. R. Kubena, M. H. Elissalde, H. H. Casper, G. E. Rottinghaus, and J. R. Tuck. 1996. Effects of dietary fumonisin B_1-containing culture material, deoxynivalenol-contaminated wheat, or their combination on growing barrows, *Am. J. Vet. Res.*, 57:1790.

Harvey, R. B., T. S. Edrington, L. F. Kubena, M. H. Elissalde, and G. E. Rottinghaus. 1995. Influence of aflatoxin and fumonisin B_1-containing culture material on growing barrows, *Am. J. Vet. Res.*, 56:1668.

Harvey, R. B., M. H. Elissalde, L. F. Kubena, E. A. Weaver, D. E. Corrier, and B. A. Clement. 1992. Immunotoxicity of ochratoxin A to growing gilts, *Am. J. Vet. Res.*, 53:1966.

Harvey, R. B., W. E. Huff, L. F. Kubena, and T. D. Phillips. 1989a. Evaluation of diets cocontaminated with aflatoxin and ochratoxin fed to growing pigs, *Am. J. Vet. Res.*, 50:1400.

Harvey, R. B., L. F. Kubena, M. H. Elissalde, D. E. Corrier, W. E. Huff, G. E. Rottinghaus, and B.A. Clement. 1991. Cocontamination of swine diets by aflatoxin and diacetoxyscirpenol, *J. Vet. Diagn. Invest.*, 3:155.

Harvey, R. B., L. F. Kubena, M. H. Elissalde, D. E. Corrier, and T. D. Phillips. 1994a. Comparison of two hydrated sodium calcium aluminosilicate compounds to experimentally protect growing barrows from aflatoxicosis, *J. Vet. Diagn. Invest.*, 6:88.

Harvey, R. B., L. F. Kubena, M. H. Elissalde, G. E. Rottinghaus, and D. E. Corrier. 1994b. Administration of ochratoxin A and T-2 toxin to growing swine, *Am. J. Vet. Res.*, 55:1757.

Harvey, R. B., L. F. Kubena, W. E. Huff, D. E. Corrier, D. E. Clark, and T. D. Phillips. 1989b. Effects of aflatoxin, deoxynivalenol, and their combinations in the diets of growing pigs, *Am. J. Vet. Res.*, 50:602.

Harvey, R. B., L. F. Kubena, W. E. Huff, D. E. Corrier, G. E. Rottinghaus, and T. D. Phillips. 1990. Effects of treatment of growing swine with aflatoxin and T-2 toxin, *Am. J. Vet. Res.*, 51:1688.

Haschek, W. M., G. Motelin, D. K. Ness, K. S. Harlin, W. F. Hall, R. F. Vesonder, R. E. Peterson, and V. R. Beasley. 1992. Characterization of fumonisin toxicity in orally and intravenously dosed swine, *Mycopathologia*, 117:83.

Helsper, J. P. F. G. 1998. Recent developments on the improvement of ANF levels in legume seeds by breeding. In *Recent Advances of Research in Antinutritional Factors in Legume Seeds and Rapeseed*, Jansman, A. J. M., G. D. Hill, J. Huisman, and A. F. B. van der Poel, Eds., Wageningen Pers, The Netherlands, 351.

Herkelman, K. L., G. L. Cromwell, T. S. Stahly, T. W. Pfeiffer, and D. A. Knabe. 1992. Apparent digestibility of amino acids in raw and heated conventional and low-trypsin-inhibitor soybeans for pigs, *J. Anim. Sci.*, 70:818.

Hill, G. D., and B. Pastuszewska. 1993. Lupin alkaloids and their role in animal nutrition. In *Recent Advances of Research in Antinutritional Factors in Legume Seeds*, van der Poel, A. F. B., J. Huisman, and H. S. Saini, Eds., Wageningen Pers, The Netherlands, 343.

Huff, W. E., L. F. Kubena, R. B. Harvey, and J. A. Doerr. 1988. Mycotoxin interactions in poultry and swine, *J. Anim. Sci.*, 66:2351.

Huisman, J. 1989. Antinutritional factors (ANFs) in the nutrition of monogastric farm animals. In *Nutrition and Digestive Physiology in Monogastric Farm Animals*, van Weerden, E. J., and J. Huisman, Eds., Pudoc, Wageningen, The Netherlands, 17.

Huisman, J. 1990. Antinutritional Effects of Legume Seeds in Piglets, Rats and Chickens, Ph.D. dissertation, Agricultural University, Wageningen, The Netherlands.

Huisman, J., and A. J. M. Jansman. 1991. Dietary effects and some analytical aspects of antinutritional factors in peas (*Pisum sativum*), common beans (*Phaseolus vulgaris*) and soyabeans (*Glycine max* L.) in monogastric farm animals. A literature review, *Nutr. Abstr. Rev. Ser. B*, 61:901.

Huisman, J., A. J. M. Jansman, A. F. B. van der Poel, and M. C. Blok. 1998. Antinutritionele factoren en de darmverteerbaarheid van eiwit en aminozuren bij varkens. CVB documentatierapport 21, Lelystad, The Netherlands.

Jansman, A. J. M. 1993. Tannins in feedstuffs for simple-stomached animals, *Nutr. Res. Rev.*, 6:209.

Jansman, A. J. M., and M. Longstaff. 1993. Nutritional effects of tannins and vicine/convicine in legume seeds. In *Recent Advances of Research in Antinutritional Factors in Legume Seeds*, van der Poel, A. F. B., J. Huisman, and H. S. Saini, Eds., Wageningen Pers, The Netherlands, 301.

Jansman, A. J. M., M. W. A. Verstegen, and J. Huisman. 1993. Effects of dietary inclusion of hulls of faba beans (*Vicia faba* L.) with a low and high content of condensed tannins on digestion and some physiological parameters in piglets, *Anim. Feed Sci. Technol.*, 43:239.

Jansman, A. J. M., M. W. A. Verstegen, J. Huisman, and J. W. O. van den Berg. 1995. Effects of hulls of faba beans (*Vicia faba* L.) with a low or high content of condensed tannins on the apparent ileal and fecal digestibility of nutrients and the excretion of endogenous protein in ileal digesta and feces of pigs, *J. Anim. Sci.*, 73:118.

Jansman, A. J. M., J. Huisman, G. M. Beelen, and J. Wiebenga. 1998. Effects of soya trypsin inhibitors on faecal nutrient digestibility and nitrogen retention in young piglets. In *Recent Advances of Research in Antinutritional Factors in Legume Seeds and Rapeseed*, Jansman, A. J. M., G. D. Hill, J. Huisman, and A. F. B. van der Poel, Eds., Wageningen Pers, The Netherlands, 331.

Jondreville, C., F. Grosjean, G. Buron, C. Peyronnet, and J. L. Beneytout. 1992. Comparison of four pea varieties in pig feeding through digestibility and growth performance results, *J. Anim. Phys. Anim. Nutr.*, 68:113.

Keeler, R. F. 1989. Quinolizidine alkaloids in range and grain lupins. In *Toxicants of Plant Origin*, Vol. I, Cheeke, P. R., Ed., CRC Press, Boca Raton, FL.

Krogh, P. 1991. Porcine nephropathy associated with Ochratoxin A. In *Mycotoxins and Animal Foods*, Smith, J. E., and R. S. Henderson, Eds., CRC Press, Boca Raton, FL, chap. 26.

Krogh, P., N. H. Axelsen, F. Elling, N. Gyrd-Hansen, B. Hald, J. Hyldgaard-Jensen, A. E. Larsen, A. Madsen, H. P. Mortensen, T. Moller, O. K. Petersen, V. Ravnsko, M. Rostgaard, and O. Aalund. 1974. Experimental porcine nephropathy. Changes of renal function and structure induced by ochratoxin A contaminated feed, *Acta Pathol. Microbiol. Scand. Sect. A Suppl.*, 246:1.

Lallès, J. P., and A. J. M. Jansman. 1998. Recent progress in the understanding of the mode of action and effects of antinutritional factors from legume seeds in non-ruminant farm animals. In *Recent Advances of Research in Antinutritional Factors in Legume Seeds and Rapeseed*, Jansman, A. J. M., G. D. Hill, J. Huisman, and A. F. B. van der Poel, Eds., Wageningen Pers, The Netherlands, 219.

Lallès, J. P., H. Salmon, N. P. M. Bakker, and G. H. Tolman. 1993. Effects of dietary antigens on health, performance and immune system of calves and piglets. In *Recent Advances of Research in Antinutritional Factors in Legume Seeds*, van der Poel, A. F. B., J. Huisman, and H. S. Saini, Eds., Wageningen Pers, The Netherlands, 253.

Le Guen, M. P., and Y. Birk. 1993. Protein protease inhibitors from legume seeds: nutritional effects, mode of action and structure-function relationship. In *Recent Advances of Research in Antinutritional Factors in Legume Seeds*, van der Poel, A. F. B., J. Huisman, and H. S. Saini, Eds., Wageningen Pers, The Netherlands, 157.

Liener, I. E. 1994. Implications of antinutritional components in soybean foods, *Crit. Rev. Food Sci. Nutr.*, 34:31.

Lindemann, M. D., D. J. Blodgett, E. T. Kornegay, and G. G. Schurig. 1993. Potential ameliorators of aflatoxicosis in weanling/growing swine, *J. Anim. Sci.*, 71:171.

Lopez-Garcia, R., and D. L. Park. 1998. Effectiveness of postharvest procedures in management of mycotoxin hazards. In *Mycotoxins in Agriculture and Food Safety*, Sinha, K. K., and D. Bhatnagar, Eds., Marcel Dekker, New York, chap. 13.

Madsen, A., H. P. Mortensen, and B. Hald. 1982. Feeding experiments with ochratoxin A contaminated barley for bacon pigs. 1. Influence on pig performance and residues, *Acta Agric. Scand.*, 32:225.

Makkink, C. A., and T. Heinz. 1991. Endogenous N losses at the terminal ileum of young piglets fed diets based on either skimmilk powder or soybean meal. In *Digestive Physiology in Pigs*, Verstegen, M. W. A., J. Huisman, and L. A. den Hartog, Eds., Pudoc, Wageningen, The Netherlands, 196.

Marquardt, R. R., and A. A. Frohlich. 1992. A review of recent advances in understanding ochratoxicosis, *J. Anim. Sci.*, 70:3968.

Melcion, J.-P., and A. F. B. van der Poel. 1993. Process technology and antinutritional factors: principles, adequacy and process optimization. In *Recent Advances of Research in Antinutritional Factors in Legume Seeds*, van der Poel, A. F. B., J. Huisman, and H. S. Saini, Eds., Wageningen Pers, The Netherlands, 419.

Merrill, A. H., Jr., E.-M. Schmelz, E. Wang, D. L. Dillehay, L. G. Rice, F. Meredith, and R. T. Riley. 1997. Importance of sphingolipids and inhibitors of sphingolipid metabolism as components of animal diets, *J. Nutr.*, 127:830S.

Miller, B. G., C. T. Whittemore, C. R. Stokes, and E. Telemo. 1994. The effect of delaying weaning on the development of oral tolerance to soya-bean protein in pigs, *Br. J. Nutr.*, 71:615.

Miller, D. M., B. P. Stuart, W. A. Crowell, J. R. Cole, Jr., A. J. Goven, and J. Brown. 1978. Aflatoxicosis in swine: its effect on immunity and relationship to salmonellosis, *Am. Assoc. Vet. Lab. Diagn.*, 21:135.

Miller, D. M., B. P. Stuart, and W. A. Crowell. 1981. Experimental aflatoxicosis in swine: morphological and clinical pathological results, *Can. J. Comp. Med.*, 45:343.

Mocchegiani, E., A. Corradi, L. Santarelli, A. Tibaldi, E. DeAngelis, P. Borghetti, A. Bonomi, N. Fabris, and E. Cabassi. 1998. Zinc, thymic endocrine activity and mitogen responsiveness (PHA) in piglets exposed to maternal aflatoxicosis B_1 and G_1, *Vet. Immunol. Immunopathol.*, 62:245.

Motelin, G. K., W. M. Haschek, D. K. Ness, W. F. Hall, K. S. Harlin, D. J. Schaeffer, and V. R. Beasley. 1994. Temporal and dose-response features in swine fed corn screenings contaminated with fumonisin mycotoxins, *Mycopathologia*, 126:27.

Nelson, C. E. 1993. Strategies of mold control in dairy feeds, *J. Dairy Sci.*, 76:898

Osweiler, G. D., K. J. Schwartz, and J. A. Roth. 1993. Effect of fumonisis-contaminated corn on growth and immune function in swine, *J. Anim. Sci.*, 71(Suppl. 1):63 (Abstr.).

Overnes, G., T. Matre, T. Sivertsen, J. S. Larsen, W. Langseth, L. J. Reitan, and J. H. Jansen. 1997. Effects of diets with graded levels of naturally deoxynivalenol-contaminated oats on immune response in growing pigs, *J. Vet. Med. Ser. A*, 44:539.

Panangala, V. S., J. J. Giambrone, U. L. Diener, N. D. Davis, F. J. Hoerr, A. Mitra, R. D. Schultz, and G. R. Wilt. 1986. Effects of aflatoxin on the growth performance and immune responses of weanling swine, *Am. J. Vet. Res.*, 47:2062.

Pemberton, A. D., and T. J. Simpson. 1991. The chemical degradation of mycotoxins. In *Mycotoxins and Animal Foods*, Smith, J. E., and R. S. Henderson, Eds., CRC Press, Boca Raton, FL, chap. 35.

Pier, A. C. 1987. Aflatoxicosis and immunosuppression in mammalian animals. In *Proc. of the Workshop Aflatoxin in Maize*, Zuber, M. S., E. B. Lillehoj, and B. L. Renfro, Eds., CIMMYT, El Batan, Mexico, 58.

Pier, A. C. 1991. The influence of mycotoxins on the immune system. In *Mycotoxins and Animal Foods*, Smith, J. E., and R. S. Henderson, Eds., CRC Press, Boca Raton, FL, chap. 22.

Pusztai, A. 1989. Antinutrients in rapeseeds, *Nutr. Abstr. Rev., Ser. B*, 59:427.

Pusztai, A. 1991. *Plant Lectins*, Cambridge University Press, Cambridge, U.K.

Rackis, J. J., W. J. Wolf, and E. C. Baker. 1986. Protease inhibitors in plant foods: content and inactivation. In *Nutritional and Toxicological Significance of Enzyme Inhibitors in Foods*, Friedman, M., Ed., Plenum Press, New York, 299.

Rafai, P., A. Bata, A. Vanyi, Z. Papp, E. Brydl, L. Jakab, S. Tuboly, and E. Tury. 1995. Effect of various levels of T-2 toxin on the clinical status, performance and metabolism of growing pigs, *Vet. Rec.*, 136:485.

Rainey, M. R., R. C. Tubbs, L. W. Bennett, and N. M. Cox. 1990. Prepubertal exposure to dietary zearalenone alters hypothalamo-hypophysial function but does not impair postpubertal reproductive function of gilts, *J. Anim. Sci.*, 68:2015.

Ramos, A. J., and E. Hernandez. 1997. Prevention of aflatoxicosis in farm animals by means of hydrated sodium calcium aluminosilicate addition to feedstuffs: a review, *Anim. Feed Sci. Technol.*, 65:197.

Richard, J. L. 1991. Mycotoxins as immunomodulators in animal systems. In *Mycotoxins, Cancer, and Health*, Vol. 1, Bray, G. A., and D. H. Ryan, Eds., Louisiana State University Press, Baton Rouge, 197.

Riley, R. T. 1998. Mechanistic interactions of mycotoxins: theoretical considerations. In *Mycotoxins in Agriculture and Food Safety*, Sinha, K. K., and D. Bhatnagar, Eds., Marcel Dekker, New York, chap. 7.

Riley, R. T., N. Y. An, J. L. Showker, H. S. Yoo, W. P. Norred, W. J. Chamberlain, E. Wang, A. H. Merrill, Jr., G. Motelin, V. R. Beasley, and W. M. Haschek. 1993. Alteration of tissue and serum sphiganine to sphingosine ratio: an early biomarker in pigs of exposure to fumonisin-containing feeds, *Toxicol. Appl. Pharmacol.*, 118:105.

Ross, P. F., L. G. Rice, G. D. Osweiler, P. E. Nelson, J. L. Richard, and T. M. Wilson. 1992. A review and update of animal toxicoses associated with fumonisin-contaminated feeds and production of fumonisins by Fusarium isolates, *Mycopathologia*, 117:109.

Rotter, R. G., B. K. Thompson, H. L. Trenholm, D. B. Prelusky, K. E. Hartin, and J. D. Miller. 1992. A preliminary examination of potential interactions between deoxynivalenol (DON) and other selected Fusarium metabolites in growing pigs, *Can. J. Anim. Sci.*, 72:107.

Rotter, B. A., B. K. Thompson, M. Lessard, H. L. Trenholm, and H. Tryphonas. 1994. Influence of low-level exposure to Fusarium mycotoxins on selected immunological and hematological parameters in young swine, *Fundam. Appl. Toxicol.*, 23:117.

Rotter, B. A., B. K. Thompson, and M. Lessard. 1995. Effects of deoxynivalenon-contaminated diet on performance and blood parameters in growing swine, *Can. J. Anim. Sci.*, 75:297.

Rotter, B. A., D. B. Prelusky, and J. J. Pestka. 1996. Toxicology of deoxynivalenol (vomitoxin), *J. Toxicol. Env. Health*, 48:1.

Rotter, B. A., D. B. Prelusky, A. Fortin, J. D. Miller, and M. E. Savard. 1997. Impact of pure fumonisin B_1 on various metabolic parameters and carcass quality of growing-finishing swine — preliminary findings, *Can. J. Anim. Sci.*, 77:465.

Samarajeewa, U. 1991. *In situ* degradation of mycotoxins by physical methods. In *Mycotoxins and Animal Foods*, Smith, J. E., and R. S. Henderson, Eds., CRC Press, Boca Raton, FL, chap. 34.

Schaeffer, J. L., and P. B. Hamilton. 1991. Interactions of mycotoxins with feed ingredients. Do safe levels exist? In *Mycotoxins and Animal Foods*, Smith, J. E., and R. S. Henderson, Eds., CRC Press, Boca Raton, FL, chap. 37.

Schell, T. C., M. D. Lindemann, E. T. Kornegay, and D. J. Blodgett. 1993a. Effects of feeding aflatoxin-contaminated diets with and without clay to weanling and growing pigs on performance, liver function and mineral metabolism, *J. Anim. Sci.*, 71:1209.

Schell, T. C., M. D. Lindemann, E. T. Kornegay, D. J. Blodgett, and J. A. Doerr. 1993b. Effectiveness of different types of clay for reducing the detrimental effects of aflatoxin-contaminated diets on performance and serum profiles of weanling pigs, *J. Anim. Sci.*, 71:1226.

Schulze, H., J. Huisman, M. W. A. Verstegen, and P. van Leeuwen. 1993a. Physiological effects of isolated soya trypsin inhibitors (sTI) on pigs. In *Recent Advances of Research in Antinutritional Factors in Legume Seeds*, van der Poel, A. F. B., J. Huisman, and H. S. Saini, Eds., Wageningen Pers, The Netherlands, 191.

Schulze, H., M. W. A. Verstegen, J. Huisman, P. van Leeuwen, and J. W. O. van den Berg. 1993b. Nutritional effects of isolated soya trypsin inhibitors (sTI) on pigs. In *Recent Advances of Research in Antinutritional Factors in Legume Seeds*, van der Poel, A. F. B., J. Huisman, and H. S. Saini, Eds., Wageningen Pers, The Netherlands, 195.

Schulze, H., H. S. Saini, J. Huisman, M. Hessing, W. van den Berg, and M. W. A. Verstegen. 1995. Increased nitrogen secretion by inclusion of soya lectin in the diets of pigs, *J. Sci. Food Agric.*, 69:501.

Sharma, R. P. 1993. Immunotoxicity of mycotoxins, *J. Dairy Sci.*, 76:892.

Silvotti, L., C. Petterino, A. Bonomi, and E. Cabassi. 1997. Immunotoxicological effects on piglets of feeding sows diets containing aflatoxins, *Vet. Rec.*, 141:469.

Smith, G. W., P. D. Constable, A. R. Smith, C. W. Bacon, F. I. Meredith, G. K. Wollenberg, and W. M. Haschek. 1996. Effects of fumonisin-containing culture material on pulmonary clearance in swine, *Am. J. Vet. Res.*, 57:1233.

Smith, J. E. 1997. Aflatoxins. In *Handbook of Plant and Fungal Toxicants*, D'Mello, J. P. F., Ed., CRC Press, Boca Raton, FL, chap. 19.

Smith, T. K. 1992. Recent advances in the understanding of Fusarium trichothecene mycotoxicoses, *J. Anim. Sci.*, 70:3989.

Smith, T. K., E. G. McMillan, and J. B. Castillo. 1997. Effect of feeding blends of Fusarium mycotoxin-contaminated grains containing deoxynivalenol and fusaric acid on growth and feed consumption of immature swine, *J. Anim. Sci.*, 75:2184.

Swanson, S. P., and R. A. Corley. 1989. The distribution, metabolism, and excretion of trichothecene mycotoxins. In *Trichothecene Mycotoxicosis: Pathophysiologic Effects*, Vol. II, Beasley, V. R., Ed., CRC Press, Boca Raton, FL, 37.

Tapia, M. O., and A. A. Seawright. 1984. Experimental ochratoxicosis A in pigs, *Aust. Vet. J.*, 61:219.

Tapia, M. O., and A. A. Seawright. 1985. Experimental combined aflatoxin B_1 and ochratoxin A intoxication in pigs, *Aust. Vet. J.*, 62:33.

Taylor, D. R. 1999. Mycotoxin binders: what are they and what makes them work? *Feedstuffs*, January 18:41.

Taylor, M. J., V. F. Pang, and V. R. Beasley. 1989. The immunotoxicity of trichothecene mycotoxins. In *Trichothecene Mycotoxicosis: Pathophysiologic Effects*, Vol. II, Beasley, V. R., Ed., CRC Press, Boca Raton, FL, 1.

Trenholm, H. L., B. C. Foster, L. L. Charmley, B. K. Thompson, K. E. Hartin, R. W. Coppock, and M. A. Albassam. 1994. Effects of feeding diets containing Fusarium (naturally) contaminated wheat or pure deoxynivalenol (DON) in growing pigs, *Can. J. Anim. Sci.*, 74:361.

Trugo, L. C., and D. von Baer. 1998. Analytical methods for the analysis of antinutritional factors in legume seeds. In *Recent Advances of Research in Antinutritional Factors in Legume Seeds and Rapeseed*, Jansman, A. J. M., G. D. Hill, J. Huisman, and A. F. B. van der Poel, Eds., Wageningen Pers, The Netherlands, 11.

van der Poel, A. F. B. 1990. Effect of processing on antinutritional factors and protein nutritional value of dry beans (*Phaseolus vulgaris* L.). A review, *Anim. Feed Sci. Technol.*, 29:179.

van Heugten, E., J. W. Spears, M. T. Coffey, E. B. Kegley, and M. A. Qureshi. 1994. The effect of methionine and aflatoxin on immune function in weanling pigs, *J. Anim. Sci.*, 72:658.

Wang, E., W. P. Norred, C. W. Bacon, R. T. Riley, and A. H. Merrill, Jr. 1991. Inhibition of sphingolipid biosynthesis by fumonisins: implications for diseases associated with Fusarium moniliforme, *J. Biol. Chem.*, 266:14486.

Wannemacher, R. W., Jr., D. L. Bunner, and H. A. Neufeld. 1991. Toxicity of trichothecenes and other related mycotoxins in laboratory animals. In *Mycotoxins and Animal Foods*, Smith, J. E., and R. S. Henderson, Eds., CRC Press, Boca Raton, chap. 23.

Wareham, C. N., J. Wiseman, and D. J. A. Cole. 1994. Processing and antinutritive factors in feedstuffs. In *Principles of Pig Science*, Cole, D. J. A., J. Wiseman, and M. A. Varley, Eds., Nottingham University Press, Loughborough, U.K., 141.

Weaver, G. A., H. J. Kurtz, F. Y. Bates, M. S. Chi, C. J. Mirocha, J. C. Behrens, and T. S. Robison. 1978a. Acute and chronic toxicity of T-2 mycotoxin in swine, *Vet. Rec.*, 103:531.

Weaver, G. A., H. J. Kurtz, C. J. Mirocha, F. Y. Bates, and J. C. Behrens. 1978b. Acute toxicity of the mycotoxin diacetoxyscirpenol in swine, *Can. Vet. J.*, 19:267.

Weaver, G. A., H. J. Kurtz, C. J. Mirocha, F. Y. Bates, J. C. Behrens, and T. S. Robison. 1978c. Effect of T-2 toxin on porcine reproduction, *Can. Vet. J.*, 19:310.

West, D. I., and L. B. Bullerman. 1991. Physical and chemical separation of mycotoxins from agricultural products. In *Mycotoxins and Animal Foods*, Smith, J. E., and R. S. Henderson, Eds., CRC Press, Boca Raton, FL, chap. 33.

Wilson, D. M., E. W. Sydenham, G. A. Lombaert, M. W. Trucksess, D. Abramson, and G. A. Bennett. 1998. Mycotoxin analytical techniques. In *Mycotoxins in Agriculture and Food Safety*, Sinha, K. K., and D. Bhatnagar, Eds., Marcel Dekker, New York, chap. 5.

Wood, G. E. 1992. Mycotoxins in foods and feeds in the United States, *J. Anim. Sci.*, 70:3941.

Wood, G. E., and M. W. Trucksess. 1998. Regulatory control programs for mycotoxin-contaminated food. In *Mycotoxins in Agriculture and Food Safety*, Sinha, K. K., and D. Bhatnagar, Eds., Marcel Dekker, New York, chap. 15.

26 Intestinal Bacteria and Their Influence on Swine Growth

H. Rex Gaskins

CONTENTS

I. Introduction 585
II. Who Comprises the Normal Microbiota? 586
III. Where Are They? 588
IV. What Are They Doing? 589
    A. Cooperative or Beneficial Effects 589
        1. Colonization Resistance 589
        2. The Intestinal Immune System 590
            a. The Mucus Layer 591
            b. The Intestinal Epithelium 592
            c. The Lamina Propria 592
            d. Intestinal T Lymphocytes 593
            e. Secretory IgA 593
        3. Nutritional Contributions 594
    B. Competitive or Negative Effects 595
        1. Amino Acid Catabolites 596
            a. Amines 596
            b. Ammonia 597
            c. Phenols and Indoles 597
        2. Bile Acid Biotransformation 598
        3. Mucin Degradation 599
V. Molecular Ecology 600
VI. Summary and Outlook 602
References 603

I. INTRODUCTION

The gastrointestinal (GI) tract of the pig harbors a numerically dense and metabolically active microbiota comprising mainly bacteria. Indeed, all animals have, and seemingly require, long-term cooperative associations with indigenous bacteria in the GI tract. Studies with gnotobiotic animal models demonstrate most conclusively that indigenous bacteria stimulate the normal maturation of host tissues and provide key defense and nutritional functions. This commensal relationship has been selected over evolutionary time resulting in a stable microbiota in mature animals that is generally similar in composition and function in a diverse range of animal species.

Despite evolutionary stability, the intestinal microbiota develops in individual animals in a characteristic successional pattern that requires substantial adaptation by the host during early life periods. The impact of the developing microbiota as well as the metabolic activities of climax communities require special consideration when viewed in the context of pig production in which efficiency of animal growth is a primary objective.

The epithelial lining of the GI tract is characterized by a high cell turnover rate and the constant production of a protective mucus coat. Together these two physiological processes provide effective innate defense against luminal threats, including those emanating from normal gut bacteria. In fact, epithelial cell turnover and secretory activity are both profoundly affected by the numbers, kinds, and spatial distribution of GI bacteria, with the latter microbial features being influenced by both exogenous and endogenous (host-derived) nutrients. Innate defense functions afforded by the epithelium are provided at the expense of animal growth efficiency. Specifically, GI tissues represent only 5% of body weight (approximate) but they receive a disproportionate fraction of cardiac output, and they contribute 15 to 35% of whole-body oxygen consumption and protein turnover because of inherently high rates of epithelial cell turnover and metabolism (McNurlan and Garlick, 1980; Edelstone and Holzman, 1981; Ebner et al., 1994). Only 10% of the total protein synthesized by the GI tract is accumulated as new mass (Reeds et al., 1993); most proteins are lost in sloughed epithelial cells or as secreted products such as mucus.

The high rate of epithelial cell turnover and secretory activity presumably evolved as a defensive response to the microbial load in the intestine. Carriage of microbial populations capable of utilizing refractory plant components enabled feral pigs to exploit distinct habitats, thereby enhancing survival and reproductive success. Animal growth efficiency is, however, a concept introduced only upon domestication of the pig as a food animal. These issues provoke consideration of an optimal gut microbiota for intestinal health vs. its effects on the efficiency of gastrointestinal and whole-body growth throughout the productive life cycle of a pig. However, the normal microbiota of the pig intestine has received surprisingly little attention from an animal growth perspective.

Most of the attention afforded the intestinal microbiota of the pig has been influenced by the much better understood rumen microbial ecosystem. Because of similarities between the rumen microbial ecosystem and the colonic microbiota of hindgut fermenters, pig intestinal microbiology research reflects an apparent colonic bias with an emphasis on defining the beneficial effects of resident fermentative bacteria. Deserving equal or perhaps greater attention is the small intestinal microbiota because of its potential to compete with the pig for nutrients, stimulate epithelial cell turnover, or add to the secretory demands placed on the small intestine via accelerated mucus production. Even in the colon, a site at which undigested nutrients may be salvaged for host use through bacterial fermentation, the optimal density and complexity of the microbiota should be considered in a cost/benefit scenario when improvement of animal growth efficiency is a goal.

Much new knowledge is needed before the concept of an optimal gut microbiota for pig growth can be transferred to practical applications for the pig industry. Robert E. Hungate, the father of intestinal microbial ecology, proposed that "the ultimate aim of ecology is to understand the relationships of all organisms to their environment" (Hungate, 1960). He suggested that at least three principal questions must be answered to achieve such an objective (Table 26.1). Hungate's principles of intestinal microecology apply to any complex microbial ecosystem and are now widely used as framework by microbial ecologists studying a variety of diverse environments. This chapter summarizes current knowledge of the pig intestinal microbiota and features host–microbe interactions that likely impact the efficiency of intestinal and subsequent whole-animal growth. Topics are organized according to Hungate's principles of intestinal microecology, namely: who comprises the normal microbiota, where are they, and what are they doing? Limitations in knowledge of the pig microbiota and of host response pathways that preclude theoretical or practical consideration of an optimal gut microbiota are noted throughout.

II. WHO COMPRISES THE NORMAL MICROBIOTA?

Throughout the GI tract, the microbiota is characterized by its high population density, extensive diversity, and complexity of interactions. Bacteria are predominant, but all major groups of microbes

TABLE 26.1
Hungate's Principles of Intestinal Microecology

Three major questions must be answered to understand complex microbial ecosystems:
1. What kinds and numbers of organisms are present? This involves identification, classification, and enumeration.
2. What are their activities? Food and metabolic products must be identified, and habit of growth, reproduction, and death known. A complete determination of activities necessitates a complete knowledge of the environment.
3. To what extent are their activities performed? This involves quantitative measurement of the entire complex as well as its individual components.

Source: Hungate, R. E., *Bacteriol. Rev.*, 24:353, 1960. With permission.

are represented. Bacterial populations as high as 10^{10} to 10^{11}/g contents belonging to as many as 400 different species have been found in the hindgut of mammals (Savage, 1977a; Lee, 1984). In most cases, these numbers have been derived from fecal samples and may not accurately represent the colonic microbiota, let alone the small intestinal microbiota. The prominent role played by anaerobic bacteria in the large intestine is obvious from the fact that more than 99% of the bacteria isolated are unable to grow in the presence of oxygen (Savage, 1977a). Importantly, bacterial cells outnumber animal cells by a factor of 10 and have a profound influence on immunological, nutritional, physiological, and protective processes in the host (Berg, 1996; Gaskins, 1997).

A distinction between indigenous (autochthonous) and nonindigenous (allochthonous) bacteria is crucial for an ecological understanding of colonization, succession, and mechanisms of host interactions. This distinction is especially difficult in neonatal animals where bacteria are acquired transiently from the sow and its surrounding environment during and immediately after the birth process. The terms *autochthonous* and *indigenous* are generally considered synonyms and are used to describe bacteria that have coevolved with the host and that colonize all habitats and niches available in the GI ecosystem (Dubos et al., 1965; Savage, 1977b). On the other hand, allochthonous species may pass through specific microhabitats, being derived from food, water, or another gut habitat, but do not colonize the GI tract (Dubos et al., 1965; Savage, 1977b). Colonization describes the process by which a GI bacterial population becomes stable in size, over time, without the need for periodic reintroduction of the bacteria. Thus, colonizing bacteria multiply in a particular intestinal habitat at a rate that equals or exceeds their rate of washout or elimination at that site (Freter, 1992). Pathogens can be autochthonous or allochthonous to the gut ecosystem and generally cause disease when the ecosystem is disturbed in some way, affecting their site of residence or growth potential.

At present, for the pig, the major bacterial groups in distinct regions of the GI tract have been reasonably described, albeit with the data subject to the biases associated with conventional cultivation-based techniques. In other words, current knowledge of microbial diversity and ecology in the pig GI tract is based largely on anaerobic culture techniques. These techniques enable phenotypic characterization of cultivable isolates according to their metabolic activities and on morphology according to light and electron microscopic examination. Cultivation-based microbial ecology techniques are limited by three major factors. First, one can only culture those organisms for which nutritional and growth requirements are known. Second, phenotypic criteria do not reliably enable phylogenetic identification. Third, cultivation techniques are, by design, tedious, imprecise, and impractical for studying ecosystems characterized by extensive microbial diversity. Molecular-based methods that examine microbial diversity independent of any cultural bias are being increasingly used (Mackie et al., 1999). The major bacterial groups that have been cultivated or isolated from pig feces are (in order of prominence): *Streptococcus, Lactobacillus, Eubacterium, Fusobacterium,*

Bacteroides, Peptostreptococcus, Bifidobacterium, Selenomonas, Clostridium, Butyrivibrio, Escherichia (Moore et al., 1987, as cited by Stewart, 1997). A recent study of microbial diversity in the mucosal layer of the pig colon with molecular analysis compared with culture-based methods demonstrated that Streptococci and Lactobacilli comprised the majority of isolates (54%) recovered from the colon wall by culturing, whereas this group accounted for only one third of the sequence variation for the same sample from random cloning (Pryde et al., 1999). In addition, 59% of randomly cloned sequences showed less than 95% similarity to database entries or sequences from cultivated organisms. These data clearly demonstrate the problem of cultivation bias and illustrate the need for reassessment of the pig intestinal ecosystem using more objective molecular-based analyses. This exercise will ideally be undertaken by multiple groups using a range of available molecular or noncultivation-based techniques.

III. WHERE ARE THEY?

The stomach and proximal small intestine contain relatively low numbers of microbes (10^3 to 10^5 bacteria/g or ml of contents) because of low pH and rapid flow. In the small intestine, the rate of digesta flow and thus the rate of bacterial washout, exceeds the maximal growth rates of most bacterial species. Accordingly, this gut region is colonized typically by bacteria that adhere to the mucus layer or epithelial cell surface. Acid-tolerant lactobacilli and streptococci are thought to predominate in the upper small intestine (Fewins et al., 1957).

The distal small intestine (ileum) maintains a more diverse microbiota and higher bacterial numbers (10^8/g or ml of contents) than the upper intestine, and it is considered a transition zone preceding the large intestine. In a study of microbial gas production in various gastrointestinal regions, Jensen and Jørgensen (1994) reported that the highest H_2 concentrations and production rates were found in the distal small intestine in pigs. This indication for substantial microbial activity in the pig ileum was substantiated in their study by dense populations of culturable anaerobic bacteria and the detection of high-ATP concentrations.

The large intestine (cecum and colon) is a major site of microbial colonization because of slow digesta turnover, and it is characterized by large numbers of bacteria (10^{10} to 10^{11}/g or ml of content), low redox potential, and relatively high short-chain fatty acid (SCFA) concentrations. The composition of the hindgut microbiota is both diverse and stable. Several hundred anaerobic bacterial species and strains appear to coexist without one or a few becoming dominant (Fewins et al., 1957; Smith and Jones, 1963; Allison et al., 1979; Robinson et al., 1981; 1984; Varel et al., 1984; Anugwa et al., 1989; Butine and Leedle, 1989; Pryde et al., 1999). At least three independent cultivation studies (Salanitro et al., 1977; Russell, 1979; Robinson et al., 1981) have demonstrated that Gram-positive bacteria predominate the colonic and fecal microbiota of the pig. On the other hand, a study by Robinson and co-workers (1981) demonstrated that about 80% of the culturable bacteria from the pig cecum were Gram negative, with *Bacteroides* and *Selenomonas* species being most prominent.

The balanced diversity of the hindgut microbiota reflects, in part, the variety of nutrient substrates found in the environment. The diversity of bacterial populations within a particular ecosystem is directly related to the number of limiting nutrients, because each limiting nutrient will support the one bacterial species or strain that is most efficient in utilizing it. The stability of the hindgut microbiota, on the other hand, is likely a function of inhibition of bacterial multiplication by compounds such as SCFA, hydrogen sulfide, deconjugated bile salts, and bacteriocins. It has been proposed that these bacterial metabolites may prolong the lag phase of allochthonous bacteria such that they are excreted from the local environment before they have a chance to colonize (Freter, 1983).

In addition to an increasing gradient of indigenous microbes from the stomach to the colon, characteristic radial distributions of organisms are found within each gut compartment. Specifically, at least four microhabitats have been described: the intestinal lumen, the unstirred mucus layer or gel that covers the epithelium of the entire tract, the deep mucus layer found in intestinal crypts, and the surface of intestinal epithelial cells (Lee, 1984). The bacterial groups residing within these specific microhabitats have not been adequately described for any animal species, due in part to the technical challenges that define the task.

Development of microbial populations in the mammalian GI tract commences soon after birth and involves complex successional changes until dense, stable populations colonize characteristic regions of the gut. Microbial succession during the first few postnatal weeks is remarkably similar among mammalian species (Mackie et al., 1999). Immediately after birth, aerobic and facultative anaerobes including clostridia, lactobacilli, coliforms, and streptococci predominate. It is generally proposed that these bacteria are responsible for the creation of a reduced environment favorable for later colonization by anaerobic genera, which constitute the predominant bacteria of the climax microbiota, at least in the large intestine (Mackie et al., 1999). Additional data are needed to define clearly microbial succession in distinct gastrointestinal regions during conventional growth phases of production pigs. Two recent reviews (Stewart, 1997; Mackie et al., 1999) contain more-detailed discussion of the numbers and distribution of specific bacterial groups during early gut development and the weaning transition.

There is a general belief that the early and abrupt weaning practices that typify modern production strategies compromise the normal microbiota and thereby increase susceptibility to enteric diseases. Accordingly, considerable efforts have been expended to develop weaning strategies that promote the growth of so-called "beneficial" bacteria at weaning via the provision of readily fermentable substrates. Interest in this strategy has been further heightened by increasing regulatory concerns surrounding the use of feed-grade antibiotics. The benefits derived from this prophylactic practice will likely vary according to the prevalence of enteric pathogens within nursery environments. Moreover, a decision on the efficacy of fermentable fibers as an alternative to antibiotics awaits a better understanding of their sites of fermentation in the pig gut, and of the animal growth costs associated with the promotion of bacterial growth in the intestine.

IV. WHAT ARE THEY DOING?

Domestic pigs used in modern production are encumbered with host adaptations derived in response to a complex gut microbiota, although their environment, diets, and lifestyle differ substantially from those of ancestral feral pigs. Notwithstanding, the commensal microbiota of the pig, and mammals in general, is viewed typically as a beneficial entity for the host. While it is certain that both nutritional and defensive functions are provided by the gut microbiota, it is also clear that the host animal invests substantially in defensive efforts first to sequester gut microbes away from the epithelial surface (pathogens and nonpathogens alike) and, second, to mount inflammatory and immune responses quickly against those organisms that manage to breech epithelial defenses. Accordingly, the concept of détente may more accurately describe the relationship between gut bacteria and their host than the more commonly used symbiosis concept. A state of détente provides the microbiota a stable niche and provides for the host the protection afforded by the symbiont (i.e., colonization resistance). The protective adaptations mounted by the host enable homestasis between the two carya but carry costs that become most apparent when considered in the context of animal growth efficiency. The beneficial vs. competitive or *costly* interactions that characterize the relationship between domestic pigs and their gut microbiota are featured in the remainder of the chapter.

A. COOPERATIVE OR BENEFICIAL EFFECTS

1. Colonization Resistance

As the first tier of defense, the normal microbiota interferes with intestinal colonization by nonidigenous organisms, including pathogens. This phenomenon has been described variously as bacterial antagonism (Freter, 1956), competitive exclusion (Lloyd et al., 1977), bacterial interference

(Aly and Shinefield, 1982), and colonization resistance (van der Waaij et al., 1971; Rolfe, 1997). Proposed mechanisms by which indigenous bacteria prevent colonization by nonindigenous bacteria include direct competition for nutrients or mucosal attachment sites (mucus or epithelial surface), or through alteration of the local growth environment via the production of antimicrobial compounds, volatile fatty acids, and chemically modified bile acids (Rolfe, 1997). The best evidence that the normal intestinal microbiota provides an important defense barrier comes from a multitude of studies demonstrating heightened sensitivity to enteric infections in germfree animals (Gordon et al., 1966; Bealmear, 1980).

The related concept of *competitive exclusion* has received considerable attention recently as a possible means to prevent enteric disease in pigs, poultry, and dairy calves (Nisbet, 1998). The applied practice consists of providing to newborn animals oral supplements of either defined or undefined mixed bacterial cultures with the objective of outcompeting pathogenic gut bacteria through the variety of mechanisms suggested to underlie colonization resistance. Most of the work has been conducted with poultry species, but recent experimental work has also been conducted with swine and cattle (Nisbet, 1998). The competitive exclusion strategy is likely to be most efficacious in animal herds carrying significant pathogen loads, and it may represent a potential growth cost in clean or noninfected herds via intestinal responses to bacterial colonization. Specific mechanisms generally remain undefined.

2. The Intestinal Immune System

The anatomic organization of the intestine provides a stratification of defense functions, beginning with the direct protective functions of the normal microbiota as discussed above. Commensal gut bacteria also indirectly benefit the host by stimulating development of host defenses including the unstirred mucus layer, the epithelial monolayer, and the underlying lamina propria, home of multiple immune cell types (McCracken and Gaskins, 1999). That nonpathogenic bacteria stimulate development of both innate and acquired components of immunological defense illustrates their antigenic nature and confirms the view that détente best describes the relationship between the host and its intestinal microbiota.

Studies with germfree animals demonstrate conclusively that in the absence of the normal microbiota, intestinal morphology is altered and the local immune system is underdeveloped (Table 26.2). For example, the cecum in germfree rodents can be up to eight times the size of the cecum of conventional animals, a result of increased numbers of mucus-producing goblet cells in the small

TABLE 26.2
Physiological Characteristics of the Germfree State

Variable	% Conventional Animals	Variable	% Conventional Animals
Amino acid absorption	>200	Cecum	
Arterial blood flow to liver	50	Wet weight with content	550
Basal metabolic rate	80–85	Ammonia concentration	10
Bile acid hydrolysis	0	Ileocecal lymph nodes	40–60
Blood		Lamina propria area	85
Peripheral NH_3 concentration	70	Lamina propria cellularity	100
Portal NH_3 concentration	25	Small intestine	
Blood volume	78	Mucosal surface area	67
Cardiac output	68	Epithelial cell renewal rate	60–70
		Water content	90
		Urea hydrolysis	0

Source: Modified from Visek (1978).

intestine and mucus accumulation in the absence of a mucus-degrading microbiota (Wostmann and Bruckner-Kardoss, 1959). Alterations of immune parameters in germfree animals include a striking decrease in total lymphocyte numbers, skewed intestinal lymphocyte and antibody profiles, and underdeveloped Peyer's patches and mesenteric lymph nodes lacking germinal centers and plasma cells (Thorbecke, 1959; McCracken and Gaskins, 1999). When germfree animals are associated with indigenous bacteria by transfer to a conventional animal facility, gut morphology and distinct components of the intestinal immune system develop quickly (McCracken and Gaskins, 1999).

a. The mucus layer

The mucus gel layer is an integral structural component of the gut mucosal surface, acting as a medium for protection, lubrication, and transport between luminal contents and the epithelial lining. Mucus is a heterogeneous mixture of secretions comprising approximately 95% water and containing electrolytes (Na^+, K^+, Mg^{2+}, and Ca^{2+}), carbohydrates, proteins, amino acids, and lipids (Verdugo, 1990). The viscoelastic, polymer-like properties of mucus are derived from the major gel-forming glycoprotein components called mucins (Forstner et al., 1995). Mucins consist of a peptide backbone containing alternating glycosylated and nonglycosylated domains, with glycosylated regions comprising 70 to 80% of the polymer. The oligosaccharide side chains are linked to the peptide core by O-glycosidic bonds between threonine or serine on the peptide core and N-acetylgalactosamine on the sugar chains (Forstner et al., 1995). N-Acetylglucosamine, N-acetylgalactosamine, galactose, and fucose are the four main mucin oligosaccharides (Forstner et al., 1995). Terminal sulfate or sialic acid groups are often added to the oligosaccharide chains, which accounts for the polyanionic nature of mucins at neutral or near neutral pH (Forstner et al., 1995). Secretory mucins in the small and large intestine are synthesized and secreted by specialized columnar epithelial cells called goblet cells, so-named by their characteristic "goblet" shape (Forstner et al., 1995).

Protection of the epithelium against intestinal microbes lies in the capacity of mucin carbohydrates to either repel or bind to microbial adhesions (Belley et al., 1999). The ability to bind to mucin carbohydrates enables some bacterial groups to colonize the mucus layer. Bacteria unable to bind mucus have either evolved growth characteristics that enable their survival in the mixed luminal contents or are excreted via peristalsis and defecation. There is a general belief that mucus-resident bacteria prevent the attachment of pathogenic organisms by occupying available binding sites. While supporting *in vitro* evidence exists, much additional *in situ* data are needed to verify or refute that postulate. For example, there is little information on the taxonomy or the temporal or spatial distribution of bacterial groups that preferentially reside within intestinal mucus. The extent and especially the complexity of the mucus layer are just beginning to be revealed through the development of histological techniques allowing its preservation (Matsuo et al., 1997).

Ontogenic changes in the composition of the mucus layer that correlate with successional changes in the intestinal microbiota and with maturation of acquired immune functions in the intestine are consistent with the postulate that mucus-secreting goblet cells play a crucial role in intestinal homeostasis (Neutra and Forstner, 1987; Turck et al., 1993). Changes in both the number of goblet cells and the chemical composition of intestinal mucus are consistently detected in response to diverse luminal insults (Neutra et al., 1982; Olubuyide et al., 1984; Dunsford et al., 1991; Forstner et al., 1995; Sharma and Schumaker, 1995; Ganessunker et al., 1999).

The authors have observed an increase in goblet cell numbers in the small intestine of neonatal pigs fed parenterally (intravenously) vs. enterally from birth, as well as an increase in sulfomucin-secreting goblet cells within ileal crypts of parenterally fed animals (Ganessunker et al., 1999). Changes in goblet cell populations in this total parenteral nutrition (TPN) piglet model correlate with alterations in microbial population profiles, enhanced inflammation, and decreased integrity of the mucosal barrier in response to the lack of enteral nutrition (Ganessunker et al., 1999; Vidal and Gaskins, unpublished obervations). All indications are that the mucus layer should be considered a dynamically bioactive component of intestinal defense rather than a static, viscous barrier simply imparting physical protective functions. Full adoption of such a view awaits the discovery of regulatory networks that interface with mucus-producing goblet cells.

The nature of the microbiota comprising the intestinal mucus biofilm is essentially undefined for all animal species. This limitation in present knowledge derives from both the difficulties associated with preservation of the mucus layer during tissue fixation and from the inherent biases of cultivation-dependent microbiological techniques (Mackie et al., 1999). A recent study demonstrating conclusively that an intestinal bacterium (*Bacteroides thetaioataomicron*) is capable of signaling the host epithelial cell to alter its glycosylation program likely reflects the general dynamic nature of host–microbe interactions in the mucus biofilm (Bry et al., 1996). An understanding of the extent and nature of those interactions requires identification of the mucus-associated microbiota and description of the ecology and physiology of the contributing microbes. Better defined are bacteria that contribute to mucin degradation, at least for humans and laboratory rodents (not pigs). The potential consequences of bacteria-mediated erosion of the intestinal mucus layer is considered in a later section addressing negative effects of the normal microbiota.

b. The intestinal epithelium

The outermost epithelial cell monolayer underlying the mucus layer is organized into two morphologically and functionally distinct compartments, the crypt regions containing stem cells and Paneth cells, and the villi (small intestine) or epithelial cuffs (large intestine) containing one of several terminally differentiated epithelial cell types (Gaskins, 1997). The formation of tight junctions between adjacent epithelial cells in mature epithelia provides a crucial physical barrier to the external environment. The process of continual desquamation and renewal of the gut epithelium further limits opportunities for pathogens to colonize epithelial cells (Potten and Loefler, 1990). In addition to these important innate functions, intestinal epithelial cells are endowed with immunological functions, including antigen presentation via major histocompatibility complex (MHC) molecules, and the ability to synthesize and secrete numerous inflammatory and regulatory cytokines (Gaskins, 1997). Bioactive cytokines produced by epithelial cells, principally those that are also produced by macrophages, enable the transduction of information on the relative state of intestinal health to intraepithelial T lymphocytes and immune cells in the underlying lamina propria.

The complex communication networks that exist between epithelial and submucosal cells in the intestine are best reflected by the concerted inflammatory responses to luminal insults (Gaskins, 1997). For example, in response to bacterial toxins or food antigens, activated lamina propria cells secrete cytokines and bioactive lipids, which collectively increase motility and blood flow to the intestine, while inhibiting absorption and stimulating water and ion secretion by intestinal epithelial cells. When integrated, these physiological responses culminate in secretory diarrhea, the common and major symptom of intestinal inflammation, regardless of the precipitating insult (Hinterleitner and Powell, 1991). The severity of a secretory response will determine the length and cost of recovery in terms of epithelial restitution. The biochemical or *growth* costs associated with epithelial maintenance and recovery from various insults both need to be defined for the pig.

Intestinal epithelial-derived cytokines also likely play key roles in the cellular and functional development of the intraepithelial T lymphocyte and lamina propria compartments; however, the specific cytokines involved and their modes of action have yet to be identified. Very little research has been communicated on the crucial topic of intestinal epithelial cell cytokines in livestock animal species. Most knowledge of epithelial cell production of and epithelial responsiveness to cytokines in vertebrate species comes from studies with immortalized cell lines. Those studies and issues relating to epithelial responses to intestinal bacteria are summarized in a recent review by McCracken and Gaskins (1999).

c. The lamina propria

Diffuse populations of T lymphocytes, B lymphocytes, plasma cells, macrophages, mast cells, eosinophils, and smaller numbers of dendritic cells and neutrophils, as well as biologically active fibroblasts, reside beneath the epithelial cell monolayer in the lamina propria (Hinterleitner and Powell, 1991). The lamina propria is also well vascularized and densely innervated with a rich plexus of enteric nerves playing a critical role in gut motility, an important innate defense function. The variety of cell types found in the lamina propria almost certainly reflects the dynamic nature of this gut compartment; however, once again, there is much yet to learn about the lamina propria in the pig and other livestock species.

Using conventional and germfree pigs of different ages, Rothkötter and co-workers (1994) reported useful data on the influence of age and the gut microbiota on the cellular composition of the intestinal immune system. Crude separations of epithelial and lamina propria compartments demonstrated that total yield of immune cells from intestine of young pigs (5 days old) was only 10% of that obtained from older pigs (45 days old), and that intestinal lymphocyte numbers of 9-month-old pigs were about 50% lower than those from 14-month-old pigs. Cell yield and lymphocyte subset patterns from the intestine of 45-day-old germfree pigs were comparable with those of 5-day-old conventional animals. These data once again indicate that the commensal microbiota is a major stimulus for the postnatal development of immune cell compartments in the intestine.

d. Intestinal T lymphocytes

Intestinal T lymphocytes, residing at sites of first contact with enteric pathogens, are considered key defensive components. Intestinal T cell populations include the intraepithelial T lymphocytes, lamina propria T cells, and those residing in Peyer's patches (Guy-Grand et al., 1993). In addition to their anatomic locale, intestinal T-cell subsets can be distinguished by their pattern of ontogenic appearance, their site of maturation, the expression of surface cell differentiation (CD) molecules, and by TCR ($\alpha\beta$ or $\gamma\delta$) subtype (Zuckermann and Gaskins, 1996; Gaskins, 1997). The aggregate of growth factors and cytokines found in particular intestinal microenvironments are thought to influence the phenotype of resident intestinal T cells (Croitoru and Ernst, 1993); however, the validity of this concept needs to be confirmed through additional experimentation. Although peripheral T-cell populations are generally well described, intestinal T-cell biology is just beginning to be addressed in the pig.

The authors have observed significant expansion of lamina propria T-cell subsets in response to both total parenteral nutrition and weaning anorexia in separate pig models (Ganessunker et al., 1999; McCracken et al., 1999). In both cases, T-cell expansion was associated with epithelial nutrient deprivation, and correlated with significant compromises in small intestinal morphology and local inflammation. Compromised epithelial integrity resulting from the lack of enteral stimulation is thought to promote bacterial translocation and subsequent local T-cell expansion in response to both TPN and weaning anorexia. At present, mechanisms underlying integrated epithelial responses to luminal nutrients remain undefined, including the regulatory cascade(s) controlling T-cell expansion in compromised states, the temporal sequence of the response, and the extent to which T-cell expansion affects epithelial functions. The hypothesis that apparent effects of luminal nutrients on the intestinal immune system are instead mediated through microbial shifts in response to exogenous nutrient availability should also be rigorously examined.

e. Secretory IgA

Secretory IgA is the best-described immunological barrier in the intestine. Secretory IgA is synthesized by B lymphocytes that originate in bone marrow and migrate to Peyer's patches, a collection of organized germinal centers found in the intestine (Mestecky, 1987; Kraehenbuhl and Neutra, 1992; Kagnoff, 1993). Initially, luminal antigens are transported through specialized epithelial cells (membranous or M cells) overlying Peyer's patches into an interfollicular area where they are presented by resident antigen-presenting cells to helper T cells. The helper T cells, in turn, secrete cytokines that stimulate B lymphocytes to undergo immunoglobulin class-specific switching to an IgA$^+$ phenotype (Kagnoff, 1993). After leaving Peyer's patches and passing through the systemic circulation, IgA$^+$ B lymphocytes migrate or "home" to mucosal surfaces, where upon reexposure to the pathogen, plasma cells secrete antigen-specific IgA, which is transported back across the epithelium by a specialized receptor (secretory component), and released onto the mucosal surface (Mostov, 1994). Mucosal IgA antibodies provide protection primarily by preventing the adherence of bacteria or toxins to epithelial cells, a process often referred to as *immune exclusion* (Stokes and Bourne, 1989; Kraehenbuhl and Neutra, 1992; Kagnoff, 1993).

The homing of differentiated IgA$^+$ B lymphocytes from Peyer's patches to other mucosal sites including the lungs, female reproductive tract, and mammary glands provides a mechanism whereby exposure to a pathogen at one mucosal site can result in widespread immunity at other mucosal surfaces. This concept is often referred to as the "common mucosal immune system." Similar to all vertebrate species, the secretory IgA system of the pig has been described in more detail than other mucosal immune components. The reader is referred to the review by Stokes and Bourne (1989) for details.

The influence of luminal antigens and particularly the intestinal microbiota on postnatal development of secretory IgA has been highlighted in animal studies demonstrating that both the size and number of Peyer's patches are reduced significantly in germfree pigs (Pabst et al., 1988; Rothkötter and Pabst, 1989; Rothkötter et al., 1991). This phenomenon has been studied in more depth in rodents where it has been demonstrated that monoassociation of germfree animals with certain commensal bacteria can restore normal development of the secretory IgA system (Cebra et al., 1980; McCracken and Gaskins, 1999). The elucidation of mechanisms whereby commensal bacteria stimulate host intestinal immune development may present novel means of precociously stimulating development of active immunity in neonatal pigs.

3. Nutritional Contributions

Indigenous gut bacteria provide the mammalian host with nutrients, including SCFA, vitamin K, B vitamins, and amino acids (Savage, 1986; Wostmann, 1996). Research interest in the nutritional benefits provided by the intestinal microbiota of the pig has focused on the types and distribution of anaerobic bacteria in the pig cecum and colon and on their production of SCFA and gases (hydrogen, methane) in response to various dietary energy sources (Fewins et al., 1957; Salanitro et al., 1977; Allison et al., 1979; Russell, 1979; Robinson et al., 1981; 1984; Moore et al., 1987; Jensen and Jørgensen, 1994). The reader is referred to Chapter 7 for a complete discussion of complex carbohydrate fermentation in the pig GI tract and to the recent review by Stewart (1997) for a summary of bacterial species residing in the pig large intestine. The collective data demonstrate that the colonic environment of the pig and the nutritional features of the more numerous and functionally more important bacteria are similar to the more completely described rumen and human colon ecosystems.

Briefly, fermentation of nonstarch polysaccharides and oligosaccharides in the voluminous colon of the pig results in the production of high SCFA concentrations (70 to 100 mM) with a typical ratio of 60 acetate:25 propionate:15 butyrate (Grieshop et al., 2000). Both SCFA and water are rapidly absorbed as the digesta move distally. Because water absorption in the intestine is partly dependent on the nature of the solute present, the absorption of SCFA contributes to body fluid conservation as well as providing a readily available source of additional energy to the pig. The contribution of SCFA to maintenance energy requirement of the pig has been estimated to vary between 5 and 28% (Grieshop et al., 2000). The degree to which energy derived from SCFA contributes to whole-animal metabolism vs. self maintenance of the colon is not certain. However, the energy obtained from microbial fermentation is used less efficiently than the energy obtained through direct digestion and absorption of carbohydrates by the host (Livesay, 1992). The production of heat, fecal SCFA, and various gases represent additional fermentative costs. Fecal excretion of fat and nitrogen in the form of microbial biomass may also reduce the retention of dietary energy (Tetens et al., 1996; Lærke and Jensen, 1999).

Once again, the concept of an optimal microbiota for efficiency of pig growth is engendered. The domestic pig is in effect encumbered with gut adaptions (i.e, a voluminous fermentation vat) that enabled ancestral feral pigs to survive and reproduce by exploiting unique dietary niches. In extant domestic animals, the nature of the diet determines the utility of maintaining a fermentative organ, with the greatest value being imparted to pigs fed by-product feedstuffs with high fiber concentrations.

Relative to complex carbohydrates, little attention has been given to the digestion and metabolism of proteins and peptides by intestinal bacteria of the pig, or to the ecological and physiological significance of these substances as carbon, nitrogen, and energy sources. Two important issues emerge.

First, the extent to which microbial protein contributes to the amino acid needs of the pig is unclear. It has generally been thought that nonruminant animals derive little value from microbial protein based on the recognition that microbial populations are greatest in the cecum and colon, whereas the major site of amino acid absorption is the small intestine. Although it is certain that microbial populations are more dense in the cecum and colon of the pig than in the small intestine, the concentration of small intestinal bacteria is nonetheless substantial ($\sim 10^8$/g contents), particularly in the ileum (Clemens et al., 1975; Robinson et al., 1989; Jensen and Jørgensen, 1994). The extent of microbial nitrogen metabolism in the small intestine of the pig should be rigorously examined.

Evidence also exists that the pig large intestine is capable of amino acid absorption and that absorption capacity declines with age (Fuller and Reeds, 1998). With the extent of amino acid absorption being much greater in germfree vs. conventional animals, the decline in amino acid absorption from the large intestine of the pig may reflect the corresponding increase in microbial colonization. Accordingly, amino acid absorption from the small intestine may also be influenced by the degree of bacterial colonization. If that were the case, the ability of oral antibiotics to improve amino acid absorption from the small intestine (Weldon, 1997) might reflect a relative decontamination of that gut region in response to the antimicrobial effects. That issue is but one of many relating to bacterial effects on amino acid supply that require additional experimentation for answers. In the meantime, the reader is referred to a recent review article that summarizes the growing evidence that microbial protein does contribute significantly to the amino acid nutrition of nonruminant species (Fuller and Reeds, 1998).

A second issue relating to proteolytic activities of intestinal bacteria is discussed later and concerns the effects on the host of toxic catabolites generated from the digestion and metabolism of proteins and peptides.

B. Competitive or Negative Effects

Much of the structure and many of the functions of the mammalian intestine seem to have evolved to enable the host to tolerate the antigenic and chemical challenges associated with the carriage of a complex microbial ecosystem. Accordingly, the benefits of the normal microbiota discussed above are provided at the cost of intestinal adapations. A cost–benefit analysis considering the animal's age, environment, and diet is thus required to define accurately the full contributory value of the intestinal microbiota. For example, the growing pig is advantaged substantially by an intestinal immune system comprising multiple tiers of both innate and acquired immune functions. Bacterial antigens derived from the normal microbiota provide the primary stimulus for the ordered development of those defense capabilities. Enteric infections would prove consistently fatal in the absence of a fully competent intestinal immune system. However, enteric infections can be controlled to some degree by the stockman through sanitary practices and vaccination. In that case, it would be useful to understand precisely the bacterial cues required for local development of immune competence. Immune competence could possibly be engendered without incurring the full metabolic costs associated with carriage of a dense gut microbiota. Similarly, it would be useful to understand better the energetic contributions of SCFA to whole-animal metabolism vs. their use for maintenance of a voluminous colon densely populated by fermentative bacteria.

It is not possible at present to perform a cost–benefit analysis of host–microbe interactions in the pig gut because neither bacterial cues nor host-response pathways are defined. As but one example, the chemical cues leading to enhanced turnover of the epithelium in conventional vs. germfree animals are not defined. As pertains to nutrient utilization, quantitative data are also generally lacking for the collective effects of the intestinal microbiota on macro- or micronutrient availability for the host. It is apparent from germfree research that most of the host-response pathways activated by bacterial cues will be costly to the animal in terms of growth efficiency, perhaps with the exception of SCFA utilization (see Table 26.2). Thus, defining biochemical activities of gut bacteria that negatively impact pig growth should become a primary objective.

Gut bacteria impart both direct and indirect competitive or negative effects. For example, the production of lactic acid from glucose by lactobacilli in the small intestine would represent a direct competition between bacteria and host epithelial cells for a readily available nutrient substrate. Because lactic acid increases gut motility (Saunders and Sillery, 1982), bacterial lactic acid production would also indirectly have a negative impact if nutrient utilization was affected by an increase in digesta passage rate. Similarly, bacterial degradation of amino acids will limit their availability to the host and generates a variety of catabolites that negatively impact epthelial functions or regenerative efficiency.

1. Amino Acid Catabolites

Knowledge of the proteolytic activities of gut bacteria of the pig is extremely poor. Because the types and metabolic activities of anaerobes in the large intestine seem to be generally similar across mammalian species, it is possible to consider potential consequences of bacterial metabolism of peptides and amino acids from data obtained from such ecoystems. However, direct work needs to be conducted with pigs, particularly in the small intestine where ecological characteristics and host cell consequences may differ significantly from hindgut scenarios described for humans and rodents.

Protein substrates available for bacterial hydrolysis are derived from dietary residues, GI and pancreatic secretions including enzymes, mucins, and other glycoproteins, desquamated epithelial cells, and bacterial secretions. Determining bacterial contributions to proteolysis and protein degradation in the intestine is difficult because of the presence of variable concentrations of pancreatic and small intestinal peptidases mixed with bacterial enzymes. In humans, this complication is largely restricted to the colon because bacterial numbers in the small intestine are generally low and proteolytic activities are derived largely from host enzymes. Bacterial proteolysis in the human colon has been reasonably characterized, resulting in considerable information on the predominant proteolytic bacteria and their enzymatic activities (Macfarlane and Macfarlane, 1995). Comparable data do not exist for the pig and are crucial for accurate accounting of the nitrogen economy throughout the intestinal tract, including the small intestine.

Numerous bacterial species use peptides and amino acids as carbon, nitrogen, and energy sources with certain species being obligate amino acid fermenters (Loesche and Gibbons, 1968; Russell, 1983; Macfarlane and Macfarlane, 1995). Amino acid degradation by small intestinal bacteria diminishes their availability to the pig and produces a range of end products having nutritional or physiological significance for the host. Of particular interest are amino acid catabolites that are potentially toxic and thereby affect growth or differentiation of intestinal epithelial cells.

a. Amines

A number of intestinal bacterial groups including *Bacteroides* (Allison and Macfarlane, 1989), *Clostridium* (Allison and Macfarlane, 1989), *Enterobacterium* (Morris and Boeker, 1983), *Lactobacillus* (Sumner et al., 1985), and *Streptococcus* (Babu et al., 1986) possess the ability to produce amines via decarboxylation of amino acids and breakdown of polyamines. Amines found in the human colon include agmatine, cadaverine, dimethlamine, histamine, piperidine, putrescine, pyrrolidine, and tyramine (Drasar and Hill, 1974; Allison and Macfarlane, 1989). Normally amines are rapidly absorbed from the colon and are either detoxified by the gut mucosa or liver, or are excreted in urine. Cadaverine, histamine, putrescine, and tyramine are pharmacologically active in the gut (Drasar and Hill, 1974). Increased amine production by intestinal bacteria was associated with diarrhea at weaning in pigs with putrescine and cadaverine concentrations being particularly high (Porter and Kenworthy, 1969).

Wilson (1954) examined intestinal and urinary histamine in normal rats and rats treated with antibiotics (aureomycin, chloramphenicol, penicillin, phthalylsuphathiazole). Histamine concentrations were 45% less in antibiotic-treated rats compared with their normal counterparts. Histamine concentrations in the mucosa and lumen were also significantly lower in germfree mice than in conventional or monoassociated mice (Beaver and Wostmann, 1962). Histamine is vasoactive and in the intestine causes smooth muscle contraction and increases gastric acid secretion, mucosal blood flow, goblet cell secretion, and intestinal permeability. There are multiple mechanisms whereby these effects either singularly or in combination might affect intestinal functions pertinent to animal growth efficiency, none of which has been examined in that regard.

b. Ammonia

Ammonia is a toxic catabolite of microbial amino acid deamination and urea hydrolysis (Visek, 1981; 1984). Approximately 40% of the urea synthesized by the liver is hydrolyzed to ammonia by bacterial urease (Drasar and Hill, 1974). A wide range of intestinal bacteria exhibit urease activity and there is indication that urea hydrolysis is carried out by epitheliam-associated organisms as is the case for bacterial urease in the rumen (Suzuki et al., 1979). Detailed studies have not been conducted in the pig. Ammonia is normally absorbed from the colon and detoxified via reconversion to urea in the liver. However, ammonia concentrations in the colon of conventional animals are several times that required for cytopathic effects, indicating that ammonia produced by bacterial urease could have substantial physiological effects at concentrations occurring naturally (Visek, 1978a). Indeed, there is evidence that microbial hydrolysis of urea and the resulting high concentrations of ammonia depress growth. Ammonia increases epithelial cell turnover by affecting cellular intermediary metabolism and DNA synthesis (Visek, 1972; 1978b). Urea hydrolysis does not occur in germfree animals (Levenson et al., 1959) and portal ammonia concentrations were only 25% of that found in conventional control animals (Warren and Newton, 1959). Mucosal cell turnover is also substantially reduced in germfree animals (Galjaard et al., 1972). Rats and chicks immunized against urease have lower *in vivo* urease activity, lower ammonia concentrations, and faster growth than nonimmunized controls (Dang and Visek, 1960). Growth efficiency was also improved in pigs fed ion-exchange resins capable of adsorbing ammonia (Pond and Yen, 1987; Veldman and Van der Aar, 1997). Visek (1978b) proposed that reduction of microbially produced ammonia is a primary mechanism for the growth response induced by feed antibiotics. Ammonia is preferentially used as a nitorgen source by a number of anaerobic bacteria in the presence of fermentable carbohydrate (Bryant and Robinson, 1962; Bryant, 1974). Accordingly, the provision of fermentable carbohydrates increases ammonia use by gut bacteria thereby reducing lumen concentrations of ammonia (Weber, 1979; Weber et al., 1987).

c. Phenols and indoles

A range of phenolic and indolic compounds are produced by intestinal bacteria from the aromatic amino acids phenylalanine, tyrosine, and tryptophan (Macfarlane and Macfarlane, 1995). *Bacteroides*, *Lactobacillus*, *Clostridium*, and *Bifidobacterium* are thought to be the major intestinal genera that metabolize aromatic amino acids (Macfarlane and Macfarlane, 1995). It has long been known that gut bacteria are capable of producing, via tyrosine metabolism, several highly toxic phenolic compounds including phenol itself, *p*-cresol, 4-ethylphenol, and hydroxylated phenol-substituted fatty acids (Baumann, 1879; Folin and Denis, 1915; Bakke and Midtvedt, 1970). Phenolic compounds are usually absorbed in the colon and detoxified via glucuronide and sulfate conjugation in the colonic mucosa or the liver, and then excreted in urine (Ramakrishna et al., 1989; 1991). In humans, a range of 50 to 160 mg of volatile phenols are excreted per day, with p-cresol being the major urinary phenol (Schmidt, 1949). A quantitative relationship between dietary protein intake, and specifically dietary tyrosine, and urinary phenol excretion has been demonstrated repeatedly (Folin and Denis, 1915; Bernhardt and Zilliken, 1958; Geypens et al., 1997). However, urinary phenol and p-cresol concentrations were unchanged in response to fasting (Bures et al., 1990). Thus, urinary phenol and p-cresol excretion does not depend entirely on oral dietary protein intake, but may also reflect metabolism of endogenous substrates by intestinal bacteria. A negative correlation between urinary p-cresol concentrations and body weight gain was observed in weanling pigs, suggesting that microbially-produced p-cresol may decrease growth (Yokoyama et al., 1982). Also, fecal and urinary excretion of phenolic and aromatic compounds, particularly p-cresol, were decreased in weanling pigs fed an antibiotic mixture (aureomycin, sulfamethazine, penicillin; Yokoyama et al., 1982), and treatment of rats with oral neomycin resulted in a 96% reduction in urinary phenol excretion (Bakke, 1969). Similarly, an inverse relationship between volatile phenol excretion and weight gain in rats fed a 10% tyrosine-supplemented diet was reversed in rats also receiving chlortetracycline (Bernhardt and Zilliken, 1958). Reduced bacterial production of phenolic compounds is therefore a potential mechanism underlying growth promotion by antibiotics. Most of the basic questions relating to the effects of microbial production of phenols in the pig intestine remain unanswered, including the taxonomy, ecology, and metabolic properties of target bacteria. Additional growth trials specifically addressing the hypothesis that bacterially-generated tyrosine catabolites may decrease growth potential would also be useful and should perhaps precede efforts to describe microbiological contributions precisely.

Phenylacetate and phenylpropionate are produced from phenylalanine, whereas indole (indican) and 3-methylindole (skatole) are the principal end products of tryptophan metabolism. Skatole has received considerable attention because of its primary contribution to "boar taint." Skatole is partially absorbed from the intestine (Agergaard and Laue, 1993, as cited by Jensen et al., 1995) and subsequently degraded in the liver, with the degradation products being excreted in urine (Friis, 1993, as cited by Jensen et al., 1995). Undegraded skatole is deposited in fat and muscle, and in high concentrations accounts for the unpleasant smell and taste of meat from uncastrated male pigs (Lundstrom et al., 1988). Jensen et al. (1995) demonstrated that skatole production depends on the amount of protein entering the large intestine and the proteolytic activity of the intestinal microbiota.

2. Bile Acid Biotransformation

Primary bile acids (e.g., cholic acid and chenodeoxycholic acid) are synthesized from cholesterol in the liver and are conjugated to either glycine or taurine. The types and proportions of bile acids vary widely among animal species (Baron and Hylemon, 1997). Under physiological conditions, conjugated and free bile acids exist as their sodium or potassium salts. The bile salts are crucial for fat absorption. Greater than 95% of the bile acids secreted in bile are absorbed from the ileum into the hepatic portal venous system by an active transport mechanism after transit through the small intestine (Lack and Weiner, 1961). Those bile acids escaping active absorption are biotransformed by bacterial enzymes during passage through the distal intestine. For example, fecal bile acids are completely deconjugated and contain, in addition to small amounts of primary bile acids, a range of secondary bile acids, generated by bacterial oxioreduction of the hydroxyl groups (yielding keto bile acids and the β-hydroxylated bile acids) and by bacterial dehydroxylation (Hill and Aries, 1971). Some deconjugated or free bile acids may be absorbed by passive diffusion from the small or large intestine (Samuel et al., 1968) and are subsequently reconjugated in the liver and resecreted in the bile.

Bile acids are not deconjugated in the gut of germfree animals, demonstrating the important role of intestinal bacteria in this process (Madsen et al., 1976). Further, the half-life of cholic acid in the bile acid pool is five times longer in germfree than in normal rats, and colonization of germfree rats with deconjugated and dehyroxylating strains of bacteria restores secondary bile acids in feces (Gustafsson et al., 1968). Microbial deconjugation and dehydroxylation of bile both impairs lipid absorption by the host animal (DeSomer et al., 1963; Eyssen, 1973) and produces toxic degradation products (Baron and Hylemon, 1997) that can impair growth (Eyssen and DeSomer, 1963a). Because bile acid hydrolysis products are reduced or abolished by antibiotics, it has been suggested that inhibition of microbial bile acid biotransformation in the gut is an important mechanism whereby antibiotics enhance animal growth (Visek, 1978a; Feighner and Dashkevicz, 1987; 1988). Using chicks, Eyssen and DeSomer (1963b) first suggested that bile acid transformation products might represent bacterial products that decrease growth. Fuller and co-workers (1984) provided additional evidence, also from chick studies, that bile acid deconjugation by gut bacteria causes a decrease in growth that is reversible by antibiotic supplementation. Decreased concentrations of lithocholic acid and corresponding increases in average daily gain and feed efficiency were also demonstrated in antibiotic-treated pigs, consistent with work reported for poultry (Tracy and Jensen, 1987).

Although other bacteria, such as *Bacteroides*, *Bifidobacterium*, and *Clostridium* spp. possess bile salt hydrolase activity, lactobacilli inhabiting the small intestine seem to be largely responsible for bile salt hydrolysis (reviewed by Baron and Hylemon, 1997). For example, elimination of lactobacilli from the microbiota reduced ileal bile salt hydrolase activity in conventional mice by 86%, and by greater than 98% when both lactobacilli and enterococci were eliminated (Tannock et al., 1989). The microbiology and physiology of bile acid transformation in pigs is yet another area in need of enhanced research efforts.

Bile salts have been found recently to stimulate mucin secretion from epithelial cell lines in a dose-dependent fashion according to their degree of hydrophobicity (Klinkspoor et al., 1999). Hydrophobic bile salts were found to be more potent than hydrophilic bile salts. Therefore, unconjugated bile salts were more effective in stimulating mucin secretion. It has been suggested that regulation of mucin secretion by bile salts might be a common mechanism by which the epithelium protects itself from the toxic action of bile salts to which they are exposed throughout the GI tract (Klinkspoor et al., 1999). The possibility that microbial bile acid transformation may indirectly stimulate mucin secretion heightens the importance of identifying the bacterial groups and mechanisms involved.

3. Mucin Degradation

Bacterially mediated degradation of the intestinal mucus layer not only compromises the defensive properties of this important physical barrier to luminal antigens, but it also represents a cost in the energy and nitrogen budgets of the growing intestine. Specifically, it is estimated that in the small intestine alone, at least 30% of the overall protein synthetic activity is devoted to the production of proteins, including the mucins and digestive enzymes, that are lost into the intestinal lumen (Simon et al., 1982; de Lange et al., 1990; Reeds et al., 1993). Further, goblet cell loss and renewal contribute significantly to the high degree of daily epithelial turnover, estimated as 25% of the villus epithelium (Reeds et al., 1993). It has been argued (Reeds, 1990) that the failure to recapture intestinal secretions not only represents a continual protein synthetic drain but also may influence the specificity of amino acid requirements, particularly in the case of the mucins, which contain a disproportionate content of serine, threonine, and proline residues. Although it is not known if goblet cell numbers or mucus secretion are increased directly in response to bacterially mediated attrition, the sensitive nature of goblet cells, in general, to luminal perturbations such as inflammation is becoming clear (Ganessunker et al., 1999). Certainly, host efforts to reconstitute or reinforce the mucus barrier in response to bacterial translocation into the lamina propria and subsequent subepithelial inflammation is easily perceived as being a beneficial response pathway. In fact, the so-called state of physiological inflammation that is manifest constitutively in the intestine may well explain the high degree of cell and mucus turnover via epithelial and goblet cell responses to cytokines or other bioactive molecules expressed by resident lamina propria cells.

Mucin degradation is a multistep process that begins with proteolysis of the nonglycosylated "naked" regions of mucin glycoproteins via host and microbial proteases (reviewed by Quigley and Kelly, 1995). This initial step markedly reduces mucin gelation and viscosity and results in the accumulation of highly glycosylated subunits (≥ 500 kDa) that are resistant to further proteolytic attack. Mucin glycopeptides are then degraded by a variety of bacterial enzymes corrresponding to the complexity of the oligosaccharide chains, which differ in size, degree of branching, type of linkage, and the presence of terminal sialic acid or sulfate groups. For example, terminal sulfate and sialic acid residues are cleaved by bacterial sialidases and glycosulfatases, and oligosaccharide side chains are degraded by linkage-specific glycosidases (Salyers et al., 1977; Hoskins, 1992). It is generally thought, although not well documented, that mucin degradation *in vivo* is performed by bacterial consortia comprising various genera that together provide the range of hydrolytic enzymes required.

Of particular interest is evidence from humans that resident mucolytic bacteria may differ among individuals according to the specific carbohydrate composition of intestinal mucins (e.g., terminal sugars or branching patterns), which seems to vary by genetic background (Hoskins et al., 1985). Evidence of host genetic background influencing bacterial community profiles has not been reported for other mammalian species. However, such a finding would be consistent with increasing evidence of stable and host-specific microbial community profiles (McCartney et al., 1996; Zoetendal et al., 1998), and with evidence that endogenous substrates may have a greater influence on the spatial pattern of bacterial population profiles along the GI tract than exogenous nutrients (Deplancke et al., 2000). Because of its complexity, the microbiology of mucus colonization and degradation will most efficiently be defined through the use of novel molecular ecology techniques.

V. MOLECULAR ECOLOGY

Two major problems faced by microbiologists studying the intestinal ecosystem are the unavoidable bias introduced by culture-based enumeration and characterization techniques, and the lack of a phylogentically based classification scheme. Modern molecular techniques that are based on sequence comparisons of nucleic acids can be used to provide molecular characterization, while at the same time providing a classification system that predicts natural evolutionary relationships (Woese et al., 1990; Stahl, 1993; Pace, 1997). The field of molecular microbial ecology is defined as the application of molecular technology, usually based on comparative nucleic acid sequence information, to identify specific microorganisms in a particular environment, to assign functional roles to these specific microorganisms, and to assess their significance or contribution to specific environmental processes.

Molecular ecology methods are most often based on comparative sequence analysis of small subunit ribosomal RNA (16S rRNA) molecules (Amann et al., 1995; Figure 26.1). Extensive comparative sequence analysis of 16S rRNA molecules representing a wide diversity of microorganisms has revealed that different regions of the molecule vary in sequence conservation. The variable regions allow the design of general and specific oligonucleotide hybridization probes. Oligonucleotides complementing regions of universally conserved 16S rRNA sequence (universal probes) are useful for quantifying the 16S rRNA from any source, whereas oligonucleotides complementing more variable regions of sequences are useful as selective probes (species-, genus-, or phylogenetic group-specific probes). A rRNA-based analysis of a microbial population or community relies on the techniques of nucleic acid amplification, cloning, and sequencing to acquire data on rRNA sequences directly from environmental samples (e.g., intestinal sample). The sequence information obtained is compared with an existing sequence database to place the novel sequence (bacterial group or species) within existing phylogenetic classification schemes. Subsequently, specific oligonucleotide probes can be designed and used for detection, quantification of cell abundance and activity, and the study of spatial and temporal distributions of newly identified organisms.

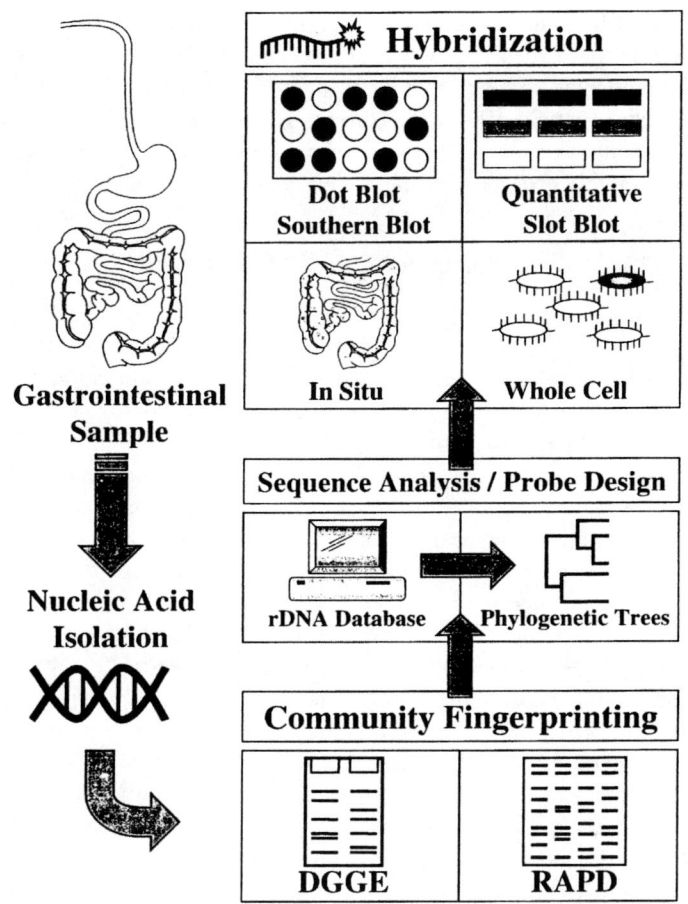

FIGURE 26.1 Diagram of molecular approaches for the detection and phylogenetic identification of microbial groups or species in gastrointestinal microbial ecosystems. Molecular microbial ecology techniques are based typically on the informational content inherent in RNA molecules. Refer to the reviews by Woese et al. (1990), Stahl (1993), Amann et al. (1995), and Pace (1997) for details. Abbreviations: DGGE, denaturing gradient gel electrophoresis; RAPD, random amplified polymorphic DNA. (From Mackie, R. I. et al., *Am. J. Clin. Nutr.*, 69:1035S, 1999. With permission.)

A new approach for directly determining the genetic diversity of complex microbial populations is based on electrophoresis of polymerase chain reaction–amplified 16S rRNA fragments in polyacrylamide gels containing a linear gradient of denaturants. In denaturing gradient gel electrophoresis (DGGE), DNA fragments of the same length but different base-pair sequences can be separated (Muyzer et al., 1993). This procedure has been applied to the analysis of polymerase chain reaction fragments derived from the variable regions of 16S rRNA (Muyzer et al., 1993). These fragments can be obtained after amplification of 16S rRNA genes from genomic DNA from uncharacterized mixtures of microorganisms. The utility and limitations of the DGGE technique for the study of the intestinal microbiota of the pig is considered in depth in a recent paper by Simpson et al. (1999).

Microscopic visualization of individual population members *in situ* has used fluorescent-dye or enzyme-conjugated oligonucleotide probes (Amann et al., 1995). After hybridization to fixed whole cells, the probes are specifically retained by those cells containing complementary rRNA molecules. Cells that retain labeled probes can be visualized by fluorescence microscopy, even in a complex community background. In addition, the amount of fluorescence conferred to single-cells by probe hybridization can be quantified using flow cytometry or digital microscopy. Quantification of single cell fluorescence can be used to estimate the *in situ* growth rate of natural populations because ribosome number, and, consequently, the rRNA content, varies in proportion to growth rate (Langendijk et al., 1995). By combining the use of several oligonucleotide probes, specific for different populations of interest and labeled with different fluorescent dyes, the spatial positioning of various members of a microbial community also can be studied (Amann et al., 1995).

VI. SUMMARY AND OUTLOOK

The intestinal microbiota provides important protective functions for its host. Indigenous bacteria are capable of directly blocking enteric pathogens from colonizing the intestine, and they are the primary stimuli for the development and maintenance of a local and multitiered defense system comprising a full array of innate and acquired immunological functions. The intestinal microbiota also contributes to host nutrition through the production of SCFA, vitamins, and amino acids. However, the cooperative or beneficial effects of the normal microbiota come at a cost to the host in terms of nutrient utilization, epithelial and mucus turnover, detoxification of bacterial catabolites, and the continual production of resident inflammatory and immune cells. The costs of maintaining a balanced relationship, or state of détente, between the host and its intestinal microbiota becomes a key consideration when maximizing the efficiency of animal growth is a primary objective.

Numerous management practices likely directly or indirectly destabilize host–microbiota relationships, resulting in intestinal inflammation and possibly disruption of normal growth. Management practices having a direct influence on the microbiota include diet changes associated with life cycle feeding strategies and the inclusion of oral antibiotics in animal diets. Indeed, the growth-promoting effects of antibiotics are consistent with the possibility that the normal microbiota negatively impacts the energetics of animal growth. However, surprisingly little is known about the effects of subtherapeutic levels of antibiotics on the normal gut microbiota. Management practices possibly having an indirect influence on microbial stability in the gut include those that disrupt normal feed and water intake patterns because of the stresses associated with herd rearrangement or relocation through the production life cycle. Often, herd rearrangement and diet changes are implemented concurrently and accompanied by overt intestinal inflammation.

These issues bring to mind the concept of an optimal microbiota for intestinal health vs. the efficiency of gastrointestinal and whole-body growth throughout the productive life cycle of a pig. However, many key questions require answers before the concept of an optimal gut microbiota for animal growth can be transferred to practical applications for the pig industry. For example, little is known about either bacterial cues or host-response pathways that underlie host–microbe homeostasis. The microbial groups colonizing the mucus layer and the epithelial surface remain undefined. There is no information on animal-to-animal variation in microbiota profiles, particularly in relation to individual variation in growth efficiency among animals. The stability of microbial population profiles within individual pigs throughout the production life cycle is unknown. The influence of diet on microbial populations is poorly understood, particularly those habitats (e.g., small intestine) that may compete with the host for nutrients or otherwise decrease growth. The nutritional costs to the host of the microbiota at various developmental stages remain undefined, as does the energetic costs associated with intestinal inflammation in response to disruption of normal host–microbe relationships. The arrival of molecular-based microbial ecology techniques provides exciting new options for finally addressing such questions. Answers should enable careful reconsideration of the role of the intestine as a growth-regulating organ. Novel strategies to enhance the efficiency of growth in livestock species may be identified in the process.

REFERENCES

Agergaard, N., and A. Laue. 1993. Absorption from the gastrointestinal tract and liver turnover of skatole. In *Measurement and Prevention of Boar Taint in Entire Male Pigs*, Institut de la Recherche Agronomique, Bonneau, M., Ed., colloques 60, Roskilde, Denmark, 107–111.

Allison, C., and G. T. Macfarlane. 1989. Influence of pH, nutrient availability and growth rate on amine production by *Bacteroides fragilis* and *Clostridium perfringens* in batch and continuous culture, *Appl. Environ. Microbiol.*, 55:2894.

Allison, M. J., I. M. Robinson, J. A. Bucklin, and G. D. Booth. 1979. Comparison of bacterial populations of the pig cecum and colon based upon enumeration with specific energy sources, *Appl. Environ. Microbiol.*, 37:1142.

Aly, R., and H. R. Shinefield. 1982. *Bacterial Interference*, CRC Press, Boca Raton, FL.

Amann, R. I., W. Ludwig, and K.-H. Schleifer. 1995. Phylogenetic identification and *in situ* detection of individual microbial cells without cultivation, *Microbiol. Rev.*, 59:143.

Anugwa, F. O. I., V. H. Varel, J. S. Dickson, W. G. Pond, and L. P. Krook. 1989. Effects of dietary fiber and protein concentration on growth, feed efficiency, visceral organ weights and large intestine microbial populations of swine, *J. Nutr.*, 119:879.

Babu, S., H. Chandler, U. K. Batish, and K. L. Bhatia. 1986. Factors affecting amine production in *Streptococcus cremoris*, *Food Microbiol.*, 3:359.

Bakke, O. M. 1969. The effect of neomycin and experimental coprostasis on the excretion of simple phenols in the rat, *Scand. J. Gastroenterol.*, 4:419.

Bakke, O. M., and T. Midtvedt. 1970. Influence of germ-free status on the excretion of simple phenols of possible significance in tumor production, *Experientia*, 26:519.

Baron, S. F., and P. B. Hylemon. 1997. Biotransformation of bile acids, cholesterol, and steroid hormones. In *Gastrointestinal Microbiology*, Vol. 1, Mackie, R. I., B. A. White, and R. E. Isaacson, Eds., Chapman & Hall, New York.

Baumann, E. 1879. Über die Bildung von Hydroparacumarsäure aus Tyrosin, *Ber. Itsch. Chem. Ges.*, 12:1450.

Bealmear, P. M. 1980. Host defense mechanisms in gnotobiotic animals. In *Immunologic Defects in Laboratory Animals*, Vol. 2, Gershwin, E., and B. Marchant, Eds., Plenum Press, New York.

Beaver, H. M., and B. S. Wostmann. 1962. Histamine and 5-hydroxytryptamine in the intestinal tract of germfree animals, animals harbouring one microbial species and conventional animals, *Br. J. Pharmacol.*, 19:385.

Belley, A., K. Keller, M. Goettke, and K. Chadee. 1999. Intestinal mucins in colonization and host defense against pathogens, *Am. J. Trop. Med. Hyg.*, 60:10.

Berg, R. D. 1996. The indigenous gastrointestinal microflora, *Trends Microbiol.*, 4:430.

Bernhardt, F. W., and A. Zilliken. 1958. Effect of dietary carbohydrate and chlortetracycline on growth and excretion of phenols in rats fed extra tyrosine, *Arch. Biochem. Biophys.*, 82:462.

Bry, L., P. G. Falk, T. Midtvedt, and J. I. Gordon. 1996. A model of host-microbial interactions in an open mammalian system, *Science*, 273:1380.

Bryant, M. P. 1974. Nutritional features and ecology of predominant anaerobic bacteria of the intestinal tract, *Am. J. Clin. Nutr.*, 27:1313.

Bryant, M. P., and I. M. Robinson. 1962. Some nutritional characteristics of predominant culturable ruminal bacteria, *J. Bacteriol.*, 84:605.

Bures, J., Z. Jergeova, L. Sobotka, B. Cervenka, F. Malir, J. Horacek, Z. Zadak, O. Komarkova, and B. Fixa. 1990. Excretion of phenol and p-cresol in the urine in fasting obese individuals and in persons treated with total enteral nutrition, *Cas. Lek. Cesk.*, 129:1166.

Butine, T. J., and J. A. Z. Leedle. 1989. Enumeration of selected anaerobic bacterial groups in cecal and colonic contents of growing-finishing pigs, *Appl. Environ. Microbiol.*, 55:1112.

Cebra, J. J., P. J. Gearhart, J. F. Halsey, J. L. Hurwitz, and R. D. Shahin. 1980. Role of environmental antigens in the ontogeny of the secretory immune response, *J. Reticuloendothelial Soc.*, 28:61s.

Clemens, E. T., C. E. Stevens, and M. Southworth. 1975. Sites of organic acid production and pattern of digesta movement in the gastrointestinal tract of swine, *J. Nutr.*, 105:759.

Croitoru, K., and P. B. Ernst. 1993. Intraepithelial lymphocyte lineage and function. In *Mucosal Immunology: Intraepithelial Lymphocytes*, Kiyono, H., and J. R. McGhee, Jr., Eds., Raven Press, New York.

Dang, H. C., and W. J. Visek. 1960. Effect of urease injection on body weights of growing rats and chicks, *Proc. Soc. Exp. Biol. Med.*, 105:164.

de Lange, C. F. M., W. B. Souffrant, and W. C. Sauer. 1990. Real ileal and amino acid digestibilities in feedstuffs from growing pigs as determined with the ^{15}N-isotope dilution technique, *J. Anim. Sci.*, 68:409.

Deplancke, B., K. R. Hristova, H. A. Oakley, V. J. McCracken, R. I. Aminov, R. I. Mackie, and H. R. Gaskins. 2000. Molecular ecological analysis of I. the succession and diversity of sulfate-reducing bacteria in the mouse gastrointestinal tract, *Appl. Environ. Microbiol.*, 66:2166.

DeSomer, P., H. Eyssen, and E. Evard. 1963. The influence of antibiotics on fecal fats in chickens. In *Biochemical Problems of Lipids*, Frazer, A. C., Ed., Elsevier/North Holland, Amsterdam.

Drasar, B. S., and M. J. Hill. 1974. *Human Intestinal Flora*, Academic Press, London.

Dubos, R., R. W. Schaedler, R. Costello, and P. Hoet. 1965. Indigenous, normal and autochthonous flora of the gastrointestinal tract, *J. Exp. Med.*, 122:67.

Dunsford, B. R., W. E. Haensly, and D. A. Knabe. 1991. Effects of diet on acidic and neutral goblet cell populations in the small intestine of early-weaned pigs, *Am. J. Vet. Res.*, 52:1743.

Ebner, S., P. A. Schoknecht, P. J. Reeds, and D. G. Burrin. 1994. Growth and metabolism of gastrointestinal and skeletal muscle tissues in protein-malnourished neonatal pigs, *Am. J. Physiol.*, 267:R221.

Edelstone, D. I., and I. R. Holzman. 1981. Gastrointestinal tract O_2 uptake and regional blood flows during digestion in conscious newborn lambs, *Am. J. Physiol.*, 241:G289.

Eyssen, H. 1973. Role of gut microflora in metabolism of lipids and sterols, *Proc. Nutr. Soc.*, 32:59.

Eyssen, H., and P. DeSomer. 1963a. Toxicity of lithocholic acid for the chick, *Poult. Sci.*, 42:1020.

Eyssen, H., and P. DeSomer. 1963b. The mode of action of antibiotics in stimulating growth in chicks, *J. Exp. Med.*, 117:127.

Feighner, S. D., and M. P. Dashkevicz. 1987. Subtherapeutic levels of antibiotics in poultry feeds and their effects on weight gain, feed efficiency, and bacterial cholyltaurine hydrolase activity, *Appl. Environ. Microbiol.*, 53:331.

Feighner, S. D., and M. P. Dashkevicz. 1988. Effect of dietary carbohydrates on bacterial cholyltaurine hydrolase in poultry intestinal homogenates, *Appl. Environ. Microbiol.*, 54:337.

Fewins, B. G., L. G. M. Newland, and C. A. E. Briggs. 1957. The normal intestinal flora of the pig. III. Qualitative studies of lactobacilli and streptococci, *J. Appl. Bacteriol.*, 20:234.

Folin, O., and W. Denis. 1915. The excretion of free and conjugated phenols and phenol deriviatives, *J. Biol. Chem.*, 22:309.

Forstner, J. F., M. G. Oliver, and F. A. Sylvester. 1995. Production, structure, and biologic relevance of gastrointestinal mucins. In *Infections of the Gastrointestinal Tract*, Blaser, M. J., P. D. Smith, J. I. Ravdin, H. D. Greenberg, and R. L. Guerrant, Eds., Raven Press, New York.

Friis, C. 1993. Distribution, metabolic fate and elimination of skatole in the pig. In *Measurement and Prevention of Boar Taint in Entire Male Pigs*, Bonneau, M., Ed., Colloques 60, Institut de la Recherche Agronomique, Roskilde, Denmark, 113–115.

Freter, R. 1956. Experimental enteric *Shigella* and *Vibrio* infections in mice and guinea pigs, *J. Exp. Med.*, 104:411.

Freter, R. 1983. Mechanisms that control the microflora in the large intestine. In *Human Intestinal Microflora in Health and Disease*, Hentges, D. J., Ed., Academic Press, New York.

Freter, R. 1992. Factors affecting the microecology of the gut. In *Probiotics — The Scientific Basis*, Fuller, R., Ed., Chapman & Hall, New York.

Fuller, M. F., and P. J. Reeds. 1998. Nitrogen cycling in the gut, *Annu. Rev. Nutr.*, 18:385.

Fuller, R., C. B. Cole, and M. E. Coates. 1984. The role of *Streptococcus faecium* in antibiotic-relieved growth depression in chickens. In *Antimicrobials and Agriculture*, Woodbine, M., Ed., Butterworths, London.

Galjaard, H., W. van der Meer-Fieggen, and J. Giesen. 1972. Feedback control by functional villus cells on cell proliferation and maturation in intestinal epithelium, *Exp. Cell Res.*, 73:197.

Ganessunker, D., H. R. Gaskins, F. A. Zuckermann, and S. M. Donovan. 1999. Total parenteral nutrition alters intestinal immune cell composition in neonatal piglets, *J. Parenter. Enteral Nutr.*, 23:337.

Gaskins, H. R. 1997. Immunological aspects of host/microbiota interactions at the intestinal epithelium. In *Gastrointestinal Microbiology*, Vol. 2, Mackie, R. I., B. A. White, and R. E. Isaacson, Eds., Chapman & Hall, New York.

Geypens, B., D. Claus, P. Evenepoel, M. Hiele, B. Maes, M. Peeters, P. Rutgeerts, and Y. Ghoos. 1997. Influence of dietary protein supplements on the formation of bacterial metabolites in the colon, *Gut*, 41:70.

Gordon, H. A., E. Bruckner-Kardoss, T. E. Staley, M. Wagner, and B. S. Wostmann. 1966. Characteristics of the germfree rat, *Acta Anat.*, 64:367.

Grieshop, C. M., D. E. Reese, and G. C. Fahey, Jr. 2000. Nonstarch polysaccharides and oligosaccharides in swine nutrition. In *Swine Nutrition*, Lewis, A. J., and L. L. Southern, Eds., CRC Press, Boca Raton, FL.

Gustafsson, J.-A. 1968. Steroids in germ free and conventional rats. Identification of C_{19} and C_{21} steroids in faeces from conventional rats, *Eur. J. Biochem.*, 6:248.

Guy-Grand, D., B. Rocha, and P. Vassalli. 1993. Origin and development of gut intraepithelial lymphocytes. In *Mucosal Immunology: Intraepithelial Lymphocytes*, Kiyono, H., and J. R. McGhee, Eds., Raven Press, New York.

Hill, M. J., and V. C. Aries. 1971. Faecal steroid composition and its relationship to cancer of the large bowel, *J. Pathol.*, 104:129.

Hinterleitner, T. A., and D. W. Powell. 1991. Immune system control of intestinal ion transport, *Proc. Soc. Exp. Biol. Med.*, 197:249.

Hoskins, L. C. 1992. Mucin degradation in the human gastrointestinal tract and its significance to enteric microbial ecology, *Eur. J. Gastroenterol. Hepatol.*, 5:205.

Hoskins, L. C., M. Augustines, W. B. McKee, E. T. Boulding, M. Kriaris, and G. Niedermeyer. 1985. Mucin degradation in human colon ecosystems. Isolation and properties of fecal strains that degrade ABH blood group antigens and oligosaccharides from mucin glycoproteins, *J. Clin. Invest.*, 75:944.

Hungate, R. E. 1960. Microbial ecology of the rumen, *Bacteriol. Rev.*, 24:353.

Jensen, B. B., and H. Jørgensen. 1994. Effect of dietary fiber on microbial activity and microbial gas production in various regions of the gastrointestinal tract of pigs, *Appl. Environ. Microbiol.*, 60:1897.

Jensen, M. T., R. P. Cox, and B. B. Jensen. 1995. Microbial production of skatole in the hind gut of pigs given different diets and its relation to skatole deposition in backfat, *Anim. Sci.*, 61:293.

Kagnoff, M. F. 1993. Immunology of the intestinal tract, *Gastroenterology*, 105:1275.

Klinkspoor, J. H., K. S. Mok, B. J.-W. Van Kilinken, G. N. J. Tygat, S. P. Lee, and A. K. Groen. 1999. Mucin secretion by the human colon cell line LS174T is regulated by bile salts, *Glycobiology*, 9:13.

Kraehenbuhl, J.-P., and M. R. Neutra. 1992. Molecular and cellular basis of immune protection of mucosal surfaces, *Physiol. Rev.*, 72:853.

Lack, L., and I. M. Weiner. 1961. *In vitro* absorption of bile salts by small intestine of rats and guinea pigs, *Am. J. Physiol.*, 200:313.

Lærke, H. N., and B. B. Jensen. 1999. D-Tagatose has low small intestinal digestibility but high large intestinal fermentability in pigs, *J. Nutr.*, 129:1002.

Langendijk, P., F. Schut, G. J. Jansen, G. C. Raangs, G. R. Camphuis, M. F. Wilkinson, and G. W. Welling. 1995. Quantitative fluorescence *in situ* hybridization of *Bifidobacterium* spp. with genus-specific 16S rRNA-targeted probes and its application in fecal samples, *Appl. Environ. Microbiol.*, 61:3069.

Lee, A. 1984. Neglected niches: the microbial ecology of the gastrointestinal tract. In *Advances in Microbial Ecology*, Marshall, K., Ed., Plenum Press, New York.

Levenson, S. M., L. V. Crowley, R. E. Horowitz, and O. J. Malm. 1959. The metabolism of carbon-labeled urea in the germfree rat, *J. Biol. Chem.*, 234:2061.

Livesay, G. 1992. The energy values of dietary fibre and sugar alcohols for man, *Nutr. Res. Rev.*, 5:61.

Lloyd, A. B., R. B. Cummings, and R. D. Kent. 1977. Prevention of *Salmonella typhimurium* infection in poultry by pretreatment of chickens and poults with intestinal extracts, *Aust. Vet. J.*, 53:82.

Loesche, W. J., and R. J. Gibbons. 1968. Amino acid fermentation by *Fusobacterium nucleatum*, *Arch. Oral Biol.*, 13:191.

Lundström, K., B. Malmfors, G. Malmfors, S. Stern, H. Petersson, A. B. Mortensen, and S. E. Sørenson. 1988. Skatole, androstenone and taint in boars fed two different diets, *Livest. Prod. Sci.*, 18:55.

Macfarlane, S., and G. T. Macfarlane. 1995. Proteolysis and amino acid fermentation. In *Human Colonic Bacteria: Role in Nutrition, Physiology, and Pathology*, Gibson, G. R., and G. T. Macfarlane, Eds., CRC Press, Boca Raton, FL.

Mackie, R. I., A. Sghir, and H. R. Gaskins. 1999. Developmental microbial ecology of the neonatal gastro-intestinal tract, *Am. J. Clin. Nutr.*, 69:1035S.

Madsen, D., M. Beaver, L. Chang, E. Bruckner-Kardoss, and B. S. Wostmann. 1976. Analysis of bile acids in conventional and germfree rats, *J. Lipid Res.*, 17:107.

Matsuo, K., H. Ota, T. Akamatsu, A. Sugiyama, and T. Katsuyama. 1997. Histochemistry of the surfus mucous layer of the human colon, *Gut*, 40:782.

McCartney, A., W. Wenzhi, and G. Tannock. 1996. Molecular analysis of the composition of the bifidobacterial and *Lactobacillus* microflora of humans, *Appl. Environ. Microbiol.*, 62:4608.

McCracken, V. J., and H. R. Gaskins. 1999. Intestinal microbes and the immune system. In *Probiotics: A Critical Review*, Tannock, G. W., Ed., Horizon Scientific Press, Norfolk, U.K.

McCracken, B. A., M. E. Spurlock, M. A. Roos, F. A. Zuckermann, and H. R. Gaskins. 1999. Weaning anorexia induces local inflammation in the piglet small intestine, *J. Nutr.*, 129:613.

McNurlan, M. A., and P. J. Garlick. 1980. Contribution of liver and gastrointestinal tract to muscle: competitors or collaborators, *Proc. Nutr. Soc.*, 52:57.

Mestecky, J. 1987. The common mucosal immune system and current strategies for induction of immune response in external secretions, *J. Clin. Immunol.*, 7:265.

Moore, W. E. C., L. V. H. Moore, E. P. Cato, T. D. Wilkins, and E. T. Kornegay. 1987. Effect of high-fiber and high-oil diets on the fecal flora of swine, *Appl. Environ. Microbiol.*, 53:1638.

Morris, D. R., and E. A. Boeker. 1983. Biosynthetic and biodegradative ornithine and arginine decarboxylase from *Escherichia coli*, *Meth. Enzymol.*, 94:125.

Mostov, K. E. 1994. Transepithelial transport of immunoglobulins, *Annu. Rev. Immunol.*, 12:63.

Muyzer, G., E. C. de Waal, and A. G. Uitterlinden. 1993. Profiling of complex microbial populations by denaturing gradient gel electrophoresis analysis of polymerase chain reaction-amplified genes coding for 16S rRNA, *Appl. Environ. Microbiol.*, 59:695.

Neutra, M. R., and J. F. Forstner. 1987. Gastrointestinal mucus: synthesis, secretion and function. In *Physiology of the Gastrointestinal Tract*, 2nd ed., Johnson, L. R., Ed., Raven Press, New York.

Neutra, M. R., L. J. O'Malley, and R. D. Specian. 1982. Regulation of intestinal goblet cell secretion. II. A survey of potential secretagogues, *Am. J. Physiol.*, 242:G380.

Nisbet, D. J. 1998. Use of competitive exclusion in food animals, *JAVMA*, 213:1744.

Olubuyide, I. O., R. C. Williamson, J. B. Bristol, and A. E. Read. 1984. Goblet cell hyperplasia is a feature of the adaptive response to jejunoileal bypass in rats, *Gut*, 25:628.

Pabst, R., M. Geist, H. J. Rothkötter, and F. J. Fritz. 1988. Postnatal development and lymphocyte production of jejunal and ileal Peyer's patches in normal and gnotobiotic pigs, *Immunology*, 64:539.

Pace, N. R. 1997. A molecular view of microbial diversity and the biosphere, *Science*, 276:734.

Pond, W. G., and J. T. Yen. 1987. Effect of supplemental carbadox, an antibiotic combination, or clinoptilolite on weight gain and organ weights of growing swine fed maize or rye as the grain sources, *Nutr. Rep. Int.*, 35:801.

Porter, P., and R. Kenworthy. 1969. A study of intestinal and urinary amines in pigs in relation to weaning, *Res. Vet. Sci.*, 10:440.

Potten, C. S., and M. Loefler. 1990. Stem cells: attributes, cycles, spirals, pitfalls and uncertainties: lessons for and from the crypt, *Development*, 110:1001.

Pryde, S. E., A. J. Richardson, C. S. Stewart, and H. J. Flint. 1999. Molecular analysis of the microbial diversity present in the colonic wall, colonic lumen, and cecal lumen of a pig, *Appl. Environ. Microbiol.*, 65:5372.

Quigley, M. E., and S. M. Kelly. 1995. Structure, function, and metabolism of host mucus glycoproteins. In *Human Colonic Bacteria: Role in Nutrition, Physiology, and Pathology*, Gibson, G. R., and G. T. Macfarlane, Eds., CRC Press, Boca Raton, FL.

Ramakrishna, B. S., D. Gee, P. R. Pannal, I. C. Roberts-Thomson, and W. E. W. Roediger. 1989. Estimation of phenolic conjugation by colonic mucosa, *J. Clin. Pathol.*, 42:620.

Ramakrishna, B. S., I. C. Roberts-Thomson, P. R. Pannal, and W. E. W. Roediger. 1991. Impaired sulphation of phenol by the colonic mucosa in quiescent and active ulcerative colitis, *Gut*, 32:46.

Reeds, P. J. 1990. Amino acid needs and protein scoring patterns, *Proc. Nutr. Soc.*, 49:17.

Reeds, P. J., D. G. Burrin, T. A. Davis, and M. L. Fiorotto. 1993. Postnatal growth of gut and whole-body protein synthesis in the rat, *Biochem. J.*, 186:381.

Robinson, I. M., M. J. Allison, and J. A. Bucklin. 1981. Characterization of the cecal bacteria of normal pigs, *Appl. Environ. Microbiol.*, 41:950.

Robinson, I. M., S. C. Whipp, J. A. Bucklin, and M. J. Allison. 1984. Characterization of predominant bacteria from the colons of normal and dysenteric pigs, *Appl. Environ. Microbiol.*, 48:964.

Robinson, J. A., W. J. Smolenski, M. L. Ogilive, and J. P. Peters. 1989. *In vitro* total-gas, CH_4, H_2, volatile fatty acid, and lactate kinetic studies on luminal contents from the small intestine, cecum and colon of the pig, *Appl. Environ. Microbiol.*, 55:2460.

Rolfe, R. 1997. Colonization resistance. In *Gastrointestinal Microbiology*, Vol. 2, Mackie, R. I., B. A. White, and R. E. Isaacson, Eds., Chapman & Hall, New York.

Rothkötter, H. J., and R. Pabst. 1989. Lymphocyte subsets in jejunal and ileal Peyer's patches of normal and gnotobiotic minipigs, *Immunology*, 67:103.

Rothkötter, H. J., H. Ulrich, and R. Pabst. 1991. The postnatal development of gut lamina propria lymphocytes: number, proliferation, and T and B cell subsets in conventional and germ-free pigs, *Pediatr. Res.*, 29:237.

Rothkötter, H. J., T. Kirchhoff, and R. Pabst. 1994. Lymphoid and non-lymphoid cells in the epithelium and lamina propria of intestinal mucosa of pigs, *Gut*, 35:1582.

Russell, E. G. 1979. Types and distribution of anaerobic bacteria in the large intestine of pigs, *Appl. Environ. Microbiol.*, 37:187.

Russell, J. B. 1983. Fermentation of peptides by *Bacteroides ruminicola* B14, *Appl. Environ. Microbiol.*, 45:1566.

Salanitro, J. P., I. G. Blake, and P. A. Muirhead. 1977. Isolation and identification of fecal bacteria from adult swine, *Appl. Environ. Microbiol.*, 33:79.

Salyers, A. A., J. R. Vercellotti, S. E. H. West, and T. D. Wilkins. 1977. Fermentation of mucin and plant polysaccharides by strains of *Bacteroides* from the human colon, *Appl. Environ. Microbiol.*, 33:319.

Samuel, P., G. M. Saypol, E. Meilman, E. H. Mosbach, and M. Chaftzadeh. 1968. Absorption of bile acids from large bowel in man, *J. Clin. Invest.*, 47:2070.

Saunders, D. R., and J. Sillery. 1982. Effect of lactate on structure and function of the rat intestine, *Dig. Dis. Sci.*, 27:33.

Savage, D. C. 1977a. Microbial ecology of the gastrointestinal tract, *Annu. Rev. Microbiol.*, 31:107.

Savage, D. C. 1977b. Interactions between the host and its microbes. In *Microbial Ecology of the Gut*, Clarke, R. T. J., and E. Bauchop, Eds., Academic Press, New York.

Savage, D. C. 1986. Gastrointestinal microflora in mammalian nutrition, *Annu. Rev. Nutr.*, 6:155.

Schmidt, E. G. 1949. Urinary phenols: simultaneous determination of phenol and *p*-cresol in urine, *J. Biol. Chem.*, 179:211.

Sharma, R., and U. Schumaker. 1995. Morphometric analysis of intestinal mucins under different dietary conditions and gut flora in rats, *Dig. Dis. Sci.*, 40:2532.

Simon, O., H. Bergner, R. Munchmeyer, and T. Zebrowska. 1982. Studies on the range of tissue protein synthesis in pigs, the effect of thyroid hormones, *Br. J. Nutr.*, 48:571.

Simpson, J., V. J. McCracken, B. A. White, H. R. Gaskins, and R. I. Mackie. 1999. Optimization of denaturant gradient gel electrophoresis for the analysis of the porcine gastrointestinal microbiota, *J. Microbiol. Meth.*, 36:167.

Smith, H. W., and J. E. T. Jones. 1963. Observation on the alimentary tract and its bacterial flora in healthy and diseased pigs, *J. Pathol. Bacteriol.*, 86:387.

Stahl, D. A. 1993. The natural history of microorganisms, *ASM News*, 59:609.

Stewart, C. S. 1997. Microorganisms in hingut fermentors. In *Gastrointestinal Microbiology*, Vol. 2, Mackie, R. I., B. A. White, and R. E. Isaacson, Eds., Chapman & Hall, New York.

Stokes, C. R., and J. F. Bourne. 1989. Mucosal immunity. In *Veterinary Clinical Immunology*, Halliwell, R. E. W., Ed., Harcourt Brace Jovanovich, Philadelphia.

Sumner, S., M. Speckland, E. Somers, and S. Taylor. 1985. Isolation of histamine-producing *Lactobacillus buchneri* from Swiss cheese implicated in food poisoning outbreak, *Appl. Environ. Microbiol.*, 50:1094.

Suzuki, K., Y. Benno, T. Mitsuoka, S. Takebe, K. Kobashi, and J. Hase. 1979. Urease-producing species of intestinal anaerobes and their activities, *Appl. Environ. Microbiol.*, 37:379.

Tannock, G. W., M. P. Dashkevicz, and S. D. Feighner. 1989. Lactobacilli and bile salt hydrolase in the murine intestinal tract, *Appl. Environ. Microbiol.*, 55:1848.

Tetens, I., G. Livesay, and B. O. Eggum. 1996. Effects of the type and level of dietary fibre supplements on nitrogen retention and excretion patterns, *Br. J. Nutr.*, 75:461.

Thorbecke, G. J. 1959. Some histological and functional aspects of lymphoid tissue in germfree animals, *Ann. N.Y. Acad. Sci.*, 78:237.

Tracy, J. D., and A. H. Jensen. 1987. Effects of a dietary antimicrobial (carbadox) on liver cholesterol 7 alpha-hydroxylase activity and bile acid patterns in the young pig, *J. Anim. Sci.*, 65:1013.

Turck, D., A. S. Feste, and C. H. Lifschitz. 1993. Age and diet affect the composition of porcine colonic mucins, *Pediatr. Res.*, 33:564.

van der Waaij, D., J. M. Berghuis-de Vries, and J. E. C. Lekkerkerk-van der Wees. 1971. Colonization resistance of the digestive tract in conventional and antibiotic-treated mice, *J. Hyg.*, 69:405.

Varel, V. H., S. J. Fryda, and I. M. Robinson. 1984. Cellulolytic bacteria from the pig large intestine, *Appl. Environ. Microbiol.*, 47:219.

Veldman, A., and P. J. Van der Aar. 1997. Effects of dietary inclusion of a natural clinoptilolite (mannelite) on piglet performance, *Agribiol. Res.*, 50:289.

Verdugo, P. 1990. Goblet cell secretion and mucogenesis, *Annu. Rev. Physiol.*, 52:157.

Visek, W. J. 1972. Effects of urea hydrolysis on cell life-span and metabolism, *Am. J. Clin. Nutr.*, 31:S216.

Visek, W. J. 1978a. The mode of growth promotion by antibiotics, *J. Anim. Sci.*, 46:1447.

Visek, W. J. 1978b. Diet and cell growth modulation by ammonia, *Fed. Proc.*, 30:1760.

Visek, W. J. 1981. The influence of urea hydrolysis and ammonia on animals, *Adv. Vet. Med.*, S33:64.

Visek, W. J. 1984. Ammonia: its effects on biological systems, metabolic hormones, and reproduction, *J. Dairy Sci.*, 67:481.

Warren, K. S., and W. L. Newton. 1959. Portal and peripheral ammonia concentrations in germ-free and conventional rats, *Am. J. Physiol.*, 197:717.

Weber, F. L. 1979. The effect of lactulose on urea metabolism and nitrogen excretion in cirrohotic patients. *Gastroenterology*, 77:518.

Weber, F. L., J. G. Banwell, K. M. Fresard, and J. H. Cummings. 1987. Nitrogen in fecal bacteria, fiber and soluble fractions of patients with cirrohosis: effects of lactulose and lactulose plus neomycin, *J. Lab. Clin. Med.*, 110:259.

Weldon, W. C. 1997. Tylosin: effects on nutrient metabolism. In *Proc. of World Pork Exposition Swine Research Review*, Elanco Animal Health, Greenfield, IN.

Wilson, C. W. M. 1954. The metabolism of histamine as reflected by changes in its urinary excretion in the rat. *J. Physiol.* (London), 125:534.

Woese, C. R., O. Kandler, and L. Wheelis. 1990. Towards a natural system of organisms: proposal for the domains Archaea, Bacteria, and Eucarya, *Proc. Natl. Acad. Sci. U.S.A.*, 87:4576.

Wostmann, B. S. 1996. Nutrition. In *Germfree and Gnotobiotic Animal Models*, Wostmann, B. S., Ed., CRC Press, Boca Raton, FL.

Wostmann, B. S., and E. Bruckner-Kardoss. 1959. Development of cecal distention in germ-free baby rats, *Am. J. Physiol.*, 197:1345.

Yokoyama, M. T., C. Tabori, E. R. Miller, and M. G. Hogberg. 1982. The effects of antibiotics in the weanling pig diet on growth and excretions of volatile phenolic and aromatic bacterial metabolites, *Am. J. Clin. Nutr.*, 35:1417.

Zoetendal, E., A. Akkermans, and W. deVos. 1998. Temperature gradient gel electrophoresis analysis of 16S rRNA from human fecal samples reveals stable and host-specific communities of active bacteria, *Appl. Environ. Microbiol.*, 64:3854.

Zuckermann, F. A., and H. R. Gaskins. 1996. Distribution of porcine CD4/CD8 double positive T lymphocytes in mucosa-associated lymphoid tissues, *Immunology*, 87:493.

27 Swine Nutrition and Environmental Pollution and Odor Control

E. T. Kornegay† and Martin W. A. Verstegen

CONTENTS

I. Introduction 609
II. Background of Problem and Challenges 610
III. Nutrition and Feeding Strategies to Reduce Excretion of Nutrients 611
    A. Have Accurate Knowledge of Nutrient Requirements and Composition and Bioavailability of Nutrients in Feed Ingredients 614
    B. Formulate Diets Based on Bioavailability Estimates 614
    C. Reduce Nutrient Excesses That Are Fed 614
    D. Use of Crystalline Amino Acids and High-Quality Protein 616
    E. Enhance Nutrient Utilization through Processing and Additions of Enzymes and Other Feed Additives 617
    F. Use Genetically Modified Feedstuffs 619
    G. Use of Phase Feeding and Split-Sex Feeding 619
    H. Reduce Feed Waste 620
    I. Follow the Principles of Diminishing Returns to Use Optimal Levels of Nutrients 621
IV. Nutrition and Feeding Strategies to Reduce Odors 622
    A. Reduce Nitrogen Levels and Improve Amino Acid Balance to Reduce pH and Total N, Ammonia, and Water Excretion 623
    B. Manipulate Diets by Adding Nonstarch Polysaccharides and Dietary Acid–Base Balance toward Acidifying the Urine, Feces, and Excreta. 624
    C. Manipulate Microbes to Alter Odor Emission 624
V. Summary 625
References 626

I. INTRODUCTION

In various parts of the world pig production has become highly specialized, industrialized, and concentrated geographically. Expansion and specialization have enabled productivity at the farm level to increase. New housing systems with slatted floors and anaerobic storage of manure beneath the slats have been introduced to increase the efficiency and volume of pork production and labor

---

† Deceased

productivity. This process of expansion and specialization has, without doubt, improved farmers' living standards in recent decades.

From the mid-1980s onward, environmental concerns have become issues in animal agriculture. Manure disposal and odor control are particularly important to swine production in many countries. The goal of swine producers and nutritionists has traditionally been to maximize performance. Diets, most with a "safety margin," were formulated to accomplish this goal. There often was little or no regard to the nutrients excreted and odors produced. Swine nutritionists must now formulate diets and develop feeding programs that optimize production not only in terms of profitability, but also in terms of minimizing nutrients excreted and odors produced. During the past decade, the number of pigs produced generally has not changed, but the number of farms has decreased and the size and intensity of production have increased sharply with some very large production units. As a result, in some situations, if land application of the manure is the method of recycling nutrients there are too many pigs on a given land area. Land application of manure is still the most economical way of recycling nutrients because of its fertilizing value, and it is also the most natural and sustainable method. Odors are concentrated when production is intensified. Land application of nutrients, such as manure, in excessive amounts will lead to surface water and groundwater contamination and also to accumulation of minerals in the soil. Intake of certain nutrients can also contribute to odors. Furthermore, many people now want to live in the countryside, and they often are not very knowledgeable about or tolerant of modern animal agriculture.

Manure management in intensive swine production units will be a greater challenge in the future than in the past, because of the volume of manure and the need to develop sustainable systems of production. Two equally important approaches must be taken in dealing with this challenge. First, the amount of nutrients being excreted must be reduced; second, the nutrients that are excreted must be recycled in a manner that is sustainable and that is not damaging to air and/or groundwater, soil fertility, and soil microbiology. Even in the best situations, pigs utilize much less then 100% of nutrients consumed, but it is possible to reduce the amount of nutrients excreted and odors produced. Several strategies are discussed in this chapter. Table 27.1 summarizes some efficiencies.

TABLE 27.1
Efficiency of Some Minerals for Different Animals (%)

	Nitrogen	Phosphorus	Potassium	Carbon
Cattle	15	21	4	13
Pigs	29	28	5	22
Poultry	31	20	7	14

Source: Booms-Prins, E. R. et al., NRLO Report 94/5, 1996. With permission.

II. BACKGROUND OF PROBLEM AND CHALLENGES

Because of the high nutrient content of manure and, thus, its fertilizing value, land application has been the major means of using manure. However, the overall quality of water, both surface and ground, can be negatively affected by land application of excess nitrogen and phosphorus (Correll, 1999), and perhaps other nutrients. Excess nitrogen application can lead to increases in nitrate content of groundwater and to potential runoff of nitrates into surface water. Excess phosphorus applications result in excess buildup of phosphorus in the soil that can lead to the movement of phosphorus during soil erosion and in surface runoff water into streams, lakes, and rivers.

Phosphorus generally does not leach into groundwater because most of it is absorbed into soil particles. Only a small portion of the phosphorus is soluble. Phosphorus is the most limiting nutrient that regulates aquatic plant growth, so as the level of phosphorus in these bodies of water increases, so does the growth of algae and other aquatic vegetation (Pierzynski et al., 1994; Sharpley et al.,

1994). Decomposition of such vegetation can lead to general deterioration of water quality, a process called "eutrophication" (Crenshaw and Johanson, 1995).

High phosphorus levels in the soil have been reported for many U.S. states. Findings of a recent survey reveal that several states had found greater than 50% of the soil samples tested for crop production to be rated high or excessive in phosphorus (Sims, 1993). These states included Maine, Connecticut, Delaware, Maryland, Michigan, Minnesota, Virginia, North Carolina, South Carolina, Ohio, Iowa, Indiana, Illinois, Utah, Wisconsin, Wyoming, Arizona, and Washington. Five of the top swine-producing states are on the list.

In most countries, especially countries of the European Union, nitrogen is used as the base to regulate the amount of manure that can be applied to the land. Because the ratio of nitrogen to phosphorus in manure is narrower than required by the crop grown, there is often an accumulation of phosphorus in the soil. Until recently, P accumulation was used to regulate the amounts in other countries, e.g., The Netherlands. For example, soil analyses of a Sampson County (North Carolina) bermudagrass pasture that was fertilized with swine lagoon effluent to satisfy the nitrogen requirement showed approximately a fourfold increase in phosphorus and zinc, a threefold increase in copper, and a onefold increase in potassium to a depth of 91 cm during the 3-year period of application (Mueller et al., 1994). The effects of 16 annual land applications of copper-rich pig manure (primarily feces from pigs fed 255 ppm copper or copper sulfate) at an average annual rate of 179 tons/ha (22.4% dry matter, DM) to three soil types increased the soil (Mehlich-3) extractable concentration of copper, zinc, and phosphorus in the Ap and upper B horizon (D. C. Martens and E. T. Kornegay, unpublished data). The average annual rate of application per hectare was 20.6 kg of copper, 6.7 kg of zinc, and 355.1 kg of phosphorus. The application of a similar amount of copper from copper sulfate resulted in similar increases in copper. Results of high-quality deep core soil samples taken in the spring of 1996 revealed that increases varied based on soil type and treatment (Table 27.2). The copper (1.6 to 2.7 ppm DM) and zinc (16.8 to 20.3 ppm DM) concentrations of the grain grown on these soils were not changed. Corn ear leaf tissue had a slightly higher copper concentration (113 to 172% of controls), but zinc concentrations were similar. Phosphorus was not measured in plant tissue and grain. Grain yields were not affected by copper application on the three soil types during any year.

Because of accumulations of phosphorus when only nitrogen-based nutrient management guidelines are used, there is increasing legislature effects at both state and federal levels to implement nutrient management plans that include both nitrogen and phosphorus. The accumulation of copper and zinc in some soil following long-term application of manure is of concern in some states for certain crops, e.g., peanuts.

Even in the best situations, pigs do not utilize 100% of nutrients consumed. A review of balance data for growing–finishing pigs fed commercial feedstuffs is summarized in Table 27.3. Although more than 50% of several macrominerals including nitrogen is digested, the average retention is usually much less than 50%, with values about 25% for trace minerals. The digestion and retention coefficients are usually lower for gestating–lactating sows. Therefore, as a percentage of intake, 45 to 90% of nitrogen, 50 to 80% of calcium and phosphorus, and 60 to 95% of potassium sodium, magnesium, copper, zinc, manganese, and iron is excreted. An example of nitrogen flow is given in Figure 27.1.

III. NUTRITION AND FEEDING STRATEGIES TO REDUCE EXCRETION OF NUTRIENTS

The implementation of nutrition and feeding strategies discussed in this chapter will significantly reduce nutrient excretion, but they are not a total solution to the amount of manure produced by large numbers of animals housed on a small land area, since 100% utilization of a diet is not possible. However, nutrient excretion can be reduced up to 50% with reasonable attention given to

TABLE 27.2
Mehlich-3 Extractable Cu, Zn, and P Concentrations in Three Soil Types after 16 Annual Applications of Cu-Rich Manure and CuSO$_4$

Horizon	Depth (cm)	Class[a]	Copper (ppm)[b]			Zinc (ppm)			Phosphorus (ppm)		
			Control	Cu Manure	Cu Sulfate	Control	Cu Manure	Cu Sulfate	Control	Cu Manure	Cu Sulfate
Bertie											
A$_p$	0–29	fsl	4.3^y	35.3^x	42.1^x	15.8^y	32.7^x	15.1^y	295.0^y	697.5^x	295.0^y
Upper B	30–61	fsl	0.4^y	2.2^x	1.5^x	0.8^y	1.6^x	0.8^y	9.1^y	230.2^x	11.9^y
Lower B	62–86	fsl	0.4^x	0.3^x	0.3^x	0.5^x	0.4^x	0.6^x	0.8^x	11.4^x	0.1^x
Upper C	87–112	sil	0.3^x	0.2^x	0.4^x	0.4^x	0.4^x	0.4^x	0.1^x	0.9^x	0.1^x
Lower C	113–133	sil	0.2^x	0.5^x	0.4^x	0.4^x	0.6^x	0.5^x	0.1^x	0.9^x	0.1^x
Guernsey											
A$_p$	0–25	sil	3.1^y	59.6^x	62.2^x	19.5^y	49.4^x	21.2^y	176.3^y	1011.7^x	199.1^y
Upper B	26–50	sic	0.6^y	3.0^x	1.6^{xy}	1.1^y	2.2^x	0.8^y	15.4^y	83.2^x	19.1^y
Middle B	51–75	sicl	1.1^x	0.7^x	0.7^x	0.9^x	0.5^x	0.5^x	1.9^x	1.2^x	3.6^x
Lower B	76–100	sic	0.6^x	1.2^x	1.4^x	0.5^x	0.7^x	0.7^x	0.1^x	0.1^x	0.1^x
Starr-Dyke											
A$_p$	0–11	sicl	14.8^x	53.7^x	54.2^x	16.9^y	43.2^x	23.1^y	38.3^y	447.9^x	77.2^y
A$_2$	12–25	sic	1.8^y	9.8^x	9.2^x	2.5^y	7.6^x	3.4^y	0.2^y	130.7^x	0.3^y
Upper B	26–50	c	1.0^x	1.1^x	1.2^x	1.0^x	0.9^x	0.8^x	0.1^x	2.0^x	0.1^x
Middle B	51–75	c	0.5^x	0.5^x	0.5^x	0.5^x	0.4^x	0.4^x	0.1^x	0.1^x	0.1^x
Lower B	76–100	c	0.8^x	0.6^x	0.7^x	1.0^x	0.5^y	0.7^{xy}	0.1^x	0.1^x	0.1^x

Note: Means on the same line followed by different superscripts are different ($P < 0.05$).

[a] fsl = fine sandy loam, sil = silt loam, sicl = silty clay loam, and c = clay.
[b] ppm = mg/dm^3. Multiply mg/dm^3 (ppm) by 1.78 to get lb/acre.

TABLE 27.3
Digestion and Retention of Nutrients by Growing-Finishing Pigs

	Percentage of Intake[a]	
Mineral	Digested	Retained
Nitrogen	75–88	40–50
Calcium	40–75	25–70
Phosphorus	20–70	20–60
Magnesium	20–45	15–38
Sodium	35–70	13–25
Potassium	60–80	10–20
Zinc	10–40	b
Copper	10–25	b
Iron	5–35	b
Manganese	8–40	b

[a] Most values are lower for sows.
[b] Usually very similar to digested values because only very small amounts of these trace minerals are excreted in urine.

Source: Adapted from Kornegay and Harper (1997).

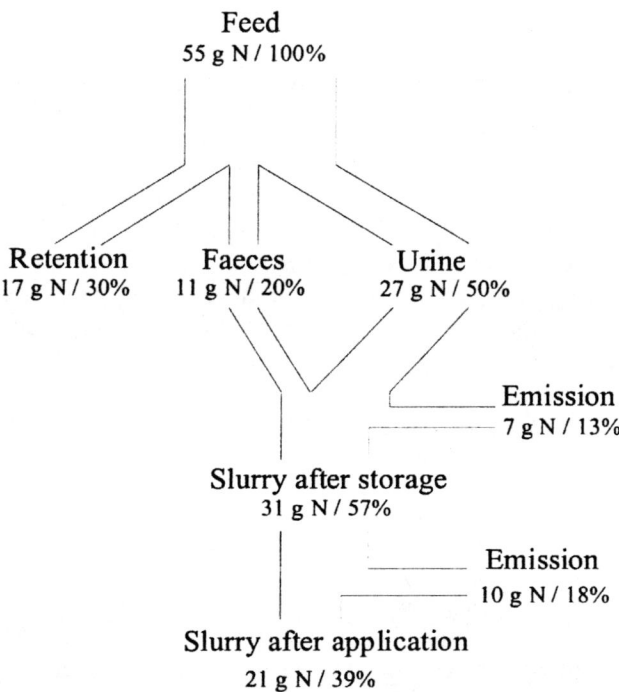

FIGURE 27.1 Nitrogen chain for growing-finishing pigs in housing with partially slatted floor and with surface application of the slurry. The N intake is assumed to be 55 g/pig/day. (From Aarnink, A. J. A., Ph.D. thesis, Agricultural University, Wageningen, The Netherlands, 1997.)

nutrition and feeding programs. The amount of a nutrient excreted can be influenced by several factors, including quality, source, and level of the nutrient fed; the level and proportion of other nutrients; processing methods; age, class, and nutritional status of animals; and environmental factors. Jongbloed and Henkens (1996) reported that for growing pigs in the Netherlands from 1973 to 1995 phosphorus excretion was reduced 58% and nitrogen excretion was reduced by 12%.

A. Have Accurate Knowledge of Nutrient Requirements and Composition and Bioavailability of Nutrients in Feed Ingredients

The successful implementation of most of the strategies that follow for reducing nutrient excretion depends on accurate estimates of the available nutrient requirements of the class of pig in question, on the accuracy of compositional information, and on bioavailability of nutrients in the feed ingredients to be used. In addition, a safety margin is usually included with regard to contents compared with requirements. Recommended nutrient requirements have been published for the various classes of pigs in a number of countries including the United States (NRC, 1998), United Kingdom (ARC, 1981), Australia (SCA, 1987), Netherlands (CVB, 1993; 1994), Germany (GFE, 1987), and France (INRA, 1984). These recommendations often vary and, in some cases, are only estimates for an "average" type of pig produced under "average" environmental conditions. The estimated nutrient requirement may be influenced by the animals genetic potential, feeding methods, environmental conditions, the ingredients used, and animal response criteria. With the exception of phosphorus and amino acids, nutrient requirements are generally based on total nutrients rather than available nutrients.

Pig type has changed during the last decade because of strong consumer pressure for leaner, heavier-muscled carcasses. The nutrient requirements of these pigs may be higher, but published data are extremely limited. Daily intake could influence the percentage composition of nutrients required, and it may be necessary to adjust percentage composition to meet daily nutrient needs.

B. Formulate Diets Based on Bioavailability Estimates

The available nutrient requirement of pigs, if known, can only be met if the compositional data of feed ingredients are expressed as available nutrient composition. With the exception of phosphorus and amino acids, estimates of the available nutrient requirement of pigs are not published, and generally are not known. The same is true for nutrient availability data for feed ingredients. Do not confuse relative bioavailability values for certain nutrients, mainly minerals, when referring to comparisons between source of ingredients or nutrients. In this chapter availability and bioavailability refer to absolute amount of nutrient utilized by the pig. The use of more precise data on composition and nutrient availability for feed ingredients and better-defined requirements would allow nutritionists to formulate the needs of animals at the various stages of production.

C. Reduce Nutrient Excesses That Are Fed

A portion of the nutrients excreted by the pig is a direct result of feeding excessive levels of nutrients — the greater the excess, the greater the portion of nutrients excreted. Results of surveys of the nutrient composition of diets indicate that diets commonly include excessive amounts of certain nutrients. These excesses are included in the diet as a "safety factor" to allow for the variability of nutrient composition of feed ingredients or to compensate for uncertainty about the availability of the nutrients. Results of surveys (Table 27.4) reported by Cromwell (1989) of calcium and phosphorus recommendations of several universities and feed companies showed that the average range of university recommendations was 110 to 120% of National Research Council (1988) requirements, whereas the average range of industry recommendations was 120 to 130% of these requirements. Spears (1996) reported that the mineral concentrations of finishing pig diets analyzed by the North Carolina Feed Testing Laboratory were greatly in excess of

TABLE 27.4
Comparison of Calcium and Phosphorus Requirements and Allowances Recommended by Universities and Feed Companies[a]

	Growing-Finishing		Gestation	Lactation
	20–50 kg	50–100 kg		
	Calcium			
NRC (1988)	0.60	0.50	0.75	0.75
1986 Survey[a]				
Universities ($n = 25$)	0.66	0.59	0.82	0.79
Feed industry ($n = 35$)	0.74	0.63	0.95	0.93
1988 Survey[b]				
Universities ($n = 7$)	0.64	0.58	0.84	0.84
Feed industry ($n = 21$)	0.73	0.62	0.93	0.90
	Phosphorus			
NRC (1988)	0.50	0.40	0.60	0.60
1986 Survey[a]				
Universities ($n = 25$)	0.55	0.49	0.66	0.63
Feed industry ($n = 35$)	0.60	0.52	0.77	0.76
1988 Survey[b]				
Universities ($n = 7$)	0.54	0.49	0.68	0.68
Feed Industry ($n = 21$)	0.60	0.52	0.76	0.74

[a] Overfield (1986) reported by Cromwell (1989).
[b] Survey conducted in 1988 (Cromwell, 1989).

recommended requirements (Table 27.5). Compared with the National Research Council (1988) requirements for finishing pig diets, the median levels were from 1.55 to 1.92 times higher for calcium, phosphorus, and sodium; 4.0 to 4.23 times higher for magnesium and potassium; and 2.98 to 31.0 times higher for copper, iron, manganese, and zinc. The excesses for the sows were

TABLE 27.5
Mineral Concentration in 17 Finishing Swine Diets[a]

Minerals	Requirement	Range	Median[b] Requirement
Ca (%)	0.50	0.57–1.38	1.92
P (%)	0.40	0.45–0.78	1.55
Na (%)	0.10	0.13–0.29	1.90
Mg (%)	0.04	0.13–0.21	4.00
K (%)	0.17	0.48–0.93	4.23
Cu (ppm)	3	9–281	6.67
Fe (ppm)	40	131–503	7.76
Mn (ppm)	2	37–160	31.0
Zn (ppm)	50	103–205	2.98

[a] Analysis conducted at the NC Feed Testing Laboratory ($n = 17$).
[b] The median level for each mineral indicates that 50% of the samples analyzed were below and 50% were above the median value.

Source: Spears, J. W., in *Nutrient Management of Food Animals to Enhance and Protect the Environment*, Kornegay, E. T., Ed., CRC Press, Boca Raton, FL, 1996, 259. With permission.

a little lower than for finishing pigs. Other surveys have reported similar findings of diets containing excess levels of nutrients.

High dietary levels of copper fed as a growth promotant and zinc fed to enhance postweaning performance also significantly increase the amount of copper and zinc that is excreted. In a study by Apgar and Kornegay (1996), 71-kg barrows excreted 6.7 times more copper when fed diets containing 218 vs. 32 ppm copper. Calculations based on data reported by Adeola et al. (1995) for 15- to 18-kg pigs fed diets with 23 or 123 ppm zinc from $ZnSO_4$ indicated that pigs fed the low-zinc diet excreted 16 mg zinc/day, whereas pigs fed the high-zinc diet excreted 61 mg zinc/day, a 3.8-fold increase in the amount of zinc excreted. When diets containing 2500 to 3000 ppm zinc are fed to weanling pigs, as is commonly done for growth promotion (Hahn and Baker, 1993; LeMieux et al., 1995; Smith et al., 1995; Hill et al., 1996), approximately 90 to 95% of the zinc will be excreted. Although these high levels would be fed for a period of only a few weeks, the total amount of zinc excreted could approach or exceed the total amount of zinc excreted during the entire growing-finishing period by pigs fed diets containing approximately 100 ppm zinc. Excretion of minerals could be markedly reduced simply by reducing these excessive levels of nutrients in diets, and avoiding the uses of high levels of trace minerals such as copper and zinc as mineral supplements.

D. Use of Crystalline Amino Acids and High-Quality Protein

Lowering the dietary protein level and supplementing with certain crystalline amino acids is a well-established method of formulating diets to achieve a more ideal amino acid pattern and is very effective in reducing nitrogen excretion. Also, using highly "digestible" feedstuffs and a high-quality protein source with superior amino acid balance and formulating diets to achieve an ideal protein basis reduces the excretion of nitrogen and other nutrients. Both procedures reduce excesses of unneeded amino acids, which otherwise are degraded and excreted as urea nitrogen.

Lysine supplementation of cereal grain/plant protein-based diets has been widely used and has generally led to about two percentage units reduction in crude protein, which results in a 17 to 22% reduction in nitrogen excretion (Gatel and Grosjean, 1992; Henry and Dourmad, 1992; Van der Honing et al., 1993; Gatel, 1994; Cromwell, 1994). A further reduction in nitrogen excretion has resulted when the crude protein level was reduced four percentage units and the diets were supplemented with three or four of the following amino acids: lysine, threonine, tryptophan, and methionine (Kephart and Sherritt, 1990; Bridges et al., 1995; Kerr and Easter, 1995; Carter et al., 1996). Total nitrogen excretion reductions ranged from 28 to 40%. The major component of reductions in nitrogen excretion that occur when the crude protein level is reduced is a large reduction in urinary nitrogen excretion (Table 27.6). There may be only small changes in fecal nitrogen losses.

Based on a review of several papers, Kerr and Easter (1995) suggested that for each one percentage unit reduction in dietary crude protein combined with amino acid supplementation, total nitrogen losses (fecal and urinary) could be reduced by approximately 8%. Although the application of crystalline amino acids in practical situations is generally straightforward, it is recognized that there will be limits to their use, in comparison with intact protein. For example, nitrogen retained is often less when amino acids are supplemented and the crude protein level is reduced, especially when three or more amino acids replace four percentage units of crude protein.

The use of highly digestible feedstuffs in diets is an effective means of reducing excretion of nitrogen and other nutrients. As cited by Van Heugten and Van Kempen (1999), FEFANA (1992) estimated that nutrient excretion in waste could be reduced about 5% by selecting highly digestible ingredients. Conversely, the use of low-quality protein sources (e.g., hydrolyzed hog hair meal) markedly increases nitrogen excretion (Kornegay, 1978b). Also, the inclusion of high levels of crude fiber in the diet reduces the efficiency of nitrogen utilization (Kornegay, 1978a).

TABLE 27.6
Effect of Reducing Dietary Protein and Supplementing with Amino Acids on Nitrogen Excretion[a]

	Diets		
	14% CP	12% CP +0.15% Lys	10% CP + 0.30% Lys + 0.08% Thr + 0.03% Trp
N intake (g/day)	46.9	40.2	35.2
N digested (g/day)	42.3	36.0	30.3
N excreted in feces (g/day)	4.5	4.3	4.9
N excreted in urine (g/day)	17.7	13.7	10.9
N excreted, total (g/day)	22.2	18.0	15.8
N retained (g/day)	24.6	22.3	19.5
Reduction in N excretion (%)	—	18.9	28.8

[a] Average of experiments 1 and 2 reported by Bridges et al. (1995). Body weights initially were 66.1 and 101.7 kg, respectively, for experiments 1 and 2.

E. Enhance Nutrient Utilization through Processing and Additions of Enzymes and Other Feed Additives

A number of feed-processing methods are known to enhance feed intake and feed efficiency (see Chapter 21 for a complete discussion of these). Improvements of 3 to 5% have been reported for grinding of cereal grains (Liptrap and Hogberg, 1991). Hancock et al. (1996), based on a summary of eight pelleting trials for swine, reported that pelleting resulted in an average 6% improvement in average daily gain and a 7% improvement in feed efficiency. Wondra et al. (1995) reported a 23% decrease in DM excretion and a 22% decrease in nitrogen excretion when finishing diets were pelleted.

Improvements in overall feed efficiency can produce a major reduction in the excretion of nutrients. Coffey (1992) reported that a reduction in the feed-to-gain ratio of 0.25 of ratio units (i.e., 3.00 vs. 3.25), would reduce nitrogen excretion by 5 to 10%. Henry and Dourmad (1992) reported for growing-finishing pigs that for each 0.1 percentage unit decrease in feed-to-gain ratio there was a 3% decrease in nitrogen output.

Several feed additives including anti- and promicrobial agents, performance enhancing-substances, and nutraceuticals are known to enhance overall feed efficiency (see Chapters 18 and 19). The use of supplemental microbial phytase is perhaps the best example of the use of an enzyme to enhance nutrient utilization. Proteases, lipases, and various carbohydrases have not consistently improved nutrient utilization, especially in corn-based diets.

In corn–soybean meal diets, two thirds of the phosphorus is bound as phytic acid and is poorly available to the pig (Cromwell and Coffey, 1991); hence, much of the phosphorus is excreted. The amount excreted can be significantly decreased by the inclusion of microbial phytase in the diet, which releases some of the bound phosphorus making it available to the pig. Thus, the amount of inorganic phosphorus that must be added to meet the available phosphorus requirement is reduced, and phosphorus excretion can be decreased. Phosphorus digestibilities were generated using 52 pig experiments representing 32 references in a review reported by Kornegay et al. (1998). A nonlinear response of supplemental phytase on phosphorus digestibility for pigs was observed (Figure 27.2). The magnitude of the response per unit of phytase was much greater at the lower phytase levels for pigs.

Digested phosphorus resulting from microbial phytase supplementation was calculated by multiplying the total phosphorus content of the low-phosphorus diet (negative control) by the increase in phosphorus digestibility or phosphorus retention resulting from phytase supplementation (Table 27.7). These values were similar to estimated phosphorus equivalency values of phytase

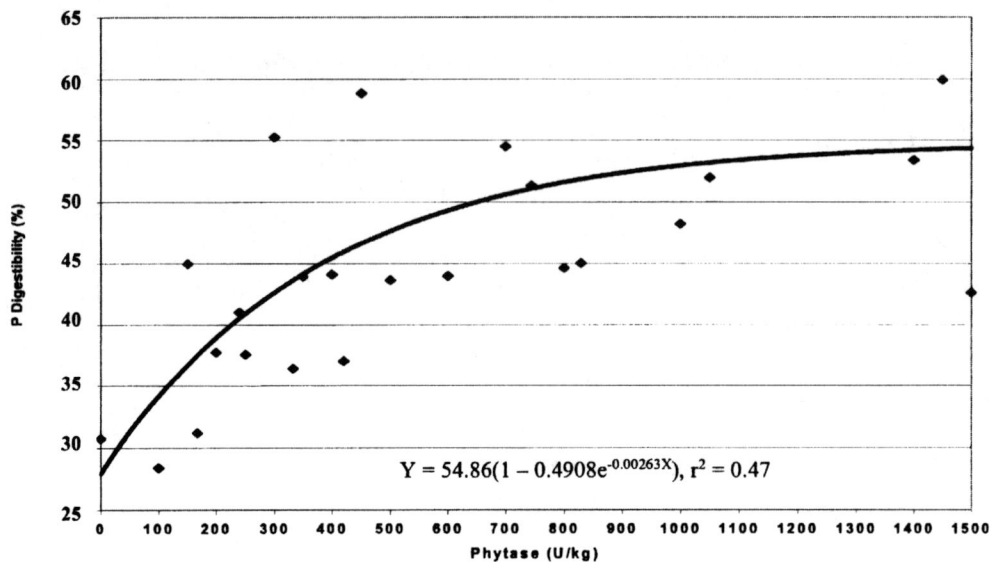

FIGURE 27.2 Phosphorus digestibility in pigs fed low-P, low-phytase activity, plant-based diets supplemented with microbial phytase. (From Kornegay, E. T. et al., Paper presented at BASF Technical Symposium, 1998. With permission.)

TABLE 27.7
Predicted P Digestibility, P Digested, and Percentage Reduction in P Excretion Based on Data Generated from Pig Data Set

Supplemental Phytase (U/kg)	Total P Digestibility (%)[a]	P Digestibility by Phytase (%)[b]	P Digested by Phytase (%)[c]	Total P Excreted (%)[d]	Decreased P Excretion (%)[e]
0	27.9	0	0	0.275	8.3
200	38.9	11.0	0.042	0.233	22.3
300	42.6	14.7	0.056	0.219	27.0
400	45.5	17.5	0.067	0.208	30.6
500	47.6	19.7	0.075	0.200	33.2
600	49.3	21.4	0.081	0.193	35.5
800	51.6	23.6	0.090	0.184	38.4
1000	52.9	25.0	0.095	0.179	40.1

[a] Generated from the equation given in Figure 27.2 [$54.86(1 - 0.4908e^{-0.00263X})$].
[b] Calculated by subtracting P digestibility of basal diet without phytase from coefficients at each phytase level.
[c] Calculated by multiplying the P digestibility due to phytase by the average P content (0.381% total P) of the basal diet. The equation for these data is = $0.1026(1 - e^{-0.00263X})$, where X = phytase level.
[d] Calculated by subtracting total P digestibility coefficients from 100 and multiplying the product by the average P content (0.381% total P) of the basal diet.
[e] Based on an inorganic P digested equation ($Y = -0.167 + 0.755X$, $r^2 = 0.24$, where X = %P from inorganic source); 0.0245% P was excreted for the 0.1% unit of added inorganic P above the basal diet making the total P excreted by the positive control diet (0.481% total P) equal to 0.2995% P (0.275 + 0.0245). Decreased P excretion was calculated by subtracting the total P excreted by the phytase supplemented diets from the P excreted by the positive control diet (0.2995%) and then dividing by the P excreted by positive control diet and multiplying by 100. For example, at 500 U/kg of phytase, 33.2% = [(0.2995 − 0.200)/(0.2995) × 100].

Source: Data from Kornegay et al., BASF Technical Symposium, Durham, NC, 1998, 125.

when equivalency values were adjusted downward by the estimated digestibility of inorganic phosphorus that would be replaced by phytase.

Based on calculations using the digestibility equation from the pig data set, phosphorus excretion can be reduced 33.2% when 500 U/kg of phytase is added to a low-phosphorus diet compared with a positive control diet (0.481% P), which is 0.1% units phosphorus higher in P. Simply lowering the dietary phosphorus level 0.1% will decrease phosphorus excretion about 8.3% in pigs.

Based on the similarity of digested phosphorus values calculated from phosphorus equivalency estimates, and values derived from equations generated in the pig data set, the estimates of phosphorus excretion should be accurate for a range of situations. However, a larger response than observed in these data sets is possible if careful attention is given to ingredient composition and diet formulation (optimal calcium and phosphorus levels), and if quality processing procedures are followed. The magnitude of the response to microbial phytase has been shown to be influenced by the source of phosphorus, dietary level of available phosphorus, the amount of phytase added, and the ratio of calcium to phosphorus (Lei et al., 1994; Kornegay, 1996; Liu et al., 1998). Microbial phytase also releases calcium (Mroz et al., 1994; Radcliffe et al., 1995), zinc (Lei et al., 1993; Pallauf et al., 1994), as well as some amino acids (Mroz et al., 1994; Kemme, 1998; Kornegay et al., 1998) that may be bound by phytic acid.

F. Use Genetically Modified Feedstuffs

The availability of genetically modified feedstuffs that have a more desirable nutrient balance and more highly available nutrients is an emerging area with only experimental data currently available. Several studies conducted with low phytic acid (LPA) corn (a nonlethal genetic mutation-Ipa1 (Raboy et al., 1994) indicate that the phosphorus in LPA corn is from 55 to 70% available compared with 10 to 15% for phosphorus in normal corn (Spencer et al., 1998; Baxter et al., 1998; Cromwell et al., 1998; Veum, 1998; Pierce et al., 1998a,b). Phosphorus reductions of 20 to 25% have been reported when LPA corn replaced normal corn and the diet was formulated based on an available phosphorus basis. Other modifications of corn are under development. Yield and grain quality continue to be of concern. This area holds great promise for producing feed ingredients that have an ideal balance of highly available nutrients. Not all aspects of genetically modified feedstuffs and their use, however, have been extensively evaluated.

G. Use of Phase Feeding and Split-Sex Feeding

The requirement of animals for most available amino acids and minerals, expressed as a percentage of the total diet, decreases as the animals grow heavier. Thus, frequent changes in diet formulation can meet the nutrient needs of the pig more efficiently. Frequent adjustments in diets can result in reduced intake of nutrient and, thus, reduced excretion of nutrients. Phase feeding, as some have described, is a way to meet the nutrient needs of growing and finishing pigs more precisely. This concept applied to dietary crude protein (CP) is illustrated in Table 27.8 and Figure 27.3. It is known that nutrient requirements change (perhaps weekly) as pigs grow; if a producer is able to change the formulation of the diet as the nutrient requirements change, then the nutrient needs of the animal can be met more precisely, thereby reducing the total quantity of nutrients excreted. These changes, however, should not be so large that the digestive system requires time to adapt to the new diets. Henry and Dourmad (1993) reported that nitrogen excretion could be reduced approximately 15% when the feeding of 14% CP diet was initiated at 60 kg body weight, rather than the continuous feeding of 16% CP grower diet to market weight. In a further study, Chauvel and Ganier (1996) reported a 9% reduction in nitrogen excretion between a multiphase system where the proportions of an 18.9 and 14.9% CP (4.1 and 2.6 g digestible lysine/MJ net energy, respectively) were changed weekly from 24 to 107 kg vs. a two-phase system, where an 18.1% CP (0.85 g lysine/MJ net energy) diet was fed to 66 kg and a 16.1% CP (7.4 g lysine/MJ net

TABLE 27.8
Effect of Feeding Strategy during the Growing-Finishing Period (25 to 105 kg) on N Output

	Single-Feed 17% CP	Two-Feeds[a] 17–15% CP	Three-Feeds[b] 17–15–13% CP
N output (g/day)	31.9	29.0	26.7
Percentage of two-feed strategy	110	100	92

[a] Crude protein changed at 55 kg.
[b] Crude protein changed at 50 and 75 kg.

Source: Adapted from Henry and Dourmad (1993).

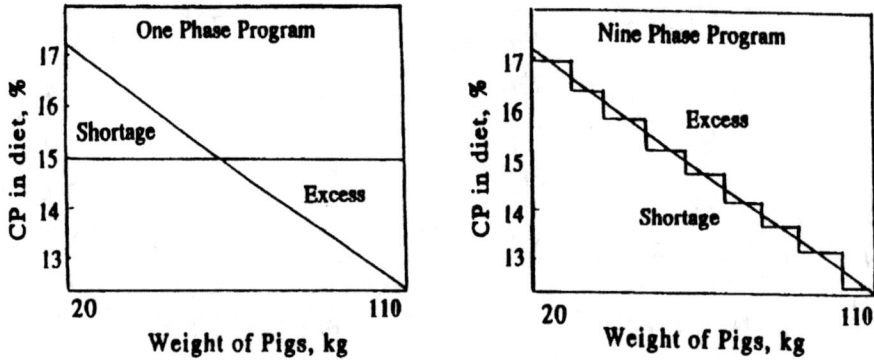

FIGURE 27.3 Example of a one-phase and a nine-phase feeding program for the growing and finishing phase. (From Kornegay, E. T., and Harper, A. F., *Prof. Anim. Sci.*, 13:99, 1997. With permission.)

energy) diet was fed to 107 kg. Also, the excretion of phosphorus and other minerals would be reduced a similar amount, if the finishing diet contained a lower level of these minerals. Henry and Dourmad (1993) suggested that this change could be made gradually by changing the ratio in which a "high" protein and phosphorus (and other minerals) grower diet is mixed with a "low" protein and phosphorus (and other minerals) finishing diet. A 14.7% reduction in urinary nitrogen excretion was reported when a multiphase feeding program was compared with a two-phase feeding program (Vander Peet-Schwering et al., 1996). Also ammonia omission was reduced 16.8%. This trial multiphase feeding program was achieved by mixing, on a weekly basis, a high-protein diet with a low-protein diet in decreasing proportions as pigs grew.

Separate-sex or split-sex feeding of swine can further improve feed efficiency. It is well established that gilts consume less feed on an *ad libitum* basis and require greater diet nutrient density than barrows (Cromwell et al., 1993). By penning and feeding gilts and barrows separately, producers can more precisely formulate diets for specific sexes and avoid overfortification and excessive excretion of nutrients. Furthermore, increased fat deposition and decreased rate of lean deposition occur at an earlier growth stage in barrows than in gilts; therefore, dietary protein and amino acid levels can be more precisely changed at different growth stages for each sex. Under such precise feeding conditions, the total quantity of nitrogen and other minerals fed and excreted can be reduced.

H. REDUCE FEED WASTE

Another simple, yet sometimes difficult and overlooked way to improve feed efficiency is to improve design and operation of feeders, so that feed waste is minimized. Researchers in several countries

TABLE 27.9
Feed Waste Impacts on Nutrient Management[a]

Feed Waste (%)	Feed Loss per Pig (kg)	Income Loss per Pig ($)	Feed N Waste per Pig (g)	Feed P Waste per Pig (g)
1	2.8	0.36	63	18
3	8.2	1.07	195	50
5	13.6	1.77	327	82
7	19.1	2.48	459	114

[a] Based on growing-finishing pigs from 22.7 to 113.5 kg body weight, 3:1 feed:gain ratio, 2.4% N and 0.60% P in the diet, and $0.13/kg diet cost.

Source: Adapted from Harper (1994).

have estimated feed waste and have quoted values of 2 to 12% in the United States, 1.5 to 20% in Great Britain, and 3 to 5% in Denmark (Van Heugten and Van Kempen, 1999). Table 27.9 shows the impact that feed waste has on feed efficiency and income loss, as well as the amount of nitrogen and phosphorus excreted in pigs. A 5% level of feed waste can result in an income loss of $1.77/market pig depending on market condition, and an additional 327 g of nitrogen and 82 g of phosphorus excreted per pig. The use of proper feeder designs, regular maintenance, and careful adjustment of feeders is essential for the prevention of excessive feed waste.

I. FOLLOW THE PRINCIPLES OF DIMINISHING RETURNS TO USE OPTIMAL LEVELS OF NUTRIENTS

The efficiency of animal performance follows the principle of diminishing returns in response to nutrient input (Heady et al., 1954; Combs et al., 1991a,b; Gahl et al., 1995). Heady et al. (1954) reported that in 14 of 16 years swine diets formulated using the diminishing return concept would have produced greater profits than diets formulated for maximum gain. As the cost of disposing of nitrogen and phosphorus increases, the nutrient levels fed to pigs will probably decrease. In the future, nutritionists may formulate diets to achieve 95 to 98% rather than 100% of maximum response, because the benefit from adding a unit of nutrient increases at a decreasing rate, and nutrient costs increase at an increasing rate as the animal reaches maximum performance.

In the future, diets can be formulated so that animals perform at slightly less than maximum because the benefit of adding additional units of a nutrient to achieve maximum performance produces benefits at a decreasing rate. This practice increases nutrient costs per unit of performance improvement at an increasing rate as the animal approaches maximum performance. As the maximum response is reached, or as the performance curve reaches a plateau, a greater amount of the nutrient is required to effect a change in the response. In a series of three trials, Combs et al. (1991a) fit asymptotic models of the effect of total Ca + P intake (varied above and below NRC recommended requirement) and days on test (weaning to market). Diminishing returns in response to Ca – P input are shown in Figure 27.4 for performance measurements. This principle of diminishing returns in response to nutrient input is not new. Heady et al. (1954) reported that in 14 of 16 years swine diets formulated using the diminishing return concept would have produced greater profits than diets formulated for maximum gain. Diminishing returns were also observed when Kornegay (1986) fit asymptotic models to combined data from a number of research trials conducted from 1969 to 1986 to evaluate the Ca + P needs of growing-finishing swine. More recently, Gahl et al. (1995) demonstrated that the most economical daily weight gain does not occur when daily weight gain is maximized and would change as feedstuffs and input costs change. Diminishing returns for nitrogen gain of pigs fed six levels of lysine from three supplemental sources

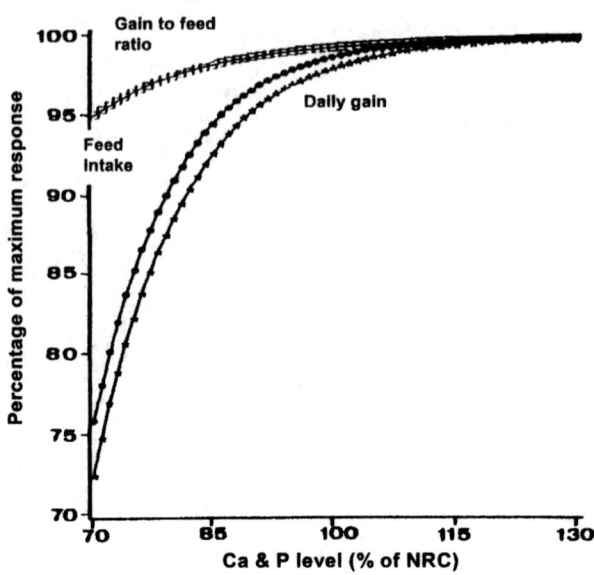

FIGURE 27.4 Percentage of maximum average daily gain (∗), average daily feed intake (•), and gain:feed ratio (ƒ) associated with each increase in average daily Ca and P intake for growing-finishing pigs. (From Combs, N. R. et al., *J. Anim. Sci.*, 69:673, 1991. With permission.)

(Figure 27.5) has been demonstrated by Gahl et al. (1995); their paper includes a useful discussion of the diminishing returns in response to nutrient input.

Another consideration in evaluating nutrient addition is the response criteria measured. It is well known that the amount of phosphorus required to maximize growth is less than the amount required to maximize bone integrity (NRC, 1988). Perhaps, from the perspective of animal well-being, attempts to maximize bone integrity are most important, but from an environmental perspective, attempts to maximize bone integrity result in excessive excretion of phosphorus (Crenshaw and Johanson, 1995). Combs et al. (1991b) observed that growing-finishing pigs fed diets that provided NRC (1988) requirements for calcium and phosphorus maintained approximately 100% of maximum growth and feed efficiency, but approximately 120 to 130% of the NRC (1988) calcium and phosphorus requirement was required to maximize bone development. Although maximizing bone development is not necessary for the production of a market pig, a more difficult question is how much bone development is required to prevent damage to the carcass during mechanical processing that occurs during slaughter. As the cost of phosphorus disposal increases, the calcium and phosphorus levels fed will decrease. In the future, nutritionists will formulate for 95 to 98% of maximum response rather than trying to approach 100% of maximum response. Therefore, the industry will feed below, rather than above, the nutrient requirements of animals to maximize growth and bone development. How much of a safety margin will be desirable will depend upon the availability of accurate knowledge of the requirements and compositional information for the feedstuffs used.

IV. NUTRITION AND FEEDING STRATEGIES TO REDUCE ODORS

Pig manure is a mixture of excreta (urine and fecal matter). It is composed of undigested dietary components, endogenous components, and products from indigenous microorganism and biomass of those microorganisms itself. Some odorous volatile components (VOC) short-chain volatile fatty acids (VFA) and other volatile carbon–nitrogen and sulfur-containing compounds from microbial fermentation in the gastrointestinal tract can be emitted immediately. Others are emitted within the

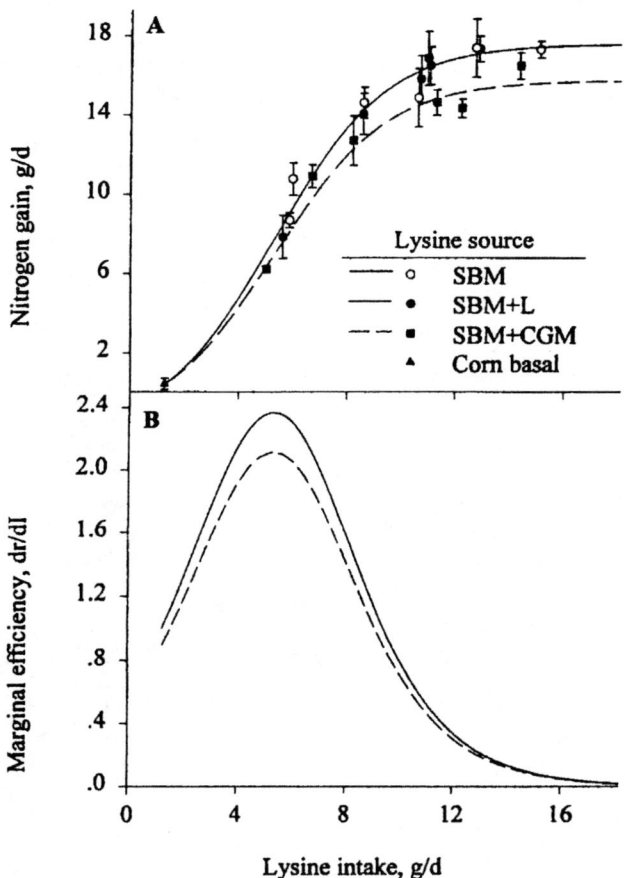

FIGURE 27.5 Diminishing returns in nitrogen gain (g/day) of pigs fed diets with graded concentrations of lysine. (A) Predicted curves estimated using a logistic equation. Data points ±SE ($n = 4$) for each treatment group. (B) Marginal efficiency of nitrogen gain with respect to lysine intake calculated as the first derivative of the predicted curves in A. Marginal efficiency is defined as the incremental response in nitrogen gain to an incremental unit of lysine intake. (From Gahl, M. J. et al., *J. Anim. Sci.*, 73:3177, 1995. With permission.)

varying time after excretion. Until recently, the effect of diet composition on excretion products related to odorous compounds was not studied extensively (Sutton et al., 1999). In Table 27.10 a short overview is given of some volatile components formed from microbial activity in manure. This is only a short list of the many possible compounds. Research reports have identified more than 200 compounds. It should be pointed out that the sensitivity of the individual compounds by olfactometry threshold detection varies widely (see Aarnink, 1997, and Sutton et al., 1999). Tables of threshold values are given in these papers and also by Tamminga (1992).

A. REDUCE NITROGEN LEVELS AND IMPROVE AMINO ACID BALANCE TO REDUCE pH AND TOTAL N, AMMONIA, AND WATER EXCRETION

Use of phase feeding reduced nitrogen excretion by 4.4% (Boisen et al., 1991) and multiphase feeding (Vander Peet-Schwering et al., 1996) resulted in reductions of NH_3 emission that ranged from 3.5 to 16.8% in studies with practical feeding methods and regimens.

Similarly, Aarnink (1997) showed in model calculations that a 9% reduction of ammonium N content in slurry could be reached with a reduction of dietary protein content (CP) with 10 g/kg

TABLE 27.10
Overview of the Volatile Products Formed by Microbial Activity in Manure from the Main Components in Urine and Feces

Excreta	Component	Conversion Products in Manure
Urine	Urea	Ammonia
	Glucuronides	Glucuronic acid
	Hippuric acid	Benzoic acid
	Sulfate	Hydrogen sulfide
Feces	Protein	Volatile fatty acids
		Phenoles
		Indole
		Skatole
		Ammonia
		Amines
		Mercaptans
	Carbohydrates (mainly (hemi-)cellulose)	Volatile fatty acids
		Alcohols
		Aldehydes

Source: Adapted from Spoelstra (1979a).

and Sutton et al. (1998) confirmed this in their studies. They reduced CP from 13 to 10% or from 18 to 10% and at the same time they added synthetic amino acids. Reduction in emission with each 1% reduction in CP is less than pointed out here if housing systems are such that high emission floors are used.

B. Manipulate Diets by Adding Nonstarch Polysaccharides and Dietary Acid–Base Balance Toward Acidifying the Urine, Feces, and Excreta

In recent years a new approach has been tested, which implies that ammonia emission can be lowered if the pH of manure is reduced by dietary composition. Geisting and Easter (1986) summarized studies using various dietary components. They reviewed studies using citric acid, hydrochloric acid, propionic acid, fumaric acid, and sulfuric acid at different inclusion levels (1 to 4%). The results concerning the effects on pH in digesta were variable and not always consistent. Other studies have investigated additions of bentonite and zeolite materials. These components are used because of their capacity to bind with NH_3. It is then hypothesized that less NH_3 is released into the atmosphere. Kreiger et al. (1993) in a study with clinoptilolite did not find any effects. Much more promising for reducing ammonia emission into the air, however, are the effects of decreasing the dietary electrolyte balance (base excess) and/or increasing the nonstarch polysaccharide content in the diet of pigs (Canh et al., 1997; 1998a,b,c), as depicted in Figure 27.6. Similarly, one can alter pH of slurry by adding various Ca salts. Mroz et al. (1998) showed that increasing Ca salt levels by adding calcium benzoate (2.4 and 8 g/kg diet) reduced pH in urine from sows from 7.7 to 5.8 and at the same time led to 53% less NH_3 emission.

C. Manipulate Microbes to Alter Odor Emission

In their review, Sutton et al. (1999) studied literature in which microbe species and number can be altered by dietary manipulation. Microbes are associated with odorous compounds, which may change as a result of changes in microbes. This is based on the premise that several microbial species can be involved with, e.g., indol and skatol production (Yokohama and Carlson, 1979).

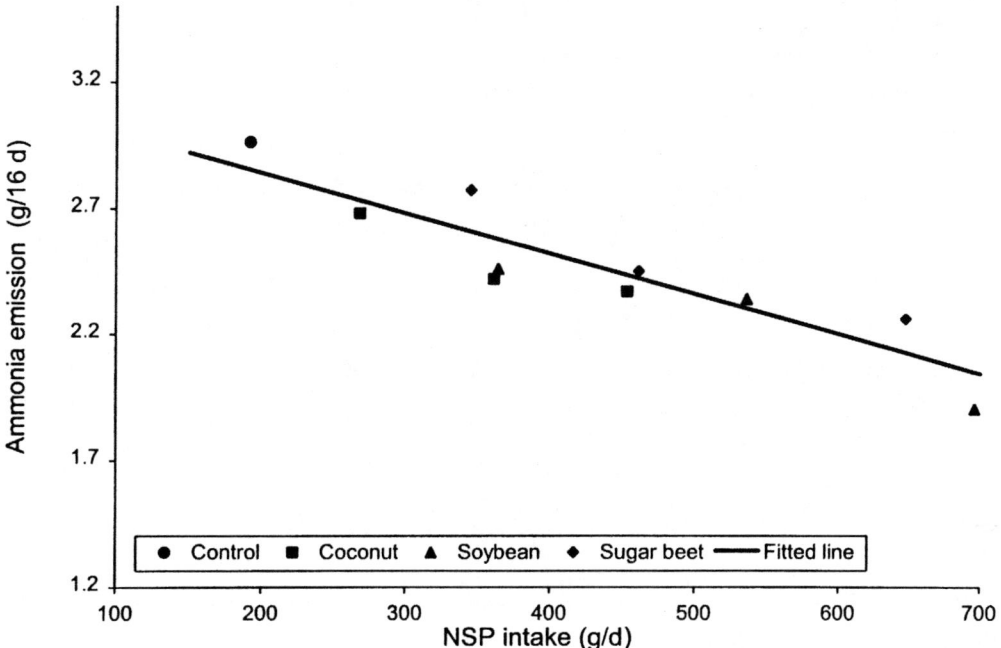

FIGURE 27.6 Ammonia emission from the slurry related to daily intake of nonstarch polysaccharides. (From Canh, T. T. et al., *J. Anim. Sci.*, 76:1887, 1998. With permission.)

Existing microflora in the gastrointestinal tract of pigs are manipulated by introducing substrates in the diet or by introducing specific cultures to the digestive system (Miner, 1995). Nondigestible oligosaccharides, e.g., fructose oligosaccharides, can alter VFA patterns in the lower gastrointestinal tract. In particular, the ratio of acetate to propionate was reduced (Houdijk, 1998) or odorous compounds from manure were reduced (Hidaha et al., 1986). The same principle can be applied if antibiotics are used to influence microbes. Yokohama et al. (1982) showed that pigs fed several antibiotics had less *p*-cresol in the urine. Sutton et al. (1999) reviewed a list of studies showing effects of dietary manipulation on microbes and potential odorous compounds in excreta. Kemme et al. (1993) used specific compounds that are said to bind to odorous components, but they could not find a clear effect.

V. SUMMARY

In recent decades many sectors of agriculture, especially the non-land-using sectors such as pig production systems, have changed dramatically as the result of farm size, specializations, and intensifications. Environmental concerns have led to the study of ways to reduce nutrients excreted with the manure. Nutritional means of achieving these reductions are as follows:

- Better knowledge of nutrient requirements of animals and adjusting diets accordingly; this can diminish N and odor in P and from excreta considerably (5 to 15%)
- Use of bioavailable nutrients in diets (variable effects)
- Diminishing excesses or safety margins in the diet (5 to 10%)
- Processing (variable effects)
- Phase feeding (variable effects)
- Use diets with absence of factors that reduce digestibility and/or availability
- Reduced wastage of feed

- Formulation of diets that are thought to give 95 to 80% of maximum response rather than the maximum response (100%)
- Reduction of odors in feeding strategies by lowering crude protein content
- Changing directly or indirectly the microbial population and activity in the gastrointestinal tract, which will change odor
- Altering the acid–base balance in diets to lower pH of excreta
- Shifting N from urine to fecal matter by using nonstarch polysaccharides in diet.
- Using special products that bind odorous compounds

REFERENCES

Aarnink, A. J. A., 1997. Ammonia Emission from Houses for Growing Pigs as Affected by Pen Design, Indoor Climate and Behaviour, Ph.D. thesis, Agricultural University Wageningen, The Netherlands.

Aarnink, A. J. A., T. T. Canh, and M. W. A. Verstegen. 1994. Influence of dietary factors on pH and ammonia emission from fattening pigs, *J. Anim. Sci.*, Vol. 72, (suppl. 1): 324 (Abstr. 1248).

Adeola, O., B. V. Lawrence, A. L. Sutton, and T. R. Cline. 1995. Phytase-induced changes in mineral utilization in zinc-supplemented diets for pigs, *J. Anim. Sci.*, 73:3384.

Apgar, G. A., and E. T. Kornegay. 1996. Mineral balance of finishing pigs fed copper sulfate or a copper lysine complex as growth stimulating levels, *J. Anim. Sci.*, 74:1594.

ARC. 1981. The Nutrient Requirements for Farm Livestock. III. *Pigs*, Agricultural Research Council, London.

Baxter, C. A., B. C. Joern, and O. Adeola. 1998. Dietary P management to reduce soil P loading from pig manure. In *Proc. of the 28th North Central Extension-Industry Soil Fertility Conference*, St. Louis, MO, Nov. 11–12, 14:104–109.

Boisen, S., J. A. Fernandez, and A. Madsen. 1991. Studies on ideal protein requirement of pigs from 20 to 95 kg live weight. *Proc. 6th Int. Symp. Protein Metabolism Nutr.*, Hering, Denmark, p. 299.

Booms-Prins, E. R., H. G. van der Meer, J. Sanders, S. Tamminga, and F. van Vugt, 1996. [Drastic improvement of nutrient utilisation in Animal Production]. In NRLO Report 94/3, The Hague, The Netherlands, 1–10.

Bridges, T. C., L. W. Turner, G. L. Cromwell, and J. L. Pierce. 1995. Modeling the effects of diet formulation on nitrogen and phosphorus excretion in swine waste, *Appl. Eng. Agric.*, 11(5):731.

Canh, T. T., M. W. A. Verstegen, A. J. A. Aarnink, and J. W. Schrama. 1997. Influence of dietary factors on nitrogen partitioning and composition of urine and feces of fattening pigs, *J. Anim. Sci.*, 75:700.

Canh, T. T., A. J. A. Aarnink, Z. Mroz, A. W. Jongbloed, J. W. Schrama and M. W. A. Verstegen, 1998a. Influence of dietary electrolyte balance and acidifying Ca-salts in the diet of growing-finishing pigs on urinary pH, slurry pH and ammonia volatilisation, *Livest. Prod. Sci.*, 56:1.

Canh, T. T., A. J. A. Aarnink, M. W. A. Verstegen, and J. W. Schrama. 1998b. Influence of dietary factors on the pH and ammonia emission of slurry from growing-finishing pigs, *J. Anim. Sci.*, 76:1123.

Canh, T. T., A. L. Sutton, A. J. A. Aarnink, M. W. A. Verstegen, J. W. Schrama, and G. C. M. Bakker. 1998c. Dietary carbohydrates alter the fecal composition and pH and the ammonia emission from slurry of growing pigs, *J. Anim. Sci.*, 76:1887.

Carter, S. D., G. L. Cromwell, M. D. Lindemann, L. W. Turner, and T. C. Bridges. 1996. Reducing N and P excretion by dietary manipulation in growing and finishing pigs, *J. Anim. Sci.*, 74(Suppl. 1):59 (Abstr.).

Chauvel, J., and R. Granier. 1996. Effet de l'alimentation multiphase sur la croissance et les rejets azotes du porc charcutier, *J. Rec. Porcine Fr.*, 28:249.

Coffey, M. T. 1992. An industry perspective on environmental and waste management issues: challenge for the feed industry, *Ga. Nutr. Conf.*, 144.

Combs, N. R., E. T. Kornegay, M. D. Lindemann, and D. R. Notter. 1991a. Calcium and phosphorus requirement of swine from weaning to market weight: 1. Development of response curves for performance, *J. Anim. Sci.*, 69:673.

Combs, N. R., E. T. Kornegay, M.D. Lindemann, D. R. Notter, J. H. Wilson, and J. P. Mason. 1991b. Calcium and phosphorus requirement of swine from weaning to market weight: II. Development of response curves for bone criteria and comparison of bending and shear bone testing, *J. Anim. Sci.*, 69:682.

Correll, D. L. 1999. Phosphorus: a rate limiting nutrient in surface waters, *Poult. Sci.*, 78:674.

Crenshaw, T. D., and J. C. Johanson. 1995. Nutritional strategies for waste reduction management: minerals. In *New Horizons in Anim. Nutr. and Health*, Longenecker, J. B., and J. W. Spears, Eds., The Institute of Nutrition of The University of North Carolina, Chapel Hill, Nov. 7 and 8.

Cromwell, G. L. 1989. An evaluation of the requirements and biological availability of calcium and phosphorus for swine. In *Feed Phosphates in Monogastric Nutrition*, Texasgulf Nutrition Symposium, May 23, Raleigh, NC.

Cromwell, G. L. 1994. Feeding strategies urged as techniques to decrease pollution from hog manure, *Feedstuffs*, 66:9.

Cromwell, G. L., and R. D. Coffey. 1991. Phosphorus — a key essential nutrient, yet a possible major pollutant — its central role in animal nutrition. In *Biotechnology in the Feed Industry*, Lysons, T. P., Ed., Alltech Technical Publications, Nicholasville, KY, 133–145.

Cromwell, G. L., T. R. Cline, J. D. Crenshaw, T. D. Crenshaw, R. C. Ewan, C. R. Hamilton, A. J. Lewis, D. C. Mahan, E. R. Miller, J. E. Pettigrew, L. F. Tribble, and T. L. Veum. 1993. The dietary protein and/or lysine requirements of barrows and gilts, *J. Anim. Sci.*, 71:1510.

Cromwell, G. L., J. L. Pierce, T. E. Sauber, D. W. Rice, D. S. Ertl, and V. Raboy. 1998. Bioavailability of phosphorus in low-phytic acid corn for growing pigs, *J. Anim. Sci.*, 76(Suppl. 2):58.

CVB (Centraal Veevoeder Bureau). 1993. [Shortened table. Nutrient requirements of livestock and feeding value of feedstuffs], Centraal Veevoederbureau, Lelystad, The Netherlands.

CVB (Centraal Veevoeder Bureau). 1994. [Table for Feedstuffs. Data on the chemical composition, digestibility and feeding value of feed ingredients], Centraal Veevoederbureau, Lelystad, The Netherlands.

FEFANA (Federation Europeenne des Fabricants d'Adjuvants pour la Nutrition Animale). 1992. Improvements in the environments: possibilities for the reduction of nitrogen and phosphorus pollution caused by animal production, FEFANA, Brussels, Belgium.

Gahl, M. J., T. D. Crenshaw, and N. J. Benevenga. 1995. Diminishing returns in weight, nitrogen, and lysine gain of pigs fed six levels of lysine from three supplemental sources, *J. Anim. Sci.*, 73:3177.

Gatel, F. 1994. Low protein, amino acid supplemented diets for pigs, *Feed Mix*, 2:32.

Gatel, F., and F. Grosjean. 1992. Effect of protein content of the diet on nitrogen excretion by pigs, *Livest. Prod. Sci.*, 31:109.

Geisting, D. W., and R. A. Easter. 1986. Acidification status in swine diets, *Feed Manage.*, 37:8.

GFE, Ausschuss für Bedarfsnormen der Gesellschaft für Ernährungsphysiologie 1987: Energie- und Nährstoffbedarf landwirtschaftlicher Nutztiere. No. 4: Schweine. DLG-Verlag, Frankfurt, 153 pp.

Hahn, J. D., and D. H. Baker. 1993. Growth and plasma zinc responses of young pigs fed pharmacologic levels of zinc, *J. Anim. Sci.*, 71:3020.

Hancock, J. D., K. J. Wondra, S. L. Traylor, and I. Mavromichalis. 1996. Feed processing and diet modifications affect growth performance and economics of swine production, *Carolina Swine Nutrition Conference, Proceedings*, Nov. 1996, 90–109.

Harper, A. F. 1994. Feeding technologies to reduce excess nutrients in swine diets. In *Proc. Meeting the Challenge of Environmental Management on Hog Farms*, Second Annual Virginia Tech Swine Producers Seminar, Carson, VA, Aug. 4, 44–51.

Heady, E. O., R. Woodworth, D. R. Catron, and G. C. Ashton. 1954. New procedures in estimating feed substitution rates and in determining economic efficiency in pork production. Agric. Exp. Sta. Res. Bull., Iowa State College, Ames, 893–976.

Henry, Y., and J. Y. Dourmad. 1992. Protein nutrition and N pollution, *Feed Mix*, May, 25–28.

Henry, Y., and J. Y. Dourmad. 1993. Feeding strategies for minimizing nitrogen outputs in pigs. In Nitrogen flow in pig production and environmental consequences. *Proc. First Int. Symposium on Nitrogen Flow in Pig Production and Environmental Consequences*, EAAP Publication 69, 137 pp.

Hidaka, H., T. Eida, T. Takizawa, T. Tokanaga and Y. Tashiro. 1986. Effect of fructooligo-saccharides on intestinal flora and human health, *Bifidobact. Microflora*, 5:37–50.

Hill, G. M., G. L. Cromwell, T. D. Crenshaw, R. C. Ewan, K. A. Knabe, A. J. Lewis, D. C. Mahan, G. C. Shurson, L. L. Southern, and T. L. Veum, NCR-42 and S-145 Regional Swine Nutrition Committees. 1996. Impact of pharmacological intakes of zinc and/or copper on performance of weanling pigs, *J. Anim. Sci.*, 74(Suppl. 1):181 (Abstr.).

Houdijk, J. G. M. 1998. Effects of Non-Digestible Oligosaccharides in Young Pig Diets, Ph.D. thesis, Wageningen, The Netherlands, 1–184.

INRA. 1984. L'alimentation des animaux monogastriques, porc, lapin, volailles, Institut National de la Recherche Agronomique, Paris.

Jongbloed, A. W., and C. H. Henkens. 1996. Environmental concerns of using animal manure — The Dutch case. In: *Nutrient Management of Food Animals to Enhance and Protect the Environment*, Kornegay, E. T., Ed., CRC Press, Boca Raton, FL, 315–333.

Kemme, P. A. 1998. Phytate and phytases in Pig Nutrition. Impact on Nutrient Digestibility and Factors Affecting Phytase Efficacy, Ph.D. thesis, University of Utrecht, The Netherlands.

Kemme, P. A., A. W. Jongbloed, B. M. Dellaert, and F. Krol-Kramer. 1993. The use of a Yucca Schidigera extract as 'urease inhibitor' in pig slurry. In *Nitrogen Flow in Pig Production and Environmental Consequences*, Verstegen, M. W. A., L. A. den Hartog, G. J. M. van Kempen, and J. H. M. Metz, Eds., EAAP Publ. 69, Pudoc Wageningen, The Netherlands, 330–335.

Kephart, K. B., and G. W. Sherritt. 1990. Performance and nutrient balance in growing swine fed low-protein diets supplemented with amino acids and potassium, *J. Anim. Sci.*, 68:1999.

Kerr, B. J., and R. A. Easter. 1995. Effect of feeding reduced protein, amino acid-supplemented diets on nitrogen and energy balance in grower pigs, *J. Anim. Sci.*, 73:3000.

Kornegay, E. T. 1978a. Feeding value and digestibility of soybean hulls for swine, *J. Anim. Sci.*, 47:1272.

Kornegay, E. T. 1978b. Protein digestibility of hydrolyzed hog hair meal for swine, *Anim. Feed Sci. Technol.*, 3:323.

Kornegay, E. T. 1986. Calcium and phosphorus in swine nutrition. In *Calcium and Phosphorus in Swine Nutrition*, National Feed Ingredients Association, Des Moines, IA, 1–102.

Kornegay, E. T. 1996. Nutritional, environmental and economical considerations for using phytase in pig diets. In *Nutrient Management of Food Animals to Enhance and Protect the Environment*, Kornegay, E. T., Ed., CRC Press, Boca Raton, FL, 279–304.

Kornegay, E. T., and A. F. Harper. 1997. Environmental nutrition: nutrient management strategies to reduce nutrient excretion of swine, *Prof. Anim. Sci.*, 13:99–111.

Kornegay, E. T., J. S. Radcliffe, and Z. Zhang. 1998. Influence of phytase and diet composition on phosphorus and amino acid digestibilities, and phosphorus and nitrogen excretion in swine, BASF Technical Symposium, Durham, NC, Nov. 16, pp. 125–155.

Kreiger, R., J. Hartung, and A. Pfeiffer. 1993. Experiments with a feed additive to reduce ammonia emissions from pig fattening housing — preliminary results. In Verstegen, M. W. A., L. A. den Hartog, G. J. M. van Kempen, and J. H. M. Metz, Eds., *Nitrogen Flow in Pig Production and Environmental Consequences*, EAAP Publ. 69, Wageningen, The Netherlands, 295–300.

LeMieux, F. M., L. V. Ellison, T. L. Ward, L. L. Southern, and T. D. Bidner. 1995. Excess dietary zinc for pigs weaned at 28 days, *J. Anim. Sci.*, 73(Suppl. 1):72.

Lei, X. G., P. Ku, E. R. Miller, D. E. Ullrey, and M. T. Yokoyama. 1993. Supplemental microbial phytase improves bioavailability of dietary zinc to weanling pigs, *J. Nutr.*, 123:117.

Lei, X. G., P. K. Ku, E. R. Miller, M. T. Yokoyama, and D. E. Ullrey. 1994. Calcium level affects the efficacy of supplemental microbial phytase in corn–soybean meal diets of weanling pigs, *J. Anim. Sci.*, 72:139.

Liptrap, D. O., and M. G. Hogberg. 1991. Physical forms of feed: feed processing and feeder design and operation. In *Swine Nutrition*, Miller, E. R., D. E. Ullrey, and A. J. Lewis, Eds., Butterworth-Heinemann, Boston, MA, 373–386.

Liu, J., D. W. Bollinger, K. Zyla, D. R. Ledoux, and T. L. Veum. 1998. Lowering the dietary calcium to total phosphorus ratio increases phosphorus utilization in low-phosphorus corn–soybean meal diets supplemented with microbial phytase for growing-finishing pigs, *J. Anim. Sci.*, 76:808.

Miner, J. R. 1995. Nature and control of odors from pork production facilities. A review of literature, National Pork Producers Council, Des Moines, IA.

Mroz, Z., A. W. Jongbloed, and P. A. Kemme. 1994. Apparent digestibility and retention of nutrients bound to phytate complexes as influenced by microbial phytase and feeding regimen in pigs, *J. Anim. Sci.*, 72:126–132.

Mroz, Z., W. Krasucki, and E. Grela. 1998. Prevention of bacteriuria and ammonia emission by adding sodium benzoate to diets for pregnant sows. In *Proc. Annual Meeting EAAP*, Vienna, Austria.

Mueller, J. P., J. P. Zublena, M. H. Poore, J. C. Barker, and J. T. Green. 1994. Managing pasture and hay fields receiving nutrients for anaerobic swine waste lagoons, N.C. Cooperative Ext. Service, AG-506.

NRC (National Research Council). 1988. *Nutrient Requirements of Swine*, 9th rev. ed., National Academy Press, Washington, D.C.

NRC (National Research Council). 1998. *Nutrient Requirements of Swine*, 10th rev. ed., National Academy Press, Washington, D.C.

Overfield, J. J., J. Krug, and R. Adkins. 1986. Swine Nutrient Requirement Survey, A report prepared for the Swine Committee of the AFIA Nutrition Council.

Pallauf, J., G. Rimbach, S. Pippig, B. Schindler, and E. Most. 1994. Effect of phytase supplementation to a phytate-rich diet based on wheat, barley and soya on the bioavailability of dietary phosphorus, calcium, magnesium, zinc and protein in piglets, *Agribiol. Res.*, 47:39.

Pierce, J. L., G. L. Cromwell, and V. Raboy. 1998a. Nutritional value of low-phytic acid corn for finishing pigs, *J. Anim. Sci.*, 76(Suppl. 1):177.

Pierce, J. L., G. L. Cromwell, T. E. Sauber, D. W. Rice, D. S. Ertl, and V. Raboy. 1998b. Phosphorus digestibility and nutritional value of low-phytic acid corn for growing pigs, *J. Anim. Sci.*, 76(Suppl. 2):54.

Pierzynski, G. M., J. T. Sims, and G. F. Vance. 1994. *Soils and Environmental Quality*, CRC Press, Boca Raton, FL, 313.

Raboy, V., K. Young, and P. Gerbasi. 1994. Maize low phytic acid (1pa) mutants, 4th International Congress of Plant Molecular Biology, No. 1827.

Radcliffe, J. S., E. T. Kornegay, and D. E. Conner, Jr. 1995. The effect of phytase on calcium release in weanling pigs fed corn–soybean meal diets, *J. Anim. Sci.*, 73(Suppl. 1):173.

SCA. 1987. Feeding Standards for Australian Livestock. V. Pigs, Editorial and Publishing Unit, CSIRO, East Melbourne, Australia.

Sharpley, A. N., S. C. Chapra, R. Wedepohl, J. T. Sims, T. C. Daniel, and K. R. Reddy. 1994. Managing agricultural phosphorus for protection of surface waters: issues and options, *J. Environ. Qual.*, 23:437.

Sims, J. T. 1993. Environmental soil testing for phosphorus, *J. Prod. Agric.*, 6:501.

Smith, II, J. W., M. D. Tokach, R. D. Goodband, J. L. Nelssen, W. B. Nessmith, Jr., K. Q. Owen, and B. T. Richert. 1995. The effect of increasing zinc oxide supplementation on starter pig growth performance, *J. Anim. Sci.*, 73(Suppl. 1):72.

Spears, J. W. 1996. Optimizing mineral levels and sources for farm animals. In *Nutrient Management of Food Animals to Enhance and Protect the Environment*, Kornegay, E. T., Ed., CRC Press, Boca Raton, FL, 259–276.

Spencer, J. D., G. L. Allee, A. Leytem, R. L. Mikkelsen, T. E. Sauber, D. S. Ertl, and V. Raboy. 1998. Phosphorus availability and nutritional value of a genetically modified low phytate corn for pigs. Animal Production Systems and the Environment, Des Moines, IA, July 19–22, pp. 61–66.

Spoelstra, S. F. 1979a. Vluchtige verbindingen in anaeroob bewaarde varkensdrijfmest [Volatile compounds in anaerobically stored piggery wastes], *Landbouwkd. Tijdschr.*, 91(8): 227.

Sutton, A. L., K. B. Kephart, J. A. Patterson, R. Mumma, D. T. Kelley, E. Bogus, D. D. Jones, and A. Heber. 1997. Dietary manipulation to reduce ammonia and odorous compounds in excreta and anaerobic manure storage. In International Symposium on Ammonia and Odour Control from Animal Production Facilities, Voermans, J. A. M., and G. J. Monteny, Eds., Praktijkonderzoek Varkenshouderij, Rosmalen, The Netherlands, 245–252.

Sutton, A. L., K. B. Kephart, M. W. A. Verstegen, T. T. Canh, and P. J. Hobbs. 1999. Potential for reduction of odorous compounds in swine manure through diet modification, *J. Anim. Sci.*, 77:430.

Tamminga, S.. 1992. Gaseous pollutants produced by farm animal enterprices. In *Farm Animals and the Environment*, Phillips, C., and D. Piggins, Eds., CAB International, Wallingford, U.K., 345–357.

Van der Honing, Y., A. W. Jongbloed, and N. P. Lenis. 1993. Nutrition management to reduce environmental pollution by pigs. VII World Conf. on Anim. Prod., Edmonton, Alberta (Abstr.).

Vander Peet-Schwering, C. M. C., and M. Voermans. 1996. Effect van voeding en huisvesting op de ammoniakemissie uit vleesvarkensstallen, *Praktijkonderzoek Varkenshouderij Jaargang*, 10:17.

Vander Peet-Schwering, C. M. C., N. Verdoes, M. P. Voermans, and G. M. Beelen. 1996. Effect of feeding and housing on the ammonia emission of growing and finishing pig facilities, Research Institute of Pig Husbandry Rep. P. 5. 3, pp. 27–28.

Van Heugten, E., and T. Van Kempen. 1999. Methods may exist to reduce nutrient excretion, *Feedstuffs*, April 1, 6 pp.

Veum, T., V. Raboy, D. Ertl, and D. Ledoux. 1998. Low phytic acid corn improves calcium and phosphorus utilization for growing pigs, *J. Anim. Sci.*, 76(Suppl. 1):177.

Wondra, K. J., J. D. Hancock, K. C. Behnke, R. H. Hines, and C. R. Stark. 1995. Effects of particle size and pelleting on growth performance, nutrient digestibility, and stomach morphology in finishing pigs, *J. Anim. Sci.*, 73:757.

Yokoyama, M. T., and J. R. Carlson. 1979. Microbial metabolites of tryptophan in the intestinal tract with special reference to skatole, *Am. J. Clin. Nutr.*, 32:173–178.

Yokoyama, M. T., C. Tabori, E. R. Miller, and M. G. Hogberg. 1982. The effects of antibiotics in the weanling pig diet on growth and excretion of volatile phenolic and aromatic bacterial metabolites, *Am. J. Clin. Nutr.*, 43:1417–1424.

28 Swine Nutrition, the Conversion of Muscle to Meat, and Pork Quality

Eric P. Berg

CONTENTS

I. Introduction 632
II. Physicochemical Factors Affecting the Conversion of Muscle to Meat...............................632
    A. Biochemical..632
    B. Molecular 633
    C. Physiological 633
        1. Stress 633
        2. Muscle Physiology 634
            a. Fast-Twitch MHC Isoforms 635
            b. Slow-Twitch MHC Isoforms 635
    D. Structural 635
        1. Protein 635
        2. Protein–Water Interactions 636
        3. Fat 636
III. Early Post-Mortem Conditioning Effects on Pork Quality...637
IV. Feeding for Quality..638
    A. Preslaughter Feed Withdrawal 639
    B. Preslaughter Feed Restriction 640
    C. Manipulating Preslaughter Carbohydrate Intake..640
    D. Manipulation of Preslaughter Protein and/or Amino Acids......................................641
    E. Dietary Fat Source and Fatty Acid Profile of Pork Fat 642
        1. General 642
        2. Conjugated Linoleic Acid 644
    F. Vitamins and Minerals 645
        1. Vitamin D..645
        2. Vitamin E 646
        3. Magnesium 647
        4. Chromium 647
        5. Copper 654
V. Conclusion...654
References 654

I. INTRODUCTION

Marsh (1970) wrote that muscle is a machine for translating chemical energy into physical movement. Like most machines, muscle has a supporting structure, an energy store, a fuel entry, and a waste exhaust system. What makes muscle different from a machine is that at the end of its working life it is both edible and nutritious and a valuable item of commerce. The primary reason for feeding pigs is to increase the quantity of the edible product (meat). For meat to remain a valuable item of commerce, the entire meat production chain must strive to produce a high-quality product that consumers will repeatedly purchase. Athletes and sports enthusiasts know that the diet that they consume in preparation for an athletic event will influence the performance of their muscles or (to carry the analogy further) improve the effectiveness of the "machine." Athletes and trainers have long known that the type and quantity of nutrients consumed will influence the physicochemical factors of muscle performance, energy utilization, and tissue composition. Similarly, nutrients consumed by meat-producing animals will ultimately affect the physicochemical factors responsible for the conversion of living muscle to meat and influence meat quality.

The objective of this chapter is to provide an overview of the biochemical and physiological (physicochemical) factors that influence the conversion of muscle to high-quality meat and to provide scientific evidence regarding the role of preharvest nutrition on this conversion process.

II. PHYSICOCHEMICAL FACTORS AFFECTING THE CONVERSION OF MUSCLE TO MEAT

A. BIOCHEMICAL

The extent of myofibrillar post-mortem change is dependent on the synthesis, degradation, and availability of high-energy phosphate compounds. Adenosine triphosphate (ATP), adenosine diphosphate (ADP), and creatine phosphate (CP) provide immediate sources of energy for muscle contraction. Creatine phosphate provides a source of high-energy phosphate and serves to rephosphorylate ADP to form ATP. Contraction begins when ATP binds within the myosin globular head and is degraded by myofibrillar actomyosin adenosine triphosphatase (mATPase) to ADP·Pi. With the release of Pi, a weak bond is formed between myosin and actin. Release of ADP initiates the power stroke and formation of a rigor (actomyosin; AM) bond (Huxley and Simmons, 1971). The AM bond is released when ATP rebinds myosin, allowing myosin to release from actin and reactivate for another contraction. The pathways for glycolysis and the tricarboxylic acid (TCA) cycle produce the bulk of myofibrillar ATP. The energy for powering glycolysis and the TCA cycle is glucose, which is stored by the body as the readily available branched polymer glycogen. The main storage sites of glycogen are the liver and muscle, where it occupies (on average) approximately 4 and 0.7% of the tissue mass, respectively. Because of its larger total mass, muscle glycogen represents three to four times more stored glycogen than is available from the liver (Mayes, 1993). The liver is almost entirely depleted of glycogen after 12 to 18 h of fasting, whereas muscle glycogen is only depleted significantly after a period of prolonged, vigorous exercise.

Glucose-1-phosphate released from muscle glycogen begins the conversion of muscle to meat. After exsanguination, cessation of blood circulation shifts muscle metabolism from aerobic to anaerobic. Mayes (1993) reports that when muscle contracts in an anaerobic environment, glycogen disappears and lactic acid becomes the principal end product of glycolysis (as opposed to the aerobic production of pyruvate). Under aerobic conditions lactic acid does not accumulate because it is oxidized to CO_2 and water or is removed by the circulatory system for disposal by the liver. One molecule of glucose will generate 3 mol of ATP via anaerobic glycolysis. This will provide the high-energy phosphates necessary for post-mortem (anaerobic) muscle contraction. Creatine phosphate is rapidly depleted as a result of post-mortem metabolism, yet ATP may be maintained for several hours from anaerobic glycolysis. Accumulation of lactic acid in post-mortem muscle reduces the localized pH and muscle is converted to meat. Conversion of glycogen to lactic acid will continue to lower muscle pH until the glycogen (or ATP stores) are depleted or until the contractile proteins cease to function as a result of low intramuscular pH.

B. Molecular

The primary molecules involved in muscle contraction are Ca^{2+}, ATP, ADP, Pi, actin, and myosin. Myosin possesses two binding sites on its large globular (S1) head; one binds ATP and has a myofibrillar ATPase that regulates speed of contraction by the rate of ATP hydrolysis. The other site binds actin to allow for the subsequent contraction stroke. Calcium ions aid in activation of the rigor (actomyosin) bond by binding to the troponin C molecule (on actin) causing a structural change to expose the myosin-binding site. Muscle contraction (myosin binding to actin) is regulated by Ca^{2+} levels inside the muscle cell (sarcoplasm). An efferent signal from the brain initiates the release of Ca^{2+} from the storage organelle called the sarcoplasmic reticulum. To cease contraction (relaxation), Ca^{2+} is returned to the sarcoplasmic reticulum via an ATP-driven calcium pump, which rapidly lowers Ca^{2+} concentrations within the sarcoplasm to levels that will not induce contraction.

High levels of sarcoplasmic Ca^{2+} in post-mortem muscle will also affect myosin activation (early post-mortem muscle contraction) and influence post-mortem activity of Ca^{2+}-dependent proteases, such as phosphorylase kinase (a regulatory enzyme of glycogenolysis; Louis et al., 1993) and the calpain proteolytic system (which play a direct role in post-mortem structural protein denaturation resulting in improved tenderness; Koohmaraie, 1992).

C. Physiological

1. Stress

The pig's physiological response to stress plays a significant role in the conversion of muscle to meat. Stressors that trigger a physiological response can be of short term (such as a loud noise, unfamiliar environment, fighting, or goading with an electric prod) or long term (sickness, dehydration, or malnourishment). The physiological response to stress is mediated by the autonomic nervous system whereby the brain sends messages through its projections (efferent nerves) to invoke a response. These nerve projections carry messages to muscles, capillaries, and/or the heart that are involuntary and essentially automatic. The sympathetic and parasympathetic nervous systems are the two components of the autonomic nervous system. Response and recovery from a stressor involves a balance between these two systems.

The sympathetic nervous system mediates vigilance, arousal, activation, and mobilization and is typically characterized by the physiological response to fight, fright, and flight. The catecholamines epinephrine (adrenaline) and norepinephrine (noradrenaline) are released from the adrenal medulla in response to activation of the sympathetic nervous system. The sympathetic nervous system stimulates a cascade of reactions to generate energy rapidly in response to the stressor while at the same time inhibiting energy storage, digestion, and immune function. Epinephrine stimulates glycogenolysis and lipolysis whereby glucose is mobilized from glycogen stores in the liver and muscle and fatty acids are released from fat cells. Epinephrine also stimulates an increase in heart rate and/or blood pressure and invokes peripheral vasodilatation to increase blood flow to the extremities for delivery of metabolites (such as oxygen and glucose) to the muscle to facilitate "escape" from the stressor. Similarly, the increased blood flow removes metabolic waste products such as lactic acid (which induce fatigue) and provides for heat dissipation produced as a result of muscle contraction. Sympathetic release of norepinephrine also stimulates lipolysis in response to stress; however, it does not affect glycogenolysis. Furthermore, norepinephrine stimulates peripheral vasoconstriction. Temperature is a positive modulator of chemomechanical coupling of muscle contractile proteins. Elevated muscle temperature increases the rate of shortening, increases contractile force, increases maximum tension, and enhances Ca^{2+} sensitivity of the contractile proteins.

Peripheral vasoconstriction inhibits external heat loss during the initial response to stress allowing for muscles to "warm up," maximizing muscle efficiency.

Epinephrine and norepinephrine are neurotransmitters produced and released from the nervous tissue that comprises the adrenal medulla responding immediately to a stress situation. Epinephrine and norepinephrine will continue to be released during prolonged stimulation of the sympathetic nervous system; however, both have very short half-lives in circulation (1 to 2 min). Prolonged exposure to stress will result in release of glucocorticoids from the adrenal cortex. The adrenal cortex comprises epithelial tissue (tissue similar to the gonads) and produces the stress steroid hormones cortisol and corticosterone. These glucocorticoids have a longer half-life in circulation (~20 min) and are often quantified as a stress indicator in stress physiology trials. During prolonged activation of the sympathetic nervous system, glucocorticoids will stimulate the process of gluconeogenesis and proteolysis. The prolonged release of glucocorticoids ultimately results in muscle tissue wasting as gluconeogenic amino acids are obtained from degraded muscle proteins, converted to glucose in the liver, and returned to the muscle for use as energy.

The parasympathetic nervous system mediates calm, relaxed state (everything but fight, fright, and flight). This system promotes growth, energy storage, digestion, absorption, and tissue repair. The two systems of the autonomic nervous system work in balance with one another. The sympathetic nervous system speeds up heart rate while the parasympathetic slows it down. The sympathetic system mobilizes energy from storage, whereas the parasympathetic promotes digestion, absorption, and energy storage, depositing glucose as glycogen and fatty acids as triglycerides.

2. Muscle Physiology

Different isoforms of contractile proteins are associated with differing degrees of muscle fiber response to physiological factors, such as a localized reduction of pH (Moss et al., 1995). The protein myosin is the largest member of the contractile apparatus in skeletal muscle fibers. The metabolic activity for differentiation between muscle fiber types is largely determined by the type and concentration of myosin isoform that constitutes the myofiber (muscle cell). The myosin molecule is responsible for contractile speed of the fiber, is susceptible to acid or alkaline sensitivity of mATPase activity, and contains the enzymes of oxidative or glycolytic metabolism.

Muscle fiber types are identified by differences in metabolic activity of mATPase based on staining intensity at specified tissue pH or by the presence of specific enzymes of anaerobic and aerobic energy metabolism. Type I muscle fibers have a slow mATPase activity, are oxidative, and constitute slow, fatigue resistant motor units. Type IIB myofibers possess a fast mATPase, a low aerobic (oxidative) capacity, and a high glycolytic metabolism. Type IIB myofibers constitute fast-fatigue motor units associated with great bursts of strength. Type IIA myofibers possess a fast mATPase yet are distinguished form IIB fibers by a higher aerobic (oxidative) capacity and are associated with fast, fatigue-resistant motor units capable of greater endurance. Schiaffino et al. (1989) identified an additional fast fiber type IIX (sometimes referred to as IID) which has an mATPase activity similar to type IIB after acid preincubation yet is distinguished from IIB after alkaline preincubation (Pette and Staron, 1990). The myofiber type IIX (IID) possesses an aerobic oxidative enzymatic activity intermediate between that of the fast myofiber types IIB and IIA.

Conversion of muscle to meat depends on the physiology of individual muscle fibers and will affect the length of the post-mortem biochemical activity. Muscle fiber types IIB and IID have been reported to be more stable under acid conditions (Pette and Staron, 1990). Fast muscle types exhibit a glycolytic metabolism that is necessary for rapid and strong bursts of power. These fiber types will propel glycogenolysis to lactic acid formation longer under the anaerobic conditions of post-mortem muscle. Essen-Gustavsson et al. (1992) reported that type I (slow, oxidative, fatigue-resistant) and type IIA (fast, higher oxidative capacity) muscle fibers from pig longissimus muscle were depleted of glycogen at slaughter, while type IIB (fast, lower oxidative capacity, higher glycolytic) fibers still retained some glycogen. Muscle tissue with a high concentration of fast IIB muscle fibers has the potential for a rapid reduction in post-mortem pH while the carcass temperature remains high, which could result in protein denaturation and a reduction in meat quality.

Muscle fiber type is characterized by (1) speed of contraction, (2) rate of *m*ATPase activity (rate of ATP hydrolysis), (3) acid or alkaline sensitivity of *m*ATPase, (4) myosin isoform composition, (5) mitochondrial (oxidative) or glycolytic energy metabolism; and/or (6) a combination of all (Pette and Staron, 1990). All of these characteristics can be attributed to the type and concentration of myosin heavy-chain (MHC) isoform associated within the muscle fiber. The physiology of a specific MHC isoform will affect the rate and level of pH decline as a result of post-mortem conversion of glycogen to lactic acid. Early post-mortem conditioning is ultimately influenced by the distinctive physiology and metabolic activity of myosin isoforms.

a. Fast-twitch MHC Isoforms

The first two fast types to be identified in the literature were MHCIIa and MHCIIb. The fast type, MHCIIa, is the principal isoform present in type IIA muscle fibers. This isoform has a higher oxidative capacity for greater endurance and is often referred to as fast oxidative-glycolytic (FOG). The fast MHCIIb is the principal heavy-chain isoform associated with the muscle type IIB, which are fast-fatigue motor units. Myosin heavy chain IIb has a low oxidative and higher glycolytic energy metabolism and is associated with greater strength of contraction. This isoform is often referred to as fast glycolytic (FG). Recently, Schiaffino et al. (1989) reported discovery of another fast MHC isoform: MHC IIx. This isoform, associated with fast motor units capable of sustained activity, was found in large concentrations in diaphragm muscle and tentatively named MHCIId. Several studies have reported increased expression of MHC IIx (d) in muscles undergoing transition from strength to endurance by chronic electrostimulation (Bär and Pette, 1988; Schiaffino et al., 1989; Termin et al., 1989). Pette and Staron (1990) reported that independent analysis suggests that MHCIIx and MHCIId are identical.

b. Slow-twitch MHC Isoforms

The slow myosin isoform MHC I is equivalent to the βMHC_{card} isoform of cardiac muscle. This isoform is associated with slow-twitch muscle fibers capable of sustained use. Myosin heavy chain I is the principal isoform found in slow, fatigue-resistant motor units predominated by type I muscle fiber types. During post-mortem conversion of muscle to meat, the muscle pH will range between 5.3 and 6.7 (Pearson et al., 1987). Type I fibers are capable of maintaining a strong *m*ATPase activity at low pH levels; however, glycogen is rapidly depleted in these fibers and post-mortem activity cannot be maintained because of the lack of glucose for conversion to ATP. Hydrolysis of ATP by *m*ATPase is necessary for myosin to bind and to release from myosin binding sites on actin. Without ATP, myosin cannot bind to actin to generate a power stroke, nor can it release from actin once bound. Post-mortem depletion of ATP stores within the muscle is the first step in the formation of the permanent actomyosin (rigor) bond.

D. STRUCTURAL

Protein, water, and fat are the three main components that give meat its unique flavor, texture, and overall palatability. The structural orientation of protein and fat content of muscle foods directly influences the moisture content. The following discussion focuses on how the structural integrity of meat influences pork quality.

1. Protein

Moss et al. (1995) provide an excellent review of the contractile properties of skeletal muscle fibers. Skeletal muscle is considered striated because arrays of dark and light bands are easily observed when a longitudinal cross section of a muscle fiber is viewed under polarized light by an electron microscope. The dark and light bands are a result of overlapping thick and thin filaments (Figure 28.1). The

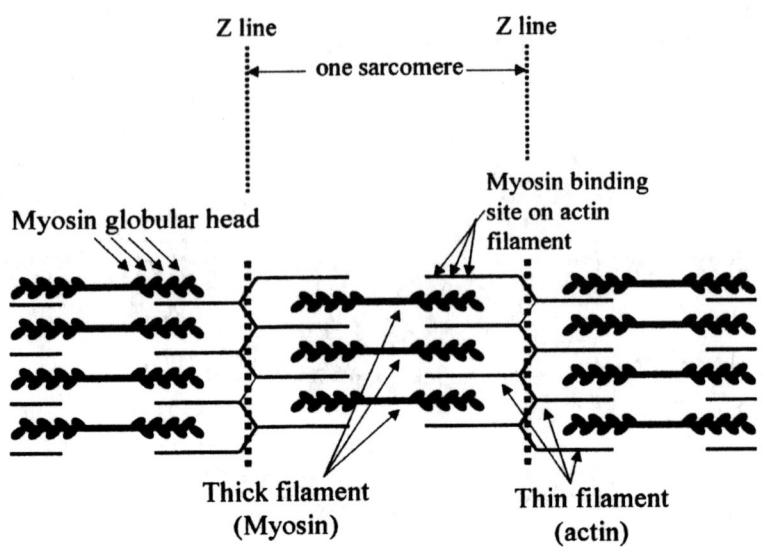

FIGURE 28.1 A simplified adaptation of the ultrastructural arrangement of the myofilaments forming the contractile lattice of the muscle fiber.

contractile protein myosin is the principal component of the thick filament and actin comprises the thin filament. The *sliding filament model* proposed by Huxley (1953) is the most widely accepted theory regarding muscle contraction. As described in Section II.A, muscles contract when the globular head of myosin binds actin forming an actomyosin bond. The hydrolysis of ATP by the *m*ATPase generates a power stroke, which pulls the thin filament over the thick filament. The distance between sarcomeres (Figure 28.1) is shortened due the "row boat" action of myosin, and muscles contract. Myosin is released from actin when an ATP molecule reinserts into the ATP binding site on the myosin globular head. Rebinding of ATP to myosin results in a conformational shift of the myosin S1 head allowing myosin to detach from actin and reactivate for another power stroke.

In post-mortem muscle, a rigor bond (*rigor mortis*) is formed when myosin and actin bind forming a permanent structure. The rigor bond is formed as a result of depletion of ATP. Without ATP, myosin cannot release from actin. The formation of this permanent actomyosin bond is vital in the conversion of muscle to meat and significantly influences the ability of meat to retain moisture.

2. Protein–Water Interactions

Prerigor muscle contains approximately 75% water. When muscle converts to meat, 0.8 to 2.0% of this water is bound covalently to molecules within the muscle. Another 4 to 12% is bound via electrostatic attraction to meat contractile and structural proteins and is dependent on the net charge of meat proteins and the intramuscular pH. The remaining 60 to 70% of this moisture is held by capillary forces within the ultrastructure of the myofilaments (NPPC, 2000). The amount of "free water" maintained within meat depends on the amount of space between the myofilaments. Expulsion or retention of moisture is largely dependent on the amount of space between the thick and thin filaments. Thus, a reduction of space between thick and thin filaments could be likened to wringing out a sponge. Water would be expelled (NPPC, 2000).

3. Fat

The structural composition of meat is not all protein and water. The fat found in meat contributes to the unique flavor, juiciness, and tenderness of meat. The majority of external fat (subcutaneous) is typically removed from wholesale and retail cuts of pork. Fat found between muscles (intermuscular or seam fat) is also removed from pork whenever it is convenient to do so. The fat is trimmed away because today's consumer is very conscious of the amount of total fat that is consumed and will typically avoid meat high in fat. Still, fat provides 1 to 10% of the total composition of pork (excluding bacon) providing 10 to 50% of the total calories. The amount of fat in pork depends on the degree of inter- and intramuscular (marbling) fat present in pork (Pettigrew and Esnaola, 2000). Even though consumers tend to avoid purchasing fresh pork containing high levels of fat (as external, intermuscular, or marbling), they will consistently prefer cooked pork that contains 2 to 6% fat when evaluated in blind taste panel analysis (Miller and Meisinger, 1998). Consumers like the flavor and palatability provided from pork containing a higher percentage fat, yet will avoid purchasing it at the retail case for fear of possible adverse health implications. Therefore, pork containing a greater amount of marbling may find its niche in the restaurant trade (where consumers expect a good "eating experience") and leaner pork would be sold at the retail case.

A growing amount of research has shown that fat in general does not possess the adverse health implications generally perceived by the consuming public. The energy provided from pork fat may even be beneficial for individuals in need of higher-energy requirements. The energy provided from fat can be detrimental when consumed in excess and can lead to increased risk for coronary heart disease (CHD) and obesity (Pettigrew and Esnaola, 2000). More specifically, the type and quantity of certain fatty acids have been linked to development of CHD. Certain saturated fatty acids have been shown to increase an individual's risk for CHD, whereas polyunsaturated fatty acids may be protective against it. Generally speaking, the fatty acid content of pork is approximately one half oleic acid (C18:1). This monounsaturated fatty acid is considered neutral in terms of CHD. Approximately one quarter of the fatty acid profile of pork is palmitic acid (C16:0), a saturated fatty acid largely considered detrimental in terms of heart health. Stearic acid (C18:0), a saturated fatty acid considered neutral in terms of CHD, is also found in lesser quantities in pork (Pettigrew and Esnaola, 2000). From a human nutrition standpoint, it would be beneficial to reduce the proportion of saturated fatty acids in pork and increase the proportion of unsaturated fatty acids. This, however, may not be practical because as pork fat becomes more unsaturated it becomes softer. Soft fat will affect the overall appearance of the fresh pork product because it often leads to a very unappealing separation of lean from fat. Soft fat makes pork difficult to process and reduces the slicing yield of bacon. Highly unsaturated pork used in further processing smears during processing, producing an unattractive product. Unsaturated fat is also more susceptible to lipid oxidation (oxidative rancidity), reducing the shelf life of fresh pork (Pettigrew and Esnaola, 2000). A proper balance of fatty acids is, therefore, desirable.

III. EARLY POST-MORTEM CONDITIONING EFFECTS ON PORK QUALITY

The physicochemical components involved in the conversion of muscle to meat interact to generate acceptable or unacceptable pork. Post-mortem metabolism of porcine muscle is more rapid than that of beef or lamb (Marsh et al., 1972). Metabolism of intramuscular glycogen plays the primary role in the conversion of muscle to meat and the expression of different quality attributes of fresh pork. The level and extent of post-mortem pH decline is glycogen dependent because anaerobic conversion of glycogen to glucose-6-phosphate to lactic acid (as described above) results in the achievement of an acceptable (or unacceptable) meat pH.

The two most common quality concerns with fresh pork are pale, soft, and exudative (PSE) and dark, firm, and dry (DFD) lean. Both are a result of post-mortem glycogen metabolism. The PSE condition occurs when intramuscular lactic acid (localized acidosis) accumulates very rapidly (<1 h) while the carcass temperature is still high. The initiation of glycolysis could be attributed to many things: (1) genetic predisposition (high concentration of glycolytic muscle fiber types); (2) elevated metabolism or "excitability" from overstimulation of the sympathetic nervous system (Grandin, 1994); (3) preslaughter stress (activation of sympathetic nervous system); and/or

(4) combinations of all. Activation of the sympathetic nervous system just prior to exsanguination initiates glycolysis and leads to the production of heat, elevating the pig's body temperature. Early studies conducted by Briskey (1964) reported that the ultimate condition of pork muscle is influenced by skeletal muscle pH drop as a function of time, *in vivo* temperature patterns, carcass chilling rate, and the conditions at the onset of rigor mortis. The rate of post-mortem pH decline is approximately three times faster in carcasses that ultimately produce PSE meat. This rapid pH drop while the carcass temperature is >37°C leads to denaturation and shrinkage of the myofibrillar proteins that bind water (Penny, 1969).

Conditions that affect the structural integrity of post-mortem muscle will ultimately affect overall meat quality and functionality. The myofibrillar proteins actin and myosin are the major proteins associated with formation of the myofibrillar protein lattice. In fresh meat, the mobility of water is determined by the spatial arrangement of the muscle proteins. The extent of myosin denaturation has been reported to affect drip loss and softness associated with PSE meat (van Laack and Solomon, 1995). Offer (1991) reported the rapid decline of pH at a higher muscle temperature caused a denaturation (shrinkage) of the myosin S1 heads and a compression of the myofibrillar lattice causing the expulsion of free water held between the myofibrils. The reduction in lateral spacing between the thick and thin filaments affects the scattering and absorbance of light (appearing paler in color) and increases the softness associated with PSE lean.

Cannon et al. (1995) reported that 75% of pork is used for production of processed meat products. The structural integrity of muscle protein is critical for formation of a protein lattice and water binding of processed meat products. Myofibrillar denaturation that occurs in PSE lean results in poor binding of added moisture and ingredients within processed meats. Monin and Sellier (1985) reported that weight gain during "pickling" was lowest for PSE-type ham muscles. Honkavaara (1990) reported that 1.5% more lean trim was necessary from PSE pork to absorb the same amount of added water as normal pork.

Actin and myosin are the two most important meat proteins with regard to formation of the protein lattice necessary for binding water and fat in further processed meat products. The average isoelectric point (pI) of actin and myosin is near 5.0 (actin 4.7, myosin 5.4; Wismer-Pedersen, 1987). At a muscle pH of 5.0, the net charge of actin and myosin is at a minimum; therefore, the water-holding capacity of the meat is at its lowest. The post-mortem changes of PSE meat rapidly drop the muscle pH near its pI, which leads to increased exudate (drip loss).

The opposite set of conditions occur in the case of DFD meat where the water-holding capacity is greatly improved (Wismer-Pedersen, 1987). Dark, firm, and dry lean is a result of sustained activation of the sympathetic nervous system, which results in nearly total depletion of muscle glycogen prior to slaughter. Sustained muscle activity or sickness prior to slaughter reduces muscle glycogen leaving little substrate for post-mortem glycogenolysis to convert to lactic acid. Dark, firm, and dry lean has an ultimate pH nearer physiological (7.0) and a high water-binding capacity. This high water-binding capacity is beneficial for further processing as added moisture and ingredients are more tightly held within the meat; however, the dark appearance of fresh pork is considered unacceptable to consumers. It is perceived as originating from an old animal or thought to have been held in the retail case for an extended period of time.

IV. FEEDING FOR QUALITY

Nutrients consumed or withheld from the pig's diet prior to slaughter have been found to influence the physicochemical factors that ultimately affect pork quality. Some dietary strategies target the endocrine system in an effort to reduce the deleterious influence of sympathetic nervous system activation. Other components are fed to buffer early post-mortem pH decline and lactic acid accumulation. Specific nutrients have been evaluated for their antioxidant properties to attempt to reduce lipid oxidation, improve pork color, and extend shelf life. Still other strategies strive to improve fresh pork palatability by improving water-holding capacity or enhancing levels of intramuscular fat (marbling). The remainder of this chapter will focus on the role nutrition plays on the biochemical, molecular, physiological, and structural characteristics affecting the conversion of muscle to meat relative to the sensory and technical qualities of pork. Many of the dietary strategies discussed will influence more than one of the physicochemical traits presented above. Therefore, they will be presented in order of nutritional input. Pettigrew and Esnaola (2000) and Ellis and McKeith (1999) provide excellent reviews of nutritional influence on pork quality.

A. Preslaughter Feed Withdrawal

It is generally accepted that a period of fasting before slaughter will reduce the amount of total carbohydrate available for post-mortem conversion of glycogen to glucose to lactic acid (De Smet et al., 1996). Jones et al. (1985) reported that overnight fasting at the slaughter plant resulted in increased ultimate meat pH, improved meat color, and increased water-holding capacity. Eikelenboom et al. (1991) found that pigs held off feed (but not water) for a minimum of 12 h before slaughter exhibited fewer PSE carcasses. Murray et al. (1989) reported that a 24- or 48-h fast significantly reduced the frequency of PSE in stress-susceptible (porcine stress syndrome) pigs. However, the finding that feed restriction is beneficial has not been universal. De Smet et al. (1996) found overnight feed withdrawal to have no effect on meat quality for all PSE-related traits. Becker et al. (1989) found no relationship between pigs fasted up to 72 h and ultimate pork quality but did note that meat tenderness was enhanced by transport and fasting.

The effect of preslaughter fast is often difficult to discern because meat quality is largely influenced by the concentration of glycogen within muscle prior to fasting. The combination of preslaughter stress and fasting can influence the ultimate pork quality. For example, Barton-Gade (1997) reported that hot weather would result in a larger number of PSE carcasses delivered to market, whereas cold weather will severely reduce muscle glycogen stores and the increase incidence of DFD carcasses. The Rendement Napole (RN) gene is a condition associated with pigs possessing elevated levels of muscle glycogen. Muscle from RN pigs has a high glycolytic potential (GP) and an increased capacity for post-mortem production of lactic acid (Ellis and McKeith, 1999). A series of trials conducted by Bidner et al. (1999a,b) examined the effect of preslaughter fast on pigs that tested positive for the RN gene (high glycogen levels) compared with control pigs (low glycogen levels). Table 28.1 reports the results of two experiments. In the first experiment (Bidner et al., 1999b) pigs were mixed prior to slaughter and in the second (Bidner et al., 1999a) pigs were not mixed. Bidner et al. (1999b) found that fasting for up to 60 h before slaughter did not adequately reduce muscle glycogen levels of RN pigs to raise the ultimate pH of the longissimus (loin) muscle, whereas fasting for 36 h was adequate to raise pH in controls (Table 28.1). This trial concluded that preslaughter fast may not be effective for improving ultimate pH of pigs possessing the RN gene. It is interesting to note that in the second trial (Bidner et al., 1999b), fasting for 36 h prior to slaughter had no effect on ultimate loin pH. This would suggest that fasting alone may not provide adequate stress to reduce intermuscular glycogen levels of pigs possessing (so-called) normal intramuscular glycogen levels.

Eilert (1997) suggested that producers include the approximate transit time and holding time at the plant when they determine length of feed withdrawal. Hyun et al. (1997) stated that an adequate preslaughter fast could be achieved by closing feeders in the evening before early morning transport to market. Pigs consume very little at night (provided they are not heat stressed or overcrowded); thus, a preslaughter fast may be self-imposed. Feed restriction of market pigs has a practical application even if one ignores the effect on pork quality. Eilert (1997) suggested that a 16- to 24-h feed withdrawal period is consistently advantageous to the packer because of the greater ease of carcass evisceration, reduced waste handling at the plant, and reduced incidence of broken viscera on the slaughter floor.

TABLE 28.1
Effect of Preslaughter Fast on Meat Quality of Pigs Possessing Low or High Intramuscular Glycogen Levels[a]

	Low Glycogen Levels[b] Time Off Feed (hrs)			High Glycogen Levels[c] Time Off Feed (hrs)		
Source/Measurement	12	36	60	12	36	60
Bidner et al., 1999b pigs mixed						
Ultimate pH	5.45[d]	5.59[e]	5.65[e]	5.36[d]	5.34[d]	5.36[d]
Purge loss (%)	4.10	2.46	2.37	4.48	4.66	4.05
Drip loss (%)	4.17	3.11	3.50	5.49	6.22	5.25
Light reflectance (Hunter L*-value)	55.54[d]	53.08[e]	51.76[e]	55.33[d]	55.55[d]	55.48[d]
Bidner et al., 1999a pigs not mixed						
Ultimate pH	5.48	5.51	—	5.46	5.42	—
Drip loss (%)	7.32	6.94	—	7.31	7.96	—
Light reflectance (Hunter L*-value)	55.3	54.4	—	52.5	53.2	—

Note: Means within rows with different superscripts differ ($P < 0.05$).

[a] Originally summarized by Ellis and McKeith (1999).
[b] Pigs without the RN gene.
[c] Pigs with the RN gene.

B. Preslaughter Feed Restriction

Ellis et al. (1996) found that the eating quality of pork was improved when pigs had *ad libitum* access to feed vs. pigs restricted in feed intake. Table 28.2 provides a comparison of two trials (Warkup et al., 1990; Ellis et al., 1996) as summarized by Ellis and McKeith (1999).

C. Manipulating Preslaughter Carbohydrate Intake

Pettigrew and Esnaola (2000) stated that the amount of glycogen stored in skeletal muscle is influenced by the amount of starch that is consumed relative to the energy demands of the tissues.

TABLE 28.2
Effects of *ad libitum* Access to Feed and Restricted Feeding Regimens on Organoleptic Properties of Fresh Pork[a]

	Advantage of *ad libitum* vs. Restricted Feeding Regimens	
Trait	Trial A[c] Feeding Duration ~30–85 kg BW	Trial B[d] Feeding Duration ~80–120 kg BW
Tenderness	0.30**	0.47*
Juiciness	0.26**	0.19*
Flavor	0.00	0.15
Odor	0.12**	0.02
Overall acceptability	0.19**	—

[a] Originally summarized by Ellis and McKeith (1999).
[b] Eight-point scale with lower values equivalent to poorer quality.
[c] Ellis et al. (1996).
[d] Warkup et al., 1990 (as cited by Ellis and McKeith, 1999).
* *Ad libitum* access differs from restricted feeding at $P < 0.05$.
** *Ad libitum* access differs from restricted feeding at $P < 0.001$.

They suggested that the length of time necessary for preslaughter fast may be shortened if levels of starch are reduced in the diet prior to the preslaughter fast, thus lowering intramuscular glycogen levels before the fast is applied. Anderson et al. (1998) found that reducing the amount of starch in the diet for 3 weeks prior to slaughter significantly raised 24-h pH values and resulted in darker meat (lower light reflectance; L-values) than controls.

Pettigrew and Esnaola (2000) cited work conducted by Pethick et al. (1997) whereby pigs at risk of reduced intramuscular glycogen levels (cold-stressed or frightened pigs) were supplemented sugar solutions to restore glycogen and reduce the chance of generating DFD pork. Pettigrew and Esnaola (2000) concluded that U.S. producers are not likely to adopt this production practice because the risk of producing PSE pork is much greater (and a larger problem for the packing industry) than the risk of producing DFD meat.

D. Manipulation of Preslaughter Protein and/or Amino Acids

The results of the 1994 *National Consumer Preference Study* found that consumer taste panelists served broiled unseasoned pork loin chops preferred pork chops containing >3% intramuscular fat (Melton, 1995). Goodwin (1995) concluded from the study that the value of the total lipid content in pork was actually very high and that the increased selection for lean genetics had led to decreased marbling content of pork. The target level of intramuscular fat for improving palatability traits has been suggested to be between 2 and 4% (NPPC, 1998).

Ellis and McKeith (1999) suggested that the simplest means to increase intramuscular fat levels of pork is via feeding protein-deficient diets. Table 28.3 summarizes literature reviewed by Ellis and McKeith (1999). The majority of the trials reported in Table 28.3 were conducted during the growing and finishing phases of production. These protein-deficient diets succeeded in increasing levels of intramuscular fat yet they also generated a large increase in external fat levels, reduced feed efficiency, decreased growth rates, and increased the cost of production. Recent data released from the National Pork Producers Council's *Quality Lean Growth Modeling Project* have also shown an increase in loin intramuscular fat. The four diets provided constant

TABLE 28.3
Influence of Feeding Protein Deficient Diets on Intramuscular Fat Content of the Longissimus (Loin) Muscle[a]

Dietary Protein/Lysine Level (%)		Intramuscular Fat (%)		Weight Range (kg)	Ref.
Adequate	Deficient	Adequate	Deficient		
18.5/0.96	13.1/0.64	1.5[d]	2.5[e]	to 103	Essen-Gustavsson et al., 1994
17.6/0.81	11.9/0.48	1.4[d]	3.5[e]	25–98	Castell et al., 1994
25.0	10.0	3.4[d]	9.4[e]	30–98	Goerl et al., 1995
16.0/0.82	12.0/0.55	5.5[d]	11.2[e]	10–100	Kerr et al., 1995
20.5/1.05	16.6/0.70	1.2[d]	2.4[e]	39–90	Blanchard et al., 1999
14.0/0.56	10.0/0.40	3.8[d]	5.7[e]	80–110	Cisneros et al., 1996
				Weeks Deficient[b]	
10.4/0.64	10.0/0.40	2.93	3.22	1	Ellis and McKeith, 1999
10.4/0.64	10.4/0.48	3.05	3.08	3	Ellis and McKeith, 1999
10.4/0.64	9.9/0.56	2.82	3.34	5	Ellis and McKeith, 1999

Note: Means within rows with different superscripts differ ($P < 0.05$).

[a] Originally summarized by Pettigrew and Esnaola (2000).
[b] Number of weeks deficient diets were fed before slaughter.

TABLE 28.4
Diet Program and Percent Intramuscular Fat for Overall Test and Three Different Endpoints Obtained from the Quality Lean Growth Modeling Project

Metabolizable Energy (kcal)	Pig Weight (kg)	Added Fat (%)	Lysine Levels[a] per Diet (%)			
			1	2	3	4
3516	41–64	5	1.25	1.10	0.95	0.80
3432	64–86	3	1.10	0.95	0.80	0.65
3302	86–109	0	0.95	0.80	0.65	0.50
3304	109–132	0	0.80	0.65	0.50	0.35
3304	132–150	0	0.80	0.65	0.50	0.35
	End Weight		Intramuscular Fat (%) by Diet			
	Overall		2.64[c]	2.73[c]	2.79[c]	3.37[d]
	113		2.44[c]	2.52[c]	2.57[c]	3.01[d]
	132		2.66[c]	2.66[c]	2.82[c]	3.49[d]
	150		2.82[c]	3.01[c]	2.98[c]	3.60[d]

Note: Means within rows with different superscripts differ ($P < 0.05$).

[a] Diets 1, 2, and 3 considered adequate for lysine content.

Source: Goodwin, personal communication, results of the 1998 NPPC Quality Lean Growth Modeling Project.

energy, minerals, and vitamins within a predetermined weight range of pigs and differed in levels of lysine. Table 28.4 contains the diet programs for each stage of production whereby Diets 1, 2, and 3 were considered adequate and Diet 4 deficient (Goodwin, personal communication). Feeding Diet 4 succeeded in increasing loin intramuscular fat levels at each of the three end weights and (similar to other trials) overall carcass fatness was also increased. The improvement in lipid in the QLGM class was not associated with other aspects of loin quality. The data from the QLGM trial are unique in the fact that loin chops from Diet 4 had significantly more drip loss (lower water-holding capacity) and produced paler-colored meat (higher L-values and lower visual scores).

Cisneros et al. (1999) evaluated the effects of short-duration amino acid deficiency in an effort to identify the maximum time deficient diets need be fed to enhance levels of intramuscular fat and minimize the other negative consequences (see Table 28.3). Deficient diets were fed for 1, 3, and 5 weeks prior to slaughter. A numeric increase of intramuscular fat was observed in the loin muscle, but the increase was not statistically significant.

Production situation, swine genotype, environmental factors, and pig health will all influence levels of amino acids required to maximize protein accretion. Lower levels of essential amino acids reduce carcass leanness, but levels higher than necessary will not make pigs leaner (Pettigrew and Esnaola, 2000).

E. Dietary Fat Source and Fatty Acid Profile of Pork Fat

1. General

Body fat is a highly efficient means to store metabolic energy. Adipocytes (fat cells) are specialized for the synthesis and storage of triacylglycerols. Triacylglycerols comprise three fatty acids bound to a glycerol backbone and serve as energy reservoirs within adipocytes of animal fat. The fatty acid profile of triacylglycerides (and, thus, pork fat) is a result of endogenous fatty acid production and/or fatty acids obtained from the diet. For more details on the biological effects of dietary fat, refer to Chapter 6.

Fatty acids obtained from the diet will inhibit endogenous production of similar fatty acids (particularly polyunsaturated fatty acids) and be incorporated (stored) within the adipocyte. The composition and fatty acid profile of body fat can thus be manipulated by changing the fatty acid profile of the feed. For example, pigs fed high levels of seed oils (such as soybean oil) will deposit high concentrations of linoleic acid (18:2) in their fat cells (Ellis and Isbell, 1926). Oils and fat are sometimes added to the diets of pigs to increase their energy intake. The deposition of unsaturated fatty acids into different fat depots will cause the fat to be soft and of poorer quality. Table 28.5 shows how it is possible to alter body fat composition by supplementation of different fat sources (Pettigrew and Esnaola, 2000).

The emphasis placed on production of lean hogs has resulted in a decrease in the quantity and quality of pork fat. The quality of pork fat is very important to bacon and sausage processors (NPPC, 2000). A firm, saturated fat improves slicing and ensures definition of individual slices. On the other hand, pork fat that is too hard will become brittle and shatter during slicing. Sliced bacon from soft fat will flatten together, has an unappealing wet or oily appearance or is translucent and gray, and will oxidize (become rancid) at a faster rate (NPPC, 2000). Soft fat is a result of high concentrations of unsaturated fatty acids, which lower the melting point of the fat. Long-chain saturated fatty acids such as stearic (C18:0) and palmitic acid (C16:0) have higher melting points (above body temperature). Monounsaturated and polyunsaturated fatty acids, such as oleic (C18:1) and linoleic acid (C18:2) have lower melting points (below body temperature). Saturated fatty acids

TABLE 28.5
The Effect of Dietary Fat Source on Fatty Acid Profile and Organoleptic Properties of Pork Longissimus Muscle (Loin) and Bacon[a]

	Fat Source in the Diet				
	Canola	Sunflower	Safflower	Animal Fat	Control
Loin fat composition[b]					
% Oleic acid (18:1)	45.9[g]	51.7[j]	48.8[i]	44.6[f]	47.4[h]
% Linoleic acid (18:2)	12.3[j]	8.4[h]	10.4[i]	11.5[i]	6.7[g]
% Linolenic acid (18:3)	3.0[j]	1.5[i]	1.4[i]	1.6[i]	1.5[i]
Organoleptic evaluation[b]					
Flavor[d]	4.7[j]	5.4[i]	5.3[i]	5.4[i]	5.2[i]
Overall palatability[c]	4.6[j]	5.1[ij]	5.2[ij]	5.3[i]	5.1[ij]
Off-flavor percentage[d]	28.6	17.5	19.6	18.8	19.0
Bacon fat composition[e]					
% Oleic acid (18:1)	50.3[h]	60.8[j]	55.2[i]	46.0[g]	45.4[g]
% Linoleic acid (18:2)	16.4[j]	9.2[g]	12.8[h]	14.3[i]	8.1[f]
% Linolenic acid (18:3)	4.8[j]	0.0[i]	0.0[i]	0.3[i]	0.0[i]
Organoleptic evaluation[e]					
Flavor[d]	2.9[j]	5.1[hi]	5.2[hi]	4.6[i]	5.6[h]
Overall palatability[c]	2.8[j]	4.8[i]	4.7[i]	4.5[i]	5.5[h]
Off-flavor percentage[d]	65.1[j]	10.6[hi]	11.5[hi]	23.4[i]	5.7[h]

Note: Means within rows followed by different superscripts differ ($P < 0.05$).

[a] Originally summarized by Pettigrew and Esnaola (2000).
[b] Miller et al. (1990).
[c] Numeric scale from 1 to 8 whereby 1 = extremely unflavorful/unpalatable and 8 = extremely flavorful/palatable.
[d] Percentage of taste panelists detecting off-flavors.
[e] Shackelford et al. (1990).

have higher melting points because the fatty acid molecules contain no double bonds and are more compact than unsaturated fatty acids that possess one or more double bonds.

According to Pork Composition and Quality Assessment Procedures (NPPC, 2000), quality pork fat must have <15% polyunsaturated fatty acids, >15% stearic acid (18:0; a saturated fatty acid), and an iodine number less than 70 mg iodine/100 g of fat. The iodine number measures the number of carbon–carbon double bonds in the fatty acids of the pork fat sample. Pork fat containing >14% linoleic acid (C18:2; a di-unsaturated fatty acid) is associated with soft fat. The amount of stearic acid present in pork fat is believed to be the most important indicator of optimum fat quality. The degree of pork fat saturation is affected by the amount of unsaturated fatty acids in the pig's diet and by the thickness of the animal's backfat (NPPC, 2000).

2. Conjugated Linoleic Acid

Conjugated linoleic acid (CLA) is a unique polyunsaturated fatty acid found naturally in meat from ruminant animals and dairy products at levels of approximately 0.5 to 1.5% of the total fatty acids (Fogarty et al., 1988). The structural configuration of CLA differs from that of other C18:2 fatty acids because a single carbon–carbon bond separates the constituent double bonds. Linoleic acid (C18:2) contains two *cis* carbon–carbon double bonds at the 9 and 12 carbon, whereas the principal biological isoform of CLA has a *cis*-9 and *trans*-11 double-bond configuration (Figure 28.2).

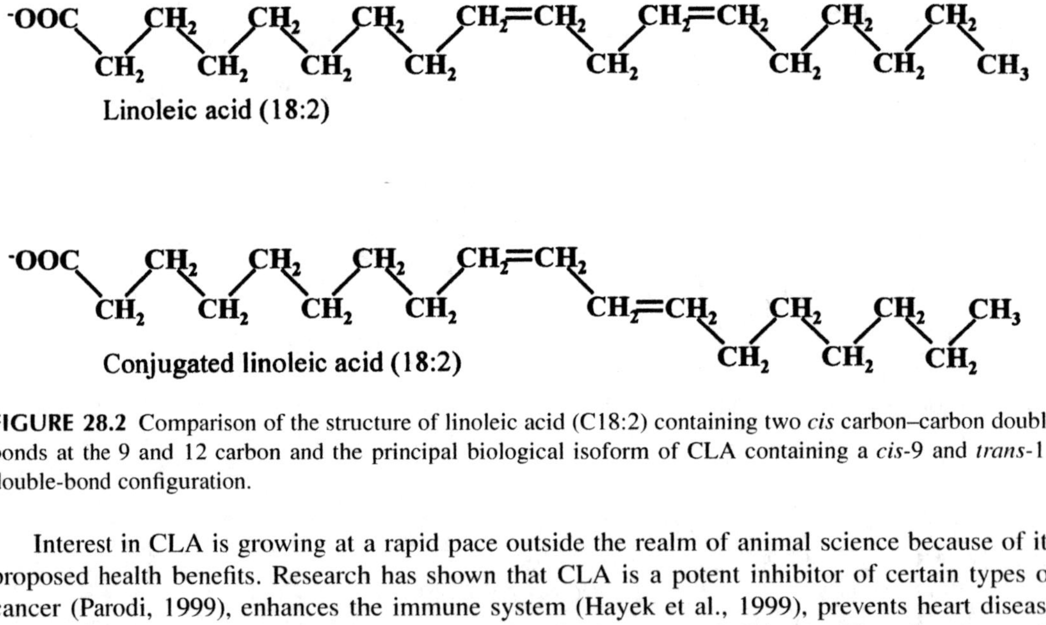

FIGURE 28.2 Comparison of the structure of linoleic acid (C18:2) containing two *cis* carbon–carbon double bonds at the 9 and 12 carbon and the principal biological isoform of CLA containing a *cis*-9 and *trans*-11 double-bond configuration.

Interest in CLA is growing at a rapid pace outside the realm of animal science because of its proposed health benefits. Research has shown that CLA is a potent inhibitor of certain types of cancer (Parodi, 1999), enhances the immune system (Hayek et al., 1999), prevents heart disease (Belury and Vanden Heuvel, 1997), prevents the development of diabetes (Houseknecht et al., 1998), and (probably of greatest interest to meat animal scientists) alters fat metabolism such that body fat is reduced while muscle mass is increased (Delany et al., 1999).

Few refereed publications are available regarding the effect of CLA supplementation on growth, meat production, or meat quality. Dugan et al. (1997) found that pigs fed a diet containing 2% CLA from 61.5 to 106 kg live weight deposited less subcutaneous fat and gained more lean than pigs fed a diet containing 2% sunflower oil. Using the same experimental group, Dugan et al. (1999) reported that CLA-fed pigs had higher subjective marbling scores, greater chemically determined intramuscular fat levels, and a higher chroma value (color saturation) within the loin, considered positive meat quality attributes. No differences were observed for light reflectance (L^*-value), shear force (loin toughness), or drip loss (water-holding capacity).

A large amount of recent research has evaluated the effects of feeding CLA; however, access to the results is limited to abstract form. Pettigrew and Esnaola (2000) review the current CLA research abstracts as they pertain to pork quality. What is interesting to note is that although CLA-fed pigs were consistently leaner, subjective evaluation of marbling content was higher from the CLA-fed pigs, ether extractable intramuscular loin fat was greater, and bellies were firmer. Of the abstracts reviewed by Pettigrew and Esnaola (2000), two reported no difference in marbling content. With regard to other pork quality attributes, water-holding capacity was either improved or unchanged, ultimate meat pH and meat tenderness were not affected, and sensory characteristics were generally unaffected by feeding CLA to pigs. Evaluation of fresh pork color (objective or subjective evaluation) was generally unaffected by CLA, yet Pettigrew and Esnaola (2000) concluded from their review that CLA supplementation probably results in subtle improvements in color intensity of fresh pork. Only one abstract found pork chops from CLA-supplemented pigs to be less juicy than those from controls.

The high cost of synthetic CLA has brought questions about the economic practicality of feeding this nutrient. The growing interest in CLA as a feed ingredient has resulted in identification of alternative sources of CLA. Modified tall oil is a by-product of kraft paper manufacturing, and this by-product contains isomers of CLA. Modified tall oil is considerably less expensive than synthetic forms of CLA or CLA derived from sunflower oil. The physiological activity of CLA and the exact mechanism by which CLA improves carcass composition, fat firmness, and marbling have yet to be determined. More basic research is necessary to determine the mode of action of CLA and to identify the specific isoforms that possess the greatest physiological activity.

F. Vitamins and Minerals

The physiological role of vitamins and minerals fed to swine has been covered in previous chapters. However, supplementation of certain vitamins and minerals at elevated levels prior to slaughter (below toxic levels of intake) has been shown to influence pork quality, sometimes in a positive and sometimes in a negative manner. Vitamins are among the nutrients necessary for a number of essential physiological functions. A number serve as enzyme cofactors and vitamins E and C function as biological antioxidants. Several act as cofactors in metabolic oxidation–reduction reactions and vitamins A and D can function as hormones (Combs, 1998). Like vitamins, all living organisms require inorganic elements (minerals) for normal life processes. Minerals are necessary in the feed at macro or trace amounts because they cannot be synthesized by the animal. Minerals act as structural components of body organs and tissues (such as the skeleton), maintain acid–base and water balance, regulate osmotic pressure, regulate membrane permeability, and play a regulatory role in muscle contractions and nerve excitability (McDowell, 1992).

1. Vitamin D

Miller and Meisinger (1998) suggested that the rapid move toward high lean growth genetics has resulted in tougher, dryer pork. Nutritional interventions for improved pork palatability have taken a cue from the beef industry. Solutions of calcium chloride ($CaCl_2$) have been injected into beef carcasses to activate calcium-dependent proteases. Section II.B described that a particular group of Ca^{2+}-dependent proteases (calpains) degrade muscle proteins during post-mortem aging. The objective of using $CaCl_2$ injections is to activate fully the calpains and maximize their activity relative to post-mortem meat tenderization through increased level of calcium substrate (Wheeler et al., 1997).

Beitz et al. (1998) describe how manipulation of Ca^{2+} levels in post-mortem muscle can influence meat tenderness. Calcium levels within the muscle cell are strictly regulated by the ATP-driven calcium pump. Maintaining low intracellular Ca^{2+} levels prevents protein denaturation by Ca-dependent proteases such as calpains. It is desirable to activate calpain enzymes post-mortem to initiate proteolysis and improve meat tenderness. Live animal blood calcium levels are regulated by parathyroid hormone, calcitonin, and 1,25-dihydroxyvitamin D (Bietz et al., 1998). 1,25-Dihydroxyvitamin D is synthesized from 25-hydroxyvitamin D, which is synthesized from vitamin D. The cumulative action of 1,25-dihydroxyvitamin D is to elevate blood concentrations of calcium significantly. Beitz et al. (1998) suggested that large intakes of vitamin D would increase blood calcium by actions of additional 1,25-dihydroxyvitamin D. It has therefore been proposed that feeding high levels of vitamin D before slaughter will result in an increased availability of Ca^{2+} for early activation of calpains in muscle before their enzymatic activity is inhibited by post-mortem pH decline (Beitz et al., 1998). Swanek et al. (1999) found that cattle fed up to 7.5 million IU of vitamin D_3 for 10 days prior to slaughter had increased blood calcium levels and improved tenderness.

There are limited data regarding supplementation of vitamin D to swine to improve pork quality; however, positive results observed from beef research merits its discussion. A review of current abstracts and university swine reports by Pettigrew and Esnaola (2000) reported that supplementation of vitamin D_3 at a level of 500,000 IU per day for 3 days before slaughter increased serum concentrations of calcium but had no effect on tenderness or post-mortem pH decline (Sparks et al., 1999). Enright et al. (1998) also found that high levels of vitamin D_3 supplementation (176,000 IU/kg) had no effect on pork tenderness but color and water-holding capacity were improved. Feeding elevated levels of vitamin D to swine may not be practical in production because both trials evaluated by Pettigrew and Esnaola (2000) showed a marked reduction in feed intake and growth rate in the vitamin D_3-supplemented pigs. The evaluation of the effects of vitamin D on pork quality is still in its infancy and requires further investigation.

2. Vitamin E

An antioxidant inhibits oxidation and prevents oxidation reactions such as the conversion of polyunsaturated fatty acids (PUFA) to fatty hydroperoxides. According to Combs (1998) vitamin E is a generic descriptor for all tocopherol and tocotrienol derivatives that exhibit similar qualitative actions of α-tocopherol. Vitamin E is a hydrophobic, fat-soluble vitamin that serves as a lipid-soluble biological antioxidant. Vitamin E incorporates into the lipid membrane near areas prone to lipid peroxidation and is therefore important for the maintenance of membrane integrity of basically every cell in the body (Combs, 1998). Polyunsaturated fatty acids of lipid membranes are particularly susceptible to attack by free radicals or so-called reactive oxygen species. Vitamin E protects PUFA from peroxidation, preventing or inhibiting loss of membrane integrity or (in the case of meat) oxidative rancidity.

Pettigrew and Esnaola (2000) reviewed current literature regarding the effects of supplementing high levels of vitamin E relative to pork quality. The reviewers suggested two possible reasons improved oxidative stability of pork may enhance pork quality. The first is that antioxidants present in meat may inhibit the conversion of oxymyoglobin (responsible for the acceptable pinkish-red color of fresh pork) to metmyoglobin (responsible for the brown, oxidized color of pork with prolonged exposure to oxygen or light). Antioxidant improvements to the color stability of myoglobin may reduce the conversion of oxymyoglobin to metmyoglobin, prolonging color acceptability during storage. The second reason is that antioxidant maintenance of lipid membrane integrity may reduce fluid leakage (reducing drip loss increasing water-holding capacity) and slow development of oxidative rancidity.

The most common chemical measurement of lipid oxidation in meat is the thiobarbituric acid reacting substances (TBARS) assay (Decker, 1998). Table 28.6 presents the results of several vitamin E trials showing a very consistent reduction in TBARS (lipid oxidation) for pork from pigs supplemented with high levels of vitamin E for various lengths of time before slaughter. Table 28.7 has the results from several research projects showing an increase in Hunter a*-values (measure of the "redness" of fresh pork) as a result of vitamin E supplementation. Table 28.8 lists research findings regarding the effects of vitamin E on drip loss (water-holding capacity).

According to the *Nutrient Requirements of Swine* (NRC, 1998), the dietary requirement for vitamin E (to prevent deficiency symptoms) is 11 mg/kg of feed of DL-α-tocopherol. Ullrey (1981) recommended increased levels of 30 mg/kg or higher in situations where relatively high levels of unsaturated fats were fed. Research trials examining the influence of dietary vitamin E regarding improved pork quality fed much higher levels of DL-α-tocopherol at a range spanning 100 to 800 mg/kg of feed. Pettigrew and Esnaola (2000) pointed out that there is essentially no obstacle to prevent supplementing high levels of vitamin E to swine because there is little danger of toxicity at these elevated levels. However, the increase in feed cost for supplementing vitamin E to a level necessary to improve pork quality is cost-prohibitive. It is highly unlikely that supplementing vitamin E to improve pork quality will be adopted for large-scale production until price incentives are in place for doing so.

3. Magnesium

Magnesium is an important metabolic nutrient necessary for optimal growth, immunity, muscle contraction, red blood cell survival, collagen metabolism, and sodium and potassium metabolism (McDowell, 1992). Swine are rarely deficient in Mg because adequate amounts are present in cereal grains and/or oilseed meals. However, the signs of Mg deficiency (in order of appearance) are hyperirritability, muscular twitching, reluctance to stand, weak pasterns, loss of equilibrium, tetany, and ultimately death (McDowell, 1992). The first symptom of deficiency, hyperirritability, may be attributed to an increased release of the stress hormones epinephrine and norepinephrine (as discussed in Section II.C.1). As stated previously, activation of the pig's sympathetic nervous system prior to slaughter has a deleterious influence on pork quality because of an increase in body temperature and increased glycogenolysis (which can lead to rapid pH decline post-mortem). It has been suggested that supplementation of high levels of Mg before slaughter will reduce sympathetic catecholamine release, reduce stress, and therefore improve pork quality (D'Souza et al., 1998). Table 28.9 summarizes the results of three research projects (originally summarized by Pettigrew and Esnaola, 2000) where magnesium was supplemented as magnesium aspartate (MgAsp), magnesium sulfate ($MgSO_4$), or magnesium chloride ($MgCl_2$) in various quantities for 5 days preslaughter.

Supplementation of high levels of Mg for several days prior to slaughter seems to be an effective means of eliminating the occurrence of PSE pork (Table 28.9). Continued research is necessary to determine the appropriate dose, duration, and source of magnesium and to identify an appropriate means of delivery acceptable to commercial practice (Pettigrew and Esnaola, 2000).

4. Chromium

Chromium seems to be an essential trace element because of its activity as an insulin potentiator. Chromium forms a complex between insulin and the insulin receptor on the tissue membrane that facilitates the uptake of insulin into tissues (McDowell, 1992). Anderson (1998) suggested that chromium is an integral part of a glucose tolerance factor (GTF) and may regulate carbohydrate storage into muscle or adipose tissue through improved insulin sensitivity. A considerable body of research has evaluated supplementation of chromium (primarily as chromium picolinate) to swine diets focusing mostly on the proposed benefits to growth and carcass composition and, therefore, merits discussion in this chapter with regard to its influence on meat quality. In theory, the influence of chromium regarding insulin sensitivity should enhance the deposition of dietary protein and carbohydrate (glucose) within the muscle cell. Both would have advantages in terms of increasing muscle mass; yet the increased deposition of glucose into muscle cells as glycogen could increase the glycolytic potential and provide more carbohydrate for post-mortem conversion to lactic acid (glycogen to glucose to lactic acid). With the focus of chromium supplementation being on improvements in growth, limited data exist pertaining to the effects of improved insulin sensitivity

TABLE 28.6
Effects of Elevated Levels of Dietary Vitamin E on Occurrence of Thiobarbituric Acid Reactive Substances[a] (TBARS)

Source/Description	Feeding Duration	Storage Days	Basal	Level of Vitamin E Supplementation[b] (mg/kg diet)			
				100		200	
			TBARS[c]	TBARS[c]	p[d]	TBARS[c]	p[d]
Asghar et al. (1991)	~98 days						
Frozen pork chops		0	0.28	0.27	NS	0.27	NS
		3	1.54	0.56	<0.05	0.35	<0.05
		6	2.96	0.94	<0.05	0.58	<0.05
		10	5.17	2.96	NS	1.33	<0.05
Ground pork		1	1.34	0.36	<0.05	0.22	<0.05
		4	3.49	1.13	<0.05	0.41	<0.05
		8	5.38	3.27	<0.05	1.59	<0.05
Monahan et al. (1994)	30–98 kg BW						
Refrigerated pork chops		0	0.20	—	—	0.17	<0.05
		2	0.37	—	—	0.19	<0.05
		4	0.38	—	—	0.20	<0.05
		6	0.51	—	—	0.21	<0.05
		8	0.78	—	—	0.13	<0.05
Lanari et al. (1995)	105 days						
Longissimus lumborum		0	0.19	—	—	0.07	<0.01
Display in air		2	0.48	—	—	0.11	<0.01
		4	0.70	—	—	0.11	<0.01
		6	0.72	—	—	0.18	<0.01
		8	0.74	—	—	0.21	<0.01
		10	0.74	—	—	0.42	<0.01
Cannon et al. (1996)	84 days						
Fresh loin chops		0 and 1[e]	0.30	0.32	NS	—	—
		0 and 3	0.51	0.30	<0.05	—	—
		0 and 5	0.74	0.41	<0.05	—	—
		14 and 1	0.50	0.50	NS	—	—
		14 and 3	0.72	0.52	<0.05	—	—

Study / Treatment	Duration[b]	Days[e]	Basal[c]	Supp[c]	P[d]	Supp[c]	P[d]
Houben et al. (1998)	72 days						
Minced pork at 7°C							
Packaged in foil		14 and 5	0.75	0.49	<0.05	—	—
		28 and 1	0.38	0.36	NS	—	—
		28 and 3	0.59	0.43	<0.05	—	—
		28 and 5	0.92	0.60	<0.05	—	—
		56 and 1	0.40	0.37	NS	—	—
		56 and 3	0.72	0.53	<0.05	—	—
		56 and 5	0.93	0.60	<0.05	—	—
Gas package storage		0	0.02	—	—	0.07	NS
		3	0.06	—	—	0.08	NS
		9	0.13	—	—	0.05	NS
		11	0.24	—	—	0.17	NS
		0	0.05	—	—	0.07	NS
		3	0.18	—	—	0.07	<0.05
		9	0.60	—	—	0.09	<0.05
		11	1.20	—	—	0.10	<0.05
Hoving-Bolink et al. (1998)	84 days						
Fresh longissimus lumborum		0	0.07	—	—	0.06	NS
		3	0.29	—	—	0.10	<0.05
		6	0.53	—	—	0.19	<0.05
Frozen longissimus lumborum		0	0.17	—	—	0.10	<0.05
		3	0.62	—	—	0.15	<0.05
		6	1.07	—	—	0.24	<0.05

[a] Originally summarized by Pettigrew and Esnaola (2000.).
[b] Approximate amount of vitamin E added to basal diet containing <12 IU supplemented vitamin E; duration varied.
[c] TBARS expressed in mg malonaldehyde/kg tissue.
[d] Statistical significance (P-value) expressed as the difference between supplemented and basal.
[e] Number of days stored under vacuum at 7°C and days in retail display.

TABLE 28.7
Effects of Elevated Levels of Dietary Vitamin E on Hunter a*-Values (Redness)[a]

Source/Description	Feeding Duration	Storage Days	Basal a*-val[c]	Level of Vitamin E Supplementation[b] (mg/kg diet)			
				100		200	
				a*-val[c]	P[d]	a*-val[c]	P[d]
Asghar et al. (1991)							
Frozen pork chops	~98 days	0	10.7	11.6	NS	12.6	<0.05
		3	10.1	11.1	NS	12.4	<0.05
		6	7.0	9.3	<0.05	10.0	<0.05
		10	7.0	7.9	NS	8.7	NS
Lanari et al. (1995)	105 days						
Experiment 1							
Longissimus lumborum		0	7.0	—	—	8.7	—
Display in air		2	6.0	—	—	7.8	—
		4	5.0	—	—	7.2	—
		6	2.9	—	—	6.3	—
		8	1.9	—	—	5.2	—
		10	1.3	—	—	4.8	—
Displayed 80% O_2, 20%CO_2		0	7.5	—	—	8.3	—
		2	6.8	—	—	7.5	—
		4	5.0	—	—	7.5	—
		6	3.2	—	—	5.7	—
		8	1.8	—	—	4.1	—
		10	1.2	—	—	3.2	—
Overall Exp. 1		—	—	—	—	—	<0.01
Experiment 2							
Illuminated display		0	8.0	—	—	8.2	—
		1	10.7	—	—	9.1	—
		2	7.0	—	—	7.2	—
		4	6.1	—	—	7.0	—
		6	4.0	—	—	6.3	—
		8	3.1	—	—	5.4	—
		10	2.0	—	—	4.3	—

Swine Nutrition, the Conversion of Muscle to Meat, and Pork Quality

Item	Day						P-value
Overall		—	—	—	—	—	<0.05
Dark Display	0	8.0	—	—	—	9.0	—
	1	10.4	—	—	—	10.4	—
	2	8.1	—	—	—	8.3	—
	4	8.0	—	—	—	8.5	—
	6	6.2	—	—	—	7.1	—
	8	6.0	—	—	—	7.1	—
	10	6.5	—	—	—	7.3	—
Overall		—	—	—	—	—	NS
Houben et al. (1998)	72 days						
Minced pork at 7°C							
Packaged in foil	0	16.4	—	—	—	16.7	NS
	3	13.5	—	—	—	11.7	<0.05
	6	12.6	—	—	—	10.8	NS
	9	12.7	—	—	—	10.9	NS
Gas package storage	0	16.4	—	—	—	16.7	NS
	3	14.8	—	—	—	14.2	NS
Hoving-Bolink et al. (1998)	84 days						
Fresh longissimus lumborum	1	10.2	—	—	—		NS
	2	10.2	—	—	—		NS
	3	9.9	—	—	—		NS
	4	9.3	—	—	—		NS
	6	8.3	—	—	—		<0.05
Frozen longissimus lumborum	1	9.2	—	—	—	9.3	NS
	2	8.6	—	—	—	8.9	NS
	3	8.1	—	—	—	8.4	NS
	4	7.7	—	—	—	8.1	NS
	5	7.4	—	—	—	8.0	NS
	6	6.9	—	—	—	7.8	<0.05

[a] Originally summarized by Pettigrew and Esnaola (2000).
[b] Approximate amount of vitamin E added to basal diet containing < 20 IU supplemented vitamin E.
[c] Hunter a*-values signifying degree of redness (higher values indicate more red color).
[d] Statistical significance (P-value) expressed as the difference between supplemented and basal.

TABLE 28.8
Effects of Elevated Levels of Dietary Vitamin E on Drip Loss (Water-Holding Capacity)[a]

Source/Description	Feeding Duration	Storage Days[c]	Basal % Drip Loss[d]	100 % Drip Loss[d]	100 P[e]	200 % Drip Loss[d]	200 P[e]
Asghar et al. (1991)	~98 days						
Frozen pork chops		3	19.0	16.2	—	10.2	<0.05
		6	20.1	19.5	—	12.2	<0.05
		10	21.3	21.2	—	14.1	<0.05
Monahan et al. (1994)	30–98 kg BW						
		2	5.1	—	—	2.9	<0.05
		4	8.0	—	—	3.1	<0.05
		6	8.7	—	—	5.3	<0.05
		8	11.6	—	—	6.1	<0.05
Cannon et al. (1996)	84 days	0	5.01	4.76	NS	—	—
		14	3.81	3.30	NS	—	—
		28	2.96	2.68	NS	—	—
		56	2.35	2.40	NS	—	—
Hoving-Bolink et al. (1998)	84 days						
Fresh longissimus lumborum		2	6.9	—	—	6.9	NS
Frozen longissimus lumborum		2	10.9	—	—	11.4	NS
Fresh psoas major		2	2.4	—	—	2.4	NS
Cheah et al. (1995)[f]	46 days						
Longissimus thoracis							
Genotype NN[g]		2	6.9	—	—	3.2	<0.01
Genotype Nn[h]		2	9.1	—	—	5.0	<0.01

[a] Originally summarized by Pettigrew and Esnaola (2000).
[b] Approximate amount of vitamin E added to basal diet containing <20 IU supplemented vitamin E.
[c] Previous treatment of meat samples and storage conditions varied.
[d] Methods for determining percentage moisture loss (% drip loss) varied among laboratories.
[e] Statistical significance (P-value) expressed as the difference between supplemented and basal.
[f] Vitamin E supplemented at 500 IU/kg.
[g] Porcine stress syndrome genotype; NN = stress negative.
[h] Porcine stress syndrome genotype; Nn = stress carrier.

TABLE 28.9
Effects of Elevated Levels of Dietary Magnesium on Various Measurements of Fresh Pork Quality[a]

Source/Measurement	Mg Dose[c]	Mg Source	Initial pH (40 or 45 m PM[b]) Control	Initial pH (40 or 45 m PM[b]) Mg	Ultimate pH (24 h PM[b]) Control	Ultimate pH (24 h PM[b]) Mg	Minolta L*-value Control	Minolta L*-value Mg	% Drip Loss Control	% Drip Loss Mg	% PSE Occurrence[d] Control	% PSE Occurrence[d] Mg
Schaefer et al. (1993)[e]												
Block 1	25 mg	Aspartate	5.84	5.82	5.46	5.45	59.4	58.7	5.0	5.0	NA	NA
Block 2	50 mg	Aspartate	5.90	5.96	5.33	5.35	55.5	54.8	4.2	3.6[j]	NA	NA
D'Souza et al. (1998)												
Longissimus thoracis												
Minimal handling[f]	3.2 g	Aspartate	6.60	6.79	5.48	5.61	48.7	45.2	4.0	3.5	8	0
Negative handling[g]	3.2 g	Aspartate	6.59	6.69	5.51	5.57	49.1	47.4	6.4	3.5	33	0
Biceps femoris												
Minimal handling	3.2 g	Aspartate	6.54	6.62	5.53	5.58	44.0	44.0	3.0	2.2	NA	NA
Negative handling	3.2 g	Aspartate	6.42	6.49	5.50	5.54	45.7	45.3	4.8	4.7	NA	NA
Probabilities[h]												
Diet				0.02		0.02		0.04		0.05		0.05
Diet x muscle				NS		0.03		0.02		NS		—
Diet x muscle x handling				NS		NS		NS		0.03		—
D'Souza et al. (1999)												
	3.2 g	Aspartate	6.48	6.70	5.55	5.56	48.7	47.8	5.8[j]	3.2	17	0
	3.2 g	Sulfate	—	6.62	—	5.53	—	49.1	—	2.8	—	0
	3.2 g	Chloride	—	6.52	—	5.56	—	48.8	—	3.1	—	0

[a] Originally summarized by Pettigrew and Esnaola (2000).
[b] Measurements of pH specified in minutes or hours post-mortem (PM).
[c] Magnesium supplemented daily for 5 days before slaughter.
[d] PSE defined as L* > 50 and drip loss > 5%.
[e] Stress genotypes pooled (positive, carriers, and normal); measurements obtained in longissimus muscle.
[f] Pigs handled gently before slaughter.
[g] Pigs goaded with electric prod before slaughter.
[h] Significant effects involving diet are shown ($P < 0.06$).
[i] Mg supplemented differs from control ($P < 0.06$).
[j] Control differs from Mg supplemented ($P < 0.05$).

regarding elevated glycolytic potential and the possible influence on fresh pork quality. Research trials that did evaluate quality traits do not lend overwhelming support to this theory. Recent abstracts reviewed by Pettigrew and Esnaola (2000) suggest that subjective color scores of pork from pigs supplemented with chromium were paler; however, no statistical differences were observed with regard to other measurement of pork quality.

5. Copper

It is a common production practice to increase concentrations of dietary copper in starting pig diets to enhance growth. Endogenous unsaturated fatty acids are produced by a group of desaturase enzymes possessing specificity for various fatty acyl chain lengths. Copper is a substrate for activation of these fatty acyl desaturase enzymes. The addition of elevated levels of copper to pigs as a growth promoter has shown a negative effect on the overall quality of carcass fat, resulting in softer fat that is more unsaturated (Pettigrew and Esnaola, 2000). Research summarized by Pettigrew and Esnaola (2000) shows overwhelming evidence that added levels of copper in swine rations increases unsaturated fatty acid concentration and decreases the melting point of subcutaneous pork fat. The added dietary copper may influence pork fat quality in two ways. The increased concentration of unsaturated fat is more susceptible to oxidative rancidity (reducing shelf stability). Also, copper may act as a pro-oxidant, hastening fatty acid and iron oxidation, which will also result in a shorter shelf life.

Copper is a key component necessary to maintain the structural integrity and function of Complex IV (cytochrome c oxidase) of the electron transport chain. Reactions occurring during oxidative metabolism are driven by electron transport in the mitochondria (mediated by Complex IV), which constitutes an essential step in cellular respiration (Voet et al., 1999). Copper plays a key role in iron absorption and mobilization and is necessary for both hemoglobin and myoglobin synthesis. Trace amounts of copper are necessary as a catalyst before the body can utilize iron for myoglobin formation. Copper is necessary for the oxidation of iron, permitting it to bind to the Fe-transport protein transferrin (McDowell, 1992). Therefore, supranutritional levels of copper may potentiate the actions of electron transport enhancing post-mortem oxidation resulting in poorer color and fatty acid stability. For these reasons it is prudent to restrict the use of nutriceutical levels of copper to the starting period.

V. CONCLUSION

The increased demand for high-quality pork both domestically and worldwide has sparked an increase in research evaluating the biochemical, physiological, molecular, and structural components of high-quality pork. Honkavaara (1989) suggested that preslaughter treatments are much easier to control than post-mortem biochemical reactions. A growing interest has focused on nutritional treatments as a means of controlling post-mortem biochemical reactions. Dietary strategies have been developed that influence the ultimate quality of pork; however, widespread incorporation of these strategies into common production is not likely until greater economic incentive is provided for the production and delivery of high-quality pork.

REFERENCES

Anderson, K. R., J. S. Petersen, H. Johansen, S. K. Jensen, A. Karlsson, and H. Andersen. 1998. Feed-induced muscle glycogen changes in slaughter pigs and their influence on meat quality. In *Proc. 44th Int. Cong. of Meat Sci. and Technol.*, Barcelona, Spain, 276.

Anderson, R. 1998. Effects of chromium on body composition and weight loss, *Nutr. Rev.*, 56:266.

Asghar, A., J. I. Gray, A. M. Booren, E. A. Gomaa, M. M. Abouzied, and E. R. Miller. 1991. Effects of supranutritional dietary vitamin E levels on subcellular deposition of -tocopherol in the muscle and on pork quality, *J. Food Agric.*, 57:31.

Bär, A., and D. Pette. 1988. Three fast myosin heavy chains in adult fast skeletal muscle. *FEBS Lett.*, 235:153.

Barton-Gade, P. 1997. The effect of pre-slaughter handling on meat quality in pigs. In *Manipulating Pig Production VI*, Cranwell, P. D., Ed., Australasian Pig Science Association, Attwood, Victoria, Australia, pp. 100–115.

Becker, B. A., H. F. Mayes, G. L. Hahn, J. A. Nienaber, G. W. Jesse, M. E. Anderson, H. Heymann, and H. B. Hedrick. 1989. Effect of fasting and transport on various physiological parameters and meat quality of slaughter hogs, *J. Anim. Sci.*, 67:334.

Beitz, D. C., J. C. Sparks, B. R. Weigand, F. C. Parrish, R. C. Ewan, R. L. Horst, and A. H. Trenkle. 1998. Effects of vitamin D on pork quality. In *Proc. Pork Quality and Safety Summit*, National Pork Producers Council, Des Moines, IA, 137.

Belury M. A., and J. P. Vanden Heuvel. 1997. Protection against cancer and heart disease by the dietary fat, conjugated linoleic acid: potential mechanisms of action, *Nutr. Dis. Update J.*, 1:58.

Bidner, B. S., M. Ellis, K. D. Miller, M. Hemann, D. Campion, and F. K. McKeith. 1999a. Effect of the RN gene and feed withdrawal prior to slaughter on fresh longissimus quality and sensory characteristics, *J. Anim. Sci.*, 77(Suppl. 1):49 (Abstr.).

Bidner, B. S., M. Ellis, D. P. Witte, M. England, D. Campion, and F. K. McKeith. 1999b. Influence of dietary lysine content, feed withdrawal period, and RN genotype on fresh longissimus quality and sensory characteristics, *J. Anim. Sci.*, 77(Suppl. 1):49 (Abstr.).

Blanchard, P. J., M. Ellis, C. C. Warkup, B. Hardy, J. P. Chadwick, and G. A. Deans. 1999. The influence of rate of lean and subcutaneous fat tissue development on pork eating quality, *Anim. Sci.*, 68:477.

Briskey, E. J. 1964. Etiological status and associated studies of pale, soft, exudative porcine musculature, *Adv. Food Res.*, 13:89.

Cannon, J. E., J. B. Morgan, J. Heavner, F. K. McKeith, G. C. Smith, and D. L. Meeker. 1995. Pork quality audit: a review of the factors influencing pork quality, *J. Muscle Foods*, 6:369.

Cannon, J. E., J. B. Morgan, G. R. Schmidt, J. D. Tatum, J. N. Sofos, G. C. Smith, R. J. Delmore, and S. N. Williams. 1996. Growth and fresh meat quality characteristics of pigs supplemented with vitamin E, *J. Anim. Sci.*, 74:98.

Castell, A. G., R. I. Cliplef, L. M. Paste-Flynn, and G. Butler. 1994. Performance carcass and pork characteristics of castrates and gilts self-fed diets differing in protein content and lysine:energy ratio, *Can. J. Anim. Sci.*, 74:519.

Cheah, K. S., A. M. Cheah, and D. I. Krausgrill. 1995. Effect of dietary supplementation of vitamin E on pig meat quality, *Meat Sci.*, 39:255.

Cisneros, F., M. Ellis, D. H. Baker, R. A. Easter, and F. K. McKeith. 1996. The influence of short-term feeding of amino acid-deficient diets and high dietary leucine levels on the intramuscular fat content of pig muscle, *Anim. Sci.*, 63:517.

Combs, G. F. 1998. *The Vitamins. Fundamental Aspects in Nutrition and Health*, 2nd ed., Academic Press, New York.

Decker, E. A. 1998. TBA as an index of oxidative rancidity in muscle foods. In *Proc. 51st Rec. Meat Conf.*, 51:66.

Delany, J. P., F. Blohm, A. A. Truett, J. A. Scimeca, and D. B. West. 1999. Conjugated linoleic acid rapidly reduces body fat content in mice without affecting energy intake, *Comp. Physiol.*, 45:R1172.

De Smet, S. M., H. Pauwels, S. De Bie, D. I. Deymeyer, J. Callewier, and W. Eeckhout. 1996. Effect of halothane genotype, breed, feed withdrawal, and lairage on pork quality of Belgian slaughter pigs, *J. Anim. Sci.*, 74:1854.

D'Souza, D. N., R. D. Warner, B .J. Leury, and F. R. Dunshea. 1998. The effect of dietary magnesium aspartate supplementation on pork quality, *J. Anim. Sci.*, 76:104.

D'Souza, D. N., R. D. Warner, F. R. Dunshea, and B. J. Leury. 1999. Comparisons of different dietary magnesium supplements on pork quality, *Meat Sci.*, 51:221.

Dugan, M. E. R., J. L. Aalhus, A. L. Schaefer, and J. K. G. Kramer. 1997. The effect of conjugated linoleic acid on fat to lean repartitioning and feed conversion in pigs, *Can. J. Anim. Sci.*, 77:723.

Dugan, M. E. R., J. L. Aalhus, L. E. Jeremiah, J. K. G. Kramer, and A. L. Schaefer. 1999. The effects of feeding conjugated linoleic acid on subsequent pork quality, *Can. J. Anim. Sci.*, 79:45–51.

Eikelenboom, G., A. H. Bolink, and W. Sybesma. 1991. Effects of feed withdrawal before delivery on pork quality and carcass yield, *Meat Sci.*, 29:25.

Eilert, S. J. 1997. What quality controls are working in the plant? In *Proc. Pork Quality Summit*, National Pork Producers Council, Des Moines, IA, 59.

Ellis, M., A. J. Webb, P. J. Avery, and I. Brown. 1996. The influence of terminal sire genotype, sex, slaughter weight, feeding regime and slaughter-house on growth performance and carcass and meat quality pigs and on the organoleptic properties of fresh pork, *Anim. Sci.*, 62:521.

Ellis, M., and F. K. McKeith. 1999. Nutritional influence on pork quality. National Pork Producers Council Fact Sheet 04422, Des Moines, IA.

Ellis, N. R., and H. S. Isbell. 1926. Soft pork studies. The effect of food fat upon body fat, as shown by the separation of the individual fatty acids of the body fat, *J. Biol. Chem.*, 69:239.

Enright, K. L, B. K. Anderson, M. Ellis, F. K. McKeith, L. L. Berger, and D. H. Baker. 1998. The effects of feeding high levels of vitamin D_3 on pork quality, *J. Anim. Sci.*, 76(Suppl. 1):149 (Abstr.).

Essen-Gustavsson, B., K. Karlstrom, and A. Lundtrum. 1992. Muscle fibre characteristics and metabolic response at slaughter in pigs of different halothane genotypes and their relation to meat quality, *Meat Sci.*, 31:1.

Essen-Gustavsson, B., A. Karlsson, K. Lundstrom, and A. C. Enfalt. 1994. Intramuscular fat and muscle fibre lipid contents in halothane-gene-free pigs fed high or low protein diets and its relation to meat quality, *Meat Sci.*, 38:269.

Fogarty, A. C., G. L. Ford, and D. Svornos. 1988. Octadeca 9,11-dienoic acid in foodstuffs and in the lipids of human blood and breast milk, *Nutr. Rep. Int.*, 38:937.

Goerl, K. F., S. J. Eilert, R. W. Mandigo, H. Y. Chen, and P. S. Miller. 1995. Pork characteristics as affected by two populations of swine and six crude protein levels, *J. Anim. Sci.*, 73:3621.

Goodwin, R. 1995. Economic values of pork product traits in pork production. In Proc. Terminal Sire Line NGEP, National Pork Producers Council, Des Moines, IA, 173.

Goodwin, R. 2000. Personal communication.

Grandin, T. 1994. Methods to reduce PSE and bloodsplash. In *Proc. Allen D. Leman Swine Conf.*, University of Minnesota, 21:206.

Hayek M. G., S. N Han, D. Y. Wu, B. A. Watkins, M. Meydani, J. L. Dorsey, D. E. Smith, and S. N. Meydani. 1999. Dietary conjugated linoleic acid influences the immune response of young and old C57BL/6NCrlBR mice, *J. Nutr.*, 129:32.

Honkavaara, M. 1989. Influence of carcass temperature, glycogenolysis and glycolysis 45 min postmortem on the development of PSE pork, *J. Agric. Sci. Finl.*, 61:433.

Honkavaara, M. 1990. Effect of PSE pork on the processing properties of cooked meat products, *Fleischwirtsch. Int.*, 2:20.

Houben, J. H., G. Eikelenboom, and A. H. Hoving-Bolink. 1998. Effect of the dietary supplementation with vitamin E on colour stability and lipid oxidation in packaged, minced pork, *Meat Sci.*, 48:265.

Houseknecht, K. L., J. P. Vanden Heuvel, S. Y. Moya-Camarena, C. P. Portocarrero, L. W. Peck, K. P. Nickel, and M. A. Belury. 1998. Dietary conjugated linoleic acid normalizes impaired glucose tolerance in the Zucker diabetic fatty *fa/fa* rat, *Biochem. Biophys. Res. Commun.*, 244:678.

Hoving-Bolink, A. H., G. Eikelenboom, J.T. M. van Diepen, A. W. Jongbloed, and J. H. Houben. 1998. Effect of dietary vitamin E supplementation on pork quality, *Meat Sci.*, 49:205.

Huxley, A. F., and R. M. Simmons. 1971. Proposed mechanism of force generation in striated muscle, *Nature*, 233:533.

Huxley, H. E. 1953. The double array of filaments in cross-striated muscle, *J. Biophys. Biochem. Cytol.*, 3:631.

Hyun, Y., M. Ellis, F. K. McKeith, and E. R. Wilson. 1997. Feed intake pattern of group-housed growing-finishing pigs monitored using a computerized feed intake recording system, *J. Anim. Sci.*, 75:1443.

Jones, S. D. M., R. E. Rompala, and C. R. Haworth. 1985. Effects of fasting and water restriction on carcass shrink and pork quality, *Can. J. Anim. Sci.*, 65:613.

Kerr, B. J., F. K. McKeith, and R. A. Easter. 1995. Effect on performance and carcass characteristics of nursery to finisher pigs fed reduced crude protein, amino acid-supplemented diets, *J. Anim. Sci.*, 73:433.

Koohmaraie, M. 1992. The role of Ca^{2+}-dependent proteases (calpains) in postmortem proteolysis and meat tenderness, *Biochimie*, 74:239.

Lanari, M. C., D. M. Schaefer, and K. K. Scheller. 1995. Dietary vitamin E supplementation and discoloration of pork bone and muscle following modified atmosphere packaging, *Meat Sci.*, 41:237.

Louis, C. F., W. E. Rempel, and J. R. Mickelson. 1993. Porcine stress syndrome: biochemical and genetic basis of this inherited syndrome of skeletal muscle. In *Proc. Recip. Meat Conf.*, 46:89.
Marsh, B. B. 1970. Introduction. In *Proc. the Physiology and Biochemistry of Muscle as a Food*, Briskey, E. J., R. G. Cassens, and B. B. Marsh, Eds., Wisconsin Press, Madison, 1.
Marsh, B. B., R. G. Cassens, R. G. Kauffman, and E. J. Briskey. 1972. Hot boning and pork tenderness, *J. Food Sci.*, 37:179.
Mayes, P. A. 1993. Metabolism of glycogen. In *Harpers Biochemistry*, 23rd ed., Appleton and Lange, Stamford, CT.
McDowell, L. R. 1992. *Minerals in Animal and Human Nutrition*, Academic Press, New York.
Melton, B. 1995. Economic values of pork product traits in pork production. In *Proc. Terminal Sire Line NGEP*, National Pork Producers Council, Des Moines, IA, 201.
Miller, M. F., S. D. Shackelford, K. D. Haydon, and J. O. Reagan. 1990. Determination of the alteration in fatty acid profiles, sensory characteristics and carcass traits of swine fed elevated levels of monounsaturated fats in the diet, *J. Anim. Sci.*, 68:1624.
Miller, R. K., and D. J. Meisinger. 1998. Pork quality Issues. In *Proc. Pork Quality and Safety Summit*, National Pork Producers Council, Des Moines, IA, 29.
Monahan, F. J., J. I. Gray, A. Asghar, A. Haug, G. M. Strasburg, D. J. Buckley, and P. A. Morrissey. 1994. Influence of diet on lipid oxidation and membrane structure in porcine muscle microsomes, *J. Agric. Food Chem.*, 42:59.
Monin, G., and P. Sellier. 1985. Pork of low techological quality with a normal rate of muscle pH fall in the immediate post-mortem period: the case of the Hampshire breed, *Meat Sci.*, 13:49.
Moss, R. L., G. M. Diffie, and M. L. Greaser. 1995. Contractile properties of skeletal muscle fibers in relation to myofibrillar protein isoforms, *Rev. Physiol. Biochem. Pharmacol.*, 116:1.
Murray, A. C., S. D. M. Jones, and A. P. Sather. 1989. The effects of preslaughter feed restriction and genotype for stress susceptibility on pork lean quality and composition, *Can. J. Anim. Sci.*, 69:83.
NPPC. 1998. Pork Quality Targets, National Pork Producers Council Fact Sheet 04366, Des Moines, IA.
NPPC. 2000. Pork fat quality. In *Pork Carcass Composition and Quality Assessment Procedures*, Berg, E. P., Ed., National Pork Producers Council, Des Moines, IA, 32.
NRC. 1998. *Nutrient Requirements for Swine*, 10th ed., National Academy Press, Washington, D.C.
Offer, G. 1991. Modeling the formation of pale, soft and exudative meat: effects of chilling regime and rate and extent of glycolysis, *Meat Sci.*, 30:157.
Parodi, P. W. 1999. Conjugated linoleic acid and other anticarcinogenic agents of bovine milk fat, *J. Dairy Sci.*, 82:1339.
Pearson, A. M. 1987. Muscle function and *postmortem* changes. In *The Science of Meat and Meat Products*, Price, J. F., and B. S. Schwiegert, Eds., Food and Nutrition Press, Westport, CT, 155
Penny, I. F. 1969. Protein denaturation and water holding capacity in pork muscle, *J. Food Technol.*, 4:269.
Pethick, D. W., R. D. Warner, D. N. D'Souza, and F. D. Dunshea. 1997. Nutritional manipulation of meat quality. In *Manipulating Pig Production VI*, Cranwell, P. D., Ed., pp. 91–99.
Pette, D., and R. S. Staron. 1990. Cellular and molecular diversities of mammalian skeletal muscle, *Rev. Physiol. Biochem. Pharmacol.*, 116:2.
Pettigrew, J. E., and M. A. Esnaola. 2000. Swine nutrition and pork quality, National Pork Producers Council Fact Sheet 04458, Des Moines, IA.
Schaefer, A. L., A. C. Murray, A. K. W. Tong, S. D. M. Jones, and A. P. Sather. 1993. The effect of ante mortem electrolyte therapy on animal physiology and meat quality in pigs segregating at the halothane gene, *Can. J. Anim. Sci.*, 73:231.
Schiaffino, S., L. Gorza, S. Sartore, L. Saggin, S. Ausoni, M. Vianello, K. Gundersen, and T. Lomo. 1989. Three myosin heavy chain isoforms in type 2 skeletal muscle fibres, *J. Muscle Res. Cell Motil.*, 10:197.
Shackelford, S. D., M. F. Miller, K. D. Haydon, N. V. Lovegren, C. E. Lyon, and J. O. Reagan. 1990. Acceptability of bacon as influenced by the feeding of elevated levels of monounsaturated fats to growing-finishing swine, *J. Food Sci.*, 55:621–624.
Sparks, J. C., B. R. Wiegand, F. C. Parrish, Jr., and J. A. Love. 1999. Effects of length of feeding conjugated linoleic acid (CLA) on growth and body composition of pigs, *J. Anim. Sci.*, 77(Suppl. 1):178 (Abstr.).
Swanek, S. S., J. B. Morgan, F. N. Owens, D. R. Gill, C. A. Strasia, H. G. Dolezal, and F. K. Ray. 1999. Vitamin D_3 supplementation of beef steers increases longissimus tenderness, *J. Anim. Sci.*, 77:874.

Termin, A., R. S. Staron, and D. Pette. 1989. Changes in myosin heavy chain isoforms during chronic low-frequency stimulation of rat fast hindlimb muscles — a single fiber study, *Eur. J. Biochem.*, 186:749.

Ullrey, D. E. 1981. Vitamin E for swine, *J. Anim. Sci.*, 53:1939.

van Laack, R. L. J. M., and M. B. Solomon. 1995. The affect of postmortem temperature on pork color and water holding capacity. In *Proc. 41st Int. Cong. Meat Sci. Technol.*, Vol. II, San Antonio, TX, 650.

Voet, D., J. G. Voet, and C. W. Pratt. 1999. *Fundamentals of Biochemistry*, John Wiley & Sons, New York.

Warkup, C. C., A. W. Dilworth, A. J. Kempster, and J. D. Wood. 1990. The effect of sire type, company source, feeding regime and sex on eating quality of pig meat, *Anim. Prod.*, 50:560 (Abstr.).

Warkup, C. C., and A. J. Kempster. 1991. A possible explanation of the variation in tenderness and juiciness in pig meat, *Anim. Prod.*, 52:559 (Abstr.).

Wheeler, T. L., M. Koohmaraie, and S. D. Shackelford. 1997. Effect of postmortem injection time and postinjection aging time on the calcium-activated tenderization process in beef, *J. Anim. Sci.*, 75:2652.

Wismer-Pedersen, J. 1987. Chemistry of animal tissue — Part 5. Water. In *The Science of Meat and Meat Products*, Price, J. F., and B. S. Schweigert, Ed., Food and Nutrition Press, Westport, CT, 141

29 Nutrient Effects on Gene Expression

Jess L. Miner, Alan S. Robertson, and Karen L. Houseknecht

CONTENTS

I. Introduction 659
    A. Transcription 659
    B. Translation 661
    C. Post-Translational Protein Modification 661
II. Examples 661
    A. A Mineral Example: Metallothionein 661
    B. A Carbohydrate Example: Fatty Acid Synthase 662
    C. A Lipid Example: Peroxisome Proliferator-Activated Receptors 663
        1. PPAR: Key Regulators of Differentiation 663
        2. Role of PPAR in Nutritional Regulation of Gene Expression 663
III. Summary 665
References 665

I. INTRODUCTION

Nutritional variation mediates dramatic effects on growth, development, reproduction, and health of animals. Specific nutrients are now known to influence the expression of genes. The future holds bright promise that more-detailed understanding of how genes are influenced by nutrition will lead to improved animal products and greater efficiency of production. The objective of this chapter is to introduce the general mechanistic model of gene expression and to present some examples of nutrient regulation of gene expression.

The structure and function of living cells is largely determined by the proteins synthesized in those cells. Gene expression is the production of functional protein. In the past 50 years, intensive biological research unearthed a basic dogma for how cells store the information for building complex proteins. The information is stored in genes composed of specific sequences of deoxyribonucleic acid (DNA) located in the cell nucleus. Genes are transcribed (copied) into messenger ribonucleic acid (mRNA), and translated into protein with remarkable fidelity. The process of protein synthesis described below is simplistic, but it illustrates many areas for regulatory intervention, the initiation of transcription, mRNA stability, translational control, and protein turnover are a few examples. More details about the various processes are given in texts such as Mathews (1996).

A. TRANSCRIPTION

Transcription is the process of making an RNA copy of a DNA template. Refer to Figure 29.1 for details. It is initiated by the binding of transcription factors to DNA operator elements upstream

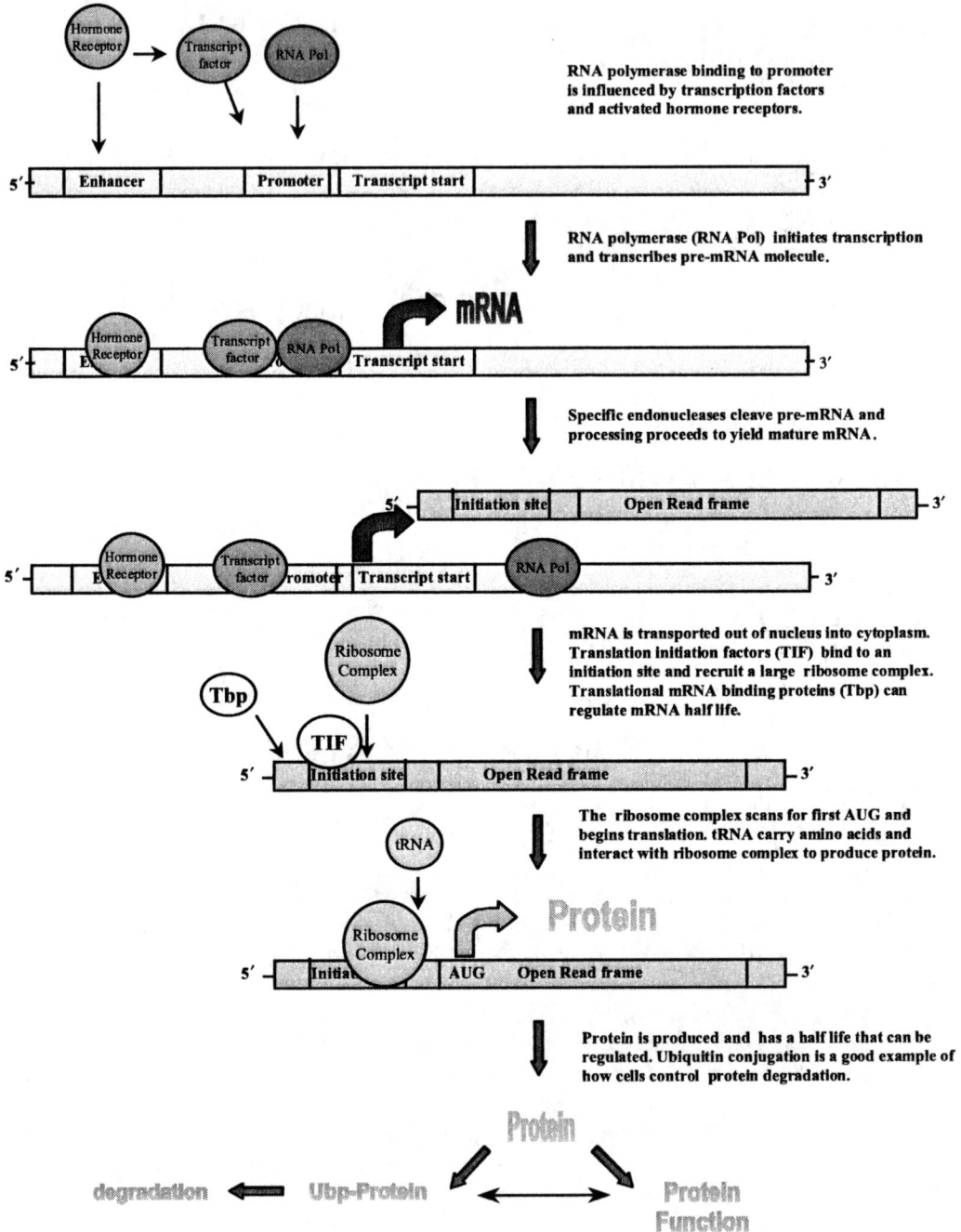

FIGURE 29.1 Graphic representation of the processes of transcription and translation.

of the transcription start site. These factors induce an RNA polymerase complex to bind to a promoter sequence (a DNA site upstream of the transcription start site) and initiate DNA transcription to mRNA in a 5′ to 3′ directional manner. Activated hormone receptors or signaling molecules can bind to transcription factors or directly to DNA enhancer sequences and influence binding of the RNA polymerase complex to the promoter. This regulation can either increase transcription initiation or repress it. The RNA polymerase complex incorporates 5′-ribonucleoside triphosphates into the growing RNA molecule. The transcription is terminated at specific 3′ terminal DNA sequences, producing a pre-mRNA molecule. The pre-mRNA is processed into mature mRNA by eliminating noncoding sections and splicing together coding sections. Alternative splicing of the pre-mRNA can produce different mature mRNA specifying several different protein products. Once properly processed, the mature mRNA is transported out of the nucleus into the cytoplasm of the cell. The production of mRNA can therefore be regulated at the stages of transcription or mRNA processing and transport (Conaway and Conaway, 1994).

B. Translation

Once the mature mRNA is transported into the cytoplasm, translation initiation factors bind to specific mRNA sequences and recruit ribosome complexes that initiate translation to make protein. The ribosomal unit scans nucleotides in a 5′ to 3′ direction until it locates the first AUG start codon (3′ sequential ribonucleotide base pairs). The AUG codon specifies a methionine residue. A methionine specific transfer RNA complexes with the ribosome unit and incorporates the first amino acid on the amino terminus. This marks the beginning of the open reading frame (ribonucleotide sequence that corresponds to translated protein sequence). The ribosome unit continues to scan codons in a 5′ to 3′ direction of the mRNA template while specific transfer RNAs shuttle the specified amino acids to the ribosomal complex. Amino acid transferase catalyzes the joining of amino acids to the growing polypeptide chain in a directional manner. The amino group of each amino acid is joined to the carboxyl end of the growing polypeptide. Termination of translation is mediated by one of three stop codons.

Translation is primarily regulated by binding of specific proteins to the mature mRNA (Hershey et al., 1996). These binding proteins can stabilize and enhance translation, sequester the mRNA and inhibit translation, or catalyze mRNA degradation. The synthesis of protein from mRNA can therefore be regulated via translation rate of mRNA or by half-life of mRNA.

C. Post-Translational Protein Modification

Post-translational modifications can dramatically influence protein activity. Depending upon the sequence of a protein and upon the cell in which it is produced, the protein may be glycosylated, acetylated, digested into smaller fragments, and/or covalently linked between cysteine disulfide bonds. In addition to the effect of these modifications on function, some are important determinants of half-life. Ubiquitin often plays a key role in protein turnover. Ubiquitin is an enzyme found in all eukaryotic cells. It conjugates to cytosolic proteins nonspecifically (on primary amino groups, such as the amino terminus of protein or lysine groups) thereby marking the protein for ubiquitin-specific protease degradation.

II. EXAMPLES

A. A Mineral Example: Metallothionein

Metallothionein is a cysteine-rich protein that sequesters elements such as zinc, copper, mercury, and cadmium. Metallothionein gene expression is clearly influenced by diet. Durnam and Palmiter (1981) first showed that injection of mice with one of the above elements would enhance transcription of metallothionein between 10- and 370-fold in liver and kidney. They also observed a twofold increase in mRNA stability. Of additional interest is the fact that these scientists ultimately used the metallothionein promoter to drive expression of heterologous genes, such as growth hormone, which stimulated tremendous interest in transgenics (Hammer et al., 1984) and demonstrated that growth hormone production in pigs could be enhanced with this new technology (Hammer et al., 1986). Ouellette et al. (1982) extended the early observations of Durnam and Palmiter (1981). They demonstrated that addition of zinc or cadmium to the diet would also increase transcription of metallothionein in intestinal tissue. Thus, the production of metallothionein protein is enhanced by dietary metals via an effect on transcription rate. Furthermore, mRNA stability is also increased by dietary metals. De et al. (1991) determined that cadmium can prolong the half-life of metallothionein mRNA in hepatocytes by 2.5-fold.

The effect of metals on transcription rate is mediated by binding of the metal to a transcription factor (MTF), thereby causing the interaction of the MTF with a metal response element in the upstream promoter region of the metallothionein gene (Magis et al., 1996).

B. A Carbohydrate Example: Fatty Acid Synthase

Animals synthesize triacylglycerol (triglyceride) for storage when energy intake exceeds expenditure. This lipid synthesis mostly occurs in hepatic and adipose tissues, which express a number of lipogenic enzymes. Fatty acids derived from the diet may be esterified directly, but these tissues also synthesize fatty acids from the metabolic intermediate, acetyl coenzyme A (CoA). Two enzymes catalyze fatty acid synthesis: acetyl CoA is carboxylated to malonyl CoA by acetyl CoA carboxylase; and fatty acid synthase (FAS) catalyzes seven sequential reactions which convert malonyl CoA and acetyl CoA into fatty acid, two carbons at a time, resulting in production of palmitate. Although the enzymatic activity of acetyl CoA carboxylase is regulated partly by allosteric interactions, FAS activity is governed completely at the level of gene expression. Expression of the FAS gene is regulated at the level of transcription rate, and to a lesser extent, by variable transcript stability (Katsurada et al., 1990). Dietary carbohydrate and dietary fat have a profound effect on FAS gene expression. Dietary fat reduces FAS expression, possibly via peroxisome proliferator-activated receptors (discussed in Section II.C). Dietary carbohydrate stimulates FAS expression, and much has recently been learned about how this is mediated.

Consumption of a fat-free, high-carbohydrate meal by rats after a 24-h fast increases FAS transcription rate by 39-fold at 6 h after the meal (Sul and Wang, 1998; Fukuda et al., 1999). Of course, it has long been recognized that carbohydrate consumption is followed by insulin secretion, and it seems that at least some of the effect that carbohydrate exerts on FAS expression is mediated by the action(s) of insulin. Administration of insulin to streptozotocin-treated rats (lacking insulin-secreting pancreatic B cells) also increased FAS transcription (19-fold). Insulin may mediate the effect of carbohydrate on FAS transcription by two general mechanisms. First, insulin promotes uptake of glucose by cells and promotes glucose metabolism. Glucose-6-phosphate, or, more likely, xylulose-5-phosphate, is thought to interact with proteins that bind regulatory regions of the FAS gene (Dorion et al., 1996). Second, insulin-stimulated intracellular signaling molecules may interact with the FAS gene directly, independent of carbohydrate metabolites.

The FAS gene contains multiple regulatory regions upstream of the transcription start site. Of special interest is an E-box located at position –65 in the FAS promoter. An E-box is a regulatory region of DNA with the consensus sequence CANNTG. This region of DNA can be bound by upstream stimulatory factors (USF1 and USF2) and by sterol response element binding protein 1 (SREBP1), as reported by Casado et al. (1999). These authors determined that the response of FAS transcription to dietary carbohydrate depends on both USF1 and USF2. These two proteins seem to heterodimerize and interact with the E-box after carbohydrate consumption. Perhaps a metabolite of carbohydrate metabolism enhances this heterodimerization. At any rate, this laboratory also demonstrated that whereas FAS transcription is impaired in carbohydrate-fed USF1- and USF2-knockout mice, SREBP1 expression is normal and FAS transcription response to insulin is normal. Insulin, in addition, seems to mediate an effect on FAS transcription via the phosphoinositol 3-kinase signaling pathway and by interacting with insulin response sequences in the FAS gene (Wang and Sul, 1998). The details of how insulin, or hormones such as glucagon, growth hormone, and triiodothyronine, mediate effects on FAS transcription are not yet complete. However, it is clear that carbohydrate, independently and through insulin, mediates a profound effect on transcription of FAS.

C. A Lipid Example: Peroxisome Proliferator-Activated Receptors

Dietary fat content has been shown to regulate gene expression in metabolic tissues; often effects observed are tissue-specific. For example, consumption of high-fat diets leads to whole-body insulin resistance in rodents, and the mechanisms underlying this insulin resistance involve the insulin responsive glucose transporter, GLUT4. Increased dietary fat (not increased calories) downregulates GLUT4 protein expression in adipose tissue but not skeletal muscle (Kahn, 1994) and expression is linked to arachidonic acid metabolites, presumably via activation of PPARγ (see below; Long and Pekala, 1996). In contrast, high-fat diets alter GLUT4 translocation to the plasma membrane and insulin signaling but not gene expression in skeletal muscle (Zierath et al., 1997). Consumption of high-fat diets has been reported to increase leptin gene expression in adipose tissue of rodents (see reviews by Caro et al., 1996; Houseknecht et al., 1998a); however, many studies are confounded by differences in caloric intake. In fact, when specific dietary fatty acids are supplemented to swine diets (balanced for caloric density), there is no effect of dietary fatty acids on leptin gene expression in adipose tissue (Spurlock et al., 1999).

Specific fatty acids are now implicated in the regulation of gene expression. Raclot et al. (1997) reported that consumption of dietary n-3 polyunsaturated fatty acids (n-3 PUFA) downregulated (40 to 75% compared with control) expression of genes involved in lipid metabolism, adipogenesis, and food intake regulation in retroperitoneal but not subcutaneous adipose tissue. Genes regulated by n-3 PUFA in retroperitoneal adipose tissue included leptin, CEBP/α, FAS, lipoprotein lipase, hormone-sensitive lipase, and phosphoenolpyruvate carboxykinase. Regulation of the aP2 fatty acid–binding protein by PUFA may also be important because it has been implicated in the targeting of fatty acids to regulatory elements in the nucleus (Hertzel and Bernlohr, 1998).

Clearly, dietary fatty acids can have profound effects on gene expression. However, the mechanisms underlying the hormonal actions of fatty acids on gene expression and protein function have not been fully elucidated. Nuclear receptors mediate at least some of the fatty acid effects on gene expression by influencing transcription. Nuclear receptors that have received considerable attention in this regard are the peroxisome proliferator-activated receptors (PPAR).

1. PPAR: Key Regulators of Differentiation

The PPAR subfamily of nuclear hormone receptors include PPARα, β, and γ, which are encoded by distinct genes (Schoonjans et al., 1996). The PPARγ gene contains three promoters that yield three isoforms, γ1, γ2, and γ3, by alternative promoter usage and splicing (Zhu et al., 1993; 1995; Tontonoz et al., 1994b; Fajas et al., 1998). Expression of the various PPAR are tissue dependent (Braissant et al., 1996). PPARα is expressed in liver, cardiac myocytes, enterocytes, and proximal tubule of the kidney. PPARβ is ubiquitously expressed, whereas PPARγ is expressed in adipose tissue and the immune system. PPAR function by binding ligands (such as fatty acids), forming heterodimeric complexes with other transcription factors (e.g., retinoic X receptor-α) binding to peroxisome proliferator response elements (PPRE) on DNA, and subsequently activating transcription (Figure 29.2; Tontonoz et al., 1994a). The PPAR class of nuclear receptors has been shown to drive differentiation in multiple cell types. Expression and activation of PPARγ is sufficient to drive differentiation of fibroblasts into adipocytes (Tontonoz et al., 1994c; Hu et al., 1995).

2. Role of PPAR in Nutritional Regulation of Gene Expression

Many fatty acids activate PPAR (reviewed by Vanden Heuvel, 1999), and PPAR are implicated in the anticancer effects of diverse fatty acids. In addition to anticancer effects of dietary fatty acids, evidence is mounting that PPARγ and its ligands play an important role not only in the regulation of adipogenesis, but also in the regulation of obesity and whole-body insulin action (Saltiel and Olefsky, 1996). Regulation of PPARγ can occur at the level of gene expression, ligand availability (both endogenous and pharmacological ligands), and at the level of PPARγ activity (phosphorylation

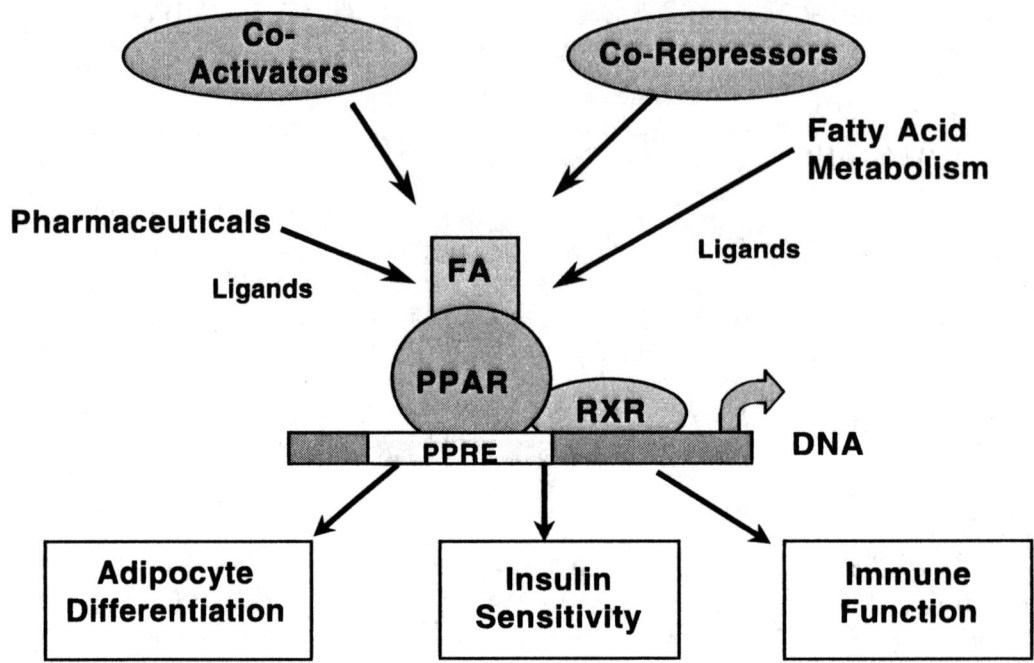

FIGURE 29.2 Illustration of the roles of PPARs.

status; Hu et al., 1996). A limited body of evidence suggests that PPARγ expression is nutritionally regulated in rodents, humans, and livestock. In rodents, adipose tissue PPARγ expression is regulated by insulin (Vidal-Puig et al., 1996; 1997) and nutrition (high-fat diets, fasting; Vidal-Puig et al., 1996; Rousseau et al., 1997), but not by obesity (Vidal-Puig et al., 1996).

PPARγ has been cloned in pigs (Grindflek et al., 1998; Houseknecht et al., 1998b) and cattle (Sunvold et al., 1997). The nucleic acid sequence of porcine PPARγ was highly conserved with the cow, human, and mouse sequences; the amino acid identities ranged from 96 to 98% for all species (Houseknecht et al., 1998b). Both PPARγ 1 and PPARγ 2 isoforms are highly expressed in porcine adipose tissue, although the γ1 isoform predominates (Houseknecht et al., 1998b). To date, the γ3 isoform has not been identified in livestock. Porcine PPARγ abundance in subcutaneous adipose tissue is regulated by nutritional status (Houseknecht et al., 1998b). Expression of porcine PPARγ2 but not PPARγ1 mRNA is significantly reduced in fasting animals or in animals allowed restricted feed intake compared with control animals allowed *ad libitum* access to feed (Houseknecht et al., 1998b). The pig data are consistent with the findings of Vidal-Puig et al. (1996) who reported that fasting reduced PPARγ2 mRNA abundance more significantly than PPARγ1 in the mouse. Recently, it was found that dietary fatty acids also regulate PPARγ2 expression in swine; expression in porcine subcutaneous adipose tissue is upregulated by dietary supplementation of 18:2 but not 16:0, 18:0, or n-3 fatty acids (Spurlock et al., 1999). The mechanisms underlying differential regulation of PPARγ2 vs. PPARγ1 gene expression are not well understood. It is tempting to speculate that nutritional, metabolic, and/or endocrine factors that are modified by feed restriction, fasting, and other nutritional/physiological/pathological states differentially modulate γ1, γ2, and γ3 gene expression and/or activity. Further research is needed to determine the functional importance of the splice variants and to delineate mechanisms that regulate their expression and activation.

In addition to regulating the gene expression of PPARγ, dietary fatty acids are also able to activate PPAR and promote diet-induced changes in gene expression in metabolically important tissues. Conjugated linoleic acid (CLA) is a group of geometric and positional isomers of linoleic acid found in ruminant meats and milks that has anticancer, antiobesity, antiatherogenic, and antidiabetic properties. CLA is a potent activator of PPARγ (Belury et al., 1997); CLA activation of PPARγ has been implicated in the anticancer effects in mammary, colon, skin, and stomach (Vanden Heuvel, 1999). CLA induces apoptosis in adipocytes (Evans et al., 2000; Miner et al., 2000; Tsuboyama-Kasaoka et al., 2000). Evidence for the diabetic and antidiabetic effects and link to PPARγ was provided by Houseknecht et al. (1998c) and Tsuboyama-Kasaoka et al. (2000). When a mixture of CLA isomers was fed to Zucker (ZDF) prediabetic rats for 14 days, impaired glucose tolerance was normalized and serum triglycerides and insulin were reduced, similar to effects seen with thiazolidinedione treatment (Houseknecht et al., 1998c). Furthermore, CLA treatment induced expression of the PPARγ-responsive aP2 gene in adipose tissue (Houseknecht et al., 1998c), uncoupling protein 1 (UCP1) gene expression in brown adipose tissue (Portocarrero et al., 1999), and UCP2 gene expression in skeletal muscle (Portocarrero et al., 1999). Additionally, CLA was able to transactivate PPARγ response elements in transfection experiments (Houseknecht et al., 1998c). These data suggest that CLA can activate PPARγ, and recent work by these authors indicates that the antidiabetic effects may be specific to certain CLA isomers (Ryder et al., 1999a,b). In swine, dietary CLA has been shown to have antiobesity and nutrient repartitioning effects as well. Dugan et al. (1997) reported that supplementation of swine diets with 2% CLA caused a reduction in feed intake and adipose tissue mass with a corresponding increase in lean growth and feed efficiency.

Presumably the effects of CLA in swine are mediated via PPAR; further research is needed to confirm this hypothesis.

III. SUMMARY

The role of nutrients in animal biology is not constrained to their nutritional contribution. Many nutrients also have specific effects on expression of genes. How is this relevant to the livestock industry? Although it is not possible to know all the ways these phenomena may be relevant, there are already some clear indications. For example, the fact that glucogenic amino acids stimulate the expression of threonine dehydratase, which breaks down threonine, may explain why overfeeding protein could induce a threonine deficiency, even when threonine intake was deemed adequate. Second, the almost pharmaceutical benefits of CLA in human diets, mediated by its effect on gene expression, may ultimately result in meat producers striving to enhance the CLA content of their products.

REFERENCES

Belury, M. A., S. Y. Moya-Camarena, L. L. Liu, and J. P. Vanden Heuvel. 1997. Dietary conjugated linoleic acid induces peroxisome-specific enzyme accumulation and ornithine decarboxylase activity in mouse liver, *J. Nutr. Biochem.*, 8:579.

Braissant, O., F. Foufelle, C. Scotto, M. Dauca, and W. Wahli. 1996. Differential expression of peroxisome proliferator-activated receptors (PPARs): tissue distribution of PPAR-alpha, -beta, and -gamma in the adult rat, *Endocrinology*, 137:354.

Caro, J. F., M. K. Sinha, J. W. Kolaczynski, P. L. Zhang, and R. V. Considine RV. 1996. Leptin — the tale of an obesity gene, *Diabetes*, 45:1455.

Casado, M., V. S. Vallet, A. Kahn, and S. Vaulont. 1999. Essential role *in vivo* of upstream stimulatory factors for a normal dietary response of the fatty acid synthase gene in the liver, *J. Biol. Chem.*, 274:2009.

Conaway, R. C., and J. W. Conaway. 1994. *Transcription: Mechanism and Regulation*, Raven Press, New York.

De, S. K., G. C. Enders, and G. K. Andrews. 1991. Metallothionein mRNA stability in chicken and mouse cells, *Biochim. Biophys. Acta*, 1090:223.

Dorion, B., M. H. Cuif, R. Chen, and A. Kahn. 1996. Transcriptional glucose signaling through the glucose response element is mediated by the pentose phosphate pathway, *J. Biol. Chem.*, 271:5321.

Dugan, M. E. R., J. L. Aalhus, A. L. Schaefer, and J. K. G. Kramer. 1997. The effect of conjugated linoleic acid on fat to lean repartitioning and feed conversion in pigs, *Can. J. Anim Sci.*, 77:723.

Durnam, D. M., and R. D. Palmiter. 1981. Transcriptional regulation of the mouse metallothionein-I gene by heavy metals, *J. Biol. Chem.*, 256:5712.

Evans, M., C. Geigerman, J. Cook, L. Curtis, B. Kuebler, and M. McIntosh. 2000. Conjugated linoleic acid suppresses triglyceride accumulation and induces apoptosis in 3T3-L1 preadipocytes, *Lipids*, 35:899.

Fajas, L., J. C. Fruchart, and J. Auwerx. 1998. PPAR-gamma-3 mRNAA distinct PPAR gamma mRNA subtype transcribed from an independent promoter, *FEBS Lett.*, 438:55.

Fukuda, H., N. Iritani, T. Sugimoto, and H. Ikeda. 1999. Transcriptional regulation of fatty acid synthase gene by insulin/glucose, polyunsaturated fatty acid and leptin in hepatocytes and adipocytes in normal and genetically obese rats, *Eur. J. Biochem.*, 260:505.

Grindflek, E., H. Sundvold, H. Klungland, and S. Lien. 1998. Characterization of porcine peroxisome proliferator-activated receptors γ1 and γ2: detection of breed and age differences in gene expression, *Biochem. Biophys. Res. Commun.*, 249:713.

Hammer, R. E., R. D. Palmiter, and R. L. Brinster. 1984. Partial correction of murine hereditary growth disorder by germ-line incorporation of a new gene, *Nature*, 311: 65.

Hammer, R. E., V. G. Pursel, C. E. Rexroad, Jr., R. J. Wall, D. J. Bolt, R. D. Palmiter, and R. L. Brinster. 1986. Genetic engineering of mammalian embryos, *J. Anim. Sci.*, 63: 269.

Hershey, J. W. B., M. B. Mathews, and N. Sonenberg, Eds. 1996. *Translational Control*, Cold Spring Harbor Laboratory Press, Cold Spring Harbor, NY.

Hertzel, A. V., and D. A. Bernlohr. 1998. Regulation of adipocyte gene expression by polyunsaturated fatty acids, *Mol. Cell. Biochem.*, 188:33.

Houseknecht, K. L., C. A. Baile, R. L. Matteri, and M. E. Spurlock. 1998a. The biology of leptin: a review, *J. Anim. Sci.*, 76:1405.

Houseknecht, K. L., C. A. Bidwell, C. P. Portocarrero, and M. E. Spurlock. 1998b. Expression and cDNA cloning of porcine peroxisome proliferator-activated receptor gamma (PPAR gamma), *Gene*, 225:89–96.

Houseknecht, K. L., J. P. Vanden Heuvel, S. Y. Moyacamarena, C. P. Portocarrero, L. W. Peck, K. P. Nickel, and M. A. Belury. 1998c. Dietary conjugated linoleic acid normalizes impaired glucose tolerance in the Zucker Diabetic Fatty FA/FA rat, *Biochem. Biophys. Res. Commun.*, 244:678.

Hu, E., P. Tontonoz, and B. M. Spiegelman. 1995. Transdifferentiation of myoblasts by the adipogenic transcription factors PPARγ and C/EBPa, *Proc. Natl. Acad. Sci. U.S.A.*, 92:9856.

Hu, E. D., J. B. Kim, P. Sarraf, and B. M. Spiegelman. 1996. Inhibition of adipogenesis through MAP kinase-mediated phosphorylation of PPAR-gamma, *Science*, 274:2100.

Kahn, B. B. 1994. Dietary regulation of glucose transporter gene expression: tissue specific effects in adipose cells and muscle, *J. Nutr.*, 124:1289S.

Katsurada, A., N. Iritani, H. Fukuda, Y. Matsumura, N. Nishimoto, T. Noguchi, and T. Tanaka. 1990. Effects of nutrients and hormones on transcriptional and post-transcriptional regulation of fatty acid synthase in rat liver, *Eur. J. Biochem.*, 190:427.

Long, S. D., and P. H. Pekala, P.H. 1996. Regulation of GLUT4 gene expression by arachidonic acid. Evidence for multiple pathways, one of which requires oxidation to prostaglandin E2, *J. Biol. Chem.*, 271:1138.

Magis, W., S. Fiering, M. Groudine, and D. I. K. Martin. 1996. An upstream activator of transcription coordinately increases the level and epigenetic stability of gene expression, *Proc. Natl. Acad. Sci. U.S.A.*, 93:13914.

Mathews, V. H. 1996. *Biochemistry*, Benjamin/Cummings, Redwood City, CA.

Miner, J. L., C. A. Cederberg, M. K. Nielsen, X. Chen, and C. A. Baile. 2000. Conjugated linoleic acid (CLA), body fat, and apoptosis in mice, *FASEB J.*, 14:A479.

Ouellette, A. J., L. Aviles, C. A. Burnweit, D. Frederick, and R. A. Malt. 1982. Metallothionein mRNA induction in mouse small bowel by oral cadmium and zinc, *Am. J. Physiol.*, 243:G396.

Portocarrero, C. P., D. E. Bauman, D. M. Barbano, J. Zierath, and K. L. Houseknecht. 1999. Regulation of UCP1 and UCP2 gene expression by dietary conjugated linoleic acid (CLA) in Zucker Diabetic Fatty (ZDF) rats, *Diabetes*, 48(Suppl. 1):A5.

Raclot, T., R. Groscolas, D. Langin, and P. Ferre. 1997. Site-specific regulation of gene expression by n-3 polyunsaturated fatty acids in rat white adipose tissues, *J. Lipid Res.*, 38:1963.

Rousseau, V., D. J. Becker, L. N. Ongemba, J. Rahier, J. C. Henquin, and S. M. Brichard. 1997. Developmental and nutritional changes of ob and PPARγ2 gene expression in rat white adipose tissue, *Biochem. J.*, 321:451.

Ryder, J., D. E. Bauman, C. P. Portocarrero, X. Song, M. Yu, J. R. Zierath, and K. L. Houseknecht. 1999a. Dietary conjugated linoleic acid (CLA) improves glucose tolerance and glucose uptake into skeletal muscle of Zucker Diabetic Fatty (ZDF) rats, *Diabetes*, 48(Suppl. 1):A308.

Ryder, J., D. E. Bauman, C. P. Portocarrero, X. Song, M. Yu, J. R. Zierath, and K. L. Houseknecht. 1999b. Anti-diabetic effects of dietary conjugated linoleic acid (CLA): Isomer-specific effects on glucose tolerance and skeletal muscle glucose transport, *J. Anim Sci.*, 77(Suppl. 1):119.

Saltiel, A., and J. M. Olefsky. 1996. Thiazolidinediones in the treatment of insulin resistance and Type II diabetes, *Diabetes*, 45:1661.

Schoonjans, K., B. Staels, and J. Auwerx. 1996. The peroxisome proliferator activated receptors (PPARs) and their effects on lipid metabolism and adipocyte differentiation, *Biochem. Biophys. Acta*, 1302:93.

Spurlock, M. E., K. L. Houseknecht, C. P. Portocarrero, S. G. Cornelius, and G. M. Willis, 1999. Regulation of PPARγ but not leptin gene expression by dietary fatty acid supplementation, *J. Anim. Sci.*, 77 (Suppl. 1):159.

Sul, H. S., and D. Wang. 1998. Nutritional and hormonal regulation of enzymes in fat synthesis: studies of fatty acid synthase and mitochondrial glycerol-3-phosphate acyltransferase gene transcription, *Annu. Rev. Nutr.*,18:331.

Sundvold, H., A. Brzozowska, and S. Lien. 1997. Characterization of bovine peroxisome proliferator-activated receptors γ1 and γ2: genetic mapping and differential expression of the two isoforms, *Biochem. Biophys. Res. Commun.*, 239:857.

Tontonoz, P., R. A. Graves, A. Budavari, H. Erdjument-Bromage, M. Lui, E. Hu, P. Tempst, and B. M. Spiegelman. 1994a. Adipocyte-specific transcription factor ARF 6 is a heterodimeric complex of two nuclear hormone receptors, PPARγ and RXRa, *Nucl. Acid Res.*, 22:5628.

Tontonoz, P., E. Hu, R. A. Graves, A. I. Budavari, and B. M. Spiegelman. 1994b. mPPARγ2: tissue-specific regulator of an adipocyte enhancer, *Genes Dev.*, 8:1224.

Tontonoz, P., E. Hu, and B. M. Spiegelman. 1994c. Stimulation of adipogenesis in fibroblasts by PPARγ, a lipid-activated transcription factor, *Cell*, 79:1147.

Tsuboyama-Kasaoka, T., M. Takahashi, K. Tanemura, H. Kim, T. Tange, H. Okuyama, M. Kasai, S. Ikemoto, and O. Ezaki. 2000. Conjugated linoleic acid supplementation reduces adipose tissue by apoptosis and develops lipodystrophy in mice, *Diabetes*, 49:1534.

Vanden Heuvel, J. P. 1999. Peroxisome proliferator-activated receptors: a critical link among fatty acids, gene expression and carcinogenesis, *J. Nutr.*, 129:575S.

Vidal-Puig, A., M. Jimenez-Linan, B. B. Lowell, A. Hamann, E. Hu, B. M. Spiegelman, J. S. Flier, and D. E. Moller. 1996. Regulation of PPARγ gene expression by nutrition and obesity in rodents, *J. Clin. Invest.*, 97:2553.

Vidal-Puig, A., R. V. Considine, M. Jimenez-Linan, A. Werman, W. J. Pories, J. F. Caro, and J. S. Flier. 1997. Peroxisome proliferator-activated receptor gene expression in human tissues. Effects of obesity, weight loss, and regulation by insulin and glucocorticoids, *J. Clin. Invest.*, 99:2416.

Wang, D., and H. S. Sul. 1998. Insulin stimulation of fatty acid synthase promoter is mediated by the phosphatidylinositol 3-kinase pathway, *J. Biol. Chem.*, 273:25420.

Zhu, Y., K. Alvares, Q. Huang, M. S. Rao, and J. Reddy. 1993. Cloning of a new member of the peroxisome proliferator-activated receptor gene family from mouse liver, *J. Biol. Chem.*, 268:26817.

Zhu, Y., C. Qi, J. R. Korenbergm X. N. Chen, D. Noya, M. S. Rao, and J. K. Reddy. 1995. Structural organization of mouse peroxisome proliferator-activated receptor gamma (mPPARgamma) gene: alternative promoter use and different splicing yield two mPPAR gamma isoforms, *Proc. Natl. Acad. Sci. U.S.A.*, 92:7921.

Zierath, J. R., K. L. Houseknecht, L. Gnudi, and B. B. Kahn. 1997. High fat feeding impairs insulin-stimulated GLUT4 recruitment via an early insulin-signaling defect, *Diabetes*, 46:215.

Part IV

Applied Feeding of Swine

30 Feeding Neonatal Pigs

Trygve L. Veum and Jack Odle

CONTENTS

I. Introduction 671
II. Advantages of Artificial Rearing 672
III. Disadvantage of Artificial Rearing 673
IV. Environmental Requirements..673
V. Passive Immunity and Milk-Borne Bioactive Agents 674
VI. Nutrient Requirements 674
VII. Development of the Digestive Enzyme System 675
    A. Pancreatic Enzymes. 675
    B. Intestinal Enzymes 676
VIII. Protein Sources and Utilization 677
IX. Carbohydrate Sources and Utilization 678
X. Fat Sources and Utilization...679
XI. Feeding Management..680
XII. The Effect of Nutrition on Diarrhea...680
XIII. Liquid Diets for Segregated Early-Weaned Pigs..681
XIV. Subsequent Performance 681
XV. Summary 682
References 682

I. INTRODUCTION

The term *neonatal* is defined as the first 4 weeks of life (*Dorland's Illustrated Medical Dictionary*, 23rd ed., W. B. Saunders Co.). Most mammalian neonates rely on milk as the primary source of nutrition during this period. The sow is best suited to provide this nutrition support in modern pig production. However, management for optimal production efficiency has led to the development of early-weaning systems that mandate removal of the pigs from the dam between 0 and 14 days of age. Three distinct management applications are noteworthy:

1. Weaning on day 0. The desire to wean immediately at birth (either via cesarean section or attended natural farrowing) is required for the establishment of foundation herds that are free of specific pathogens. The primary challenge with this application stems from denying the pig access to sow colostrum.
2. Weaning on day 1. Pigs are allowed to receive colostrum from the dam and then are removed to an artificial rearing system.
3. Weaning on day 10 to 14. Known as segregated early weaning, this management strategy removes the pig from the sow early enough to reduce disease transfer, but the pigs are older and better able to withstand the stressors of weaning and the transition to dry feed.

Because of the rapid changes that occur in the development of the digestive system of the baby pig, all these management schemes are dependent to varying degrees on diets containing large amounts of milk-derived ingredients and/or smaller amounts of animal plasma–derived ingredients. Furthermore, liquid diets (milk replacers) are required to achieve maximal performance of the pig in each case (Lecce et al., 1979). An earlier review on the nutrition of early-weaned pigs is available (Jones, 1972).

Whereas the majority of the pigs produced commercially are weaned between 2 and 3 weeks of age, pigs can be removed from the sow at 1 to 3 days of age and reared successfully. However, pigs weaned at 1 to 3 days of age are usually reared in units designed specifically for this purpose, as described later in this chapter (Section XI). Most of these rearing devices utilize liquid feeding systems that feed continuously or at specific intervals daily. Rearing neonatal pigs with these mechanical feeding devices is generally referred to as "artificial rearing."

II. ADVANTAGES OF ARTIFICIAL REARING

1. Saving entire litters when extensive lactation failure occurs such that cross-fostering is not possible.

2. Saving pigs from large litters as an option to cross-fostering when the sow cannot nurse them all, especially the smaller pigs that often get pushed away and starve (Lecce, 1971).

3. Reducing neonatal death losses that occur from environmental causes (Figure 30.1).

Preweaning death losses of pigs born alive in the United States declined from 11.6% in 1990 to 9.4% in 1995 (USDA, 1997). Stillbirths and mummies also declined from 8.4% of the total litter number born in 1990 to 6.5% in 1995. This represents consistent significant improvement in reducing preweaning death losses compared with the high losses of earlier decades. Most of the preweaning death losses occur during the first 3 to 4 days postfarrowing and decline thereafter to weaning (Fahmy and Bernard, 1971; Nielsen et al., 1974; Gastonbury, 1976).

Low birth weight is an important factor contributing to pig mortality (Gardner et al., 1989), with the most predominant causes of death being sow overlay, starvation, and scours (Leman et al., 1972; Gastonbury, 1977; USDA, 1997). Diarrhea has become more significant as a cause of pig morbidity (Caple, 1989; Dewey et al., 1995). The six most common pathogens causing diarrhea in newborn pigs include rotavirus, *Escherichia coli*, transmissible gastroenteritis virus, *Clostridium perfringens*, *Lsospora suis*, and *Enterococcus durans* (Johnson et al., 1992).

In contrast to the high death losses incurred with natural rearing, artificial rearing of pigs removed from the sow at 1 day of age has been accomplished with death losses below 5% thereafter

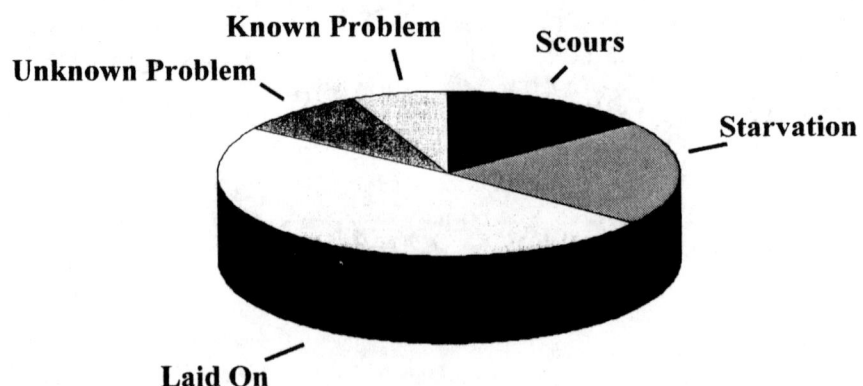

FIGURE 30.1 Cause of death for preweaning pigs (USDA, 1997) observed in the National Swine Survey conducted by the National Animal Health Monitoring System. Graph shows percentage of total deaths attributed to various causes.

(Lecce, 1969; 1975; Veum and Bowman, 1973; Sherry et al., 1978a,b; Mateo and Veum, 1980a,b; Lauxen and Veum, 1982).

4. Early rebreeding of the sow to increase the litters per sow per year is a potential advantage, but currently is not an advantage because of the delayed and erratic return to estrus and the smaller litter size that results from weaning at a few days of age (Moody and Speer, 1971; Pay, 1973; Svajgr et al., 1974; Walker and Eddie, 1974). However, early weaning may have economic value in a farrowing system utilizing only gilts, where the pigs are weaned and reared artificially after nursing colostrum and the dams shipped to slaughter.

5. Improving feed efficiency by feeding the pigs directly in contrast to feeding the sow, who in turn nurses the pigs.

6. Utilizing the neonatal pig as a model for human infant nutrition research due to the biological and physiological similarities of pigs and humans (Book and Bustad, 1974; Tumbleson, 1986; Miller and Ullrey, 1987; Shulman et al., 1988; Moughan et al., 1992; Reeds and Odle, 1996).

7. Elimination of specific pathogens by cesarean section. When establishing specific pathogen-free foundation herds, there is a need to rear pigs artificially that are delivered by cesarean section.

III. DISADVANTAGE OF ARTIFICIAL REARING

1. The lower fertility rate of sows weaned at 1 day of age compared with weaning at 2 to 3 weeks of age. This disadvantage in itself is of sufficient economic importance to prevent the widespread use of artificial rearing except for saving pigs as described above.

2. The high level of management and extra labor required to operate an artificial rearing unit successfully (Van der Hyde, 1972).

3. The initial economic investment in a rearing facility, caging, and feeding equipment for pigs 1 to 2 days old.

4. Sow milk contains antibodies capable of neutralizing the enterotoxigenic effects of *Escherichia coli* organisms (Svendsen and Larson, 1977) as well as other enteric pathogens (Bourne, 1973; Wilson, 1974; Yabiki et al., 1974). Deprivation of colostrum thus poses the primary challenge to rearing pigs weaned immediately at birth. Even pigs weaned on day 1 that have consumed an adequate amount of colostrum are deprived of this continuous source of specific milk immunoglobulins. For this reason, if sanitation is marginal, death rates of artificially reared pigs can exceed those reared naturally.

IV. ENVIRONMENTAL REQUIREMENTS

Early-weaned pigs require a warm, dry, draft-free environment. Artificial rearing units usually house pigs individually in some type of caging with wire or slatted flooring for waste removal. Individual caging is preferred to allow precise feeding and observation of each pig and to prevent undesirable social behaviors such as ear and navel sucking (Van der Hyde, 1972) due to the strong nursing instinct that exists at birth. As pigs age, the need for individual housing decreases such that by 10 to 14 days of age pigs may be successfully reared with group housing.

The perinatal and postnatal environmental requirements of pigs have been reviewed by Curtis (1970; 1974) and Pond and Houpt (1978). The lower critical temperature of the perinatal pig is approximately 34°C (Bianca and Blaxter, 1961; Mount, 1963a). The perinatal pig has little thermal insulation or pelage. Thus, when the effective environmental temperature falls to 34°C the pig must raise its heat-production rate above the minimum or suffer a reduction in body temperature. However, severe cold stress leads to hypothermia in the newborn pig, not due to a lack of energy mobilization from stores but from a defect in glucose utilization (Duee et al., 1988). The lack of full expression of gluconeogenesis in hepatocytes isolated from fasted newborn pigs was not due to a limitation in fatty acid oxidative capacity (Lepine et al., 1993). Pig thermostability improves rapidly during the first 2 days postpartum (Curtis et al., 1967).

The ambient temperature preferred by pigs housed singly the first day of life is approximately 32°C (Mount, 1963b), and this drops to 29 or 30°C by 1 day of age and remains at that temperature throughout the neonatal period for pigs housed singly or in groups of five. In addition to air temperature, other important environmental factors such as airflow (draft), humidity, flooring, and group size must be considered in providing an appropriate environment for the neonatal pig (Curtis, 1970). For example, moving single newborn pigs from a concrete floor to a wooden box containing 10 cm of straw and 10°C had the same thermal effect as raising the ambient temperature to 18°C (Stephens, 1971).

V. PASSIVE IMMUNITY AND MILK-BORNE BIOACTIVE AGENTS

In addition to supplying highly digestible nutrients, colostrum and milk are rich in a variety of substances that may aid development of the pig postnatally (reviewed by Odle et al., 1996). Of primary importance are the colostral immunoglobulines that confer passive immunity (Brown et al., 1961; Lecce, 1972; Bourne, 1973) to the pig that is otherwise immunologically naive at birth (see Chapter 24 on nutrition and immunity) (Hammerberg et al., 1989; Schwager and Schulze, 1997). While it is possible to rear colostrum-deprived pigs, weaned at day 0 into sterile incubators (Coalson et al., 1973) or into highly sanitary isolation units (Lecce, 1969; Ziljstra et al., 1994; 1996; Gomez, 1997), these systems are not practical for routine use in production agriculture. When attempting to rear colostrum-deprived pigs in nonsterile production environments, the animals should be supplemented with immunoglobulins (Scoot et al., 1972; McCallum et al., 1977a). While bovine-derived immunoglobulins may be efficacious (Gomez et al., 1998), porcine immunoglobulins are preferred (Kennelly et al., 1979; Drew and Owen, 1988; Arthington et al., 1997).

If pigs are allowed to obtain colostrum from the sow, a prolonged period of nursing is not needed; 1 to 2 h of good nursing may be adequate (Coalson and Lecce, 1973a). This is best achieved by farrowing in such a manner that all the pigs are placed with the sow simultaneously for the first nursing. However, pigs reared in unsanitary conditions and/or exposed to disease organisms may benefit from a longer nursing of colostrum before removing for artificial rearing (Coalson and Lecce, 1973b). The small intestine has a reduced capacity to absorb antibodies (macromolecules) by 1 to 1.5 day of age in pigs reared naturally or artificially (Speer et al., 1959; Asplund et al., 1962; Lecce, 1973). However, closure can be delayed considerably by subjecting the pigs to starvation at birth (Lecce and Morgan, 1962), which may explain in part why underprivileged pigs show enhanced uptake of macromolecules (Svendsen et al., 1990).

In addition to immunoglobulins, mammary secretions contain several other bioactive peptides, such as insulin-like growth factors, epidermal growth factor, etc. These peptides may be important for gastrointestinal tract development (see Odle et al., 1996, and Burrin, 1997, for reviews), which occurs at an accelerated pace after birth (Widdowson et al., 1976; Zhang et al., 1997, 1998). Because bioactivity is largely destroyed by heat processing, consideration has been given to fortification of commercial formulas and milk replacers with bioactive agents postprocessing. Although biological efficacy of various bioactive peptides has been documented (Zijlstra et al., 1994; Burrin et al., 1996; 1997; Houle et al., 1997), current economics limit practical application in production agriculture.

VI. NUTRIENT REQUIREMENTS

The National Research Council (NRC, 1988) has published the minimum nutrient requirements for baby pigs as small as 3 kg in weight. Diets for pigs of this age are expected to contain a substantial amount (25 to 75%) of milk products. It should be noted that feed intake and growth performance estimates by the NRC reflect the feeding of dry diets. It is well established that feed intake and growth of young pigs is superior when diets are offered in liquid form (reviewed by Odle and Harrell, 1998).

VII. DEVELOPMENT OF THE DIGESTIVE ENZYME SYSTEM

Maturation of the gastrointestinal tract begins *in utero* in preparation for the transition from placental to enteral nutrition, with dramatic postnatal intestinal growth and development occurring during the first 6 h of nursing colostrum (Zhang et al., 1997; 1998). Jensen et al. (1997) have reported the ontogeny of gastric lipase activity in the pig, which increased slightly during nursing and then leveled off after weaning. Regardless of age, gastric lipase represented a small fraction (e.g., 1/1000) of pancreatic lipase activity. Gastric proteolytic enzyme activity per gram of tissue and total activity are low the first 2 weeks of life before rapidly increasing with age (Lindemann et al., 1986).

Digestive organ growth and development during the neonatal period has been described (Walker, 1959b; Aumaitre, 1972; Corring et al., 1978; Aumaitre and Corring, 1978), including changes in pH (Walker, 1919b), dry matter flow, and retention times as affected by milk and soybean proteins (Braude et al., 1970b; Wilson and Leibholz, 1981b). Colostrum and mature milk are both effective in promoting gastrointestinal tissue development in the newborn pig (Simmens et al., 1990). Gastrin, a peptide hormone produced by cells in the stomach and duodenum beginning in early gestation, may be involved in gastrointestinal maturation in fetal and neonatal pigs (Xu and Cranwell, 1991; 1992). Polyamines are also necessary for intestinal growth and development, and supplementation of neonatal pig diets containing soy proteins with amines (ethylamine or putrescine) may enhance intestinal absorption and enterocyte proliferation (Grant et al., 1990).

In general, the digestive enzymes produced by the exocrine pancreas hydrolyze a major fraction of the ingested food compared with that hydrolyzed by the intestinal enzymes (Corring, 1977). Changes do occur with age, however, with pancreatic protease representing 70 to 80% of the total activity up to 6 weeks of age, and declining to 50% thereafter (Shields et al., 1980). The pancreatic contribution to amylase activity is reversed, contributing 30% at birth then increasing to 70% by 4 weeks of age. Similar changes occurred in the digestive enzyme activities of weaned vs. unweaned pigs from birth through 8 weeks of age for most enzymes (Hartman et al., 1961). Neither age at weaning (2 vs. 4 weeks) nor feeding method (paste form vs. dry meal) influenced enzyme development or pig performance to 10 weeks of age (Shields et al., 1980).

The development of the digestive enzyme system in neonatal pigs has been reviewed (Aumaitre, 1972; Pond and Houpt, 1978). A brief review of pancreatic and intestinal mucosa enzyme activities and total enzyme production is presented here.

A. PANCREATIC ENZYMES

Fresh pancreatic tissue weight increases rapidly during the neonatal period in pigs nursing sows (Lindemann et al., 1986). From birth to 4 weeks of age pancreatic growth occurs by hyperplasia, and after 4 weeks by hyperplasia and hypertrophy (Corring et al., 1978). The pancreas also adapts readily to changes in diet with corresponding changes in digestive enzyme production (Corring, 1977). This adaptation requires 5 to 7 days in pigs. For example, pancreatic juice volume was doubled and the pancreatic activities of amylase, protease, and lipase increased fivefold in pigs fed soybean protein compared with milk protein from 3 to 7 weeks of age (Pekas et al., 1966). Evidence indicates that pancreatic enzyme production is more important in the digestion of soybean protein than milk protein (Pekas et al., 1964).

The pancreatic enzymes lipase, amylase, chymotrypsin, and trypsin are present at birth (Kitts et al., 1956; Hartman et al., 1961; Corring et al., 1978; Lindemann et al., 1986). Enzymatic development varies according to the enzyme considered. Pancreatic lipase activities are high at birth, drop transiently with the onset of suckling (J. Odle, unpublished observations) and weaning (Lindemann et al., 1986; Jensen et al., 1997), and then increase with age (Kitts et al., 1956; Aumaitre, 1972; Jensen et al., 1997). Weaning at 1 week of age caused a marked reduction in tributyrinase activity levels, which did not return to nonweaned pig levels until 6 or 7 weeks of age (Hartman et al., 1961). The specific pancreatic activities (per milligram of protein) for the proteolytic enzymes chymotrypsin and trypsin declined from birth to 2 or 3 weeks of age, respectively, before increasing to 6 or 8 weeks of age, respectively (Corring et al., 1978), in the 8-week experiment. Chymotrypsin and trypsin activities per gram of tissue and total activities dropped transiently with weaning at 4 weeks of age (Lindemann et al., 1986). Pigs weaned at 2 weeks of age had higher pancreatic protease activities at 10 weeks of age than pigs weaned at 4 weeks of age (Shields et al., 1980). Pancreatic amylase activity is very low at birth and increases rapidly with age (Kitts et al., 1956; Walker, 1959a; Hartman et al., 1961). Pigs fed diets containing wheat had higher pancreatic amylase activities than pigs fed diets containing lactose (Leibholz, 1982b).

B. Intestinal Enzymes

Of the disaccharidases, only mucosal lactase activities are high at birth (Walker, 1959a; Hartman et al., 1961; Dahlqvist, 1961a; Manners and Stevens, 1972) reaching a maximum at 1 week before declining at 6 or 8 weeks of age (Dahlqvist, 1961b; Aumaitre and Corring, 1978; Kidder and Manners, 1980; James et al., 1987; Shulman et al., 1988). Mucosal lactase activities from jejunum of neonatal pigs were about 20-fold greater than the activities from colon (Murray et al., 1991), with lactose removal from the colon without apparent cleavage by lactase. Replacing lactose with a mixture of maltodextrin and sucrose (MDS) in a diet fed to artificially reared pigs had no effect on carrier-mediated uptake of glucose, galactose, or fructose, although the pigs fed MDS scoured initially and grew more slowly (Vega et al., 1992). However, pigs fed diets containing about 52% lactose maintained higher intestinal mucosal activity levels of lactose than did pigs fed diets containing wheat (Leibholz, 1982b). Maltase activity, which is low in intestinal mucosa at birth (Bailey et al., 1956; Hartman et al., 1961; Dahlqvist, 1961a), increases gradually from birth to 6 or 8 weeks of age (Aumaitre and Corring, 1978; Shulman et al., 1988), and is higher in pigs fed diets containing wheat compared with lactose (Leibholz, 1982b). Maltose was readily digested by pigs 2 to 5 days of age (Cunningham and Brisson, 1957b). Sucrase activity was not found at birth by Dahlqvist (1961a), Hartman et al. (1961), or Aumaitre and Corring (1978), although activity was present by 1 week of age (Manners and Stevens, 1972; Shulman et al., 1988). Intestinal sucrase levels increase rapidly with age (Dahlqvist, 1961a), reaching appreciable levels by 2 weeks of age (Bailey et al., 1956; James et al., 1987). The activities of all the intestinal disaccharidases were low in the duodenum. Sucrase activity first appeared in the jejunum and ileum at 1 week and in the duodenum at 6 weeks (Aumaitre and Corring, 1978). There was considerable fluctuation in activity for all the mucosal enzymes along the intestinal tract (Stevens and Kidder, 1972). Weaning at 3 weeks of age results in a rapid drop in lactase activity, with sucrase activity declining temporarily before recovering (Hampton and Kidder, 1986).

Mucosal amylase activities are low at birth and increase with age (Kitts et al., 1956; Walker, 1959b; Hartman et al., 1961), although the increase in activity is not as dramatic as in pancreatic tissue (Leibholz, 1982b). Mucosal amylase activities were similar from proximate to distal end of the small intestine (Kidder and Manners, 1980; Shields et al., 1980; Leibholz, 1982b; Shulman et al., 1988).

Lactobacilli from the environment colonize the gastrointestinal tract of the baby pig on the day of birth, and gradually increase to ten times the initial number in 10 days (Pedersen and Tannock, 1989). Lactobacilli in the proximal digestive tract may be beneficial to the pig by producing lactic acid, because little gastric hydrochloric acid is produced early in the neonatal period (Ratcliffe, 1985). Strains of lactobacilli that degrade the mixed-linked β-D-glucans found in barley have also been found in the stomach of neonatal pigs (Johnson and Hemmingsson, 1991). The β-glucan degrading lactobacilli decreased significantly in number during nursing and increased again when the pigs started eating substantial amounts of dry feed containing barley.

VIII. PROTEIN SOURCES AND UTILIZATION

The utilization of soybean and milk proteins by neonatal pigs reared artificially has been reviewed (Veum et al., 1986). Soybean proteins were inferior to milk proteins for pig growth (Schneider and Sarett, 1969; Pond et al., 1971b; Newport, 1980; Wilson and Leibholz, 1981a; Leibholz, 1982a). Soy flour was less acceptable to pigs 10 days old than milk protein (Bayley and Holmes, 1972). The type of milk protein also influences neonatal pig performance, as dried skim milk was superior to skim milk hydrolyzate and sodium caseinate plus sweet dried whey (Pettigrew et al., 1977a,b).

About 50% of the dried skim milk protein could be replaced with soybean meal for pigs reared artificially starting at 1 or 2 days of age (Sherry et al., 1978a; Zamora and Veum, 1978; Zamora et al., 1979). These pigs were fed by machine every 90 min (16 times daily in slurry form), which may have improved performance of the pigs fed diets containing 50% soybean meal protein compared with the less favorable results of earlier investigators where the pigs were only fed three to five times daily. The level of soybean meal protein in the diet could be increased with increasing age, suggesting rapid adaptation of the digestive system (Sherry et al., 1978a; Zamora and Veum, 1979). About one half of the dried skim milk protein could be replaced by an isolated soy protein without impairing neonatal pig performance, although complete replacement with a soy isolate resulted in scours, reduced growth, and a high death loss (Newport, 1980). A soy concentrate decreased pig performance even more than the soy isolate (Newport and Keal, 1982).

Pigs fed diets containing soybean meal have a reduced villus height, higher serum anti-soy-IgG titers, and increased skin-fold thickness compared with pigs fed diets containing dried skim milk (Li et al., 1991b). When comparing soy protein sources, daily gain of young pigs fed a diet containing moist extruded soy protein concentrate was higher than the daily gains of pigs fed diets containing soybean meal, soy protein concentrate, or soy protein isolate (Li et al., 1991a). Ingestion of textured vegetable protein by neonatal pigs did not elicit an immune response compared with ingestion of milk proteins, as measured by total and specific serum IgG concentrations (Hankins et al., 1992). Hydrolyzed soy protein was better digested and absorbed than isolated soy protein, although the casein-whey protein was digested and absorbed more rapidly than the soy proteins (Zijlstra et al., 1996).

Soybean meal contains sucrose and the oligosaccharides stachyose and raffinose, which cause flatulence and digestive disturbances in baby pigs (Hartwig et al., 1997). Selection for higher seed protein content may reduce the concentration of these oligosaccharides in soybeans, increasing the quality of soybean protein for baby pigs.

Dried skim milk tended to produce greater pig performance than casein, whereas both milk proteins were clearly superior to isolated soy protein as evaluated by pig performance, nutrient digestibilities, and nitrogen retention (Mateo and Veum, 1980c; Leibholz, 1982a,b). Other studies have found casein to be superior to isolated soy protein (Maner et al., 1961; Pond et al., 1971b), with the protein quality of isolated soy protein plus methionine about 85% compared with that of milk proteins for baby pigs (Schneider and Sarett, 1969; Wilson and Leibholz, 1981a). Pond et al. (1971a) concluded that the inferior performance of pigs fed isolated soy protein compared with casein was not due to an insufficiency of the pancreatic enzymes chymotrypsin, trypsin, amylase, or lipase, but some other contributing factor(s). Casein also produces a faster postprandial decrease in gastric content pH and a slower rate of passage through the small intestine than isolated soy protein (Maner et al., 1962). The buffering action of isolated soy protein delays the activation of pepsinogen in the stomach, which reduces the efficiency of protein digestion. Additional studies have compared milk and soy proteins with regard to digesta retention times, pH, and nitrogen digestibilities over the entire tract, and amino acid digestibilities and nitrogen retention from the small intestine in pigs between 7 and 35 days of age (Leibholz, 1981; Wilson and Leibholz, 1981b,c,d,e).

Based on amino acid profile, chicken egg albumen should be an excellent source of protein for neonatal pigs (Cotterill et al., 1977). However, casein produced greater growth and N balance than spray-dried egg albumen (DA), DA supplemented with amino acids, or dry autoclaved DA, while wet autoclaved DA was similar to casein (Watkins and Veum, 1986). Injecting the pigs fed DA or autoclaved DA with 100 µg biotin/day did not improve performance. Uncooked egg albumen was found to be an unsatisfactory protein source for neonatal pigs (Pettigrew and Harmon, 1977), which is related to the avidin–biotin complex causing a biotin deficiency (Gyorgy and Ross, 1941; Cunha et al., 1946). Egg albumen also contains trypsin and chymotrypsin inhibitors (Kassell, 1970). Although avidin and the protease inhibitors are inactivated by heating (Green, 1970; Kassell, 1970), the protein and lysine availabilities are also easily reduced by heating (Kelly and Scott, 1968; Hurrell and Carpenter, 1976). Excessive heating of whole milk (88°C for 30 min) prior to spray-drying increased protein denaturation and reduced pig performance compared with heating to a lower temperature (66°C) and drying immediately (Braude et al., 1971).

Fish protein concentrate was equal to casein in supporting neonatal pig performance when diet consumption and growth of all the pigs was low (Pond et al., 1971b). However, with high dietary intakes, the performance of pigs fed diets containing dried skim milk protein or 50% dried skim milk protein and 50% fish protein concentrate (plus dried whey) were similar, whereas total replacement of the dried skim milk with fish protein concentrate plus dried whey greatly reduced pig performance (Newport, 1979). Further research indicated a linear decline in pig performance with each increase in a functional fish protein concentrate (plus dried whey) as a replacement for dried skim milk (Newport and Keal, 1983). Fish meal produced pig performance similar to that of isolated soy protein and soybean meal, whereas milk proteins were clearly superior (Leibholz, 1982a).

Replacement of 50% of the dried skim milk protein with a single-cell (bacterial) protein did not reduce pig performance, although higher dietary levels of the single-cell protein reduced performance (Newport and Keal, 1980).

IX. CARBOHYDRATE SOURCES AND UTILIZATION

The utilization of carbohydrates by neonatal pigs has been reviewed (Veum and Mateo, 1986). Artificially reared neonatal pigs utilized the monosaccharide glucose and the disaccharide lactose equally well starting at 1 day of age when the diets contained either isolated soy protein or casein as the protein source (Mateo and Veum, 1980a,c), which confirmed earlier research with these sugars (Becker et al., 1954; Aherne et al., 1969). There is a proximal-to-distal gradient of glucose absorption from the intestine of the nursing pig (Cherbuy et al., 1997). The rates of intestinal transport of glucose, galactose, and fructose are highest at birth with a sharp decline after the onset of nursing (Puchal and Buddington, 1992). The galactose moiety of lactose may be important in the regeneration of liver glycogen in the neonatal pig (Bird and Hartmann, 1994). Lactose increased the biological value of the protein sources in diets fed to rats compared with diets without lactose (Eggum, 1973; Forsum, 1975). The addition of lactose to an isolated soy protein diet improved the performance of pigs ≥21 days of age (Sewell and West, 1965).

Sucrose is utilized about as well as glucose by pigs starting about 1 week of age (Mateo and Veum, 1980b; Veum and Mateo, 1981). However, pigs do not utilize sucrose well at less than 1 week of age (Becker et al., 1954; Kidder et al., 1963a; Aherne et al., 1969) because newborn pigs do not produce adequate amounts of intestinal sucrase (Johnson, 1949). Pigs reared artificially and fed diets containing sucrose adapted physiologically by increasing intestinal production of sucrase compared with pigs nursing sows (Manners and Stevens, 1972).

Pigs fed diets containing cornstarch do not grow well as a result of a lower diet consumption even though starch digestibility was not reduced (Cunningham and Brisson, 1957a; Cunningham, 1959; Mateo and Veum, 1980b; Veum and Mateo, 1981). Diet consumption and growth was also low for neonatal pigs fed diets containing wheat starch compared with lactose, while apparent digestibilities were similar (Leibholz, 1982b). Pigs weaned at 2 weeks of age and fed a cereal-based diet adjusted physiologically as evidenced by a greater total amylase activity, primarily due to greater pancreatic activity, compared with pigs weaned at an older age (Shields et al., 1980). The baby pig is not able to utilize xylose (Wise et al., 1954) or fructose (Johnson, 1949; Becker et al., 1954; Aherne et al., 1969), with improvement in fructose utilization with age (Kidder et al., 1963b; Aherne et al., 1969; Steele et al., 1971).

X. FAT SOURCES AND UTILIZATION

Sow's milk contains 30 to 40% fat on a dry matter basis (deMann and Bowland, 1963), which emphasizes the importance of adequate levels of digestive lipase. The growth of pigs from 3 to 24 days of age was improved when corn oil or coconut oil was included in the diet (Veum et al., 1974). Pigs from 3 to 5 or 6 weeks of age can utilize fat calories from corn oil (Allee et al., 1971), corn oil and peanut oil (Cline et al., 1977), and fish oil (Chiang et al., 1989), as efficiently as carbohydrate calories. Dietary essential fatty acid supply affects pig phospholipid composition and ecosanoid synthesis (Huang and Craig-Schmidt, 1996). Positional distribution of fatty acids within the triglyceride molecule also may affect absorption and systemic distribution within the pig (Innis et al., 1997).

The metabolizable energy of colostrum is very efficiently utilized by the newborn pig (Le Dividich et al., 1994). However, bottle feeding newborn pigs removed from the sow with colostrum containing increasing concentrations of fat had little effect on the total volume of colostrum consumed in 24 h (Le Dividich et al., 1997), suggesting that the mechanisms controlling energy intake are not fully developed at birth. Nonetheless, it is suggested that formulation methods be used to maintain a constant nutrient:calorie ratio when incorporating fat into the diet of the young pig (Allee et al., 1971). Hoffman et al. (1993) found that neonatal pigs fed diets containing isolated soy protein and soy oil utilized fat calories as efficiently as carbohydrate calories. However, several reports suggested that young pigs (weaned at 2 to 3 weeks) did not utilize fat calories efficiently (Asplund et al., 1960; Eusebio et al., 1965; Frobish et al., 1969; 1970; 1971; Leibbrandt et al., 1975a,b), possibly because of inadequate intakes of other nutrients (e.g., lysine:calorie ratio). The protein:calorie ratio for neonatal pigs should be at least 67 g protein/Mcal of digestible energy when soybean meal and dried skim milk each provide 50% of the dietary protein (Sherry et al., 1978b). Daily gains and protein deposition rates of young pigs increased linearly with increasing lysine content up to about 0.23 g lysine/kcal gross energy, and remained constant thereafter when the diets contained milk proteins and lactose (Auldist et al., 1997).

Fatty acid chain length (molecular weight) had a greater effect on fat digestibility than degree of unsaturation, with short-chain fatty acids being more digestible than the longer-chain fatty acids (Lloyd and Crampton, 1957; Lloyd et al., 1957; Leibbrandt et al., 1975b). An inverse relationship between melting point (unsaturation) and digestibility (Bayley and Lewis, 1965; Hamilton and McDonald, 1969) also exists for fats fed to neonatal pigs (Sherry et al., 1978b). Pig digestibilities of corn oil and lard were considerably greater than those for tallow (Carlson and Bayley, 1968).

Medium-chain triglycerides represent a readily available energy source for the newborn pig (reviewed by Odle, 1998). The substitution of medium-chain triglycerides for soybean oil in the diet did not improve neonatal pig performance or nitrogen retention (Newport et al., 1979). In a comparison of dietary fat sources, pig performance and apparent fat digestibilities indicated that soybean oil was equal to butterfat for pigs from 2 to 28 days of age, whereas butterfat was slightly superior to coconut oil and far superior to tallow (Braude and Newport, 1973). From 2 to 7 days of age, however, butterfat was superior to all the fat sources. The digestion of oleic and linoleic acids was higher than that of palmitic and stearic acids (Braude et al., 1976).

In comparison with sows milk wherein lipids are packaged into well-emulsified lipid droplets, commercial milk replacers typically provide fat agglomerated with other ingredients to render a product easily dispersed in water. However, fat concentrations in commercial milk-replacers seldom exceed 20% because of limits in emulsification. Although the ontogeny of bile salt production in the pig has not been well studied, it is clear that poor emulsification of dietary fat can lead to reduced lipid digestibility (Wieland et al., 1993). In suckling calves, addition of emulsifying agents such as monoglycerides, diglycerides, and lecithin improved milk-replacer fat digestibility, and homogenization to produce particles to ≤3 to 4 µm also was beneficial (Raven, 1970).

Carnitine, a metabolite required for transporting long-chain fatty acids across the inner mitochondrial membrane for subsequent oxidation, may become limiting (Baltzell et al., 1987) if pigs are deprived of colostrum (Kempen and Odle, 1993) and reared on diets devoid of milk products. Sow milk provides ample carnitine for the suckling pig (Kerner et al., 1984). Supplementation of a diet containing isolated soy protein and soy oil with L-carnitine did not improve the utilization of metabolizable energy by neonatal pigs (Hoffman et al., 1993).

XI. FEEDING MANAGEMENT

A majority of the automated systems developed for artificial rearing have fed pigs individually in bowls or cups (Braude et al., 1969; Lecce, 1969; 1975; Sherry, 1978a), although McCallum et al. (1977b) developed an automated nipple feeding system to reduce wastage. The frequency of cleaning the feeding equipment could be reduced by adding formalin (a preservative) to the diet (Robertson et al., 1971; Menge and Frobish, 1976), especially when the diets were refrigerated prior to feeding.

The liquid feeding systems developed provided diet continuously (Pettigrew and Harmon, 1977; Pettigrew et al., 1977a,b; Zijlstra et al., 1996), twice daily (Braude et al., 1970a), four times daily (Pond et al., 1961), every 90 min (Veum and Bowman, 1973; Veum and Mateo, 1986; Veum et al., 1986), or hourly (Braude et al., 1970a; Braude and Newport, 1973). Pigs fed their daily ration in 24 portions (hourly) were less likely to develop diarrhea when challenged with enteropathogenic *Escherichia coli* and rotavirus than pigs consuming their daily ration in three meals (Lecce et al., 1983).

Braude et al. (1970a) found that pigs weaned at 2 days of age and fed either a cow's milk (12.5% total solids) diet or a reconstituted cow's milk diet (20% total solids) at high levels had faster growth rates than those of pigs nursing sows, which was accomplished by rearing the pigs in individual cages with sterilization of the feeding equipment twice daily and the cages twice weekly. Pigs weaned at 2 days of age and individually fed their diet in a liquid form consumed more dry matter and gained considerably more weight to 28 days than pigs kept in groups and fed the same diet in pelleted form from 7 to 28 days (Braude and Newport, 1977). The earlier that artificially reared neonatal pigs are changed from a liquid feeding regimen to a dry feeding regimen, the more severe the depression in growth rate (Lecce et al., 1979), indicating the importance of frequent or continuous feeding of liquid diets to pigs ≤30 days of age.

Pigs weaned at 1 to 3 days of age and given *ad libitum* access to a liquid diet with dried skim milk as the protein source gained in excess of 200 g/days (Pettigrew and Harmon, 1977; Pettigrew et al., 1977a). Good growth has also been obtained with diets fed in mash or dry meal form for the purposes of measuring growth (Menge and Frobish, 1976) and conducting mineral balance studies (Miller and Ullrey, 1987). In a majority of the experimental studies conducted with neonatal pigs, however, individual pig growth was lower than that generally obtained by pigs nursing sows. This is primarily due to nutrient limitations in the experimental diets and/or restricted diet intake based on the feeding regimen utilized, such as equalizing nutrient intake across treatments in balance and bioavailability experiments (Veum and Mateo, 1986; Veum et al., 1986; Watkins and Veum, 1986).

XII. THE EFFECT OF NUTRITION ON DIARRHEA

Enteric diseases and diarrhea are most prevalent during the neonatal suckling period (Lecce, 1986; USDA, 1997). Bacterial (e.g., *Colibacillosis, Treponema hyodysenteriae;* Moon and Kohler, 1994;

Harris et al., 1993), viral (e.g., rotavirus, transmissible gastroenteritis; Saif et al., 1987; Woods et al., 1996) and protozoal (*Cryptosporidia*) infections of the intestinal tract lead to secretory and/or malabsorptive diarrhea, which rapidly become life-threatening to the pig. Negative nutrient balance, including electrolyte depletion and dehydration rapidly drain the limited reserves of the pig. Furthermore, structural damage to the intestinal lining may reduce digestive capacity (contributing to nutrient malabsorption) and can lead to bacterial invasion, general septicemia, and death. Nutritional therapy involves all or partial discontinuation of milk replacer feeding and substitution of oral rehydration solutions containing iso-osmotic electrolytes and glucose (Rhoads et al., 1996). Glutamine (Mareskes et al., 1999) and bioactive peptides such as epidermal growth factor (Zijlstra et al., 1994) also have been examined as agents to accelerate recovery with no or marginal benefits at best. After the severity of the diarrhea passes, it is important to resume enteral nutrition; otherwise the recovery period may be prolonged (Zijlstra et al., 1997; 1999).

XIII. LIQUID DIETS FOR SEGREGATED EARLY-WEANED PIGS

The widespread application of medicated/segregated early weaning (SEW; Alexander et al., 1980) as a management strategy to limit disease transfer from sow to pig with concomitant enhancement of postweaning health status and growth performance has prompted renewed interest in liquid-based transition diets (see reviews by Azain, 1998, and Odle and Harrell, 1998). Because SEW pigs are typically 10 to 14 days of age, the husbandry challenge of rearing these animals is less formidable than of rearing pigs at 0 or 1 day of age (see Chapter 31). Although it is possible to rear these pigs without the use of liquid diets, recent studies reconfirm previous research (see Odle and Harrell, 1998) documenting the superior growth performance of liquid vs. dry-fed pigs at this age. Odle and co-workers have documented growth rates of milk-replacer-fed SEW pigs in excess of twofold greater than those of dry-fed controls (Zijlstra et al., 1996; Heo et al., 1999; Kim et al., 1999) due principally to increased feed intake. Although growth advantages have been reported when liquid diets were fed to 3-week-old pigs via complete (Geary et al., 1996; Russell et al., 1996) or split weaning (Pluske and Williams, 1996), enhancements are generally less impressive.

Improvements in growth have been associated with greater accretion of both protein and fat and have been linked to longer intestinal villi compared with both sow-nursed and dry-fed controls (Pluske et al., 1996a,b; Zijlstra et al., 1996). Furthermore, improvements in weight gains during early life can be maintained to market weight (Mahan et al., 1998; Kim et al., 1999). Thus, beyond the possible economic advantage of accelerated growth, if liquid feeding was selectively applied to the smallest 20 to 30% of SEW pigs, additional returns may be gleaned from decreased sort-loss caused by high variation in days to market weight.

XIV. SUBSEQUENT PERFORMANCE

Most of the negative effects of nutritional deprivation on growth and development during the neonatal period seem to be reversible in the pig. Carcass traits were unaffected by early dietary treatments, and decreases in total muscle RNA and DNA that resulted from suboptimal neonatal nutrition were completely reversed by 6 months of age (Martin et al., 1974).

Neonatal pigs fed diets containing $\leq 25\%$ of milk protein as a percentage of the dietary protein had severely decreased postneonatal growth from 23 to 51 or 65 days of age compared with pigs fed neonatal diets in which $\geq 45\%$ of the protein was milk protein (Sherry et al., 1978a). However, in nutrition studies with neonatal pigs where the diets contained $\geq 50\%$ milk protein (as a percentage of the dietary protein) postneonatal pig performance was similar for all the pigs fed the same diet from 3 to 11 weeks of age (Zamora and Veum, 1978; 1979; Zamora et al., 1979). Evaluation of various carbohydrate sources for neonatal pigs also indicated that the neonatal diet fed did not influence postneonatal pig performance from 3 to 9 weeks of age when all the pigs were fed the same diet (Mateo and Veum, 1980a,b,c; Veum and Mateo, 1981).

Pigs weaned at 2 days of age and reared artificially on a high-calorie liquid diet for 5 weeks, followed by dry feeding, reached slaughter weight earlier than control pigs weaned at 8 weeks of age (Horakova et al., 1971). Pigs reared artificially from 1.8 to 6.5 kg and fed a high-calorie liquid diet also reached 20 and 75 kg faster than pigs weaned at 6.5 kg (Campbell and Dunkin, 1983). These results indicate that artificial rearing does not have a detrimental effect on subsequent performance when the nutritional and environmental requirements are optimized during the neonatal rearing period.

XV. SUMMARY

The rearing of neonatal pigs artificially by removal from the sow at 1 or 2 days of age has been shown to be a very effective way of rearing pigs that would otherwise be lost as a result of starvation due to lactation failure or insufficient milk glands for nursing large litters. Diets should contain ≥50% milk protein as a percentage of the dietary protein. Neonatal pigs utilize fat, glucose, lactose, and corn syrup calories effectively. The nutrition and management procedures for successful artificial rearing of neonatal pigs are well described. The main limitation to the practical use of artificial rearing systems in swine production, however, is the reduction in sow fertility associated with such early weaning. The neonatal pig is an excellent model for human infant nutrition research because of the biological and physiological similarities of the two species.

REFERENCES

Aherne, F., V. W. Hayes, R. C. Ewan, and V. C. Speer. 1969. Absorption and utilization of sugars by baby pigs, *J. Anim. Sci.*, 29:444.

Alexander, T. I. L., K. Thornton, G. Boon, R. J. Lysons, and A. F. Gush. 1980. Medicated early weaning to obtain pigs free from pathogens endemic in the herd of origin, *Vet. Rec.*, 106:114.

Allee, G. L., D. H. Baker, and G. A. Leveille. 1971. Fat utilization and lipogenesis in the young pig, *J. Nutr.*, 101:1415.

Arthington, J., E. Weaver, F. Chi, and L. Russell. 1997. The use of concentrated spray-dried plasma protein in the preweaned/neonatal pig, *Am. Assoc. Swine Pract.*, 1:123.

Asplund, J. M., R. H. Grummer, and P. H. Phillips. 1960. Stabilized white grease and corn oil in the diet of baby pigs, *J. Anim. Sci.*, 19:709.

Asplund, J. M., R. H. Grummer, and P. H. Phillips. 1962. Absorption of colostral gamma-globulins and insulin by the newborn pig, *J. Anim. Sci.*, 21:412.

Auldist, D. E., F. L. Stevenson, M. G. Kerr, P. Eason, and R. H. King. 1997. Lysine requirements of pigs from 2 to 7 kg liveweight, *Anim. Sci. (Br. Soc.)*, 65:501.

Aumaitre, A. 1972. Development of enzyme activity in the digestive tract of the suckling pig: nutritional significance and implications for weaning, *World. Rev. Anim. Prod.*, 9(3):54.

Aumaitre, A., and T. Corring. 1978. Development of digestive enzymes in the piglet from birth to 8 weeks. 2. Intestine and intestinal disaccharidases, *Nutr. Metab.*, 22:244.

Azain, M. J. 1998. Young pig nutrition, use of liquid diets examined, *Feedstuffs*, 70(8):12.

Bailey, C. B., W. D. Kitts, and A. J. Wood. 1956. The development of the digestive enzyme system of the pig during its pre-weaning phase of growth. B. Intestinal lactase, sucrase and maltase, *Can. J. Agric. Sci.*, 36:51.

Baltzell, J. K., F. W. Bazer, S. G. Miguel, and P. R. Borum. 1987. The neonatal piglet as a model for human neonatal carnitine metabolism, *J. Nutr.*, 117:754.

Bayley, H. S., and J. H. G. Holmes. 1972. Protein sources for early weaned pigs, *J. Anim. Sci.*, 35:1101 (Abstr.).

Bayley, H. S., and D. Lewis. 1965. The use of fats in pigs feeding. II. The digestibility of various fats and fatty acids, *J. Agric. Sci.*, 64:373.

Becker, D. E., D. E. Ullrey, S. W. Terrill, and R. A. Notzold. 1954. Failure of the newborn pig to utilize dietary sucrose, *Science*, 120:345.

Bianca, W., and K. L. Blaxter. 1961. The influence of the environment on animal production and health under housing conditions. In *Proc. VIIth Int. Congr. Anim. Prod.*, Vol. 1, Hamburg, E. Ulmer, Stuttgart, 113.

Bird, P. H., and P. E. Hartmann. 1994. The response in the blood of piglets to oral doses of galactose and glucose and intravenous administration of galactose, *Br. J. Nutr.*, 4:553.

Book, S. A., and L. K. Bustad. 1974. The fetal and neonatal pig in biomedical research, *J. Anim. Sci.*, 38:997.

Bourne, F. J. 1973. Symposium on nutrition of the young farm animal. The immunoglobulin system of the suckling pig, *Proc. Nutr. Soc.*, 32:205.

Braude, R. and M. J. Newport. 1973. Artificial rearing of pigs. 4. The replacement of butterfat in a whole-milk diet by either beef tallow, coconut oil or soya-bean oil, *Br. J. Nutr.*, 29:447.

Braude, R., and M. J. Newport. 1977. A note on a comparison of two systems for rearing pigs weaned at 2 days of age, involving either a liquid or a pelleted diet, *Anim. Prod.*, 24:271.

Braude, R., K. G. Mitchell, and S. F. Suffolk. 1969. The Shinfield unit for artificial rearing of baby pig with automatic feeding, *J. Inst. Anim. Tech.*, 20:43.

Braude, R., K. G. Mitchell, M. J. Newport, and J. W. G. Porter. 1970a. Artificial rearing of pigs. 1. Effect of frequency and level of feeding on performance and digestion of milk proteins, *Br. J. Nutr.*, 24:501.

Braude, R., M. J. Newport, and J. W. G. Porter. 1970b. Artificial rearing of pigs. 2. The time course of milk protein digestion and proteolytic enzyme secretion in the 28-day-old pig, *Br. J. Nutr.*, 24:827.

Braude, R., M. J. Newport, and J. W. G. Porter. 1971. Artificial rearing of pigs. 3. The effect of heat treatment on the nutritive value of spray-dried whole-milk powder for the baby pig, *Br. J. Nutr.*, 25:113.

Braude, R., H. D. Keal, and M. J. Newport. 1976. Artificial rearing of pigs. 5. The effect of different portions of beef tallow or soya-bean oil and dried skim milk in the diet on growth, feed utilization, apparent digestibility and carcass composition, *Br. J. Nutr.*, 35:253.

Brown, H., V. C. Speer, L. Y. Quinn, V. W. Hays, and D. V. Catron. 1961. Studies on colostrum-acquired immunity and active antibody production in baby pigs, *J. Anim. Sci.*, 20:323.

Burrin, D. G. 1997. Is milk-borne insulin-like growth factor-I essential for neonatal development? *J. Nutr.*, 127:S975.

Burrin, D. G., T. J. Wester, T. A. Davis, S. Amick, and J. P. Heath. 1996. Orally administered IGF-I increases intestinal mucosal growth in formula-fed neonatal pigs, *Am. J. Physiol.*, 207:R1085.

Burrin, D. G., T. A. Davis, M. L. Fiorotto, and P. J. Reeds. 1997. Role of milk-borne vs. endogenous insulin-like growth factor I in neonatal growth, *J. Anim. Sci.*, 75:2739.

Campbell, R. G., and A. C. Dunkin. 1983. The influence of nutrition in early life on growth and development of the pig. 2. Effects of rearing method and feeding level on growth and development to 75 kg, *Anim. Prod.*, 36:425.

Caple, I. W. 1989. Neonatal viral diarrhoeas, *Aust. Vet. J.*, 66:407.

Carlson, W. E., and H. S. Bayley. 1968. Utilization of fat by baby pigs: fatty acid composition of ingesta in different regions of the digestive tract and apparent and corrected digestibilities of corn oil, lard and tallow, *Can. J. Anim. Sci.*, 48:315.

Cherbuy, C., B. Darcy-Vrillon, L. Posho, P. Vaugelade, M. T. Morel, F. Bernard, A. Leturque, L. Penicaud, and P. H. Duee. 1997. GLUT2 and hexokinase control proximodistal gradient of intestinal glucose metabolism in the newborn pig, *Am. J. Physiol.*, 272:G1530.

Chiang, S.-H., J. E. Pettigrew, S. D. Clarke, and S. G. Cornelius. 1989 Digestion and absorption of fish oil by neonatal piglets, *J. Nutr.*, 119:1741.

Cline, T. R., J. A. Coalson, J. G. Lecce, and E. E. Jones. 1977. Utilization of fat by baby pigs, *J. Anim. Sci.*, 44:72.

Coalson, J. A., and J. G. Lecce. 1973a. Influence of nursing intervals on changes in serum proteins (immunoglobulins) in neonatal pigs, *J. Anim. Sci.*, 36:381.

Coalson, J. A., and J. G. Lecce. 1973b. Herd differences in the expression of fatal diarrhea in artificially reared piglets weaned after 12 hours vs. 36 hours of nursing, *J. Anim. Sci.*, 36:1114.

Coalson, J. A., C. V. Maxwell, J. C. Hiller, E. C. Nelson, I. L. Anderson, and L. D. Corley. 1973. Techniques for rearing cesarean section derived colostrum free piglets, *J. Anim. Sci.*, 36:259.

Corring, T. 1977. Possible role of hydrolysis products of the dietary components in the mechanisms of the exocrine pancreatic adaptation to the diet, *World Rev. Nutr. Diet.*, 27:132.

Corring, T., A. Aumaitre, and G. Durane. 1978. Development of digestive enzymes in the piglet from birth to 8 weeks. I. Pancreas and pancreatic enzymes, *Nutr. Metab.*, 22:231.

Cotterill, O. J., J. Glauert, and G. W. Froning. 1977. Nutrient composition of commercially spray-dried egg products. *Poult. Sci.*, 57:439.

Cunha, T. J., D. C. Lindley, and M. E. Ensminger. 1946. Biotin deficiency syndrome in pigs fed desiccated egg white, *J. Anim. Sci.*, 5:219.

Cunnningham, H. M. 1959. Digestion of starch and some of its degradation products by newborn pigs, *J. Anim. Sci.*, 18:964.

Cunningham, H. M., and G. J. Brisson. 1957a. The effect of amylases on the digestibility of starch by baby pigs, *J. Anim. Sci.*, 16:370.

Cunningham, H. M., and G. J. Brisson. 1957b. The utilization of maltose by newborn pigs, *J. Anim. Sci.*, 16:574.

Curtis, S. E. 1970. Environmental–thermoregulatory interactions and neonatal piglet survival, *J. Anim. Sci.*, 31:576.

Curtis, S. E. 1974. Responses of the piglet to perinatal stressors, *J. Anim. Sci.*, 38:1031.

Curtis, S. E., C. J. Heidenreich, and R. B. Harrington. 1967. Age dependent changes of thermostability in neonatal pigs, *Am. J. Vet. Res.*, 28:1887.

Dahlqvist, A. 1961a. Intestinal carbohydrases of a new-born pig, *Nature*, 190:31.

Dahlqvist, A. 1961b. The location of carbohydrases in the digestive tract of the pig, *Biochem. J.*, 78:282.

deMann, J. M., and J. P. Bowland. 1963. Fatty acid composition of sow's colostrum, milk and body fat as determined by gas-liquid chromatography, *J. Dairy Res.*, 30:339.

Dewey, C. E., T. E. Wittum, H. S. Hurd, D. A. Dargatz, and G. W. Hill. 1995. Herd- and litter-level factors associated with the incidence of diarrhea morbidity and mortality in piglets 4–14 days of age, *Swine Health Prod.*, 3:105.

Drew, M. D., and B. D. Owen. 1988. The provision of passive immunity to colostrum-deprived piglets by bovine or porcine serum immunoglobulins, *Can. J. Anim. Sci.*, 68:1277.

Duee, P. H., J. P. Pegorier, J. Dividich, and J. Girard. 1988. Metabolic and hormonal response to acute cold exposure in newborn pig, *J. Dev. Physiol.*, 10:371.

Eggum, B. O. 1973. The influence of lactose on protein utilization. A study of certain factors influencing protein utilization in rats and pigs, Landhusholdningsselskabets Forlag, Copenhagen, 120.

Eusebio, J. A., V. W. Hays, V. C. Speer, and J. T. McCall. 1965. Utilization of fat by young pigs, *J. Anim. Sci.*, 24:1001.

Fahmy, M. H., and C. Bernard. 1971. Causes of mortality in Yorkshire pigs from birth to 20 weeks of age, *Can. J. Anim. Sci.*, 51:351.

Forsum, E. 1975. Effect of dietary lactose on nitrogen utilization of a whey protein concentrate and its corresponding amino acid mixture, *Nutr. Rep. Int.*, 11:419.

Frobish, L. T., V. W. Hays, V. C. Speer, and R. C. Ewan. 1969. Effect of diet form and emulsifying agents on fat utilization by young pigs, *J. Anim. Sci.*, 29:320.

Frobish, L. T., V. W. Hays, V. C. Speer, and R. C. Ewan. 1970. Effect of fat source and level on utilization of fat by young pigs, *J. Anim. Sci.*, 30:197.

Frobish, L. T., V. W. Hays, V. C. Speer, and R. C. Ewan. 1971. Effect of fat source on pancreatic lipase activity and specificity and performance on baby pigs, *J. Anim. Sci.*, 33:385.

Gardner, I. A., D. W. Hird, and C. E. Franti. 1989. Neonatal survival in swine: effects of low birth weight and clinical disease, *Am. J. Vet. Res.*, 50:792.

Gastonbury, J. R. W. 1976. A survey of preweaning mortality in the pig, *Austr. Vet. J.*, 52:272.

Gastonbury, J. R. W. 1977. Preweaning mortality in the pig. The prevalence of various causes of preweaning mortality and the importance of some contributory factors, *Austr. Vet. J.*, 53:315.

Geary, T. M., P. H. Brooks, D. T. Morgan, A. Campbell, and P. J. Russell. 1996. Performance of weaner pigs fed *ad libitum* with liquid feed at different dry matter concentrations, *J. Sci. Food Agric.*, 72:17.

Gomez, G. G. 1997. The colostrum-deprived, artificially-reared, neonatal pig as a model animal for studying rotavirus gastroenteritis, *Front. Biosci.*, 2:471.

Gomez, G. G., O. Phillips, and R. A. Goforth. 1998. Effect of immunoglobulin source on survival, growth and hematological and immunological variables in pigs, *J. Anim. Sci.*, 76:1.

Green, N. M. 1970. Purifications of avidin. In *Methods in Enzymology XVIIA*, McCormick, D. B. and L. D. Weight, Eds., Academic Press, New York, 414–417.

Gyorgy, P., and C. S. Ross. 1941. Egg white injury as a result of non absorption or inactivation of biotin, *Science*, 94:477.

Hamilton, R. M. G., and B. E. McDonald. 1969. Effect of dietary fat source on the apparent digestibility of fat and the composition of fecal lipids of the young pig, *J. Nutr.*, 97:33.

Hammerberg, C., G. G. Schurig, and D. L. Ochs. 1989. Immunodeficiency in young pigs, *Am. J. Vet. Res.*, 50:868.

Hampton, D. J., and D. E. Kidder. 1986. Influence of creep feeding and weaning on bush border enzyme activities in the piglet small intestine, *Res. Vet. Sci.*, 40:24.

Hankins, C. C., P. R. Noland, A. W. Burks, Jr., C. Connaughton, G. Cockrell, and C. L. Metz. 1992. Effect of soy protein on total and specific immunoglobulin G concentrations in neonatal porcine serum measured by enzyme-linked immunosorbent assay, *J. Anim. Sci.*, 70:3096.

Harris, D. L., R. D. Glock, L. Joens, and T. B. Stanton. 1993. Swine dysentery, In *Pork Industry Handbook*, PIH-56, North Carolina Cooperative Extension Service, 1–4.

Hartman, P. A., V. W. Hays, R. O. Baker, L. H. Neagle, and D. V. Catron. 1961. Digestive enzyme development in the young pig, *J. Anim. Sci.*, 20:114.

Hartwig, E. E., T. M. Kuo, and M. M. Kenty. 1997. Seed protein and its relationship to soluble sugars in soybean, *Crop Sci.*, 37:770.

Heo, K. N., J. Odle, W. Oliver, J. H. Kim, I. K. Han, and E. Jones. 1999. Effects of milk replacer and ambient temperature on growth performance of 14-day-old early-weaned pigs, *Asian-Aust, J. Anim. Sci.*, 12(12):980.

Hoffman, L. A., D. J. Ivers, M. R. Ellersieck, and T. L. Veum. 1993. The effect of L-carnitine and soybean oil on performance and nitrogen and energy utilization by neonatal and young pigs, *J. Anim. Sci.*, 71:132.

Horakova, U., A. Holub, and J. Zezula. 1971. Lasting effects of weaning at two to three days after birth in pigs, *Acta Vet. Brno*, 40(Suppl. 2):29.

Houle, V. M., E. A. Schroeder, J. Odle, and S. M. Donovan. 1997. Small intestinal disaccharidase activity and ileal villus height are increased in piglets consuming formula containing recombinant human insulin-like growth factor-I, *Pediatr. Res.*, 42:78.

Huang, M. C., and M. C. Craig-Schmidt. 1996. Arachidonate and decosahexaenoate added to infant formula influence fatty acid composition and subsequent eicosanoid production in neonatal pigs, *J. Nutr.*, 126:2199.

Hurrell, R. F., and J. K. Carpenter. 1976. Mechanisms of heat damage in proteins. 7. The significance of lysine-containing isopeptides and lanthionine in heated proteins, *Br. J. Nutr.*, 35:383.

Innis, S. M., R. A. Dyer, and E. L. Lien. 1997. Formula containing randomized fats with palmitic acid (16:0) in the 2-position increases 16:0 in the 2-position of plasma and chylomicron triglycerides in formula-fed piglets to levels approaching those of piglets fed sow's milk, *J. Nutr.*, 127:1362.

James, P. S., M. W. Smith, D. R. Tivey, and T. V. G. Wilson. 1987. Epidermal growth factors selectively increases maltase and sucrase activities in neonatal piglet intestine, *J. Physiol.*, 393:583.

Jensen, M. S., S. K. Jensen, and K. Jakobsen. 1997. Development of the digestive enzymes in pigs with emphasis on lipolytic activity in the stomach and pancreas, *J. Anim. Sci.*, 75:437.

Johnson, E., and S. Hemmingsson. 1991. Establishment in the piglet gut of lactobacilli capable of degrading mixed-linked beta-glucans, *J. Appl. Bacteriol.*, 70:512.

Johnson, M. W., G. R. Fitzgerald, M. W. Weler, and C. J. Welter. 1992. The six most common pathogens responsible for diarrhea in newborn pigs, *Vet. Med.*, 87:382.

Johnson, S. R. 1949. Comparison of sugars in the purified diets of baby pigs, *Fed. Proc.*, 8:387.

Jones, A. A. 1972. Problems of nutrition and management of early-weaned piglets, *Proc. Br. Soc. Anim. Prod.*, 1:19.

Kassell, B. 1970. Proteinase inhibitors from egg white. In *Methods in Enzymology XIX*, Perlmann, G. E., and L. Lorand, Eds., Academic Press, New York, 890–906.

Kelly, M., and H. M. Scott. 1968. Autoclaving time in relation to the nutritional quality of dried egg white, *Poult. Sci.*, 47:850.

Kennelly, J. J., R. O. Ball, and F. X. Aherne. 1979. Influence of porcine immunoglobulin administration on survival and growth of pigs weaned at two and three weeks of age, *Can. J. Anim.*, 59:693.

Kempen, T. A. T. G. van, and J. Odle. 1993. Medium-chain fatty acid oxidation in colostrum-deprived newborn piglets: stimulatory effect of L-carnitine supplementation, *J. Nutr.*, 123:1531.

Kerner, J., J. A. Froseth, E. R. Miller, and L. L. Bieber. 1984. A study of the acylcarnitine content of sows' colostrum, milk and serum and newborn piglet tissues: demonstration of high amounts of isovaleryl-carnitine in colostrum and milk, *J. Nutr.*, 114:854.

Kidder, D. E., and M. J. Manners. 1980. The level of distribution of carbohydrases in the small intestine mucosa of pigs from 3 weeks of age to maturity, *Br. J. Nutr.*, 43:141.

Kidder, D. E., M. J. Manners, and M. R. McCrea. 1963a. The digestion of sucrose by the piglet, *Res. Vet. Sci.*, 4:131.

Kidder, D. E., M. J. Manners, M. R. McCrea, and B. M. Q. Weaver. 1963b. Fructose utilization in the piglet, *Res. Vet. Sci.*, 4:145.

Kim, J. H., J. Odle, K. N. Heo, I. K. Han, and R. J. Harrell. 1999. Liquid diets accelerate growth of early-weaned pigs and effects are maintained until market weight, *J. Anim. Sci.*, 77(Suppl. 1):185.

Kitts, W. D., C. B. Bailey, and A. J. Wood. 1956. The development of the digestive enzyme system of the pig during its pre-weaning phase of growth. A. Pancreatic amylase and lipase, *Can. J. Agric. Sci.*, 36:45.

Lauxen, R. C., and T. L. Veum. 1982. Piglet survival and performance as influenced by exposure to sow manure, *Nutr. Rep. Int.*, 26:415.

Lecce, J. G. 1969. Rearing colostrum-free pigs in an automatic feeding device, *J. Anim. Sci.*, 28:27.

Lecce, J. G. 1971. Rearing neonatal piglets of low birth weight with an automatic feeding device, *J. Anim. Sci.*, 33:47.

Lecce, J. G. 1972. Health and vigor in neonatal pigs, *World Rev. Anim. Prod.*, 8:45.

Lecce, J. G. 1973. Effect of dietary regimen on cessation of uptake of macromolecules by piglet intestinal epithelium (closure) and transport to the blood, *J. Nutr.*, 103:751.

Lecce, J. G. 1975. Rearing piglets artificially in a farm environment: a promise unfullfilled, *J. Anim. Sci.*, 41:659.

Lecce, J. G. 1986. Diarrhea: the nemesis of the artificially reared early weaned piglet and a strategy for defense, *J. Anim. Sci.*, 63:1307.

Lecce, J. G., W. D. Armstrong, P. C. Crawford and G. A. Ducharme. 1979. Nutrition and management of early weaned piglets: liquid vs. dry feeding, *J. Anim. Sci.*, 48:1007.

Lecce, J. G., D. A. Clare, R. K. Balsbaugh, and D. N. Collier. 1983. Effect of dietary regimen on rotavirus-*Escherichia coli* weanling diarrhea of piglets, *J. Clin. Micro.*, 17:689.

Lecce, J. G., and D. O. Morgan. 1962. Effect of dietary regimen on cessation of intestinal absorption of large molecules (closure) in the neonatal pig and lamb, *J. Nutr.*, 78:263.

Le Dividich, J., P. Herpin, and R. M. Rosario-Ludovino. 1994. Utilization of colostral energy by the newborn pig, *J. Anim. Sci.*, 72:2082.

Le Dividich, J., P. Herpin, E. Paul, and F. Strullu. 1997. Effect of fat content of colostrum on voluntary colostrum intake and fat utilization in newborn pigs, *J. Anim. Sci.*, 75:707.

Leibbrandt, V. D., R. C. Ewan, V. C. Speer, and D. R. Zimmerman. 1975a. Effect of age and calorie:protein ratio on performance and body composition of baby pigs, *J. Anim. Sci.*, 40:1070.

Leibbrandt, V. D., V. W. Hays, R. C. Ewan, and V. C. Speer. 1975b. Effect of fat on performance of baby and growing pigs, *J. Anim. Sci.*, 40:1081.

Leibholz, J. 1981. Digestion in the pig between 7 and 35 d of age. 6. The digestion of hydrolyzed milk and soya-bean proteins, *Br. J. Nutr.*, 46:59.

Leibholz, J. 1982a. Utilization of casein, fish meal and soya bean proteins in dry diets for pigs between 7 and 28 days of age, *Anim. Prod.*, 34:9.

Leibholz, J. 1982b. Wheat starch in the diet of pigs between 7 and 28 days of age, *Anim. Prod.*, 35:199.

Leman, A. D., C. Knudson, H. E. Rodeffer, and A. G. Mueller. 1972. Reproductive performance of swine on 76 Illinois farms, *J. Am. Vet. Med. Assoc.*, 161:1248.

Lepine, A. J., M. Watford, R. D. Boyd, D. A. Ross, and D. M. Whitehead. 1993. Relationship between hepatic fatty acid oxidation and gluconeogenesis in the fasting neonatal pig, *Br. J. Nutr.*, 70:81.

Li, D. F., J. L. Nelssen, P. G. Reddy, F. Blecha, R. D. Klemm, D. W. Giesting, J. D. Hancock, G. L. Allee, and R. D. Goodband. 1991a. Measuring suitability of soybean products for early-weaned pigs with immunological criteria, *J. Anim. Sci.*, 69:3299.

Li, D. F., J. L. Nelssen, P. G. Reddy, F. Blecha, R. Klemm, and R. D. Goodband. 1991b. Interrelationship between hypersensitivity to soybean proteins and growth performance in early-weaned pigs, *J. Anim. Sci.*, 69:4062.

Lindemann, M. D., S. G. Cornelius, S. M. El Kandelgy, R. L. Moser, and J. E. Pettigrew. 1986. Effect of age, weaning and diet on digestive enzyme levels in the piglet, *J. Anim. Sci.*, 62:1298.

Lloyd, L. E., and E. W. Crampton. 1957. The relationship between certain characteristics of fats and oils and the apparent digestibility by young pigs, young guinea pigs and pups, *J. Anim. Sci.*, 16:377.

Lloyd, L. E., E. W. Crampton, and V. G. MacKay. 1957. The digestibility of ration nutrients by three- vs. seven-week old pigs, *J. Anim. Sci.*, 16:283.

Mahan, D. C., G. L. Cromwell, R. C. Ewan, C. R. Hamilton, and J. T. Yen. 1998. Evaluation of the feeding duration of a phase 1 nursery diet to three-week-old pigs to two weaning weights, *J. Anim. Sci.*, 76:578.

Maner, J. H., W. G. Pond, and J. K. Loosli. 1961. Utilization of soybean protein by baby pigs and by rats, *J. Anim. Sci.*, 20:614.

Maner, J. H., W. G. Pond, J. K. Loosli, and R. S. Lowrey. 1962. Effect of isolated soybean protein and casein on the gastric pH and rate of passage of food residues in the baby pigs, *J. Anim. Sci.*, 21:49.

Manners, M. J., and J. A. Stevens. 1972. Changes from birth to maturity in the pattern of distribution of lactase and sucrase activity in the mucosa of the small intestine in pigs, *Br. J. Nutr.*, 28:113.

Mareskes, C., G. Gomez, B. Black, J. Odle, O. Phillips and R. Goforth. 1997. Therapeutic effects of oral rehydration solution (ORS) and L-glutamine (GLN) on porcine rotaviral enteritis, *FASEB J.* 11:A401.

Martin, R. J., M. Ezekwe, J. H. Herbein, G. W. Sherritt, J. L. Gobble, and J. H. Ziegler. 1974. Effects of neonatal nutritional experiences on growth and development of the pig, *J. Anim. Sci.*, 39:521.

Mateo, J. P., and T. L. Veum. 1980a. Utilization of glucose vs lactose in an isolated soya bean protein diet by neonatal pigs reared artificially, *Anim. Prod.*, 30:407.

Mateo, J. P., and T. L. Veum. 1980b. Utilization of glucose, sucrose and corn starch with isolated soybean protein by 15-day-old pigs reared artificially, *Nutr. Rep. Int.*, 22:419.

Mateo, J. P., and T. L. Veum. 1980c. Utilization of casein or isolated soybean protein supplemented with amino acids and glucose or lactose by neonatal pigs reared artificially, *J. Anim. Sci.*, 50:869.

McCallum, I. M., J. I. Elliot, and B. D. Owen. 1977a. Survival of colostrum-deprived neonatal piglets fed gamma-globulins, *Can. J. Anim. Sci.*, 57:151.

McCallum, I. M., B. D. Owen, and M. J. Farmer. 1977b. An automated nipple feeding system for artificially rearing colostrum-deprived neonatal piglets, *Can. J. Anim. Sci.*, 57:489.

Menge, H., and L. T. Frobish. 1976. Nutritional studies with the early weaned neonatal pig, *J. Anim. Sci.*, 42:99.

Miller, E. R., and D. E. Ullrey. 1987. The pig as a model for human nutrition, *Annu. Rev. Nutr.*, 7:361.

Moody, N. W., and V. C. Speer. 1971. Factors affecting sow farrowing interval, *J. Anim. Sci.*, 23:510.

Moon, J. W., and E. M. Kohler. 1994. Colibacillosis. *Pork Industry Handbook*, PIH-30, North Carolina Cooperative Extension Service, 1–4.

Moughan, P. J., M. J. Birtles, P. D. Cranwell, W. C. Smith, and M. Pedraza. 1992. The piglet as a model animal for studying aspects of digestion and absorption in milk-fed human infants. In *Nutritional Triggers for Health and in Disease*, Simopoulos, A. P., Ed., Karger, Basel, 67:40–113.

Mount, L. E. 1963a. Responses to thermal environments in newborn pigs, *Fed. Proc.*, 22:818.

Mount, L. E. 1963b. Environmental temperature preferred by the young pig, *Nature*, 199:1212.

Murray, R. D., A. H. Ailabouni, P. A. Powers, H. J. McClung, B. U. K. Li, L. A. Heitlinger, and H. R. Sloan. 1991. Absorption of lactose from colon of newborn piglet, *Am. J. Physiol.*, 261:G1.

Newport, M. J. 1979. Artificial rearing of pigs. 9. Effect of replacement of dried skim milk by fish protein concentrate on performance and digestion of protein, *Br. J. Nutr.*, 41:103.

Newport, M. J. 1980. Artificial rearing of pigs. 11. Effect of replacement of dried skim milk by an isolated soya-bean protein on the performance of the pigs and digestion of protein, *Br. J. Nutr.*, 44:171.

Newport, M. J., and H. D. Keal. 1980. Artificial rearing of pigs. 10. Effect of replacing dried skim milk by a single-cell protein (Pruteen) on performance and digestion of protein, *Br. J. Nutr.*, 44:161.

Newport, M. J., and H. D. Keal. 1982. Artificial rearing of pigs. 12. Effect of replacement of dried skim milk by either a soy protein isolate or concentrate on the performance of the pigs and digestion of protein, *Br. J. Nutr.*, 48:89.

Newport, M. J., and H. D. Keal. 1983. Artificial rearing of pigs. 13. Effect of replacement of dried skim milk by a functional fish protein concentrate on the performance of the pigs and digestion of protein, *Br. J. Nutr.*, 49:43.

Newport, M. J., J. E. Story, and B. Tuckley. 1979. Artificial rearing of pigs. 7. Medium chain triglycerides as a dietary source of energy and their effect on live-weight gain, feed:gain ratio, carcass composition and blood lipids, *Br. J. Nutr.*, 41:85.

Nielsen, N. C., K. Christensen, N. Bille, and J. K. Larsen. 1974. Preweaning mortality in pigs. 1. Herd investigations, *Nord. Vet. Med.*, 26:137.

NRC. 1998. *Nutrient Requirements for Swines*, 10th ed, National Academy Press, Washington, D.C.

Odle, J. 1998. Medium-chain triglycerides: a unique energy source for neonatal pigs, *Pig News Info.*, 20:25.

Odle, J., and R. J. Harrell. 1998. Nutritional approaches for improving neonatal piglet performance: is there a place for liquid diets in commercial production? *Asian-Aust. J. Anim. Sci.*, 11:774.

Odle, J., T. R. Zijlstra, and S. M. Donovan. 1996. Intestinal effects of milkborne growth factors in neonates of agricultural importance, *J. Anim. Sci.*, 74:2509.

Pay, M. G. 1973. The effect of short lactations on the productivity of sows, *Vet. Rec.*, 92:255.

Pedersen, K., and G. W. Tannock. 1989. Colonization of the porcine gastrointestinal tract by lactobacilli, *Appl. Environ. Microbiol.*, 55:279.

Pekas, J. C., V. W. Hays, and A. Thompson. 1964. Exclusion of the exocrine pancreatic secretion: effect on digestibility of soybean and milk protein by baby pigs at various ages, *J. Nutr.*, 82:277.

Pettigrew, J. E., and B. G. Harmon. 1977. Milk proteins for artificially reared piglets. 1. Comparison to egg white protein and effect of added immunoglobulins, *J. Anim. Sci.*, 44:374.

Pettigrew, J. E., B. G. Harmon, S. E. Curtis, S. G. Cornelius, H. W. Norton, and A. H. Jensen. 1977a. Milk proteins for artificially reared piglets. III. Efficacy of sodium caseinate and sweet dried whey, *J. Anim. Sci.*, 45:261.

Pettigrew, J. E., B. G. Harmon, J. Simon, and D. J. Baker. 1977b. Milk proteins for artificially reared piglets. II. Comparison to a skim milk hydrolysate, *J. Anim. Sci.*, 44:383.

Pluske, J. R., and I. H. Williams. 1996. Split weaning increases the growth of light piglets during lactation, *Aust. J. Agric. Res.*, 47:515.

Pluske, J. R., I. H. Williams, and F. X. Aherne. 1996a. Maintenance of villous height and crypt depth in piglets by providing continuous nutrition after weaning, *Anim. Sci.*, 62:131.

Pluske, J. R., I. H. Williams, and F. X. Aherne. 1996b. Villous height and crypt depth in piglets in response to increases in the intake of cows' milk after weaning, *Anim. Sci.*, 62:145.

Pond, W. G., and K. A. Houpt. 1978. *The Biology of the Pig*, Cornell University Press, Ithaca, NY.

Pond, W. G., S. J. Roberts, J. A. Dunn, J. M. King, J. H. Maner, R. S. Lowrey, and P. Olafson. 1961. Eradication of atrophic rhinitis and virus pig pneumonia from a swine herd, *J. Anim. Sci.*, 20:88.

Pond, W. G., J. T. Snook, D. A. McNeill, W. Snyder, and B. R. Stillings. 1971a. Pancreatic enzyme activities of pigs up to three weeks of age, *J. Anim. Sci.*, 33:1270.

Pond, W. G., W. Snyder, E. F. Walker, Jr., B. R. Stillings, and V. Sidwell. 1971b. Comparative utilization of casein, fish protein concentrate and isolated soybean protein in liquid diets for growth of baby pigs, *J. Anim. Sci.*, 33:587.

Puchal, A. A., and R. K. Buddington. 1992. Postnatal development of monosaccharide transport in pig intestine, *Am. J. Physiol.*, 262:G895.

Ratcliffe, B. 1985. The influence of the gut microflora on the digestive process. In *Digestive Physiology in the Pig*, Just, A., H. Jorgensen, and J. A. Fernandez, Eds., National Institute of Animal Science, Copenhagen, Denmark, 245–267.

Raven, A. M. 1970. Fat in milk replacers for calves, *J. Sci. Food Agric.*, 21:352.

Reeds, P. J., and J. Odle. 1996. Pigs as models for nutrient functional interaction. In *Advances in Swine in Biomedical Research*, Tumbleson, M., and L. Schnook, Eds., Plenum Press, New York.

Rhoads, J. M., G. G. Gomez, W. Chen, R. Goforth, R. A. Argenzio, and M. J. Neylan. 1996. Can a super oral rehydration solution stimulate intestinal repair in acute viral enteritis? *J. Diarrhoeal Dis. Res.*, 14:175.

Robertson, V. A. W., A. S. Jones, M. F. Fuller, and F. W. H. Elsley. 1971. A pig herd established by hysterectomy. 1. The techniques for rearing hysterectomy-derived piglets to 5 weeks of age, *Res. Vet. Sci.*, 12:59.

Russell, P. J., T. M. Geary, P. H. Brooks, and A. Campbell. 1996. Performance, water use and effluent output of weaner pigs fed *ad libitum* with either dry pellets or liquid feed and the role of microbial activity in the liquid feed, *J. Sci. Food Agric.*, 72:8.

Saif, L. J., J. G. Lecce, and A. Torres. 1987. Rotaviral diarrhea in pigs. In *Pork Industry Handbook*, PIH-61, North Carolina Cooperative Extension Service, 1–4.

Schneider, D. L., and H. P. Sarett. 1969. Growth of baby pigs fed infant soybean formulas, *J. Nutr.*, 98:279.

Schwager, J., and J. Schulze. 1997. Maturation of the mitogen responsiveness, IL2 and IL6 production by neonatal swine leukocytes, *Vet. Immunol. Immunopathol.*, 57:105.

Scoot, A., B. D. Owens, and J. L. Agar. 1972. Influence of orally administered porcine immunoglobulins on survival and performance of newborn colostrum-deprived pigs, *J. Anim. Sci.*, 35:1201.

Sewell, R. F., and J. P. West. 1965. Some effects of lactose on protein utilization in the baby pig, *J. Anim. Sci.*, 24:239.

Sherry, M. P., M. K. Schmidt, and T. L. Veum. 1978a. Performance of neonatal piglets mechanically fed diets containing corn, soybean meal and milk protein, *J. Anim. Sci.*, 46:1250.

Sherry, M. P., M. K. Schmidt, and T. L. Veum. 1978b. Dietary protein to calorie ratios and fat sources for neonatal piglets reared artificially with subsequence performance. I. Performance, *J. Anim. Sci.*, 46:1259.

Shields, E. G., Jr., K. E. Ekstrom, and D. C. Mahan. 1980. Effect of weaning age and feeding methods on digestive enzyme development in swine from birth to ten weeks, *J. Anim. Sci.*, 50:257.

Shulman, R. J., S. J. Henning, and B. L. Nicols. 1988. The miniature pig as an animal model for the study of intestinal enzyme development, *Pediatr. Res.*, 23:311.

Simmens, F. A., K. R. Cera, and D. C. Mahan. 1990. Stimulation by colostrum or mature milk of gastrointestinal tissue development in newborn pigs, *J. Anim. Sci.*, 68:3596.

Speer, V. C., H. Brown, L. Quinn, and D. V. Catron. 1959. The cessation of antibody absorption in the young pig, *J. Immunol.*, 83:632.

Steele, N. C., L. T. Frobish, L. R. Miller, and E. P. Young. 1971. Certain aspects on the utilization of carbohydrates by the neonatal pig, *J. Anim. Sci.*, 33:983.

Stephens, D. B. 1971. The metabolic rates of newborn pigs in relation to floor insulation and ambient temperature, *Anim. Prod.*, 13:303.

Stevens, J. A., and D. E. Kidder. 1972. The distribution of trehalase, sucrase, amylase, glucoamylase and lactase (β-galactosidase) along the intestine of five pigs, *Br. J. Nutr.*, 28:129.

Svajgr, A. J., V. W. Hays, G. L. Cromwell, and R. H. Dutt. 1974. Effect of lactation duration on reproductive performance of sows, *J. Anim. Sci.*, 38:100.

Svendsen, J., and J. L. Larsen. 1977. Studies of the pathogenesis of enteric *E. coli* infections in weaned pigs, *Nord. Vet. Med.*, 29:533.

Svendsen, L. S., B. R. Westrom, J. Svendsen, A.-C. Olsson, and B. W. Karlsson. 1990. Intestinal acromolecular transmission in underprivileged and unaffected newborn pigs: implication for survival of underprivileged pigs, *Res. Vet. Sci.*, 48:184.

Tumbleson, M. E., Ed. 1986. *Swine in Biomedical Research*, Vols. 1, 2, and 3, Plenum Press, New York.

USDA. 1997. National Animal Health Monitoring System, Amimal and Plant Health Inspection Service, Veterinary Services. Part III: Changes in the U.S. Pork Industry 1990–1995.

Van der Hyde, H. 1972. A practical assessment of early weaning, *Proc. Br. Soc, Anim. Prod.*, 1:33–36.

Vega, Y. M., A. A. Puchal, and R. Buddington. 1992. Intestinal amino acid and monosaccharide transport in suckling pigs fed milk replacers with different sources of carbohydrate, *J. Nutr.*, 122:2430.

Veum, T. L., and G. L. Bowman. 1973. *Saccharomyces cervisiae* yeast culture in diets for mechanically-fed neonatal piglets and early rowing self-fed pigs, *J. Anim. Sci.*, 37:67.

Veum, T. L., and J. P. Mateo. 1981. Utilization of glucose, sucrose or cornstarch with casein or isolated soybean protein supplemented with amino acids by 8-day-old pigs reared artificially, *J. Anim. Sci.*, 53:1027.

Veum, T. L., and J. P. Mateo. 1986. A review of utilization of lactose, glucose, sucrose and cornstarch by neonatal piglets reared artificially. In *Swine in Biomedical Research*, Vol. 2, Tumbleson, M. E., Ed., Plenum Press, New York, 735–743.

Veum, T. L., M. K. Schmidt, D. Wilson, and D. P. Hutcheson. 1974. Energy sources for neonatal piglets, *J. Anim. Sci.*, 39:984 (Abstr.).

Veum, T. L., R. G. Zamora, and M. P. Sherry. 1986. Utilization of soybean and milk proteins by neonatal pigs reared artificially. In *Swine in Biomedical Research*, Vol. 2, Tumbleson, M. E., Ed., Plenum Press, New York, 1113–1124.

Walker, D. M. 1959a. The development of the digestive system of the young animal. II. Carbohydrase enzyme development in the young pig, *J. Agric. Sci.* (Cambridge), 52:357.

Walker, D. M. 1959b. The development of the digestive system of the young animal. I. Tissue weights, dry matter of tissues, total acidity and chloride content of stomach contents in the young pig, *J. Agric. Sci.*, 52:352.

Walker, N., and S. M. Eddie. 1974. The effect of sow productivity on estrus suppression following a two-day lactation, *Anim. Prod.*, 18:153.

Watkins, K. L., and T. L. Veum. 1986. Utilization of spray-dried egg albumen vs. casein by neonatal pigs reared artificially. In *Swine in Biomedical Research*, Vol. 2, Tumbleson, M. E., Ed., Plenum Press, New York, 1125–1135.

Widdowson, E. M., V. E. Colombo, and C. A. Artavanis. 1976. Changes in the organs of pigs in response to feeding for the first 24 h after birth. II. The digestive tract, *Biol. Neonate*, 28:272.

Wieland, T. M., X. Lin, and J. Odle. 1993. Emulsification and fatty acid chain length affect the utilization of medium-chain triglycerides by neonatal piglets, *J. Anim. Sci.*, 71:1869.

Wilson, M. R. 1974. Immunologic development of the neonatal pig, *J. Anim. Sci.*, 38:1018.

Wilson, R. H., and J. Leibholz. 1981a. Digestion in the pig between 7 and 35 days of age. 1. The performance of pigs given milk and soya bean proteins, *Br. J. Nutr.*, 45:301.

Wilson, R. H., and J. Leibholz. 1981b. Digestion in the pig between 7 and 35 days of age. 2. The digestion of dry matter and the pH of digesta in pigs given milk and soya-bean proteins, *Br. J. Nutr.*, 45:321.

Wilson, R. H., and J. Leibholz. 1981c. Digestion in the pig between 7 and 35 days of age. 3. The digestion of nitrogen in pigs given milk and soya-bean proteins, *Br. J. Nutr.*, 45:337.

Wilson, R. H., and J. Leibholz. 1981d. Digestion in the pig between 7 and 35 days of age. 4. The digestion of amino acids in pigs given milk and soya-bean proteins, *Br. J. Nutr.*, 45:347.

Wilson, R. H., and J. Leibholz. 1981e. Digestion in the pig between 7 and 35 days of age. 5. The incorporation of amino acids absorbed in the small intestines into empty-body gain of pigs given milk or soya-bean proteins, *Br. J. Nutr.*, 45:359.

Wise, M. B., E. R. Barrick, G. H. Wise, and J. C. Osborne. 1954. Effects of substituting xylose for glucose in a purified diet for pigs, *J. Anim. Sci.*, 13:365.

Woods, R. D., L. J. Saif, E. O. Haelterman, and E. H. Bohl. 1996. Transmissible gastroenteritis (TGE). In *Pork Industry Handbook*, PIH-47, North Carolina State Extension Service, 1–5.

Xu, R. J., and P. D. Cranwell. 1991. Gastrin in fetal and neonatal pigs, *Comp. Biochem. Physiol.*, 98B:615.

Xu, R. J., and P. D. Cranwell. 1992. Gastrin metabolism in neonatal pigs and grower pigs, *Comp. Biochem. Physiol.*, 101A:177.

Yabiki, T., M. Kashiwazaki, and S. Namioka. 1974. Quantitative analysis of three classes of immunoglobulins in serum of newborn pigs and milk of sows, *Am. J. Vet. Res.*, 35:1483.

Zamora, R. G., and T. L. Veum. 1978. Various levels of soybean meal as replacement for dried skim milk for artificially reared neonatal pigs, *Nutr. Rep. Int.*, 18:495.

Zamora, R. G., and T. L. Veum. 1979. The effects of increasing the levels of soybean protein in the diets for artificially reared neonatal pigs, *Nutr. Rep. Int.*, 19:49.

Zamora, R. G., M. K. Schmidt, and T. L. Veum. 1979. Equal levels of soybean and milk proteins in diets for artificially reared neonatal pigs, *Philipp. Agric.*, 62:191.

Zhang, H., C. Malo, and R. K. Buddington. 1997. Suckling induces rapid intestinal growth and changes in brush border digestive functions of newborn pigs, *J. Nutr.*, 127:418.

Zhang, H., C. Mao, C. R. Boyle, and R. K. Buddington. 1998. Diet influences development of the pig (Sus scrofa) intestine during the first 6 hours after birth, *J. Nutr.*, 128:1302.

Zijlstra, R. T., J. Odle, W. F. Hall, B. W. Petschow, H. B. Gelberg, and R. E. Litove. 1994. Effect of orally administered epidermal growth factor on intestinal recovery of neonatal pigs infected with rotavirus, *J. Pediatr. Gastroenterol. Nutr.*, 19:382.

Zijlstra, R. T., A. M. Mies, B. A. McCracken, J. Odle, H. R. Gaskins, E. L. Lien, and S. M. Donovan. 1996a. Short-term metabolic responses do not differ between neonatal piglets fed formulas containing hydrolyzed or intact soy proteins, *J. Nutr.*, 126:913.

Zijlstra, R. T., K.-Y. Whang, R. A. Easter, and J. Odle. 1996b. Effect of feeding a milk replacer to early-weaned pigs on growth, body composition and small intestinal morphology, compared with suckled littermates, *J. Anim. Sci.*, 74:2948.

Zijlstra, R. T., S. M. Donovan, J. Odle, H. B. Gelberg, B. W. Petschow, and H. R. Gaskins. 1997. Protein-energy malnutrition delays small-intestinal recovery in neonatal pigs infected with rotavirus, *J. Nutr.*, 127:1118.

Zijlstra, R. T., B. A. McCracken, J. Odle, S. M. Donovan, H. B. Gelberg, B. W. Petschow, F. A. Zuckerman, and H. R. Gaskins. 1999. Malnutrition modifies pig small intestinal inflammatory responses to rotavirus, *J. Nutr.*, 129:838.

31 Feeding the Weaned Pig

Charles V. Maxwell, Jr. and Scott D. Carter

CONTENTS

I. Introduction 692
II. Digestive Capacity 692
III. Nutrient Requirements 693
    A. Energy 693
    B. Amino Acids 693
    C. Minerals 694
    D. Vitamins 694
    E. Water 694
IV. Factors Affecting Nutrient Requirements 695
    A. Weaning Age 695
    B. Effect of Antigen Exposure on Performance and Nutrient
        Requirements of Pigs 695
    C. Sex and Genotype Effects on Nutrient Requirements 696
V. Diet Composition 696
    A. Energy Sources 696
        1. Lactose 696
        2. Other Carbohydrate Sources 697
        3. Fats and Oils 698
    B. Protein Sources 698
        1. Plasma Protein 698
        2. Other Animal Sources 699
        3. Plant Sources 700
    C. Minerals 701
    D. Vitamins 702
    E. Feed Additives 702
        1. Antibiotics 702
        2. Copper 702
        3. Zinc 703
        4. Microbial Supplements 703
        5. Enzymes 703
        6. Organic Acids 703
VI. Feeding the Weaned Pig 704
    A. Performance Estimates 704
    B. Recommended Ingredients and Feeding Practices
        for a Phased-Feeding Program 704
    C. Diet Forms 706
VII. Summary 706
References 706

I. INTRODUCTION

The swine industry continues to move to earlier weaning with pigs in conventional intensive swine production systems routinely weaned as early as 17 days of age, and those produced in off-site segregated early-weaning systems are weaned as early as 12 to 14 days of age. This trend is driven by economic factors, such as improving the number of pigs per sow per year and the need to minimize the capital cost of swine farrowing facilities by moving more sows through the facilities. Furthermore, recent studies have shown that early weaning and removal of pigs to a second isolated site for rearing can reduce the potential for disease transfer from the dam. An additional benefit to off-site production is that the lower immune system activation permits increased partitioning of nutrients to growth, allowing pigs to grow much faster and more efficiently. Tremendous strides have been made in improving performance in early-weaned pigs in the last decade. These advances are the result of rapid development and implementation of advanced technologies in the areas of nursery facilities, improved feeding programs, increased weaning weight, and the development of innovative management systems. Research in systems with these improved technologies has produced a better understanding of requirements for optimum performance of early-weaned pigs.

II. DIGESTIVE CAPACITY

The digestive system in the young pig before weaning and in the newly weaned pig is adapted to secreting the digestive enzymes necessary for the digestion of milk but not other feedstuffs, particularly plant sources. Therefore, lactase activity is high and the activity of lipases and proteases is sufficient to digest the fat and protein in milk. Immediately after weaning, the digestive system of the pig has to adapt to a new feeding regime with respect to enzyme secretion. At weaning, enzyme activity is as much as ninefold lower than at 4 weeks postweaning, and weaning is accompanied by as much as a twofold reduction in subsequent enzyme activity (Jensen et al., 1997; Table 31.1). These data are consistent with the observations of Lindemann et al. (1986) and Makkink et al. (1994) who observed a decrease in pancreatic enzyme activity in the weaned pig compared with the suckling pig. Cranwell and Moughan (1989) concluded that gastrointestinal system development of the young pig is far from complete, even by 4 weeks of age, and that it has to undergo a period of adaptation to develop the capacity to cope satisfactorily with the postweaning diet. Postweaning performance can be enhanced in the early-weaned pig by ensuring that dietary ingredients provided at weaning are compatible with the established pattern of enzyme secretion, and ease of digestion must be considered when choosing nursery diet ingredients.

TABLE 31.1
The Effect of Age of Pig and Weaning on Enzyme Activity (µmol substrate hydrolyzed/min)[a]

Age (days)	Trypsin	Chymotrypsin	Amylase
3	14.6	0.94	2,076
7	22.0	3.52	14,666
14	33.8	4.91	21,916
21	32.1	6.99	26,165
28	55.6	9.49	65,051
35	42.1	3.90	24,730
56	515.0	14.30	182,106

[a] Pigs were weaned at 28 days of age.

Source: Adapted from Jensen et al. (1997).

III. NUTRIENT REQUIREMENTS

A. ENERGY

The NRC (1998) publication on nutrient requirements of swine indicates that diets fed to pigs weighing 3 to 20 kg should contain 3265 kcal metabolizable energy (ME)/kg. Estimated daily ME requirements for the 4-, 7.5-, and 15-kg pig are 820, 1620, and 3265 kcal/day, respectively. These estimates were made by a modification of the NRC (1986) equation for pigs weighing less than 20 kg body weight, and they are based upon limited data. McNutt and Ewan (1984) estimates that the ME requirement for maintenance for the 4-week-old weaned pig was (115 kcal/day)/(kg$^{0.75}$).

Maintaining feed intake in the young pig during the early postweaning period is challenging. High-health, newly weaned pigs do not consume enough energy to meet their needs for rapid protein deposition, particularly during the first few days after weaning. A young pig that just maintains body weight may be losing as much as 50 g fat/day to satisfy its energy requirement, matched by a gain of a similar weight of water (Whittemore, 1984). Thus, as a practical matter, a young-weaned pig will grow well only when fed a high-nutrient-dense complex diet composed of ingredients that are highly digestible and appropriate for the pig's stage of physiological development. Unfortunately, dietary fat addition is not very beneficial, because pigs at this stage of development do not utilize fat very well (see Section V.A.E on fats and oils). Therefore, suitable energy for optimum performance in the newly weaned pig can only be supplied by providing part of the energy as readily available carbohydrates, including lactose, glucose, or sucrose (for additional information concerning energy sources, see Chapters 5, 6, and 7, and the section in this chapter on energy sources).

B. AMINO ACIDS

Lysine has long been considered the limiting amino acid in swine diets (Southern, 1991; Kerr, 1993). Most research has indicated that pigs, particularly those reared under high-health conditions, will respond with higher growth rate and improved feed efficiency at higher lysine levels than those recommended by NRC (1998). Owen et al. (1995d) reported that segregated early-weaned (SEW) pigs required between 1.65 and 1.80% lysine (Figure 31.1). This response is consistent with the requirement of at least 1.75% lysine in SEW pigs (Chung et al., 1996). Pigs in SEW systems seem to have higher lean tissue gain and, as expected, have a higher lysine requirement than convention-

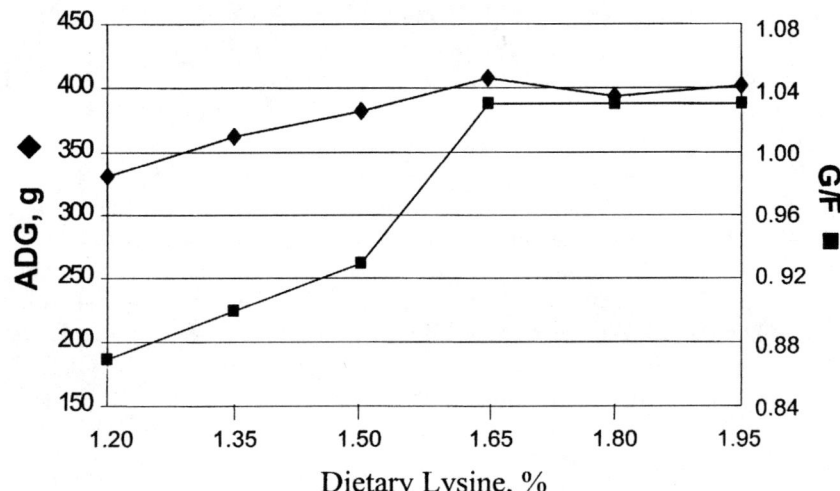

FIGURE 31.1 Lysine requirements of segregated early-weaned (SEW) pigs (0 to 14 days).

ally weaned pigs (Williams et al., 1997). Davis et al. (1996), however, reported that the lysine requirement for conventionally weaned pigs was greater than 1.60% lysine using whey protein concentrate as a lysine source. Nam and Aherne (1994) and Auldist et al. (1997) reported that weanling pigs require 0.95 g lysine/MJ digestive energy (DE) and 1.07 g lysine/MJ GE, respectively.

There is some evidence that the ratio of other amino acids to lysine may be different in the young pig than the ratio for growing-finishing pigs. Owen et al. (1995c) reported that a diet with 1.60% lysine containing spray-dried blood products should contain 0.41 to 0.42% methionine. Subsequently, Owen et al. (1995a) reported that methionine should be 27.5% of dietary lysine during the first 21 days postweaning. Bergstrom et al. (1997a) reported that the digestible isoleucine requirement was not greater than 60% of the lysine requirement immediately after weaning, and then it drops to 50% of lysine in 10-kg pigs (Bergstrom et al., 1997b). Bergstrom et al. (1996a) reported that the digestible threonine requirement was no more than 45% of lysine for the first 2 weeks after weaning in pigs weaned at 10 days of age. The optimum digestible threonine requirement was 55% of lysine for pigs from 11.4 to 22.7 kg (Bergstrom et al., 1996b). Han et al. (1993) reported that the tryptophan requirement was 0.16% lysine for pigs weighing 10 to 20 kg. Based on these data, the ratio of isoleucine, methionine, and threonine to lysine for the SEW pig is 60, 27.5, and 45, respectively, whereas the ratio in the 10- to 20-kg pig is 50, 27.5, and 55, respectively. In the growing-finishing pig, the recommended ratio of isoleucine, methionine, and threonine to lysine for protein accretion is 54, 27, and 60, respectively (NRC, 1998).

C. MINERALS

The NRC (1998) lists requirements for 12 minerals. Practical weanling pig diets should be supplemented with calcium, phosphorus, sodium, chloride, copper, iodine, iron, manganese, selenium, and zinc because typical diets fed to young pigs are deficient in these minerals. Typically, salt levels are reduced in nursery diets containing milk products because these products are relatively high in sodium. Mahan et al. (1996a,b), however, reported that weanling pigs fed diets high in whey and plasma (which are both high in sodium) respond to added sodium as sodium chloride or sodium phosphate and to added chloride as hydrochloric acid. These results suggest that the sodium and chloride requirement for the early-weaned pig is higher than previously thought. For additional information concerning mineral requirements, see Chapters 10, 11, 12, 14, and 16.

D. VITAMINS

The NRC (1998) lists requirements for 13 vitamins. Those that should be routinely added to weanling pig diets include the fat-soluble vitamins A, D, E, and K, as well as the B vitamins, riboflavin, niacin, pantothenic acid, and B_{12}. Choline, biotin, folic acid, thiamin, and vitamin C are added to many nursery diets, although their requirement is not well documented. Recent studies suggest that greater concentrations of specific vitamins may improve performance in young pigs. Stahly et al. (1995a) suggested that young pigs with a high capacity for lean tissue growth required greater than 470% of NRC (1988) requirements for the B vitamins to maximize growth performance. Similarly, this same laboratory (Stahly and Cook, 1996) reported that pigs with a high or moderate antigen exposure require greater concentrations of B vitamins than NRC (1988) estimates. Woodworth et al. (1998) and Matte et al. (1998) reported that the requirement for pyridoxine in weanling pigs was greater than current estimates (NRC, 1998). These data suggest that under certain conditions, the B vitamin requirements for weanling pigs may be greater than NRC (1998) estimates. For additional information concerning vitamin requirements, see Chapters 13 through 16.

E. WATER

Although the requirement for water has not been well documented, the importance of water intake cannot be overstated in the weaned pig. Availability of good-quality water affects the amount of water consumed, and this in turn affects voluntary feed intake and subsequent performance (Barber et al., 1989). These researchers also noted that the young pig will not always increase drinking time to compensate for restricted water delivery rates, even though the total time spent drinking was less than 4 min/day under the most restricted regime. Restricted water flow reduced feed intake by approximately 15% in pigs from 3 to 6 weeks of age, and it had a similar effect on weight gain (Toplis and Tibble, 1994). These researchers recommend a minimum water flow rate of 570 ml/min in water nipples in the nursery. For additional information concerning water requirements see Chapter 17.

IV. FACTORS AFFECTING NUTRIENT REQUIREMENTS

A. Weaning Age

Weaning as early as 3 weeks of age has been accomplished for a number of years by the use of diets containing high levels of milk products (e.g., dried skim milk, dried whey, cheese by-product), fish meal, and refined soybean protein as the primary protein sources. The earlier pigs are weaned, the greater the need for a complex diet to minimize poor postweaning performance. This response was demonstrated some time ago by Okai et al. (1976). In their study, diets varying in complexity were fed to pigs weaned at 3 or 5 weeks of age. A more complex diet was required to maximize postweaning performance in pigs weaned at 3 weeks of age than in those weaned at 5 weeks of age. More recently, weaning as early as 2 weeks of age has become routine in large production complexes with three site production systems. Dritz et al. (1996) observed that increasing diet complexity increased gain more in pigs weaned at 9 days of age than in those weaned at 19 days of age. More complex diets containing higher levels of plasma protein and very little unprocessed carbohydrate are required for consistent excellent performance in this young pig.

B. Effect of Antigen Exposure on Performance and Nutrient Requirements of Pigs

Early weaning at less than 21 days of age and removal of pigs to a second isolated site, which is commonly referred to as SEW, has been shown to reduce disease transfer from the dam substantially (Fangman et al., 1997). Pigs reared in isolation after weaning have been shown to have reduced immunological stress (Johnson, 1997), resulting in a substantial improvement in growth and efficiency of feed utilization compared with those reared in conventional farrow-to-finish systems (Williams et al., 1997). The approximately 21.3% improvement in gain in SEW pigs (across all lysine levels) compared with those reared in conventional systems is thought to be in response to reduced pathogens. However, Patience et al. (1997) evaluated the impact of site of weaning on pig performance in pigs derived from a breeding herd free of infectious respiratory disease, internal and external parasites, and most infectious gastrointestinal diseases, and they still observed an 18.8% improvement in pig weight at 56 days of age in pigs reared in off-site facilities. These studies suggest that differences in performance may be due to changes in both pathogenic and nonpathogenic immune challenges.

Activation of the immune system has a major impact on pig performance during the nursery phase, which is not surprising. Exposure of animals to antigens has been shown to result in the release of cytokines that activate the immune system (Dinarello, 1984; Spurlock, 1997). Proinflammatory cytokines produce a major alteration in the metabolic processes (Klasing, 1988; Spurlock, 1997), resulting in decreased protein synthesis (Jepson et al., 1986) and an increased protein degradation in skeletal muscle (Zamir et al., 1994). Therefore, pigs exposed to antigens, which activate the immune system, would be expected to exhibit reduced feed intake and weight gain. A second important feature of the inflammatory response is an increased synthesis of acute-phase proteins in the liver. Synthesis of some acute-phase proteins may increase several 100-fold. These acute-phase proteins are synthesized at the expense of degradation of skeletal muscle protein because nutrients are directed away from tissue growth in support of immune function. Thus, immunological stress is linked by proinflammatory cytokines to enhanced hepatic acute-phase protein synthesis, and decreased muscle protein synthesis and/or increased muscle protein degradation.

An additional impact that immune system activation has on pig performance is to alter nutrient requirements. Reeds et al. (1994) estimated that to provide sufficient amounts of phenylalanine, the limiting amino acid for acute-phase protein synthesis, it would require more than a twofold increase in degradation of muscle protein. This changes nutrient requirements, such as amino acid requirements, from a system driven by rate of lean tissue synthesis, to a system driven by the demands of the immune system. This effect is illustrated by Williams et al. (1997) who observed a greater growth response to increasing dietary lysine in SEW pigs than in conventionally reared pigs, with a 31.5% improvement in gain at the highest lysine intake. This response is also consistent with the greater rate of protein accretion observed in SEW pigs than in conventional pigs.

C. Sex and Genotype Effects on Nutrient Requirements

For the most part, sex and genotype effects on nutrient requirements of the weanling pig have been ignored. However, it seems that sex and genotype can impact the nutrient requirements of weanling pigs. Hansen et al. (1995) reported greater growth rates for gilts than barrows during the nursery phase. In a summary of 58 weanling pig experiments involving 3621 barrows and 3525 gilts, Cromwell et al. (1996) reported that gilts gained 4.7% faster than barrows and were heavier at the end of the experiments. However, the NRC (1998) does not list separate requirements for gilts and barrows at this young age.

With the increase in lean growth potential of growing-finishing pigs in recent years, there has come a need to examine the effect of lean growth potential on nutrient requirements of weanlings pigs. An increased lean growth potential of weanling pigs has been reported to increase the lysine (Stahly et al., 1994a), available phosphorus (Frederick and Stahly, 2000), and B vitamin requirements (Stahly et al., 1995a). Because of the effect of lean growth potential on the nutrient requirements of weanling pigs, dietary specifications should be targeted to the lean growth potential of weanling pigs.

V. DIET COMPOSITION

A. Energy Sources

1. Lactose

Early-weaned pigs have insufficient pancreatic amylase and intestinal disaccharidases (Cunningham, 1959; Sewell and Maxwell, 1966) for optimum performance when they are fed cereal starches as the primary energy source. Research in the last decade has indicated that lactose in the diet the first few days after weaning is essential for success in feeding pigs weaned at less than 3 weeks of age. Several sources of lactose, including whey, whey permeate, deproteinized whey, or crystalline lactose, have been shown to be very effective sources in the initial nursery diet (Dritz et al., 1993; Owen et al., 1993b; Touchette et al., 1995; Nessmith et al., 1997a). Spray-dried whey, because of the very limited time the product is exposed to heat during the drying process, has been the preferred source of whey since heat treatment of milk products has been identified as the most critical factor affecting milk product quality (Tomkins, 1989). This response is consistent with the observations of Pollmann et al. (1983), Sohn et al. (1993), and Pettigrew et al. (1977) who reported that spray-dried whey was superior to roller-dried whey, which is heated to a high temperature for a longer duration. However, Crenshaw (1997) reported that there was no difference between roller-dried and spray-dried whey in diets for pigs weaned at 11 or 20 days of age. These studies demonstrate differences among dried whey sources and the importance of selecting high-quality ingredients. Yang et al. (1997) reported that a milk chocolate product could replace a portion of the whey in early-weaned pig diets without affecting growth performance.

Several studies have attempted to determine the optimum level of lactose in diets for early-weaned pigs. Mahan and Newton (1993) demonstrated increases in growth performance of weanling pigs fed up to 35% simple carbohydrates, including lactose or dextrose, but not cornstarch. Dritz et al. (1993) reported that gain was maximized in pigs at the highest inclusion level of 20% dried whey. Touchette et al. (1995) fed increasing levels of lactose from 0 to 40%, at the expense of skim milk and whey, and they reported maximum growth and feed efficiency at the 40% inclusion level (Figure 31.2). In a second experiment Touchette et al. (1996) observed a quadratic response to the inclusion of lactose from 0 to 30%. This response is consistent with the linear increases in growth performance with increasing lactose from 7 to 23% reported by Owen et al. (1993b). Based on these and other results, it is generally recommended that SEW and Phase I diets for early-weaned pigs contain from 15 to 25% lactose for optimum performance. Response to lactose also has been demonstrated in the second and third week postweaning (Crow et al., 1995), and 10 to 15% lactose is generally recommended in Phase 2 diets of early-weaned pigs.

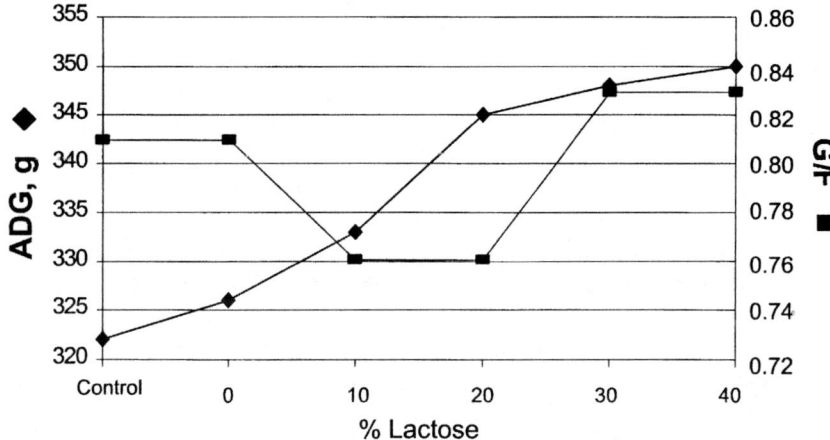

FIGURE 31.2 Lactose substitution for skim milk and whey in diets fed for 2 weeks postweaning.

Changes in milk supply as well as increased alternative markets for milk-based by-products, which could substantially increase the cost and decrease the availability of the high-lactose-containing by-products, have led to research seeking alternative ingredients. Effective substitutes that could replace all or a portion of the lactose in Phase 1 and/or Phase 2 diets include a carbohydrate by-product (Kim and Allee, 1997), dextrose (Mahan and Newton, 1993; Richert et al., 1996), and a product containing a high level of sucrose (de Rodas et al., 1998b). Dove and Usry (1996) reported that lactose and crystalline amino acids could replace all but 5% of the whey in diets fed to pigs weaned at 10 days of age.

2. Other Carbohydrate Sources

Most complex carbohydrates, such as starch present in grains, are utilized less efficiently than lactose by the young pig during the early postweaning period (Mahan and Newton, 1993). The focus of research has been to identify highly digestible carbohydrates for use as a replacement for corn in high-nutrient-dense nursery diets. Although a number of innovative carbohydrate sources have been tested, these research efforts have met with limited success, beyond the lactose and simple sugar substitutes discussed above. Giesting et al. (1985) reported that pigs fed diets containing cornstarch or hydrolyzed cornstarch had lower gains than pigs fed diets containing lactose. Although oat products have long been considered an excellent energy source for young pigs, Rantanen et al. (1995) observed little difference in performance in early-weaned pigs fed corn or oat products, including whole oats, oat groats, flour, or roasted oats. Similarly, Hongtrakul et al. (1996) reported similar gain and gain:feed in pigs fed diets that contained cornstarch, wheat flour, grain sorghum, or rice. Kerr et al. (1998) reported that substituting a modified potato starch for corn can improve gain and feed intake of weanling pigs compared with corn, but it only had a feeding value between that of corn and lactose. Additional ingredients that have been tested that had little effect on improving performance in the newly weaned pig include cooked cereal (Lawlor et al., 1998), sorghum-based distillers grains (Senne et al., 1997), high-oil corn (Bergstrom et al., 1997c), naked oat (Landblom and Poland, 1997), and potato chip scraps (Rahnema et al., 1997). Extrusion of corn (Deluca et al., 1995) or replacing corn with naked oat (Whitney et al., 1997) or hard red winter wheat (de Rodas et al., 1997) improved performance of early-weaned pigs.

3. Fats and Oils

The value of added fat to the early-weaned pig diet has been variable. Pettigrew and Moser (1991) summarized data from 92 comparisons of fat addition for pigs from 5 to 20 kg and found that fat addition reduced growth rate and feed intake, whereas feed efficiency was improved. The number of positive (37) and negative responses (38) were similar. It seems that utilization of fat may be dependent on pancreatic enzymes (Borgström, 1993), although gastric lipase may also play a major role in the hydrolysis of triglycerides in the young pig (Newport and Hawarth, 1985; Jensen et al., 1997). Lindemann et al. (1986) and Cera et al. (1990) observed up to a 60% decrease in pancreatic lipase after weaning. This decrease is consistent with the observation that, although performance can be improved in pigs fed high-fat diets over the entire nursery phase, the response to fat addition during the first weeks postweaning is very small or even negative (Howard et al., 1990; Mahan, 1991). Utilization of fat in the early-weaned pig is enhanced in lipid sources with a high concentration of short-chain fatty acids or long-chain unsaturated fatty acids compared with sources rich in long-chain saturated fatty acids (Lawrence and Maxwell, 1983; Cera et al., 1988; Partridge and Gill, 1993). Medium-chain triglycerides have been shown to increase growth performance substantially in the postweaning pig, because they are readily hydrolyzed and absorbed from the digestive tract and transported to the liver via the portal vein, thereby enhancing the opportunity for hepatic uptake (de Rodas and Maxwell, 1990). For additional information concerning fat utilization and medium-chain triglyceride utilization in the neonatal pig, see Chapters 6 and 30, respectively.

Some factors that may increase fat utilization in the early-weaned pig have been identified. Fat utilization is increased by 250 ppm copper addition (Dove, 1993), which has been shown to increase intestinal lipase and phospholipase activity leading to an increase in fat digestibility (Luo and Dove, 1996). Owen et al. (1996) observed increased nursery performance in the first 2 weeks postweaning by the addition of 1000 ppm of L-carnitine.

Despite poor utilization of fat by the early-weaned pig, 3 to 6% fat is typically added in the diet to enhance pelleting of diets high in milk-based ingredients.

B. Protein Sources

1. Plasma Protein

Weaning as early as 2 weeks of age, with an average weaning age of about 17 days of age, has become routine in large production complexes with three site production systems. At this age, pigs are very sensitive to the source of dietary protein. Many dietary proteins produce allergic reactions, in which diarrhea, reduced growth, and increased mortality can occur (Bimbo and Crowther, 1992). Various protein sources have been tested in diets for early-weaned pigs in an attempt to overcome these problems and to decrease diet cost. Spray-dried plasma protein is the most exciting protein product to be tested in recent years. Improved handling of blood products, and the utilization of the spray-drying process dramatically improved the quality and subsequent use of blood protein products in nursery diets. Spray-dried plasma protein has consistently improved performance of early-weaned pigs when included in Phase 1 (day 0 to 14 postweaning) diets at the expense of dried skim milk (Hansen et al., 1993; Kats et al., 1994a; de Rodas et al., 1995), soybean meal (Fakler et al., 1993; Coffey and Cromwell, 1995; de Rodas et al., 1995), whey (Hansen et al., 1993), or spray-dried blood meal (Hansen et al., 1993; de Rodas et al., 1995). A summary of studies evaluating plasma protein as a protein source is presented in Table 31.2. These studies indicate that plasma protein consistently improves feed intake (35.9%) and gain (46.9%) in young pigs.

In studies to determine the fraction of plasma protein responsible for improved performance, growth performance of pigs consuming a diet containing the high-molecular-weight fraction (globular proteins) was similar to that of pigs fed the spray-dried plasma protein diet (Cain, 1995; Owen et al., 1995b; Pierce et al., 1995). Growth of pigs fed the medium-molecular-weight (albumin) or low-molecular-weight fractions was not different from that of the negative control. Thus, it seems likely that the high-molecular-weight fraction in the plasma has a biological function beyond simply meeting nutritional requirements.

TABLE 31.2
A Summary of Recent Experiments Evaluating Spray-Dried Porcine Plasma as a Protein Source for Weanling Pigs[a]

Ref.	Protein in Control Diet	Percent Improvement over Pigs Fed Control Diet		
		Daily Gain	Daily Feed	Feed:Gain
Hansen et al., 1990	Skim milk	+42	+37	−3.6
Gatnau and Zimmerman, 1991	Soybean meal	+102	+76	+12.0
Kats et al., 1994a	Skim milk	+41	+35	+5.3
deRodas et al., 1995	Skim milk	+29	+24	+1.2
Gatnau et al., 1991	Soybean meal	+82	+34	+59.5
Hansen et al., 1993				
Exp. 1	Skim milk	+2	0	+0.03
Exp. 2	Skim milk	+27	+27	+0.01
Gatnau et al., 1990	Skim milk	+50	+54	+29.3

[a] All experiments were conducted for 2 weeks postweaning.

Also consistent with the concept that passive immunity via the globular fraction in plasma protein is involved in the improved performance in early-weaned pigs fed plasma protein is the finding of a protein source by environment interaction. Coffey and Cromwell (1995) reported a much greater improvement in performance in pigs fed plasma protein in a challenging, conventional environment compared with those fed plasma protein in a temperature- and humidity-controlled, off-site environment (Figure 31.3). This study suggests that other approaches may be used to obtain improved performance in pigs without the inclusion of plasma protein. The U.S. swine industry is pursuing a program of earlier weaning (as early as 14 days) with all-in, all-out placement of nursery pigs by site as a means of improving performance.

2. Other Animal Sources

Milk proteins have historically been considered excellent protein sources for early-weaned pigs since Speer et al. (1954) and Diaz et al. (1959) demonstrated that pigs weaned at 1 to 2 weeks of age could be successfully reared on dry diets containing 40% dried skim milk plus other highly digestible

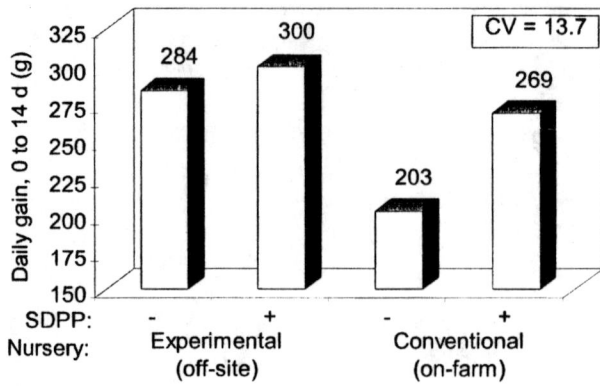

FIGURE 31.3 The effect of nursery environment on growth response to spray-dried porcine plasma. Dietary inclusion of spray-dried porcine plasma improved daily gain in the conventional nursery ($P < 0.001$) but not in the experimental nursery ($P = 0.25$). (From Coffey, R. D. and Cromwell, G. L., *J. Anim. Sci.*, 73:2532, 1995. With permission.)

ingredients. Early-weaned pigs fed milk-based diets have generally performed better than those fed other protein sources (Fitzpatrick and Bayley; 1977; Wilson and Leibholz, 1981a,b,c; Walker et al., 1986). Recent research has been directed at attempts to identify other protein sources that can be efficiently substituted for the more expensive milk proteins, or which can be fed in combination with milk proteins to improve performance. Select-grade menhaden fish meal that has been properly processed and preserved seems to be one of the most widely utilized protein sources in young pig diets because of a combination of consistent quality and competitive price. Stoner et al. (1990) demonstrated that select menhaden fish meal could be successfully used at levels up to 20% in diets for weanling pigs, although breakpoint analysis indicated that the optimum fish meal level for daily gain was between the 4 and 8% inclusion level. Blood meal is another protein source that with proper processing is an excellent source of available lysine for pigs (Parsons et al., 1975). Kats et al. (1994b) indicated that the optimum level of spray-dried blood meal was 2% of the diet when fed from 7 to 28 days postweaning, and de Rodas et al. (1995) observed increased feed intake and gain in pigs fed 2.75% blood meal as a replacement for 10% dried skim milk in Phase 1 nursery diets formulated to maintain equivalent levels of lactose. Dried porcine solubles is a product resulting from processing porcine mucosa and small intestines, which produces a liquid peptone product rich in amino acids.

This protein product potentially can be used to effectively replace a portion of the more expensive proteins in diets for early-weaned pigs (Zimmerman et al., 1997; Lindemann et al., 1998). A product combining hydrolyzed porcine proteins and porcine plasma protein has been shown to replace plasma effectively (Wright et al., 1998). Similarly, a spray-dried rendered peptide product produced from beef muscle and manufactured using an enzymatic hydrolysis process has been shown to be an excellent protein source in Phase 1 nursery diets (de Rodas et al., 1998a,d). Other animal protein sources that have shown promise as alternative protein sources for the early-weaned pig include spray-dried egg (Owen et al., 1993a; Nessmith et al., 1995), poultry by-products (Sohn et al., 1993; Veum and Haque, 1994), avian spray-dried blood meal (Dritz et al., 1993), and spray-dried bovine globulin (Pierce et al., 1996).

3. Plant Sources

Growth rate and efficiency of feed utilization of early-weaned pigs are much better with milk proteins than with soybean proteins (Wilson and Leibholz, 1981a; Veum et al., 1986; Walker et al., 1986; Sohn et al., 1994). Reduced performance in pigs fed soybean proteins has been associated with reduced protein digestibility (Wilson and Leibholz, 1981b; Walker et al., 1986; Sohn et al.,

1994; Qin et al., 1996). This decreased digestibility should not be surprising because pigs develop transient hypersensitivity to soybean products (Li et al., 1990; 1991; Friesen et al., 1993a; Qin et al., 1996). The native storage globulins, particularly glycinin and β-conglycinin, as well as possibly antinutritional factors like protease inhibitors and lectin, have been implicated (Lallès, 1999).

Steam-heated soybean products such as soybean meal and soybean flour have very low levels of trypsin inhibitors and lectin, and they can be utilized very effectively by most animals. However, young pigs have poor growth and digestive disorders when fed soybean meal (Lallès, 1993). Further processing of soybean proteins by solvent extraction of oligosaccharides and protein isolation to produce soy protein isolate and isolated soy protein, respectively, resulted in only a marginal increase in growth performance of young pigs. However, additional technologies, including alcohol denaturation and extrusion of these products, have resulted in improved performance (Friesen et al., 1993b; Sohn et al., 1994). Excellent performance also can be attained in high-health early-weaned pigs fed diets containing 15 to 22% soybean meal, if plasma protein is also a dietary component of the diet (Friesen et al., 1993a). Lactose also seems to have a positive effect on performance of high-health pigs fed diets high in soybean meal (Nessmith et al., 1997b).

C. Minerals

Minerals may be supplied in the diets of weanling pigs in inorganic or organic forms. For the most part, inorganic sources have been utilized to meet the mineral requirements of weanling pigs. However, in recent years, organic forms of trace minerals have become more prevalent. Organic forms of copper, zinc, and iron are available for use in weanling pig diets. Organic forms are often compared with inorganic forms based on bioavailability of the mineral in question, response criteria, and cost.

The growth-promoting activity of supplemental copper fed in the form of copper sulfate to weanling pigs is well documented (see Chapters 12 and 18 for additional information). Coffey et al. (1994) compared the response of pigs fed 200 ppm copper as copper sulfate or as a copper–lysine complex. The response to copper–lysine was equal to or greater than that for copper sulfate. Apgar and Kornegay (1996) also compared the efficacy of a copper–lysine complex to copper sulfate for stimulating growth performance in weanling pigs. These authors also reported that the response to copper–lysine was equal to that of copper sulfate. Other organic sources of copper, such as copper–methionine (Bunch et al., 1965) and copper complexed with EDTA (Stansbury et al., 1990), have been reported to be as efficacious as copper sulfate in stimulating growth performance in weanling pigs. Thus, it seems that organic forms of copper are equally as effective as copper provided via copper sulfate in stimulating growth performance in weanling pigs.

Another trace mineral that has received attention in recent years is zinc. The addition of 1000 to 3000 ppm zinc, provided as zinc oxide or zinc sulfate, in the diet of weanling pigs improves growth performance. Other forms of zinc available for inclusion in weanling pig diets include organically complexed forms such as zinc–lysine, zinc–methionine, and other zinc–amino acid complexes. However, unlike copper, the responses to organic forms of zinc compared with zinc oxide or zinc sulfate have been variable. Hahn and Baker (1993) compared 3000 ppm zinc from zinc oxide, zinc sulfate, or zinc–methionine. Growth rate and feed intake were not affected by zinc source, but there tended to be a slight improvement in gain:feed ratios when pigs were fed zinc–methionine compared with zinc sulfate. Swinkels et al. (1996) reported no difference in growth performance of pigs fed 45 ppm of zinc from zinc sulfate or a zinc–amino acid chelate. Similarly, Cheng et al. (1998) found no difference in growth performance of young pigs fed zinc sulfate or a zinc–lysine complex. For additional information concerning the effect of zinc source on immune function and bioavailability, see Chapters 12 and 16, respectively.

Organic forms of trace minerals often are promoted as having a higher biological availability of the mineral than inorganic forms. However, research supporting this contention is lacking. Wedekind et al. (1994) reported the following rankings for zinc bioavailability: zinc sulfate > zinc–methionine > zinc–oxide > zinc–lysine. However, Schell and Kornegay (1996) reported that the bioavailability of zinc relative to zinc sulfate was lowest for zinc oxide, followed by zinc–lysine and zinc–methionine. Equivalent bioavailabilities, based on plasma concentrations of zinc, have been reported for zinc sulfate, zinc–lysine, and zinc–methionine (Hahn and Baker, 1993).

Ward et al. (1996) reported that the growth response of weanling pigs was similar between those fed 250 ppm of zinc from a zinc–methionine complex or 2000 ppm zinc from zinc oxide, which suggests an increase in the bioavailability of zinc in zinc–methionine. However, more recent studies have not been able to repeat this response. McCalla et al. (1999) and Woodworth et al. (1999) reported that the growth response of weanling pigs was greater for pigs fed diets supplemented with 3000 ppm of zinc from zinc oxide than for those fed 100 to 500 ppm of zinc from a zinc–amino acid complex.

The response of weanling pigs to organic forms of iron compared with iron sulfate is variable. Lewis et al. (1995) reported that the iron in iron–methionine was less bioavailable than the iron in ferrous sulfate. However, this same laboratory reported that the bioavailability of iron in two iron proteinates was similar to that for the iron in ferrous sulfate (Lewis et al., 1999).

D. Vitamins

Limited data exist concerning the forms of vitamins to include in weanling pig diets. One exception to this is vitamin C. The NRC (1998) lists no requirement for vitamin C for weanling pigs, and Chiang et al. (1985) reported no response to supplemental vitamin C in weanling pigs. However, several researchers have reported a response to supplemental vitamin C (Yen and Pond, 1981; Mahan et al., 1994). Recently, de Rodas et al. (1998c) reported that supplementation of the diet with L-ascorbyl-2-polyphosphate, a stable form of vitamin C, increased performance of pigs weaned at 2 weeks of age. Thus, the response to vitamin C may be dependent on the stress level, environment, and stability of the vitamin C source.

E. Feed Additives

1. Antibiotics

Young pigs respond markedly to antibiotic supplementation of the diet. A summary of 1194 experiments indicated that antimicrobials improved growth rate by 16.4% in weanling pigs (Hays, 1978; Zimmerman, 1986; Cromwell, 1991). Furthermore, the response to antibiotics may be twice as great under commercial conditions compared with those observed in a research environment (Cromwell, 1991).

The impact of antibiotics on growth response of weanling pigs also may be dependent on the lean growth potential and immune system activation of pigs. Stahly et al. (1996) reported that pigs with a high capacity for lean tissue deposition responded more to Carbadox than those of a low lean growth genotype. Additionally, these researchers reported that pigs with a high level of immune system activation responded more to Tylosin (Stahly et al., 1995b) or Carbadox (Stahly et al., 1994b) than pigs with a low level of immune stimulation. It seems that the magnitude of response to antibiotics in weanling pigs is dependent on the health status of the pigs, environment ("dirty" vs. "clean"), and lean growth potential. For more information on antimicrobials, the reader is referred to Chapter 18.

2. Copper

Supplementation of weanling pig diets with copper has consistently increased pig growth performance (Braude, 1967; Cromwell et al., 1989). Furthermore, the improvement in pig performance with supplementation of copper is independent and additive to that for antibiotics (Roof and Mahan, 1982; Cromwell, 1991). The reader is referred to Chapter 18 for more information.

3. Zinc

Poulsen (1989) reported a growth performance response of weanling pigs to supplementation of the diet with 3000 ppm of zinc from zinc oxide. Several recent studies have confirmed this response (Hahn and Baker, 1993; Hill et al., 1996; Smith et al., 1997). Unlike copper, the response to zinc does not seem to be additive to that for antimicrobials. In a recent regional study, Mahan et al. (2000) reported that weanlings pigs fed 3000 ppm zinc with or without Carbadox responded to zinc supplementation, but the increase in growth performance was not additive to that observed with Carbadox supplementation.

Because both copper and zinc increase performance in weanling pigs, there has been interest in determining if the response to zinc and copper is additive. Smith et al. (1997) and Hill et al. (1996) demonstrated an improvement in growth performance of weanling pigs fed copper or zinc, but the responses were not additive.

4. Microbial Supplements

There are many reports in the popular press concerning the efficacy of probiotics in the diets of weanling pigs. However, the scientific literature to support these claims is lacking. Pollmann et al. (1980) reported that supplementation of the diet of weanling pigs with *Lactobacillus acidophilus* culture increases growth performance slightly. However, Kornegay et al. (1995) reported no improvement in growth performance of weanling pigs when yeast was added to a corn–soybean meal diet. An increase in growth performance of pigs fed diets supplemented with yeast was reported by Mathew et al. (1998). However, these authors reported no effect of yeast on ileal microflora or short-chain fatty acid concentrations. Improvements in growth performance of young pigs in response to supplementation of the diet with strains of *Bacillus cereus* have been reported (Kirchgessner et al., 1993; Zani et al., 1998). The inconsistent response of weanling pigs to microbial supplementation of the diet most likely depends on whether colonization of organisms in the intestine occurs.

5. Enzymes

The response of weanling pigs to enzyme supplementation of the diet has been variable. Phytase is an enzyme that has received a great deal of attention in recent years. An increase in performance and availability of phosphorus in the diet of weanling pigs with phytase supplementation has been reported (Lei et al., 1993; Biehl and Baker, 1996; Radcliffe et al., 1998). Positive responses to the enzyme, β-glucanase, in diets containing barley have been reported by Li et al. (1996). The lack of information concerning the efficacy of other enzymes, such as arabinoxylanase, xylanase, and amylase, in the diet of weanling pigs makes conclusions regarding these enzymes difficult. Mavromichalis et al. (1998) reported that arabinoxylanse addition to wheat-based diets for weanling pigs did not improve performance. The efficacy of specific enzymes, with the exception of phytase, in improving digestibility of feedstuffs for weanling pigs has promise, but more research is needed in order to determine the conditions where positive responses will be observed.

6. Organic Acids

Research on the use of organic acids to promote gastric acidification in young pigs has established a basis for the use of acids in weaning pig diets. The digestive system of the early-weaned pig is not sufficiently developed to handle the transition from diets based on milk proteins to those based on plant proteins. Part of the problem could be the lack of protein denaturation, which could be a consequence of a higher gastric pH than the acidic pH values (pH 2.0 to 3.5) of mature pigs (Kidder and Manners, 1978). Acid secretion does not reach appreciable levels until 3 to 4 weeks postweaning (Cranwell and Moughan, 1989). Easter (1988) discussed the strategies used by the nursing pig to overcome the limitations of gastric acid secretion. These include the conversion of lactose to lactic acid by lactobacilli bacteria in the stomach and the frequent ingestion of small meals, thereby reducing the demand for high levels of acid secretion. The failure to maintain a low gastric pH has major implications for the performance of early-weaned pigs, in addition to protein denaturation. These include decreased digestion by pepsin, control of gastric emptying, and bacteriocidal effects on certain microorganisms (Ravindran and Kornegay, 1993). The evidence suggests, however, that reducing pH does not seem to be one of the primary effects of acidification (Burnell et al., 1988; Sutton et al., 1989; Sweet et al., 1990; Risley et al., 1992; Roth et al., 1992).

In spite of the lack of evidence of a direct effect of dietary acidifiers on pH, acidifiers have been shown to have an impact in controlling digestive scouring (White et al., 1969) and reducing the associated coliform burden along the gastrointestinal tract (Cole et al., 1968; Thomlinson and Lawrence, 1981; Bolduan et al., 1988; Bokori et al., 1989; Mathew et al., 1991; Eckel et al., 1992; Johnson, 1992). Mathew et al. (1991) observed that lactobacilli popoulation was reduced to almost zero within 2 days of weaning whereas the coliform population increased. This change was associated with an increased pH in the ileal contents.

Although efficacy of acidifiers has been demonstrated in numerous studies, responses have been inconsistent with all types of acidifiers. Ravindran and Kornegay (1993) published a review of studies summarizing the effects of numerous acidifiers on pig performance. They suggested that variables that influence efficacy of acidifiers include type of diet, age of pigs, type and dosage of acidifier, and existing environmental conditions.

VI. FEEDING THE WEANED PIG

A. Performance Estimates

Fowler and Gill (1989) calculated that the 21-day-old pig before weaning has a live-weight gain of 280 g/day. After weaning, voluntary feed intake has typically been insufficient to meet maintenance requirements (Robertson et al., 1985; Bark et al., 1986; Pluske, 1993), much less support weight gain at preweaning levels. This response is in spite of the fact that the gain potential is much greater than that observed in the preweaning pig (Hodge, 1974; Lecce et al., 1979). Pluske et al. (1995) calculated from the data of Bark et al. (1986) that the estimated energy requirement for maintenance was not met until the fifth day after weaning at 21 days of age.

Recent studies suggest that rearing pigs under high-health conditions and fed high-nutrient-dense diets containing plasma protein and an adequate level of simple carbohydrates produces a much higher level of performance, although gain is still less than the demonstrated potential. A summary of growth performance of pigs under conditions that meet these criteria is presented in Table 31.3. These selected studies demonstrate that growth in the early-weaned pig fed dry diets can approach or exceed the rate of gain observed in the preweaning pig (Fowler and Gill, 1989), and that gain:feed under these circumstances can exceed 1.00.

B. Recommended Ingredients and Feeding Practices for a Phased-Feeding Program

Nutritional requirements for optimum performance of the early-weaned pig are changing rapidly during the early postweaning period. They change from a requirement for an energy-dense, highly palatable, highly digestible diet in the newly weaned pig to a rather simple grain–soybean meal diet by 3 to 4 weeks after weaning. Newly weaned pigs, particularly those weaned at less than 17 days of age, perform well only when given a complex diet appropriate for their stage of development. These diets are very expensive, but intake of this initial diet is so little that the contribution to the overall cost of production is not excessive. Complex diets with plasma protein and a good-quality lactose source are needed to achieve maximum feed intake and gain during week 1 postweaning in early-weaned pigs. A phased-feeding program with feeding programmed

TABLE 31.3
Performance of Pigs Fed Plasma-Based Complex Diets

		Day 0–7		Day 0–14	
Experiment	% Total Lys.	ADG (g)	G:F	ADG (g)	G:F
Hansen et al., 1993[a]	1.55	221	1.02	266	0.80
Hansen et al., 1993[b]	1.40	365	1.04	414	0.86
de Rodas et al., 1995[c]	1.40	280	1.02	360	0.90
Owen et. al., 1995d[d]	1.80	348	1.21	394	1.04
Davis et al., 1996[e]	1.60	294	1.18	376	1.05
Chung et al, 1996[f]	1.75	229	1.10	337	1.05
Chung et al., 1996[f]	1.90	266	1.26	365	1.16

[a] Mean of four pens of 15 to 16 pigs/pen, Conventional system, 6.4 kg initial wt, 24 days of age at weaning.
[b] Mean of 20 pens of five pigs/pen, Conventional system, 5.9 kg initial wt, 21 days of age at weaning.
[c] Mean of eight pens of six pigs/pen, Conventional system, 7.2 kg initial wt, 24 days of age at weaning.
[d] Mean of six pens of four pigs/pen, SEW system, 4.6 kg initial wt, 14 to 18 days of age at weaning.
[e] Mean of six pens of six pigs/pen, Conventional system, 6 kg initial wt, 20 days of age at weaning.
[f] Mean of five pens of four pigs/pen, SEW system, 4.3 kg initial wt, 14 days of age at weaning.

for a maximum period or a maximum quantity of intake is essential to optimize performance and to get pigs to a grain–soybean meal diet as quickly as possible to minimize costs. A summary of recommended feeding practices and ingredients for a phased-feeding program in early-weaned pigs is presented in Table 31.4 (Shurson et al., 1995; Goodband et al., 1995; Thacker, 1998). Typically, pigs weaned at 17 days of age or weighing less than 5 kg are offered a very complex SEW diet as the initial diet followed by the Phase 1 diet. Pigs weaned at greater than 17 days of age or weighing more than 5 kg are offered the Phase 1 diet as the initial diet followed by the Phase 2 diet. Pigs weaned at 10 to 21 days of age should be fed the initial diet for 7 to 10 days postweaning, whereas pigs weaned at greater than 21 days of age should receive the initial diet for only 3 to 4 days, if at all. Many nutritionists prefer to eliminate soybean products from the SEW or Phase 1 diets and follow a program of a reduced rate of the decrease of complexity

TABLE 31.4
Summary of Recommended Feeding Practices for Early-Weaned Pigs

	SEW	Phase 1	Phase 2	Phase 3
Pig weight range (kg)	3.0–5.0	5.0–7.0	7.0–11.0	11.0–23.0
Duration diet fed	1 week	1 week	2 weeks	2–3 weeks
Lysine (%)	1.6–1.8	1.5–1.6	1.35–1.45	1.25–1.35
Digestible lysine (%)	1.4–1.5	1.25–1.35	1.10–1.20	1.05–1.15
Methionine (%)	0.48–0.50	0.42–0.44	0.37–0.40	0.34–0.37
Lactose (%)	15–25	15–20	5–10	None
Spray-dried porcine plasma (%)	5–8	4–6	None	None
Spray-dried blood meal (%)	1–2	2–2.5	0–2.5	None
Fish meal (%)	4–8	4–8	0–5	None
Soybean meal (%)	0–15	10–20	As required	As required
Added fat (%)	4–6	3–5	0–5	None
Additional energy source	Corn/wheat/ oats	Corn/wheat/ oats	Corn/wheat/ oats	Corn/wheat/ oats
Growth promotant	Cu or Zn	Cu or Zn	Cu	Cu
Diet form	Pellet	Pellet	Pellet/Meal	Meal

Source: Adapted from Shurson et al. (1995), Goodband et al. (1995), and Thacker (1998).

of subsequent nursery diets. Such a system will enhance performance under varying environmental conditions, but costs are increased.

The Phase 2 diet is designed to contain some of the palatability factors (substituting spray-dried blood meal or other alternative quality proteins for plasma protein) present in the Phase 1 diet and get the pig exposed to higher levels of soybean proteins. It seems that 1 to 2 weeks of this diet is sufficient in most early weaning situations; however, a longer period of time may be required for lighter pigs.

The Phase 1 and 2 diets can then be followed by the less complex Phase 3 diet essentially devoid of the more expensive alternative protein sources. Some researchers suggest that the Phase 3 diet should contain some whey and/or fish meal; however, very good results have been obtained with a 1.2 to 1.4% lysine level in a corn–soybean meal diet starting at 21 to 28 days postweaning. This diet can be fed until pigs reach 20 to 22 kg and are switched to a grower diet.

C. Diet Forms

Although there is not a large body of published data concerning the preference of weanling pigs for either a pellet or meal diet, it generally is assumed that young pigs prefer a pelleted diet over a meal diet. Jensen and Becker (1965) reported that young pigs, when given a choice, prefer a pelleted diet over a diet fed in meal form. Vanschoubroek et al. (1971) reported that crumbled diets were preferred over pelleted diets for the young pig. Hardness of pellet also can affect acceptance by the young pig (Jensen and Becker, 1965). More recently, feed companies have introduced small pellets coated with milk flavors to increase feed intake in the young pig. For further information regarding pelleting, the reader is referred to Chapter 21.

VII. SUMMARY

The process of weaning invariably produces challenges, which the pig previously has not experienced. These include an abrupt change in diet, usually to ingredients that the pig has limited ability to digest, and a new social structure. Combined, these effects disrupt nutrient intake, which is necessary to maintain gut integrity. These disruptive effects on growth performance are further exacerbated by an immature immune system, which creates susceptibility to digestive upsets and diarrhea. Developments during the past decade have resulted in major improvements in performance of the newly weaned pig. First, the movement to off-site facilities has reduced the immune challenge, producing an improvement in growth performance. This has demonstrated, if nothing else, the growth potential of the young postweaning pig. Secondly, the development of two dietary components was essential for the consistent success of weaning pigs at less than 3 weeks of age. These are an adequate supply of simple carbohydrates, such as good-quality lactose or whey, and spray-dried animal plasma. An understanding of why these components work and a better understanding of the environment by diet interaction in the newly weaned pig should lead to further improvements in growth performance of the weanling pig.

REFERENCES

Apgar, G. A., and E. T. Kornegay. 1996. Mineral balance of finishing pigs fed copper sulfate or a copper-lysine complex at growth-stimulating levels, *J. Anim. Sci.*, 74:1594.

Auldist, D. E., F. L. Stevenson, M. G. Kerr, P. Eason, and R. H. King. 1997. Lysine requirements of pigs from 2 to 7 kg liveweight, *Anim. Prod.*, 65:501.

Barber, J., P. H. Brooks, and J. L. Carpenter. 1989. The effect of water delivery rate on the voluntary food intake, water use and performance of early-weaned pigs from 3 to 6 weeks of age. In *The Voluntary Feed Intake of Pigs*, British Society of Animal Production, Edinburgh, 103.

Bark, L. J., T. D. Crenshaw, and V. D. Leibbrandt. 1986. The effect of meal intervals and weaning on feed intake of early weaned pigs, *J. Anim. Sci.*, 62:1233.

Bergstrom, J. R., J. L. Nelssen, M. D. Tokach, R. D. Goodband, K. Q. Owen, and W. B. Nessmith. 1996a. Determining the optimal threonine:lysine ratio in starter diets for the segregated early weaned pig, *J. Anim. Sci.*, 74(Suppl. 1):56 (Abstr.).

Bergstrom, J. R., J. L. Nelssen, M. D. Tokach, R. D. Goodband, K. Q. Owen, B. T. Richert, and W. B. Nessmith. 1996b. Determining the optimal threonine:lysine ratio in starter diets for the phase III nursery pig, *J. Anim. Sci.*, 74(Suppl. 1):56 (Abstr.).

Bergstrom, J. R., C. J. Samland, J. L. Nelssen, M. D. Tokach, and R. D. Goodband. 1997c. The effects of high oil corn and fat level on nursery pig growth performance, *J. Anim. Sci.*, 75(Suppl. 1):71 (Abstr.).

Bergstrom, J. R., J. L. Nelssen, M. D. Tokach, and R. D. Goodband. 1997a. Determining the optimum isoleucine:lysine ratio for the segregated early-weaned pig weighing 5 to 8 kg, *J. Anim. Sci.*, 75(Suppl. 1):60 (Abstr.).

Bergstrom, J. R., J. L. Nelssen, M. D. Tokach, and R. D. Goodband. 1997b. Determining the optimum isoleucine:lysine ratio for the SEW-reared 10 to 20 kg pig, *J. Anim. Sci.*, 75(Suppl. 1):60 (Abstr.).

Biehl, R. R., and D. H. Baker. 1996. Efficacy of supplemental 1 alpha-hydroxycholecalciferol and microbial phytase for young pigs fed phosphorus- or amino acid-deficient corn–soybean meal diets, *J. Anim. Sci.*, 74:2960.

Bimbo, A. P., and J. B. Crowther. 1992. Fish meal and oil: current uses, *J. Am. Oil Chem. Soc.*, 69:221.

Bokori, J., P. Galfi, and I. Boros. 1989. Swine experiment with a feed containing Na-*n*-butyrate, *Magy. Allatorv. Lapja*, 44:501.

Bolduan G., H. Jung, R. Schneider, J. Block, and B. Klenke. 1988. Effect of propionic and formic acids in piglets, *J. Anim. Physiol. Anim. Nutr.*, 59:72.

Borgström, B. 1993. Luminal digestion of fats. In *The Pancreas: Biology, Pathobiology and Disease*, Go, V. L. W., E. P. Dimagno, J. D. Gardner, E. Lebenthal, H. A. Reber, and G. A. Scheele, Eds., Raven Press, New York, 475.

Braude, R. 1967. Copper as a stimulant in pig feeding (cuprum pro pecunia), *World Rev. Anim. Prod.*, 3:69.

Bunch, R. J., J. T. McCall, V. C. Speer, and V. W. Hays. 1965. Copper supplementation for weanling pigs, *J. Anim. Sci.*, 24:995.

Burnell, T. W., G. L. Cromwell, and T. S. Stahly. 1988. Effects of dried whey and copper sulfate on the growth responses to organic acid in diets for weaning pigs, *J. Anim. Sci.*, 66:1100.

Cain, C. 1995. Mode of action of spray-dried porcine plasma in weanling pigs. In *Proceedings of American Assoc. of Swine Practitioners*, Omaha, NE, 225.

Cera, K. R., D. C. Mahan, and G. A. Reinhart. 1988. Weekly digestibilities of diets supplemented with corn oil, lard, or tallow by weanling swine, *J. Anim. Sci.*, 66:1430.

Cera, K. R., D. C. Mahan, and G. A. Reinhart. 1990. Effect of weaning, week postweaning and diet composition on pancreatic and small intestinal luminal lipase response in young swine, *J. Anim. Sci.*, 68:384.

Cheng, J., E. T. Kornegay, and T. Schell. 1998. Influence of dietary lysine on the utilization of zinc from zinc sulfate and a zinc-lysine complex by young pigs, *J. Anim. Sci.*, 76:1064.

Chiang, S. H., J. E. Pettigrew, R. L. Moser, S. G. Cornelius, K. P. Miller, and T. R. Heeg. 1985. Supplemental vitamin C in swine diets, *Nutr. Rep. Int.*, 31:573.

Chung, J., B. Z. de Rodas, C. V. Maxwell, and M. E. Davis. 1996. The effect of increasing whey protein concentrate as a lysine source on performance of segregated early-weaned pigs, *J. Anim. Sci.*, 74(Suppl. 1):195 (Abstr.).

Coffey, R. D., and G. L. Cromwell. 1995. The impact of environment and antimicrobial agents on growth response of early-weaned pigs to spray-dried porcine plasma, *J. Anim. Sci.*, 73:2532.

Coffey, R. D., G. L. Cromwell, and H. J. Monegue. 1994. Efficacy of a copper-lysine complex as a growth promotant for weanling pigs, *J. Anim. Sci.*, 72:2880.

Cole, B. J. A., R. M. Beal, and J. R. Luscombe. 1968. The effect on performance and bacterial flora of lactic acid, propionic acid, calcium propionate and calcium acrylate in the drinking water of weaned pigs, *Vet. Rec.*, 83:459.

Cranwell, P. D., and P. J. Moughan. 1989. Biological limitations imposed by the digestive system to the growth performance of weaned pigs. In *Manipulating Pig Production II*, Barnett, J. L., and D. P. Hennessy, Eds., Australasian Pig Science Association, Werribee, Australia, 140.

Crenshaw, T. D. 1997. Relative nutritional value of roller-dried versus spray-dried whey for pigs weaned at 11 or 20 days, *J. Anim. Sci.*, 75(Suppl. 1):60 (Abstr.).

Cromwell, G. L. 1991. Antimicrobial agents. In *Swine Nutrition*, Miller, E. R., D. E. Ullrey, and A. J. Lewis, Eds., Butterworth-Heinemann, Stoneham, MA, 297.

Cromwell, G. L., T. S. Stahly, and H. J. Monegue. 1989. Effects of source and level of copper on performance and liver copper stores in weanling pigs, *J. Anim. Sci.*, 67:2996.

Cromwell, G. L., R. D. Coffey, D. K. Aaron, M. D. Lindemann, J. L. Pierce, H. J. Monegue, V. M. Rupard, D. E. Cowen, M. B. Parido, and T. M. Clayton. 1996. Differences in growth rate of weanling barrows and gilts, *J. Anim. Sci.*, 74(Suppl. 1):186 (Abstr.).

Crow, S. D., K. J. Touchette, G. L. Allee, and M. B. Newcomb. 1995. Late nursery pigs respond to lactose (day 7–21 postweaning), *J. Anim. Sci.*, 73(Suppl. 1):71 (Abstr.).

Cunninghan, H. M. 1959. Digestion of starch and some of its degradation products by newborn pigs, *J. Anim. Sci.*, 18:964.

Davis, M. E., B. Z. de Rodas, C. V. Maxwell, and J. Chung. 1996. Effect of increasing level of dietary whey protein concentrate (77%) as a protein source on pig performance during phase 1 of the nursery period, *J. Anim. Sci.*, 74(Suppl. 1):172 (Abstr.).

DeLuca, D. D., T. L. Veum, D. W. Bollinger, F. H. Hsieh, H. Huff, and M. Ellersieck. 1995. Extrusion of the corn, soybeans or soybean meal in diets for early weaned pigs, *J. Anim. Sci.*, 73(Suppl. 1):175 (Abstr.).

de Rodas, B. Z., and C. V. Maxwell. 1990. The effect of fat source and medium-chain triglyceride level on performance of the early-weaned pig, Okla. Agric. Exp. Sta. Res. Rep. MP-129:278.

de Rodas, B. Z., K. S. Sohn, C. V. Maxwell, and L. J. Spicer. 1995. Plasma protein for pigs weaned at 19 and 24 days of age: effect on performance and plasma insulin-like growth factor 1, growth hormone, insulin, and glucose concentrations, *J. Anim. Sci.*, 73:3657.

de Rodas, B. Z., W. G. Luce, and C. V. Maxwell. 1997. Efficacy of wheat based diets for early weaned pigs, *J. Anim. Sci.*, 75(Suppl. 1):15 (Abstr.).

de Rodas, B. Z., C. V. Maxwell, M. E. Davis, J. Chung, E. Broekman, and C. R. Hamilton. 1998a. Efficacy of Peptide Plus™ in phase 1 diets for segregated early weaned pigs, *J. Anim. Sci.*, 76(Suppl. 2):47 (Abstr.).

de Rodas, B. Z., C. V. Maxwell, M. E. Davis and W. G. Luce. 1998b. Lactose equivalent-80 as a lactose alternative in the diets of phase 2 nursery pigs, *J. Anim. Sci.*, 76(Suppl. 2):63 (Abstr.).

de Rodas, B. Z., C. V. Maxwell, M. E. Davis, S. Mandali, E. Broekman, and B. J. Stoecker. 1998c. L-Ascorbyl-2-phosphate as a vitamin C source for segregated and conventionally weaned pigs, *J. Anim. Sci.*, 76:1636.

de Rodas, B. Z., C. V. Maxwell, W. Luce, E. Broekman, M. E. Davis, and C. R. Hamilton. 1998d. Efficacy of Peptide Plus™ in phase 1 diets for conventionally reared nursery pigs, *J. Anim. Sci.*, 76(Suppl. 2):65 (Abstr.).

Diaz, F., V. C. Speer, P. G. Homeyer, V. W. Hays, and D. V. Catron. 1959. Comparative performance of baby pigs fed infant and baby pig diets, *J. Nutr.*, 68:131.

Dinarello, C. A. 1984. Interleukin-1, *Rev. Infect.*, 44:105.

Dove, C. R. 1993. The effect of adding copper and various fat sources to the diets of weanling swine on growth performance and serum fatty acid profiles, *J. Anim. Sci.*, 71:2187.

Dove, C. R., and J. Usry. 1996. Substitution of lactose and amino acids for whey in diets of pigs weaned at 10 days, *J. Anim. Sci.*, 74(Suppl. 1):56 (Abstr.).

Dritz, S. S., M. D. Tokach, J. L. Nelssen, R. D. Goodband, and L. J. Katz. 1993. Optimal whey level in starter diets containing spray dried blood meal and comparison of avian and bovine spray-dried blood meals, *J. Anim. Sci.*, 71(Suppl. 1):57 (Abstr.).

Dritz, S. S., K. Q. Owen, J. L. Nelssen, R. D. Goodband, and M. D. Tokach. 1996. Influence of weaning age and nursery diet complexity on growth performance and carcass characteristics and composition of high-health status pigs from weaning to 109 kilograms, *J. Anim. Sci.*, 74:2975.

Easter, R. A. 1988. Acidification of diets for pigs. In *Recent Advances in Animal Nutrition*, Haresign, W., and D. J. A. Cole, Eds., Butterworths, London, 61.

Eckel, B., M. Kirchgessner, and F. X. Roth. 1992. Influence of formic acid on daily weight gain, feed intake, feed conversion rate and digestibility. 1. Communication: Investigations about the nutritive efficacy of organic acids in the rearing of piglets, *J. Anim. Physiol. Anim. Nutr.*, 67:93.

Fakler, T. M., C. M. Adams, and C. V. Maxwell. 1993. Effect of dietary fat source on performance and fatty acid absorption in the early-weaned pig, *J. Anim. Sci.*, 71(Suppl. 1):174 (Abstr.).

Fangman, T. J., M. S. Roderick, and C. Tubbs. 1997. Segregated early weaning, *Swine Health Prod.*, 5:195.

Fitzpatrick, D. W., and H. S. Bayley. 1977. Evaluation of blood meal as protein source for young pigs, *Can. J. Anim. Sci.*, 57:745.

Fowler, V. R., and B. P. Gill. 1989. Voluntary food intake in the young pig. In *The Voluntary Food Intake of Pigs*, Forbes, J. M., M. A. Varley, and T. L. J. Lawrence, Eds., British Society of Animal Production, Edinburgh, 51.

Frederick, B. R., and T. S. Stahly. 1999. Dietary available phosphorus needs of high lean pigs, *J. Anim. Sci.*, 78:(Suppl. 1):59 (Abstr.).

Friesen, K. G., R. D. Goodband, J. L. Nelssen, F. Blecha, D. N. Reddy, P. G. Reddy, and L. J. Kats. 1993a. The effect of pre- and post-weaning exposure to soybean meal on growth performance and the immune response in the early-weaned pig, *J. Anim. Sci.*, 71:2089.

Friesen, K. G., J. L. Nelssen, R. D. Goodband, K. C. Behnke, and L. J. Kats. 1993b. The effect of moist extrusion of soy products on growth performance and nutrient utilization in the early-weaned pig, *J. Anim. Sci.*, 71:2099.

Gatnau, R., and D. R. Zimmerman. 1990. Spray dried porcine plasma (SDPP) as a source of protein for weanling pigs, *J. Anim. Sci.*, 68(Suppl. 1):374 (Abstr.).

Gatnau, R., and D. R. Zimmerman. 1991. Spray dried porcine plasma (SDPP) as a source of protein for weanling pigs in two environments, *J. Anim. Sci.*, 69(Suppl.1):103 (Abstr.).

Gatnau, R., D. R. Zimmerman, T. Diaz, and J. Johns. 1991. Determination of optimum levels of inclusion of spray-dried porcine plasma (SDPP) in diets for weanling pigs, *J. Anim. Sci.*, 69(Suppl.1):369 (Abstr.).

Giesting, D. W., R. A. Easter, and B. A. Roe. 1985. A comparison of protein and carbohydrate sources of milk and plant origin, *J. Anim. Sci.*, 61(Suppl. 1):299 (Abstr.).

Goodband, R. D., M. D. Tokach, S. S. Dritz, and J. L. Nelssen. 1995. Practical nutrition for the segregrated early weaned pig. In *Proc. of Saskatchewan Pork Industry Symp.*, Saskatoon, Saskatchewan. 15.

Hahn, J. D., and D. H. Baker. 1993. Growth and plasma zinc responses of young pigs fed pharmacologic levels of zinc, *J. Anim. Sci.*, 71:3020.

Han, Y., T. K. Chung, and D. H. Baker. 1993. Tryptophan requirement of pigs in the weight category 10 to 20 kilograms, *J. Anim. Sci.*, 71:139.

Hansen, E. L., C. R. Hamilton, G. W. Libal, and D. N. Peters. 1995. Effects of dietary level of whey, skim milk and protein on separate sex feeding of gilts, barrows and boars in the nursery phase, *J. Anim. Sci.*, 73(Suppl. 1):71 (Abstr.).

Hansen, J. A., R. D. Goodband, J. L. Nelssen, and T.L. Weeden. 1990. Effect of substituting spray-dried plasma protein for milk products in starter pig diets, *Kans. Swine Day Proc.*, p. 30.

Hansen, J. A., J. L. Nelssen, R. D. Goodband, and T. L. Weeden. 1993. Evaluation of animal protein supplements in diets of early-weaned pigs, *J. Anim. Sci.*, 71:1853.

Hays, V. W. 1978. Effectiveness of feed additive usage of antibacterial agents in swine and poultry production, Report to the Office of Technology Assessment, U.S. Congress, U.S. Government Printing Office, Washington, D.C.

Hill, G. M., G. L. Cromwell, T. D. Crenshaw, R. C. Ewan, D. A. Knabe, A. J. Lewis, D. C. Mahan, G. C. Shurson, L. L. Southern, and T. L. Veum. 1996. Impact of pharmacological intakes of zinc and/or copper on performance of weanling pigs, *J. Anim. Sci.*, 74(Suppl. 1):181 (Abstr.).

Hodge, R. W. 1974. Efficiency of food conversion and body composition of the pre-ruminant lamb and the young pig, *Br. J. Nutr.*, 32:113.

Hongtrakul, K., J. R. Bergstrom, R. D. Goodband, K. C. Behnke, W. B. Nessmith, M. D. Tokach, and J. L. Nelssen. 1996. The effect of carbohydrate source and extrusion processing on growth performance of early-weaned pigs, *J. Anim. Sci.*, 74(Suppl. 1):169 (Abstr.).

Howard, K. A., D. M. Forsyth, and T. R. Cline. 1990. The effect of adaptation period to soybean oil additions in the diet of young pigs, *J. Anim. Sci.*, 68:678.

Jensen, A. H., and D. E. Becker. 1965. Effect of pelleting diets and dietary components on the performance of young pigs, *J. Anim. Sci.*, 24:392.

Jensen, M. S., S. K. Jensen, and K. Jakobsen. 1997. Development of digestive enzymes in pigs with emphasis on lipolytic activity in the stomach and pancreas, *J. Anim. Sci.*, 75:437.

Jepson, M. M., J. M. Pell, P. C. Bates, and D. J. Millward. 1986. The effects of endotoxemia on protein metabolism in skeletal muscle and liver of fed and fasted rats, *Biochem. J.*, 235:329.

Johnson, R. 1992. Role of acidifiers and enzymes in assuring performance and health of pigs post-weaning. In *Biotechnology in the Feed Industry. Proc. Alltech's Eighth Annu. Symp.*, Alltech Technical Publications, Nicholasville, KY, 139.

Johnson, R. W. 1997. Explanation for why sick pigs neither eat well nor grow well. In *Proc. Thirteenth Annual Carolina Swine Nutr. Conf.*, p. 49.

Kats, L. J., J. L. Nelssen, M. D. Tokach, R. D. Goodband, J. A. Hansen, and J. L. Laurin. 1994a. The effect of spray-dried porcine plasma on growth performance in the early-weaned pig, *J. Anim. Sci.*, 72:2075.

Kats, L. J., J. L. Nelssen, M. D. Tokach, R. D. Goodband, T. L. Weeden, S. S. Dritz, J. A. Hansen, and K. G. Friesen. 1994b. The effect of spray-dried blood meal on growth performance of the early-weaned pig, *J. Anim. Sci.*, 72:2860.

Kerr, B. J. 1993. Optimizing lean tissue deposition in swine, BioKyowa Technical Review 6, Nutri Quest, Chesterfield, MO.

Kerr, C. A., R. D. Goodband, M. D. Tokach, J. L. Nelssen, S. S. Dritz, B. T. Richert, and J. R. Bergström. 1998. Evaluation of enzymatically modified potato starches in diets for weanling pigs, *J. Anim. Sci.*, 76:2838.

Kidder, D. E., and M. J. Manners. 1978. *Digestion in the Pig*, Kingston, Bath, U.K.

Kim, I. B., and G. L. Allee. 1997. Effect of carbohydrate source in phase 1 and phase 2 starter diets, *J. Anim. Sci.*, 75(Suppl. 1):58 (Abstr.).

Kirchgessner, M., F. X. Roth, U. Eidelsburger, and B. Gedek. 1993. The nutritive efficiency of *Bacillus cereus* as a probiotic in the raising of piglets. 1. Effect on the growth parameters and gastrointestinal environment. *Arch. Tierernähr.*, 44:111.

Klasing, K. C. 1988. Nutritional aspects of leukocytic cytokines, *J. Nutr.*, 118:1436.

Kornegay, E. T., D. Rhein-Welker, M. D. Lindemann, and C. M. Wood. 1995. Performance and nutrient digestibility in weanling pigs as influenced by yeast culture additions to starter diets containing dried whey or one of two fiber sources, *J. Anim. Sci.*, 73:1381.

Lallès, J. P. 1993. Nutritional and antinutritional aspects of soyabean and field pea proteins used in veal calf production: a review, *Livest. Prod. Sci.*, 34:181.

Lallès, J. P. 1999. Soy products as protein sources for preruminants and young pigs. In *Soy in Animal Nutrition Symposium, Proc. Global Soy Forum*, Chicago, IL.

Landblom, D. G., and W. W. Poland. 1997. Replacement value of Paul naked oat in weanling pig starter diets, *J. Anim. Sci.*, 75(Suppl. 1):58 (Abstr.).

Lawlor, P. G., P. B. Lynch, and P. J. Caffrey. 1998. Effect of cereal cooking on the performance of newly weaned pigs fed a diet with a high or low level of dairy products, *J. Anim. Sci.*, 76(Suppl. 1):166 (Abstr.).

Lawrence, N. J., and C. V. Maxwell. 1983. Effect of dietary fat source and level on the performance of neonatal and early-weaned pigs, *J. Anim. Sci.*, 57:936.

Lecce, J. G., W. D. Armstrong, P. C. Crawford, and G. A. Ducharme. 1979. Nutrition and management of early weaned piglets: liquid vs. dry feeding, *J. Anim. Sci.*, 48:1007.

Lei, X. G., P. K. Ku, E. R. Miller, and M. T. Yokoyama. 1993. Supplementing corn–soybean meal diets with microbial phytase linearly improves phytate phosphorus utilization by weanling pigs, *J. Anim. Sci.*, 71:3359.

Lewis, A. J., P. S. Miller, and C. K. Wolverton. 1995. Bioavailability of iron in iron methionine for weanling pigs, *J. Anim. Sci.*, 73(Suppl. 1):172 (Abstr.).

Lewis, A. J., H. Y. Chen, and P. S. Miller. 1999. Bioavailability of iron in iron proteinate for weanling pigs, *J. Anim. Sci.*, 77:(Suppl. 1)61 (Abstr.).

Li, D. F., J. L. Nelssen, P. G. Reddy, F. Blecha, J. D. Hancock, G. L. Allee, R. D. Goodband, and R. D. Klemm. 1990. Transient hypersensitivity to soybean meal in the early-weaned pig, *J. Anim. Sci.*, 68:1790.

Li, D. F., J. L. Nelssen, P. G. Reddy, F. Blecha, R. D. Klemm, and R. D. Goodband. 1991. Interrelationship between hypersensitivity to soybean proteins and growth performance in early-weaned pigs, *J. Anim. Sci.*, 69:4062.

Li, S., W. C. Sauer, S. X. Huang, and V. M. Gabert. 1996. Effect of β-glucanase supplementation to hulless barley- or wheat-soybean meal diets on the digestibilities of energy, protein, β-glucans, and amino acids in young pigs, *J. Anim. Sci.*, 74:1649.

Lindemann, M. D., S. G. Cornelius, S. M. El Kandelgy, R. L. Moser, and J. E. Pettigrew. 1986. Effect of age, weaning, and diet on digestive enzyme levels in the piglet, *J. Anim. Sci.*, 62:1298.

Lindemann, M. D., J. L. G. van de Ligt, H. J. Monegue, G. Keller, and G. L. Cromwell. 1998. Evaluation of dried porcine solubles (DPS) as a feed ingredient for weanling pigs, *J. Anim. Sci.*, 76(Suppl. 1):181 (Abstr.).

Luo, X. G., and C. R. Dove. 1996. Effect of copper and fat on nutrient utilization, digestive enzyme activities, and tissue mineral levels in weanling pigs, *J. Anim. Sci.*, 74:1888.

Mahan, D. C. 1991. Efficacy of initial postweaning diet and supplemental coconut oil or soybean oil for weanling swine, *J. Anim. Sci.*, 69:1397.

Mahan, D. C., and E. A. Newton. 1993. Evaluation of feed grains with dried skim milk and added carbohydrate sources on weanling pig performance, *J. Anim. Sci.*, 71:3376.

Mahan, D. C., A. J. Lepine, and K. Dabrowski. 1994. Efficacy of magnesium-L-ascorbyl-2-phosphate as a vitamin C source for weanling and growing-finishing swine, *J. Anim. Sci.*, 72:2354.

Mahan, D. C., E. A. Newton, and K. R. Cera. 1996a. Effect of supplemental sodium chloride, sodium phosphate, or hydrochloric acid in starter pig diets containing dried whey, *J. Anim. Sci.*, 74:1218.

Mahan, D. C., E. M. Weaver, and L. E. Russell. 1996b. Improved postweaning performance responses by adding NaCl or HCl to diets containing animal plasma, *J. Anim. Sci.*, 74(Suppl. 1):58 (Abstr.).

Mahan, D. C., S. D. Carter, G. C. Cromwell, G. M. Hill, R. L. Harrold, A. J. Lewis, and T. L. Veum. 2000. Efficacy of added zinc oxide levels with and without an antibacterial agent in the postweaning diets of pigs, *J. Anim. Sci.* 78 (Suppl. 2):61 (Abstr.).

Makkink, C. A., P. J. M. Berntsen, B. M. L. op den Kamp, B. Kemp, and M. A. Verstegen. 1994. Gastric protein breakdown and pancreatic enzyme activities in response to two different dietary protein sources in newly weaned pigs, *J. Anim. Sci.*, 72:2843.

Mathew, A. G., A. L. Sutton, A. B. Scheidt, D. M. Forsyth, J. A. Patterson, and D. T. Kelly. 1991. Effects of a propionic acid containing feed additive on performance and intestinal microbial fermentation of the weanling pig. In *Proc. Sixth Int. Symp. on the Digestive Phys. in Pigs*, Wageningen, The Netherlands, 464.

Mathew, A. G., S. E. Chattin, C. M. Robbings, and D. A. Golden. 1998. Effects of a direct-fed yeast culture on enteric microbial populations, fermentation acids, and performance of weanling pigs, *J. Anim. Sci.*, 76:2138.

Matte, J. J., A. Giguere, and C. L. Girard. 1998. Vitamin B_6 in early-weaned piglets: a need to revise the requirement? *J. Anim. Sci.*, 76(Suppl. 1):190 (Abstr.).

Mavromichalis, I., J. D. Hancock, B. W. Senne, H. Cao, and R. H. Hines. 1998. Arabinoxylanase supplementation and particle size of wheat-based diets in nursery and finishing pigs, *J. Anim. Sci.*, 81(Suppl. 2):62 (Abstr.).

McCalla, J. M., D. D. Gallaher, L. J. Johnston, M. H. Whitney, and G. C. Shurson. 1999. Evaluation of the optimal growth promoting level of dietary Zn from a Zn amino acid complex for weanling pigs, *J. Anim. Sci.*, 78:(Suppl. 1):64 (Abstr.).

McNutt, S. D., and R. C. Ewan. 1984. Energy utilization of weaning pigs raised under pen conditions, *J. Anim. Sci.*, 59:738.

Nam, D. S., and F. X. Aherne. 1994. The effects of lysine:energy ratio on the performance of weanling pigs, *J. Anim. Sci.*, 72:1247.

Nessmith, W. B., M. D. Tokach, R. D. Goodband, J. L. Nelssen, J. R. Bergström, J. W. Smith, K. Q. Owen, and B. T. Richert. 1995. The effects of substituting spray-dried whole egg from grading plants only for spray-dried animal plasma in phase 1 diets, *J. Anim. Sci.*, 73(Suppl. 1):171 (Abstr.).

Nessmith, W. B., Jr., J. L. Nelssen, M. D. Tokach, R. D. Goodband, and J. R. Bergström. 1997a. Effects of substituting deproteinized whey and/or crystalline lactose for dried whey on weanling pig performance, *J. Anim. Sci.*, 75:3222.

Nessmith, W. B., Jr., J. L. Nelssen, M. D. Tokach, R. D. Goodband, J. R. Bergström, S. S. Dritz, and B. T. Richert. 1997b. Evaluation of the interrelationships among lactose and protein sources in diets for segregated early-weaned pigs, *J. Anim. Sci.*, 75:3214.

Newport, M. J., and G. L. Hawarth. 1985. Contribution of gastric lipolysis to the digestion of fat in the neonatal pig. In *Proc. 3rd Int. Seminar on Dig. Physiol. in the Pig*, Just, A., H. Jørgensen, and J. A. Fernandez, Eds., Copenhagen, Denmark, 143.

NRC (National Research Council). 1986. *Predicting Feed Intake of Food-Producing Animals*, National Academy Press, Washington, D.C., 85.

NRC. 1988. *Nutrient Requirements of Swine*, 9th ed., National Academy Press, Washington, D.C.

NRC. 1998. *Nutrient Requirements of Swine*, 10th ed., National Academy Press, Washington, D.C.

Okai, D. B., F. X. Aherne, and R. T. Hardin. 1976. Effects of creep and starter composition on feed intake and performance of young pigs, *Can. J. Anim. Sci.*, 56:573.

Owen, K. Q., J. L. Nelssen, M. D. Tokach, R. D. Goodband, S. S. Dritz, and L. J. Katz. 1993a. Spray-dried egg protein in diets for early-weaned starter pigs. In *Proc. Kansas State University Swine Day*, p. 50.

Owen, K. Q., J. L. Nelssen, M. D. Tokach, R. D. Goodband, S. S. Dritz, and L. J. Katz. 1993b. The effect of increasing level of lactose in a porcine plasma-based diet for the early weaned pig, *J. Anim. Sci.*, 71(Suppl. 1):175 (Abstr.).

Owen, K. Q., R. D. Goodband, J. L. Nelssen, M. D. Tokach, and S. S. Dritz. 1995a. The effect of dietary methionine and its relationship to lysine on growth performance of the segregated early-weaned pig, *J. Anim. Sci.*, 73:3666.

Owen, K. Q., J. L. Nelssen, R. D. Goodband, M. D. Tokach, K. G. Friesen, J. W. Smith, and L. E. Russell. 1995b. Effects of various fractions of spray-dried porcine plasma on performance of early-weaned pigs, *J. Anim. Sci.*, 73(Suppl. 1):81 (Abstr.).

Owen, K. Q., J. L. Nelssen, R. D. Goodband, M. D. Tokach, L. J. Katz, and K. G. Friesen. 1995c. Added methionine in starter diets containing spray-dried blood products, *J. Anim. Sci.*, 73:2647.

Owen, K. Q., J. L. Nelssen, R. D. Goodband, M. D. Tokach, B. T. Rickert, K. G. Friesen, J. W. Smith, J. R. Bergström and S. S. Dritz. 1995d. Dietary lysine requirements of segregated early-weaned pigs, *J. Anim. Sci.*, 73(Suppl. 1):68 (Abstr.).

Owen, K. Q., J. L. Nelssen, R. D. Goodband, T. L. Weeden, and S. A. Blum. 1996. Effect of L-carnitine and soybean oil on growth and body composition of early-weaned pigs, *J. Anim. Sci.*, 74:1612.

Partridge, I. G., and B. P. Gill. 1993. New approaches with pig weaner diets. In *Recent Advances in Animal Nutrition*, Nottingham University Press, Loughborough, U.K., 221.

Parsons, M. J., E. R. Miller, W. G. Bergen, P. K. Ku, F. F. Green, and D. E. Ullrey. 1975. Bioavailability of lysine in blood meal for swine, *J. Anim. Sci.*, 41:325 (Abstr.).

Patience, J. F., H. W. Gonyou, E. Beltranena, D. L. Whitington, and C. S. Rhodes. 1997. The impact of age and site of weaning on pig performance under high health conditions, *J. Anim. Sci.*, 75(Suppl. 1):246 (Abstr.).

Pettigrew, J. E., Jr., and R. L. Moser. 1991. Fat in swine nutrition. In *Swine Nutrition*, Miller, E. R., D. E. Ullery, and A. J. Lewis, Eds., Butterworth-Heinemann, Stoneham, MA, 133.

Pettigrew, J. E., B. G. Harmon, S. E. Curtis, S. G. Cornelius, H. W. Norton, and A. H. Jensen. 1977. Milk proteins for artificially reared piglets III. Efficacy of sodium caseinate and sweet dried whey, *J. Anim. Sci.*, 45:261.

Pierce, J. L., G. L. Cromwell, M. D. Lindemann, and R. D. Coffey. 1995. Assessment of three fractions of spray-dried porcine plasma on performance of early-weaned pigs, *J. Anim. Sci.*, 73 (Suppl. 1):81 (Abstr.).

Pierce, J. L., G. L. Cromwell, M. D. Lindemann, H. J. Moneque, E. M. Weaver, and L. E. Russel. 1996. Spray-dried bovine globulin for early weaned pigs, *J. Anim. Sci.*, 74 (Suppl. 1):171 (Abstr.).

Pluske, J. R. 1993. Psychological and Nutritional Stress in Pigs at Weaning: Production Parameters, the Stress Response, and Histology and Biochemistry of the Small Intestine, Ph.D. thesis, University of Western Australia, Perth, Australia.

Pluske, J. R., I. H. Williams, and F. X. Aherne. 1995. Nutrition of the neonatal pig. In *The Neonatal Pig, Development and Survival*, Varley, M. A., Ed., CAB International, Wallingford, U.K.

Pollmann, D. S., D. M. Danielson, and E. R. Peo, Jr. 1980. Effects of microbial feed additives on performance of starter and growing-finishing pigs, *J. Anim. Sci.*, 51:577.

Pollmann, D. S., G. L. Allee, and S. Pope. 1983. Effects of weaning age, source of whey, and lysine level on performance of starter pigs, *J. Anim. Sci.*, 57(Suppl. 1):86 (Abstr.).

Poulsen, H. D. 1989. Zinkoxid til grise i fravaenningsperioden [Zinc oxide for pigs during weaning], Meddelelse [English summary]. *Statens Husdyrbrugsforsøg* (Denmark), 746.

Qin, G., E. R. ter Elst, M. W. Bosch, and A. F. B. van der Poel. 1996. Thermal processing of whole soya beans: studies on the inactivation of antinutritional factors and effects on ileal digestibility in piglets, *Anim. Feed Sci. Technol.*, 57:313.

Radcliffe, J. S., Z. Zhang, and E. T. Kornegay. 1998. The effects of microbial phytase, citric acid, and their interaction in a corn–soybean meal diet for weanling pigs, *J. Anim. Sci.*, 76:1880.

Rahnema, S., M. A. Barrieklow, R. H. Ellis, and T. Meek. 1997. Potato chip scrap as a source of energy in the diet of nursery pigs, *J. Anim. Sci.*, 75(Suppl. 1)58 (Abstr.).

Rantanen, M. M., R. H. Hines, J. D. Hancock, M. R. Cabrera, and L. L. Burnham. 1995. Influence of oat products on growth performance of weanling pigs, *J. Anim. Sci.*, 73(Suppl. 1):78 (Abstr.).

Ravindran, V., and E. T. Kornegay. 1993. Acidification of weaner pig diets: a review, *J. Sci. Food Agric.*, 62:313.

Reeds, P. J., C. R. Field, and F. Jahoor. 1994. Do the differences between the amino acid composition of acute-phase and muscle proteins have a bearing on nitrogen loss in traumatic stress? *J. Nutr.*, 124:906.

Richert, B. T., K. R. Cera, and A. P. Schinckel. 1996. Effect of carbohydrate source and level on early-weaned pig performance, *J. Anim. Sci.*, 74(Suppl. 1):169 (Abstr.).

Risley, C. R., E. T. Kornegay, M. D. Lindemann, C. M. Wood, and W. N. Eigel. 1992. Effect of feeding organic acids on selected intestinal content measurements at various times postweaning in pigs, *J. Anim. Sci.*, 70:196.

Robertson, A. M., J. J. Clark, and J. M. Bruce. 1985. Observed energy intake of weaned piglets and its effect on temperature requirements, *Anim. Prod.*, 40:475.

Roof, M. D., and D. C. Mahan. 1982. Effect of carbadox and various dietary copper levels for weanling swine, *J. Anim. Sci.*, 55:1109.

Roth, F. X., B. Eckel, M. Kirchgessner, and U. Eidelsburger. 1992. Influence of formic acid on pH value, dry matter content, concentrations of volatile fatty acids and lactic acid in the gastrointestinal tract. 3. Communication: Investigations about the nutritive efficacy of organic acids in the rearing of piglets, *J. Anim. Physiol. Anim. Nutr.*, 67:148.

Schell, T. C., and E. T. Kornegay. 1996. Zinc concentration in tissues and performance of weanling pigs fed pharmacological levels of zinc from ZnO, Zn–methionine, Zn–lysine, or $ZnSO_4$, *J. Anim. Sci.*, 74:1584.

Senne, B. W., J. D. Hancock, I. Mavromichalis, S. L. Johnston, and J. R. Froetschner. 1997. Sorghum-based distillers grains in diets for nursery pigs, *J. Anim. Sci.*, 75(Suppl.1):70 (Abstr.).

Sewell, R. F., and C. V. Maxwell. 1966. Effects of various sources of carbohydrates in the diet of early-weaned pigs, *J. Anim. Sci.*, 25:796.

Shurson, J., L. Johnston, J. Pettigrew, and J. Hawton. 1995. Nutrition and the early weaned pig, *Proc. Manitoba Swine Sem.*, 9:21.

Smith, J. W., II, M. D. Tokach, R. D. Goodband, J. L. Nelssen, and B. T. Richert. 1997. Effects of the interrelationship between zinc oxide and copper sulfate on growth performance of early-weaned pigs, *J. Anim. Sci.*, 75:1861.

Sohn, K. S., B. S. de Rodas, M. L. Rose, and C. V. Maxwell. 1993. Alternative to fish meal and edible dried whey in early weaning pig diets, *J. Anim. Sci.*, 71(Suppl. 1):15 (Abstr.).

Sohn, K. S., C. V. Maxwell, D. S. Buchanan, and L. L. Southern. 1994. Improved soybean protein sources for early weaned pigs. I. Effects of performance and total tract amino acid digestibility, *J. Anim. Sci.*, 72:622.

Southern, L. L. 1991. Digestible amino acids and digestible amino acid requirements for swine. BioKyowa Technical Review 2, Nutri Quest, Chesterfield, MO.

Speer, V., G. Ashton, F. Diaz, and D. Catron. 1954. New I.S.C. Pre-starter "75," *Ia. Farm Sci.*, 8:3.

Spurlock, M. E. 1997. Regulation of metabolism and growth during immune challenge: an overview of cytokine function, *J. Anim. Sci.*, 75:1773.

Stahly, T. S., and D. R. Cook. 1996. Dietary B vitamin needs of pigs with a moderate or high level of antigen exposure, *J. Anim. Sci.*, 74(Suppl. 1):170 (Abstr.).

Stahly, T. S., N. H. Williams, and S. Swenson. 1994a. Impact of genotype and dietary amino acid regimen on growth of pigs from 8 to 25 kg, *J. Anim. Sci.*, 72(Suppl. 1):165 (Abstr.).

Stahly, T. S., N. H. Williams, and D. R. Zimmerman. 1994b. Impact of Carbadox on rate, efficiency and composition of growth in pigs with a low and high level of immune system activation, *J. Anim. Sci.*, 72(Suppl. 1):165 (Abstr.).

Stahly, T. S., N. H. Williams, S. G. Swenson, and R. C. Ewan. 1995a. Dietary B vitamin needs of high and moderate lean growth pigs fed from 9 to 28 kg body weight, *J. Anim. Sci.*, 73(Suppl. 1):193 (Abstr.).

Stahly, T. S., N. H. Williams, and D. R. Zimmerman. 1995b. Impact of Tylosin on rate, efficiency, and composition of growth in pigs with a low or high level of immune system activation, *J. Anim. Sci.*, 73(Suppl. 1):84 (Abstr.).

Stahly, T. S., N. H. Williams, and S. G. Swenson. 1996. Impact of Carbadox on rate, efficiency, and composition of growth in pigs with a high or low genetic capacity for lean growth, *J. Anim. Sci.*, 74(Suppl. 1):64 (Abstr.).

Stansbury, W. F., L. F. Tribble, and D. E. Orr, Jr. 1990. Effect of chelated copper sources on performance of nursery and growing pigs, *J. Anim. Sci.*, 68:1318.

Stoner, G. R., G. L. Allee, J. L. Nelssen, M. E. Johnston, and R. D. Goodband. 1990. Effect of select menhaden fish meal in starter diets for pigs, *J. Anim. Sci.*, 68:2729.

Sutton, A. I., D. M. Forsyth, J. A. Patterson, D. T. Kelly, and A. G. Mathew. 1989. Effect of Luprosil® NC on pig performance and microbial fermentation in the lower gastrointestinal tract, *J. Anim. Sci.*, 67(Suppl. 1):600 (Abstr.).

Sweet, L. R., E. T. Kornegay, and M. D. Lindemann. 1990. The effects of dietary Luprosil® NC on the growth performance and scouring index of weanling pigs, *Agribiol. Res.*, 43:271.

Swinkels, J. W. G. M., E. T. Kornegay, W. Zhou, M. D. Lindemann, K. E. Webb, Jr., and M. W. A. Verstegen. 1996. Effectiveness of a zinc amino acid chelate and zinc sulfate in restoring serum and soft tissue zinc concentrations when fed to zinc-depleted pigs, *J. Anim. Sci.*, 74:2420.

Thacker, P. A. 1998. Nutritional requirements for the suckling and early weaned pig. In *Proc. of the 8th World Conference on Animal Production*, Seoul National University, Seoul, Korea, 312.

Thomlinson, J. R., and T.L.J. Lawrence. 1981. Dietary manipulation of gastric pH in the prophylaxis of enteric disease in weaned pigs: some field observations, *Vet. Rec.*, 109:120.

Tompkins, T. 1989. Factors affecting the quality of milk based products and milk substitutes, and performance of the young pig. In *Proc. Carolina Nutr. Conf.*, North Carolina State University, Raleigh, 13.

Toplis, P., and S. Tibble. 1994. Improvement of post-weaning intake of piglets explored, *Feedstuffs*, 66:12.

Touchette, K. J., S. D. Crow, G. L. Allee, and M. D. Newcomb. 1995. Weaned pigs response to lactose (day 0–14 postweaning), *J. Anim. Sci.*, 73(Suppl. 1):70 (Abstr.).

Touchette, K. J., G. L. Allee, and M. D. Newcomb. 1996. The effects of plasma, lactose, and soy protein source fed in a phase 1 diet on nursery performance, *J. Anim. Sci.*, 74(Suppl. 1):170 (Abstr.).

Vanschoubroek, F. L. Coucke, and R. Van Spaendonck. 1971. The quantitative effect of pelleting feed on the performance of piglets and fattening pigs, *Nutr. Abstr. Rev.*, 41:1.

Veum, T. L., and A. K. M. Haque. 1994. Spray-dried poultry by-product as a replacement for spray-dried porcine plasma protein in weanling pig diets, *J. Anim. Sci.*, 72(Suppl. 2):60 (Abstr.).

Veum, T. L., R. G. Zamora, and M. P. Sherry. 1986. Utilization of soybean and milk proteins by neonatal pigs reared artificially. In *Swine in Biomedical Research*, Tumbelson, M. E., Ed., Plenum Press, New York, 1113.

Walker, W. R., C. V. Maxwell, F. N. Owens, D. S. Buchanan. 1986. Milk versus soybean protein sources for pigs. I. Effects on performance and digestibility, *J. Anim. Sci.*, 63:505.

Ward, T. L., G. L. Asche, G. F. Louis, and D. S. Pollmann. 1996. Zinc–methionine improves growth performance of starter pigs, *J. Anim. Sci.*, 74(Suppl. 1):182 (Abstr.).

Wedekind, K. J., A. J. Lewis, M. A. Giesemann, and P. S. Miller. 1994. Bioavailability of zinc from inorganic and organic sources for pigs fed corn–soybean meals diets, *J. Anim. Sci.*, 72:2681.

White, F., G. Wenham, G. A. M. Sharman, A. S. Jones, E. A. S. Rattray, and I. McDonald. 1969. Stomach function in relation to a scour syndrome in the piglet, *Br. J. Nutr.*, 23:847.

Whitney, M. H., R. L. Harrold, and S. D. Carter. 1997. Effects of naked oats on growth performance in early-weaned pigs, *J. Anim. Sci.*, 75(Suppl. 1):70 (Abstr.).

Whittemore, C. T. 1984. Nutrition of the sow and weaner. In *Proc. of the Colborn-Dawes Nutrition Conf.*, U.K.

Williams, N. H., T. S. Stahly, and D. R. Zimmerman. 1997. Effect of chronic immune system activation on the rate, efficiency, and composition of growth and lysine needs of pigs fed from 6 to 27 kg, *J. Anim. Sci.*, 75:2463.

Wilson, R. H., and J. Leibholz. 1981a. Digestion in the pig between 7 and 35 days. 1. The performance of pigs given milk and soyabean proteins, *Br. J. Nutr.*, 45:301.

Wilson, R. H., and J. Leibholz. 1981b. Digestion in the pig between 7 and 35 days of age. 2. The digestion of dry matter and the pH of digesta in pigs given milk and soyabean proteins, *Br. J. Nutr.*, 45:321.

Wilson, R. H., and J. Leibholz. 1981c. Digestion in the pig between 7 and 35 days of age. 3. The digestion of nitrogen in pigs given milk and soyabean proteins, *Br. J. Nutr.*, 45:337.

Woodworth, J. C., R. D. Goodband, J. L. Nelssen, M. D. Tokach, and R. E. Musser. 1998. Pyridoxine, but not thiamin improves weanling pig growth performance, *J. Anim. Sci.*, 81(Suppl. 2):50 (Abstr.).

Woodworth, J. C., M. D. Tokach, J. L. Nelssen, R. D. Goodband, P. R. O'Quinn, and T. M. Fakler. 2000. The effects of added zinc from zinc sulfate or zinc sulfate/zinc oxide combinations on weanling pig growth performance, *J. Anim. Sci.*, 77:(Suppl. 1):61 (Abstr.).

Wright, C. S., B. Z. deRodas, C. V. Maxwell, M. E. Davis, B. R. Dunsford, and J. D. Hahn. 1998. Effect of Problend™-65 in phase 1 diets for segregated early weaned pigs, *J. Anim. Sci.*, 76(Suppl. 1):165 (Abstr.).
Yang, H., J. A. Kerber, J. E. Pettigrew, L. J. Johnston, and R. D. Walker. 1997. Evaluation of milk chocolate product as a substitute for whey in pig starter diets, *J. Anim. Sci.*, 75:423.
Yen, J. T., and W. G. Pond. 1981. Effect of dietary vitamin C addition on performance, plasma vitamin C, and hematic iron status in weanling pigs, *J. Anim. Sci.*, 53:1292.
Zamir, O., W. O'Brien, R. Thompson, D. C. Bloedow, J. E. Fischer, and P. Hasselgren. 1994. Reduced muscle protein breakdown in septic rats following treatment with interleukin-1 receptor antagonist, *Int. J. Biochem.*, 26:943.
Zani, J. L., F. Weykamp de Cruz, A. Freitas dos Santos, and C. Gil-Turnes. 1998. Effect of probiotic CenBiot on the control of diarrhoea and feed efficiency in pigs, *Appl. Microbiol.*, 84:68.
Zimmerman, D. R. 1986. Role of subtherapeutic antimicrobials in pig production, *J. Anim. Sci.*, 62(Suppl. 3):6.
Zimmerman, D. R., J. C. Sparks, and C. M. Cain. 1997. Carry-over responses to an intestinal hydrolysate in weanling pigs diets, *J. Anim. Sci.*, 75(Suppl. 1):71 (Abstr.).

32 Feeding Growing-Finishing Pigs

Tilford R. Cline and Brian T. Richert

CONTENTS

I. Factors Affecting Nutrient Requirements 717
    A. Genetics 717
    B. Sex 718
    C. Stage of Maturity 718
    D. Environmental Temperature 719
    E. Herd Health 719
II. Feeding Management Considerations 719
    A. Feed Wastage 719
    B. Calcium and Phosphorus 720
    C. Specialty Grains 720
    D. Antibiotics 720
    E. Feed Budgeting 721
    F. Feed Processing and Pelleting 721
References 722

I. FACTORS AFFECTING NUTRIENT REQUIREMENTS

The growing-finishing period(s) is generally considered to encompass the weight range from 25 or 30 to 120 kg or that time between removal from the nursery to market. This period has been considered to be the least-complicated segment of swine production, but with newer genotypes and feeding strategies it is growing in complexity. Approximately 75 to 80% of the total feed used per unit of pork marketed is consumed during this period, representing approximately 50 to 60% of the total cost of pork production. Several factors can, however, affect the growing-finishing pig's nutrient requirements. Those factors of greatest influence on the pig's growth rate and nutrient requirements are genetics, sex, herd health, environmental temperature, and stage of development. The National Research Council (NRC, 1998) has included most of these factors in the computer model used to predict nutrient requirements for today's growing-finishing pigs.

A. GENETICS

Pigs differ in their genetic potential to deposit lean (muscle) and adipose tissue (lipid) and in the pattern of development of these tissues (see Chapter 4 for a detailed discussion). Some genotypes have the potential to gain both of these body-component tissues rapidly throughout the entire growing-finishing period, whereas others gain both lean and fat slowly. Other genetic lines may fit into a slow-rapid or a rapid-slow pattern of lean and fat deposition, respectively.

    The rate and composition of weight gain during the growing-finishing period can affect the amino acid and energy needs of the pig perhaps more than other nutrients. A rapid rate of lean gain increases the need for amino acids because these nutrients are used for protein synthesis, most of which is deposited as muscle tissue (Schinckel and de Lange, 1996). On the other hand, lean deposition requires less energy than fat deposition. The deposition of 1 kg of muscle requires approximately 2.23 Mcal of energy, whereas the deposition of 1 kg of body fat requires approximately 10.30 Mcal of energy or about five times the energy cost of lean tissue gain (Noblet et al., 1999).

To formulate diets accurately for different genetic lines, it is necessary to know the rate and pattern of lean accretion and the feed intake for that specific genetic line. Seed stock suppliers may provide this information to their customers. If not, the minimum amount of information required is feed intake data for 2- to 3-week intervals and subsequent slaughter data at market time. When carcass measurements are available, total lean gain (or lean gain per day) can be calculated using published formulas (NPPC, 1991; Wagner et al., 1999). Computer models used by the NRC (NRC, 1998) to estimate the nutrient requirements of growing-finishing pigs include lean accretion as an input. Feed intake can also be entered by the user, or default values can be inserted. If values for a specific genetic line are known, they can be inserted; otherwise default values are used. For more precise estimates, monthly weight gain, tenth rib loin eye area, and backfat thickness need to be collected so the operational protein accretion rate and pattern can be determined for the specific genetics used in the operation so that diet formulation can be optimized for the specific environment (Smith et al., 1997).

B. Sex

Gilts and barrows differ in their pattern of lean and fat deposition. Gilts usually have a higher daily lean gain than barrows and have larger loin eye areas and a higher percent lean in the carcass at market weight (Schinckel, 1994; Thompson et al., 1996). This difference in lean accretion between gilts and barrows is wider in some genetic lines than in others (Wagner et al., 1999). Barrows generally consume more feed, and thus energy, than gilts and, because barrows have a lower energy need for lean tissue synthesis, the extra energy is stored as fat. Consequently, because of the higher feed intake but slightly lower amount of body lean tissue, barrows require a lower concentration of amino acids in their diet than gilts.

Because of the differences in lean and fat deposition and in feed intake, the feeding of gilts and barrows separately (split-sex feeding) is recommended. This allows for more precise formulation of diets to meet the nutrient needs of the two sexes.

Because barrows fed fortified corn–soybean diets consume more energy than is needed for lean tissue synthesis, the addition of large quantities of fat (energy) to these diets should be avoided. This effect of excess energy intake is exacerbated as the barrow approaches market weight. On a practical basis, limiting feed (energy) intake should be considered during the latter stages or phases of the finishing period for barrows. Practical diet formulation for barrows may also include fibrous feedstuffs during late finishing to limit energy intake, thus decreasing lipid accumulation. Feeding high-energy diets to gilts may or may not be of value or concern depending on the propensity of the genetic line for lean accretion and feed intake.

C. Stage of Maturity

Nutrient requirements change with age or maturity. Expressed as daily needs, the requirements increase, but when expressed as a percentage of the diet, they decrease as the animal ages (grows) or matures. Although these changes theoretically occur daily, it is not feasible or necessary to reformulate the pig's diet that frequently. Feeding several diets (phase feeding) during the growing-finishing period will lower feed costs without significant negative effects on performance (Han et al., 1998; NCR-42, unpublished data).

Probably the more important considerations of phase feeding during the growing-finishing period deal with nutrient excretion. The excretion of excess nutrients, particularly but not limited to, nitrogen and phosphorus are of major concern in the environmental area (see Chapter 27 for a detailed discussion). As diets are reformulated to minimize excesses and to reflect the animals true biological needs, there will be less wastage of nutrients in the excrement (Han et al., 1998).

D. Environmental Temperature

Ambient temperature can affect feed intake and thus nutrient requirements and performance of growing-finishing pigs (see Chapter 23 for a detailed discussion). The digestion and metabolism of the major nutrient groups (carbohydrates, fats, and proteins) provide the animal with both chemical and heat energy. The heat produced is used by the pig to maintain its body temperature if housed in cold air temperatures. Cold air temperatures stimulate feed intake to facilitate heat production. On the other hand, hot environmental temperatures will bring about a reduction in feed intake as the pig attempts to decrease heat production (Lopez et al., 1991a,b).

Diet composition has an effect on "heat" production. Fiber produces more heat during digestive and metabolic processes than do fats and oils (Stahly and Cromwell, 1986). Therefore, the feeding of fats and oils to pigs housed in hot ambient temperatures will have less of a detrimental effect on feed intake than high levels of protein or fiber.

As feed intake changes, diet formulation can and should be adjusted to ensure that the animals are fed adequate, but not excessive, levels of nutrients, particularly indispensable amino acids and macrominerals. Many swine nutrition models contain environmental temperature as a variable, and the users can insert the desired value for their conditions.

E. Herd Health

It is difficult, if not impossible, to quantify the health of pigs, but pigs of a high health status gain weight more rapidly and are more efficient in feed utilization than pigs that have clinical or subclinical diseases (Clark et al., 1991). Healthy pigs are more likely to reach their genetic potential for growth. High-health-status pigs gain lean more rapidly, but they also deposit fat at a faster rate (Holck et al., 1998). The inclusion of antibiotics and other "growth-promoting" compounds in the diets of growing-finishing pigs usually elicits an improvement in gain and feed conversion. This is probably due to the control of subclinical disease (see Chapter 18 for a detailed discussion). The response usually decreases as pigs mature. Antibacterials should not be used as substitutes for good management and sanitation.

II. FEEDING MANAGEMENT CONSIDERATIONS

A. Feed Wastage

Feed wastage is difficult to measure in most pig feeding facilities; however, it is generally acknowledged that if feed is observed to be outside the feeder, at least 10% of the feed is being wasted. Commercially available feeders have been found to have feed wastage that ranges from 1 to 34% (Baxter, 1991; Payne, 1991; Kelly, 1978). The selection of a good feeder and its correct adjustment are critically important to reduce feed wastage (Gonyou and Lou, 1997). A properly adjusted feeder has approximately one quarter to one half of the bottom pan lightly covered with feed, indicating an adequate feed flow rate.

The addition of water to the feed in liquid feeding systems has been shown to reduce feed wastage and improve feed efficiency by 3 to 8% and body weight gain by 4% (Jensen and Mikkelson, 1998). Frequent feeder adjustments and the removal of wet, unused, or older feed may increase the amount of labor needed to achieve this efficiency. The addition of water to feeders and/or feed may reduce water wastage by 40 to 50% during the summer (Rantanen et al., 1995), but the growth of molds in the feeder must be closely monitored when this type of feeder is used. Wet/dry feeders have been shown to increase feed intake and body weight gain by 5 to 8% and 4 to 6%, respectively (Payne, 1991) over traditional dry feeders. The wet/dry feeders may be a practical answer to improve feed intake in low feed intake/high lean genetics to improve body weight gain. The use of wet feeding systems is easier to manage when limited feeding is practiced because feed residues are rarely present in the feeder. The best use of a liquid system is when there is a liquid by-product that can be utilized with this feeding system to reduce feed costs. Feeder design and feeding systems are discussed in more detail in Chapter 22.

B. Calcium and Phosphorus

Because of increased environmental pressure, some producers have greatly reduced the dietary level of Ca and P in the last 4 to 6 weeks of the finishing period. This practice will result in less excretion of Ca and P without adversely affecting growth performance (Lindemann et al., 1995; van de Ligt et al., 1997; Mavromichalis et. al., 1999). There have been observations in the "packing industry" that such a practice may increase the incidence of "broken backs or vertebra" occurring at the time of stunning (S. Pederson, IBP Inc., Logansport, IN, personal communication). An excess of minerals should certainly be avoided, but caution should be used in lowering available mineral levels below the requirement.

A very appropriate method to lower the P in the excrement is to add the enzyme phytase to growing-finishing feed. This subject is discussed in detail in Chapter 27, but, in general, the feeding of 300 to 500 phytase units/kg of feed increases the P availability in a corn–soybean meal diet from 20 to 25% to 45 to 50%. This allows for the use of less total P in the diet and reduces the P excreted by a sizable quantity (Harper et al., 1997; Kemme et al., 1997; O'Quinn et al., 1997).

C. Specialty Grains

The recent explosion of research in the area of genetic engineering of plants has led to the development of "new" cereal grains for use in swine feeds. (See Chapter 35 for more details.) The one product most used currently is "high-oil" corn. High-oil corn generally contains 2 to 4% additional oil, raising the total oil level from 3 to 4% to 5 to 8% (Adeola and Bajjalieh, 1997). Diets formulated with high-oil corn will contain a higher level of metabolizable energy than diets formulated with conventional corn and in most situations will result in slightly faster gains and improved feed conversion, especially in the summer heat (Kendall et al., 1999).

As discussed earlier in this chapter, high-fat, high-energy diets are well suited for feeding during periods of high environmental temperatures. Also, rapid lean gaining gilts may benefit from the higher-energy diets, but barrows, particularly as they approach market weight, may only get fatter as they consume such a diet (Smith et al., 1999).

Another specialty corn recently available commercially is a corn low in phytic acid. Most of the P in "normal" plant seeds is present as phytic acid, which is unavailable to nonruminant animals, but the P in these mutant products is highly available. The increased availability of the plant P allows diets to be formulated with significantly less total P and results in a sizable (35 to 50%) reduction in excreted P (Pierce and Cromwell, 1999a,b,c; Sugiura et al., 1999).

D. Antibiotics

The use of antibiotics as "growth promotants" during the growing-finishing period has been a common practice in the industry for over 40 years. Antibiotics are an important management tool that has been effective in treating and/or preventing diseases. In general, young pigs demonstrate the greatest response to antibiotics in improved gain and feed efficiency with a declining improvement in pig performance as the pig ages and reaches market weight (see Chapter 18 for a more detailed discussion). There is increasing pressure to discontinue subtheraputic antibiotic use in livestock to curtail the development of microbial resistance to antibiotics. A question of concern in the industry is "how can we cope with both clinical and subclinical disease problems without feed levels of antibiotics and other chemotherapeutic agents?"

The use of probiotics is discussed in Chapter 18. These types of compounds may have more applications if antibiotic use is curtailed, but it is not likely that they will completely substitute for antibiotics currently used.

The keys to profitable pork production without antibiotics are better pig management and sanitation. Most pig producers attempt to adopt management techniques that lead to fewer "disease" problems. A small percentage substitute drugs for good management. Although a reasonably high level of sanitation is practiced by most swine producers, a higher level will be required in the absence of growth-promotant levels of antibiotics. Counteracting the potential loss of antibiotics may require those in animal production to "reinvent" fumigation as a method of sterilization.

E. Feed Budgeting

As indicated previously in this chapter, it is generally recommended that growing-finishing pigs be fed several diets with decreasing concentrations of amino acids and macrominerals as they mature to meet more closely their metabolic needs and to minimize the excretion of N and P. A very practical question is when does one make changes? Scientifically, it might be more correct to make changes at given weights of pens of pigs, but this is not practical in most growing-finishing facilities.

Two feed-budgeting methods are available that do not require the routine weighing of pigs. A predetermined amount of feed per pig can be fed and then the diet can be changed. Alternatively, a diet can be fed for a predetermined time period and then the pigs can be fed the next phase diet. In both cases, a relatively accurate estimate of gain and feed conversion must be available to predict the diet composition needed at that period. Pig weights should be periodically monitored to verify that the feed amount or time period was estimated accurately.

F. Feed Processing and Pelleting

Fine grinding of feed is effective in improving feed utilization and decreasing dry matter and N and P excretion. By reducing the particle size, the surface area of the grain particles is increased, allowing for greater interaction with digestive enzymes. When particle size is reduced from 1000 to 400 μm, dry matter and N digestibility increase by approximately 5 to 6% (Hale and Thompson, 1986; Wondra et al., 1995). As particle size is reduced from 1200 to 600 μm, dry matter and N excretion are reduced by 20 and 24%, respectively. Finer grinding is a simple but effective way to reduce the swine waste concentration of dry matter and N with minimal cost to the producer. The industry-average particle size is approximately 1100 μm with the recommended size being between 650 and 750 μm. Reducing particle size further increases the energy costs of grinding and reduces the throughput of the mill below the economic returns for finer grinding as well as increasing the incidence of stomach ulcers in pigs (Healy et al., 1994).

Pelleting of diets is an effective way to improve feed efficiency for all phases of swine production. However, pelleting of diets will not likely increase feed intake or gain during most production phases. During the nursery phase where very fine ingredients are fed, a slight increase in feed intake may be observed when the diet is pelleted with a pronounced improvement in feed efficiency. Generally, a 4 to 6% improvement in feed efficiency is observed with pelleted diets compared with the meal form in most phases of production (Szabo, 1988; Wondra et al., 1995). The improved feed efficiency is due to several factors. The first is a slight reduction in feed wastage; the second is a slight improvement in digestibility of the diet because the steam heat of the pelleting process gelatinizes some of the starch, thereby increasing the susceptibility area of the diet to digestive enzyme hydrolysis. A side benefit to pelleting the diet is a 10 to 15% reduction in dry matter and N excretion caused by the reduced wastage and improved feed efficiency and digestibility. On the negative side, pelleting does increase the cost of feed. Other aspects of feed processing are discussed in Chapter 21.

REFERENCES

Adeola, O., and N. L. Bajjalieh. 1997. Energy concentration of high-oil corn varieties for pigs, *J. Anim. Sci.*, 75:430.

Baxter, M. R. 1991. The design of the feeding environment for pigs, in *Manipulating Pig Production III*, Batterham, E. S., Ed., Australasian Pig Science Association, Attwood, Australia, p. 150.

Clark, L. K., A. B. Schedit, C. N. Armstrong, K. Knox, and V. B. Mayrose. 1991. The effect of all-in/all-out management on pigs from a herd with enzootic pneumonia, *Vet. Med.*, 86:946.

Gonyou, H. W., and Z. Lou. 1997. Grower/finisher feeders: design, behavior and performance, Prairie Swine Center Monograph, 97-01, p. 24.

Hale, O. M., and L. M. Thompson. 1986. Influence of particle size of wheat on performance of finishing swine, *Nutr. Rep. Int.*, 33:307.

Han, I. K., J. H. Kim, K. S. Chu, Z. N. Xuan, K. S. Sohn, and M. K. Kim. 1998. Effect of phase feeding on the growth performance and nutrient utilization in finishing pigs, *AJAS*, 11(5):559.

Harper, A. F., E. T. Kornegay, and T.C. Schell. 1997. Phytase supplementation of low phosphorus growing-finishing pig diets improves performance, phosphorus digestibility, and bone mineralization and reduces phosphorus excretion, *J. Anim. Sci.*, 75:3174.

Healy, B. J., J. D. Hancock, G. A. Kennedy, P. J. Bramel-Cox, K. C. Behnke, and R. H. Hines. 1994. Optimum particle size of corn and hard and soft sorghum for nursery pigs, *J. Anim. Sci.*, 72:2227.

Holck, J. T., A. P. Schinckel, J. L. Coleman, V. M. Wilt, M. K Senn, B. J. Thacker, E. L. Thacker, and A. L. Grant. 1998. The influence of environment on the growth of commercial finisher pigs, *Swine Health Prod.*, 6 (4):141.

Jensen, B. B., and L. L. Mikkelsen. 1998. Feeding liquid diets to pigs. In *Recent Advances in Animal Nutrition 1998*, Garnsworthy, P. C., and J. Wiseman, Eds., Nottingham University Press, Thrumpton, Nottingham, 107.

Kelly, M. 1978. Feed wastage in flat-decks, *Pig Farm.*, 27(12):62.

Kemme, P. A., J. S. Radcliffe, A. W. Jongbloed, and Z. Mroz. 1997. Factors affecting phosphorus and calcium digestibility in diets for growing-finishing pigs, *J. Anim. Sci.*, 75:2139.

Kendall, D. C., K. A. Bowers, B. T. Richert, and T. R. Cline. 1999. Evaluation of high-oil corn feeding straegies for grow-finish pigs, *J. Anim. Sci.*, 77(Suppl. 1):65 (Abstr.).

Lindemann, M. D., G. L. Cromwell, G. R. Parker, and J. H. Randolph. 1995. Relationship of length of time of inorganic phosphate removal from the diet on performance and bone strength of finishing pigs, *J. Anim. Sci.*, 73(Suppl. 1):174 (Abstr.).

Lopez, J., G. W. Jesse, B. A. Becker, and M. R. Ellersieck. 1991a. Effects of temperature on the performance of finishing swine: I. Effects of a hot, diurnal temperature on average daily gain, feed intake, and feed efficiency, *J. Anim. Sci.*, 69:1843.

Lopez, J., G. W. Jesse, B. A. Becker, and M. R. Ellersieck. 1991b. Effects of temperature on the performance of finishing swine: II. Effects of a cold, diurnal temperature on average daily gain, feed intake, and feed efficiency, *J. Anim. Sci.*, 69:1850.

Mavromichalis, I., J. D. Hancock, I. H. Kim, B. W. Senne, D. H. Kropf, G. A. Kennedy, R. H. Hines, and K. C. Behnke. 1999. Effects of omitting vitamin and trace minerals premixes and/or reducing inorganic phosphorus additions on growth performance, carcass characteristics, and muscle quality in finishing pigs, *J. Anim. Sci.*, 77:2700.

Noblet, J., C. Karege, S. Dubois, and J. van Milgen. 1999. Metabolic utilization of energy and maintenance requirements in growing pigs: effects of sex and genotype, *J. Anim. Sci.*, 77:1208.

NPPC. 1991. *Procedures to Evaluate Market Hogs*, 3rd ed., National Pork Producers Council, Des Moines, IA.

NRC. 1998. *Nutrient Requirements of Swine*, 10th ed., National Academy Press, Washington, D.C.

O'Quinn, P. R., D. A. Knabe, and E. J. Gregg. 1997. Efficacy of Natuphos® in sorghum-based diets of finishing swine, *J. Anim. Sci.*, 75:1299.

Payne, H. G. 1991. The evaluation of single-space and wet-and-dry feeders for the Australian environment, *Manipulating Pig Production III*, Batterham, E. S., Ed., Australasian Pig Science Association, Attwood, Australia, p. 158.

Pierce, J. L., and G. L. Cromwell. 1999a. Effects of phytase on bioavailability of phosphorus in normal and low-phytic acid corn, *J. Anim. Sci.*, 77(Suppl. 1):60 (Abstr.).

Pierce, J. L., and G. L. Cromwell. 1999b. Performance and phosphorus excretion of growing-finishing pigs fed low-phytic acid corn, *J. Anim. Sci.*, 77(Suppl. 1):60 (Abstr).

Pierce, J. L., and G. L. Cromwell. 1999c. Phytase addition to normal corn- and low phytic acid corn–soybean meal diets for chicks and pigs, *J. Anim. Sci.*, 77(Suppl. 1):175 (Abstr.).

Rantanen, M. M., J. D. Hancock, R. H. Hines, and I. H. Kim. 1995. Effects of feeder design and pelleting on growth performance and water use in finishing pigs, *Kan. Exp. Sta. Rep.*, 746:112.

Schinckel, A. P. 1994. Nutrient requirements of modern pig genotypes. In *Recent Advances in Animal Nutrition*, Garnsworthy, P. C., and D. J .A. Cole, Eds., University of Nottingham Press, Nottingham, U.K., p. 133.

Schinckel, A. P., and C. F. M. de Lange. 1996. Characterization of growth parameters needed as inputs for pig growth models, *J. Anim. Sci.*, 74:2021.

Smith, J. W., II, M. D. Tokach, A. P. Schinckel, S. S. Dritz, J. L. Nelssen, and R. D. Goodband. 1997. Farm specific modeling of growth, protein and fat accretion, and nutrient requirements of finishing pigs on commercial swine farms, *J. Anim. Sci.*, 75(Suppl. 1):48 (Abstr.).

Smith, J. W., II, M. D. Tokach, P. R. O'Quinn, J. L. Nelssen, and R. D. Goodband. 1999. Effects of dietary energy density and lysine: Calorie ratio on growth performance and carcass characteristics of growing-finishing pigs, *J. Anim. Sci.*, 77:3007.

Stahly, T. S., and G. L. Cromwell. 1986. Responses to dietary additions of fiber (alfalfa meal) in growing pigs housed in a cold, warm or hot thermal environment, *J. Anim. Sci.*, 67:1870.

Sugiura, S. H., V. Raboy, K. A. Young, F. M. Dong, and R. W. Hardy. 1999. Availability of phosphorus and trace elements in low-phytate varieties of barley and corn for rainbow trout (*Oncorhynchus mykiss*), *Aquaculture*, 170 (3/4):285.

Szabo, P. 1988. Effect of consistency of feed mixtures on fattening performance, *Allattenyesztes-es-Takarmanyozas*, 37:39.

Thompson, J. M., F. Sun, T. Kuczek, A. P. Schinckel, and T. S. Stewart. 1996. The effect of genotype and sex on the patterns of protein accretion in pigs, *Anim. Sci.*, 63:265.

van de Ligt, C. P. A., M. D. Lindemann, and G. L. Cromwell. 1997. Effect of inorganic phosphorus withdrawal on absorption and retention of phosphorus and bone traits in finishing pigs, *J. Anim. Sci.*, 75(Suppl. 1):189 (Abstr.).

Wagner, J. R., A. P. Schinckel, W. Chen, J. C. Forrest, and B. L. Coe. 1999. Analysis of body composition changes of swine during growth and development, *J. Anim. Sci.*, 77:1442.

Wondra, K. J., J. D. Hancock, K. C. Behnke, R. H. Hines, and C. R. Stark. 1995. Effects of particle size and pelleting on growth performance, nutritent digestibility, and stomach morphology in finishing pigs, *J. Anim. Sci.*, 73:757.

33 Feeding Gilts during Development and Sows during Gestation and Lactation

Nathalie L. Trottier and Lee J. Johnston

CONTENTS

I. Introduction 726
II. Developing Gilts 726
    A. Objectives of Gilt Feeding Program 726
    B. Nutrition and Longevity 727
        1. Lean and Fat Accretion 727
        2. Body Condition and Feeding Intensity on Reproductive Performance 727
        3. Nutrition and Locomotor Problems 728
        4. Nutrient Needs and Practical Feeding Recommendations 729
    C. Occurrence of Puberty 730
        1. Nutrition and Hormone Interactions 731
        2. Dietary Nutrient Supply and Occurrence of Puberty 732
    D. Nutrition Pre- and Postmating 733
        1. Flushing 733
        2. Embryo Survival 733
    E. Practical Considerations 733
III. Gestating Sows 735
    A. Objectives 735
    B. Feeding Systems 735
    C. Feeding Strategies 735
        1. Constant Feeding Level 736
        2. Phase Feeding 736
        3. Interval Feeding 737
        4. Metabolic Disorders Associated with Excess Gestational Feed Intake and Weight Gain 738
    D. Mammary Development 738
    E. Modeling Nutrient Requirements 739
        1. Maintenance 739
        2. Fetal Growth 740
        3. Maternal Weight Gain 740
IV. Lactating Sows 742
    A. Objectives 742
    B. Feeding Strategies 743
        1. Postfarrowing Appetite Depression and Factors That Affect Lactation Feed Intake 743
        2. Maximizing Feed Intake 744

    C. Lactation and Body Weight Loss 744
        1. Composition of Weight Loss 745
        2. Nutrition and Reproduction Interaction...745
    D. Milk Production 746
        1. Milk Production and Nutrient Composition..746
        2. Nutrient Uptake by the Mammary Gland..749
    E. Modeling Amino Acids and Energy Needs for Lactation...750
        1. Amino Acid Requirements...750
        2. Energy Requirement...752
V. Feed Ingredients and Diet Composition..754
    A. Common Feed Ingredients..754
    B. Use of Dietary Fiber 755
    C. Selected Aspects of Mineral Nutrition 757
        1. Calcium and Phosphorus 757
        2. Calcium and Magnesium 757
        3. Chromium...757
        4. Selenium and Vitamin E 758
    D. Dietary Fat...758
VI. Practical Considerations of Gestation and Lactation Feeding Programs 759
    A. Economics 759
    B. Implementation Issues..759
VII. Feeding from Weaning to Rebreeding...760
References 761

I. INTRODUCTION

Nutrition of the gilt and the sow has evolved rapidly over the past 20 years. The importance of formulating diets according to genetic potential and production level is now recognized. This recognition has arisen from research addressing problems at a factorial and mechanistic level as well as from models integrating the last 20 years of empirical data. This chapter covers applied and biological aspects of nutrition for the replacement gilt, gestating, lactating, and dry sow. Feeding practices at each production stage have specific objectives. However, because of the interrelation between each production stage, feeding practices must be geared to a long-term beneficial reproductive outcome. The way the replacement gilt is nutritionally managed during growth will impact reproductive longevity. Feeding of pregnant sows is not only concerned with optimizing fetal survival and growth but also with maximizing voluntary feed intake during lactation. While the short-term objective of feeding lactating sows is to maximize litter growth rate, the long-term objective is to minimize the weaning-to-estrus interval during the dry period and maximize ovulation rate for the following pregnancy. These issues are discussed using the current literature with an emphasis on nutrient requirements.

II. DEVELOPING GILTS

A. OBJECTIVES OF GILT FEEDING PROGRAM

Nutrition of the gilt during rearing may have short- and long-term effects on reproduction. Thus, the objectives behind a gilt's feeding program are to optimize reproductive productivity and longevity. In this first section of the chapter, the nutrition of the growing and prepubertal gilt will be covered with special interest in the influence of nutrition during rearing on reproduction and longevity.

B. NUTRITION AND LONGEVITY

1. Lean and Fat Accretion

The tremendous capacity of swine to accumulate fat during their prepubertal life is characteristic of the gilt. The prepubertal period represents the time of most rapid weight gain, particularly in lean body mass, followed by an increasing propensity to fatten. The percentage of body fat in the growing gilt relative to body weight has been shown to reach 25, 32, 34, and 38% at live weight of 23, 68, 91, and 114 kg, respectively, while the percentage of lean tissue mass decreases to 62, 58, 56, and 52%, respectively (Richmond and Berg, 1971).

2. Body Condition and Feeding Intensity on Reproductive Performance

The body condition at which gilts enter their productive life is one of the many factors that affect sow longevity. High culling rate may be related to low body fat stores (Whittemore et al., 1980; Esbenshade et al., 1986). In general, as parity increases, culling rate for anestrus and failure to breed decreases while culling rate for other reasons such as decreased productivity increases (Trottier, 1991). Thus, culling for reproductive reasons is mostly restricted to young sows (replacement gilts, primiparous and second parity). With the combined effects of genetic selection for leaner pigs and earlier mating, modern gilts begin their breeding lives with lower fat reserves. Whether the lower body fat reserve is related to the short breeding life (fewer than three parity) of modern sows remains speculative. It has been suggested that selection for reduced backfat depth may have an adverse effect of long-term reproductive performance of sows. In a large study using 1072 Large White sows, the effect of backfat depth at selection on first litter and lifetime reproductive performance was investigated (Gaughan et al., 1995). Backfat depth at mating was related positively to lifetime productivity of sows (Table 33.1).

Few studies have investigated the effect of feeding level during rearing and body condition at puberty on subsequent reproductive performance and longevity of breeding sows. Gueblez et al. (1985) demonstrated that the level of backfat at 100 kg live weight was highly correlated with the breeding longevity. In sows having over 20 mm of backfat, 46% reached the fourth parity, compared to 28% of the sows with 14 mm and less of backfat. On the other hand, the number of piglets born alive and weaned tended to be greater in the leaner sows at 100 kg live weight for the first two parities. Similar results were reported by Vangen (1980). Sorensen et al. (1993) conducted a study where gilts were fed either a control diet restricted to allow for maintenance and growth, a diet fed at 75% of control, and a diet providing *ad libitum* access twice per day for 30 min. This resulted

TABLE 33.1
Lifetime Reproductive Productivity for Sows Selected for Different Leanness at Mating

| | Selection Group | | | |
Item	Lean	Moderate	Fat	Significance
Litters per sow	2.81	3.47	3.75	$p < 0.05$
Total pigs born per sow	27.47	34.85	37.55	$p < 0.05$
Piglet birth weight (kg)	1.51	1.34	1.32	$p < 0.05$
Total pigs born alive per sow	24.03	30.86	32.76	$p < 0.05$
Piglet weaning weight (kg)	6.87	6.71	6.47	$p < 0.05$
Total pigs weaned per sow	21.91	27.63	30.08	$p < 0.01$
Piglet mortality (%)	24.27	25.15	22.76	

Source: Adapted from Gaughan et al. (1995).

TABLE 33.2
Effect of Rearing Intensity on Litter Size and Litter Weight Averaged through Parity 1 to 4

Item	Rearing Intensity			Significance (P value)
	75% Control	Control	Semi-*ad libitum*	
Litter size				
Live born	9.1	10.1	9.9	0.26
Live weaned	8.6	9.4	9.3	0.19
Litter weight (kg)				
At birth	15.4	17.3	16.6	0.57
At weaning	72.2	75.6	75.8	0.51

Source: Adapted from Sorensen et al. (1993).

in significantly different feed intake level between 6 weeks of age to mating (286, 401, and 456 kg, for 75% control, control, and semi-*ad libitum*, respectively). Gilts were studied from mating throughout the subsequent four parities. Despite the differential feed intake during rearing and weight at mating (109, 129, and 134 kg, for restricted, control, and semi-*ad libitum*, respectively), milk yield, litter size, and interval between weaning and estrus at each production cycle were not significantly different. However, number of pigs born alive and weaned tended to be lower in the gilts fed 75% control and tended to be higher in gilts fed control (Table 33.2). Similar benefits of restricted feeding were reported by den Hartog and Verstegen (1990) where gilts fed a restricted dietary regimen during rearing produced more litters compared with gilts provided *ad libitum* access to feed. A feeding level during rearing of 2.5 times maintenance energy requirements or higher decreased reproductive performance (den Hartog, 1984). In a recent study, energy restriction to 90 and 75% of *ad libitum*-fed gilts between 13 and 25 weeks of age increased the number of live embryos at 30 days of gestation (Klindt et al., 1998). In another study using several modern genetic lines, gilts were assigned to various development diets at 120 days of age, i.e, a high-energy, high-protein (18%) diet provided on an *ad libitum* scheme or restricted, and a high-energy, low-protein (13%) diet provided *ad libitum* until 180 days of age (Long et al., 1998). Although the various development diets had no influence on first-parity reproductive performance, the probability of gilts farrowing a litter was highest for gilts fed on a restricted basis, and the gilts receiving *ad libitum* access to the high-energy, high-protein diet had the poorest stayability through four parities (Long et al., 1998). In contrast, one study looking at the effect of body composition at first breeding on long-term sow productivity and longevity over three parities did not show any response (Rozeboom et al., 1996).

3. Nutrition and Locomotor Problems

Structural soundness of the developing gilt's legs is a critical component of sow longevity. The annual culling rate due to locomotor problems in gilts and sows is 13 and 11%, respectively (Dewey et al., 1992), but much higher percentages have been reported, up to 20 and 45% in sows (D'Allaire et al., 1992). Locomotor problems refer to a number of conditions, such as lameness, injury, posterior paralysis, fracture, and downer sow syndrome (D'Allaire et al., 1992). Causes of lameness are osteochondrosis, foot rot, infectious arthritis, osteomalacia, and fractures (Hill et al., 1986). Osteochondrosis is the major cause of leg weakness among young, breeding age swine and sows (Martin et al., 1987; Dewey et al., 1993). Because many factors can contribute to lameness, such as floor designs, bedding and floor condition, environmental conditions, rearing system, and genetics, the role of nutrition in the etiology of leg weakness or lameness is poorly understood and often conflicting. For example, earlier studies (Vaughan,

1971; Grondalen, 1974) have shown that fast-growing pigs would appear to be more prone to locomotor problems while others did not show such a relationship (Nakano and Aherne, 1977; Nakano et al., 1979). In addition, studies designed to address the effect of nutrition on leg weakness in gilts and its impact on sow longevity require long-term experiments involving large numbers of animals, which are difficult criteria to meet (Dourmad et al., 1994). Therefore, it is difficult to make precise nutritional recommendations for the growing gilt to ensure structural soundness throughout her reproductive life. Few studies have been conducted to determine the macromineral and vitamin needs of the developing skeleton for gilts destined for breeding. Similarly, limited information is available regarding the importance of protein nutrition, or interactions between minerals and energy. Restricting energy intake to 78% of the energy consumed in gilts allowed *ad libitum* access to feed, and increasing calcium and phosphorus to 150% of NRC (1973) recommendations did not improve structural soundness in growing gilts and in sows kept for three parities (Calabotta et al., 1982; Arthur et al., 1983). A few studies have investigated the effect of dietary energy, feeding level, and body condition throughout development and reproductive cycles on leg disorders and lameness. The incidence of leg disorders after the fourth parity in gilts reared under various levels of nutritional intensity (semi-*ad libitum*, control, and 75% control) was examined (Sorensen et al., 1993). Significantly higher incidence of leg disorders was found in gilts fed at a levels higher (semi-*ad libitum*) than required for maintenance and moderate growth (Table 33.3). Incidence of leg disorders was lowest in gilts fed for growth and maintenance (control) or restricted to 75% of control.

TABLE 33.3
Effect of Rearing Intensity on Leg Weakness Traits[a]

Trait	Rearing Intensity			Significance (P value)
	75% Control	Control	Semi-*ad libitum*	
Sum of all traits	22.15	22.46	23.55	0.002
Selected traits				
Fore legs,				
Weak pasterns	1.68	1.5	1.94	0.53
Accessory digits	1.11	1.24	1.36	0.05
Hind legs,				
Weak pasterns	1.41	1.44	1.66	0.09
Legs turned out	1.76	1.87	1.89	0.22
Stiffness	1.43	1.51	1.53	0.09
Swaying hind quarters	1.2	1.3	1.39	0.48
Lameness	1.2	1.18	1.29	0.58

[a] Data are uncorrected means of leg soundness scores at 6 months of age and in first to fourth parity.

Source: Adapted from Sorensen et al. (1993).

4. Nutrient Needs and Practical Feeding Recommendations

The nutrient needs of the replacement gilt are similar to that of the growing-finishing pig prior to entering the gilt pool, around 6 months of age. Some macromineral, trace mineral, and vitamin dietary requirements may be different for the gilt destined for breeding (Table 33.4), although research conducted in this area is lacking. Vitamin and mineral fortification should be the same as for the gestating sow diet. Maternal lines classified as high lean or high producing will be fed to maximize lean gain during the first 6 months; thus, the amino acid needs during that period will reflect the lean gain potential of the gilt. A moderate restriction in feed intake which will slow growth rate of gilts in the late finishing and prebreeding phases seems to be the most prudent

TABLE 33.4
Modified Nutrient Recommendations for Replacement Gilt Development

	Weight Range (kg)			
Item	20–45	45–70	70–90	90–110
Macro-minerals[a]				
Calcium, total (%)	0.85	0.8	0.75	0.75
Phosphorus total (%)	0.75	0.7	0.65	0.65
Phosphorus available (%)	0.49	0.45	0.4	0.4
Trace minerals[b]				
Copper (ppm)	15	15	15	15
Zinc (ppm)	150	150	150	150
Selenium (ppm)	0.3	0.3	0.3	0.3
Vitamin E (IU/kg)[b]	44	44	44	66

Note: These nutrients are considered as modifications for replacement gilts.

[a] Values are total dietary levels unless denoted otherwise.
[b] Values are supplemental levels.

Source: Adapted from Tri-State Nutrition Guide (1998).

strategy. A target weight of 110 to 120 kg at mating on the second estrus is a reasonable target. In many instances with rapidly growing pigs, moderate feed restriction in late finishing and prebreeding will be necessary to prevent gilts from getting too heavy and fat; however, the specific approach may vary from farm to farm depending on genetics and management practices. Restricting feed intake to 2.25 to 2.5 kg/day of a diet that contains about 3230 kcal metabolizable energy (ME)/kg and 0.8% total lysine will provide 7.3 to 8.0 Mcal ME and 18 to 20 g lysine daily. This level of restriction should allow continued growth of body tissues without excessive fattening, while having little or no negative effects on age at puberty. In some production systems restricting feed intake is not feasible. Use of low-energy feed ingredients that dilute the energy content of the diet may be a reasonable alternative.

In gilts with less lean potential, a recommended feeding strategy is to reduce the ration, hence to feed gilts on a restricted basis to ensure a moderate increase in fatness. So far, there has been no dietary recommendation to meet specifically the energy requirement of the gilt selected for breeding. As discussed above, gilts fed a high plane of nutrition at various periods during rearing are more inclined to be culled due to locomotor problems. On the other hand, gilts entering their breeding life with insufficient fat cover may have a reduced productivity and a shorter reproductive life. In both cases, the consequence is decreased longevity. Gilts raised outside will require higher intake of energy. Table 33.5 shows feed intake and nutritional adjustments recommended for gilts raised under various environmental temperatures.

C. Occurrence of Puberty

Puberty in gilts usually occurs between 200 and 220 days of age; however, this range can be as wide as 102 to 350 days (Hughes, 1982). Factors such as genetic line, social environment, season, boar exposure, growth rate, body composition, and age have all been shown to influence onset of puberty in gilts (Hughes, 1982). It is not surprising that such a wide range in age at puberty is observed given the many and varied factors that influence its occurrence. Many of the factors mentioned above result from the production and management system chosen to produce pigs and are beyond the scope of this book. However, growth rate, body composition, and age are intimately interrelated with each other and the nutritional program implemented for gilts.

TABLE 33.5
Feed Intake and Nutritional Adjustments for Nonpregnant Gilts under Cold Stress

Effective Environmental Temperature (°C)		Feed Intake to Meet ME Needs (kg)	Percent Lysine Needed for 12 g/day Intake	Percent Calcium Needed for 16 g/day Intake	Percent Total Phosphorus Needed for 14.2 g/day Intake	Percent Available Phosphorus Needed for 8.4 g/day Intake[a]
18.3	(65°F)	1.5	0.8	1.07	0.95	0.56
10	(50°F)	2	0.6	0.8	0.71	0.42
4.4	(40°F)	2.2	0.55	0.73	0.65	0.38
−1	(30°F)	2.5	0.48	0.64	0.57	0.34
−7	(19°F)	2.8	0.43	0.57	0.51	0.3
−12	(10°F)	2.9	0.41	0.55	0.49	0.29

Note: Based on a corn–soybean meal mixture containing 3265 kcal ME/kg.

[a] Corn–soybean meal diets should be formulated to meet available P needs of gilts. At feed intakes of 2.5 kg or greater, formulating on a total P requirement will not provide enough available P for animal health and growth.

Source: Adapted from the Tri-State Nutrition Guide (1998).

Researchers have attempted to separate the effects of age, body weight, and body composition on occurrence of puberty with conflicting results. If the specific effects of each factor are known, then feeding and management systems could be devised easily to achieve given targets for each factor that have been shown to elicit puberty in gilts. One theory is that gilts must achieve a given body weight or composition before they will express their first estrus. This minimal threshold concept was advanced by research that demonstrated puberty did not occur in girls until a threshold level of fatness was achieved (Frisch, 1988). Armstrong and Britt (1987) rehabilitated nutritionally anestrous gilts and reported that body weight was higher when estrous cycles resumed compared with when gilts became anestrous but backfat depth was similar. This observation suggests that cessation and resumption of estrous cycles occurred at different body compositions. Rozeboom et al. (1993a) imposed varying degrees of dietary energy restriction on cyclic gilts and measured body composition at anestrous. They reported wide variation in body composition of individual gilts when they became anestrous regardless of degree of energy restriction. These two studies suggest that body composition alone is not the primary determinant of the onset of puberty.

A second theory is that chronological age is a primary determinant for onset of puberty. This approach holds that, as gilts achieve a given age, they are sufficiently developed to express pubertal estrus and that body composition has minimal impacts on the age at which pubertal estrus is expressed. It is difficult to determine the effects of age independent of body weight or composition because as the gilt ages it also increases in body weight and changes in body composition. The most likely trigger(s) for expression of pubertal estrus is a combination of thresholds for age and body composition. Thresholds are more conceptual in nature as opposed to definite, quantifiable levels. Achieving these thresholds does not guarantee expression of pubertal estrus but rather plays a permissive role in the onset of puberty (Kirkwood and Aherne, 1985). Once the thresholds have been achieved, they no longer serve as a factor limiting expression of pubertal estrus. Consequently, other factors assume more prominent roles in determining onset of puberty. Burnett et al. (1988) demonstrated that interval from boar exposure to pubertal estrus decreased and became less variable as gilts aged. Additionally, increasing live weight at a given age reduced the interval to expression of first estrus.

1. Nutrition and Hormone Interactions

An obvious question related to thresholds of age and body composition is how does the gilt's reproductive system know that these thresholds have been achieved? In other words, what is the body's signal to the reproductive system that reproduction can proceed normally? Metabolic condition of the gilt may be a more important and direct controller of pubertal onset than body weight or composition. Body weight or composition may simply be a correlated result of the gilt's metabolic condition with little or no direct impact on expression of estrus (Rozeboom et al., 1993a). Availability of metabolic fuels such as glucose and fatty acids significantly influences the continuation of estrous cycles in female hamsters (Schneider and Wade, 1989). Inhibiting metabolism of glucose or fatty acids individually did not affect estrous cycles in food-deprived hamsters but concurrent inhibition of glucose and fatty acid metabolism during food deprivation stopped estrous cycles. Evidently, the reproductive system monitors the availability of metabolic fuels to determine if reproduction is possible. Quantity of nutrients supplied in the diet and nutrient balance of the gilt directly influence availability of metabolic fuels. Restricting feed intake of gilts decreases episodic release of luteinizing hormone, a critical signal to initiate estrus, and refeeding restores the pulsatility of LH secretion (Armstrong and Britt, 1987; Booth, 1990). Infusing glucose in restricted-fed gilts elicited LH secretion identical to that observed in full-fed control gilts indicating that the metabolic fuel, glucose, can signal the reproductive system to function (Booth, 1990). Insulin, a metabolic hormone related to nutrient intake, has been suggested as an important signal that communicates the metabolic state of the female to the reproductive system (Johnston, 1988; Pettigrew and Tokach, 1993). In addition to metabolites and metabolic hormones, the reproductive system may monitor the degree of body fatness through circulating levels of leptin (Kiess et al., 1999). Leptin is secreted by adipocytes. Circulating leptin levels in blood are positively correlated with degree of body fat content (Kiess et al., 1999). A definitive role for leptin in reproduction of the gilts or sows has not been established.

2. Dietary Nutrient Supply and Occurrence of Puberty

Many studies have been conducted to determine the ideal nutritional program for development of gilts. Effects of dietary nutrient supply on occurrence of puberty is difficult to separate from effects of changes in body composition and weight that result from a given nutritional regimen. Nonetheless, producers and nutritionists must establish a feeding program that results in optimal development of gilts to enter the breeding herd. Kirkwood and Aherne (1985) reviewed scientific literature published to that date and concluded that "severe overfeeding or underfeeding will delay puberty, but between these, as yet, undefined limits, the effect of nutrition on puberty onset is unclear." More than 15 years later, there still is no definitive answer on the ideal feeding program for gilt development.

Restriction of energy (den Hartog, 1984) or protein intake (Jones and Maxwell, 1974; Wahlstrom and Libal, 1977) during rearing (about 30 to 100 kg body weight) of gilts can delay age at puberty. den Hartog and van Kempen (1980) determined from literature reports that age at puberty declined as average daily gain during the rearing period increased. In contrast, Rozeboom et al. (1995) found no significant relationship between lifetime average daily gain of gilts and age at puberty. However, they did report a negative relationship between daily gain of lean tissue and age at puberty. Considered collectively, these results suggest that gilts should be fed for rapid growth rate during the rearing period to encourage early expression of pubertal estrus. Restricting feed intake after achievement of puberty and establishment of regular estrous cycles may be necessary to prevent gilts from becoming too fat before breeding.

The degree of restriction may have important influences on breeding performance. Feeding high levels (2.7 times maintenance) during the early rearing period followed by restricted feeding (1.65 times maintenance) during the finishing period and before mating decreased the proportion of gilts expressing spontaneous estrus and conceiving to first insemination and increased age at puberty compared with gilts that were not fed restrictively (den Hartog and Verstegen, 1990). den Hartog (1984) found that high feeding levels (2.5 to 3.0 times maintenance needs) reduced conception rate of gilts compared with lower feeding levels (1.8 to 2.1 times maintenance) during the rearing period. It appears that a delicate balance must be achieved between high feeding levels needed to attain early puberty and restricted feeding after puberty to control weight gain if optimal reproductive performance of the gilt is to be realized.

D. Nutrition Pre- and Postmating

1. Flushing

Offering elevated levels of feed 10 to 14 days before mating to increase the number of ova ovulated is called flushing (Aherne and Kirkwood, 1985). The ovulation rate response is due primarily to increases in energy intake rather than elevated protein intake (Aherne and Kirkwood, 1985). Anderson and Melampy (1972; as cited by Aherne and Kirkwood, 1985) suggested that about 6 Mcal of additional ME are necessary to elicit optimal ovulation rates in restricted-fed gilts. About 1.8 kg of a typical corn–soybean meal diet containing 3200 kcal ME/kg will satisfy the increased nutrient needs for flushing. Alternatively, 1.8 to 2.0 kg of additional corn, wheat, sorghum or other similar high energy feedstuff will be as effective as feeding additional quantities of complete feed. Ovulation rate typically increases two to three eggs in response to flushing, but larger increases have been reported (Flowers et al., 1989). The intent of flushing is to have direct, short-term impacts on ovulation rate without substantial influence on growth rate or body composition, although the additional feed often increases body weight gain of gilts. Flushing increases gonadotropic support of the ovaries through increased frequency of luteinizing hormone (LH) pulses (Flowers et al, 1989; Beltranena et al., 1991) and increased concentration of follicle-stimulating hormone (FSH) in blood (Flowers et al., 1989). Simultaneously, circulating concentrations of insulin are increased with elevated feed intake of flushed gilts (Cox et al., 1987b; Beltranena et al., 1991) and could have positive effects on ovulation rate. Insulin can have gonadotropic effects on the ovary (Poretsky and Kalin, 1987).

Flushing may not increase ovulation rate over that normally expected but rather correct a depression of ovulation rate imposed by dietary restriction since most gilts experience some level of dietary restriction between puberty and mating. The benefits achieved by restricting feed intake to control weight gain outweigh the detrimental effects on ovulation rate when a flushing program is instituted. Increases in ovulation rate do not guarantee increases of similar magnitude in litter size at the subsequent farrowing. However, the number of eggs ovulated sets the upper limit of litter size and increases the likelihood that more total eggs will be fertilized, develop into fetuses, and survive to parturition.

2. Embryo Survival

Embryo survival during early pregnancy may be influenced by feed intake during the early postmating period. Several reports indicate that high feed intake similar to that used for flushing during the first month of gestation decreases embryo survival (den Hartog and van Kempen, 1980). However, this effect is inconsistent (Rozeboom et al., 1993b; Cassar et al., 1994). Decreased embryo survival erases any potential improvements in litter size achieved by flushing-induced increases in ovulation rate.

Embryo survival is not compromised if flushing levels of feed intake are reduced to near-maintenance levels of intake on the first day after mating (Figure 33.1) (Jindahl et al., 1996). High-level feeding during the first few days of pregnancy likely increases hepatic blood flow and clearance of progesterone resulting in depressed concentration of progesterone in blood (Jindahl et al., 1996; 1997). Adequate levels of circulating progesterone aid in orchestrating the synchronous development of the embryos and preparation of the uterus for pregnancy (Jindahl et al., 1997).

E. Practical Considerations

Successful gilt development programs begin early in the gilt's life to ensure complete preparation for a long productive life in the breeding herd. Gilts should be housed so that specially formulated

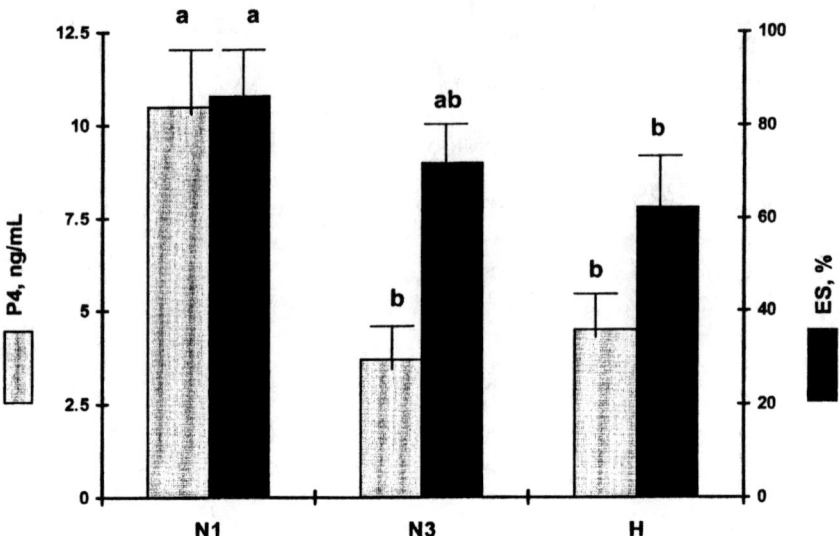

FIGURE 33.1 Embryonal survival (ES) at day 28 of pregnancy and plasma progesterone (P4) concentration on day 3 in gilts fed either 1.5× maintenance from day 1 (N1) or 3 (N3) or 2× maintenance from day 1 (H) of pregnancy. Bars with unlike superscripts differ at $P < 0.05$. (Adapted from Jindal et al., 1996.)

gilt development diets can be fed to potential replacement females without feeding this more expensive diet to slaughter hogs. Feeding gilts for efficient, rapid lean gain allows accurate assessment of the female's growth potential and enables sufficient development of body tissues that will be needed later in the female's reproductive life. Beginning at 45 kg body weight, dietary calcium and phosphorus should be increased by 0.1% above typical grow-finish diets to enhance skeletal development of gilts.

Controlled growth is the target once females enter the gilt pool at about 150 days of age. Dietary restrictions of energy will slow body growth and more importantly reduce deposition of fat tissue while allowing continued growth of lean body mass which will be beneficial to reproductive performance and longevity. Diets for females in the gilt pool contain the same vitamin and mineral fortifications as the diets for older sows in the breeding herd. Since feed intake is restricted upon entering the gilt pool, gilts must receive a flushing level of feed intake 10 to 14 days before anticipated mating to maximize ovulation rates. Feed intake must be reduced to preflushing levels immediately after breeding to avoid high rates of embryo mortality common with high postbreeding feed intake. This is easiest to accomplish with gilts that are fed and housed individually. If gilts are housed in groups and stay in groups after mating, the timing of this reduction in feed intake postbreeding is difficult because not all gilts will display estrus and be mated on the same day. Breeding barn managers will likely reduce feed intake for the entire group after the first 10 to 20% of the gilts are mated. This approach allows the majority of the gilts to be flushed effectively while minimizing the potential for reduced embryo survival. The synchrony of estrus in the group of gilts will greatly impact the timing of reduction in feed intake postbreeding.

Economic considerations of a gilt development program are difficult to determine because the biological impacts of nutritional programs for gilts in early life up to breeding on long-term reproductive performance of the female are not fully understood. It would seem intuitive that modest but necessary additional investment in nutrition and management of developing gilts is warranted since there are long-term implications for the breeding herd. It is hoped that breeding managers will become more proficient at making these economic decisions as understanding of gilt development and nutrition improves.

III. GESTATING SOWS

A. OBJECTIVES

Feeding and management during gestation focuses on preparing the sow for parturition and lactation. In the very early stages of gestation immediately after conception, the first objective is to provide conditions that will ensure maximal survival of embryos and favor a large litter size at the subsequent farrowing. Growth of the developing fetuses and increasing nutrient stores in the sow's body through growth of young sows toward their mature body size or replenishment of stores lost during the previous lactation are the main objectives during mid-gestation (day 30 to 75). In late gestation, fetal growth continues at a very rapid rate, and mammary development occurs in preparation for the upcoming lactation.

The desired outcome of a successful gestation feeding program is a large, vigorous litter of pigs and a healthy sow equipped with the adequate mammary development and body stores of nutrients to produce large quantities of milk for the suckling litter.

B. FEEDING SYSTEMS

Every feeding system has strengths and weaknesses that must be considered in light of the nutrition program, production system, and management practices. Housing sows in groups requires a very different feeding system compared with individually housed sows. The increased freedom of movement and social interaction of group-housed sows is perceived to be more "welfare-friendly" than housing sows individually. This approach to housing may decrease chronic stress experienced by sows (Barnett et al., 1987) and speed the farrowing process (Ferket and Hacker, 1985). However, the same social interactions create challenges with feeding management. Dominant sows often consume more feed than desired at the expense of sows lower on the social hierarchy. This problem, commonly referred to as the "boss sow" syndrome, increases the variability of weight gain and body condition of sows within a group. Even when sows are grouped uniformly by size, parity, and condition and close attention is paid to feeding practices, it is difficult to avoid the boss sow syndrome.

One way to control the variability of sows in groups is to install a computerized feeding station. These stations identify sows individually via an electronic ear tag or collar when the sow freely enters the station. A programmed amount of feed based on sow weight, condition, and/or stage of pregnancy is offered daily. Each sow receives her daily allotment of feed when the system is working properly and sows are accustomed to using the feeding station. A computerized feeding station greatly increases capital costs over a more conventional group-feeding system, with the advantage of controlling the boss sow problem.

Housing sows individually requires relatively inexpensive feeding equipment but increased costs for individual penning. The primary advantage of individual housing is that each sow can be handled differently if necessary, to satisfy individual nutritional requirements, effectively eliminating the boss sow syndrome. Managers can be assured that sows consume the desired amount of feed with this feeding system.

A perfect feeding system has not been developed that is well adapted to all production situations. A variety of feeding systems can work quite effectively if managed properly. Comparisons of computerized feeding with hand feeding of sows housed in individual gestation stalls revealed no significant differences in farrowing (Singleton, 1989; Blair et al., 1994) or lactation performance (Singleton, 1989) of sows.

C. FEEDING STRATEGIES

Several feeding strategies have been implemented to feed gestating sows. Three of the most common approaches are discussed below.

1. Constant Feeding Level

This approach sets a constant feeding level throughout gestation. Obviously, the initial selection of a feeding level is critical to the success of this method. Although this method is easy to implement, it does not provide flexibility to adjust nutrient intake based on body condition of the sow. This approach is based on earlier research that suggested that the total amount feed offered during gestation is a more important controller of sow performance than the pattern of feed intake (Elsley et al., 1971). However, more recent evidence suggests that modern sows may catabolize maternal tissues during the late phases of gestation (Shields and Mahan, 1983; Trottier, 1991). The impact of this catabolic state during late gestation on sow performance has not been determined.

2. Phase Feeding

Phase-feeding strategies adjust feed intake of sows to mimic nutrient needs of the developing litter *in utero*. The nutrient demands of the fetuses are very small during the first two thirds of gestation so that any adjustments in feed intake are implemented to accommodate desired changes in condition and weight gain of the sow. However, Dwyer et al. (1994) theorized that increasing feed intake of sows during the period of muscle fiber hyperplasia in growing fetuses might influence pre- and postnatal muscle development of piglets. These researchers doubled feed intake of pregnant sows from day 25 to 50, day 50 to 80, or day 25 to 80 postcoitum and reported a significant increase in the ratio of secondary to primary muscle fibers. This ratio is an indicator of muscularity in pigs. In addition, rate and efficiency of growth for pigs from sows receiving supplemental feed during the 25- to 80-day period was significantly improved compared with pigs from control sows. Under field conditions, Musser et al. (1998) reported a small but significant increase in lean content of the gilt but not barrow carcasses when sows received additional feed during mid-gestation. Many more studies under commercial conditions will be needed to determine if adjusting feed intake during this phase of the gestation period will consistently influence performance and carcass composition of offspring.

Fetal growth rate in the last trimester of pregnancy increases dramatically compared with early and mid-gestation (Figures 33.2 and 33.3). During this same period, sows may catabolize maternal tissues if maintained on a constant feeding level that satisfied their nutritional needs in earlier portions of gestation (Shields and Mahan, 1983; Trottier, 1991). These two observations have prompted many nutritionists and producers to increase feed intake during late gestation to accommodate the increased nutrient demands of rapid fetal growth. A 75% increase in feed intake during the last 23 days of gestation increased gain in sow body weight, increased birth weight of piglets, and produced larger litter size at birth and 21 days postpartum (Cromwell et al., 1989). Energy intake >6 Mcal ME/day in thermoneutral conditions is usually reflected in an increase in maternal weight gain with little influence on piglet birth weights. It is not clear if the positive responses observed in this study were the result of strategically offering extra feed in late gestation or more total feed consumed throughout the entire gestation period. In contrast, Pond et al. (1981) doubled the energy intake of sows from day 100 of gestation until parturition and observed no significant effects on piglet birth weight, survival rate of piglets, feed intake of sows during lactation, or weight gain of nursing pigs. The majority of weight gain in the products of conception in late gestation is attributable to water gain. Consequently, the energy and amino acid needs of the developing litter can be satisfied by about 0.45 kg of a typical corn–soybean meal gestation diet (Noblet et al., 1985). For less-nutrient-dense diets, >0.45 kg will be needed to meet the nutrient needs of the developing fetuses. Large increases in feed intake (1.0 to 2.25 kg/day) often employed in commercial conditions do not seem justified based on nutrient needs of the developing litter. One must be cautious of large increases in feed intake in late gestation. Such increase can have negative impacts on mammary development, and the excessive sow weight gains that result may depress feed intake during the subsequent lactation. Some aspects of excessive feed intake and weight gain on metabolism and mammary gland development are discussed later in this chapter.

Feeding Gilts during Development and Sows during Gestation and Lactation

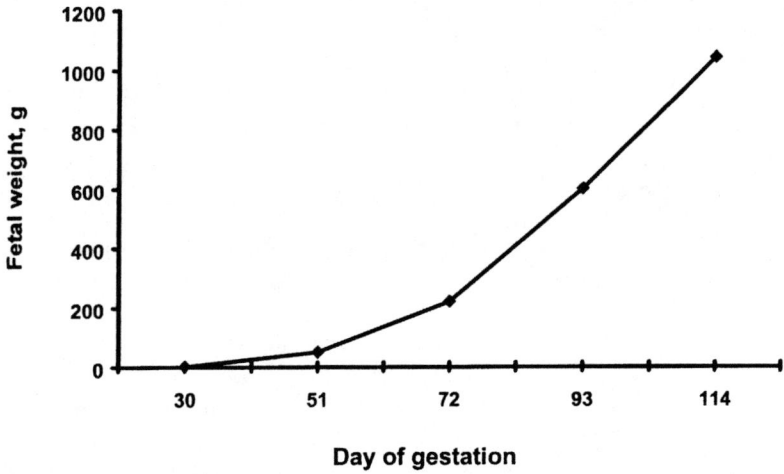

FIGURE 33.2 Relationship of fetal weight to day of gestation. (Adapted from Ullrey et al., 1965.)

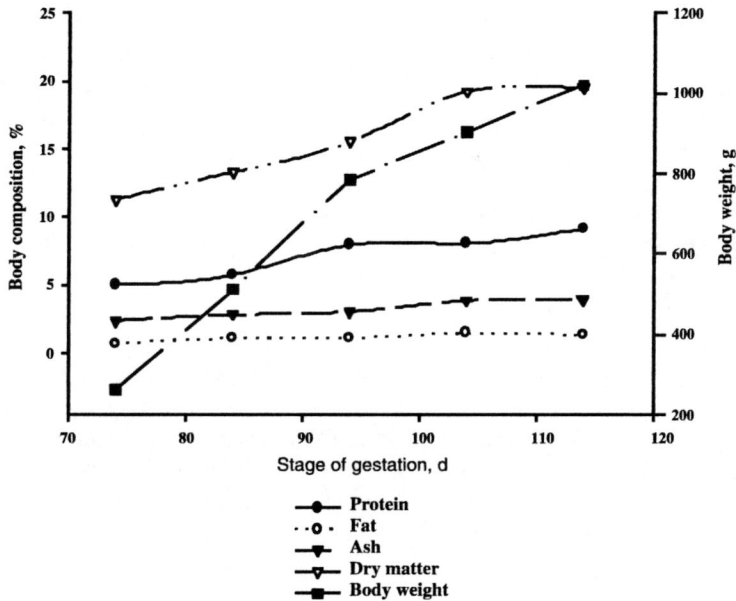

FIGURE 33.3 Relationship of fetal body composition and day of gestation. (Adapted from Padalikova and Jerkova, 1984.)

3. Interval Feeding

Some management systems implement interval feeding of gestating sows as a way to reduce labor requirements of feeding. Interval feeding programs are designed to provide feed to sows every second or third day rather than daily. The total amount of feed offered over a 3-day period is the same in either an interval or daily feeding program. For instance, sows offered 1.8 kg/day in a daily feeding program would be offered 5.4 kg every third day. Michel et al. (1980) reported no difference in gestation weight gain or reproductive performance for sows fed every third day compared with a daily feeding regimen. In contrast, gilts fed every third day suffered lower gestation weight gains and fewer, lighter live pigs at birth compared with daily feeding. Typically, gilts are better suited to an interval feeding program that provides feed every other day. Interval-fed sows were less active, exhibiting less sham chewing, licking, and drinking behaviors compared with sows fed daily (Douglas et al., 1998). These behavioral differences may suggest a greater degree of well-being for interval-fed sows compared with sows fed daily. Greater inactivity of interval-fed sows may improve efficiency because energy is not being expended for behaviors that do not translate directly into useful products. Regardless of the feeding system employed, animal caretakers must monitor daily the health and well-being of each sow.

4. Metabolic Disorders Associated with Excess Gestational Feed Intake and Weight Gain

In the sow, glucose levels rise when approaching parturition. This rise in glucose concentration may be due to a slight increase in insulin resistance toward the end of gestation or to a decrease in glycemic stimuli to the pancreas. Increased placental degradation of insulin was shown in the gestating rat, potentiating the elevation of blood glucose (Frienkel, 1980). Shaefer et al. (1991) observed that pregnant swine exhibit diabetes tendencies. These mechanisms may have a significant effect in preparing the sow for parturition and giving the mammary gland priority for glucose utilization. However, excessive energy and/or feed intake during gestation can exacerbate gestational diabetes as indicated by glucose and insulin kinetics, and postfarrowing performance, such as depressed appetite and increased body protein and fat degradation rate (Weldon et al., 1994a,b; Trottier and Easter, 1995; Revell et al., 1998a).

Another consequence of excessive gestational feeding levels is decreased milk production (Weldon et al., 1994a) or periparturient hypogalactic syndrome (PHS). Excessive energy intake during gilt development has been associated with udder hypoplasia as a result of excessive fat infiltration of the alveoli, thus restricting circulation to the mammary system and leading to udder edema. An edematous udder is more susceptible to infection and consequently poor lactation. In addition, excessively obese sows tend to have more farrowing difficulties due to increased exhaustion and susceptibility to heat and environmental stress, predisposing them to lactation failure. Although limiting feed intake during the last 1 or 2 weeks of gestation has been demonstrated to decrease the incidence of PHS in some herds, it is not known whether this is due to a decrease in total energy, protein concentration, or a combination of both. In practice, decreasing feed consumption during late gestation such as the last 3 weeks seems to be most effective in herds with a high incidence of PHS (>30 to 35%) (Martineau et al., 1992). On the other hand, one must be aware of the consequence of decreasing feed intake on body condition of the sow and subsequent litter performances, as discussed previously. Postpartum feeding methods on the other hand do not affect the incidence of PHS (Moser et al., 1987).

D. MAMMARY DEVELOPMENT

Body composition in late gestation may affect mammary development and ultimately milk production in the subsequent lactation. Very little mammary development occurs during gestation until day 75 postmating. After day 75, there is an exponential growth in the concentration (Kensinger et al., 1982) and total quantity (Weldon et al., 1991) of DNA and RNA in the mammary gland. DNA is a measure of the total number of cells, whereas RNA provides an indication of the protein synthetic capacity of a tissue. No differences in the weight and chemical composition of mammary glands collected from pregnant, obese, and lean gilts were observed (Head and Williams, 1991); however, obese gilts had a significantly lower concentration of cells in dry, defatted mammary tissue compared with lean gilts (Head and Williams, 1991; Head et al., 1991). Unfortunately, specific characteristics of body composition such as backfat depth or percent body fat of obese and lean gilts were not well described. Weldon et al. (1991) increased energy intake of gilts from 5.75 to 10.5 Mcal ME daily after day 75 of gestation and observed a significant reduction in the weight of parenchymal tissue. They also reported reductions in total DNA and RNA of parenchymal tissues, indicating potentially reduced capacity for milk synthesis. It is not clear if these differences in cell numbers will translate into differences in milk production after farrowing. In contrast to the effects of elevated energy intake, altering protein intake of gilts during late gestation had no influence on mammary development (Weldon et al., 1991; King et al., 1996). Increasing lysine intake from severely deficient (4 g/day) to liberal (16 g/day) levels (NRC, 1998) had no effect on number of milk secreting cells in the mammary gland (Kusina et al., 1999b) but did increase milk production (Kusina et al., 1999a) in the subsequent lactation. Increased milk production may have resulted from elevated synthetic capacity of the mammary tissue rather than increases in the total amount of mammary tissue involved in milk production or some other factor related to nutrient balance of the sow. On the other hand, Kim et al. (1999) found that lysine is required for mammary growth during lactation, suggesting that lactating sows may need more lysine than currently recommended by NRC (1998).

E. Modeling Nutrient Requirements

Variations in body size, productivity, and environmental conditions dictate different daily rations of nutrients be fed to satisfy the sow's requirements. Without accurate data to compensate for these differences, nutritionists historically have estimated the nutrient needs of the "average" sow under average conditions, then formulated diets with elevated levels of nutrients as a margin of safety. This approach often meets the biological needs of the pregnant sow but may compromise the economic and environmental health of the breeding operation. Slim profit margins in pork production and concern over environmental impacts of the swine industry encourage producers and nutritionists to fine-tune diets to minimize excess nutrient concentrations in diets. Conducting a scientific experiment in every possible production setting to determine the nutrient requirements for sows in that production system is one way to fine-tune gestating sow diets. Obviously, this approach is not economical or practical.

Mathematical models are an increasingly useful approach to estimating nutrient requirements of pigs. These models use mathematical relationships between inputs (e.g., feed intake and environmental temperature) and outputs (maternal body weight gain, fetal growth, and mammary tissue growth) to estimate the nutrient requirements under a given set of conditions. The model assumes a constant relationship between inputs and outputs, so that nutrient requirements under a wide range of conditions can be predicted without conducting a physical experiment. Unfortunately, very few validated mathematical models are available currently in the public sector for prediction of nutrient requirements of gestating sows. The NRC (1998) published a model that predicts energy and amino acid requirements of gestating sows. However, this model has not been thoroughly validated because of insufficient published data suitable for this purpose. Interest in mathematical models for gestating sows is less intense than that for lactating sows because nutrient demands are less rigorous.

1. Maintenance

Nutrient requirements for maintenance are influenced primarily by body weight of the sow and the environment in which she is housed. Requirements are based on metabolic body size. Several exponential functions have been proposed (NRC, 1998) to describe metabolic body size but body weight raised to the 0.75 power ($BW^{0.75}$) is the most widely accepted. In addition to body weight, maintenance energy requirements are influenced by the effective ambient temperature experienced by the sow (NRC, 1981). Effective ambient temperatures below or above the sow's thermoneutral zone will increase maintenance energy requirements. The thermoneutral zone is the range of ambient temperatures within which the sow must expend no added energy above that needed for body tissue functions to maintain her core body temperature. When the effective ambient temperature falls below the thermoneutral zone, additional energy is needed to generate heat for maintenance of body temperature. Similarly, temperatures above the thermoneutral zone require extra energy be expended to dissipate heat mainly via increased respiration rates in swine. The lower and upper ends of the thermoneutral zone are referred to as the lower critical temperature and upper critical temperature, respectively. The lower critical temperature for a sow housed individually with no bedding is approximately 24°C (NRC, 1981). However, addition of bedding and housing sows in groups can reduce this benchmark at least 4°C. From a nutritional perspective, as the lower critical temperature declines, the feed required to maintain the sow also declines.

Protein requirements for maintenance are based on metabolic body weight just like maintenance energy requirements. It is not known whether effective ambient temperature directly influences estimates of protein requirements for maintenance. Therefore, maintenance protein requirements for sows housed in a cold or hot environment are assumed not to be significantly different from those of sows housed in a thermoneutral environment.

Estimates of daily maintenance energy requirements range from 100 to 125 kcal ME/kg $BW^{0.75}$ with an average of 106 kcal ME/kg $BW^{0.75}$ (NRC, 1998). Maintenance energy requirements do not change with advancing pregnancy (Noblet et al., 1990). The true ileal digestible lysine requirement for maintenance was estimated by NRC (1998) to be 36 mg/kg $BW^{0.75}$. Maintenance requirements for vitamins and minerals have not been established separately but are part of the total requirements for these nutrients.

2. Fetal Growth

Growth of the products of conception and the associated nutrient needs for that growth are fairly resistant to nutritional manipulations at feed intakes typical of production settings. Noblet et al. (1985) reported increasing feed intake of pregnant primiparous sows from 5 to 7.5 Mcal digestible energy (DE) daily significantly increased total weight of fetuses at the end of gestation. In contrast, Dourmad et al. (1996) reported no influence of gestation feeding levels for multiparous sows ranging from 7.4 to 10.4 Mcal DE/day on live weight of fetuses at 112 days postmating. Under conditions of adequate energy intakes ranging from 6 to 10 Mcal ME daily (Noblet et al., 1990), changes in weight of fetuses are relatively small. In addition, feeding level had little (Noblet et al., 1990) or no (Noblet et al., 1985) influence on body composition of fetuses.

3. Maternal Weight Gain

Maternal body composition is influenced heavily by nutrient requirements for maintenance, growth of the products of conception, and the quantity of nutrients supplied to the sow. The sow's daily ration of nutrients is allocated to maintain normal bodily functions; growth of fetal, placental, uterine, and mammary tissues; and deposition in maternal body tissues. Maintenance of the sow and growth of the conceptus receive the highest priority for nutrients; however, this prioritization likely is not absolute. Conceptually, once these two high-priority needs are satisfied, any "extra" nutrients are deposited in maternal tissues. Any conditions that alter the requirements for maintenance or fetal growth will influence the quantity of nutrients available for deposition in maternal tissues. The components of primary importance to the reproducing sow that are stored in maternal tissue include energy as fat and amino acids as proteins stored in muscle and other proteinaceous tissues.

Protein and energy available, after requirements for maintenance and fetal growth are satisfied, can be deposited in maternal tissues. Consequently, one must consider the energy and protein supplied by the diet above that needed for maintenance and fetal growth when discussing effects of nutrition on body composition. Several studies have demonstrated that increasing intake of feed during pregnancy increases maternal weight gain, resulting in a heavier sow at the beginning of lactation (Mullan and Williams, 1989; 1990; Yang et al., 1989). This increase in maternal body weight is due primarily to increases in fat and proteinaceous tissues, with only minor increases in ash content of the empty body (Mullan and Williams, 1990).

Varying the amount of energy and protein above that required for maintenance and fetal growth can influence composition of the maternal weight gain. Feeding a low-protein, high-energy diet yielded sows that were significantly fatter but of similar body weight at farrowing to sows that received a high-protein, low-energy diet (Table 33.6; Revell et al., 1998a). Similarly, feeding a constant amount of protein with increasing intakes of energy increased nitrogen retention and muscle weight in addition to maternal body weight and dissectable fat (Dourmad et al., 1996). Conversely, feeding a constant amount of energy with increasing intakes of protein to pregnant gilts increased nitrogen retention (King and Brown, 1993). Improved nitrogen retention likely corresponds to increases in muscle mass of the sow; however, this was not measured directly. These results suggest that manipulation of energy or protein supply can significantly influence the composition of maternal body weight gain (Pettigrew and Yang, 1997). Differences in maternal body composition at the end of pregnancy could have important effects on parturition and the following lactation.

TABLE 33.6
Influence of Protein and Energy Intake during Gestation on Body Composition of Primiparous Sows

Trait	Crude Protein Intake (g/day):	133	265
	Digestible Energy Intake (Mcal/day):	8	5.9
Number of sows		16	19
Sow body wt. at mating (kg)		120.8	121.5
Backfat depth at mating (mm)		17.3	15.8
Sow body wt. at farrowing (kg)		159.1	151.7
Backfat depth at farrowing (mm)		24.3	17.9
Estimated body fat at farrowing (kg)		54.9	42.2
Estimated body lean at farrowing (kg)		96.3	101.9

Source: Revell, D. K. et al., *J. Anim. Sci.*, 76:1729, 1998a. With permission.

The most desirable amount and composition of maternal gain during pregnancy is a subject of much interest to pork producers and nutritionists. This interest is well placed when one considers the ease with which maternal gain can be influenced and the consequences of improperly managing that maternal gain. Excessive maternal gain and fatness can predispose the sow to dystocia at farrowing (Dourmad et al., 1994), decreased feed intake in the subsequent lactation (Dourmad, 1991; Weldon et al., 1994; Coffey et al., 1994), and decreased sow longevity (Dourmad et al., 1994). Hoppe et al. (1990) fed sows 6 or 9 Mcal ME daily throughout four consecutive gestation periods and observed total gestation weight gains of 37 to 55 kg. Additional dietary energy increased total gestation weight gain from 0.5 to 15 kg over the four gestation periods with no significant effects on lactation performance or longevity of sows. In contrast, insufficient maternal gain may compromise the sow's ability to sustain a successful lactation due to low body stores of nutrients, resulting in thin sows at weaning and delayed return to estrus (MacLean, 1969; Johnston et al., 1989). This scenario decreases longevity of sows in commercial conditions (Dourmad et al., 1994). Young et al. (1991) observed a higher culling rate for sows with <12 mm of backfat depth, suggesting that very low levels of body fat can compromise reproductive performance and longevity. These researchers suggested that 22 to 30 kg of total gestation weight gain are required to prevent loss of backfat during pregnancy. The old rule of thumb of 35 to 45 kg of weight gain for pregnant gilts and 30 to 40 kg gain for older sows seems to be an acceptable target. Increased total weight gain for gilts compared with older sows recognizes the fact that these young animals will increase their maternal body size at a faster rate than older animals.

TABLE 33.7
Estimated Nutrient Requirements of Gestating Sows

Total Gestation Weight Gain (kg)	ME (Mcal/d)	Crude Protein (g/day)	Lysine, Total (g/day)	Lysine, Dig[a] (g/day)
		125 kg[b]		
30	4.23	182	8.6	6.8
40	5.05	211	9.7	7.6
50	5.86	239	10.9	8.5
		150 kg[b]		
30	4.8	194	8.8	6.9
40	5.61	222	10	7.8
50	6.42	250	11.2	8.6
		175 kg[b]		
30	5.34	207	9.1	7.1
40	6.15	233	10.3	7.9
50	6.96	262	11.4	8.8
		200 kg[b]		
30	5.87	217	9.3	7.2
40	6.68	245	10.5	8
50	7.48	273	11.7	8.9

Note: Assumes a total litter size of 12 at farrowing and thermoneutral conditions.

[a] Apparent ileal digestible basis.
[b] Body weight of sow at breeding.

Source: Modified from NRC, *Nutrient Requirement of Swine*, 10th rev. ed., National Academy Press, Washington, D.C.

The metabolizable energy, crude protein, total lysine, and digestible lysine needs of the gestating sow have been estimated by NRC (1998) using a mathematical model (Table 33.7). An important feature to note is that there is not one single set of requirements for all gestating sows. A variety of factors discussed above influence the total nutrient requirement of a pregnant sow. Advances in understanding of swine nutrition are allowing nutritionists to account more accurately for the effect of these factors on nutrient requirements.

IV. LACTATING SOWS

A. OBJECTIVES

Long-term productivity of the breeding herd represents the main objective behind optimal feeding management and care of the lactating sow. Feeding the lactating sow is perhaps the most challenging dietary goal of the breeding herd. Intensification of productive demands has resulted in part from improvement in management systems and health status, combined with increased genetic selection pressure for leanness. While efforts to increase litter weights have been successful, the feed intake capacity during lactation to support the nursing progeny remains a limiting factor to milk production, mainly for the primiparous sow. Approximately 50% of preweaning deaths are related to insufficient milk production (Kertiles and Anderson, 1979); however, the extent to which nutrition directly contributes to this observation is unknown. Long-term productivity also depends on maintenance of body condition, a reflection of the nutritional status of the sow relative to its metabolic demand.

B. FEEDING STRATEGIES

Feeding strategies play an important role in maximizing voluntary feed intake, which is critical to optimize lactation output and subsequent reproductive performance. In essence, the lactating sow adjusts voluntary feed intake to match the energy requirements for milk production with the dietary supply of energy (Revell and Williams, 1993). However, this adjustment is typically affected by other physiological mechanisms that complicate prediction of feed intake. Information and research on the effect of feeding methods postpartum on sow and litter performance is limited (Moser et al., 1987).

1. Postfarrowing Appetite Depression and Factors That Affect Lactation Feed Intake

Parturition is often followed by feed intake depression for several days. Low feed intake during the early stages of lactation may affect the subsequent reproductive ability of sows (Revell et al., 1998a). Sows with either low feed intake throughout lactation or low feed intake at various times during lactation are more likely to be have lower litter size at weaning and extended postweaning anestrus (Koketsu et al., 1996a). Several factors affect feed intake during the initial phase of lactation such as postfarrowing lethargy, limited gut capacity, and stress of parturition, but the major nutritional factor is related to high feed intake level with excessive fat gain during the gestation period. This usually affects feed intake during both the initial phase and throughout lactation. In a study by Weldon et al. (1994a), sows given *ad libitum* access to feed during the last third of the gestation period voluntarily reduced their feed intake throughout the lactation period. Similarly, sows fed a high-fat diet compared with sows fed a high-fiber diet during the entire gestation period reduced their total energy intake during lactation and mobilized more body fat (Trottier, 1991). Alterations in metabolism resulting from overfeeding and fatness during gestation create a physiological condition in which the sow adjusts her feed consumption below her nutritional requirements. This response is amplified under high environmental temperature and humidity (Lynch, 1977). High concentrations of blood lipids, such as nonesterified free fatty acids, and low concentrations of branched-chain amino acids may be involved in limiting feed intake by acting at the brain centers for appetite control (Trottier and Easter, 1995). Revell et al. (1998a) showed that preprandial concentrations of glycerol and nonesterified free fatty acids during the last week of gestation were higher in fat sows compared with lean sows and voluntary feed intake during lactation was significantly lower in fat sows compared with lean sows.

Feed intake during lactation usually increases gradually until weaning, and generally increases from the first to sixth parity (O'Grady et al., 1985; Koketsu et al., 1996b). Heavier sows and multiparous sows have a higher maintenance requirement and might be expected to consume more feed compared with primiparous sows, which exhibit poor appetite in relation to requirements for maintenance, growth, and milk production (O'Grady et al., 1985). Voluntary feed intake increases with litter size, where 0.45 kg of feed is recommended for each nursing pig (Verstegen et al., 1985), and advancement of lactation, reflecting an increase in nutrient demand for milk production. Protein concentration of the diets fed during both gestation and lactation may affect voluntary feed intake during lactation. For example, feeding higher protein levels during gestation stimulates appetite during lactation (Mahan and Mangan, 1975), and this response is further amplified with feeding high-protein lactation diets. Both lean and fat sows respond to high protein lactation diets by increasing voluntary feed intake, but this response is significantly higher in lean sows and during the last third of the lactation period (Revell et al., 1998a). On the other hand, Johnston et al. (1993) found that sows fed a 14% crude protein diet during gestation did not differ in feed intake patterns when exposed to various crude protein levels during lactation.

2. Maximizing Feed Intake

Phase feeding during lactation is becoming the feeding practice of choice; however, the lack of information regarding the productivity and the variation in phase-feeding programs adapted to different herds, breeds, and environmental conditions renders recommendations difficult. The concept behind a phase-feeding program during lactation is similar, in that sows are provided a gradual and restrictive increase in feed intake during the first few days after farrowing and are allowed to reach full feeding within the first week of lactation. Typically, on the first day of lactation, levels of feed selected will provide nutrient requirements for maintenance only. A controlled increase in feed allowance will follow until day 4 or 5 of lactation. *Ad libitum* access to feed is usually allowed thereafter for the remainder of the lactation period. While this practice offers managerial advantages, such as increased attention spent per animal and decreased feed spoilage, it does not increase total feed intake or improve sow and litter performances compared with sows allowed *ad libitum* access to feed immediately after parturition (English, 1970; Stahly et al., 1979; Moser et al., 1987; Snow et al., 1997). In fact, the earlier the sows can reach a full feeding status and not experience a drop in feed intake, the more likely is earlier return to estrus postweaning (Koketsu et al., 1996a). As production systems in North America are moving toward early weaning, feeding strategies should be adjusted accordingly, as shortening of lactation length reduces average daily feed intake per sow (Koketsu et al., 1996b). In sows lactating for 28 days compared with sows lactating 10 days, average daily feed intake decreased from 5.4 to 4.1 kg. Although feeding frequencies of sows was shown to have no effect on voluntary feed intake of sows or litter performance (NRC-89, 1990), ideally lactating sows should be fed three times a day to decrease feed spoilage and increase the attention spent on sows. Factors such as water availability, feeder design, ventilation and room temperature, and monitoring feed intake are part of management practices that should be implemented first when adopting a successful feeding program.

C. LACTATION AND BODY WEIGHT LOSS

Sows usually satisfy nutrient need for milk production primarily from dietary nutrients but also from body protein and adipose tissue storage, where lean and fat represent 95% of the total body weight change during lactation (Mullan and Williams, 1990). Body weight loss is becoming a key issue and an essential parameter to consider when estimating nutrient requirements and predicting reproductive success. Today, sows require a greater amino acid supply than in the past because they have larger litters (Johnston et al., 1993), and the understanding behind body stores catabolism in support of milk production is becoming more important as feed intake may not be keeping pace with litter growth potential. Selection for leanness and for genotypes with high lean growth capacity has led to a reduced capacity for feed intake in sows (Riley, 1989).

Many studies indicate that fat losses during lactation outweigh fat gains during pregnancy, so that every production cycle represents a net loss of body fat (Whittemore et al., 1980; Esbenshade et al., 1986; Young and King, 1989; Trottier, 1991; Sorensen et al., 1993). Consequently, as sows proceed through breeding life, they become thinner and lose condition. Thus, changes in the sows' body reserves during pregnancy and lactation have become a critical tool to evaluate nutritional needs (King et al., 1986; King, 1989). Although body weight and muscle depth increase over each production cycle, backfat thickness was shown to decrease (Sorensen et al., 1993). Other reports have failed to show a decrease in backfat through succeeding parities (Whittemore and Yang, 1989; Lee and Mitchell, 1989). It is suggested that a backfat level of 10 mm represents the minimum amount of fat stored, below which the sow is resistant to further depletion of her reserves, when utilizing body resources as a supplement to dietary energy intake (Whittemore et al., 1984; Eastham et al., 1988).

1. Composition of Weight Loss

The composition of weight loss is important in determining milk production requirements for both protein and energy. Typically, the body compositional loss during lactation is affected by the dietary protein and energy intake, the body composition of the sow, and the metabolic need imposed by lactation. Compositional weight loss in sows fed typical lactation diets has been assumed to be 30% fat and 13% protein (NRC, 1988). More recent studies have found that, as a proportion of body weight loss, fat loss varies from 0.60 to 0.69 and protein from 0.09 to 0.14, showing that the loss of fat relative to lean is not constant, and is affected by the protein:energy ratio of the diet relative to milk nutrient output (Mullan, 1991). Lactating sows restricted-fed during lactation can mobilize up to 25 to 30% of their body protein stores to maintain milk production (Mullan and Williams, 1990), and further feed restriction will limit milk production and reduce pig growth rate (Clowes et al., 1998). Energy-restricted sows mobilize more fat during lactation compared with non-energy-restricted sows (Armstrong et al., 1986; Brendemuhl et al., 1989) and have elevated blood urea nitrogen concentration throughout lactation, indicating greater muscle catabolism (Reese et al., 1982; Nelssen et al., 1985). Fat sows fed a high-protein diet (19% CP) will primarily mobilize body fat, whereas fat sows fed a low-protein diet (7% CP) will readily mobilize both body protein and fat tissue (Revell et al., 1998a). The study of compositional weight loss of lactating sows has been of interest for many years because of the extended postweaning anestrous period in sows losing excessive amounts of body weight. Recently, composition of weight loss, particularly regarding body protein, has provided important insights in building a nutrient requirement model for the lactating sow (NRC, 1998). This will be discussed in a later section of this chapter.

2. Nutrition and Reproduction Interaction

Sows remain anestrus during lactation because of a reduced responsiveness of the hypothalamic pituitary unit to hormonal stimulation (Kirkwood et al., 1987). It is suggested that this inhibition decreases as lactation proceeds (Elsaesser and Parvizi, 1980). Numerous studies have demonstrated that postweaning anestrus is extended in primiparous sows either fed a low-energy diet or restricted-fed during lactation (Reese et al., 1982; King and Williams, 1984; Armstrong et al., 1986). Typically, this response has not been observed in multiparous sows. Anestrus is also highly correlated with the body weight and backfat level at weaning (Johnston et al., 1989; Mullan and Williams, 1989), whereby sows with lower body weight and backfat at weaning demonstrate a longer anestrus period. Sows that lose extensive weight in lactation remain catabolic after weaning for an extended period of time (Brooks, 1982; Reese et al., 1982). However, the composition of weight loss is in major part water (Zoiopoulos et al., 1983). Recent work indicates that the dietary energy source, such as carbohydrate vs. fat, differentially affects some of the reproductive hormones (Kemp et al., 1995). Starch-based diets increased LH surge and progesterone concentration, but did not affect the postweaning interval to estrus in multiparous sows (Kemp et al., 1995). Similarly, Zak et al. (1998) showed that LH pulse frequency and IGF-I concentration at weaning were decreased and the weaning-to-estrus interval was extended in sows subjected to a restricted feeding regimen during lactation compared with sows allowed *ad libitum* access to feed or superalimented. The etiology of estrus inhibition in response to feeding or metabolic status is unclear and the studies so far have given little clue to explain a cause-and-effect relationship (Kirkwood et al., 1987). Today, it is still debated whether the loss in body fat, body protein, or a combination of both during lactation lengthen the postweaning anestrus period.

Nutrition during lactation can influence subsequent litter size. Tritton et al. (1996) reported a positive relationship between lysine intake during a sow's first lactation and number of pigs born in the second litter. In this study, number of pigs born live in the second litter increased from a low of 9.48 to a high of 10.92 as dietary lysine intake increased from 37 to 60 g/day. The lysine intake necessary to maximize subsequent litter size was higher than that needed to maximize milk

TABLE 33.8
Effect of Dietary Lysine Concentration during First, Second, and Third Lactation on Subsequent Litter Size

Trait	Dietary Lysine Concentration during Lactation (%)				
	0.6	0.85	1.1	1.35	1.6
Litter size at second farrowing					
Lysine intake in first lactation	32.5	44.2	53.7	65.8	73.3
No. of litters	26	30	27	28	26
Born alive[a]	11	11	10.6	9.5	8.9
Total born[b]	11.7	11.9	11.4	11	10.1
Litter size at third farrowing					
Lysine intake in second lactation	39	55.2	68.8	79.3	92.9
No. of litters	19	21	19	20	19
Born alive[c]	11.8	10.1	10.3	11.2	12.4
Total born[c]	13.3	11.2	11.6	11.9	13.6
Litter size at fourth farrowing					
Lysine intake in third lactation	41.3	55.6	71.1	88.6	98.9
No. of litters	18	16	15	17	18
Born alive	11.4	10.6	11.3	11.2	12
Total born	13.7	11.9	12.3	13.6	13.5

[a] Linear effect of lysine, $P < 0.01$.
[b] Linear effect of lysine, $P < 0.10$.
[c] Quadratic effect of lysine, $P < 0.05$.

Source: Yang, H. et al., *J. Anim. Sci.*, 78:348, 2000. With permission.

production. In contrast, Touchette et al. (1998) reported that incremental additions of synthetic lysine to diets for lactating primiparous sows yielded a linear decline in number of total and liveborn pigs in the second litter. These studies focused on nutrition of primiparous lactating sows and concluded when sows farrowed their second litter. More recently, Yang et al. (2000) studied the effects of dietary lysine intake during lactation on subsequent litter size over four parities. Increases in dietary lysine were achieved without the use of synthetic lysine. They found detrimental effects of relatively high lactational lysine intakes on size of the subsequent litter in parities two and three (Table 33.8). In parity four, there seemed to be no effect of previous lactational lysine intake on litter size at farrowing. Additionally, they found no difference between the amount of lysine intake needed to maximize milk production and that required to maximize subsequent litter size in sows. Additional long-term sow experiments will be necessary to understand fully the effects of lactation nutrient intake on subsequent litter size and lactational performance.

D. Milk Production

1. Milk Production and Nutrient Composition

Milk production in the lactating sow is largely governed by demand from the litter (Sauber et al., 1994; Boyd et al., 1995) and nutrients available from the sow. Direct measurement of milk production in the lactating sow is not possible; hence various indirect methods have been used to estimate milk yield in nutritional research such as litter weight gain (3.88 g milk:1 g of pig gain; Clowes et al., 1998), deuterium oxide (Pettigrew et al., 1987; Pluske et al., 1997), and weigh-suckle-weigh (Speer and Cox, 1984). Recent research indicates that milk yield peaks as early as between day 15 and 18 of lactation (Nielsen et al., unpublished; Guan et al., unpublished; Toner et al., 1996). This is in contrast to earlier studies in which peak lactation occurred between the third and fifth week (Elsley, 1971). This may be due to genotypic differences, but also perhaps is the product of selection for rapid growth rate, hastening the onset of peak milk yield. This could be regarded as a nutritional advantage in production systems weaning at <21 days. Peak lactation corresponds to peak arteriovenous difference of amino acids and glucose across the mammary gland (Nielsen et al., unpublished; Guan et al., unpublished), indicating that the mammary gland nutrient uptake is maximized. Whether the decrease in milk production after peak milk yield is a result of decreased activity of nutrient transport systems has not been studied. It is clearly not the result of lesser nutrient availability because sow voluntary feed intake continues to increase with advancement of lactation.

Sow milk nutrient composition changes with the stage of lactation (Tables 33.9 and 33.10). Total solids are highest in colostrum during the initial 6 h after parturition. This is mainly attributed to the whey protein concentrations, specifically the concentration of immunoglobulins. Both albumin and IgG account for a major portion of the whey proteins immediately after parturition, but decline rapidly until approximately 48 h. As lactation advances, the concentration of IgA as a percentage of whey protein increases, while IgM decreases slightly and IgG decreases drastically (a 92% decrease from day 0 of lactation). Therefore, whey proteins as a percentage of total proteins decrease from 91 to 58% from parturition to the end of a 29-day lactation period. On the other hand, fat and lactose concentration increase from 5.0 to 7.1% and 3.1 to 5.6%, respectively. The transition from colostrum to normal milk is signaled by the sharp decrease in total proteins and a parallel increase in lactose concentration (Klobasa et al., 1987). The increase in lactose concentration corresponds to an increase in mammary protein synthesis and a high correlation exists between milk lactose and α-lactalbumin content (Jenness, 1974). The decrease in percentage of whey in total protein marks the increase in casein synthesis and secretion (Klobasa et al., 1987).

Milk nutrient composition can be altered by manipulating the sow's diet; however, the response is highly variable depending on the previous nutritional status of the sow, stage of production, and the adequacy of the diet being fed. Fat supplementation of the sow diet increases colostral and milk fat concentration (Pettigrew, 1978; 1981) and decreases the rate of liver glycogen disappearance in nursing pigs (Moser, 1983). After an extensive review of the literature on the effect of supplemental fat in lactating sow diets on colostral and milk fat, and piglet

TABLE 33.9
Gross Composition of Sow Colostrum

Constituents	Stage of Lactation			
	0 h	6 h	12–18 h	24–48 h
Total solids (%)	25.6	22.7	18.1	18
Fat (%)	5	4.8	5.1	6.1
Lactose (%)	3.1	3.4	4.3	4.7
Total Protein (TP) (%)	15.7	13	8.1	6.4
Whey Protein (WP) (%)	14.3	10.9	6.3	4.3
WP:TP	91.1	83.8	78.3	66.4
IgG (mg/ml)	95.6	64.8	26.9	10.3
IgM (mg/ml)	9.1	6.9	3.7	2.7
IgA (mg/ml)	21.2	15.6	8.4	5.8
Albumin (mg/ml)	20	18	9	6
IgG:WP	67.1	59.6	42.7	24.2
IgM:WP	6.4	6.3	5.9	6.4
IgA:WP	14.8	14.3	13.3	13.6
Albumin:WP	14	16.5	14.3	14.1

Source: Klobasa, F. et al., *J. Anim. Sci.*, 64:1458, 1987. With permission.

TABLE 33.10
Gross Composition of Sow Milk throughout Lactation[a]

Constituents	Concentration
Total solids (%)[b]	18.5
Fat (%)[b]	7.1
Lactose (%)[b]	5.6
Total protein (TP)(%)[b]	5.2
Whey protein (WP)(%)[b]	3
WP:TP[b]	57.9
IgG (mg/ml)[b]	1.6
IgM (mg/ml)[b]	1.7
IgA (mg/ml)[b]	5.2
Albumin (mg/ml)[b]	4.5
IgG:WP[b]	5.3
IgM:WP[b]	5.6
IgA:WP[b]	17.2
Albumin:WP[b]	14.9
Cholesterol (mg/100g)[c]	33.8
Inorganic elements (ppm)[c]	
Ca	1510.5
K	356.2
Mg	78.9
Na	390.9
P	1041.9
S	36.1
Al	1.79
B	3.45
Cu	2.01
Mn	0.1
Mo	0.1
Zn	7.35

[a] Data are nonweighted averages from day 4 to 28 of lactation.
[b] Klobasa et al. (1987); King et al. (1993a); King et al. (1993b); Pluske et al. (1998).
[c] Park et al. (1994).

survival, Moser (1983) concluded that, although the effect is small, it is large enough to offset the increase in feed cost associated with dietary fat addition. Dietary protein level can also affect milk nutrient concentrations. Increasing dietary protein levels to maximize milk yield is accompanied by an increase in milk fat, protein, and lactose content (King et al., 1993b). However, the effect on milk protein and lactose was found significant in late stage of lactation only (third week). On the other hand, Revell et al. (1995) found no effect of dietary protein on milk protein, lactose, or fat concentration.

Limit feeding sows during lactation produces milk with a substantially higher fat content and lower lactose level (Noblet and Etienne, 1986; Roos, 1990). This metabolic adaptation may have evolved as a mechanism to spare blood glucose for maternal needs. On the other hand, Pluske et al. (1998) found no effect of feeding levels (i.e., restricted vs. superalimented sows) on milk nutrient concentrations. These results are also supported by the studies of Revell et al. (1998b) who examined the effect of sow body composition (i.e., lean vs. fat) at parturition and also those of Toner et al. (1996).

2. Nutrient Uptake by the Mammary Gland

Nutrients for milk synthesis, such as amino acids, glucose, and fatty acids, are made available to the mammary gland via the arterial supply, and are of dietary and/or endogenous origin. In lactating mammals, amino acids are taken up mostly as free entities in plasma and erythrocytes (Trottier, 1997). Some evidence in the goat suggests that peptide-bound amino acids may contribute to the pool of amino acids found in milk proteins (Backwell et al., 1994). Although the control and mode of uptake is unknown in the porcine mammary gland, it is certain that the uptake of amino acids is not regulated uniformly. Arteriovenous differences of certain amino acids such as lysine, threonine, methionine, phenylalanine, tryptophan, and valine plateau with an increase in dietary concentrations of these amino acids, while the arteriovenous differences of leucine and isoleucine seem to be unregulated (Trottier, 1997; Guan et al., 1998). The nutritional significance of mammary amino acid uptake lies behind the fact that the amino acid uptake profile does not match the amino acid profile in the milk (Table 33.11), a product of differential amino acid mammary retention. This may imply that amino acid requirements during lactation may be higher than currently thought. Much interest has been given to valine since Richert et al. (1996) demonstrated a response in litter weight gain for lactating sows fed graded levels of crystalline valine. Current productive demands may in fact increase the need of certain amino acids beyond their output reflected in milk. The metabolic fate of amino acids in the mammary gland of mammals is virtually unknown, but maintenance costs associated with cellular remodeling and milk protein synthesis should be factored into the amino acid requirement estimates for lactation (Trottier, 1997).

The role of nutrition in the control of mammary nutrient uptake is certainly orchestrated with physiological and hormonal functions. The role of insulin, prolactin, and IGF-I at the mammary cellular level has never been studied in the porcine mammary gland. Recent findings (Guan et al., 1999) indicate that the blood level of insulin correlates with amino acids and glucose uptake by the mammary cell *in vivo*, but no relationships were found for prolactin and IGF-I, although the site of action at the receptor level is still lacking. An optimum carbohydrate:protein ratio may maximize the uptake of amino acid by the mammary gland via insulin action and may be a better predictor than the dietary energy:protein ratio. Nutrient uptake is not only the product of substrate availability but also of blood flow. The role of nutrition on mammary blood flow is unknown. Physiologically speaking, suckling demand per teat should be the driving force to stimulate blood flow, although excess nutrient availability may decrease blood flow. Excess nutrient availability may also reduce the rate of amino acid uptake across the mammary cell

TABLE 33.11
Amino Acid Profile in Milk and across the Porcine Mammary Gland (g/day) Relative to Lysine[a]

Amino Acid	AA:Milk[a] (g/16 g N)	AA:Lysine Milk	AA:Lysine[b] Uptake
Arginine	5.79	76	123
Histidine	3.79	50	30
Isoleucine	4.71	62	87
Leucine	8.8	116	146
Lysine	7.61	100	100
Methionine	2.34	31	32
Phenylalanine	4.42	58	66
Threonine	4.75	62	69
Tryptophan	1.3	15	20
Valine	5.8	76	96

[a] Dourmad et al. (1998); Guan et al., unpublished.
[b] Guan et al. (1998); Trottier (1995).

through transport systems saturation. This model has been proposed to explain the quadratic response in litter weight gain observed when feeding amino acids from below and to well in excess of requirements (Guan et al., 1998). Further data are essential to understand the role of nutrient interactions in optimizing production. The contribution, if any, of amino acids to *de novo* milk fat synthesis is probably insignificant.

The dynamics of glucose and other energy substrates uptake by the porcine mammary gland for milk production is clearly lacking in the literature. Studies regarding glucose utilization and kinetics across the porcine mammary gland are limited. Earlier work (Linzell et al., 1969; Spincer and Rook, 1971) has shown that plasma glucose contribution to milk fatty acid synthesis is very low, whereas 38% of the glycerol moiety found in triglycerides is derived from glucose (Spincer and Rook, 1971). Most milk triglyceride fatty acids are derived from plasma triglycerides (Spincer and Rook, 1971). On the other hand, 60 to 70% of milk lactose is synthesized from blood glucose (Spincer and Rook, 1971; White et al., 1984). The uptake of blood glucose by the mammary gland is dependent on blood glucose concentration. The role of insulin in glucose uptake by porcine mammary tissue is unknown. The insulin concentration in sows during lactation is inversely proportional to milk yield and lactose content (Reynolds and Rook, 1977). Earlier studies showed that insulin administration to lactating sows decreases milk yield (Goldobin, 1976). On the other hand, a more recent study showed that exogenous insulin increased weight gain of nursing pigs during lactation (Weldon et al., 1994b). Glucose may be dependent on insulin for mammary uptake and insulin receptor affinity on mammary tissue may be different from peripheral tissues.

E. Modeling Amino Acids and Energy Needs for Lactation

The current NRC (1998) provides in-depth coverage on modeling amino acid and energy needs of the lactating sow. It allows one to easily model the amino acid requirements on a total or digestible basis under different body loss conditions, feed intake, and environmental temperature. However, as mentioned earlier, the NRC (1998) model remains to be validated. For the purpose of this chapter, the principles and the conceptual approach of modeling amino acid and energy needs of the lactating sow will be described. Recommendations and examples are given to the reader so estimation of amino acid and energy requirements can be made.

1. Amino Acid Requirements

Requirements for all essential amino acids are based in part on the ideal protein concept and on a series of selected empirical observations from the literature (Pettigrew, 1993). For the lactating sow, both milk and body protein amino acid pattern relative to lysine are used as the basis to establish the ideal protein (Pettigrew, 1993). The following steps are used in estimating requirements. First, from a regression analysis obtained by combining selected empirical studies, Pettigrew (1993) determined that 26 g of lysine is required for each kilogram of litter weight gain per day (i.e., milk protein synthesis; Figure 33.4). Notice that the negative intercept represents the difference between maintenance requirement and lysine mobilization from body protein stores. Second, the amounts of amino acids present in milk and body protein, both expressed as grams per 16 g of nitrogen and as proportion of lysine, are used to estimate their requirements for milk production (Table 33.12). An example of amino acid requirement estimation using the values from Table 33.12, for a sow weighing 160 kg postfarrowing with an expected litter growth rate of 2000 g/day (10 pigs × 200 g body weight gain/day) is shown in Table 33.13. Lysine requirement must be calculated first, where 26 g lysine/kg of litter gain is multiplied by 2 kg of expected litter gain per day, for a total of 52 g of lysine required per day. If no body protein losses occur, the maintenance requirement for lysine is added to litter growth requirements (i.e., 2.09 g (maintenance) + 52.00 g lysine (litter growth), to obtain a total of 54.09 g lysine/day). Requirements for other amino acids are derived from their ratio relative to lysine in milk. For example, the threonine requirement is 58% of lysine

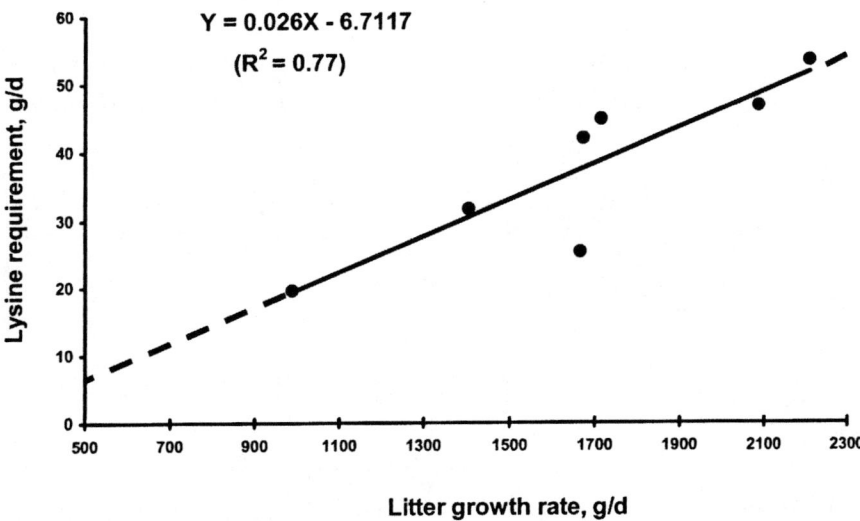

FIGURE 33.4 Relationship of lysine requirement during lactation and daily litter growth rate. (Adapted from Pettigrew, 1993.)

TABLE 33.12
Estimates of Amino Acid Requirements for Maintenance and Composition in Sow Milk and Body Protein

Amino acid	Milk Protein (g/16 g N)	Milk Protein (AA:Lysine)	Required for Maintenance (mg/kg BW$^{0.75}$)	Body Protein (g/16 g N)	Body Protein (AA:Lysine)
Arginine	4.93	0.66	0	6.81	1.05
Histidine	3.02	0.4	0	2.91	0.45
Isoleucine	4.11	0.55	20	3.25	0.5
Leucine	8.6	1.15	29	7.12	1.09
Lysine	7.5	1	49	6.51	1
Methionine	1.94	0.26	11	1.75	0.27
Total sulfur AA	3.4	0.45	61	2.91	0.45
Phenylalanine	4.12	0.55	23	3.91	0.6
Total aromatic AA	8.42	1.12	46	6.73	1.03
Threonine	4.38	0.58	41	3.76	0.58
Tryptophan	1.32	0.18	14	0.98	0.1
Valine	5.5	0.73	25	4.5	0.69

Source: Adapted from Pettigrew (1993).

requirement, because the threonine to lysine ratio in milk is 0.58 (see Table 33.12). Hence, the threonine requirement for a sow nursing a litter with a growth rate of 2 kg/day, would be 30.16 g/day (52 g lysine × 0.58), plus the maintenance requirement for threonine of 1.76 g/day, for a total of 32.12 g/day. Amino acid requirements on an ileal apparent digestible basis are calculated in the same manner, using apparent digestible amino acids required for maintenance and apparent digestible lysine required for litter growth. This is the basis on which NRC (1998) model calculates amino acid requirements of the lactating sow.

How does one take into consideration the amino acid contribution from body protein loss in sows with limited feed intake capacity and therefore an inability to maintain a zero nitrogen

TABLE 33.13
Requirements of Selected Amino Acids for a Lactating Sow with a Postfarrowing Weight of 160 kg and Expected to Produce a Litter Growth Rate of 2000 g/day

Amino Acid	Required for Maintenance (g/day)	Required for Milk Protein (g/day)	Total Required (g/day)[a]
Lysine	2.09	52.00[b]	54.09
Methionine	0.48	13.48[c]	13.96
Total sulfur AA	2.63	23.62[c]	26.25
Threonine	1.76	30.36[c]	32.12
Valine	1.07	38.15[c]	39.22
Tryptophan	0.59	9.17[c]	9.76

[a] Maintenance + milk protein.
[b] 26 g/kg growth rate × 2 kg (expected daily litter growth rate).
[c] 52 g × AA:lysine ratio in milk protein.

Source: Adapted from Pettigrew, 1993.

balance? Return to Table 13.12 and examine the amino acid profile of body protein. This profile was obtained by Pettigrew (1993) from averaging estimates of amino acid composition of body protein from three studies (Aumaitre and Duee, 1974; Zhang et al., 1986; Moughan and Smith, 1987). Each amino acid is then expressed as a ratio to lysine. Lysine contribution from body weight loss is estimated from the regression equation intercept in sows losing 20 kg during a 21-day lactation period (see Figure 33.4). The intercept (−6.71 g) and the maintenance requirements for lysine (2.09 g) constitute the daily lysine arising from body weight loss, i.e., 8.85 g lysine/day [−6.71 to 2.09 g]. Table 33.14 shows an example for amino acid requirements calculated using the NRC (1998) model for a sow weighing 160 kg postfarrow, and expected to nurse a litter with a growth potential of either 200 or 250 g/pig/day, and expected to lose either zero or 10 kg during a 21-day lactation period. The major pitfall in considering amino acids arising from body protein pool is the assumption that all amino acids are used for milk protein synthesis. As discussed earlier in this chapter, this would be relevant only in situations where energy is nonlimiting. In practice, when feed intake is limiting, both dietary amino acids and energy are limiting.

2. Energy Requirement

The current NRC (1998) provides an excellent tool to model the energy requirement of the lactating sow. Four basic pools are considered in the model (i.e., requirements for maintenance, requirements for milk production, adjustment of dietary energy requirement as affected by environmental temperature on energy intake, and adjustment of dietary energy requirement as affected by energy contribution from body weight loss). First, as for the gestating sow, the lactating sow maintenance requirement is 106 kcal ME/kg $BW^{0.75}$. Second, the energy required for milk production is obtained from an equation derived from Noblet and Etienne (1989) where milk gross energy (GE) per day = (4.92 × litter gain) − (90 × number of pigs). This amount is then converted to dietary energy, where dietary ME = milk GE × 72%, and where 72% represents the marginal efficiency of ME utilization for conversion into milk energy (Noblet and Etienne, 1987). Third, the model assumes the above requirements under thermoneutrality at 20°C. For each degree deviation from thermoneutrality, the sow adjusts her daily energy intake by 310 kcal ME. Hence, for each degree above thermoneutrality, daily dietary energy requirement should decrease by 310 kcal ME, whereby for each degree below thermoneutrality daily dietary energy requirements should increase by 310 kcal ME. Thus, energy requirements can be easily determined when no body weight change is observed.

TABLE 33.14
Amino Acid Recommendations for Lactating Sows with a Postfarrowing Weight of 160 kg Nursing Ten Pigs for 21 days

Amino Acid	Anticipated Lactational Weight Change (kg)			
	0	0	−10	−10
	Daily Weight Gain of Pigs (g)			
	200	250	200	250
Total (g/d)				
Arginine	25.52	33.93	22.1	30.51
Histidine	19.21	24.5	17.62	22.91
Isoleucine	27.03	34.33	25.22	32.52
Leucine	52.26	67.16	48.2	63.62
Lysine	48.89	62.2	45.2	58.51
Methionine	12.28	15.64	11.34	14.7
Methionine + cystine	23.66	29.7	22.03	28.07
Phenylalanine	26.04	33.27	23.98	31.22
Phenylalanine + tyrosine	53.74	68.52	50.12	64.9
Threonine	31.44	39.46	29.21	37.24
Tryptophan	8.7	11.04	8.29	10.63
Valine	41.04	52.45	38.53	49.94
Apparent Digestible (g/day)				
Arginine	21.62	28.96	18.73	26.07
Histidine	16.09	20.56	14.78	19.26
Isoleucine	22.04	28.06	20.62	26.65
Leucine	46.04	58.89	42.73	55.58
Lysine	39.52	50.52	36.71	47.71
Methionine	10.56	13.45	9.76	12.65
Methionine + cystine	19.38	24.33	18.05	23.01
Phenylalanine	21.67	27.72	19.98	26.02
Phenylalanine + tyrosine	44.93	57.33	41.95	54.35
Threonine	23.38	29.46	21.83	27.91
Tryptophan	6.59	8.41	6.34	8.15
Valine	32.91	42.1	30.93	40.12

Source: Nutrient Requirements of Swine, 10th rev. ed., National Academy Press, Washington, D.C., 1998. With permission.

It becomes more complicated when the fourth pool is taken into consideration (i.e., prediction of energy contribution from body weight loss).

As opposed to amino acid prediction from body weight loss coming solely from the body protein pool, energy contribution from body weight loss arises from three pools, i.e., protein, fat, and glycogen, hence rendering difficult the prediction of dietary energy requirement in sows expected to lose body weight during lactation. The NRC (1998) model assumes a constant body compositional loss to simplify the dietary energy requirement prediction. It combines the energy content of adipose tissue (9.4 kcal GE/g fat), the energy content of protein (5.6 kcal GE/g protein), and the amount of body protein contributing to energy (9.55%). For example, if a sow loses 1 kg of body weight, 9.42% is protein, or 0.41 kg lean tissue (lean tissue is 23% protein). The difference between lean tissue loss and total body loss is adipose tissue; hence, 1.0 − 0.41 = 0.59 kg of adipose tissue or 0.53 kg of fat (adipose tissue is 90% fat). Thus, the energy contribution from protein for each kilogram of body weight loss would be 410 g × 23% × 5.6 kcal = 528 kcal/kg and the energy contribution from adipose tissue for each kilogram of body weight loss would be 590 g × 90% ×

TABLE 33.15
Energy and Protein Recommendations for Lactating Sows with a Postfarrowing Weight of 175 kg Nursing Ten Pigs for 21 days

Items	Estimated Lactational Weight Change (kg)			
	0	0	−10	−10
	Daily Weight Gain of Pigs (g)			
	200	250	200	250
DE content of diet (kcal/kg)	3,400	3,400	3,400	3,400
ME content of diet (kcal/kg)[a]	3,265	3,265	3,265	3,265
Estimated DE intake (kcal/day)	18,205	21,765	15,680	19,240
Estimated ME intake (kcal/day)[a]	17,475	20,895	15,055	18,470
Estimated feed intake (kg/day)	5.35	6.40	4.61	5.66
Crude protein (%)	17.5	18.4	18.5	19.2

[a] Assumes that ME is 96% of DE.

Source: Nutrient Requirements of Swine, 10th rev. ed., National Academy Press, Washington, D.C., 1998. With permission.

9.4 kcal = 4991 kcal/kg. The total would then be 5519 kcal of GE for each kilogram of body weight loss (528 kcal from lean tissue and 4991 kcal from adipose tissue). Efficiency of energy utilization from mobilized tissue is approximately 88%; hence, each kilogram of body tissue loss contributes to 4856.7 kcal in milk. Table 33.15 provides an example of energy requirements estimated from the NRC (1998) model for sows with different milk production levels and various body weight loss conditions, using the numbers and equations described above.

V. FEED INGREDIENTS AND DIET COMPOSITION

A wide array of feed ingredients can be safely included in diets for gestating sows because of the low energy requirement of pregnancy relative to other phases of the reproductive cycle. This flexibility enables the use of many nontraditional feed ingredients for gestating sows that would not be acceptable for lactating sows. Factors such as nutrient content and digestibility, availability of supply, purity, freedom from antinutritional factors, physical form, and price per unit of nutrient must be evaluated when selecting feed ingredients. Ingredients that seem very inexpensive on a cost per ton basis may not be such a good deal if price is expressed on the basis of cost per unit of nutrient. If new equipment must be purchased to handle the ingredient or if the ingredient is contaminated with mycotoxins, the inexpensive ingredient suddenly becomes rather expensive relative to competing ingredients.

A. COMMON FEED INGREDIENTS

Most diets for gestating and lactating sows in North America are composed of an energy source, a source of protein to complement the amino acid deficiencies in the cereal grain, and a combination of vitamins and minerals. The primary energy sources are cereal grains such as corn, sorghum, barley, and wheat. Other grains such as oats, millet, and triticale are used less frequently. The most common protein supplement is soybean meal. Other important protein sources include canola meal, meat and bone meal, by-products of the brewing and distilling industries, whole soybeans, and sunflower meal. Local growing conditions and production systems may favor the use of field peas, lupins, peanut meal, or cull beans, but their inclusion is rather situation specific. Although corn and soybean meal are the predominate ingredients in North American swine diets, it is important to realize that pigs do not have a requirement for these ingredients. The potential ingredients listed above indicate that pigs can be fed successfully a wide range of ingredients. Complete knowledge of the advantages and disadvantages of each ingredient will ensure that optimal biological performance is achieved when these ingredients are used.

Most nutritionists supplement energy and protein ingredients with synthetic vitamins to satisfy the sow's total requirement. Natural feedstuffs do contain vitamins that are useful to the sow but for most vitamins concentration and stability are rather variable. Consequently, synthetic vitamins are supplemented to ensure sows are not deficient in any of the required vitamins. The macro- and microminerals are also supplemented in diets. Unlike the vitamins, natural feedstuffs are credited for their content of the macrominerals, calcium, phosphorus, sodium, and chloride. Macromineral deficiencies in the natural feedstuffs are corrected by the addition of supplements such as limestone, dicalcium phosphate, mono-dicalcium phosphate, bone meal, and salt. Typically, microminerals are treated similarly to vitamins in that the natural feedstuffs are assumed to contain no microminerals. These requirements are satisfied by supplementation to the diets.

Crystalline amino acids (L-isomers) can be supplemented to lactating sow diets deficient in specific amino acids. For example, L-lysine is commonly added to lactation diets formulated to meet the lysine requirement of the high-producing sow. Other amino acids can become limiting when feed ingredients other than corn and soybean meal are used. For example, threonine was shown to become limiting in sorghum-based diets. Valine has recently received much attention as a potentially limiting amino acid on its own or colimiting amino acid with lysine in corn–soybean meal diets fed to high-producing sows (Richert et al., 1996). Further research is needed before recommendation can be made, as Boyd et al. (1999) did not find any benefit from supplementing crystalline valine. Crystalline amino acids are typically not added to gestating sow diets. Amino acid requirements are met from intact proteins found in typical gestation diets. In addition, because gestating sows are typically fed either once or twice daily, the utilization of crystalline amino acids would not be maximized.

Diets for gestating and lactating sows do not routinely contain additives. However, in some situations, additives may be included for specific reasons. Some additives used in gestating and lactating sow diets include antibiotics, laxatives, yucca extracts, binders, chromium picolinate, and anthelmintics.

Water is the most important and usually the most ignored ingredient in the sow's diet. Certainly, water quality and quantity can influence performance, health, and well-being of the sow. Inadequate water intake and changes in drinking troughs between gestation and farrowing sections can be encountered in practice, thus reducing feed intake and causing poor milk production. This effect is usually noticed in an individual sow if the watering system is malfunctioning. Method of water delivery may influence health of the sow. Howell et al. (1994) reported a higher incidence of urinary tract infections when sows were offered water in intermittently filled troughs compared with nipple waterers mounted in individual gestation stalls. These authors suggested that the higher water intake of sows offered nipple waterers was responsible for the improved urinary tract health. Automatic nipple or cup waters should be checked to ensure that they are delivering at least 2 l/min. A thorough discussion of water in swine nutrition is presented in Chapter 17.

B. Use of Dietary Fiber

The gestating sow seems to be the most capable class of swine in modern production systems to utilize dietary fiber effectively. The need to limit energy intake for the control of gestation weight gain makes the gestating sow a logical choice to consume fibrous feedstuffs as part of the diet. Dietary fiber confers four primary benefits in diets for pregnant sows. Fiber increases the rate of passage for digesta in the gastrointestinal tract (Calvert, 1991) and thus serves as a laxative agent (Etienne, 1987). Control of constipation may improve sow comfort but such a benefit is difficult to document. This is further discussed below, along with the potential benefits of dietary fibers on reducing PHS.

Dietary fiber also serves to decrease the energy and bulk density of the diet because of the relatively lower concentration of usable energy in fibrous feedstuffs compared with common energy and protein sources (NRC, 1998). This energy dilution allows limited energy intake and thus controlled body weight gain without severely restricting total feed intake. Allowing sows to consume a larger quantity of feed decreases expression of stereotypic behaviors, increases level of satiety in the sow, and presumably improves well-being of the sow (Robert et al., 1993). Feeding relatively large quantities of a bulky diet throughout gestation enhances voluntary feed intake of sows during the subsequent lactation (Farmer et al., 1996; Vestergaard and Danielsen, 1998). Researchers have theorized that the gut becomes accustomed to the large quantity of feed in gestation and is physically prepared to handle the large feed intake desired in lactation (Reese, 1996). Reese (1997) reported an increase in litter size at birth ranging from 0.5 to 1.8 pigs when alfalfa hay, alfalfa haylage, corn gluten feed, oat hulls, or wheat straw was fed to sows during gestation (Table 33.16). A slight depression in live births per litter was observed when alfalfa meal or distillers grains were included in gestation diets (Reese, 1997). Evidently, source as well as level of fiber plays an important role in the litter size response. The biological mechanisms for increased litter size have not been elucidated. One reason for this lack of understanding is because there has not been a clear description of fiber used in studies reported in the literature. In addition, there is not a universally accepted method of describing dietary fiber and its components. Consequently, it is nearly impossible to establish cause-and-effect relationships from studies reported in the scientific literature.

The effect of feeding fiber on the incidence of PHS in sows has been briefly studied. Incidence of agalactia in sows fed a low-energy diet containing wheat bran and/or alfalfa during gestation and lactation is usually lower than in sows fed a normal energy diet (Nachreiner and Ginther, 1972; Wallace et al., 1974; Goransson, 1989). In addition, sows fed to low allowance in combination with free access to straw during the last 3 weeks prior to parturition have a lower incidence of PHS. Sows receiving a high-fiber diet during gestation have a markedly lower incidence of constipation and have approximately 40% faster intestinal transit time. Some evidence has suggested that endotoxins may be released from Gram-negative bacteria in the intestinal tract and be absorbed systemically (Smith, 1985). Endotoxins have been suggested to decrease prolactin release, and, consequently, the reduced level of prolactin results in a decline in milk production (Smith, 1985; Persson, 1996). That perhaps explains why constipation and low intestinal transit may be risk factors for the development of PHS.

On the other hand, dietary fibers may create some problems in certain pork production systems. The lower digestibility of fibrous feedstuffs compared with typical energy and protein sources

TABLE 33.16
Average Change in Litter Size According to Source of Dietary Fiber Fed to the Sow during Gestation

Fiber Source	Daily NDF Intake (g[a])		No. of Pigs Born Alive	No. of Pigs Weaned	No. of Litters[b]
	Control	Fiber			
Alfalfa meal	264	381	−0.4	−0.7	269
Alfalfa hay/haylage	246	721	0.5	0.8	647
Corn gluten feed	166	794	0.7	0.4	229
Distillers grains	139	418	−0.3	−0.4	118
Oat hulls/oats	260	1221	1.8	0.7	96
Wheat straw	150	368	0.5	0.7	699

[a] Average neutral detergent fiber intake by the sow consuming control and fibrous diets during gestatoin.
[b] Total number of litters produced by sows fed control and fibrous diets.

Source: Reese, D. E., Nebraska Swine Rep. EC 97-219A, University of Nebraska, 1997. With permission.

combined with the increased daily allotment of feed results in a larger quantity of fecal material being generated. This increases time and expense of manure removal from confinement production systems. In addition, the bulky nature of fecal material can slow the transfer of manure through perforated floors into storage units. This may create dirty housing conditions for sows. Increased daily feed allowance often will increase cost of feeding sows. However, Reese (1998) calculated that increased litter size at farrowing will offset any increase in gestation feed costs. These and other aspects of fiber are discussed in detail in Chapter 7.

C. Selected Aspects of Mineral Nutrition

1. Calcium and Phosphorus

Calcium and phosphorus are important to gestating sows for development of fetuses *in utero* and integrity of the sow's skeleton. Calcium and phosphorus required for fetal development can be derived from the diet or maternal stores. Severe restriction of Ca intake by the sow (0.3% dietary Ca), especially during the last trimester of pregnancy, will compromise the Ca status of fetuses (Itoh et al., 1967). A similar relationship likely exists for P. However, the sow is able to mitigate negative effects on fetal development of a moderate restriction. Mahan and Fetter (1982) fed diets ranging from 0.65 to 0.90% Ca and 0.50 to 0.70% P through three consecutive gestation and lactation periods with no effects of diet on mineral status of offspring. These researchers did note reduced bone ash of sows fed diets containing <0.9% Ca and 0.7% P at the end of the experiment. Reduction in bone mineralization may compromise longevity of sows in the breeding herd due to a higher incidence of crippling injuries and nonbreeders (Kornegay et al., 1973). Proper mineral nutrition during gestation can replenish bone mineral reserves that were depleted during lactation to satisfy the high mineral demands of milk production (Giesemann et al., 1998). Low Ca intake in late gestation may be a contributing factor to PHS during the subsequent lactation (Guan and Trottier, 1997).

Daily intakes of 14 to 18 g of Ca and 12 to 16 g of total P during gestation seem to satisfy the reproducing sow's needs during gestation. This recommendation allows for a moderate degree of mineral mobilization from bone reserves during lactation. If excessive mobilization occurs during lactation, higher levels of Ca and P intake during gestation may be required.

2. Calcium and Magnesium

Although hypocalcemia plays a very minor role in agalactia, it is nonetheless important to discuss. There are two ways that subclinical hypocalcemia could contribute to lactation failure. Hypocalcemia may have a depressant effect on the action of the mammary myoepithelium, which could lead to milk ejection failure. Hypocalcemia also decreases the strength of uterine contractions and may contribute to a prolonged farrowing, thereby increasing farrowing stress thus predisposing to lactation failure. In addition, with marginal Ca deficiency in successive lactations, the bones may become progressively weakened due to incomplete restoration of losses, making it increasingly difficult for sows to maintain milk flow. Magnesium salts are often used for their laxative effect (Bradford, 1990). Oversupplementation of Mg, however, can lead to competition with Ca for absorption sites in the gastrointestinal tract, thereby inducing a shortage of Ca and reducing milk production.

3. Chromium

Supplementation of sow diets with chromium has received considerable attention recently. Inorganic forms of chromium are so poorly absorbed by pigs that they are often used as inert markers of digesta in digestibility trials. However, organic forms, especially chromium tripicolinate, seem to have positive effects on reproductive function of sows. Chromium added to sow diets in the form of chromium

TABLE 33.17
Effect of Added Chromium Tripicolinate on Performance of Sows in Commercial Conditions[a,b]

Trait	Chromium Tripicolinate (ppb Cr)		Significance Level
	0	200	
Farrowing rate (%)	80	78.3	0.23
Sows bred within 7 days (%)	87.8	90.6	0.08
Total pigs born/litter	11.4	11.62	0.13
Pigs born live/litter	10.05	10.42	0.02
Pigs weaned/litter	8.75	9.08	0.02
Sow death rate (%)	10.9	9.4	0.09

[a] Data collected from April 1997 through March 1998.
[b] Each mean represents six 4000-sow units.

Source: Hagen, C. D. et al., in *Proc. of Use of Supplemental Chromium in Sow Diets Symp.*, Prince Agri Products, 1998, p. C-1. With permission.

tripicolinate at 200 ppb of chromium increases litter size (Lindemann et al., 1995b; Hagen et al., 1998), and farrowing rate (Campbell, 1996), and decreases mortality of sows in commercial production situations (Table 33.17; Hagen et al., 1998). Chromium tripicolinate potentiates the actions of insulin in swine (White et al., 1993). Cox et al. (1987) used exogenous insulin to increase ovulation rate in gilts. Increased litter size from sows fed chromium tripicolinate may be due to their heightened sensitivity to circulating insulin. The magnitude of reproductive response to chromium seems to be influenced by the basal litter size in the herd and the period of chromium supplementation (Campbell, 1996). An extended period of chromium supplementation seems necessary before positive effects on reproduction are demonstrable (Lindemann et al., 1995a; Purser, 1998).

4. Selenium and Vitamin E

Diets deficient in Se and vitamin E predispose sows to significantly higher incidence of PHS. The addition of either vitamin E or Se was reported to decrease the incidence of PHS (Mahan, 1994). It is well known that both vitamin E and Se function as antioxidants, protecting against the peroxidation of unsaturated fatty acids to free radicals in the cellular membranes. The free radicals and hyperperoxides cause metabolic derangement and destroy the structural integrity of cells. Besides acting as antioxidants, vitamin E and Se are involved in normal leukocyte function. Vitamin E restriction depressed peripheral blood lymphocyte and polymorphonuclear cell immune functions, where Se restriction depressed mainly polymorphonuclear cell immune function (Wuryastuti et al., 1993). Vitamin E and Se supplementation can increase the immune response of pigs to *Escherichia coli* (Wuryastuti et al., 1993). It seems that vitamin E and Se may play a role in decreasing the susceptibility of sows to coliform infections and therefore decrease the incidence of PHS.

D. Dietary Fat

The gestating sow's ability to consume feed in excess of nutrient needs precludes the need to increase energy density of the diet with supplemental fat. The primary challenge during gestation is to control energy intake and weight gain rather than increasing energy intake. However, supplemental fat in diets of pregnant sows during the late stages of gestation may improve survival rate of piglets. Pettigrew (1981) concluded that at least 1000 g of supplemental fat consumed by sows in late gestation would significantly improve survival rate of piglets in herds with a survival rate of <80% (Table 33.18). The improvement can be attributed primarily to increased fat concentration

TABLE 33.18
Effect of Adding Fat to the Sow's Gestation Diet on Percentage Survival of Piglets

Category	Estimated Survival Rate (%)		Fat Minus Control (percentage units)
	Control	Fat	
	Mean Piglet Survival Rate of Herd ≤80%		
Total prepartal fat intake (g)			
<1000	77.6	76.8	−0.8
>1000	74.6	80.8	6.2**
	Mean Piglet Survival Rate of Herd >80%		
Total prepartal fat intake (g)			
<1000	86.2	85.5	−0.7
>1000	89.1	89.9	0.8

** $P < 0.01$.

Source: Pettigrew, J. E., J. Anim. Sci., 53:107, 1981. With permission.

of colostrum and milk, which increases energy content and slightly increases carcass fat of newborn piglets. If survival rate of piglets in the herd is already rather high, supplemental fat in late gestation will be of little value.

VI. PRACTICAL CONSIDERATIONS OF GESTATION AND LACTATION FEEDING PROGRAMS

A. ECONOMICS

Economic evaluations of sow-feeding programs should include a range of inputs and outcomes. The common temptation is to focus on feed cost per pound of complete diet. A more accurate picture of feed costs is created if one considers the total daily feed costs on a per-sow basis. This accounts for differing amounts of feed offered to sows based on varying nutrient density of the diet. Low-cost feeding programs that increase the risk of compromised reproductive performance via abortions, early farrowings, reduced litter size at farrowing, or depressed milk production must be avoided. Such lapses can wreak havoc with production schedules in the sow herd, which easily impacts flow of pigs through the nursery, growing and finishing phases of the pork production system. Obviously, nutritional errors in the breeding herd can have long-lasting effects.

The cost of any feed input must be weighed against the value of any output. Obvious outputs that are fairly easy to measure are number of piglets, weight gain of piglets, and weight change of sows. Other outcomes of the feeding program that are more difficult to quantify include well-being of the sow, sow longevity, wear and tear on equipment, and the environmental consequences of nutrients in slurry generated by sows. All these factors should be considered in the development of an economically feasible feeding program.

B. IMPLEMENTATION ISSUES

The downfall of many feeding programs is failure to implement the program fully. A thorough understanding of the nutrient needs and the physiological processes of the gestating and lactating sow can lead to a biologically sound feeding program. A "perfect" feeding program designed on a nutritionist's computer can be compromised seriously with faulty implementation. The person designing the feeding program must be aware of the production conditions under which the feeding program will be used. The nutritionist must consider the capabilities and limitations of the facilities, and production schedule when designing a feeding program. For example, there is little value in striving for 1000 g of supplemental fat intake in late gestation if sows of all gestational stages are housed together in pens. People play a critical role in success of the feeding program. Be certain animal caretakers understand the program and are motivated to implement it completely. Generally, simple, easy-to-implement programs are more likely to be put into practice correctly by barn personnel. Periodic follow-up observations are crucial to success of the program. This follow-up is most valuable if there is a personal visit at the time of feeding to determine if the proper quantity and quality of feed is being fed to sows in the proper stage of gestation. In addition, an effective quality-control program for the feed manufacturing process will ensure that mixing errors do not occur. It is important not to assume that the program is being implemented as designed.

VII. FEEDING FROM WEANING TO REBREEDING

In many commercial production units, sows do not return to estrus after weaning as quickly as desired by the pork producer. Typically, this delayed return to estrus is caused by excessive loss of body weight and condition during the preceding lactation. Breeding managers are forced in these situations to implement nutritional programs and management practices attempting to hasten the return to postweaning estrus. Some producers argued that deprivation of feed and/or water for 24 to 48 h postweaning stops milk production and encourages a prompt return to estrus. MacLean (1969) reported a reduction in the interval to first estrus when feed or feed and water were withheld for 24 h postweaning. However, several researchers (Brooks and Cole, 1973; King, 1974; Tribble and Orr, 1982) reported no significant benefit of fasting to hasten estrus. Knabe and Tanksley (1982) imposed fasting treatments 48 h before weaning and reported that feed deprivation increased the interval to first estrus while water deprivation had no effect. Allrich et al. (1979) demonstrated that, as the length of fasting increased, the ovulation rate decreased.

Restricting nutrient intake was not beneficial to postweaning reproductive performance so researchers studied the effects of high nutrient intake during the postweaning period. Brooks and Cole (1972) fed primiparous sows 1.8, 2.7, or 3.6 kg/day from the day after weaning until the day after mating. They found that sows receiving 1.8 kg/day took longer to display estrus when compared with those sows receiving 2.7 or 3.6 kg/day (21.6 vs. 12.0 and 9.3 days, respectively). Brooks et al. (1975) reported a similar trend for a reduction in days to first estrus of multiparous sows as postweaning feed intake increased. Grandhi (1992) supplemented postweaning diets with fat or synthetic lysine for sows that experienced low (<14 kg) or high (>14 kg) body weight loss in the previous lactation. Added fat seemed to benefit first-parity sows with high weight loss by increasing the proportion of sows that displayed estrus by day 7 postweaning and increasing the number of normal embryos 30 days after breeding. However, older sows and young sows with low weight loss generally were unaffected by these dietary interventions.

Other researchers have found no benefits resulting from high postweaning nutrient intake. Feeding sows 1.8 or 3.6 kg of complete feed during the immediate postweaning period produced no beneficial effects on rebreeding performance (Tribble and Orr, 1982; Kirkwood and Thacker, 1991). Johnston et al. (1986) added 10% beef tallow to postweaning diets for first- and second-parity sows with no beneficial effects on postweaning interval to estrus.

Phases of the reproductive cycle are interrelated. Consequently, nutrition in one phase of the reproductive cycle not only affects sow performance in that phase but it also influences performance in subsequent phases. It seems that nutritional intervention after weaning to improve postweaning breeding performance is fairly ineffective. A much more effective approach to achieving acceptable postweaning breeding performance is to ensure that sows are fed properly during the preceding gestation and lactation periods. This approach prevents excessive lactational losses of body weight and condition by minimizing negative energy and nutrient balance in sows. It is much easier to prevent problems with postweaning breeding performance than it is to correct them once they appear.

REFERENCES

Aherne, F. X., and R. N. Kirkwood. 1985. Nutrition and sow prolificacy, *J. Reprod. Fertil. Suppl.*, 33:169.

Allrich, R. D., J. E. Tilton, J. N. Johnson, W. D. Slanger, and M. J. Marchello. 1979. Effect of lactation length and fasting on various reproductive phenomena of sows, *J. Anim. Sci.*, 48:359.

Armstrong, J. D., and J. H. Britt. 1987. Nutritionally-induced anestrus in gilts: metabolic and endocrine changes associated with cessation and resumption of estrous cycles, *J. Anim. Sci.*, 65:508.

Armstrong, J. D., J. H. Britt, and R. R. Kraeling. 1986. Effect of restriction of energy during lactation on body condition, energy metabolism, endocrine changes and reproductive performance in primiparous sows, *J. Anim. Sci.*, 63:1915.

Arthur, S. R., E. T. Kornegay, H. R. Thomas, H. P. Veit, D. R. Notter, and R. A. Barczewski. 1983. Restricted energy intake and elevated calcium and phosphorus intake for gilts during growth. III. Characterization of feet and limbs and soundness scores of sows during three parities, *J. Anim. Sci.*, 56:876.

Aumaitre, A., and P. H. Duee. 1974. Composition en acides amines des proteines corporelles du porcelet entre la naissance et l'age de huit semaines, *Ann. Zootech.*, 23:231.

Backwell, F. R., B. J. Bequette, D. Wilson, A. G. Calder, J. A. Metcalf, D. Wray-Cahen, J. C. MacRae, D. E. Beever, and G. E. Lobley. 1994. Utilization of dipeptides by the caprine mammary gland for milk protein synthesis, *Am. J. Phys.*, 267:R1.

Barnett, J. L., P. H. Hemsworth, C. G. Winfield, and V. A. Fahmy. 1987. The effects of pregnancy and parity number on behavioural and physiological responses related to the welfare status of individual and group-housed pigs, *Appl. Anim. Behav. Sci.*, 17:229.

Beltranena, E., G. R. Foxcroft, F. X. Aherne, and R. N. Kirkwood. 1991. Endocrinology of nutritional flushing in gilts, *Can. J. Anim. Sci.*, 71:1063.

Blair, R. M., D. A. Nichols, and D. L. Davis. 1994. Electronic animal identification for controlling feed delivery and detecting estrus in gilts and sows in outside pens, *J. Anim. Sci.*, 72:891.

Booth, P. J. 1990. Metabolic influences on hypothalamic-pituitary-ovarian function in the pig, *J. Reprod. Fertil., Suppl.*, 40:89.

Boyd, D., R. S. Kensinger, R. J. Harrell, and D. E. Bauman. 1995. Nutrient uptake and endocrine regulation of milk synthesis by mammary tissue of lactating sows, *J. Anim. Sci.*, 73(Suppl. 2):36.

Boyd, R. D., M. E. Johnston, J. L. Usry, and K. J. Touchette. 1999. Valine addition to a practical lactation diet did not improve sow performance, *J. Anim. Sci.*, 77(Suppl 1):51 (Abstr.).

Bradford, J. R. 1990. *Investigating and Correcting Sub-optimum Lactation Performance in Sows*, Luceville Veterinary Clinic, Luceville, IN.

Brendemuhl, J. H., A. J. Lewis, and E. R. Peo. 1989. Influence of energy and protein intake in primiparous sows during lactation on body composition of primiparous sows, *J. Anim. Sci.*, 64:1478.

Brooks, P. H. 1982. The gilt for breeding and for meat. In *Proceedings of Easter School in Agric. Science*, University of Nottingham, Butterworth, London, 211.

Brooks, P. H., and D. J. A. Cole. 1973. The effect of feed pattern in lactation and fasting following weaning on reproductive phenomena in the sow, *Vet. Rec.*, 93:276.

Brooks, P. H., and D. J. A. Cole. 1972. Studies in sow reproduction. 1. The effect of nutrition between weaning and remating on the reproductive performance of primiparous sows, *Anim. Prod.*, 15:259.

Brooks, P. H., D. J. A. Cole, and P. Rowlinson. 1975. Studies in sow reproduction. 3. The effect of nutrition between weaning and remating on the reproductive performance of multiparous sows, *Anim. Prod.*, 20:407.

Burnett, P. J., N. Walker, and D. J. Kilpatrick. 1988. The effect of age and growth traits on puberty and reproductive performance in the gilt, *Anim. Prod.*, 46:427.

Calabotta, D. F., E. T. Kornegay, H. R. Thomas, J. W. Knight, D. R. Notter, and H. P. Veit. 1982. Restricted energy intake and elevated calcium and phosphorus intake for gilts during growth. I. Feedlot performance and foot and leg measurements and scores during growth, *J. Anim. Sci.*, 54:565.

Calvert, C. C. 1991. Fiber utilization by swine. In *Swine Nutrition*, Miller, E. R., D. E. Ullrey, and A. J. Lewis, Eds., Butterworth-Heinemann, Boston, 285.

Campbell, R. G. 1996. The effects of chromium picolinate on the fertility and fecundity of sows under commercial conditions. In *Proc. 16th Annual Prince Feed Ingredient Conf.*, Quincy, IL.

Cassar, G., C. Chapeau, and G. J. King. 1994. Effects of increased dietary energy after mating on developmental uniformity and survival of porcine conceptuses, *J. Anim. Sci.*, 72:1320.

Clowes, E. J., I. H. Williams, V. E. Baracos, J. R. Pluske, A. C. Cegielski, L. J. Zak, and F. X. Aherne. 1998. Feeding lactating primiparous sows to establish three divergent metabolic states: II. Effect on nitrogen partitioning and skeletal muscle composition, *J. Anim. Sci.*, 75:1154.

Coffey, M. T., B. G. Diggs, D. L. Handlin, D. A. Knabe, C. V. Maxwell, Jr., P. R. Noland, T. J. Prince, and G. L. Cromwell. 1994. Effects of dietary energy during gestation and lactation on reproductive performance of sows: a cooperative study, *J. Anim. Sci.*, 72:4.

Cox, N. M., J. L. Ramirez, I. A. Matamoros, W. A. Bennett, and J. H. Britt. 1987a. Influence of season on estrous and luteinizing hormone responses to estradiol benzoate in ovariectomized sows, *Theriogenology*, 27:395.

Cox, N. M., M. J. Stuart, T. G. Althen, W. A. Bennett, and H. W. Miller. 1987b. Enhancement of ovulation rate in gilts by increasing dietary energy and administering insulin during follicular growth, *J. Anim. Sci.*, 64:507.

Cromwell, G. L., D. D. Hall, A. J. Clawson, G. E. Combs, D. A. Knabe, C. V. Maxwell, P. R. Noland, D. E. Orr, Jr., and T. J. Prince. 1989. Effects of additional feed during late gestation on reproductive performance of sows: a cooperative study, *J. Anim. Sci.*, 67:3.

D'Allaire, S., A. D. Leman, and R. Drolet. 1992. Optimizing longevity in sows and boars, *Swine Reprod.*, 8(3):545.

den Hartog, L. A. 1984. The Effect of Energy Intake on Development and Reproduction of Gilts and Sows, Ph.D. dissertation, Agricultural University of Wageningen, The Netherlands.

den Hartog, L. A., and G. J. M. van Kempen. 1980. Relation between nutrition and fertility in pigs, *Neth. J. Agric. Sci.*, 28:211.

den Hartog, L. A., and M. W. A. Verstegen. 1990. Nutrition of gilts during rearing, *Pig News Info.*, 11:523.

Dewey, C. E., R. M. Friendship, and M. R. Wilson. 1992. Lameness in breeding age swine: a case study, *Can. Vet. J.*, 33:747.

Dewey, C. E., R. M. Friendship, and M. R. Wilson. 1993. Clinical and postmortem examination of sows culled for lameness, *Can. Vet. J.*, 34:555.

Dourmad, J. Y. 1991. Effect of feeding level in the gilt during pregnancy on voluntary feed intake during lactation and changes in body composition during gestation and lactation, *Livest. Prod. Sci.*, 27:309.

Dourmad, J. Y., M. Etienne, A. Prunier, and J. Noblet. 1994. The effect of energy and protein intake of sows on their longevity: a review, *Livest. Prod. Sci.*, 40:87.

Dourmad, J. Y., M. Etienne, and J. Noblet. 1996. Reconstitution of body reserves in multiparous sows during pregnancy: effect of energy intake during pregnancy and mobilization during the previous lactation, *J. Anim. Sci.*, 74:2211.

Dourmad, J. Y., J. Noblet, and M. Etienne. 1998. Effect of body protein and lysine supply on performance, nitrogen balance, and body composition changes of sows during lactation, *J. Anim. Sci.*, 76:542.

Douglas, M. W., J. E. Cunnick, J. C. Pekas, D. R. Zimmerman, and E. H. von Borell. 1998. Impact of feeding regimen on behavioral and physiological indicators for feeding motivation and satiety, immune function, and performance of gestating sows, *J. Anim. Sci.*, 76:2589.

Dwyer, C. M., N. C. Strickland, and J. M. Fletcher. 1994. The influence of maternal nutrition on muscle fiber number development in the porcine fetus and on subsequent postnatal growth, *J. Anim. Sci.*, 72:911.

Eastham, P. R., W. C. Smith, C. T. Whittemore, and P. Phillips. 1988. Responses of lactating sows to food level, *Anim. Prod.*, 46:71.

Elsaesser, F., and N. Parvizi. 1980. Partial recovery of the stimulatory oestrogen feedback action on LH (luteinizing hormone) release during late lactation in the pig, *J. Reprod. Fertil.*, 59:63.

Elsley, F. W. H., E. V. J. Bathurst, A. G. Bracewell, J. M. M. Cunningham, J. B. Dent, T. L. Dodsworth, R. M. MacPherson, and N. Walker. 1971. The effect of pattern of food intake in pregnancy upon sow productivity, *Anim. Prod.*, 13:257.

English, P. R. 1970. A comparison of two sow-feeding systems from 5 days before to 7 days after farrowing, *Anim. Prod.*, 12:375 (Abstr.).

Esbenshade, K. L., J. H. Britt, J. D. Armstrong, V. D. Toelle, and C. M. Stanislaw. 1986. Body condition of sows across parities and relationship to reproductive performance, *J. Anim. Sci.*, 62:1187.

Etienne, M. 1987. Utilization of high fibre feeds and cereals by sows, a review, *Livest. Prod. Sci.*, 16:229.

Farmer, C., S. Robert, and J. J. Matte. 1996. Lactation performance of sows fed a bulky diet during gestation and receiving growth hormone-releasing factor during lactation, *J. Anim. Sci.*, 74:1298.

Ferket, S. L., and R. R. Hacker. 1985. Effect of forced exercise during gestation on reproductive performance of sows, *Can. J. Anim. Sci.*, 65:851.

Flowers, B., M. J. Martin, T. C. Cantley, and B. N. Day. 1989. Endocrine changes associated with a dietary-induced increase in ovulation rate (flushing) in gilts, *J. Anim. Sci.*, 67:771.

Frienkel, N. 1980. Of pregnancy and progeny, *Diabetes*, 29:1023.

Frisch, R. E. 1988. Fatness and fertility, *Sci. Am.*, 258:88.

Gaughan, J. B., R. D. A. Cameron, G. McL. Dryden, and M J. Josey. 1995. Effect of selection for leanness on overall reproductive performance in Large White sows, *Anim. Sci.*, 61:561.

Giesemann, M. A., A. J. Lewis, P. S. Miller, and M. P. Akhter. 1998. Effect of the reproductive cycle and age on calcium and phosphorus metabolism and bone integrity of sows, *J. Anim. Sci.*, 76:796.

Goldobin, M. I. 1976. The effect of hyperinsulinism on milk secretion and composition in sows, *Anim. Breed. Abstr.*, 44: 425.

Goransson, L. 1989. The effect of dietary crude fiber content on the frequency of post-partum agalactia in the sow, *J. Vet. Med.*, 36:474.

Grandhi, R. R. 1992. Effect of feeding supplemental fat or lysine during the postweaning period on the reproductive performance of sows with low or high lactation body weight and fat losses, *Can. J. Anim. Sci.*, 72:679.

Grondalen, T. 1974. Leg weakness in pigs. I. Incidence and relationship to skeletal lesions, feed level, protein and mineral supply, exercise and exterior conformation, *Acta Vet. Scand.*, 15:555.

Guan, X., and N. L. Trottier. 1997. Nutritional and management implications of lactation depression in the sow. In *Proc. Fifth Regional Amer. Soybean Assoc. Tech. Feed Workshop*, Bangkok, Thailand.

Guan, X., F. P. K. Ku, J. L. Snow, J. E. Pettigrew, H. Huynh, and N. L. Trottier. 1998. Dietary protein level affects amino acid concentration in porcine milk, *J. Anim. Sci.*, 76(Suppl. 1):163 (Abstract).

Guan, X. F., J. E. Pettigrew, C. Farmer, P. K. Ku, R. J. Tempelman, and N. L. Trottier. 1999. Relationship between plasma arterio-venous differences of nutrients across the porcine mammary gland and circulating insulin, prolactin, and IGF-1 concentrations, *J. Anim. Sci.*, 77(Suppl. 1):181 (Abstr.).

Gueblez, R., Gestin, J. M., and G. Le Henaff. 1985. Incidence de l'age et de l'epaisseur de lard dorsal a 100 kg sur la carriere reproductrice des truies Large White, *J. Rech. Porcine Fr.*, 17:113.

Hagen, C. D., M. D. Lindemann, and K. W. Purser. 1998. Effect of dietary chromium tripicolinate on productivity of sows under commercial conditions. In *Proc. of Use of Supplemental Chromium in Sow Diets Symp.*, Prince Agri Products, p. C-1.

Head, R. H., and I. H. Williams. 1991. Mammogenesis is influenced by pregnancy nutrition. In *Manipulating Pig Production III*, Batterham, E. S., Ed., Australasian Pig Science Association, Attword, p. 33.

Head, R. H., N. W. Bruce, and I. H. Williams. 1991. More cells might lead to more milk. In *Manipulating Pig Production III*, Batterham, E. S., Ed., Australasian Pig Science Association, Attword, p. 76.

Hill, M. A., H. D. Hilley, and R. H. C. Penny. 1986. Skeletal system. In *Diseases of Swine*, 6th ed., Leman, A. D., R. D. Glock, W. L. Mengeling, R. H. C. Penny, E. Scholl, and B. Straw, Eds., The Iowa State University Press, Ames.

Hoppe, M. K., G. W. Libal, and R. C. Wahlstrom. 1990. Influence of gestation energy level on the production of Large White × Landrace sows, *J. Anim. Sci.*, 68:2235.

Howell, S., G. Almond, and J. Stevens. 1994. Optimal water delivery systems for sow health. In *Proc. 25th Annu. Mtg. Am. Assoc. Swine Practitioners*, Chicago, IL, 342.

Hughes, P. E. 1982. Factors affecting the natural attainment of puberty in the gilt. In *Control of Pig Reproduction*, Cole, D. J. A., and G. R. Foxcroft, Eds., Butterworth Scientific, Boston, 117.

Itoh, H., S. L. Hansard, J. C. Glenn, F. H. Hoskins, and D. M. Thrasher. 1967. Placental transfer of calcium in pregnant sows on normal and limited-calcium rations, *J. Anim. Sci.*, 26:335.

Jenness, R. 1974. The composition of milk. In *Lactation: A Complete Treatise*, B. L. Larson, Ed., Iowa State University Press, Ames.

Jindahl, R., J. R. Cosgrove, F. X. Aherne, and G. R. Foxcroft. 1996. Effect of nutrition on embryonal mortality in gilts: association with progesterone, *J. Anim. Sci.*, 74:620.

Jindahl, R., J. R. Cosgrove, and G. R. Foxcroft. 1997. Progesterone mediates nutritionally induced effects on embryonic survival in gilts, *J. Anim. Sci.*, 75:1063.

Johnston, L. J. 1988. Relationship of Body Fat, Insulin and Selected Blood Borne Metabolites to Expression of Postweaning Estrus in Primiparous Sows, Ph.D. dissertation, Michigan State University.

Johnston, L. J., D. E. Orr, Jr., L. F. Tribble, and J. R. Clark. 1986. Effect of lactation and rebreeding phase energy intake on primiparous and multiparous sow performance, *J. Anim. Sci.*, 63:804.

Johnston, L. J., R. L. Fogwell, W. C. Weldon, N. K. Ames, D. E. Ullrey, and E. R. Miller. 1989. Relationship between body fat and postweaning interval to estrus in primiparous sows, *J. Anim. Sci.*, 67:943.

Johnston, L. J., J. E. Pettigrew, and J. W. Rust. 1993. Response of maternal-line sows to dietary protein concentration during lactation, *J. Anim. Sci.*, 71: 2151.

Jones, R. D., and C. V. Maxwell. 1974. Effect of protein level on growth, nitrogen balance and reproductive performance in gilts, *J. Anim. Sci.*, 39:1067.

Kemp, B., N. M. Soede, F. A. Helmond, and M. W. Bosch. 1995. Effects of energy source in the diet on reproductive hormones and insulin during lactation and subsequent estrus in multiparous sows, *J. Anim. Sci.*, 73:3022.

Kensinger, R. S., R. J. Collier, F. W. Bazer, C. A. Ducsay, and H. N. Becker. 1982. Nucleic acid, metabolic and histological changes in gilt mammary tissue during pregnancy and lactogenesis, *J. Anim. Sci.*, 54:1297.

Kertiles, L. P., and L. L. Anderson. 1979. Effect of relaxin on cervical dilation, parturition and lactation in pig, *Biol. Reprod.*, 21:57.

Kiess, W., A. Reich, K. Meyer, A. Glasow, J. Deutscher, J. Klammt, Y. Yang, G. Muller, and J. Kratzsch. 1999. A role for leptin in sexual maturation and puberty, *Horm. Res.*, 51(Suppl. S3):55.

Kim, S. W., W. L. Hurley, I. K. Han, H. H. Stein, and R. A. Easter. 1999. Effect of nutrient intake on mammary gland growth in lactating sows, *J. Anim. Sci.*, 77:3304.

King, G. J. 1974. Effects of several weaning procedures on the interval of estrus in sows, *Can. J. Anim. Sci.*, 54:251.

King, R. H. 1989. A note on the effects of nutrient intake during the later stages of rearing and early reproductive life on the subsequent reproductive efficiency of gilts, *Anim. Prod.*, 48:241.

King, R. H., and W. G. Brown. 1993. Interrelationships between dietary protein level, energy intake, and nitrogen retention in pregnant gilts, *J. Anim. Sci.*, 71:2450.

King, R. H., and I. H. Williams. 1984. The effect of nutrition on the reproductive performance of first-litter sows. I. Feeding level during lactation, and between weaning and mating, *Anim. Prod.*, 38:241.

King, R. H., E. Spiers, and P. Eckerman. 1986. A note on the estimation of the chemical body composition of sows, *Anim. Prod.*, 43:167.

King, R. H., C. J. Rayner, and M. Kerr. 1993a. A note on the amino acid composition of sow's milk, *Anim. Prod.*, 57:500.

King, R. H., M. S. Toner, H. Dove, C. S. Atwood, and W. G. Brown. 1993b. The response of first-litter sows to dietary protein level during lactation, *J. Anim. Sci.*, 71:2457.

King, R. H., J. E. Pettigrew, J. P. McNamara, J. P. McMurty, T. L. Henderson, M. R. Hathaway, and A. F. Sower. 1996. The effect of exogenous prolactin on lactation performance of first-litter sows given protein-deficient diets during the first pregnancy, *Anim. Reprod. Sci.*, 41:37.

Kirkwood, R. N., and F. X. Aherne. 1985. Energy intake, body composition and reproductive performance of the gilt, *J. Anim. Sci.*, 60:1518.

Kirkwood, R. N., and P. A. Thacker. 1991. The influence of premating feeding level and exogenous insulin on the reproductive performance of sows, *Can. J. Anim. Sci.*, 71:249.

Kirkwood, R. N., S. K. Baidoo, F. X. Aherne, and A. P. Sather. 1987. The influence of feeding level during lactation in the occurrence and endocrinology of the postweaning estrus in sows, *Can. J. Anim. Sci.*, 67:405.

Klindt, J., Yen, J. T., and R. K. Christenson. 1998. Effect of pattern of prepubertal feed level on reproductive development of gilts, *J. Anim. Sci.*, 76(Suppl.2): 51.

Klobasa, F., E. Werhahn, and J. E. Butler. 1987. Composition of sow milk during lactation, *J. Anim. Sci.*, 64:1458.

Knabe, D. A., and T. D. Tanksley, Jr. 1982. Effect of feed and water deprivation prior to weaning on subsequent reproductive performance, *J. Anim. Sci.*, 55(Suppl. 1):192 (Abstr.).

Koketsu, Y., G. D. Dial, J. E. Pettigrew, and V. L. King. 1996a. Feed intake pattern during lactation and subsequent reproductive performance of sows, *J. Anim. Sci.*, 74:2875.

Koketsu, Y., G. D. Dial, J. E. Pettigrew, W. E. Marsh, and V. L. King. 1996b. Characterization of feed intake patterns during lactation in commercial swine herds, *J. Anim. Sci.*, 74:1202.

Kornegay, E. T., H. R. Thomas, and T. N. Meacham. 1973. Evaluation of dietary calcium and phosphorus for reproducing sows housed in total confinement on concrete or in dirt lots, *J. Anim. Sci.*, 37:493.

Kusina, J., J. E. Pettigrew, A. F. Sower, M. R. Hathaway, M. E. White, and B. A. Crooker. 1999a. Effect of protein intake during gestation and lactation on the lactational performance of primiparous sows, *J. Anim. Sci.*, 77:931.

Kusina, J., J. E. Pettigrew, A. F. Sower, M. R. Hathaway, M. E. White, and B. A. Crooker. 1999b. Effect of protein intake during gestation on mammary development of primiparous sows, *J. Anim. Sci.*, 77:925.

Lee, P. A., and K. G. Mitchell. 1989. Feeding sows for specific weight gains in pregnancy and its effect on reproductive performance, *Anim. Prod.*, 48:407.

Lindemann, M. D., A. F. Harper, and E. T. Kornegay. 1995a. Further assessment of the effects of supplementation of chromium picolinate on fecundity in swine, *J. Anim. Sci.*, 73(Suppl. 1):185 (Abstr.).

Lindemann, M. D., C. M. Wood, A. F. Harper, E. T. Kornegay, and R. A. Anderson. 1995b. Dietary chromium picolinate additions improve gain:feed and carcass characteristics in growing-finishing pigs and increase litter size in reproducing sows, *J. Anim. Sci.*, 73:457.

Linzell, J. L., T. B. Mepham, E. F. Annison, and C. E. West. 1969. Mammary metabolism in lactating sows: arteriovenous differences of milk precursors and the mammary metabolism of [^{14}C]glucose and [^{14}C]acetate, *J. Nutr.*, 23:319.

Long, T. E., K. J. Stalder, R. N. Goodwin, J. Halstead, J. M. Anderson, and R. L. Wyatt. 1998. Effect of gilt development diet on stayability to fourth parity in sows, *J. Anim. Sci.*, 76(Suppl. 2):52.

Lynch, P. B. 1977. Effect of environmental temperature on lactating sows and their litters, *Ir. J. Agri. Res.*, 16:123.

MacLean, C. W. 1969. Observations on non-infectious infertility in sows, *Vet. Rec.*, 85:675.

Mahan, D. C. 1994. Effects of dietary vitamin E on sow reproductive performance over a five-parity period, *J. Anim. Sci.*, 72:2870.

Mahan, D. C., and A. W. Fetter. 1982. Dietary calcium and phosphorus levels for reproducing sows, *J. Anim. Sci.*, 54:285.

Mahan, D. C., and L. T. Mangan. 1975. Evaluation of various protein sequences on the nutritional carry-over from gestation to lactation with first-litter sows, *J. Nutr.*, 105:1291.

Martin, S. W., A. H. Meek, and P. Willeberg. 1987. *Veterinary Epidemiology. Principles and Methods*, Iowa State University Press, Ames, 51.

Martineau, G.-P., B. B. Smith, and B. Doize. 1992. Pathogenesis, prevention, and treatment of lactational insufficiency in sows, *Swine Reprod.*, 8:661–684.

Michel, E. J., R. A. Easter, H. W. Norton, and J. K. Rundquist. 1980. Effect of feeding frequency during gestation on reproductive performance of gilts and sows, *J. Anim. Sci.*, 50:93.

Moser, B. D. 1983. The use of fat in sow diets. In *Recent Advances in Animal Nutrition*, William Haresign, Ed., Butterworths, London, 78.

Moser, R. L., S. G. Cornelius, J. E. Pettigrew, H. E. Hanke, T. R. Heeg, and K. P. Miller. 1987. The influence of postpartum feeding method on performance of the lactating sow, *Livest. Prod. Sci.*, 16:91.

Moughan, P. J., and W. C. Smith. 1987. Whole body amino acid composition of the growing pig, *N.Z. J. Agric. Res.*, 30:301.

Mullan, B. P. 1991. The catabolism of fat and lean by sows during lactation, *Pig News Info.*, 12 (2):221.

Mullan, B. P., and I. H. Williams. 1989. The effect of body reserves at farrowing on the reproductive performance of first-litter sows, *Anim. Prod.*, 48:449.

Mullan, B. P., and I. H. Williams. 1990. The chemical composition of sows during their first lactation, *Anim. Prod.*, 51:375.

Musser, R. E., R. D. Goodband, D. L. Davis, S. S. Dritz, M. D. Tokach, J. L. Nelssen, J. S. Bauman, and M. Heintz. 1998. Sow and offspring performance after feeding additional diet or corn from d 30 to 50 of gestation, *J. Anim. Sci.*, 76(Suppl. 2):51 (Abstr.).

Nachreiner, R. F., and O. J. Ginther. 1972. Gestational and periparturient periods of sows: effects of altered environment, withholding of bran feeding and induced mastitis on serum chemical, hematologic and clinical variables, *Am. J. Vet. Res.*, 33:2221.

Nakano, T., and F. X. Aherne. 1977. Study of leg weakness, 56th Annu. Feeders Day Rep., University of Alberta, 18.

Nakato, T., F. X. Aherne, and J. R. Thompson. 1979. Effects of feed restriction, sex and diethylstilbestrol on the occurrence of joint lesions with some histological and biochemical studies of the articular cartilage of growing-finishing swine, *Can. J. Anim. Sci.*, 59:491.

Nelssen, J. L., A. J. Lewis, E. R. Peo, and J. D. Crenshaw. 1985. Effect of dietary energy intake during lactation on performance of primiparous sows and their litters, *J. Anim. Sci.*, 61:1164.

Noblet, J., and M. Etienne. 1986. Effect of energy level in lactating sows on yield and composition of milk and nutrient balance of piglets, *J. Anim. Sci.*, 63:1888.

Noblet, J., and M. Etienne. 1987. Metabolic utilization of energy and maintenance requirements in lactating sows, *J. Anim. Sci.*, 64:774.

Noblet, J., and M. Etienne. 1989. Estimation of sow milk nutrient output, *J. Anim. Sci.*, 67:3352.

Noblet, J., W. H. Close, R. P. Heavens, and D. Brown. 1985. Studies on the energy metabolism of the pregnant sow. 1. Uterus and mammary tissue development, *Br. J. Nutr.*, 53:251.

Noblet, J., J. Y. Dourmad, and M. Etienne. 1990. Energy utilization in pregnant and lactating sows: modeling of energy requirements, *J. Anim. Sci.*, 68:562.

NRC. 1973. *Nutrient Requirements of Swine*, 7th rev. ed., National Academy Press, Washington, D.C.

NRC. 1981. *Effect of Environment on Nutrient Requirements of Domestic Animals*, National Academy Press, Washington, D.C.

NRC. 1988. *Nutrient Requirements of Swine*, 9th rev. ed., National Academy Press, Washington, D.C.

NRC. 1998. *Nutrient Requirements of Swine*, 10th rev. ed., National Academy Press, Washington, D.C.

NCR-89 Committee on Confinement Management of Swine. 1990. Feeding frequency and the addition of sugar to the diet for the lactating sow, *J. Anim. Sci.*, 68:3498.

O'Grady, J. F., P. B. Lynch, and P. A. Kearney. 1985. Voluntary feed intake by lactating sows, *Livest. Prod. Sci.*, 12:355.

Padalikova, D., and D. Jezkova. 1984. Chemical composition of bodies and organs of pig fetuses in the last forty days of intrauterine life, *Acta Vet. Brno*, 53:19.

Park, Y. W., M. Kandeh, K. B. Chin, W. G. Pond, and L. D. Young. 1994. Concentrations of inorganic elements in milk of sows selected for high and low serum cholesterol, *J. Anim. Sci.*, 72:1399.

Persson, A. 1996. Lactational disorders in sows with special emphasis on mastitis, Commission on Pig Production, session 2: Qualitative and quantitative aspects of lactation, presented at 47th Meeting of the European Association for Animal Production, Lillehammer, Norway.

Pettigrew, J. E. 1978. Supplemental dietary fat in sow diets. In *Proc. 1978 Pacific Northwest Pork Exposition*, Spokane, WA.

Pettigrew, J. E. 1981. Supplemental dietary fat for peripartal sows: a review, *J. Anim. Sci.*, 53:107.

Pettigrew, J. E. 1993. Amino acid nutrition of gestating and lactating sows, BioKyowa Tech. Rev. 5.

Pettigrew, J. E., and M. D. Tokach. 1993. Metabolic influences on sow reproduction, *Pig News Info.*, 14:69N.

Pettigrew, J. E., and H. Yang. 1997. Protein nutrition of gestating sows, *J. Anim. Sci.*, 75:2723.

Pettigrew, J. E., S. G. Cornelius, R. L. Moser, and A. F. Sower. 1987. A refinement technique for estimating milk intake of pigs using pig serum, *Livest. Prod. Sci.*, 16:163.

Pluske, J. R., T. W. Fenton, M. L. Lorschy, J. E. Pettigrew, A. F. Sower, and F. X. Aherne. 1997. A modification to the isotope-dilution technique for estimating milk intake of pigs using pig serum, *J. Anim. Sci.*, 75:1279.

Pluske, J. R., I. H. Williams, L. J. Zak, E. J. Clowes, A. C. Cecielski, and F. X. Aherne. 1998. Feeding lactating primiparous sows to establish three divergent metabolic states: III. Milk production and pig growth, *J. Anim. Sci.*, 76:1176.

Pond, W. G., J. T. Yen, R. R. Maurer, and R. K. Christenson. 1981. Effect of doubling daily energy intake during the last two weeks of pregnancy on pig birth weight, survival, and weaning weight, *J. Anim. Sci.*, 52:535.

Poretsky, L., and M. F. Kalin. 1987. The gonadotropic function of insulin, *Endocr. Rev.*, 8:132.

Purser, K. W. 1998. Effect of supplemental chromium picolinate on productivity of sows under commercial conditions. In *Proc. Am. Assoc. Swine Practitioners*, Des Moines, 213.

Reese, D. E. 1996. Dietary fiber in sow gestation diets. In *Proc. Carolina Nutr. Conf.*, Raleigh, NC.

Reese, D. E. 1997. Dietary fiber in sow gestation diets — a review. Nebraska Swine Rep. EC 97–219A, University of Nebraska, 23.

Reese, D. E. 1998. Dietary fiber in sow gestation diets — an economic analysis. Nebraska Swine Rep. EC 98-219-A. University of Nebraska, 23.

Reese, D. E., B. D. Moser, E. R. Peo, Jr., A. J. Lewis, D. R. Zimmerman, J. E. Kinder, and W. W. Stroup. 1982. Influence of energy intake during lactation on the interval from weaning to first estrus in sows, *J. Anim. Sci.*, 5:590.

Revell, D. K., and I. H. Williams. 1993. A review — physiological control and manipulation of voluntary food intake. In *Manipulating Pig Production IV*, Batterham, E. S., Ed., Australasian Pig Science Association, Attwood, Victoria, Australia, 55–80.

Revell, D. K., I. H. Williams, B. P. Mullan, J. L. Ranford, and R. J. Smits. 1995. A high-protein diet maximizes milk output and minimizes weight loss in lactation. In *Manipulating Pig Production V*, Cranwell, P. D., and D. P. Hennessy, Eds., Australasian Pig Science Association, Werribee, Victoria, Australia, 136.

Revell, D. K., I. H. Williams, B. P. Mullan, J. L. Ranford, and R. J. Smits. 1998a. Body composition at farrowing and nutrition during lactation affect the performance of primiparous sows: I. Voluntary feed intake, weight loss, and plasma metabolites, *J. Anim. Sci.*, 76:1729.

Revell, D. K., I. H. Williams, B. P. Mullan, J. L. Ranford, and R. J. Smits. 1998b. Body composition at farrowing and nutrition during lactation affect the performance of primiparous sows: II. Milk composition, milk yield, and pig growth, *J. Anim. Sci.*, 76:1738.

Reynolds, L., and J. A. F. Rook. 1977. Intravenous infusion of glucose and insulin in relation to milk secretion in the sow, *Br. J. Nutr.*, 37:45.

Richert, B. T., M. D. Tokach, R. A. Goodband, J. L. Nelssen, J. E. Pettigrew, R. A. Walker, and L. J. Johnston. 1996. Valine requirement of the high-producing lactating sow, *J. Anim. Sci.*, 74:1307.

Richmond, R. J., and R. T. Berg. 1971. Muscle growth and distribution in swine as influenced by liveweight, breed, sex and ration, *Can. J. Anim. Sci.*, 51: 41.

Riley, J. E. 1989. Recent trends in pig production: the importance of intake. In *The Voluntary Food Intake of Pigs*, Forbes, J. M., M. A. Varley and T. J. L. Lawrence, Eds., British Society of Animal Production, Edinburg, 1–6.

Robert, S., J. J. Matte, C. Farmer, C. L. Girard, and G. P. Martineau. 1993. High-fibre diets for sows: effects on stereotypies and adjunctive drinking, *Appl. Anim. Behav. Sci.*, 37:297.

Roos, M. A. 1990. Dynamics of Energy and Protein Metabolism in the Reproducing Sow, Ph.D. thesis, University of Illinois, Urbana.

Rozeboom, D. W., R. L. Moser, S. G. Cornelius, J. E. Pettigrew, and S. M. El Kandelgy. 1993a. Body composition of postpubertal gilts at nutritionally induced anestrus, *J. Anim. Sci.*, 71:426.

Rozeboom, D. W., J. E. Pettigrew, G. D. Dial, and J. E. Wheaton. 1993b. Effect of pre- and postbreeding dietary energy intake on ovulation rate, embryo number, and percent embryo survival in gilts, *J. Anim. Sci.*, 71(Suppl. 1):67.

Rozeboom, D. W., J. E. Pettigrew, R. L. Moser, S. G. Cornelius, and S. M. El Kandelgy. 1995. Body composition of gilts at puberty, *J. Anim. Sci.*, 73:2524.

Rozeboom, D. W., J. E. Pettigrew, R. L. Moser, S. G. Cornelius, and S. M. E. Kandelgy. 1996. Influence of gilt age and body composition at first breeding on sow reproductive performance and longevity, *J. Anim. Sci.*, 74:138.

Sauber, T. E., T. S. Stahly, R. C. Ewan, and N. H. Williams. 1994. Maximum lactational capacity of sows with high and low genetic capacity for lean tissue growth, *J. Anim. Sci.*, 72 (Suppl. 1):364 (Abstr.).

Schaefer, A. L., A. K. W. Tong, A. P. Sather, E. Beltranema, A. Phaearyn, and F. X. Aherne. 1991. Preparturient diabetogenesis in primiparous gilts, *Can. J. Anim. Sci.*, 71:69.

Schneider, J. E., and G. N. Wade. 1989. Availability of metabolic fuels controls estrous cyclicity of Syrian hamsters, *Science*, 244:1326.

Shields, R. G., Jr., and D. C. Mahan. 1983. Effects of pregnancy and lactation on the body composition of first-litter female swine, *J. Anim. Sci.*, 57:594.

Singleton, W. L. 1989. Effect of gestation housing and feeding systems on sow and litter performance, *J. Anim. Sci.*, 67(Suppl. 1):470 (Abstr.).

Smith, B. B. 1985. Pathogenesis and therapeutic management of lactation failure in periparturient sows. Corvallis, Oregon, Oregon State University, *Compendum Continuing Educ.*, 7(9):S523.

Snow, J. L., P. Ku, D. Rozeboom, and N. L. Trottier. 1997. Effect of feeding strategies on feed intake response and performance in lactating sows, *J. Anim. Sci.*, 75(Suppl. 1):248 (Abstr.).

Sorensen, M. T., B. Jorgensen, and V. Danielsen. 1993. Different feeding intensity of young gilts: effect on growth, milk yield, reproduction, leg soundness, and longevity. Report No. 14/1993, National Institute of Animal Science, Denmark.

Speer, V. C., and D. F. Cox. 1984. Estimating milk yield of sow, *J. Anim. Sci.*, 59:1281.

Spincer, J., and J. A. F. Rook. 1971. The metabolism of [1-14C]glucose, [1-15C]palmitic acid and [1-14C] stearic acid by the lactating mammary gland of the sow, *J. Dairy Res.*, 38:315.

Stahly, T. S., G. L. Cromwell, and W. S. Simpson. 1979. Effects of full vs. restricted feeding of the sow immediately postpartum on lactation performance, *J. Anim. Sci.*, 49:50.

Toner, M. S., R. H. King, F. R. Dunshea, H. Dove, and C. S. Atwood. 1996. The effect of exogenous somatotropin on lactation performance of first-litter sows, *J. Anim. Sci.*, 74:167.

Touchette, K. J., G. L. Allee, M. D. Newcomb, and R. D. Boyd. 1998. The lysine requirement of lactating primiparous sows, *J. Anim. Sci.*, 76:1091.

Tribble, L. F., and D. E. Orr, Jr. 1982. Effect of feeding level after weaning on reproduction in sows, *J. Anim. Sci.*, 55:608.

Tri-State Nutrition Guide. 1998. The Ohio State University, Bulletin 869.

Tritton, S. M., R. H. King, R. G. Campbell, A. C. Edwards, and P. E. Hughes. 1996. The effects of dietary protein and energy levels of diets offered during lactation on the lactational and subsequent reproductive performance of first-litter sows, *Anim. Sci.*, 62:573.

Trottier, N. L. 1991. Relationship between Energy Intake, Backfat Thickness and Reproductive Performance of Sows, M.S. thesis, McGill University, Montreal, Quebec, Canada.

Trottier, N. L. 1995. Protein Metabolism in the Lactating Sow, Ph.D. thesis, Department of Animal Sciences, University of Illinois, Urbana.

Trottier, N. L. 1997. Nutritional control of amino acid supply to the mammary gland during lactation in the pig, *Proc. Nutr. Soc.*, 56:581.

Trottier, N. L., and R. A. Easter. 1995. Dietary and plasma branched-chain amino acids in relation to tryptophan: effect on voluntary feed intake and lactation metabolism in the primiparous sow, *J. Anim. Sci.*, 76:1086.

Ullrey, D. E., J. I. Sprague, D. E. Becker, and E. R. Miller. 1965. Growth of the swine fetus, *J. Anim. Sci.*, 24:711.

Vangen, O. 1980. Studies on a two traits selection experiment in pigs. V. Correlated response in reproductive performance, *Acta Agric. Scand.*, 30:309.

Vaughan, L. C. 1971. Leg weakness in pigs, *Vet. Rec.*, 89:81.

Verstegen, M. W. A., J. Mesu, G. J. M. van Kempen, and C. Geerse. 1985. Energy balances of lactating sows in relation to feeding level and stage of lactation, *J. Anim. Sci.*, 60:731.

Vestergaard, E. M., and V. Danielsen. 1998. Dietary fibre for sows: effects of large amounts of soluble and insoluble fibres in the pregnancy period on the performance of sows during three reproductive cycles, *Anim. Sci.*, 68:355.

Wahlstrom, R. C., and G. W. Libal. 1977. Effect of dietary protein during growth and gestation on development and reproductive performance of gilts, *J. Anim. Sci.*, 45:94.

Wallace, H. D., D. D. Thieu, and G. E. Combs. 1974. Alfalfa meal as a special bulky ingredient in the sow diet at farrowing and during lactation, Res. Rep. Dept. Anim. Sci., University of Florida, Gainesville, FL.

Weldon, W. C., A. J. Thulin, O. A. MacDougald, L. J. Johnston, E. R. Miller, and H. A. Tucker. 1991. Effects of increased dietary energy and protein during late gestation on mammary development in gilts, *J. Anim. Sci.*, 69:194.

Weldon, W. C., A. J. Lewis, G. F. Louis, J. L. Kovar, M. A. Giesemann, and P. S. Miller. 1994a. Postpartum hypophagia in primiparous sows: I. Effects of gestation feeding level on feed intake, feeding behavior, and plasma metabolite concentrations during lactation, *J. Anim. Sci.*, 72:387.

Weldon, W. C., A. J. Lewis, G. F. Louis, J. L. Kovar, and P. S. Miller. 1994b. Postpartum hypophagia in primiparous sows: II. Effects of feeding level during gestation and exogenous insulin on lactation feed intake, glucose tolerance, and epinephrine-stimulated release of nonesterified fatty acids and glucose, *J. Anim. Sci.*, 72:395.

White, C. E., H. H. Head, K. C. Bachman, and F. W. Bazer. 1984. Yield and composition of milk and weight gain of nursing pigs from sows fed diets containing fructose or dextrose, *J. Anim. Sci.*, 59:141.

White, M., J. Pettigrew, J. Zollitsch-Stelzl, and B. Crooker. 1993. Chromium in swine diets. In *Proc. Minnesota Nutr. Conf.*, University of Minnesota, Bloomington, 251.

Whittemore, C. T., and H. Yang. 1989. Physical and chemical composition of the body of breeding sows with differing body subcutaneous fat depth at parturition, differing nutrition during lactation and differing litter size, *Anim. Prod.*, 48:203.

Whittemore, C. T., M. F. Franklin, and B. S. Pearce. 1980. Fat changes in breeding sows, *Anim. Prod.*, 31:183.

Whittemore, C. T., A. G. Taylor, G. M. Hillyer, D. Wilson, and C. Stamataris. 1984. Influence of body fat stores on reproductive performance of sows, *Anim. Prod.*, 38:527.

Wuryastuti, H., H. D. Stowe, R. W. Bull, and E. R. Miller. 1993. Effects of vitamin E and selenium on immune response of peripheral blood, colostrum, and milk leukocytes of sows, *J. Anim. Sci.*, 71:2464.

Yang, H., P. R. Eastham, P. Phillips, and C. T. Whittemore. 1989. Reproductive performance, body weight and body condition of breeding sows with differing body fatness at parturition, differing nutrition during lactation, and differing litter size, *Anim. Prod.*, 48:181.

Yang, H., J. E. Pettigrew, L. J. Johnston, G. C. Shurson, and R. D. Walker. 2000. Lactational and subsequent reproductive responses of lactating sows to dietary lysine (protein) concentration, *J. Anim. Sci.*, 78:348.

Young, L. G., and G. J. King. 1989. Gestation energy levels for sows, Annual Report 1988–1989, Ontario Agricultural College, University of Guelph.

Young, L. G., G. J. King, J. Shaw, M. Quinton, J. S. Walton, and I. McMillan. 1991. Interrelationships among age, body weight, backfat and lactation feed intake with reproductive performance and longevity of sows, *Can. J. Anim. Sci.*, 71:567.

Zak, L. J., I. H. Williams, G. R. Foxcroft, J. R. Pluske, A. C. Cegielski, E. J. Clowes, and F. X. Aherne. 1998. Feeding lactating primiparous sows to establish three divergent metabolic states: I. Associated endocrine changes and postweaning reproductive performance, *J. Anim. Sci.*, 76: 1145.

Zhang, Y., I. G. Partridge, and K. G. Mitchell. 1986. The effect of dietary energy level and protein:energy ratio on nitrogen and energy balance, performance and carcass composition of pigs weaned at 3 weeks of age, *Anim. Prod.*, 42:389.

Zoiopoulos, P. E., Topps, J. H., and P. R. English. 1983. Losses in weight and body water in sows after weaning, *Br. J. Nutr.*, 50:163.

34 Feeding of Developing and Adult Boars

Bas Kemp and Nicoline M. Soede

CONTENTS

I. Introduction 771
II. Effects of Protein and Energy Intake on Reproductive Characteristics
    of Developing Boars 772
III. Effects of Protein and Energy Intake on Reproductive Characteristics
    of Adult Boars 773
    A. Effects of Protein Intake 773
    B. Effects of Energy Intake 775
IV. Energy Requirements of Breeding Boars: A Factorial Approach 777
    A. Maintenance 777
    B. Growth 778
    C. Reproduction 778
    D. Total Requirements 779
V. Vitamins and Minerals for Breeding Boars 779
    A. Vitamin E and Selenium 779
    B. Calcium, Phosphorus, and Biotin 779
    C. Vitamin A 780
    D. Zinc 780
VI. Conclusions 780
References 780

I. INTRODUCTION

Breeding boars are a relatively small part of the pig population, which is probably the reason that their nutrition has received relatively little attention. Information regarding nutritional requirements and effects of nutrition on reproductive aspects of the boar is therefore relatively scarce. Thus in this chapter, relative old literature is sometimes cited, but one should realize that the modern breeding boar is genetically a different animal from those boars used 20 to 30 years ago. The feed requirements for boars as provided by nutritionists around the world are often based on sow data. The aim of this chapter is to review the available information on the nutrition for breeding boars, which then can be incorporated into nutritional requirement settings.

Reproductive performance of a boar can be described by three characteristics: libido, number of sperm cells produced per time unit, and fertilizing capacity of the sperm cells (or semen quality). Libido is usually estimated as the number of successful mountings expressed as a proportion of the total mounting opportunities. A successful mounting means the production of an ejaculate on a sow or a dummy. More detailed measurements, such as time taken to mount a dummy or sow, amount of sexual interest, penis extension, intromission, and ejaculation, are sometimes used to describe libido in more detail (Berger et al., 1981). The number of sperm cells produced can be estimated by counting the number of sperm cells in ejaculates or by quantitative testicular and epididymal histology after slaughter. For accurate estimates of sperm output, it is important to have the experimental groups of boars on a similar mating frequency to avoid differences in mating frequency affecting sperm output. The mating frequency should be sufficiently high (e.g., two or three times a week) to avoid loss of semen through masturbation or urine. Assessment of semen quality is done in many different ways, ranging from light microscopic evaluation of movement of the sperm cells and morphology of the sperm cells to assessment of pregnancy rates and litter size after insemination.

In general, for experiments on the effects of nutrition on reproductive performance in boars, a long preliminary period is needed. According to Singh (1962), it takes 25 days before a sperm cell, which is formed from an A-type spermatogonium, appears in the epididymis. Swierstra (1968) considered 34.4 days as a reasonable approximation of the duration of spermatogenesis in boars. Sperm cells mature in the epididymis for about 10 days (Swierstra, 1968) to 14 days (Singh, 1962) after leaving the testis. Therefore, it can be concluded that feeding experiments with boars should contain a preliminary period of at least 6 weeks. When studying the effects of nutrition of developing boars on reproductive characteristics later in life, even longer experimental periods are required.

In this chapter, the effects of protein and energy intake on reproductive characteristics of developing and adult boars are discussed. Following this, a factorial approach to the energy requirements for breeding boars is presented. Finally, current information on vitamins and minerals is discussed.

II. EFFECTS OF PROTEIN AND ENERGY INTAKE ON REPRODUCTIVE CHARACTERISTICS OF DEVELOPING BOARS

Breeding boars are usually fed *ad libitum* during the growing period using protein adequate growing-finishing diets. This allows proper boar selection based on lean tissue growth rate, feed intake, feed conversion, and carcass quality. It is currently assumed that feeding boars to appetite does not impair later reproductive performance. However, after the selection period (usually at 105 kg or 5 to 6 months of age), a restricted growth is desired to prevent the boar from becoming too heavy for natural service. Although no data are available on how best to limit the growth rate that results in a moderately growing breeding boar, one can assume that growth reduction should be done by a stepwise limitation in feed intake rather than by an abrupt reduction in feed intake. This gradual change will give the boar time to adapt to the new situation.

Many feeding trials with developing boars have studied the onset of puberty. Onset of puberty is a period in which physiological and behavioral changes lead to expression of libido and a normal ejaculation with good-quality sperm cells. In most western breeds, onset of puberty occurs at 120 to 180 days of age (Lunstra et al., 1997).

Nutrition during the growing period affects weight and age at puberty. Dutt and Barnhart (1959) fed Hampshire boars from weaning to 312 days of age diets with 100, 70, and 50% of the NRC requirements (Beeson at al., 1953). Weight at puberty was 101, 78, and 61 kg, respectively, and age at puberty was 203, 212, and 219 days, respectively. Semen volume at puberty was 30% lower in the boars fed the low feeding level compared with the high feeding level, and semen concentration, percentage of motile sperm, percentage of abnormal sperm, and pregnancy rate and embryonic survival in sows inseminated with semen of the three groups of boars were similar. Kim and Lee (1975) fed Korean purebred and crossbred boars for 14 months starting at weaning 100 or 70% of the NRC (1973) requirements. Weight and age at puberty in the 100% NRC group averaged 89.0 and 79.5 kg and 215 and 179 days, for the purebred and crossbred boars, respectively. In the 70% NRC group, age at puberty was delayed by 47 and 30 days, for the purebred and crossbred boars, respectively, and weight at puberty was 15.5 and 2.0 kg lower for the purebred and crossbred boars. In agreement with the results of Dutt and Barnhart (1959), Kim and Lee (1975) found that restricted feeding resulted in a 30% lower semen volume, but it had no effect on sperm concentration or quality of the semen. Although, Dutt and Barnhart (1959) found that feeding level during rearing affected age at puberty to a lesser extent than weight at puberty, Kim and Lee (1975) seemed to find the opposite. This difference is probably breed dependent.

Protein restriction during the growing period has similar effects on weight and age at puberty and sexual development. Uzu (1979) fed boars *ad libitum* using diets with 12.0, 18.0, or 23.0% crude protein (CP). Age at puberty was reached at 193, 182, and 177 days, respectively, and weight at puberty was similar (88 kg). Semen was collected at puberty. Semen characteristics did not differ significantly, although the number of sperm cells per ejaculate was decreased about 50%, and the weight of the testes at slaughter was significantly decreased in the group fed 12.0% protein.

These data indicate that protein and energy restriction during the growing period can affect age and weight at puberty, and rate of sexual development. The question is whether restriction during growth has long-term effects on reproductive functioning of boars during their breeding life. Althen et al. (1974) fed isocaloric diets containing 10, 15, or 20% CP from weaning to 1 year of age. They found a higher follicle-stimulating hormone (FSH) and luteinizing hormone (LH) pituitary content in boars fed the higher protein diets at 230 days of age, but there were no differences between the groups at 365 days of age. This response indicates that protein restriction may retard sexual development, but that it has no lasting effects on reproductive output later in life. Dickerson et al. (1964) severely underfed boars for 1 year starting at 2 to 3 weeks of age, and then refed them. Realimentation resulted in compensatory development of the reproductive organs toward the boars fed normally.

Although information is relatively limited, it seems that nutrition during growing affects age and sexual development at puberty, but unless severely undernourished, there is no lasting effect on reproductive capacity.

III. EFFECTS OF PROTEIN AND ENERGY INTAKE ON REPRODUCTIVE CHARACTERISTICS OF ADULT BOARS

A. Effects of Protein Intake

The literature reveals a specific interest in protein nutrition of boars. Various experiments have been conducted on the effect of protein, and more specifically on the effect of the amino acids lysine and methionine plus cystine on fertility of the breeding boar. A detailed review of the older literature is given by Kemp and den Hartog (1989). In the 1960s and 1970s, many experiments were published that lacked explicit information on the level and composition of the diets. This makes it difficult to draw conclusions on protein needs for breeding boars.

In 1974, Poppe et al. conducted an experiment with 28 boars (20 boars were 8 to 9 months old and 8 boars were 12 to 13 months old at the start of the 18- to 20-week experiment). One group of boars received a low-protein diet (19.3% CP) and three other groups received a high-protein diet (28.3% CP). The boars on the three high-CP diets were supplemented with synthetic lysine (12 g L-lysine/boar/day), methionine (16 g DL-methionine/boar/day), or not supplemented. After a 6-week preliminary period, boars were kept for 6 weeks on a low semen collection frequency (one or two times a week for young and old boars, respectively). Subsequently, boars were kept on a high semen collection frequency for 6 to 8 weeks (three or four times a week for young and old boars, respectively). At the low mating frequency, the difference in sperm output between groups was not significant. However, at the high mating frequency, the sperm output in the groups of boars given synthetic amino acids was significantly higher than in the other two groups. Supplemented lysine increased the number of sperm cells ejaculated by 7%, and the supplemented methionine increased the number by 28%. No effect of diet was found on semen quality. Poppe et al. (1974) also calculated that during the period of high mating frequency, the young boars fed the low protein levels showed a decrease over time in the number of sperm cells produced, whereas sperm production in boars fed the high protein levels remained stable. This decrease over time in semen production was only observed in the young boar. Based on this research, they recommended a diet containing 28.3% CP, 1.84% total lysine, and 1.23% of total methionine plus cystine when boars were used intensively. Subsequent research has been unable to substantiate the need for these high-protein diets for breeding boars. Van der Kerk and Willems (1985) reported an experiment with 72 boars fed one of three diets for a period of 7 months. The diets used were (1) a basal diet (16.2% CP, 0.78% total lysine, and 0.59% total methionine plus cystine per day); (2) a diet containing extra methionine (16.6% CP, 0.79% total lysine, and 0.75% total methionine plus cystine, and (3) a diet containing both extra lysine and methionine (18.2% CP, 0.93% total lysine, and 0.75% methionine plus cystine). They found no effect of diet on sperm output or semen quality characteristics. Meding and Nielsen (1977) also found no effect of feeding a diet containing 18.4% CP compared with a diet containing 15.8% CP on the number of sperm cells produced. However, the mating frequency in both experiments was rather low: two times per week in the experiment of Van der Kerk and Willems (1984) and 6.4 times per month in the experiment of Meding and Nielsen (1977). Poppe et al. (1974) stated that the positive effect of protein and amino acid supplementation on sperm production is found only at high mating frequencies. Therefore, Kemp et al. (1988) conducted an experiment using 96 adult boars on a high (three times a week) or low (three to four times in 2 weeks) semen collection scheme. The boars were given a control diet, 12.56 MJ metabolizable energy (ME), 14.5% CP, 0.68% lysine, and 0.44% methionine plus cystine, or a high-protein diet, 12.56 MJ ME, 22.2% CP, 1.20% lysine, and 0.81% of methionine plus cystine. The control diet was comparable with a normal commercial sow diet. Again, no positive effects of extra protein on sperm output or on semen quality were found, regardless of mating frequency. It is therefore unlikely that very high protein levels are needed to ensure good fertility of the breeding boar.

A relevant question is what are the minimal protein requirements before reproduction is impaired. Yen and Yu (1985) measured the number of sperm cells produced by 96 1-year-old boars fed four protein levels for a period of 1 year. Daily CP, total lysine, and total methionine plus cystine levels varied between 200 to 394 g, 6.2 to 18.2 g, and 5.8 to 9.6 g, respectively. The number of sperm cells produced reached a maximum at an intake of 280 g of CP, 11.6 g lysine, and 7.2 g methionine plus cystine per day, at an energy intake of 28.0 or 33.5 MJ digestible energy (DE)/day. Yen and Yu (1985) found no effect of protein level on the percentage of deformed sperm cells. The boars used in these experiments were between 1 and 2 years old and weighed 133 to 185 kg. This is a relatively low live weight because modern breeding boars can weigh 250 kg or more at this age. Hence, the protein requirement for growth would have been lower in the boars used by Yen and Yu (1985) compared with modern breeding boars. More recently, Louis et al. (1994b) conducted an experiment with 20 1-year-old modern crossbred boars. During a 23-week period, a diet with 23.2 MJ ME containing 7.3 or 16.2% CP (0.31 or 0.83% total lysine) was fed. Feeding the low-protein diet resulted in a significantly reduced libido (in terms of time needed to mount a dummy and ejaculate), lower sperm volume per ejaculate, and a lower testis volume. The low-protein group had a 15% lower sperm output compared with the control group, but this effect was not significant. Semen quality characteristics were not affected by the low protein levels. To elucidate the effects of low protein levels on libido and semen volume output, Louis et al. (1994b) measured LH release from the pituitary before and after GnRH challenge and testosterone and estrogen levels in the boars after 23 weeks. Luteinizing hormone release before and after GnRH challenge and testosterone levels were similar among treatments. However, lower plasma estrogen levels were found in the boars fed the low-CP diets. Estrogen levels were inversely related to the time needed to mount a dummy and ejaculate. Joshi and Raeside (1973) found that supplemental estrogen after castration maintained semen volume in boars. These data suggest that decreased estrogen levels may be involved in the impaired libido and semen volume caused by low-protein diets.

In general, protein intake seems to influence libido and semen quantity, but no effects were found on semen quality. In Table 34.1 CP, total lysine, and total methionine plus cystine intake

TABLE 34.1
Ranges in Crude Protein, Lysine, and Methionine Plus Cystine in Experiments Describing Effects of Protein Intake on Reproductive Performance in Adult Boars

Ref.	CP Intake (g/day)	Total Lysine Intake (g/day)	Total Methionine + Cystine Intake (g/day)	Positive Effects of High Level[a]		
				Libido	Sperm No.	Sperm Quality
Poppe et al. (1974)	506.6–743.7	42.0–57.0	23.0–38.0	.	+	.
Van der Kerk et al. (1985)	405–455	18.5–22	15.3–19.5	.	.	.
Kemp et al. (1988)	433–666	18.4–32.4	11.9–21.9	.	.	.
Louis et al. (1994a)	160–356	6.8–18.3	—	+	Trend	.

[a] . = no effect, + = statistically significant positive effect, − = no information available

levels are summarized for experiments studying the effects of protein intake on reproductive performance in adult boars. The lowest daily intake of protein reported in the literature that did not affect reproductive output of modern boars was (expressed as lysine and methionine plus cystine) 18.3 g of total lysine and 11.9 of total methionine plus cystine (see Table 34.1). The lowest level of protein in a diet that did not affect reproductive output of modern breeding boars was in a commercial sow diet that contained 12.56 MJ ME/kg, 14.5% CP, 0.68% total lysine, and 0.44% total methionine plus cystine (Kemp et al., 1988). Levels of protein below this may compromise libido and semen quantity.

B. Effects of Energy Intake

Stevemer et al. (1961) conducted an experiment using six 22-month-old Yorkshire boars. For a period of 15.5 month two boars were fed *ad libitum* (74.5 MJ DE/day), two boars were fed according to the NRC recommendations (Beeson et al., 1959; 40.2 MJ DE/day), and two boars were fed 75% of the NRC recommendations during the first 6 months and 50% of the NRC recommendations for the remainder of the experiment. The boars on the low feeding level lost large amounts of body fat (backfat thickness decreased during the experimental period from 36 mm to a level to thin too measure). In the 15th month of the experiment, the boars on the low feeding level refused to serve the artificial vagina during a period of 2 weeks. In the other boars, no libido problems were detected. The boars fed *ad libitum* had a backfat thickness of 76 mm at the end of the experiment. These data suggest that effects of energy intake on libido are seen only when boars are in an extremely poor body condition. The sperm output per ejaculate was 35% greater in the boars fed *ad libitum* compared with boars fed the lowest level of intake. This difference was not significant because of the small number of boars and the large variation between and within boars. However, these boars were in a very good condition at the start of the experiment (backfat thickness was 36 mm). Yen and Yu (1985) conducted an experiment with 96 1-year-old breeding boars fed at two levels (28.0 MJ and 33.5 MJ DE/day) of feed intake for 1 year. They reported similar numbers of sperm cells per ejaculate (collected at 4-day intervals). These experiments on the effect of energy intake on semen characteristics in boars (Stevemer et al., 1961; Yen and Yu, 1985) showed no effects on semen quantity or quality. In rams and bulls, however, clear effects of energy intake on semen production are observed. A reduced reproductive performance was seen in rams (Alkass et al., 1982) and bulls (Keraby et al., 1983; Coulter and Kozub, 1984) fed at or below maintenance compared with animals fed well above maintenance. More-detailed information on the experiment of Yen and Yu (1985) is given by Yen et al. (1982). The 1-year-old boars had an average initial weight of 133 kg and an average final weight of 185 kg. Assuming a maintenance requirement of 447 kJ ME/kg$^{0.75}$/day (Kemp et al., 1989a), the boars fed the low level of feed were fed between 1.2 and 1.5 times the energy requirement for

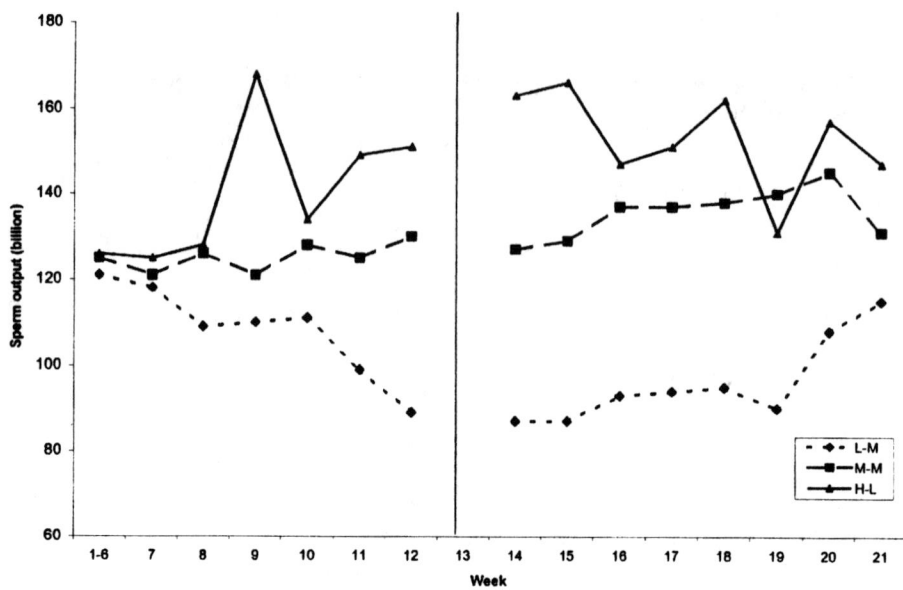

FIGURE 34.1 Number (×10^9) of ejaculated sperm cells per week for boars fed different levels of a commercial diet L = 1.92 kg/day, M = 3.62 kg/day, and H = 5.74 kg/day. At week 13, feeding levels were changed. (From Kemp, B. et al., *Anim. Reprod. Sci.*, 20:245, 1989. With permission.)

maintenance. The boars fed on the high level of feed were fed 1.5 to 1.9 times the energy requirement for maintenance. This might explain why Yen et al. (1982) found no differences in reproductive performance between the boars fed 1.2 to 1.5 and 1.5 to 1.9 times maintenance. Kemp et al. (1989a) conducted an experiment to investigate the influence of feeding level on semen quantity and quality in breeding boars. In the experiment, 42 Yorkshire boars (13 months old) were fed a protein sufficient diet for 12 weeks, either at *ad libitum* (H = 5.74 kg/day), at a medium level (M = 3.62 kg/day), or at a low feeding level (L = 1.92 kg/day). After 8 weeks, the number of ejaculated sperm cells for the boars fed the L diet was significantly lower than for boars fed the H or M diets. In the last 2 weeks of the experiment the boars fed M or H ejaculated 46 and 69% more sperm cells, respectively, compared with the L boars (Figure 34.1). Differences in sperm output were significant among all three levels of feed intake ($p < 0.05$). No effects of treatments were found on the semen quality variables: percentage of moving sperm cells in the ejaculate, vitality of the moving sperm cells, and nonreturn percentage of sows 56 days after insemination. Those boars initially receiving the L and M levels of feed were fed the M level during a second 8-week period, whereas those fed the H level were fed the L feeding level during this second period. After 7 weeks, sperm output of the initially L level group started to increase and at week 8, differences between the intitially L and M group were not significant.

Westendorf and Richter (1977) indicated in their literature review on nutrition of boars that a low feeding level should be applied because a high feeding level may induce leg weakness, resulting in libido problems. Culling of boars from commercial swine herds is primarily because boars become too heavy (D'Allaire and Leman, 1990). Low feeding levels are therefore often seen in practice. Louis et al. (1994a) conducted an experiment to study the effects of low feeding levels on fertility of boars, and the possible positive effects of higher protein levels when boars were subjected to low feeding levels. During a 27-week period, boars were fed 32.2 MJ ME, 363 g CP, and 18.1 g total lysine/day, or 25.5 MJ ME/day on two dietary protein intake levels (356 g CP and 18.1 g total lysine, or 188 g CP and 7.7 g lysine). Reduction in energy intake resulted in reduced libido and lower sperm output, and these adverse effects could only be partly compensated by increasing protein level. Semen quality was not influenced by treatments.

TABLE 34.2
Ranges in Energy Intake (in MJ and expressed as times maintenance) as Studied in Experiments Describing Effects of Feed or Energy Intake on Reproductive Performance in Adult Boars

Ref.	Energy Level (MJ)	Unit[a]	Times Maintenance[b]	Negative Effects of Low Feeding Level[c]		
				Libido	Sperm No.	Semen Quality
Stevemer et al. (1961)	20.1–30.2, 40.2, 75.4	DE	0.9–1.2, 1.4, 2.3	–	Trend	.
Yen and Yu (1985)	28.0–33.5	DE	1.4–1.8	.	.	.
Kemp et al. (1989a)	24.9–46.9, 74.4	ME	1.0–1.8–2.9	.	–	.
Louis et al. (1994b)	25.5–32.2	ME	1.2–1.5	–	–	.

[a] DE = digestible energy, ME = metabolizable energy.
[b] Maintenance = 447 kJ ME/kg$^{0.75}$ live weight/day (Kemp et al., 1989a).
[c] . = no effect, – = negative effect.

In general, it seems that a reduced feed or energy intake can affect libido and sperm output, but semen quality seems to be unaffected. In Table 34.2, the ranges in energy levels as studied in various experiments are given in megajoules of DE or ME, and also are expressed as units times maintenance. The latter figure corrects for weight differences of boars between experiments. It seems that feeding adult boars at levels below about 1.4 times maintenance has detrimental effects on sperm output and/or libido. One should bear in mind, however, that most of these data are based on boars 1 year of age. The actual energy requirements of boars will be dependent on their age. Young boars are expected to grow toward adult weight, and will therefore require higher levels of energy (relative to maintenance) compared with adult boars. Therefore, a factorial approach to the energy requirements of breeding boars is presented in the next section.

IV. ENERGY REQUIREMENTS OF BREEDING BOARS: A FACTORIAL APPROACH

Daily energy requirements for boars can be assessed using a factorial approach taking into account the following energy-demanding processes: maintenance, growth, and reproductive functions. In this section, the energy costs for each of these processes are discussed.

A. Maintenance

Maintenance requirements of an animal are usually described as a function of metabolic weight (Brody, 1945),

$$\text{Maintenance (kJ)} = a * (\text{live weight})^{0.75}/\text{day} \quad (a = \text{constant}) \quad (34.1)$$

Using data of two experiments with boars (Kemp et al., 1989b; 1990) where ME intake, live weight, and protein and fat retention were determined, Kemp (1991) calculated the maintenance requirements for boars to be 415 kJ ME/kg live weight$^{0.75}$/day. This estimate does not differ substantially from the estimated maintenance requirements of sows (430 kJ/kg live weight$^{0.75}$), which is based on an extensive review by Williams et al. (1985). Close and Roberts (1993) used data from growing-fattening boars, which were extrapolated to accommodate the breeding boar. On this basis, they calculated the maintenance requirements of a boar to be 763 kJ ME/kg live weight$^{0.665}$. In Table 34.3, daily maintenance requirements are given for boars ranging from 150 to 400 kg based on the calculation of Kemp (1991). When using maintenance

TABLE 34.3
Thermoneutral Feeding Level for Boars Based on a Factorial Approach[a]

Live weight (kg)	150	200	250	300	350	400
Weight gain (g/day)	500	400	300	200	100	50
ME for maintenance (MJ/day)[b]	17.79	22.07	26.09	29.91	33.58	37.12
ME for weight gain (MJ/day)[c]	16.40	13.11	9.83	6.55	3.28	1.64
ME total (MJ/day)	34.19	35.18	35.92	36.46	36.86	38.76
kg of diet (12.56 MJ ME/kg)	2.7	2.8	2.9	2.9	2.9	3.1

[a] Data of Kemp (1991).
[b] Maintenance = 415 kJ/kg live weight$^{0.75}$/day (see text). ME = metabolizable energy.
[c] Efficiency for growth from ME is 0.72, energy in growth = 23.6 kJ/g (see text).

requirements calculated based on the estimates of Close and Roberts (1993), daily requirements are 3.6 to 4 MJ ME/day higher.

As in pregnant sows, energy requirements for boars are influenced by ambient temperature. Kemp et al. (1989b) calculated a lower critical temperature for individually penned boars on slatted floors at 20°C. The extra thermoregulatory heat production was estimated at 16 kJ/kg$^{0.75}$/°C/day. This implies that a 250-kg boar should be given 1 MJ of extra ME daily for each degree Celsius below 20°C to account for extra thermoregulatory heat production.

B. Growth

Weight gain of breeding boars is necessary because boars are still young when they start their reproductive life. On arrival at artificial insemination centers, boars are usually 7 to 9 months old and weigh 150 kg. An adult Yorkshire boar can easily weigh over 400 kg. The desired growth rate for breeding boars is a matter of debate. On the one hand, a very restricted growth rate is desired so that boars can be used to serve young gilts for a long period without causing injury to the gilts or the boars. On the other hand, feeding levels that are too low affect libido and sperm output. There is almost no information on what the ideal growth rate of a boar should be. Combining experimental and field data reported by Close and Roberts (1993) and Kemp (1991), a growth rate of 500, 400, 300, 200, 100, and 50 g/day is suggested for boars weighing 150, 200, 250, 300, 350, and 400 kg, respectively. Because no data are available on efficiency of growth in boars, data from sows have been used. ARC (1981) estimated the energy deposition of maternal weight gain in pregnant sows to be 23.6 kJ/g. By using an efficiency (NE/ME) of energy retention of 0.72 (Close et al., 1985), the energy requirement for growth is 23.6/0.72 = 32.8 kJ ME/g growth. This estimate is used for calculation of the energy costs of growth as shown in Table 34.3.

C. Reproduction

The reproductive processes consist of the energy costs for mating and the costs of building an ejaculate. Kemp et al. (1990) measured heat production and energy and protein balances in boars at different mating frequencies. From these data, it was clear that the energy requirements for mating are approximately 18 kJ/kg metabolic weight. This means that a 200-kg breeding boar needs about 958 kJ extra ME on a mating day. Compared with the 35.18 MJ ME the boar needs for maintenance and growth at thermoneutrality, the energy costs for mating are negligible (less than 3% of maintenance and growth on a mating day). Also, the energy costs of building an ejaculate are likely to be small. Boars produce ejaculates of about 300 to 400 ml, containing 95% water, 3.4% protein, and 1.6% other products such as carbohydrates and fat (Hansel and McEntee, 1970). A boar ejaculating twice a week will have to produce 100 ml of ejaculate per day containing

3.4 g of protein and 1.6 g of other products. The energy costs of this production are negligible compared with the energy costs of maintenance and growth.

D. Total Requirements

The factorial estimate for thermoneutral energy requirements is given in Table 34.3 (Kemp, 1991). For boars of 150 and 350 kg body weight, 34.2 and 36.9 MJ ME/day should be fed, respectively. Close and Roberts (1993) also did a factorial calculation of the energy requirements for breeding boars and found comparable figures of 30.7 and 39.4 MJ ME for boars weighing 150 and 350 kg, respectively.

During a 20-week period, Kemp et al. (1991) fed boars according to the factorial estimates presented in Table 34.3 (including energy costs for extra thermoregulatory heat production), or 80% of this level of intake. The boars averaged 18 months old and weighed 271 kg at the start of the experiment. Boars fed according to the factorial approach gained 264 g/day of weight and 0.4 mm backfat per month. The 20% reduction in feed intake resulted in only 23 g weight gain/day and fat losses of 0.45 mm/month. Moreover, boars on the lower feeding levels had a 10% lower number of sperm cells, indicating that the calculated energy requirements for breeding boars are relatively close to the minimum requirements for good development and reproductive output.

V. VITAMINS AND MINERALS FOR BREEDING BOARS

Studies on the impact of vitamins and minerals on reproductive function of breeding boards are scarce. Most studies are directed to young developing boars. The available data are summarized.

A. Vitamin E and Selenium

Liu et al. (1982) indicated that a prolonged selenium (Se) deficiency in boars resulted in reduced sperm concentrations and sperm motility, and sperm with a high incidence of cytoplasmic droplets. Brezinska-Slebodzinska et al. (1995) reported that vitamin E supplementation had a protective effect against fatty acid peroxidation of boar semen, and it resulted in better semen quality. The effects of vitamin E and Se supplementation to boar diets during growth was studied by Marin-Guzman et al. (1997). Boars were fed a basal diet containing 0.63 ppm Se and 3.46 mg α-tocopherol. In a 2 × 2 factorial arrangement, 0 or 0.5 ppm Se and 0 or 220 IU vitamin E were added to the diet. The diets were fed from weaning to 9 months of age, and then during a 16-week collection period. Semen was collected three times weekly during the 16-week period. The basal diet resulted in lower motility of semen and more abnormal sperm cells compared with the supplemented groups. The effects of added Se on semen quality were more pronounced than the effects of added vitamin E. Gilts were inseminated with semen from the four groups and slaughtered at day 5 to 7 postcoitum. Selenium supplementation resulted in greater fertilization rates and higher accessory sperm counts. Marin-Guzman et al. (1997) state in their paper that the amounts of Se and α-tocopherol in their basal diet are comparable to many typical corn–soybean meal mixtures. Therefore, they recommend addition of Se and vitamin E to boar diets.

B. Calcium, Phosphorus, and Biotin

To the authors' knowledge, calcium, phosphorus, and biotin requirements have not been studied in adult boars, and no data are available on the relationship of these nutrients to semen production characteristics. However, for proper libido, sound legs and feet are a prerequisite. In developing boars, Hines et al. (1979) showed that optimum dietary levels for bone development (0.93% Ca and 0.75% P) were higher than for optimal growth (0.55% Ca and 4.5% P). The NRC (1973) recommendations for Ca and P were, respectively, 0.66 and 0.50% during the growing phase and 0.50 and 0.40% during the finishing phase. Numerous researchers have compared these recommendations with higher levels ranging from 125 to 200% of these NRC recommendations (Kornegay and Thomas, 1981; Kornegay et al.; 1981, Kesel et al., 1983; Nimmo et al., 1980a,b). In general, they found that increased levels improve bone strength and bone mineralization variables without adverse effects on growth and feed conversion.

Although no experimental data are available on the effects of biotin on boar fertility or leg soundness, Close and Roberts (1993) state in their literature review on nutrition of boars that diets should contain at least 300 µg/kg biotin, and in the event of foot problems, this level should be increased to 1000 µg/kg diet. No effects are to be expected on reproductive output, but foot problems could be prevented.

C. Vitamin A

Paufler (1993) studied the effects of supplementation of 600 mg β-carotene to adult boars on semen characteristics. Supplementation did not affect numbers of sperm cells or sperm motility after collection. However, the incidence of proximal cytoplasmic droplets was lower and motility of sperm cells after 2 days of storage at 16°C was higher in the supplemented group.

D. Zinc

Zinc deficiency results in retardation of the development of Leydig cells, a reduced response to LH, and reduced testicular steroidogenesis (Hesketh, 1982). Liao et al. (1985) compared diets ranging from 31.8 to 197 ppm Zn in 1-year-old breeding boars. The lowest level of Zn resulted in a reduced number of sperm cells and a tendency to reduce semen quality. Based on their results, they recommend Zn levels of 80 to 150 ppm for breeding boars.

VI. CONCLUSIONS

Reduced energy and protein levels delay puberty and sexual development in developing boars and sperm output and libido in adult breeding boars. Interestingly, no effect of protein or energy restriction was found on semen quality characteristics. For optimizing libido and sperm output, nutrient recommendations are given in this chapter. Literature on effects of vitamins and minerals on reproductive characteristics are scare and exemplary. Interestingly, deficiencies in vitamins and minerals also seem to affect semen quality. Because semen quality is an important characteristic of a boar, more attention to vitamin and mineral requirements for boars should be given.

REFERENCES

Alkass, J. E., M. J. Bryant, and J. S. Walton. 1982. Some effects of level of feeding and body condition upon sperm production and gonadotropin concentrations in the ram, *Anim. Prod.*, 34:256.

Althen, T. G., R. J. Gerrits, and E. P. Young. 1974. Pituitary gonadotropins in boars as affected by dietary protein and age, *J. Anim. Sci.*, 39:601.

ARC. 1981. The Nutrient Requirements of Pigs Agricultural Research Council Working Party. Commonwealth Agricultural Bureaux, London, 1–307.

Beeson, W. M., E. W. Crampton, T. J. Cunha, N. R. Ellis, and R. W. Luecke. 1953. Nutrient requirements of swine. National Research Council Publication 295.

Beeson, W. M., E. W. Crampton, T. J. Cunha, N. R. Ellis, and R. W. Luecke. 1959. Nutrient requirements of swine. National Research Council Publication 648.

Berger, T., K. L. Esbenshade, M. A. Diekman, T. Hoagland, and J. Tuite. 1981. Influence of prepubertal consumption of Zearalenore on sexual development of boars, *J. Anim. Sci.*, 53:1559.

Brody, S. 1945. *Bioenergetics and Growth, with Special Reference to the Efficiency Complex in Domestic Animals*, Reinhold, New York.

Brzezinska-Slebodzinska, E., A. B. Slebodzinski, B. Pietras, and G. Weiczorek. 1995. Antioxidant effect of vitamin A and glutathione on lipid peroxidation in boar semen plasma, *Biol. Trace Elem. Res.*, 47:67.

Close, W. H., and F. G. Roberts. 1993. Nutrition of the working boar. In *Recent Developments in Pig Nutrition*, 2nd ed., Cole, D.J.A., and W. Haresign, Eds., Nottingham University Press, Loughborough, U.K.

Close, W. H., J. Noblet, and R. P. Heavens. 1985. Studies on the energy metabolism of the pregnant sow. 2. The partitioning and utilisation of metabolisable energy intake in pregnant and non pregnant animals, *Br. J. Nutr.*, 53:267.

Coulter, G. H., and G. C. Kozub. 1984. Testicular development, epididymal sperm reserves and seminal quality in two-year-old Hereford and Angus bulls: effects of two levels of dietary energy, *J. Anim. Sci.*, 59:432.

D'Allaire, S., and A. D. Leman. 1990. Boar culling in swine breeding herds in Minnesota, *Can. Vet. J.*, 31:581.

Dickerson, J. W. T., G. A. Gresham, and R. A. McCance. 1964. The effect of undernutrition and rehabilitation on the development of the reproductive organs: pigs, *J. Endocrinol.*, 29:111.

Dutt, R. H., and C. E. Barnhart. 1959. Effect of plane of nutrition upon reproductive performance of boars, *J. Anim. Sci.*, 18:3.

Hansel, W., and K. McEntee. 1970. Male reproductive processes. In *Dukes Physiology of Domestic Animals*, 8th ed., Swenson, M.J. Ed., Cornell University Press, Ithaca, NY, 1298.

Hesketh, J. E., 1982. Effects of dietary zinc deficiency on Leydig cell ultrastructure in the boar, *J. Comp. Pathol.*, 92:239.

Hines, R. H., J. C. Greer, and G. L. Allee. 1979. Calcium and phosphorus levels for developing boars, *J. Anim. Sci.*, 49(Suppl. 1):101.

Joshi, H. S., and J. I. Raeside. 1973. Synergistic effects of testosterone and oestrogens on accessory sex glands and sexual behavior of the boar, *J. Reprod. Fertil.*, 33:411.

Kemp, B. 1991. Nutritional strategy for optimal semen production in boars, *Pig News Info.*, 12:555.

Kemp, B., and L. A. den Hartog. 1989. The influence of energy and protein intake on the reproductive performance of the breeding boar, *Anim. Reprod. Sci.*, 20:103.

Kemp, B., H. J. G. Grooten, L. A. den Hartog, P. Luiting, and M. W. A. Verstegen. 1988. The effect of a high protein intake on sperm production in boars at two semen collection frequencies, *Anim. Reprod. Sci.*, 17:103.

Kemp, B., L. A. den Hartog, and H. J. G. Grooten. 1989a. The effect of feeding level on semen quantity and quality of breeding boars, *Anim. Reprod. Sci.*, 20:245.

Kemp, B., M. W. A. Verstegen, L. A. den Hartog, and H. J. G. Grooten. 1989b. The effect of environmental temperature on metabolic rate, and partitioning of energy intake in breeding boars, *Livest. Prod. Sci.*, 23: 329.

Kemp, B., F. P. Vervoort, P. Bikker, J. Janmaat, M. W. A. Verstegen, and H. J. G. Grooten. 1990. Semen collection frequency and the energy metabolism of A.I. boars, *Anim. Reprod. Sci.*, 22:87.

Kemp, B., G. C. M. Bakker, L. A. den Hartog, and M. W. A. Verstegen. 1991. The effect of semen collection frequency and food intake on semen production in breeding boars, *Anim. Prod.*, 52:355.

Keraby, F. E., I. M. Soliman, M. K. Hathout, and S. A. Fawzy. 1983. Effect of energy intake level on semen quality of Friesian bulls, *Agric. Res. Rev.*, 58:61.

Kesel, G. A., J. W. Knight, E. T. Kornegay, H. P. Veit, and D. R. Notter. 1983. Restricted energy and elevated calcium and phosphorus intake for boars during growth. 1. Feedlot performance and bone characteristics, *J. Anim. Sci.*, 57:82.

Kim, J. K., and Y. B. Lee. 1975. A study on the development of spermatogenic function and semen quality in boar, *Korean J. Anim. Sci.*, 17:294.

Kornegay, E. T., and H. R. Thomas. 1981. Phosphorus in swine. 2. Influence of dietary calcium and phosphorus levels and growth rate on serum minerals, soundness scores and bone development in barrows, gilts and boars, *J. Anim. Sci.*, 52:1049.

Kornegay, E. T., H. R. Thomas, and J. L. Baker. 1981. Phosphorus in swine. 4. Influence of dietary calcium and phosphorus levels on feedlot performance, serum minerals, bone development, and soundness scores in boars, *J. Anim. Sci.*, 52:1070.

Liao, C. W., S. C. Chyr, and T. F. Shen. 1985. The effect of dietary zinc content on reproductive performance of the boar. In *Proc. of the 3rd EAAP Animal Science Congress*, Seoul, Korea Republic, 2:613.

Liu, C. H., Y. M. Chen, J. Z. Zhang, M. Y. Huang, Q. Su, Z. H. Lu, R. X. Yin, G. Z. Shao, D. Feng, and P. L. Zheng. 1982. Preliminary studies on influence of selenium deficiency to developments of genital organs and spermatogenesis of infancy boars, *Acta Vet. Zootech. Sinica*, 13:73.

Louis, G. F., A. J. Lewis, W. C. Weldon, P. M. Ermer, P. S. Miller, R. J. Kittok, and W. W. Stroup. 1994a. The effect of energy and protein intakes on boar libido, semen characteristics, and plasma hormone concentrations, *J. Anim. Sci.*, 72:2051.

Louis, G. F., A. J. Lewis, W. C. Weldon, P. S. Miller, R. J. Kittok, and W. W. Stroup. 1994b. The effect of protein intake on libido, semen characteristics, and plasma hormone concentrations, *J. Anim. Sci.*, 72:2038.

Lunstra, D. D., J. J. Ford, J. Klindt, and T. H. Wise. 1997. Physiology of the Meishan boar, *J. Reprod. Fertil.*, 52 (Suppl.):181.

Marin-Guzman, J., D. C. Mahan, Y. K. Chung, J. L. Pate, and W. F. Pope. 1997. Effects of dietary selenium and vitamin E on boar performance, and tissue responses, semen quality, and subsequent fertilization rates in mature gilts, *J. Anim. Sci.*, 75:2994.

Meding, A. J. H., and H. E. Nielsen. 1977. Fortskellige proteinnormers indflydelse på frugtbarheden hos orner, der anvendes til kunstig saerdoverforing, *Statens Husdyrbrugsforsøg*, 175:2.

Nimmo, R. D., E. R. Peo, Jr., B. D. Moser, P. J. Cunningham, T. D. Crenshaw, and D. G. Olsen. 1980a. Response of different genetic lines of boars to varying levels of dietary calcium and phosphorus, *J. Anim. Sci.*, 51:112.

Nimmo, R. D., E. R. Peo, Jr., B. D. Moser, P. J. Cunningham, D. G. Olsen, and T. D. Crenshaw. 1980b. Effect of various levels of dietary calcium and phosphorus on performance, blood and bone parameters in growing boars, *J. Anim. Sci.*, 51:100.

NRC. 1973. *Nutrient Requirements of Swine*, 7th ed., National Academy Press, Washington, D.C.

Paufler, S. 1993. Untersuchung der Ejakulat- and Blutparameter von Ebern während sechsmonatiger oraler Verabreichung von synthetischer Beta Katotin, Thesis, Justus-Liebig Universität, Giessen, Germany.

Poppe, S., U. Huhn, F. Kleeman, and I. Konig. 1974. Untersuchungen zur nutritiven Beeinflussung bei Jung- und Besamlungsebern, *Arch. Tierernähr.*, 6:499.

Singh, G. 1962. The labeling of boar spermatozoa with radioactive phosphorus, 32P, *in vivo*, *Ann. Biol. Anim. Biochem. Biophysiol.*, 1:403.

Stevemer, E. J., M. F. Kovacs, W. G. Hoekstra, and H. L. Self. 1961. The effect of feed intake on semen characteristics and reproductive performance of mature boars, *J. Anim. Sci.*, 20:858.

Swierstra, E. E. 1968. Cytology and duration of the cycle of the epithelium of the boar, *Anat. Rec.*, 61:171.

Uzu, G. 1979. Influence de l'alimenation azotée entre 30 et 90 kg depoids vif sur les performance de reproduction du jeune verrat, *Ann. Zootech.*, 48:431.

Van der Kerk, P. and C. M. T. Willems. 1985. Zum Einfluss der Rohprotein, Lysin und Methionine + Cysine Versorgung auf Fruchtbarkeitsmerkmale beim Eber, *Z. Tierphys. Tierernähr. Futtermittelkd.*, 53:43.

Westendorf, P., and L. Richter. 1977. Ernährung der Eber, *Übersicht. Übers. Tierern.*, 5:161.

Williams, I. H., W. H. Close, and D. J. A. Cole. 1985. Strategies for sow nutrition: predicting the response of pregnant animals to protein and energy intake. In *Recent Advances in Animal Nutrition*, Haresign, W., and D. J. A. Cole, Eds., Butterworths, London, U.K., 133.

Yen, H. T., and I. T. Yu. 1985. Influence of digestible energy and protein feeding on semen characteristics of breeding boars. In *Efficient Animal Production for Asian Welfare, Proc. of the 3rd AAAP Animal Science Congress*, Seoul, Vol. 2:610.

Yen, H. T., M. Y. Lu, H. T. You, and S. Y. Chen. 1982. The effect of feed intake and dietary protein level on semen characteristics of the boar, *J. Chinese Soc. Anim. Sci.*, 1:77.

Part V

Feedstuffs Included in Swine Diets

35 Cereal Grains and By-Products for Swine

Thomas E. Sauber and Fredric N. Owens

CONTENTS

I. Grain Production 785
II. Energy and Nutrient Content of Cereal Grains 787
    A. Energy-Yielding Constituents 788
    B. Amino Acid Content and Bioavailability 792
    C. Minerals 794
    D. Fat-Soluble Vitamins 795
    E. Water-Soluble Vitamins 795
    F. Variability in Nutrient Content of Grains 796
    G. Antinutritive Factors in Grains 796
III. Grain Processing 798
IV. Genetic Modifications to Improve Cereal Grains 798
    A. Starch Form and Availability 799
    B. Amino Acid Concentrations and Bioavailability 800
    C. Oil Concentration 800
    D. Phosphorus Bioavailability 801
V. Palatability of Cereal Grains 801
VI. Marketing and Handling of Grains with Modified Nutritional Traits 801
VII. Sustainability of Grain Production 801
References 802

The primary ingredient in most diets fed to swine in the Western Hemisphere is cereal grain. This is because cereal grains are (1) widely grown and available, (2) energy dense, (3) easily transported and handled, (4) readily consumed by swine, and, foremost, (5) usually the most economical source of metabolizable energy (ME). Energy content and availability from cereals is critically important. But in addition to energy, cereal grains provide a substantial proportion of the dietary protein (amino acids) in swine diets. Consequently, least-cost diet formulation must be based on proper estimation of available energy and amino acid content of the cereal grain(s) being fed.

I. GRAIN PRODUCTION

Grain producers typically select the type and specific hybrid that they plant based on seed cost and expected grain yields. However, specialty grains like white corn are produced where added commercial value of the grain increases economic return. The factors of prime interest for formulating economical swine diets from grains are energy (ME or net energy) content, levels and constancy of concentrations of limiting available amino acids, and absence of compounds and toxins that reduce nutritional availability or palatability. Examples of specialty grains of interest in swine production include grain hybrids with high starch content or availability, high fat content or modified fatty acid content, and grain pigmentation. Additional traits that can alter lean carcass yield, meat quality, and fat color become of interest when producing pork to meet demands of specific markets. To meet the needs of swine producers producing pork for specific markets, "identity preserved" grains can be homegrown, grown under contract, or obtained through specialty grain traders. In the future, grain varieties and composition may be customized or grain types or varieties may be blended to match requirements for specific genetic strains of swine in a fashion similar to that used today in which specific grain varieties are customized for the starch extraction, human food, and grain export markets.

The cereal grain(s) that are produced and become available locally for feeding to swine differs with region of the country, primarily due to agronomic conditions. Compared with corn grain, sorghum grain is more resistant to adverse growing conditions (hot weather and drought). In contrast, barley, wheat, and oats thrive in geographic regions with cooler weather or a shorter growing season (fewer degree-days). With development of corn grain varieties more tolerant of adverse environmental conditions, the "Corn Belt" continues to enlarge. Within each cereal grain, varieties or hybrids have been developed to match specific growing season lengths, soil fertility conditions, and predator (insect, bird, nematode, mycotoxin) pressures. And within these varieties, specific hybrids or strains may differ in protein and amino acid content, starch structure and packing, fiber and oil content, and color; these factors in turn may impact nutritional value.

A corn–soy mixture has become the standard swine diet against which other cereal grains and protein supplements generally are compared (Luce et al., 1991). The other major cereal grains fed to livestock include sorghum (typically milo), barley, wheat, and oats. Several other feed grains, grain by-products, or coproducts enjoy regional popularity. These include products of starch extraction and wet or dry milling as well as pulses (beans and peas), millet, rice, buckwheat, and even acorns. Discussions below will center on the five major cereal grains fed to swine.

As an aid to enhance uniformity of commercially marketed grain, quality standards were developed by the USDA. These standards are based largely on the five major factors involved with the stability of grain to be stored (grain density and prevalence of broken kernels, foreign matter, and heat-damaged kernels) with higher quality (lower numeric grades) being more desirable. Although each of these five factors as well as moisture content can impact storage and transport of grain, these factors have limited direct effect on nutritional value of grain (Table 35.1). Indeed, some of the properties considered desirable nutritionally (adequate moisture, fragility for processing, higher oil content) can make grain less desirable for grain storage, handling, and transport. For example, the metabolizable energy value for grade 3 corn grain may be slightly higher than grade 2 or 1 grain (Table 35.1). Grain that fails to meet the grade 1 or 2 USDA grain trading specifications (due to light test weight, sprouted, heat or water damaged, drought stressed) is discounted in grade and price even though its feeding value may equal that of grain of a superior grade. Grain discounted in price due to high moisture content also can prove to be a bargain feed if it can be handled easily and fed before mold damage occurs. Additionally, by-products of grain processing (residues from starch extraction for production of sweetener or alcohol as listed in Table 35.1) as discussed by Miller et al. (1990) are often fed to swine because of their low cost and local or regional availability. Removal of oil and starch generally decreases the ME value of the product. Because nutrient content is more directly correlated with feeding value of grains than USDA grade, direct assays for nutrient content are gradually displacing USDA grading factors as a basis for trade and commercial pricing of cereal grains.

TABLE 35.1
Metabolizable Energy (ME) Values for Swine Based on NRC (1971) for Various USDA Grades and By-Products of Corn Grain

		USDA Grade	lb/Bu	Mcal ME/kg Component			ME,% of No. 2 Yellow Dent
				U.S.	Eastern Canada	Western Canada	
Corn grain	Yellow dent	1	56	3818	3809	3785	99.9
	Yellow dent	2	54	3817	3808	3795	100.0
	Yellow dent	3	52	3853	3807	3783	100.2
	Yellow dent	4	49	3735	3800	3786	99.1
	Yellow dent	5	46	3815	3786	3753	99.4
	Yellow dent	Sample		3766			98.7
	Flint			3831			100.4
	Pop			3806			99.7
	Soft			3766			98.7
	Sweet			3807			99.7
	White			3800			99.6
By-Products	Distillers grains			3915			102.6
	Distillers solubles			3373			88.4
	Distillers stillage			3464			90.8
	Gluten feed			3523	3569		93.0
	Gluten meal			3373	3247		86.8
	Hominy feed, <5% fat			3527			92.4
	Hominy feed, >5% fat			3460			90.7
	Hominy grits			3830			100.3
	Molasses			2965			77.7
	Oil			7340			192.3
	Oil meal, 1% fat			2879			75.4
	8.5% fat			3342			87.6
	9.8% fat			3293			86.3
	Starch			4070	4070		106.8

II. ENERGY AND NUTRIENT CONTENT OF CEREAL GRAINS

Nutrient composition and bioavailability differ widely among grains and to a lesser degree within a cereal grain. These differences can be attributed to environmental conditions during grain production (soil fertility, growing conditions, maturity, yield), genetic (variety) differences, and an interaction between environment and genetics. With continued development of selected or genetically modified grains, diversity in nutrient content of grain varieties is likely to increase in the future. In addition, nutrient and energy availability can be altered by processing (drying, grinding, flaking) potentially producing a three-way interaction (environment, genetics, and processing). Combined with differences among swine (gender and selected genetic line), even more complex interactions may exist. Large variability among varieties and the potential for a plant genetics–environment interaction increases the need for analytical methods that can rapidly and accurately predict energy and available amino acid concentrations of grains and other diet ingredients. Nutrient content (moisture, protein, oil, and starch) can be rapidly quantified via near infrared (NIR) reflectance or transmission techniques. Additional techniques are needed to assess rapidly the bioavailability of energy and nutrients as well as concentrations of certain essential components (individual amino acids, minerals). Although some methods have been proposed to predict performance responses from grain analyses, animal studies to verify prediction equations have been very limited.

A. ENERGY-YIELDING CONSTITUENTS

Starch, lipid, and protein are the major sources of energy in cereal grains; dilution of these by nonenergy-yielding components (water, ash, indigestible fiber, chemically bound protein and carbohydrate) reduces the available energy value of a grain. The primary constituent of all cereal grains is starch (Figure 35.1). Among these grains, corn and oats are richest in ether extract. Available energy content of feeds will increase as ether extract (fatty acid) content increases. Fiber, measured as the residue insoluble in a neutral detergent solution or neutral detergent fiber (NDF), differs among grains, being greater for oats, barley, and sorghum grains. Energy values for individual grains based on NRC (1998) means are shown in Figure 35.2 for comparison with estimated minimum dietary energy requirements. Because corn grain tends to be less variable in chemical composition (lower coefficient of variation for protein and ether extract) than other grains, corn grain often is used as a standard for comparison. Even though barley contains more NDF than most other grains and thereby has a lower digestible energy (DE) and metabolizable energy (ME) value, the net energy of barley has been measured as being nearly equal to that of corn grain, perhaps due to greater pre-cecal digestion of barley starch. Nevertheless, DE and ME concentrations of barley remain slightly lower than recommended for growing-finishing pigs. Relative to crude protein requirements for growing pigs, all cereal grains tend to be low, although wheat is considerably richer in protein and lysine than other grains. Adequacy of available amino acids rather than of crude protein is preferable for formulating diets to meet protein requirements of pigs.

Energy values cited above (Table 35.1; Figure 35.2) are mean values for specific grains. Because the ME content of barley and oats is lower than the ME recommended for finishing pigs, these grains would be expected to produce lower rates or efficiencies of gain. Because these grains contain more fiber and thereby are more bulky, growing pigs, because of their limited feed intake capacity, are more at risk; larger as well as older pigs with greater capacity for feed intake and intestinal fiber digestion thrive with diets richer in NDF content. Nevertheless, for maximum rate of gain by younger finishing pigs, addition of fat to diets containing these specific grains or limiting the dietary

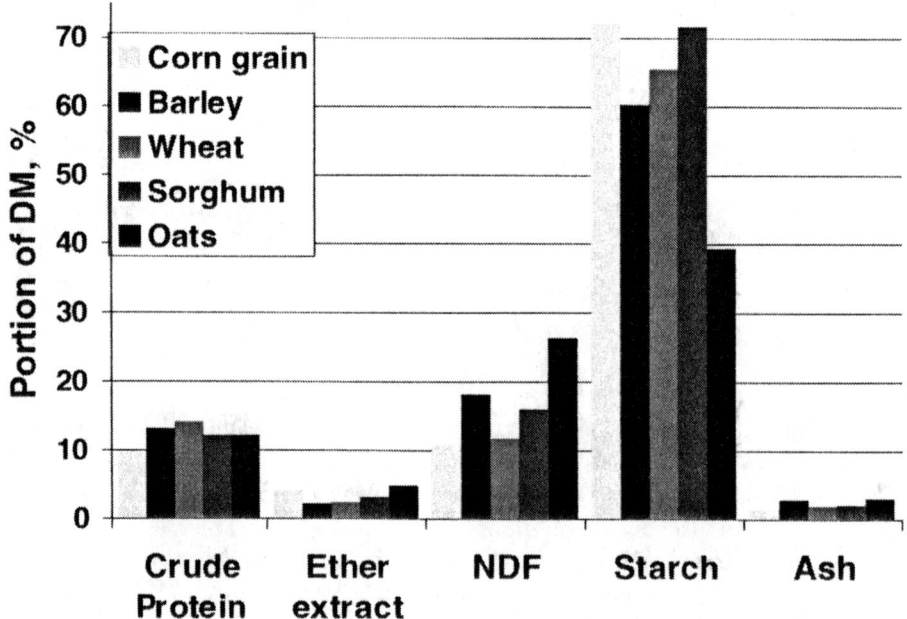

FIGURE 35.1 Chemical constituents of various cereal grains. (From NRC, *Atlas of Nutritional Data on United States and Canadian Feeds*, National Academy Press, Washington, D.C., 1971. With permission.)

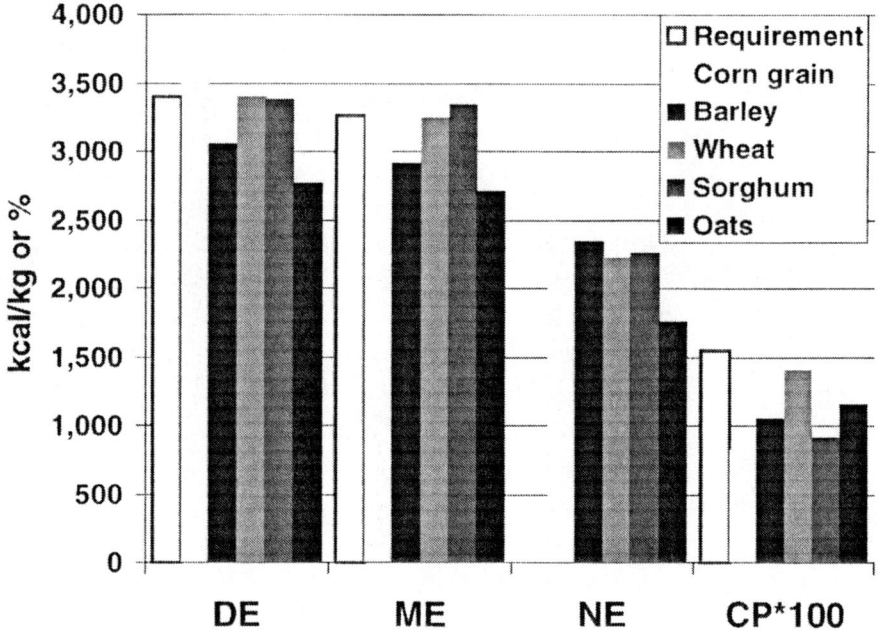

FIGURE 35.2 Energy and protein content of various cereal grains. (From NRC, *Nutrient Requirements of Swine*, 10th rev. ed., National Academy Press, Washington, D.C., 1998. With permission.)

inclusion level for these grains (Holden et al., 1991) can prove useful. Individual batches of grain may differ from this mean based on genetic makeup and environmental (growth and processing) history. Although mean values often are employed for diet formulation, deeper knowledge about the nutritional value of the grain, obtained through specified analysis or genetic history, should allow diets to be customized to take advantage of nutrient or energy differences.

Specific batches of a grain can differ in energy value for swine due to differences either in chemical composition or in availability of these chemical components. Metabolizable energy values for poultry and DE values for swine for various trials using multiple grain cultivars and diverse environmental production conditions are presented in Table 35.2. van Barneveld (1997) indicated that differences in digestibility of energy, rather than differences in chemical composition (gross energy content), were primarily responsible for differences in DE values (van Barneveld, 1997). He suggested that cultural practices including fertilization had a greater impact on DE content than cultivar, growing region, and year. Nevertheless, cultivars selected genetically for nutrient content or type (starch form and oil content) also differ from unselected grain in ME content. Among the primary cereal grains, variation among samples within a trial seems lower for wheat, corn, and sorghum grain than for barley and oats, the two grains with the highest fiber content. Surprisingly, corn variety comparisons with swine have not been published to date.

With grains as with other feeds, ether extract is correlated positively and crude fiber and ash are correlated negatively with ME. This can partially explain why ME range differs among grains, with a range of 9% for 25 samples of sorghum compared with 28% for 70 samples of wheat and 36% for 125 samples of barley (van Barneveld, 1997). In contrast, Sibbald (1986) reported that True Metabolizable Energy (TME) values for poultry for corn grain (20 samples) differed by only 8.9%. These ranges indicate that variability in energy availability among grain samples and varieties can be substantial. Among 34 samples of wheat, Sibbald and Price (1976) noted that ME values for poultry were most closely related to bulk density ($r = 0.34$) and to starch content ($r = 0.237$); among 28 oats samples, ME was most closely related to starch ($r = 0.81$) and bulk density ($r = 0.75$); among 40 samples of barley, ME was most closely related to bulk density ($r = 0.58$) and

TABLE 35.2
Energy Values (Mcal/kg) and Variability for Various Grain Sources Fed to Poultry and Swine

Grain	Samples	Type	Poultry Min ME	Poultry Max ME	Poultry Variation % of min	Swine Min DE	Swine Max DE	Swine Variation % of min	Ref.
Corn	20		3.85	4.06	5.6				Sibbald, 1986
	18		3.33	3.94	18.3				Unpublished (Chick)
	18		4.36	4.73	8.5				Unpublished (Rooster)
	13		3.83	4.04	5.5				Unpublished (Cecectomized rooster)
Barley	29		3.03	3.42	12.6				Sibbald, 1986
	23	Hulless	3.06	3.58	17.2				Sibbald, 1986
			2.93	3.23	10.2				van Barneveld, 1997
			2.48	2.91	17.3				Hughes and Choct, 1999
	16					3.12	3.72	19.1	SCA, 1987
	30					3.30	3.52	6.7	van Barneveld, 1997
	125					2.80	3.82	36.8	van Barneveld, 1997
	30					3.49	3.88	11.0	Kopinski et al., 1997
	20					2.98	3.48	16.6	Fairbairn et al., 1997
Oats	16		2.68	3.18	18.8				Sibbald, 1986
	10	Hulless	3.77	4.01	6.3				Sibbald, 1986

Grain	n							Reference
Sorghum	8				3.83	4.04	5.7	SCA, 1987
	25				3.39	3.67	8.4	Kopinski et al., 1997
	25				3.85	4.18	8.4	van Barneveld, 1997
Wheat	23	3.49	3.63	4.1				McNab, 1996
		3.44	3.73	8.3				Sibbald, 1986
		2.48	3.80	52.9				Hughes and Choct, 1999
	15				3.70	4.05	9.5	de Lange et al., 1993
	21				3.75	3.96	5.8	SCA, 1987
	31				3.86	4.32	11.7	Kopinski et al., 1997
	70				3.18	4.06	27.8	van Barneveld, 1997
	10				3.30	3.52	6.7	van Barneveld, 1998

Weighted Variation

Corn	9.6	—
Barley	14.6	26.1
Oats	14.0	—
Sorghum	—	8.0
Wheat	8.3	18.0

ether extract ($r = 0.49$). Methods to assess energy availability rapidly are needed so that feeding value of individual grain samples can be predicted both for livestock producers and grain breeders.

B. Amino Acid Content and Bioavailability

Essential amino acid content of various cereal grains expressed as a percentage of the dietary requirement for each essential amino acid for finishing swine (NRC, 1998) are presented in Figure 35.3. Based on these values, lysine is the first limiting amino acid in each of these grains followed either by tryptophan (for corn) or threonine (barley and sorghum). Although no amino acid is clearly second limiting for wheat, benefits from supplemental threonine have been observed with pigs fed lysine-supplemented wheat-based diets.

As discussed in Chapters 8 and 9 and by Tanksley et al. (1990), digestion of dietary protein to amino acids in the small intestine is not complete; disappearance of amino acids prior to the ileo-cecal junction (hereafter called ileal) often is used as an index of amino acid availability. Ileal availability values for essential amino acids from grains are shown in Figure 35.4. Of dietary amino acids in cereal grains, some 10 to 20% are recovered at the end of the small intestine and thereby may have resisted digestion. For amino acids to be released from protein, active digestive enzymes must make physical contact for some minimum time period with protein capable of being cleaved. Specific factors that limit amino acid availability from grain can include (1) presence of compounds that inhibit secretion or activity of digestive enzymes; (2) physical inaccessibility of grain protein (as with encapsulation in large feed particles); (3) stable chemical linkage of protein or amino acids with sugars, lipids, fiber, or phenolic compounds (e.g., tannins or lignin); (4) amino acid oxidation or destruction during processing; (5) insoluble or poorly digested protein classes, particularly gliadins (zein, kafrin); and (6) rapid digesta passage (e.g., diarrhea) that leads to insufficient exposure time for digestion. Note that the amino acid with lowest availability, except for oats, is lysine. Whether the low apparent availability of lysine is due to formation of complexes with the exposed epsilon amino group of lysine or merely an

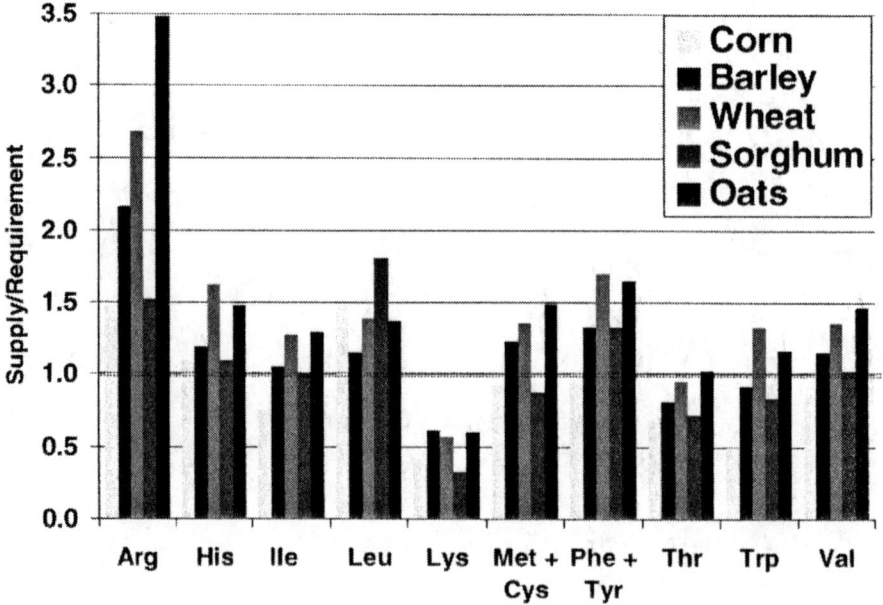

FIGURE 35.3 Total amino acid content of various cereal grains relative to amino acid requirements for finishing pigs. Dotted line represents the point where supply meets requirement. (From NRC, *Nutrient Requirements of Swine*, 10th rev. ed., National Academy Press, Washington, D.C., 1998. With permission.)

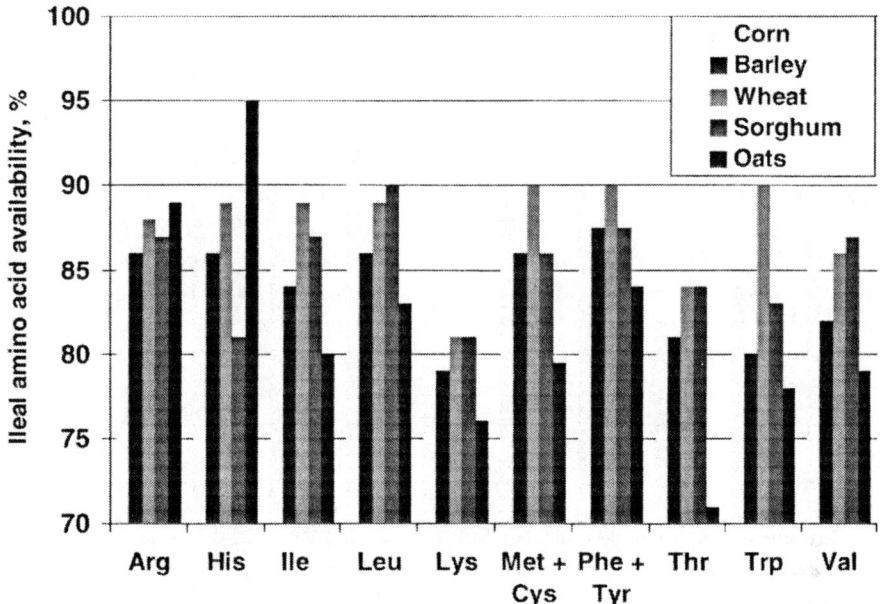

FIGURE 35.4 Availability of various amino acids from various cereal grains (From NRC, *Nutrient Requirements of Swine*, 10th rev. ed., National Academy Press, Washington, D.C., 1998. With permission.)

artifact of availability measurements (failure to account fully for endogenous lysine loss) is not clear. Ideally, swine diets should be formulated based on available amino acids rather than the total amount of each amino acid present in a feed. Unfortunately, both requirement estimates for available amino acids for various classes of swine and various growth rates as well as precise and reliable estimates of availability of amino acids from cereal grains and other dietary protein sources are lacking.

When water shortage or soil fertility, particularly N, limits grain yield, nutrient composition of grain can be altered. Generally, as fertility and growing conditions are improved, kernel (particularly endosperm) size and starch content will increase at a rate faster than protein deposition (partially dependent on germ size); this causes protein content of the kernel to decrease. Because both digestibility and biological value (lysine content) generally is lower for various proteins of the endosperm than various proteins of the germ, biological value of the total protein (or lysine as a percentage of total protein in grain) declines as endosperm size and starch content increase and total protein content decreases (Finley and Hopkins, 1985). Consequently, as grain yields increase with ideal environmental conditions, both protein content of the grain and amino acid quality of the protein decrease. These differences in amino acid content that can be attributed to alterations in the endosperm-to-germ ratio appear to be more dependent on environmental than on genetic factors with modern grain varieties. With genetic selection, the relative masses of the endosperm and the germ, and thereby their relative contributions to kernel mass, can be reduced, maintained, or increased (as with high oil corn), so higher-yielding and higher-protein grain varieties do not necessarily have less lysine. Linear regression equations relating amino acid concentrations to protein content of cereal grains have been developed to predict changes in total amino acid content of cereal grains (NRC, 1998). If dilution with starch alone were driving amino acid concentration, these equations would have no intercept. Therefore, factors in addition to dilution by starch must be involved. Unfortunately, the amino acid:protein need not always be linear. Indeed, the slope and shape of the relationship of essential amino acids to total protein would be expected to differ depending on whether the endosperm:germ ratio or the subcomponent proteins in each of these fractions is altered. Mutant strains with decreased amounts of specific zeins (corn) and inversion of kafrin (milo) have been developed. Such alterations alter amino acid content and enhance both amino acid and energy (starch) availability.

Through genetic selection or modification, grain varieties with higher nutritive value have been produced. Strains with modified traits, e.g., richer in lysine or oil, with modified starch type, lipid composition, or phosphorus availability, have been developed. In some cases, nutritional changes have been accompanied by alterations in kernel physiology, e.g., zein content of opaque-2 (high-lysine) corn grain is reduced by half; high-oil corn has much larger germ. Of total protein in grain, germ protein comprised 22% for corn grain, 10% for barley, and 8% for sorghum. Although germ protein contains only about 70% as much sulfur-amino acids as endosperm protein, germ protein is richer in most essential amino acids with two to three times more lysine and tryptophan than endosperm protein. Because lysine usually is the first limiting amino acid of grains, amino acid balance for feeding to swine should be is improved if a larger proportion of total grain protein comes from the germ.

C. Minerals

Mineral contents of various cereal grains as a fraction of the dietary requirements for growing-finishing swine are presented in Figure 35.5. Chapters 10, 11, and 12 provide more information regarding mineral nutrition of pigs. Calcium clearly is inadequate in all cereal grains. Available rather than total phosphorus is listed because much of the phosphorus in cereal grains is indelibly bound to inositol to form phytate. Availability of phosphorus in grains ranges from under 15% for corn grain to 50% for wheat, presumably being higher for wheat because of the presence of phytase in the seed. Availability of phytate phosphorus can be increased if feeds are exposed to phytase prior to being fed (as from bacterial phytase during fermentation of ensiled grain) or if active phytase is present in the digestive tract. In addition, corn grain mutants that have higher available phosphorus content and much lower phytate concentrations have been isolated. Level of supplemental dietary phosphorus can be reduced if phosphorus availability from feeds is increased. With greater phosphorus availability, swine producers can decrease the amount of phosphorus added to

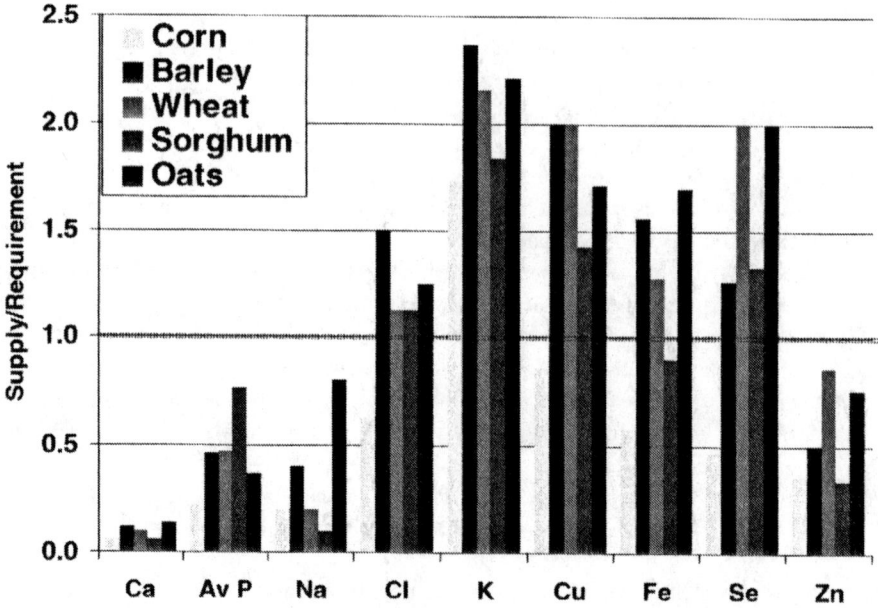

FIGURE 35.5 Adequacy of minerals and available phosphorus from various cereal grains (NRC, 1998). Dotted line represents the point where supply meets requirement.

the diet; this decreases phosphorus excretion, a major environmental concern. If a diet is simultaneously deficient in both calcium and phosphorus, supplements providing both phosphorus and calcium (dicalcium phosphate; bone meal) can be added.

Sodium also is deficient in cereal grains, so salt (sodium chloride) is added to most diets. Added salt will help to meet the chloride deficiency suggested for corn, as well. Zinc supplementation also is required with all grains. As with phosphorus, availability of zinc from both grains and plant protein sources is incomplete, being reduced by presence of phytate. Supplemental copper and iron may not be needed with cereals other than corn grain. Selenium content of grain depends on environmental (soil) conditions; compared with other grains, corn grain is more frequently grown on selenium-deficient soils. Therefore, corn is more likely to contain inadequate selenium for optimal swine performance and health than other cereal grains, although selenium content of sorghum grain can also be low.

D. Fat-Soluble Vitamins

Concentrations of vitamins in cereal grains are shown in Figure 35.6. Vitamins A, D, and E typically are added to cereal-based swine diets because cereal grains have low or unreliable concentrations of these vitamins. Although vitamin E is present in all cereal grains at harvest, vitamin E activity is lost by either oxidation or microbial fermentation during ensiled storage; added trace minerals exacerbate oxidative losses of vitamins A and E.

E. Water-Soluble Vitamins

Concentrations of marginally supplied B vitamins relative to minimal requirements for growing-finishing pigs also are presented in Figure 35.6 from NRC (1998) excluding niacin, B_{12}, biotin, thiamin, and vitamin B_6. Available niacin and vitamin B_{12} were excluded from this figure because these two vitamins are deficient in all cereal grains; values for biotin, thiamin, and vitamin B_6 were excluded because concentrations of these three vitamins in all five grains exceed the estimated

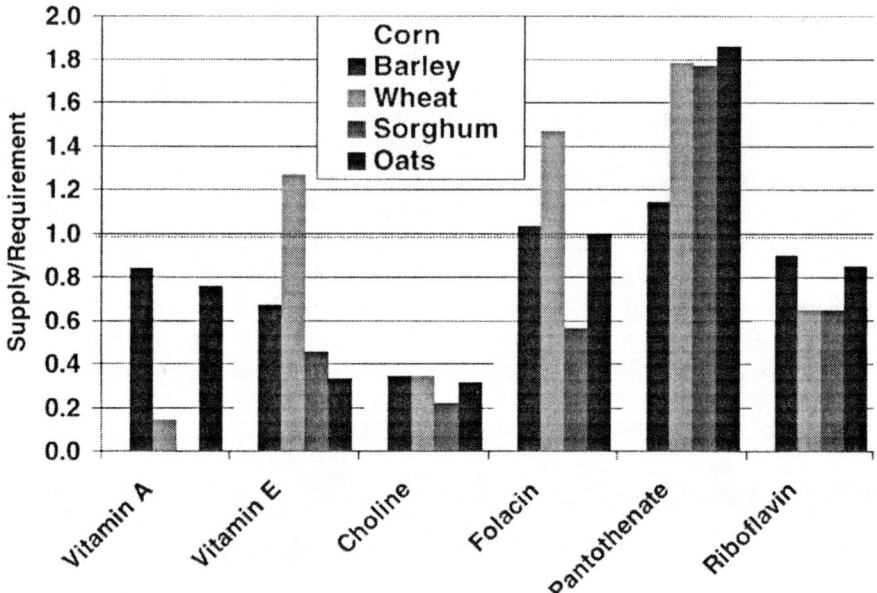

FIGURE 35.6 Adequacy of vitamins from various cereal grains (NRC, 1998). Dotted line represents the point where supply meets requirement.

requirements for growing pigs. In some studies, vitamin supplementation above minimal requirements has improved production efficiency, so minimums cited by NRC (1998) may be lower than optimal concentrations. Niacin of cereal grains and by-products, being bound in an alkali-labile complex, is virtually unavailable. Like most mammals, pigs can synthesize niacin from tryptophan although this process seems quite inefficient and relies on an excess of tryptophan, an amino acid whose supply usually is quite limited in corn-based diets.

In addition to niacin and B_{12}, choline, pantothenic acid, and riboflavin typically are added to grain-based diets because of low concentrations (see Figure 35.6) or availability of these vitamins from grain. Additional vitamins may be of concern with certain diets. For example, biotin supply in corn grain should meet requirements, particularly when combined with synthesis in the large intestine and limited coprophagy. However, when antibiotics are included in the diet, they can limit microbial synthesis of biotin in the intestine and precipitate a biotin deficiency. Although folic acid calculates to be deficient in corn and sorghum grains, performance benefits from supplementing corn–soy diets with folic acid have not been consistent, suggesting that the requirement may be overestimated.

F. Variability in Nutrient Content of Grains

Swine feeding trials have been conducted to determine the relative "nutritive value" of various cereal grains for nearly a century. Amino acid contents and availability as well as ME and net energy values for grains cited above represent a compilation of information from numerous experiments. Unfortunately, "average" values ignore localized or variety differences due to genetics and growing conditions. Examples below are drawn from experiments with corn grain, but similar patterns probably exist for other cereal grains. First, numerous genetic types of corn grain can be produced (pop, flint, dent, waxy, amylose, sweet, floury, high-oil, opaque). Although grade 2 yellow dent corn typically is used as a baseline in many nutrition experiments, the degree of flintiness in dent corn generally is greater for shorter-day hybrids. And depending on fertilization practices, genetic background, and processing, the content and availability of protein, starch, and oil can differ. A plot of oil and starch content based on NIR transmittance analysis of samples for high-oil and yellow dent corn (about 13,000 and 26,000 samples, respectively) is presented in Figure 35.7. Note that oil content of samples of normal dent grain ranges from under 2 to over 5% whereas high-oil corn ranges from 5.5 to over 10% of dry matter. As oil content increases, starch percentage decreases; the total range in starch is from about 63 to over 75% of grain dry matter. Similarly, protein content of corn grain exhibits a range from under 6 to over 12% with high-oil corn; usually protein and essential amino acid content is slightly higher for high-oil grain than grain with normal oil content (Figure 35.8) because of the larger germ of high-oil corn. This diversity in chemical composition within corn grain, a grain generally used as a base for comparison with other grains because of its assumed constancy, is discouraging from a nutritional standpoint. Fortunately, such variability ensures that potential remains for continued genetic advancement by selection. Information about the chemical and physical analysis of grain used in nutrition trials is seldom very thorough; greater analytical detail about such grains should help to undergird contrasts, improve understanding of factors limiting energy and protein availability, and speed development of rapid *in vitro* or near infrared reflectance or transmission (NIR or NIT) systems to predict nutrient value (van Barneveld, 1998).

G. Antinutritive Factors in Grains

Cereal grains contain certain compounds that prevent predation by microbes, insects, and animals. These and additional antinutritive compounds are discussed in Chapter 25. Certain strains of sorghum grain carry bitter-flavored tannins under the seed coat (testa layer); these reduce field losses of the grain to birds. Like certain strains of sorghum (milo) grain, barley contains soluble polyphenols; concentrations of phenolic compounds in wheat and corn generally are very low.

Cereal Grains and By-Products for Swine

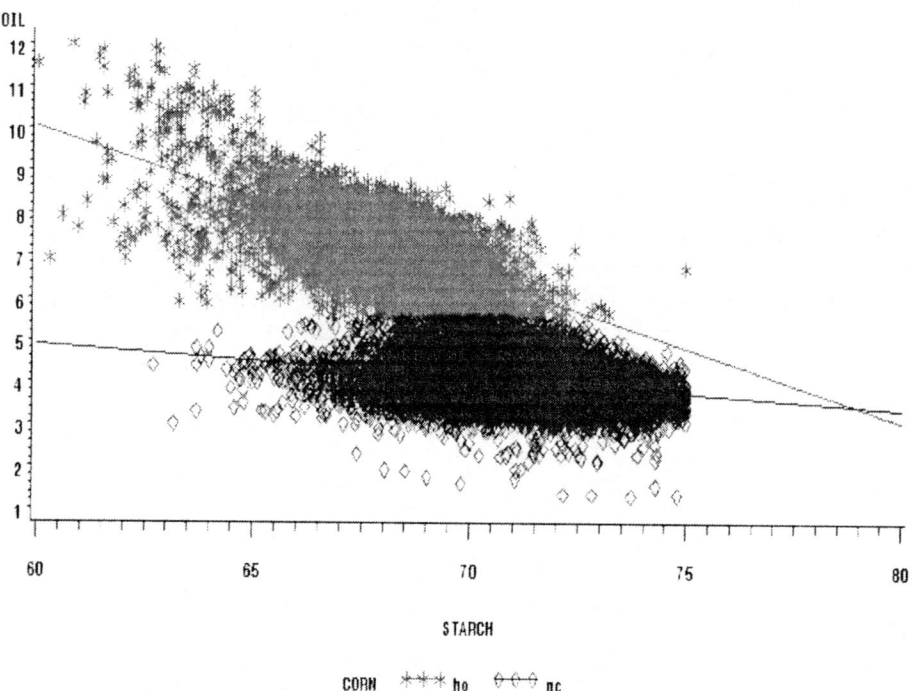

FIGURE 35.7 Oil and starch content (%) of high-oil (stars) and normal dent yellow corn grain (diamonds) based on NIR transmittance analysis of grain samples from 1996 to 1998.

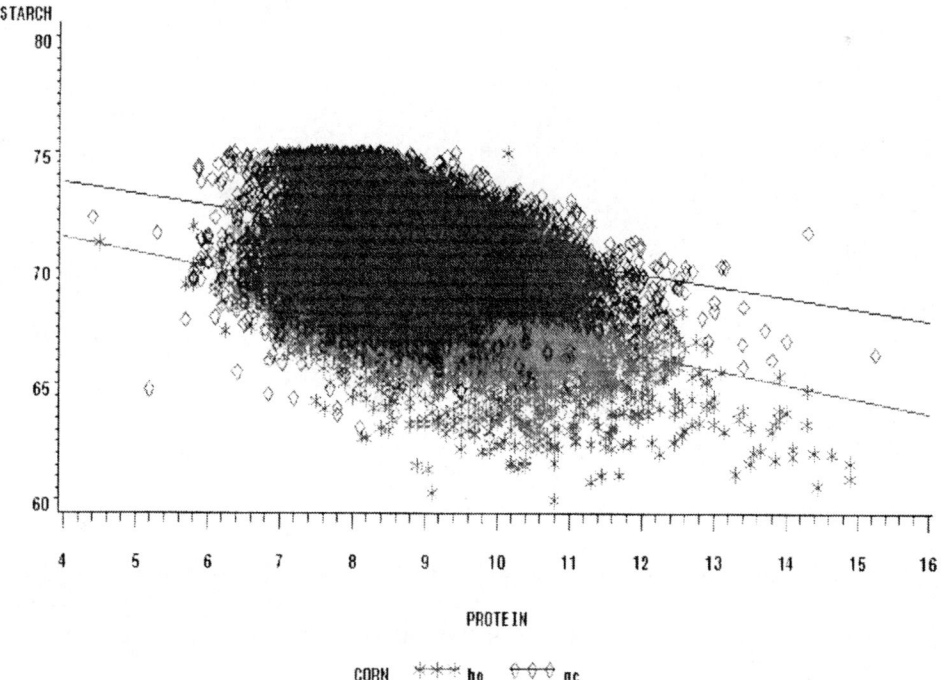

FIGURE 35.8 Starch and protein content (%) of high-oil (stars) and normal dent yellow corn grain (diamonds) based on NIR transmittance analysis of grain samples from 1996 to 1998.

Polyphenols including tannin form complexes with free amino groups so that protein digestibility by pigs is lower for sorghum grain strains that contain higher concentrations of tannins. Trypsin inhibitors, prevalent in most legume seeds, also are found in certain cereal grains including corn; concentrations will increase during insect infestation, but whether this reflects a plant response or presence of insect residues is not clear. Corn grain also contains amylase inhibitors that may reduce starch digestibility. During germination and giberillin release, amylase inhibitors disappear. Amylase released by the pericarp will degrade starch for use by the developing embryo. Certain carbohydrates also resist digestion (β-glucans in oats and barley). Polysaccharides and lectins in these same two grains will increase viscosity of intestinal chyme; this, in turn, can reduce digestibility. Lectins also can interact with the intestinal mucosa resulting in allergic reactions and thickening of the intestinal wall. Opiods present in wheat, through accelerating passage of digesta, can depress digestibility. Although heat processing of legume seeds to inactivate various inhibitors of digestive enzymes is a routine practice, heat processing of cereal grains seldom improves performance of pigs. This lack of response would suggest that levels of heat-sensitive digestion inhibitors, although detectable in cereal grains (pepsin, trypsin inhibitors), are not prevalent enough to warrant heat treatment.

III. GRAIN PROCESSING

As discussed in Chapter 21, feed efficiency typically is improved by 3 to 10% by grinding and pelleting grains. For optimum feed efficiency, corn grain usually is finely ground (geometric mean particle diameter maximum of about 800 μm). Optimum particle size represents a balance between increased energy and protein availability and the potential for adverse effects of fine grinding. An increased incidence of gastric ulcers and depressed feed intake often are noted with finely ground or gelatinized starch. When finely ground, wheat yields flour that becomes glue when chewed; this can reduce feed intake. Feeding corn grain as a paste or with liquid often increases rate but not efficiency of gain. Failure to improve efficiency is surprising because feeding a paste or liquid rather than dusty feed should decrease feed waste. Perhaps wetted grain, particularly if not finely ground, is less thoroughly chewed than dry grain; less chewing and less particle size reduction would reduce energy digestibility. More extensive grain processing (roasting, steam flaking, micronizing, and extruding) has not consistently improved rate or efficiency of gain by pigs, and excessive heat may adversely affect nutritive value. Extensive heat processing, particularly in the presence of reducing sugars, can decrease protein digestibility and reduce amino acid (particularly cystine) availability. Heat processing also can convert amylopectin into retrograde or amylase-resistant starches that may reduce ME value by reducing digestibility in the small intestine. Grains preserved through ensiling are subjected to microbial fermentation and acid solubilization of nutrients. During fermentation, some solubilized amino acids are deaminated, reducing the concentration of essential amino acids. Solubilization of vitreous starch and action of bacterial phytase during fermentation with ensiling generally increase availability of both energy and phosphorus from grains.

IV. GENETIC MODIFICATIONS TO IMPROVE CEREAL GRAINS

Many of the nutritional traits of cereal grains can be modified through selection or genetic modification. Of primary interest are increased energy content (more oil or starch) or increased availability of these components. Modified oil content of the grain also can alter fatty acid composition of depot fat of pigs fed these cereal grains. Grain varieties with increased concentrations and availability of amino acids and increased phosphorus availability are already available for production. Because varieties with modified traits require identity preservation, swine producers desiring such varieties may need to produce the grain themselves or contract with grain producers or traders to obtain grain with a specific trait of interest. Certain traits like resistance to the corn rootworm and herbicide (Roundup®) resistance have been achieved through transfer of genes from other organisms or plants; these are commonly called genetically modified (GM) plants. Other traits, such as high available phosphorus content and high oil content, are mutations inherent in the plant genome itself. Although genetically different, these varieties are not produced by transfer of external genes to the plant and thereby are classified as non-GM varieties. Although unfounded scientifically, public concerns about the food safety and environmental effects of GM crops may hinder application of new technologies that otherwise might increase nutritional value and reduce both production cost (grain productivity, resistance to insects, disease, fungi) and the widespread use of chemicals to control plant and grain pests.

A. Starch Form and Availability

Starch consists of amylose, a linear glucosan, and amylopectin, a branched glucosan. Starch is packed in microscopic granules, primarily but not exclusively in the endosperm of the grain kernel. Keys and Debarthe (1974) indicated that amylose comprised 25, 19, 22, and 20% of total starch (amylose plus amylopectin) for wheat, milo, corn and barley, respectively. In genetic mutants, the amylose-to-amylopectin ratio can differ; waxy corn and waxy milo grain are primarily amylopectin with little if any amylose. In contrast, high-amylose strains contain no amylopectin. Preileal digestibility of amylose for these grains ranged from 85 to 97%; digestibility of amylopectin was 3 to 8 percentage units lower than for amylose. With compensatory digestion in the large intestine, total tract digestion of starch for wheat and corn were over 98% and for milo and barley were about 95%. In contrast, Purser et al. (1979) observed that energy digestibility prior to the terminal ileum was greater for waxy than for normal grain sorghum. That more amylose than amylopectin reaches the large intestine for fermentation is supported by the observation that, compared with low-amylose starch, high-amylose starch increased length of the large bowel and colon in pigs and the concentrations of starch and propionate in the colon. Considering that energy and nutrients are lost during starch fermentation in the large intestine, intestinally digested starch should have a higher net energy value than fermented starch; this should give amylopectin (100% of starch in waxy grains) an advantage in energy availability over amylose starch (60 to 80% of starch in typical grains). However, most of the feeding trials comparing waxy grains have detected little if any feed efficiency advantage for the waxy grains. This is not surprising numerically. If 5% more amylose than amylopectin were fermented in the large intestine, and net energy were 20% lower, net energy would be only 1% lower for amylose than amylopectin. In a study by Rosa et al. (1977), dry matter digestibility ranked corn grain from highest to lowest those with 100, 75, and 60% of their starch as amylopectin; gain-to-feed ratios for both swine and rats ranked these varieties of corn grain in the opposite order! Unfortunately, isogenic varieties have not been used in most energy comparisons to date, so differences other than starch type, including starch vitreousness, may have been involved. With more rapid digestion of amylopectin than amylose, waxy grains may yield absorbable glucose and protein more rapidly than normal grain does and thereby alter hormonal responses and blood urea concentrations (L. Southern, personal communication.)

Starch form also may alter response to heat processing. With flaking or extruding, amylopectin that is melted and not rapidly cooled will crystallize or harden to form resistant or retrograde starch. As it is not readily solubilized, resistant starch is not readily digested by amylase but still should be fermented in the large intestine.

Starch granules within a grain kernel vary in packing density. In the corneous or vitreous endosperm, granules are packed tightly and often bound together by protein (gliadins), whereas in the floury portion of the endosperm, granules are packed loosely. Although this floury (often white) and soft portion of grain kernels is readily disrupted and dispersed, the tightly and densely packed starch granules of the corneous endosperm are more tightly and rigidly bound together. Corn grain varieties with more extensive corneous endosperm often are classified as flint types; the more rigid starch hull of flint grain prevents collapse (indenting) of the endosperm surface during drying of the grain that is characteristic of dent corn grain. Floury grains are more extensively damaged during handling and artificial drying. Presence of fines and formation of stress cracks complicates grain storage and handling by increasing susceptibility to insect and mold damage; fines also prevent the flow of air needed for drying and storing grain. Corn and milo grains, having more corneous endosperm than other grains, have as much as 50% of their endosperm protein composed of gliadin (zein and kafrin, respectively). By gluing starch granules together, these insoluble proteins reduce enzymatic access of starch granules. Fine grinding or more extensive chewing of the grain particles enhances accessibility of the starch in the corneous endosperm to digestive enzymes.

In addition to starch, other glucosans can be stored in grain with β-glucan being prevalent in oats and barley grains. Although a substantial portion of this glucosan is soluble, the β-glucan linkage is not cleaved by amylase or disaccharidases produced by animals. Exposure to the enzyme β-glucanase, either prior to feeding or in the small intestine from addition of this enzyme to the diet, will enhance small intestinal availability of β-glucan. If not digested earlier, β-glucan entering the large intestine is fermented by intestinal bacteria yielding volatile fatty acids. Mucopolysaccharides, glucans, and glutinous proteins, through increasing viscosity of digesta, also can reduce extent of digestion by reducing enzymatic attack and/or mucosal exposure of glucose for absorption. Endproduct accumulation also can reduce amylase activity. Depending on the specific sugars that are exposed, polysaccharides, acting as allergens, may cause inflammation and thickening of the intestinal wall that in turn will increase protein turnover and reduce rate and extent of nutrient absorption. Decreased β-glucan content should increase the energy value of barley and oats.

Neutral detergent fiber, the general class of polysaccharides that includes most pentosans but fails to include certain soluble fibers such as arabino-xylan, comprises plant cell walls. Resistant to digestion by animal enzymes, NDF is slowly but incompletely fermented to volatile fatty acids in the large intestine. Fecal loss of protein often increases when NDF intake increases. Although this increase might be attributed to greater sloughing of intestinal tissue and thereby an increased need for essential amino acids, fermentation of NDF or other carbohydrates in the large intestine also yields microbial protein. As it is derived largely from ammonia, microbial protein lost in feces represents a drain on reserves of nonessential nitrogen (urea), not necessarily of essential amino acids. Regardless of the NDF source, an increase in dietary NDF decreases energy availability and may increase fecal loss of nitrogen.

B. Amino Acid Concentrations and Bioavailability

Genetic mutants of corn grain enriched in lysine and tryptophan (Opaque 2; Floury) were developed several decades ago. Low grain yields and grain damage during handling decreased thier commercial acceptability. Newer corn varieties markedly enriched in free lysine and other amino acids are now being tested for future release. Decreased phytate varieties or added phytase, either through reduced inhibition of proteolytic enzymes or binding of amino acids by phytate, appear to increase ileal availability of amino acids.

C. Oil Concentration

Increased oil content of cereal grains automatically increases net energy value of the grain. This is because gross energy content of oil is more than twice that of starch; net energy value of oil for lipid deposition approaches three times that of starch because of the low heat increment of fat. With nearly twice the ether extract content of typical corn grain (7.4 vs. 4.0% of dry matter), high-oil grain has over 5% greater metabolizable energy content as well as higher concentrations of essential amino acids. Relative cost of production must be balanced against the higher amounts of ME and amino acids to calculate the economic benefit from growing or purchasing high-oil corn. In addition to higher oil content, cereal grains enriched in specific fatty acids, e.g., oleic

D. PHOSPHORUS BIOAVAILABILITY

From 80 to 90% of the phosphorus in corn grain is bound as the phytate salt. Several different recessive mutants of corn grain have been developed with 56 to 100% less phytate; phosphorus bioavailability is three- to eightfold greater from such mutants. Providing diets are formulated to take advantage of the increased phosphorus availability, phosphorus excretion can be reduced and environmental release of phosphorus can be attenuated through feeding such hybrids.

V. PALATABILITY OF CEREAL GRAINS

Pigs and other nonruminants often exhibit preferences for certain strains of grain, especially when the grain is fed whole. Although differences in palatability can be detected in research trials when animals can select from several diets, these same animals, when not given a choice, typically consume equal amounts of preferred and nonpreferred feeds. Consequently, the importance of palatability is greatest for nutritionists developing pet foods (where immediate animal acceptance is monitored) or selecting an ideal rat poison. Differences in palatability may reflect variety or strain differences in kernel texture, hardness, rate of water uptake, gumming, dustiness, or mustiness of the grain.

VI. MARKETING AND HANDLING OF GRAINS WITH MODIFIED NUTRITIONAL TRAITS

Several hurdles hinder development and utilization of improved grain hybrids for livestock feeding. An improved nutritional trait first must be incorporated into a hybrid variety with high yield potential so that grain farmers are willing to grow it. Second, the increased value must be easily and rapidly quantified and demonstrable. Third, users who benefit must share that enhanced value or somehow stimulate production of the select hybrid, and, fourth, identity must be maintained from producer to end user. These challenges can be met by cooperative efforts of progressive swine producers and innovative grain dealers.

VII. SUSTAINABILITY OF GRAIN PRODUCTION

As long as production cost remains below market price, grain will be produced. However, several factors including escalating costs of production (fertilizer, irrigation water in certain areas), deletion of governmental farm supports, and environmental restrictions that are intended to reduce soil erosion and water contamination all will increase the cost of producing grain. Some of these increased costs can be met by increased grain yields, enhanced nutritional value of the grain, and increased efficiency of swine growth. Yet, most futurists predict that social pressures will reduce grain availability. With water depletion in certain regions, corn already has been displaced by dryland wheat and sorghum grain production. Alternatives to grain as an energy source for swine include numerous by-products of industrial extraction and processing (grain residues from distilling, brewing, milling, and baking) and of human food production (waste fats and greases, by-products of milk, meat, and egg processing, sugar and starch by-products, outdated human foods, vegetable residues). When forced to formulate diets that do not contain cereal grains, producers and feed manufacturers readily learn to appreciate the nutritional consistency and the relatively simple methods of harvest, storage, handling, and processing for grains. Fortunately, economic pressures forcing grain displacement should occur gradually and regionally. The experience gained by swine producers who are feeding numerous by-products to swine today (Miller et al., 1990) will be useful if grain feeding becomes economically or environmentally prohibitive.

REFERENCES

de Lange, C. F. M., D. Gillis, L. Whittington, and J. Patience. 1993. Feeding value of various wheat samples for pigs, Ann. Res. Rep., Prairie Swine Center, Inc., Saskatoon, 27.

Fairbairn, S. L., J. F. Patience, and H. L. Classen. 1997. Defining the sources of variation in the energy content of barley, *J. Anim. Sci.*, 75:71.

Finley, J. W., and D. T. Hopkins. 1985. *Digestibility and Amino Acid Availability in Cereals and Oilseeds*, American Association of Cereal Chemists, St. Paul, MN.

Holden, P. J., G. C. Shurson, and J. E. Pettigrew. 1991. Dietary energy for swine, *Pork Industry Handbook*, Michigan State Extension Service, PIH-3.

Hughes, R. J., and M. Choct. 1999. Chemical and physical characteristics of grains related to variability in energy and amino acid availability in poultry, *Aust. J. Agric. Res.*, 50:689.

Kopinski, J. S., M. H. McGee, P. R. Martin, P. Van Melzen, and A. Pytko. 1997. Digestible energy values of wheat, sorghum and barley. In *Manipulating Pig Production VI*, Cranwell, P. D., Ed., Australasian Pig Science Association, Werribee, 234.

Keys, J. E., Jr., and J. V. Debarthe. 1974. Site and extent of carbohydrate, dry matter, energy and protein digestion and the rate of passage of grain diets in swine, *J. Anim. Sci.*, 39:57.

Luce, W. G., G. R. Hollis, D. C. Mahan, and E. R. Miller. 1991. Swine diets, *Pork Industry Handbook*, Michigan State Extension Service, PIH-23.

McNab, J. M. 1996. Factors affecting the energy value of wheat for poultry, *World Poult. Sci. J.*, 52:69.

Miller, E. R., P. J. Holden, and V. D. Liebbrandt. 1990. By-products in swine diets, *Pork Industry Handbook*, Michigan State Extension Service, PIH-108.

NRC. 1971. *Atlas of Nutritional Data on United States and Canadian Feeds*, National Academy Press, Washington, D.C.

NRC. 1998. *Nutrient Requirements of Swine*, 10th rev. ed., National Academy Press, Washington, D.C.

Purser, K. W., T. D. Tanksley, Jr., T. Zebroska, and D. A. Knabe. 1979. Effect of sorghum endosperm starch type on nutrient digestibility at the terminal ileum and over the entire tract of finishing pigs, *J. Anim. Sci.*, 49(Suppl. 1):251.

Rosa, J. G., D. M. Forsyth, D. V. Glover, and T. R. Cline. 1977. Normal, opaque-2, waxy, waxy opaque-2, sugary-2 and sugary-2 opaque-2 corn (*Zea mays* L.) endosperm types for rats and pigs. Studies on energy utilization, *J. Anim. Sci.*, 44:1004.

SCA (Standing Committee on Agriculture–Pig Subcommittee). 1987. Feeding Standards for Australian Livestock — Pigs. In Robards, G. E., and J. C. Radcliffe, Eds., Standing Committee on Agriculture, CSIRO, East Melbourne, 109.

Sibbald, I. R. 1986. The TME system of feed evaluation: methodology, feed composition data and bibliography, Contribution 85–19, Research Branch, Agriculture Canada, Ottawa, Ontario.

Sibbald, I. R., and K. Price. 1976. Relationships between metabolizable energy values for poultry and some physical and chemical data describing Canadian wheats, oats, and barleys, *Can. J. Anim. Sci.*, 56:255.

Tanksley, T. D. Jr., D. H. Baker, and A. J. Lewis. 1990. Protein and amino acids for swine, *Pork Industry Handbook*, Michigan State Extension Service, PIH-5.

van Barneveld, R. J. 1997. Characteristics of feed grains that influence their nutritive value and subsequent utilisation by pigs. In *Manipulating Pig Production VI*, Cranwell, P. D., Ed., Australasian Pig Science Association, Werribee, 193.

van Barneveld, R. J. 1998. Use of near infra-red spectroscopy to predict the energy content of feed grains. In *Proc. 19th Western Nutrition Conference*, Saskatoon, Saskatchewan, 176.

36 Protein Supplements

Lee I. Chiba

CONTENTS

I.	Introduction	804
II.	Diet Formulation	805
III.	Plant Protein Supplements	807
	A. Oilseed Meals in General	807
	B. Alfalfa Meal	809
	1. Introduction	809
	2. Nutrient Content	809
	3. Antinutritional Factors	809
	4. Feeding Alfalfa Meal to Pigs	810
	C. Canola Seed (Rapeseed) and Meal	810
	1. Introduction	810
	2. Nutrient Content	811
	3. Antinutritional Factors	811
	4. Feeding Canola Seed (Rapeseed) and Meal to Pigs	811
	D. Coconut (Copra) Meal	812
	1. Introduction	812
	2. Nutrient Content	812
	3. Antinutritional Factors	812
	4. Feeding Coconut Meal to Pigs	813
	E. Cottonseed Meal	813
	1. Introduction	813
	2. Nutrient Content	813
	3. Antinutritional Factors	813
	4. Feeding Cottonseed Meal to Pigs	814
	F. Linseed (Flax) Meal	815
	1. Introduction	815
	2. Nutrient Content	815
	3. Antinutritional Factors	815
	4. Feeding Linseed (Flax) Meal to Pigs	815
	G. Peanut Meal and Whole Peanuts	816
	1. Introduction	816
	2. Nutrient Content	816
	3. Antinutritional Factors	816
	4. Feeding Peanut Meal and Whole Peanuts to Pigs	817
	H. Safflower Meal	817
	1. Introduction	817
	2. Nutrient Content	818
	3. Antinutritional Factors	818
	4. Feeding Safflower Meal to Pigs	818

	I.	Sesame Meal 819
		1. Introduction 819
		2. Nutrient Content 819
		3. Antinutritional Factors 819
		4. Feeding Sesame Meal to Pigs 819
	J.	Soybeans and Soybean Products 819
		1. Introduction 819
		2. Nutrient Content 820
		3. Antinutritional Factors 820
		4. Feeding Soybeans and Soybean Products to Pigs 821
	K.	Sunflower Seeds and Meal 821
		1. Introduction 821
		2. Nutrient Content 822
		3. Antinutritional Factors 822
		4. Feeding Sunflower Seeds and Meal to Pigs 822
IV.	Animal Protein Supplements 823
	A.	Animal Protein Sources in General 823
	B.	Blood Meal 823
		1. Introduction 823
		2. Feeding Blood Meal to Pigs 824
	C.	Feather Meal 824
		1. Introduction 824
		2. Feeding Feather Meal to Pigs 825
	D.	Fish Meal 825
		1. Introduction 825
		2. Feeding Fish Meal to Pigs 826
	E.	Meat and Bone Meal 826
		1. Introduction 826
		2. Feeding Meat and Bone Meal to Pigs 827
	F.	Meat Meal 827
		1. Introduction 827
		2. Feeding Meat Meal to Pigs 827
	G.	Milk, Dried 828
		1. Introduction 828
		2. Feeding Dried Milk to Pigs 828
	H.	Plasma Protein 828
		1. Introduction 828
		2. Feeding Plasma Protein to Pigs 828
	I.	Poultry By-Product Meal 829
		1. Introduction 829
		2. Feeding Poultry By-Product Meal to Pigs 829
	J.	Whey, Dried 829
		1. Introduction 829
		2. Feeding Dried Whey to Pigs 830
References 830

I. INTRODUCTION

Improving the efficiency of feed utilization is important for successful pig production, simply because feed costs account for the largest economic input in most swine enterprises. This is especially true for protein sources because they account for a major portion of total feed costs (SCA, 1987). Wasteful usage of protein supplements is likely to increase the cost of production in any swine enterprise. In addition, feeding excess protein to animals can have an adverse impact on the environment (see Chapter 27 for more information). The management of wastes and odors has become a major issue facing the pig industry. Large amounts of nitrogen excreted in animal wastes can lead to contamination of water, and to odorous emissions, because many odorous compounds originate from undigested dietary protein and other nitrogenous compounds. Furthermore, the competition between humans and animals, particularly nonruminant species, for quality sources of protein is likely to increase continuously because of the ever-increasing world population. Therefore, efficient feed utilization not only improves profitability of pig enterprises and has a positive impact on the environment, but it also helps ensure continuous availability of quality sources of nutrients for future pig production.

The increased demand for protein sources for both humans and animals is likely to lead to reduced availability and increased cost. Many different protein sources can be used for pig production. Alternative feed ingredients have different feeding values because of variations in nutrient content and other factors such as bioavailability and stability, antinutritional factors, interactions among the nutrients and possibly with non-nutritive factors, and palatability. Potential alternative protein sources can be used successfully in pig diets, but only if diets are formulated correctly. Having accurate nutrient information on the protein source is, therefore, necessary to make appropriate adjustments for the formulation of cost-effective and environmentally friendly diets.

The objective of this chapter is to review briefly the major protein supplements used in pig production. For each plant protein source, the discussion is separated into the background information, nutrient content, antinutritional factors, and its value as a feed ingredient, whereas only the background information and its value as a feed ingredient are discussed for each animal protein source. The relative feeding values and suggested maximum incorporation rates of some protein supplements are presented in Table 36.1. For the complete information on the composition of feed ingredients, readers are referred to a recent NRC (1998) publication and other sources. Excellent reviews on protein supplements have been presented over the years (e.g., Cunha, 1977; Aherne and Kennelly, 1985; Thacker and Kirkwood, 1990; Seerley, 1991; and Church and Kellems, 1998).

II. DIET FORMULATION

In commercial pig production, the main objective of diet formulation and feeding strategy is to maximize profits, which does not necessarily imply maximal animal performance. To maximize economic efficiency, supplying indispensable nutrients as close as possible to meeting but not exceeding the requirements of the pig is advantageous. In addition, it will have a positive impact on today's environmentally conscious society by reducing the excretion of unutilized nutrients. Such optimum feeding strategies involve consideration of a multitude of factors, but two concepts that may contribute greatly to the formulation of "efficient and environmentally friendly" diets are (1) ideal protein concept and (2) formulation of diets based on available nutrients.

The body uses mixtures of amino acids collectively for protein synthesis; thus, the balance of amino acids is very important for optimum utilization of protein (Whittemore, 1993). Ideal protein can be described operationally as protein that cannot be improved by any substitution of a quantity of one amino acid for the same quantity of another (Fuller and Chamberlain, 1985). On a practical basis, the proportions of threonine, tryptophan, and sulfur amino acids relative to lysine are perhaps the most important, because these amino acids are likely to be limiting after lysine in most practical pig diets (Knabe, 1996). Any departure from a desirable pattern of amino acids may lead to a reduction in pig performance, at least in terms of efficiency of protein utilization (Lewis, 1991), or it may result in acute neurological aberrations and even death (D'Mello, 1994), depending on the degree of departure. Thus, consideration of the ideal protein concept in diet formulation is very beneficial.

TABLE 36.1
Relative Feeding Values and Suggested Maximum Incorporation Rates of Some Protein Sources

Ingredient	Relative Feeding Value[a,c]	Lysine (g/100 g Crude Protein)[d]	Maximum Recommended Inclusion Rate (% of Diet)[a,b]			
			Starter	Grower-Finisher	Gestation	Lactation
Alfalfa meal, dehydrated	—	4.35–4.59	0	10	25	0
Blood meal, spray-dried	220–230	8.39	3	5–6	5	5
Canola meal	70–80	5.84	0	15	15	15
Cottonseed meal	—	4.15	0	10	15	0
Fish meal, menhaden	160–170	7.72	20	6	6	6
Meat and bone meal	105–115	4.87	5	5	10	5
Meat meal	130–140	5.69	0	5	10	5
Plasma protein, spray-dried	205–215	8.77	10	¶	¶	¶
Skim milk, dried	105–115	8.27	30	¶	¶	¶
Soy protein concentrate	135–145	6.56	20	¶	¶	¶
Soy protein isolate	—	6.13	10	¶	¶	¶
Soybean meal	100	6.46	15	25	15	20
Soybean meal, dehulled	105–110	6.36	15	25	15	20
Soybeans, full-fat, heat-treated	85–95	6.31	0	20	10	10
Sunflower meal	55–65	2.84–3.77	0	20	10	0
Whey, dried	55–65	7.44	30–40	15	5	5

Sources: Reese et al. (1995) and Hill et al. (1998).

[a] ¶ indicates no nutritional limitation in a diet balanced for indispensable amino acids, minerals, and vitamins, but economical considerations may preclude the use of an ingredient for a particular class of swine.
[b] 44% CP soybean meal = 100%. Values apply when ingredients are fed at no more than maximum recommended percentage of complete diet. A range is provided to compensate for quality variation.
[c] Based on values reported by NRC (1998).

Efficiency of amino acid utilization can be increased by several methods, such as using high-quality protein sources with a desirable amino acid balance, formulating diets to achieve ideal protein, and lowering the dietary protein concentration and supplementing with certain crystalline amino acids (NRC, 1998). In commercial pig production, using high-quality protein sources to satisfy the amino acid needs may not always be possible. Thus, using a mixture of various protein sources with complementary amino acid compositions, or supplementing diets with crystalline amino acids to simulate the ideal amino acid patterns, is a more practical means to incorporate this concept into diet formulation. Pigs fed such diets should utilize amino acids more efficiently and reduce excretion of nitrogen (e.g., Hansen et al., 1993a,b; Cromwell and Coffey, 1994; Tuitoek et al., 1997).

Besides the variations in the content of nutrients in feed ingredients and the variability associated with various laboratories and analytical techniques (Wiseman and Cole, 1985; NCR-42, 1993; Patience, 1996; NCR-42 and S-145, 1997), an important factor for nonruminant species is nutrient availability. Simply because not all of the nutrients are available to pigs, expressing the requirements and formulating diets based on the available nutrients, rather than the total, would be more effective in precisely satisfying the pig's needs. However, it is questionable whether there is sufficient information on the nutritive value of individual feed ingredients to achieve this objective (Close and Fowler, 1985). Parsons (1996) indicated that amino acid digestibility values in feed ingredients determined by balance assays are often higher than amino acid availability values determined by slope-ratio growth assays, and the ileal digestibility assay overestimates the amount of amino acids available or utilizable for protein synthesis. Similarly, Batterham et al. (1990) concluded that the values for the ileal digestibility of lysine in protein concentrates are not suitable in diet formulations because a considerable portion of amino acids may be absorbed in a form that is not utilized efficiently by the pig. Therefore, there is no agreement on how to address the availability issue in practice, and a question exists regarding whether using available nutrient values will improve the precision of diet formulation enough to meet the needs of the industry (Patience, 1996).

Nevertheless, formulation of diets based on available amino acids should be an improvement over formulation on a total amino acid basis, simply because pigs can utilize only those nutrients available to them. Obviously, further progress must be made in developing procedures to describe a true nutritional value of feed ingredients. Besides amino acids, consideration of the availability of phytate P is important in pig nutrition because P is the third most expensive nutrient in the pig diet after energy and amino acids. Although other nutrients are equally important, consideration of the availability of energy, amino acids, and P in diet formulation would contribute greatly to the efficiency and economics of pig production, as well as reducing the release of unutilized nitrogen and P into the environment. Apparent ileal digestibility of indispensable amino acids and availability of P in common protein supplements are presented in a recent NRC (1998) publication and in other publications.

III. PLANT PROTEIN SUPPLEMENTS

A. OILSEED MEALS IN GENERAL

Today, the major protein sources used for animal production are oilseed meals. The production of oilseeds has increased from 228 million metric tons (MMT) in 1992 to 1993 to 287 MMT (preliminary data) in 1997 to 1998 (Foreign Agricultural Service, or FAS; U.S. Department of Agriculture, or USDA). Soybeans, peanuts, and sunflowers are grown primarily for their seeds, which produce oils for human consumption and other purposes (Church and Kellems, 1998). Rapeseed is grown for the same reason. Cottonseed is a by-product of cotton production, and its oil is widely used for food and other purposes. In the past, linseed (flax) was grown to provide fibers for linen cloth production. The invention of the cotton gin in 1792, however, made cotton more available for clothing materials (Aherne and Kennelly, 1985). The demand for linen cloth

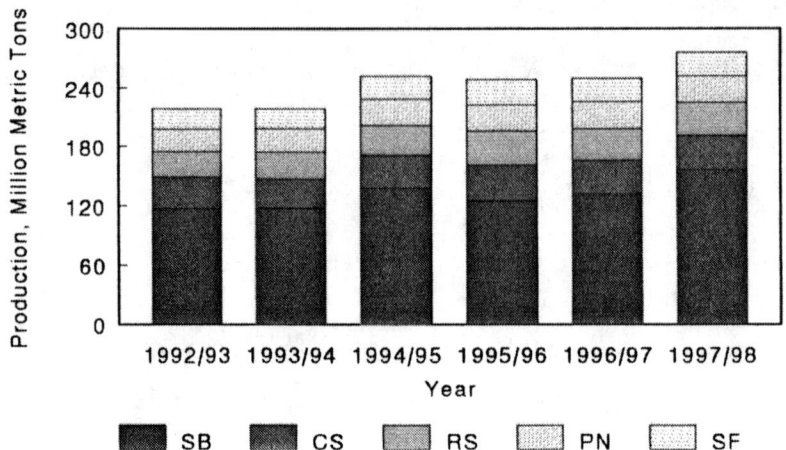

FIGURE 36.1 Annual production of major oilseeds. SB = soybean, CS = cottonseed, RS = rapeseed, PN = peanut, and SF = sunflower seed. (From Foreign Agricultural Service, USDA.)

has decreased since then, and linseed shifted its prominent position in fiber production to industrial oil production. The soybean is clearly the prominent oilseed produced in the world (Figure 36.1), and soybean meal accounted for 64.1% of the world production of protein meals in 1997 to 1998 (Table 36.2). Major producers of this important meal are presented in Table 36.3.

The process of oilseed meal production has been described briefly by Church and Kellems (1998). Moderate heating is generally required to inactivate antinutritional factors present in oilseed meals. At the same time, overheating of oilseed meals can greatly reduce the amount of digestible or available lysine. Other amino acids (arginine, histidine, and tryptophan) are usually affected to a lesser extent (Parsons, 1996; Church and Kellems, 1998). However, the potential problems are well recognized by oilseed processors, which is reflected in today's production of high-quality meals.

As a group, the oilseed meals are high in crude protein (CP) content except safflower meal with hulls (Church and Kellems, 1998). The CP content is usually standardized before marketing by dilution with hulls or other materials. Relative to the amino acid requirement of nonruminant species, most oilseed meals are low in lysine, but soybean meal is an exception (Aherne and Kennelly, 1985). The extent of dehulling will affect the protein and fiber contents, whereas the method of oil extraction will influence the ether extract content (Aherne and Kennelly, 1985), and

TABLE 36.2
World Production of Major Protein Meals (million metric tons)

Protein Meal	Year					
	1992/93	1993/94	1994/95	1995/96	1996/97	1997/98[a]
Soybean meal	76.38	81.20	87.50	89.10	91.81	100.10
Rapeseed meal	14.00	14.81	16.53	18.56	18.02	19.05
Cottonseed meal	11.46	10.67	11.74	13.10	12.23	11.86
Sunflower meal	8.55	8.33	9.50	10.12	9.94	9.83
Fish meal	5.90	6.35	6.59	6.50	6.41	5.10
Peanut meal	5.11	5.24	5.99	5.73	6.17	5.53
Total	125.08	130.53	142.12	147.40	149.32	156.05

[a] Preliminary data.

Source: Foreign Agricultural Service, USDA.

TABLE 36.3
Soybean Meal Production by Main Producers (million metric tons)

	Year					
Country	1992/93	1993/94	1994/95	1995/96	1996/97	1997/98[a]
United States	27.55	27.68	30.18	29.51	31.04	34.54
Brazil	12.17	14.50	15.87	17.04	15.72	15.73
European Union	10.98	9.85	11.49	10.91	11.62	12.01
Argentina	6.86	7.08	7.00	8.38	9.01	10.60
China	3.63	6.16	6.96	6.05	6.95	8.36
India	2.25	2.88	2.20	3.20	2.92	3.80
Japan	2.94	2.85	2.88	2.87	2.94	2.96
Mexico	2.08	2.06	1.86	1.95	2.15	2.77
Total	76.38	81.20	87.50	89.10	91.81	100.10

[a] Preliminary data.

Source: Foreign Agricultural Service, USDA.

thus the energy content of the meal. Oilseed meals are generally low in Ca, but high in P content. The biological availability of minerals in plant sources such as oilseeds are generally low, and this is especially true for P (see Chapters 10, 16, and 27 for more information).

B. Alfalfa Meal

1. Introduction

Alfalfa (*Medicago* sp.) is one of the most popular forage crops grown throughout the world (Thacker, 1990a), and it is the most widely used legume meal in pig diets (Cunha, 1977). It is an excellent source of many nutrients, and not too long ago the inclusion of alfalfa meal in the diet was considered to be essential to meet the nutrient requirements of reproducing swine. Unfortunately, alfalfa is relatively unpalatable, the protein is poorly digested, and it has a low digestible energy due to a high fiber content (Thacker, 1990a). Despite its shortcomings, there is still considerable interest in using alfalfa in pig diets. If alfalfa is to be used as a protein supplement, cutting at the early bud stage is most appropriate (Thacker, 1990a).

2. Nutrient Content

A summary of the nutrient content of alfalfa has been presented by Thacker (1990a). The CP content of alfalfa ranges from 12 to 22% and the crude fiber ranges from 25 to 30% (Seerley, 1991). The accessibility of digestive enzymes to the soluble cellular proteins is reduced by the high fiber content. Thus, the protein in alfalfa has a digestibility of approximately 60%. Alfalfa contains a reasonable level of lysine, and it has a good amino acid balance. Sun-cured alfalfa is high in Ca, and its bioavailability can be similar to Ca carbonate when fed to gestating swine (Walker et al., 1993). Alfalfa is low in P, but it is a reasonably good source of other minerals such as Mg, K, Cu, Mn, Fe, Cl, and Zn (Thacker, 1990a). Alfalfa meal is a good source of most vitamins, and it is an excellent source of vitamins A, D, E, and K, and some B vitamins such as riboflavin, pantothenic acid, biotin, and niacin (Thacker, 1990a; Seerley, 1991).

3. Antinutritional Factors

Alfalfa contains potential toxins such as saponins and tannins (Thacker, 1990a). Saponins are bitter-tasting compounds. Although a mechanism has not been elucidated, they may depress feed intake, inhibit digestive enzymes or cellular metabolism, and/or form complexes with nutrients to make them unavailable. Tannins are water-soluble polymeric phenolics that can depress protein digestibility by binding dietary protein and inhibiting digestive enzymes. Tannins may also reduce feed intake. In addition, alfalfa may contain a trypsin inhibitor and a photosensitizing agent.

4. Feeding Alfalfa Meal to Pigs

Because of its high fiber content and possible palatability problems, alfalfa meal should not be used in the diet for weanling pigs (Thacker, 1990a). It has been suggested that grower-finisher pigs can be fed 2.5 to 10% alfalfa meal (Cunha, 1977; Seerley, 1991). Rate and efficiency of weight gain were, however, decreased progressively as the content of alfalfa meal increased from 0 to 60% (Kass et al., 1980; Powley et al., 1981). Although palatability problems (Leamaster and Cheeke, 1979) and inadequate energy intake seemed to be primarily responsible for the reduced growth performance, its effect on nutrient digestibility cannot be ignored (Kass et al., 1980). In a cold environment, however, the additional heat produced during the digestion and metabolism of a fibrous ingredient such as alfalfa may be used to satisfy a portion of the pig's increased maintenance energy needs, thus possibly partitioning other nutrients for tissue growth (Stahly and Cromwell, 1986).

The use of alfalfa in gestation diets has a long history, and most research has indicated little or no detrimental effects of alfalfa on reproductive performance of sows (e.g., Danielson and Noonan, 1975; Allee, 1977). In addition, inclusion of alfalfa in sow diets has increased ovulation rate (Teague, 1955), litter size at birth (Teague, 1955; Seerley and Wahlstrom, 1965), pig survival rate (Pollmann et al., 1981), farrowing percentage (Danielson and Noonan, 1975), and longevity (Pollmann et al., 1981). The beneficial effects of alfalfa in improving litter size at birth and survival rate seem to be related to the increased ketogenic substrates in sows fed high-fiber diets. Thacker (1990a), however, cautioned that alfalfa in gestation diets may reduce birth weight of pigs, although levels as high as 60% of the diet should not pose any problems. Although alfalfa meal should not be included in the lactation diet (Thacker, 1990a), it can be fed during preparturition and early lactation to prevent or alleviate constipation.

Because of its high fiber content, alfalfa should not be used in weanling pig diets. Grower-finisher pig diets could contain 2.5 to 10% alfalfa meal, but growth performance may be reduced at higher levels. Alfalfa may have its greatest potential for use in gestation diets, and it can be used at levels as high as 60% (Thacker, 1990a) or greater depending on the economics. Although alfalfa can be fed to sows during preparturition and early lactation phase to prevent or alleviate constipation, it is not recommended for lactating sows.

C. Canola Seed (Rapeseed) and Meal

1. Introduction

World annual rapeseed production was 11.4 MMT in 1980 to 1981 (Aherne and Kennelly, 1985), and it has increased to 25.3 MMT in 1992 to 1993 and to 34.3 MMT (preliminary data) in 1997 to 1998 (FAS, USDA). The leading countries in rapeseed production are China, Canada, India, and the European Union. In the mid-1970s, Canada's rapeseed production was shifted to cultivars that contain low erucic acid levels in the oil and low glucosinolate levels in the meal. These nutritionally superior cultivars were tradenamed "Canola" types (Aherne and Bell, 1990). To be called canola, the oil must contain less than 2% erucic acid, whereas meal must contain less than 30 µmol glucosinolates/g (Thacker, 1990b). Two species now represent the main cultivated oilseed, and canola meal may be produced from a Polish (*Brassica campestris*) or an Argentine type (*B. napus*; Church and Kellems, 1998).

2. Nutrient Content

Reviews on the nutrient content of canola seed (Aherne and Bell, 1990) and canola meal (Bell, 1984; Aherne and Kennelly, 1985; Thacker, 1990b) have been presented. Generally, canola seed contains about 40% ether extract, 22% CP, and 7% crude fiber (Aherne and Bell, 1990). Compared with soybeans, canola seed is a good source of Ca, S, Se, and Zn, but it is a poor source of K and Cu. Canola seed is a good source of biotin, choline, niacin, and riboflavin, but not folic acid or pantothenic acid.

Canola meal from *B. campestris* contains about 35% CP, whereas the meal from *B. napus* contains 38 to 40% CP (Thacker, 1990b). The amino acid content of both low- and high-glucosinolate rapeseed varieties does not differ greatly (Aherne and Kennelly, 1985). The lysine content of canola meal is lower than soybean meal, but it has a comparable amino acid profile. However, canola meal generally contains less available amino acids than soybean meal (Aherne and Kennelly, 1985; Thacker, 1990b). Because of its high fiber content (>11%), canola meal contains about 15 to 25% less digestible energy than soybean meal (Thacker, 1990b). High phytic acid and fiber contents reduce the availability of many mineral elements, but canola meal is generally a better source of many minerals than soybean meal.

3. Antinutritional Factors

In the past, the presence of glucosinolates was the major factor limiting the use of rapeseed or rapeseed meal in pig diets (Bell, 1984; Aherne and Bell, 1990; Thacker, 1990b). Although glucosinolates themselves are biologically inactive, they can be hydrolyzed by myrosinase in the seed to produce goitrogenic compounds (Thacker, 1990b; Church and Kellems, 1998). Fortunately, selected cultivars of the canola seed contain only about 15% of the glucosinolates found in the old rapeseed (Bell, 1984). In addition, heat processing is likely to inactivate the myrosinase enzyme in the seed. Tannins and sinapine are two other groups of compounds found in canola seed or meal that can affect the feeding value (Thacker, 1990b), but data on their effect on performance are lacking (Aherne and Kennelly, 1985).

4. Feeding Canola Seed (Rapeseed) and Meal to Pigs

Aherne and Bell (1990) reviewed the use of rapeseed and canola seed in pig diets. The inclusion of up to 10 or 12% rapeseed resulted in reduced performance of growing pigs, and increased degree of polyunsaturation of backfat. Growth performance of starter pigs was reduced by 30% canola seed, whereas up to 10, 15, or 20% of canola seed in separate studies had no effect on performance of grower-finisher pigs. Reproductive performance of sows was reduced by feeding 15% canola seed during the lactation phase. Processing can generally improve nutrient digestibilities of rapeseed and canola seed.

Despite the reduction in glucosinolate content of canola meal, pig performance is often reduced by the use of canola meal because of other factors (Aherne and Kennelly, 1985). McIntosh et al. (1986) reported that feed intake and weight gain of pigs were reduced when diets contained more than 9% canola meal. However, digestibility coefficients of dry matter and nitrogen were not affected by the level of dietary canola meal. In a preference study, pigs consumed 2.5 to 7 times more soybean meal diet than diets containing 5 to 20% canola meal, respectively (Baidoo et al., 1986), indicating that a reduction in feed intake is perhaps responsible for decreased performance.

Growth performance of grower pigs may be reduced by including 9 to 12.5% canola meal in diets, or providing more than half the supplemental protein with canola meal (Aherne and Kennelly, 1985). Lysine supplementation had a positive effect on the apparent nutrient digestibilities and nitrogen retention, but those criteria were still lower for pigs fed canola meal diets than for those fed the soybean meal diet (Rowan and Lawrence, 1986a,b). There seems to be a considerable variation among canola meals in nutrient digestibilities. Fan et al. (1996) indicated that neutral detergent fiber content of canola meal is mainly responsible for the variation in ileal amino acid digestibilities. de Lange et al. (1998), however, reported low negative relationships between the apparent ileal amino acid digestibility and various types of fibers in the canola meal samples. Reducing fiber content generally had no effect on the apparent ileal CP or amino acid digestibility.

For finisher pigs, the majority of the published data indicate that canola meal can be used to supply all of the supplemental protein (Aherne and Kennelly, 1985: Thacker, 1990b). A complete replacement of soybean meal with canola meal seems to have no effect on growth performance or carcass quality of pigs.

There are limited data available on the use of rapeseed or canola meal in sow diets. Reproductive performance seemed to improve as the level of glucosinolates in the rapeseed meal decreased (Aherne and Kennelly, 1985). In one study, the researchers concluded that canola meal can be used as the only protein supplement for pregnant and lactating females for at least two reproductive cycles without any adverse effects on reproductive performance (Aherne and Kennelly, 1985; Thacker, 1990b).

Diets for starter and grower-finisher pigs may contain up to 15% of canola seed, but it should be limited to 10% of the diet for sows (Aherne and Bell, 1990). In his review, Seerley (1991) suggested that up to 15% of canola meal could be included in the diet for all classes of pigs, whereas Thacker (1990b) recommended an inclusion rate of up to 5% in starter diets and 10% in grower-finisher and sow diets. Some research has shown, however, that canola meal can be used to supply all the supplemental protein for finisher pigs and sows.

D. Coconut (Copra) Meal

1. Introduction

Coconut (*Cocos nucifera*) is widely distributed in many tropical areas of the world. Parts of the coconut plant may be used as food for humans, but the primary product is copra, its dry kernel, which is used as the raw material for coconut oil production (Thorne et al., 1990). The production of copra was 4.9 MMT in 1992 to 1993 and 5.5 MMT (preliminary data) in 1997 to 1998 (FAS, USDA). The leading oil-producing countries are Philippines, Indonesia, and India (Thorne et al., 1990). Coconut meal (frequently called copra meal) is produced by the expeller method. Its residual oil content is about 8% (Thorne et al., 1990), which is sometimes reduced further by solvent extraction. Coconut meal is an important feed ingredient in many tropical areas of the world (Creswell and Brooks, 1971a; Cunha, 1977). Although it is underutilized, there seems to be a potential to increase its use in pig diets, especially in combination with other feed ingredients (Thorne et al., 1990).

2. Nutrient Content

Residual oil contents of most coconut meals fall between 9 and 16%, but some meals may contain more than 20% oil (Thorne et al., 1990). Coconut oil is composed predominantly of short- and medium-chained fatty acids that can be digested easily, especially by young pigs. Coconut meal contains about 21% CP and 10% fiber (Cunha, 1977; Seerley, 1991). It is deficient in lysine and methionine, and processing methods and temperatures may affect protein digestibility and quality of the meal (Cunha, 1977; Church and Kellems, 1998). Coconut meal is a poor source of amino acids as indicated by lower amino acid digestibilities compared with other protein sources such as soybean meal, fish meal, linseed meal, and sesame meal (Kim et al., 1993).

3. Antinutritional Factors

Coconut meal can be subjected to a high incidence of mold growth such as *Aspergillus* spp. Although there have been no reports of aflatoxicosis in pigs fed high levels of coconut meal, aflatoxin contaminations in excess of that normally permitted in pig diets have been reported in the field (Thorne et al., 1990).

4. Feeding Coconut Meal to Pigs

Although there seem to be no data available on the use of coconut meal in starter pig diets, it may not be a suitable protein source for young pigs because of its deficiency in lysine, low available amino acids, and high fiber content. Growth performance of grower-finisher pigs was reduced by addition of 20 and 30% (Lekule et al., 1982) or 20 and 40% (Creswell and Brooks, 1971b) coconut meal, and carcass quality was reduced by the 40% coconut meal (Creswell and Brooks, 1971b). Similarly, as dietary coconut meal increased from 0 to 50%, pig performance decreased linearly (Thorne et al., 1990). Inclusion of coconut meal reduced protein and dry matter digestibilities (Creswell and Brooks, 1971a). Supplementation of diets with lysine and/or other amino acids (Creswell and Brooks, 1971b; Thorne et al., 1990) or increasing protein level by adding more soybean meal (Creswell and Brooks, 1971b) was not effective in alleviating the reduced pig performance. It has been suggested that the amount of coconut meal should be limited to 10 to 20% or less in pig diets for optimum performance (Cunha, 1977; Seerley, 1991).

Coconut meal is not a good protein supplement for weanling pigs. For optimum performance, the quantity of coconut meal should be limited to 10 to 20% of the diet for other classes of pigs.

E. COTTONSEED MEAL

1. Introduction

Cotton (*Gossypium* spp.) has been grown for several thousand years as a source of textile fiber, but the cotton plant also yields approximately 160 kg of cottonseed for every 100 kg of cotton fiber produced (Tanksley, 1990). Cottonseed is second in world oilseed production according to the 1997 to 1998 preliminary data (FAS, USDA). World cottonseed production reached 34.7 MMT in 1997 to 1998, and the major producers are China, the United States, India, and Pakistan with annual production of 8.28, 6.29, 5.10, and 3.00 MMT, respectively, in 1997 to 1998 (FAS, USDA). Typical yields from cottonseed processing are 50% meal, 22% hulls, 16% oil, 7% linters, with 5% loss (Tanksley, 1990). Cottonseed meal ranks third among the protein meals produced in the world (see Table 36.2). Most of the production in the United States is used in ruminant diets, but cottonseed meal can be a good source of protein for pig diets when its limitations are considered (Tanksley, 1990; Seerley, 1991).

2. Nutrient Content

The nutrient content of cottonseed meal has been summarized by Aherne and Kennelly (1985), Tanksley (1990), and Seerley (1991). The CP content of cottonseed meal may vary from 36 to 41%, depending largely on residual hulls remaining in the product. Indispensable amino acid content and amino acid digestibility of cottonseed meal are lower than soybean meal. Amino acid digestibility is especially low for lysine in the screw press and direct solvent meals (Tanksley, 1990), perhaps because of the formation of an insoluble complex between the ϵ-amino group of lysine and free gossypol. The fiber content of cottonseed meal is greater than soybean meal, and its energy value is inversely related to the fiber content. Cottonseed meal is a poorer source of minerals than soybean meal. Vitamin D and carotene are deficient in cottonseed meal, but it compares favorably with soybean meal in the B vitamin content, except biotin, pantothenic acid, and pyridoxine.

3. Antinutritional Factors

Cottonseed contains gossypol, which is a natural pigment of the plant found in the oil phase of the seed (see reviews by Cunha, 1977; Aherne and Kennelly, 1985; Tanksley, 1990; Church and

Kellems, 1998). Gossypol can be classified into bound gossypol, which is nontoxic to nonruminant species, and free gossypol, which is toxic. Toxicity signs usually occur when free gossypol levels approach 100 ppm (Knabe et al., 1979; Aherne and Kennelly, 1985; Tanksley, 1990). Although gossypol in cottonseed meal can be inactivated to some extent by heat processing, it may induce formation of insoluble, inert gossypol–protein complexes.

The Fe salts, such as ferrous sulfate, are effective in blocking the toxic effect of dietary gossypol, possibly by forming a strong complex between Fe and gossypol, thus preventing gossypol absorption. A 1:1 weight ratio of Fe to free gossypol can be used to inactivate the free gossypol in excess of 100 ppm (Aherne and Kennelly, 1985). In addition, high dietary protein may decrease the toxicity of gossypol by supplying a greater number of free ϵ-amino groups. Although glandless cotton varieties devoid of gossypol have a high nutritional value, there is essentially no glandless cottonseed meal available for livestock feeding (Tanksley, 1990) because of the lower cotton production potential of those varieties.

4. Feeding Cottonseed Meal to Pigs

Reviews on the use of cottonseed meal in pig diets have been presented by Aherne and Kennelly (1985) and Tanksley (1990). Three characteristics of commercially available glanded cottonseed meals that may contribute to the reduced pig performance are low lysine, high crude fiber, and free gossypol content (Knabe et al., 1979). There is limited information available on the use of glandless cottonseed meal in weanling pig diets. Noland et al. (1968) reported that weight gain and feed efficiency decreased as replacement of soybean meal with glandless cottonseed meal increased from 0 to 100%. Addition of 0.1% lysine to cottonseed meal diets had no effect, but supplementation with 0.4% lysine improved growth performance and nitrogen retention.

The use of glanded cottonseed meal as the only supplemental protein in cereal-based diets for grower-finisher pigs is likely to result in reduced pig performance compared with soybean meal–based diets (Knabe et al., 1979; Tanksley, 1990). Many early studies have shown clearly that excellent pig performance can be obtained when cottonseed meal is fed in combination with other high-quality protein supplements (Tanksley, 1990). Knabe et al. (1979) suggested that the reduced performance of growing pigs fed cottonseed meal diets is mostly due to low dietary lysine, but Tanksley (1990) indicated that other amino acids may also be limiting. Compared with soybean meal, the availability of ileal digestible nitrogen from cottonseed meal seems to be low (Prawirodigdo et al., 1997). The addition of lysine improved amino acid digestibility and biological value of cottonseed meal, and a further supplementation with threonine and tryptophan improved the digestibility of many amino acids, although only numerically (Feggeros et al., 1992).

As expected, digestibility of amino acids was consistently higher for glandless than glanded cottonseed meal (Tanksley, 1990). LaRue et al. (1985) observed similar or greater digestibility of nitrogen and all indispensable amino acids, except lysine, for glandless cottonseed meal compared with soybean meal. They concluded that glandless cottonseed meal supplemented with lysine could be used to replace at least 40% of the supplemental protein without affecting growing pig performance. On the other hand, Zongo and Couibaly (1993) indicated that glandless cottonseed meal supplemented with lysine could totally replace soybean meal in finisher diets without affecting pig performance.

For sows, it has been reported that cottonseed meal can replace up to one half the soybean meal in sorghum–soybean meal gestation and lactation diets (Tanksley et al., 1973; Haught et al., 1977). However, based on the lower weaning weight observed in their study (Haught et al., 1977), Tanksley (1990) suggested later that lactation diets should contain less than 50% cottonseed meal as the supplemental protein. Limiting cottonseed meal to 25% of the supplemental protein is likely to result in similar reproductive performance to those fed a grain–soybean meal lactation diet.

Because of the high fiber content of cottonseed meal and limited information on its effect on growth performance, the use of cottonseed meal in weanling pig diets should be limited. As Tanksley

(1990) suggested, cottonseed meal can supply approximately 50% of the supplemental protein in grower-finisher and gestation diets and 25% of the supplemental protein in lactation diets, but all diets should be formulated on a lysine basis. When diets contain greater than 100 ppm free gossypol, Fe should be added on a 1:1 weight basis to inactivate the free gossypol.

F. Linseed (Flax) Meal

1. Introduction

Flax (*Linum usitatissimum*) is one of the oldest crops known to humans (Aherne and Kennelly, 1985; Bowland, 1990), and it is now produced primarily for its drying oils (Church and Kellems, 1998). World production of linseed was 2.3 MMT in 1996, and Canada, China, and India are leading producers (FAO, 1997). The oil content of flaxseed ranges from 40 to 45% (Bowland, 1990), and linseed meal is a by-product of oil extraction from flaxseed. Linseed meal accounts for only a small part of the total plant proteins produced in North America (Church and Kellems, 1998), and most linseed meal is used for ruminant species and horses (Bowland, 1990).

2. Nutrient Content

The nutrient content of linseed meal has been reviewed by Bowland (1990). Linseed meal contains 5.6 and 1.4% ether extract for expeller and solvent meals, respectively. The CP content averages 35 to 36%, but may vary from 34 to 42%. Linseed meal is grossly deficient in lysine and contains less methionine than other oilseed meals (Aherne and Kennelly, 1985). Because of the hulls, which are coated with high quantities of mucilage, the crude fiber content of linseed meal is relatively high. The mucilage contains a water-dispersible carbohydrate, which has low digestibility for nonruminant species (Aherne and Kennelly, 1985; Batterham et al., 1991). The major macrominerals in linseed meal are comparable with other oilseed meals, although Ca, P, and Mg are all higher than the level found in soybean meal (Bowland, 1990). Although microminerals in linseed meal vary widely, it is a very good source of Se (Bowland, 1990). The B-complex vitamin content of linseed meal is similar to soybean meal and most other oilseed meals (Bowland, 1990).

3. Antinutritional Factors

Flaxseed or linseed meal contains a number of antinutritional factors for livestock; the main ones are linamarin and linatine (Bowland, 1990; Batterham et al., 1991). Linamarin is a cyanoglycoside, which has the potential to cause cyanide poisoning by the action of the enzyme linamarase. The enzyme is normally destroyed by heat during oil extraction. Linatine is a dipeptide that can act as an antagonist for vitamin B_6 or pyridoxine, and diets containing linseed meal may be marginally deficient in vitamin B_6 (Aherne and Kennelly, 1985; Bowland, 1990).

4. Feeding Linseed (Flax) Meal to Pigs

The use of linseed meal in pig diets has been reviewed by Bowland (1990). A low level of linseed meal (at least 3%) can be included in creep feed or early starter diets (Bowland, 1990). Recently, Richter and Kohler (1997) reported that up to 15% of linseed meal in diets had no effect on performance of pigs between 6 and 11 weeks of age. Linseed meal, however, had an antithyroid effect. A similar effect on thyroid hormones was reported by Schone et al. (1997). Richter and Kohler (1997) recommended that linseed meal should not exceed 10% of diets for young pigs.

For grower-finisher pigs, Bowland (1990) summarized studies conducted during the mid-1950s. He concluded that, if the lysine deficiency is corrected, linseed meal can be used as a major proportion of the protein supplement because up to 25% had been fed to pigs without adverse effects. In a more recent study, 5% linseed meal reduced efficiency of feed and digestible energy utilization (Bell and Keith, 1994). Batterham et al. (1991) evaluated the nutritional value of low-linolenic acid linseed meals for grower pigs (20 to 45 kg), and concluded that the nutritional value of the new cultivar was similar to conventional linseed meal.

The mucilage in linseed meal is indigestible by nonruminant species, but it can absorb a large amount of water (Bowland, 1990). Thus, linseed meal may have a laxative effect and be beneficial in preventing constipation in sows at parturition (Bowland, 1990; Seerley, 1991). There seems to be no literature on the use of linseed meal for gestating and lactating sows, but Bowland (1990) suggested that at least 10% of linseed meal could be included in sow diets if properly balanced for lysine.

Linseed meal can be fed to young pigs at low levels (3%) in the diet (Bowland, 1990; Seerley, 1991), and older pigs seem to be able to utilize higher levels. Seerley (1991) suggested that linseed meal could be used to best advantage at a level of up to 50% of the protein supplement. Because it is deficient in lysine, linseed meal should be used in combination with a complementary protein source(s) (Bowland, 1990; Seerley, 1991).

G. Peanut Meal and Whole Peanuts

1. Introduction

Peanuts (*Arachis hypogaea* L.) have been grown extensively in tropical and subtropical regions, and they were recognized as an important oilseed in Europe in the mid-1800s when France began importing them from West Africa for the oil (Aherne and Kennelly, 1985; Newton et al., 1990). As the demand for its oil increased, peanut production grew greatly, and the world production reached 17.5 MMT in 1980 to 1981 (Aherne and Kennelly, 1985). In recent years, the world production has remained relatively stable, and preliminary data indicate that it was 27.1 MMT in 1997 to 1998 (FAS, USDA). China and India are the largest producers with annual production of 9.7 and 8.0 MMT, respectively, in 1997 to 1998 (FAS, USDA). Its by-product, peanut meal, is widely used as a protein supplement in livestock diets (Aherne and Kennelly, 1985). Peanut meal is quite palatable, and pigs will consume more than they need to balance their diet when it is provided free-choice (Cunha, 1977).

2. Nutrient Content

The fat content of peanuts is more than twice that of soybeans, and it may vary widely from 36 to 54% (Newton et al., 1990). The CP content of peanut meal ranges from 41 to 50% with an average of 45 or 47% (Aherne and Kennelly, 1985; Seerley, 1991). Peanut meal is deficient in lysine and low in methionine and tryptophan (Seerley, 1991). Mechanically extracted meals may contain 5 to 7% fat, and thus tend to become rancid if stored more than 5 to 6 weeks during summer and 8 to 12 weeks during winter (Cunha, 1977; Seerley, 1991). The crude fiber content of peanut meal is three times as high as that of dehulled soybean meal (Aherne and Kennelly, 1985). The content of most minerals in peanut meal is lower than that of soybean meal, but it is a relatively good source of Mg, S, and K (Aherne and Kennelly, 1985). Peanut meal is a good source of many vitamins such as niacin, pantothenic acid, and thiamin, but it may be deficient in others such as choline, carotene, vitamin D, and vitamin E (Aherne and Kennelly, 1985; Seerley, 1991).

3. Antinutritional Factors

Newton et al. (1990) reviewed the antinutritional factors present in peanut kernels. Peanuts contain protease inhibitors and tannins. Because of their low content, these antinutritional factors are of limited concern in peanut kernels. However, tannins may be a contributing factor for low protein digestibility of peanut meals (Church and Kellems, 1998).

Peanuts are subject to the growth of certain molds, and *Aspergillus flavus*, which produces aflatoxin, can grow in peanuts and peanut meal (Cunha, 1977; Aherne and Kennelly, 1986). Aflatoxin is carcinogenic and acutely toxic to humans and animals depending on the level of contamination. Affected animals show varying degrees of liver, heart, spleen, or kidney damage (Aherne and Kennelly, 1985).

4. Feeding Peanut Meal and Whole Peanuts to Pigs

Reviews on the use of whole peanuts (Aherne and Kennelly, 1985; Newton et al., 1990) and peanut meal (Aherne and Kennelly, 1985) in pig diets have been presented. Haydon and Newton (1987) concluded that 5% roasted peanut kernels seemed to be an optimum inclusion rate for weanling pigs. The inclusion of 5% raw or roasted peanuts on an equal lysine basis (Newton and Haydon, 1988) or addition of 10, 15, or 20% full-fat peanuts (Balogun and Koch, 1979b) had no effect on growth performance or nutrient digestibilities in growing pigs. Heat processing of whole peanuts reduced trypsin inhibitor activity, but it had no effect on pig performance (Balogun and Koch, 1979a).

Pigs fed 20% whole peanuts, however, had inferior carcass quality compared with those fed the soybean meal diet (Balogun and Koch, 1979b). Nevertheless, Newton et al. (1990) concluded that peanuts are as effective as added fat in improving feed efficiency, and peanut protein can be utilized efficiently when substituted for other protein supplements on a lysine basis. For sows, Haydon et al. (1990) reported that 12% raw and roasted peanuts can be substituted for 5% animal fat in lactation diets without any effect on reproductive performance.

Replacing soybean meal completely with peanut meal resulted in lower feed intake, slower growth rate, and lower feed efficiency in pigs weaned at 15 days of age, and reduced digestion coefficients at 7 to 8 weeks of age (Combs et al., 1963). Similarly, replacing 50 or 100% of soybean meal with peanut meal in diets for 5-weeks-old starter pigs resulted in reduced growth performance (Orok et al., 1975). In their study, lysine supplementation of the peanut meal diet did not alleviate the growth depression of young pigs.

Grower-finisher pigs fed peanut meal diets without amino acid supplementation grew slower than those fed soybean meal diets (Brooks and Thomas, 1959). Supplementation with only lysine was partially effective, but supplementation with lysine and methionine alleviated the decrease in growth. In another study, weight gain and feed efficiency decreased linearly as substitution of soybean meal with peanut meal increased from 0 to 15% (cited by Aherne and Kennelly, 1985). Performance was increased with lysine and methionine supplementation, but it was considerably lower than in pigs fed the soybean meal diet. Ilori et al. (1984) reported no difference in performance of pigs fed diets containing 15 to 20% peanut meal plus 3 to 4% blood meal compared with pigs fed the soybean meal diet.

Approximately 5% of roasted peanut kernels seems to be an optimum inclusion rate in diets for weanling pigs. Grower-finisher pigs can perhaps utilize higher levels, but roasted or raw peanuts should be limited to less than 10% of the diets because of their adverse effects on carcass quality (Newton et al., 1990). Whole peanuts are an excellent source of dietary fat for sows. Peanut meal alone is not a suitable protein supplement for weanling or grower-finisher pig diets. Because of its low lysine content, using peanut meal in combination with ingredients high in lysine would be the most effective way to incorporate this protein supplement in the pig diet.

H. SAFFLOWER MEAL

1. Introduction

Safflower (*Carthamus tictorius*) is a warm-temperature plant cultivated throughout tropical climates (Darroch, 1990; Church and Kellems, 1998) that does not require as much water as many other oilseed plants (Church and Kellems, 1998). World production of safflower seed was 0.84 MMT in

1996, and India, the United States, and Mexico are major producers (FAO, 1997). Removal of the oil by a prepress solvent extraction process produces an undecorticated safflower meal with approximately 20 to 22% CP and 40% crude fiber. Decortication of this meal yields a high protein (42 to 45% CP), less fibrous (15 to 16% crude fiber) meal, which is more suitable for inclusion in pig and poultry diets (Williams and Daniels, 1973).

2. Nutrient Content

Safflower seeds are composed of approximately 40% hull and 36 to 40% oil (Seerley, 1991). The hull is removed before prepress solvent extraction to increase the efficiency of crushing (Darroch, 1990). The hull is utilized as a fiber source or incorporated into the meals to produce safflower meals with protein levels ranging from 20 to 70% (Darroch, 1990). Safflower meal is a poor source of lysine, methionine, and isoleucine for pigs, and the low level and availability of lysine are major factors contributing to the overall poor nutritive value of the protein in safflower meal (Darroch, 1990). The mineral content of safflower meal is generally less than that of soybean meal, but it is a comparable source of Ca and P (Aherne and Kennelly, 1985). Safflower meal is a rich plant source of Fe, containing about 3.5 times the level found in soybean meal (Darroch, 1990). Compared with other oilseed meals, safflower meal has a relative poor vitamin profile, but it is a good source of biotin, riboflavin, and niacin relative to soybean meal (Darroch, 1990).

3. Antinutritional Factors

Besides the high content of crude fiber, safflower meals contain two phenolic glucosides, matairesinol-β-glucoside, which gives a bitter flavor, and 2-hydroxyarctiin-β-glucoside, which has cathartic properties (Darroch, 1990). Both glucosides are associated with the protein fraction of the meal, and they can be removed by extraction with water or methanol, or by the addition of β-glucosidase.

4. Feeding Safflower Meal to Pigs

There are limited data on the use of safflower meal as a protein supplement in pig diets. A relative feeding value of the undecorticated safflower meal for pigs may be only 45 to 50% of soybean meal (Darroch, 1990). Thus, undecorticated safflower meal may not be appropriate as a protein supplement in pig diets (Williams and Daniels, 1973; Darroch, 1990). Decortication of the meal improves the nutritional value of the safflower meal for pigs, and the remaining discussion will deal with the use of dehulled meals.

Considering the high nutrient requirements of weanling pigs, their digestive capacity and the nutrient content of safflower meal, it may not be a suitable protein supplement for weanling pigs. For grower-finisher pigs, Williams and Daniels (1973) concluded that safflower meal was not suitable as the only source of protein supplement. Safflower meal should be used with a protein source high in lysine and it should be restricted to pigs weighing more than 45 kg live weight. Williams and O'Rourke (1974) reported that finisher female pigs fed safflower meal diets supplemented with amino acids had reduced growth, and a small increase was observed when safflower meal diet was supplemented with fish meal instead of lysine and methionine. It has been suggested that safflower meal should not provide more than 5 to 10% (Seerley, 1991) or 12.5% (Cunha, 1977) of the supplemental protein in the diet.

Feeding safflower meal to weanling pigs is not recommended. Safflower meal may be used to supply approximately 5 to 10% of the supplemental protein in grower-finisher pig diets. Darroch (1990), however, indicated that up to 12% of safflower meal could be included in the grower-finisher diet, especially if a lysine requirement is met. Safflower meal can be included up to 15% in the diet of pregnant females, but it should be limited to very low levels for lactating sows (Darroch, 1990).

I. Sesame Meal

1. Introduction

Sesame (*Sesamum indicum*) is one of the oldest vegetable oil crops cultivated by humans, and it has been grown in Africa, throughout Asia, and in parts of Europe for centuries (Caldwell, 1958). World production of sesame seed was 2.5 MMT in 1996 (FAO, 1997). The major producers of sesame are China and India, and these countries account for more than 40% of the world production (Ravindran, 1990; Seerley, 1991). Sesame meal is the product that remains after oil extraction of sesame seeds (Caldwell, 1958; Johnson et al., 1979), and solvent extraction produces a meal that is higher in protein and lower in oil than meals produced by the screw press or hydraulic methods (Seerley, 1991).

2. Nutrient Content

On average, sesame seeds contain 25% CP, 50% ether extract, 4% crude fiber, 5% ash, 11% nitrogen-free extract, and 5% moisture (Caldwell, 1959; Johnson et al., 1979). An average protein content of 42% and fiber content of 6.5% are typical for dehulled, expeller-extracted sesame meal (Ravindran, 1990). Sesame meal is an excellent source of methionine, cystine, and tryptophan, but it is low in lysine (Aherne and Kennelly, 1985; Ravindran, 1990). Although sesame meal is a good source of Ca, P, Mg, and others, their availability may be low because of high levels of oxalic and phytic acids in the hull (Johnson et al., 1979; Aherne and Kennelly, 1985; Ravindran, 1990). Vitamin levels in sesame meal are comparable with soybean meal and most other oilseed meals (Aherne and Kennelly, 1985; Ravindran, 1990).

3. Antinutritional Factors

Although sesame seed is not known to contain any protease inhibitors or other antinutritional factors (Caldwell, 1958), high levels of oxalic and phytic acids may have adverse effects on availability of minerals and protein (Aherne and Kennelly, 1985). Decortication of seeds almost completely removes oxalates, but it has little effect on phytate (Ravindran, 1990).

4. Feeding Sesame Meal to Pigs

The published information on the use of sesame meal in pig diets is limited. Because of its high fiber content and possible palatability problems associated with phytates and oxalates, use of sesame meal in starter diets should be limited (Ravindran, 1990). Satisfactory growth performance was observed in grower pigs fed diets containing 15% sesame meal (Squibb and Salazar, 1951). For grower-finisher pigs, Cunha (1977) and Ravindran (1990) reviewed the available data and concluded that sesame meal could be utilized successfully, but the inclusion rate would depend on the type and quantity of other protein supplements in the diet. Seerley (1991) indicated that sesame meal should be blended with other high-lysine protein supplements, and it may replace up to 10% of the soybean meal in corn–soybean meal diets for grower-finisher pigs and sows.

J. Soybeans and Soybean Products

1. Introduction

The existence of soybeans (*Glycine max*) dates back to at least 2838 B.C., but it was not until the mid-1930s that soybean meal became an accepted part of livestock and poultry diets (Aherne and Kennelly, 1985). Soybean production has increased over the years, and its world production reached 156.1 MMT in 1997 to 1998 compared with 117.3 MMT in 1992 to 1993 (FAS, USDA) and 82.2 MMT in 1980 to 1981 (Aherne and Kennelly, 1985). The United States, Brazil, Argentina, and

China are the main producers of soybeans with annual production of 73.6, 31.0, 18.7, and 14.7 MMT, respectively, in 1997 to 1998 (FAS, USDA).

Soybean meal is the most widely used protein supplement in pig diets in the United States. Soybean meal is unsurpassed by other plant protein sources in terms of its feeding value, and consequently it is the standard to which other protein sources are compared (Cromwell, 1998). Soy protein concentrate is produced from dehulled and oil-extracted soybeans and leached with water to remove most of the water-soluble nonprotein constituents, whereas soy protein isolate is the most highly refined soy protein product, in which most of the nonprotein components have been removed.

A rapidly expanding area of interest in recent years has been bioengineering of soybeans, and it may soon change the way soybeans are grown and marketed. New soybeans on the horizon include soybeans with a 80 to 100% increase in methionine, 100 to 400% increase in lysine, reduced oligosaccharide contents, and altered fatty acid contents (Haumann, 1997). These developments on soybeans, along with similar developments on cereal grains, are most likely to have significant impacts on the way the nutritional needs of animals will be satisfied in the future.

2. Nutrient Content

The nutrient content of soybeans and soybean products has been summarized (Aherne and Kennelly, 1985; Danielson and Crenshaw, 1991; Seerley, 1991; Church and Kellems, 1998; Cromwell, 1998). Whole soybeans contain 36 to 37% CP, whereas soybean meal contains 41 to 50% CP depending on the residual hulls and the oil extraction process used. Soybean meal is generally available in two forms, 44% CP meal and dehulled meal, which contains 48 to 50% CP. Soybean meal has an excellent amino acid balance. It is high in lysine, tryptophan, and threonine, which are most often deficient in cereal grains, but it is deficient in methionine. Soy protein concentrate contains about 70% CP, whereas soy protein isolate contains about 90% CP on a dry matter basis.

Whole soybeans contain 15 to 21% oil, which is usually removed by solvent extraction during preparation of the meal. Because of its low fiber content, the digestible and metabolizable energy contents of soybean meals are higher than most other oilseed meals. Soybean meal is generally low in minerals and vitamins. Phytate P accounts for about two thirds of the total P in soybean meal. Because of the formation of phytate–protein–mineral complexes during the processing, the availability of many mineral elements may be reduced.

3. Antinutritional Factors

Raw soybeans contain some biological activities that can decrease animal performance (Anderson et al., 1979), and the trypsin–chymotrypsin inhibitors are considered the most important. A genetic line of soybeans that is low in Kuniz trypsin inhibitor has been shown to be a superior protein source compared with conventional soybeans (Herkelman et al., 1992). Although heat treatment is effective in removing most of the growth-inhibitory effects, heat may reduce availability of lysine and other amino acids (Aherne and Kennelly, 1985). However, the range of heat treatments normally found among commercially available soybean meals has no effect on the nutritive value (Chang et al., 1987; Hansen et al., 1987).

Soybeans also contain antigrowth factors that are not easily deactivated by heat treatment. Certain oligosaccharides in soybean meal are indigestible and can cause excessive fermentation in the hindgut of young pigs (Cromwell, 1998). Li et al. (1990) reported that soybean meal caused transient hypersensitivity, which seemed to be caused by glycinin and β-conglycinin (Li et al., 1991). These factors can be reduced by ethanol extraction or extrusion, and the reduction in antigenic activity seems to have beneficial effects on intestinal morphology, immunology, and growth performance of weanling pigs (Li et al., 1991). (See Chapters 30 and 31 for more information.)

4. Feeding Soybeans and Soybean Products to Pigs

The use of raw and processed whole soybeans in pig diets has been reviewed by Danielson and Crenshaw (1991). The ability of pigs to utilize raw soybeans may be related to their age and changes in their relative amino acid needs. Older pigs seem to tolerate raw soybeans better than younger pigs (Cromwell, 1998). Young and grower-finisher pigs fed raw, uncooked soybeans have a reduced growth performance (Crenshaw and Danielson, 1985b; Danielson and Crenshaw, 1991). However, carcass traits were not different when diets were supplemented with appropriate amino acids (Southern et al., 1990). Although raw soybeans may have some detrimental effects during lactation (Yen et al., 1991), they can be fed to gestating sows as the only source of protein supplement without any adverse effects (Crenshaw and Danielson, 1985a; Yen et al., 1991).

Properly cooked soybeans can be used to replace soybean meal in grower-finisher and breeding herd diets (Danielson and Crenshaw, 1991; Seerley, 1991), and they may improve growth performance of growing pigs and reproductive performance of sows because of additional dietary lipids. However, whole soybeans may have adverse effects on the carcass fat of growing pigs. Although whole soybeans can be used in practical pig diets, the benefits and economics should be evaluated fully before their use in place of soybean meal (Seerley, 1991).

Soybean meal is the most widely used protein supplement in the United States, accounting for more than 85% of all protein supplements fed to pigs (Cromwell, 1998). A proper proportion of soybean meal and corn (or most other cereal grains) makes an excellent dietary amino acid pattern for pigs (Aherne and Kennelly, 1985; Seerley, 1991). Commercially available soybean meals are quite consistent in terms of nutrient content and quality, but limestone is sometimes added to improve flowability of the meal (Danielson and Crenshaw, 1991; Seerley, 1991).

Recently, several studies have shown that weanling pigs fed soy protein concentrate or soy protein isolate have excellent growth performance. Growth performance of weanling pigs fed soy protein concentrate was similar to those fed a dried skim milk–based diet (Li et al., 1991; Sohn et al., 1994a). Similarly, weanling pigs fed soy protein isolate had similar performance to those fed a dried skim milk–based diet (Dietz et al., 1988; Geurin et al., 1988; Sohn et al., 1994a). A greater digestibility of nitrogen or amino acids over soybean meal is perhaps responsible for the response (Walker et al., 1986; Sohn et al., 1994b), and moist extrusion seemed to improve the nutritional value of soy protein concentrate further (Li et al., 1991). (See Chapter 31 for more information.)

Gestating sows can perform rather well with raw soybeans as the only source of protein supplement. Properly processed whole soybeans can be used to replace soybean meal in pig diets. Soybean meal is the most widely used protein supplement, and a proper proportion of soybean meal and cereal grains makes the most balanced amino acid source for all classes of pigs. Soy protein concentrate and isolate can be used successfully in weanling pig diets as a replacement for dried skim milk and to replace some of the soybean meal.

K. SUNFLOWER SEEDS AND MEAL

1. Introduction

The development of sunflower (*Helianthus anuus*) as an oilseed occurred in Southern Europe in the 16th-century, and sunflower oil is highly valued for its stability at high temperatures (Aherne and Kennelly, 1985) and very high content of polyunsaturated fatty acids (Dinusson, 1990). In 1980 to 1981, worldwide sunflower production was 13.2 MMT (Aherne and Kennelly, 1985), but it has increased to 21.2 MMT in 1992 to 1993 and to 23.9 MMT in 1997 to 1998 (FAS, USDA). Major sunflower-producing areas are the former Soviet Union, Argentina, Eastern Europe, the United States, China, and the European Union. Sunflowers are grown for oil production, but processing plants may not be available in all areas and not all sunflower seeds are appropriate for production of oil. For this reason, sunflower seed may be available as an alternative protein source for pigs (Wahlstrom, 1990).

2. Nutrient Content

Nutrient content of sunflower seeds and/or meals has been reviewed by Aherne and Kennelly (1985), Dinusson (1990), and Wahlstrom (1990). Sunflower seeds contain approximately 38% oil, 17% CP, and 15% crude fiber. Although the additional energy provided by the oil in sunflower seeds is partially offset by the high crude fiber content, they are a good source of dietary lipids for pigs. The nutrient composition of sunflower meal varies considerably according to the quality of the seed, method of extraction, and presence of the hull. Whole sunflower meal contains about 26% CP (Dinusson, 1990), whereas the protein content of prepress solvent meal can range from 36 to 44% (Aherne and Kennelly, 1985). The lysine and other amino acid content is variable (Dinusson, 1990), but it is clear that sunflower meal is very deficient in lysine.

The fiber content of sunflower meal depends on the proportion of hulls remaining before oil extraction. The crude fiber content of whole sunflower meal can be 30% (Dinusson, 1990). With a complete decortication, the fiber content can be 12% or less (Dinusson, 1990), but its energy values are still considerably lower than in soybean meal. Calcium and P levels compare favorably with those of other plant protein sources, and sunflower meal contains relatively higher levels of Ca than phytate P (Aherne and Kennelly, 1990). Sunflower meal tends to be lower in trace elements compared with soybean meal (Aherne and Kennelly, 1985). In general, sunflower meal is high in the B vitamins and carotene (Aherne and Kennelly, 1985), but the stability of those and other vitamins during storage and mixing of diets is not known (Dinusson, 1990).

3. Antinutritional Factors

In contrast to other major oil seeds and oilseed meals, sunflower seeds and meals seem to be relatively free of antinutritional factors (Dinusson, 1990; Wahlstrom, 1990).

4. Feeding Sunflower Seeds and Meal to Pigs

Reviews on the use of sunflower seeds (Aherne and Kennelly, 1985; Wahlstrom, 1990) and sunflower meal (Aherne and Kennelly, 1985; Dinusson, 1990) in pig diets have been presented. Because of its high oil content, sunflower seeds provide a convenient method of providing additional energy to pig diets (Hartman et al., 1985), and the oil in sunflower seeds seems to be utilized well by young pigs (Adams and Jensen, 1985). Fitzner et al. (1989), however, concluded that the inclusion of sunflower seeds should be limited to 15% of the diet for weanling pigs.

As sunflower seeds increased from 0 to 60% of the diet for grower pigs, feed intake decreased and feed efficiency increased linearly (Laudert and Allee, 1975). For grower-finisher pigs, 10% sunflower seeds increased weight gain in one trial, although it was reduced slightly in another trial (Hartman et al., 1985). Improved protein digestibility with the addition of sunflower seeds (Noland et al., 1980; Marchello et al., 1984) may partially explain the beneficial effects of sunflower seeds on performance of pigs. On the other hand, 25 and 50% sunflower seeds reduced weight gain in finisher pigs (Laudert and Allee, 1975). In addition, adverse effects of sunflower seeds on carcass quality have been reported, and it has been recommended that grower-finisher diets should not contain more than 10% (Hartman et al., 1985) or 13% (Marchello et al., 1984) sunflower seeds.

Research on the use of sunflower seeds in breeding stock is limited (Wahlstrom, 1990). Percentage of milk fat increased linearly as dietary sunflower increased (0, 25, and 50%), but pig weaning weight or percentage survival was not affected (Kepler et al., 1982). Because of reduced feed intake in sows fed diets containing 50% sunflower seeds, Kepler et al. (1982) concluded that sunflower seeds should be limited to 25% of sow diets.

Very little research has been conducted on the use of sunflower meal in creep or starter diets for pigs (Dinusson, 1990). A complete replacement of soybean meal protein by sunflower meal reduced growth performance, but supplementation with lysine improved weight gain and feed efficiency slightly (Aherne and Kennelly, 1985). Wahlstrom et al. (1985) reported that tryptophan and threonine were equally limiting in corn–sunflower meal diets fortified with lysine for starter and grower pigs.

Replacing a portion or all of soybean meal with sunflower meal decreased growth performance and carcass quality of grower-finisher pigs (Diggs and Baker, 1972; Seerley et al., 1974), but lysine supplementation was effective in alleviating the reduced pig performance (Seerley et al., 1974; Baird, 1981). Therefore, although sunflower meal is very deficient in lysine, it can be used as the only source of protein for growing pigs if diets are balanced for lysine (Wahlstrom, 1985).

Sunflower meal can be used in diets for gestating females and adult boars because their lysine requirements are lower (Dinusson, 1990). In a combination with protein sources high in lysine or crystalline lysine, sunflower meal can also be used in lactation diets. Because of the lower energy content of sunflower meal, the daily feed allowance must be increased.

Sunflower seeds should not be included in starter, grower, or finisher diets at levels more than 10 to 15% of the diet. It has been suggested that sunflower meal should be limited to 20% of the soybean meal (Cunha, 1977) or one third of the protein source (Seerley, 1991) in pig diets. However, it is possible that sunflower meal can be used as the only source of protein for older pigs if diets are balanced for lysine.

IV. ANIMAL PROTEIN SUPPLEMENTS

A. Animal Protein Sources in General

Animal protein supplements are good sources of lysine and other amino acids, and the amino acid pattern is often very similar to the dietary needs of the pig. Compared with plant proteins, they are also very good sources of vitamins and minerals such as the B vitamins (especially vitamin B_{12}) and Ca and P. However, animal protein supplements are more variable in nutrient content, and they are subjected to high drying temperatures during processing for dehydration and sterilization (Cromwell, 1998). Obviously, proper heating is necessary to produce a quality product (Batterham et al., 1986a,b).

A listing by the Association of American Feed Control Officials (AAFCO) for animal products include meat meal, meat and bone meal, meat meal tankage, and meat and bone meal tankage, and there are some differences in the definitions (Cunha, 1977; Seerley, 1991; Anonymous, 1994; Church and Kellems, 1998). The only difference between meal and tankage is that the meal does not contain blood. Meat meal is distinguished from meat and bone meal based on the P content. If the product contains more than 4% P, it is considered as meat and bone meal. Meat meal tankage and meat and bone meal tankage can be differentiated similarly on the basis of P content. For all these products, the Ca level should not be more than 2.2 times the actual P level. In addition, these products should not contain more than 14% pepsin indigestible residues and not more than 11% of the CP in the product should be pepsin indigestible.

Cunha (1977) indicated that meat by-products produced in the past tended to contain more meat and internal organs; thus, they were superior nutritional products than many now being produced. Today, considerable variations in the quality of meat products can be expected depending on many factors. Clearly distinguishing one meat-product from other meat-products may be very difficult, and also there seem to be differences in the terminology used by various countries. For this reason, the description of meat meal and meat and bone meal or the discussion on the use of those products in pig diets in this chapter should be viewed with such uncertainties in mind.

B. Blood Meal

1. Introduction

In the past, blood meal was produced by subjecting clotted blood to extensive heat treatment to ensure a dry product and to eliminate any biological contaminations (Campbell, 1998). Blood meal produced by this conventional vat cooking and drying process has not been used in pig diets extensively because of poor palatability and low lysine availability (Miller, 1990). Older methods of processing may result in inconsistent products with varying degrees of contamination with other by-products of processing (Campbell, 1998). Spray-drying and flash-drying procedures have improved both the palatability and lysine availability of blood meal (Miller, 1990; Cromwell, 1998).

The composition of blood meal was reviewed by Miller (1990). Spray-dried and flash-dried blood meals contain 86 and 83% CP and 7.4 and 9.7% lysine, respectively. Lysine from conventionally dried blood meal is lower in concentration (about 20%) and availability (0 to 19.2% vs. 81.5 to 90.7%) than that from flash-dried blood meal (Parsons et al., 1985; Miller, 1990). Parsons et al. (1985) reported that the lysine availability of flash-dried porcine and bovine blood meal for young pigs ranged from 71 to 76%. Blood meal is very high in leucine, which may increase the isoleucine requirement. Isoleucine has been shown to be the first limiting amino acid in a corn–soybean meal/flash-dried blood meal diet for pigs. Mineral concentrations are quite low in flash-dried blood meal except Fe, which is highly available to pigs. Flash-dried blood meal is not a rich source of any of the vitamins required by pigs. (See Chapter 31 for more information.)

2. Feeding Blood Meal to Pigs

It has been suggested earlier that blood meal should not be used in weanling pig diets (Cunha, 1977). Hansen et al. (1993c), however, reported that spray-dried porcine blood meal (6.6%) was an effective protein source for early-weaned pigs (0 to 14 days after weaning), and it had a positive effect on subsequent performance (14 to 35 days). Similar results have been reported by Kats et al. (1994a). Palatability of spray-dried blood meal may be a problem during the initial postweaning phase, but it can actually stimulate feed intake after pigs have acclimated to the meal (Kats et al., 1994a). Weanling pigs fed 2.5% spray-dried blood meal during the 7 to 28 days postweaning had higher weight gain than those fed other protein sources (Kats et al., 1994b). Similarly, weanling pigs fed diets containing 3 or 6% flash-dried blood meal had higher nitrogen retention than those fed a soybean meal diet (Parsons et al., 1985). Blood meals of various origins (i.e., bovine, porcine, and avian) seem to be equally effective as a protein supplement for weanling pigs (Kats et al., 1994b).

Pigs fed diets containing 5% flash-dried blood meal during the starter, grower, and finisher phases performed as well as or better than those fed diets without blood meal (Miller, 1990). For grower-finisher pigs, Wahlstrom and Libal (1977) reported that rate and efficiency of weight gain were decreased when 4% conventional drum-dried blood meal replaced an equivalent amount of soybean meal, but 0.1% lysine supplementation was effective in alleviating the growth depression. They also found that replacing soybean meal with flash-dried blood meal on an equal protein basis up to 6% of the diet did not affect performance of pigs, even though blood meal supplied all of the supplemental protein during the finisher phase.

It has been recommended that dried blood should be limited to 1 to 4% of pig diets (Cunha, 1977; Wahlstrom and Libal, 1977; Cromwell, 1998). Similarly, Miller (1990) indicated that up to 2 and 5% blood meal could be used for starter pigs and older pigs, respectively. On the other hand, Seerley (1991) suggested that 6 to 8% blood meal could be used in pig diets.

C. FEATHER MEAL

1. Introduction

A review on processed chicken feathers as a feed ingredient for pigs and poultry has been presented by Papadopoulos (1985). Although this keratinous product has a high protein content, poultry feathers are virtually indigestible in their natural state. Feather keratin is very rich in disulfide bonds, which contribute to the insolubility and indigestibility of this protein. The bonds must be destroyed before feather protein can be digested by animals. The most widely used commercial feather product is hydrolyzed (autoclaved) feather meal.

Feather meal is deficient in methionine, lysine, histidine, and tryptophan, but it is rich in many other amino acids (Cupo and Cartwright, 1991; Han and Parsons, 1991). Because of differences in processing conditions and source materials, commercially prepared feather products may vary widely in nutrient composition. For example, nine feather meal samples obtained by Han and Parsons (1991) ranged from 76.4 to 87.3% in CP, 2.0 to 8.6% in ether extract, 1.3 to 4.8% in ash, 1.46 to 2.15% in lysine, 4.07 to 5.30% in cystine, and 0.45 to 0.61% in methionine. The availability of nutrients may also vary greatly. However, with the possible exception of lysine, the indispensable amino acid availability of feather meal seems to be similar to that of soybean meal in nonruminant species (Knabe et al., 1989; Han and Parsons, 1991).

2. Feeding Feather Meal to Pigs

Although feather meal has been used extensively in practical swine diets (Papadopoulos, 1985), the available data in the literature are quite limited. Replacing all the soybean meal with feather meal resulted in reduced rate and efficiency of weight gain in grower-finisher pigs (Hall, 1957). Supplementation of the feather meal diet with DL-methionine was beneficial in improving weight gain. Combs et al. (1958) reported that grower-finisher pigs fed diets containing 7.5 or 10% feather meal grew slower than those fed 0 or 5% feather meal.

The value of hydrolyzed feather meal was evaluated as a source of nonspecific nitrogen to enhance carcass quality of finisher pigs (Chiba et al., 1995). Carcass quality improved as dietary lysine and CP increased, regardless of the protein source or method of incorporating feather meal into the diets. The results indicated that feather meal was effective in enhancing carcass quality of finisher pigs. In a subsequent study, rate and efficiency of weight gain did not differ in finisher pigs fed corn–soybean meal diets containing 0 to 12% feather meal, but carcass quality was reduced with 12% feather meal (Chiba et al., 1996). The results indicated that up to 9% feather meal could be included in the finisher diet. As expected, pigs fed feather meal diets without soybean meal grew slower than those fed diets containing soybean meal. Lysine supplementation had no effect on growth performance but improved carcass quality and lean accretion. They concluded that feather meal can be used as the only source of protein supplement without decreasing carcass quality, provided that the diet is supplemented with lysine, although weight gain may be reduced.

Although it is generally recommended that feather meal should be incorporated into the pig diet based on amino acid content (Seerley, 1991), this may increase the protein content of diets and the excretion of urinary nitrogen into the environment. Supplementation with appropriate amino acids, therefore, would be a better way to use this protein source in pig diets. For optimum performance, feather meal should be limited to 5% of diets. However, older pigs may be able to utilize more feather meal if supplemented with appropriate amino acids.

D. Fish Meal

1. Introduction

Fish meal is defined as clean, dried, and ground tissues of undecomposed whole fish or fish cuttings, with or without extraction of the oil (Anonymous, 1994; Church and Kellems, 1998). World production of fish meal from 1992/1993 through 1997/1998 is presented in Table 36.2. The major producers are Peru and Chile. Fish meal must not contain more than 10% moisture or 7% salt, and the amount of salt must be specified if it is greater than 3%. Although most of the oil is removed from fish meal, the oil does not seem to affect feed intake or growth performance of weanling pigs (Newport and Keal, 1983). Antioxidants are commonly included in the meal to prevent oxidation, overheating, and molding (Church and Kellems, 1998).

Fish meals are generally high in protein (50 to 75%) and indispensable amino acids that are deficient in many cereal grains (Seerley, 1991; Church and Kellems, 1998). Most mineral elements, especially Ca and P, and B vitamins are moderate to high when compared with other protein sources (Seerley, 1991; Church and Kellems, 1998). The quality of fish meal may vary greatly depending on the quality of fish materials used, processing factors such as overheating, and oxidation of the meal (Cunha, 1977; Seerley, 1991; Wiseman et al., 1991). (See Chapter 31 for more information.)

2. Feeding Fish Meal to Pigs

Weanling pigs fed fish meal in combination with milk products or soybean meal had better growth performance than those fed processed soybeans with added lysine or soybean meal (de Moura and Fowler, 1983; Newport and Keal, 1983). Protein sources, however, generally had no effect on apparent digestibility of nitrogen and amino acids or on nitrogen retention (Newport and Keal, 1983; Viljoen et al., 1998).

Addition of 5% fish meal promoted optimum pig performance during the first 3 weeks after weaning, whereas 10% fish meal was most effective during the last 2 weeks of the 5-week baby pig study (Gore et al., 1990). Stoner et al. (1990) reported that the maximum weight gain in weanling pigs was obtained with 8% fish meal, but 12% fish meal was necessary to maximize feed intake. Nursery environment and health status may have an effect on the response of weanling pigs to fish meal. Pigs with a lower health status reared in an on-site nursery seemed to respond more to fish meal than segregated early-weaned pigs with high-health status (Bergström et al., 1997).

The effect of high-nutrient or conventional diets, both with or without 5% fish meal, on performance of pigs from 3 or 5 weeks of age until slaughter at 90 kg was evaluated (Pike et al., 1984). Overall, growth rate and feed efficiency were reduced in pigs fed the conventional diet without fish meal, but pigs fed the high-nutrient diets performed better than those fed the conventional diets with fish meal. Laksesvela (1961) reported that weight gain and feed efficiency in grower-finisher pigs were increased as dietary fish meal increased from 0 to 12%, but most of the response was obtained with the initial levels of 6 to 8% fish meal. Carcass quality was not affected by 6 to 8% fish meal or less.

In his review, Seerley (1991) indicated that addition of up to 15% fish meal increased performance of young pigs, but the results of some studies indicate that the optimum inclusion rate would be somewhere between 5 and 10% of the diet. The variations in the quality of fish meal and the economics are obviously important considerations in determining the optimum inclusion rate. In addition, Cromwell (1998) suggested that the amount of fish meal in pig diets should not exceed 6 to 7% because of its potential of causing a fishy flavor in pork, and its use should be avoided in the diets of pigs that are approaching slaughter weight.

E. Meat and Bone Meal

1. Introduction

According to AAFCO, meat and bone meal can be defined as the rendered product from mammalian tissues including bone, but exclusive of blood, hair, hoof, horn, hide trimmings, manure, and stomach and rumen contents (Anonymous, 1994). Meat and bone meal may contain 21 to 61% bone, and bone protein is 83% collagen, which contains no tryptophan (Leibholz, 1979). Collagen can be found in skin, connective tissue, cartilage, and tendon; thus, 50 to 65% of the total protein in meat and bone meal could be collagen. The CP content of such products can range from 40 to 65% (Evans and Leibholz, 1979b). In addition, largely indigestible keratin proteins may be found in the meal. The analyses of 17 different meat and bone meals indicated that they contained 42.2 to 54.6% CP, 8.2 to 15.8% Ca, 4.4 to 6.0% P, 0.20 to 0.49% tryptophan, 2.38 to 3.39% lysine, and 0.22 to 0.63% cystine (Leibholz, 1979). Ash or Ca content and the content and quality of protein are likely to influence the nutritional quality of meat and bone meal.

2. Feeding Meat and Bone Meal to Pigs

Weight gain and feed efficiency of grower pigs decreased linearly as replacement of soybean meal with meat and bone meal increased from 0 to 100% (Kennedy et al., 1974a). The addition of 8% bone meal to a soybean meal diet, high levels of Ca and P, or the source of Ca and P had no effect on pig performance. The results of a subsequent study (Kennedy et al. (1974b) may support a general assumption that meat and bone meals with a low to moderate ash content and/or a high protein content are superior protein supplements. Pigs fed a soybean meal diet, however, had better growth performance, higher organic and dry matter digestibilities, and nitrogen retention than those fed the meat and bone meal diets.

Pig performance decreased linearly as the levels of meat and bone meal in grower-finisher diets increased from 0 to 10% (Peo and Hudman, 1962). Low or high ash content of meat and bone meal had no clear effect on growth performance or nutrient digestibility (Partanen, 1998). However, grower-finisher pigs fed the soybean meal diet grew faster and more efficiently than those fed the meat and bone meal diets. In addition, weight gain decreased as dietary meat and bone meal increased. Similarly, the efficiency of nitrogen utilization in finisher pigs decreased as dietary meat and bone meal increased from 10 to 20% (Partanen and Nasi, 1994).

It has been recommended that meat by-product meals should be used at levels no higher than 3 to 10% (Cunha, 1977) or 4 to 5% (Cromwell, 1998) of pig diets. For sows, Cromwell (1998) indicated that diets may contain meat by-product meals up to one third of the protein supplement. Seerley (1991) suggested that meat and bone meal can be used to replace up to one third of the soybean meal without adversely affecting growth performance or carcass quality of pigs.

F. MEAT MEAL

1. Introduction

According to AAFCO, meat meal can be defined as the rendered product from mammal tissues, exclusive of blood, hair, hoof, horn, hide trimmings, manure, and stomach and rumen contents (Anonymous, 1994). Meat meal is mostly waste meat trimmings and organs, and the average composition of meat meal is 55% CP, 8% Ca, and 3.9% P. Tryptophan is the first limiting amino acid in meat meal, and also lysine and methionine may be limiting (Evans and Leibholz, 1979b; Cromwell et al., 1991). In addition, the bioavailability of the tryptophan is low and quite variable (Cromwell et al., 1991). Considering recent advances in the technology to produce crystalline tryptophan and other amino acids, it is possible that a protein supplement, such as meat meal that is deficient in particular amino acids, can be incorporated in the diet much more effectively, and the use of such protein supplements may increase considerably in the future.

2. Feeding Meat Meal to Pigs

Meat meal varies not only in nutrient content but also in quality depending on the processing method, temperature, and type of materials in the meal, which in turn can affect pig performance (Leibholz, 1979; Ristic et al., 1993). Weight gain, feed efficiency and apparent dry matter digestibility in weanling pigs decreased linearly as replacement of soybean meal with meat meal increased from 0 to 100%, possibly because of the high Ca content of the meat meal diets (Evans and Leibholz, 1979a). Supplementation of meat meal diets with either lysine and methionine or tryptophan increased pig performance in some studies, but supplementation with all three amino acids was necessary to improve growth performance and/or nitrogen retention of weanling pigs in other studies (Evans and Leibholz, 1979b; Leibholz, 1982).

Inclusion of 5 to 10% meat meal reduced feed intake, weight gain, and feed efficiency of grower-finisher pigs (Cromwell et al., 1991), but addition of L-tryptophan prevented the reduction in growth performance. Further supplementation with isoleucine or a combination of isoleucine and threonine did not increase pig performance further. These researchers concluded that high levels (up to 10% or even more) of meat meal can be used in corn-based diets fortified with lysine for grower-finisher pigs, provided that the diets are supplemented with tryptophan.

Meat by-product meals should be used at levels no higher than 3 to 10% (Cunha, 1977) or 4 to 5% (Cromwell, 1998) of the pig diet because of the variation in nutritional quality, palatability problems, and excess Ca and P. However, 10% or more meat meal may be included in grower-finisher diets if diets are fortified with lysine and tryptophan (Cromwell et al., 1991). Sow diets may contain meat by-product meals up to one third of the protein supplement (Cromwell, 1998).

G. Milk, Dried

1. Introduction

The benefits of drying milk have been understood for a long time (Early, 1992). After traveling to Mongolia, Marco Polo described a product made by boiling milk, skimming off the cream to be made into butter, then drying the remaining milk by leaving it in the sun. The powder was reconstituted with water and consumed as a beverage, particularly at breakfast. Dried milk products include dried whole milk and dried skim milk. The only difference between dried whole milk and dried skim milk is that most of the fat and fat-soluble vitamins are removed from the skim milk. Both milk products are very palatable and highly digestible protein supplements with an excellent balance of amino acids, and they are good sources of vitamins and minerals (Seerley, 1991; Cromwell, 1998). The only nutrients that tend to be deficient are the fat-soluble vitamins, Fe, and Cu, and, depending on the species, Mg and Mn (Seerley, 1991; Church and Kellems, 1998). Under most instances, the value of milk products in human diets makes them too valuable to be used in animal diets. (See Chapter 31 for more information.)

2. Feeding Dried Milk to Pigs

Dried milk products are almost the perfect food for very young pigs. Although they are nearly always too expensive for use as a feed ingredient, a certain amount of dried skim milk has been used in pig starter diets over the years. Research emphasis on this area has been to replace dried skim milk with alternative protein supplements in weanling pig diets rather than evaluating the value of the dried milk per se. Dried whole milk and skim milk can be fed successfully to all classes of pigs; thus, the use of these products in pig diets should be determined mostly on economical considerations (Seerley, 1991).

H. Plasma Protein

1. Introduction

The plasma fraction of blood yields a fine, light tan powder containing 78% protein (spray-dried plasma protein), whereas the blood cell fraction yields a fine, dark red powder containing 92% protein (spray-dried blood cells; Campbell, 1998). Spray-dried plasma protein is relatively high in lysine, tryptophan, and threonine, but low in methionine and isoleucine (Campbell, 1998). In addition to its amino acid content, globular proteins (including immunoglobulins) in dried plasma may stimulate feed intake and growth during the critical postweaning stage, and it has been shown to be an excellent source of protein for early-weaned pigs (Cromwell, 1998). Spray-dried plasma seems to be highly digestible, and it contains an amino acid profile that closely matches the young pig's requirements. Furthermore, it may have a positive effect on the immune system of the young pig. (See Chapter 31 for more information.)

2. Feeding Plasma Protein to Pigs

Zimmerman (1987) and Gatnau and Zimmerman (1990) reported that weanling pigs fed diets containing plasma protein had higher feed intake, weight gain, and feed efficiency than those fed a control diet. These initial reports led to further investigation of plasma protein. Campbell (1998) summarized 25 studies that evaluated the nutritional value of spray-dried plasma protein. Essentially all experiments have shown that plasma protein can improve feed intake and weight gain of early-weaned pigs and reduce the incidence of postweaning lag. Plasma protein seems to improve performance of weanling pigs because of its high palatability and resulting increased feed intake (Ermer et al., 1994).

Gatnau and Zimmerman (1992) concluded that feed intake and weight gain were maximized at 6% dietary spray-dried porcine plasma. Similarly, Kats et al. (1994a) concluded that up to 10% plasma protein could be used during the 0-to-14-day postweaning period. However, methionine may become the first limiting amino acid in diets containing more than 6% spray-dried porcine plasma (Hansen et al., 1993c; Kats et al., 1994a).

Nursery environment may affect the response of weanling pigs to plasma protein. Pigs reared in a conventional, on-farm nursery setting responded more to spray-dried porcine plasma than those in a cleaner, off-site nursery (Coffey and Cromwell, 1995; Bergström et al., 1997). Several studies indicate that the response to feeding plasma can be achieved by feeding the high-molecular-weight fraction (globulin), supporting the hypothesis that it has a biological function and affects pig performance through the gut (Campbell, 1998).

Growth performance of weanling pigs can be enhanced by spray-dried plasma protein. The degree of response is dependent on inclusion rate, age and weight of pigs, health status, and environment. Spray-dried plasma protein may be included up to 6 to 10% in the postweaning diet, but the diet may have to be supplemented with methionine if it contains more than 6% plasma protein.

I. Poultry By-Product Meal

1. Introduction

Poultry by-product meal consists of the ground, rendered, or clean parts of slaughtered poultry, such as heads, feet, undeveloped eggs, and intestines, exclusive of feathers (Anonymous, 1994; Church and Kellems, 1998). It cannot contain more than 16% ash and more than 4% acid-insoluble ash (Pesti, 1986; Church and Kellems, 1998). Poultry by-product meal contains 58% CP and 13% fat, and it has good amino acid balance and provides minerals and vitamins (Seerley, 1991). However, the composition and protein quality of poultry by-product meals may vary greatly (Pesti, 1986). Dong et al. (1993) reported that poultry by-product meals obtained from several manufacturers in North America differed in chemical composition (e.g., 55 to 74% CP, 10 to 19% lipids, and 11 to 23% ash on a dry matter basis) and protein digestibility, illustrating the range of product quality that can be expected in the marketplace.

2. Feeding Poultry By-Product Meal to Pigs

The author is not aware of any published reports on the use of poultry by-product meal in pig diets. According to Cunha (1977), however, some research demonstrated that 8.5 to 16% poultry by-product meal could be used successfully in diets for grower-finisher pigs. Seerley (1991) indicated that poultry by-product meal can replace some soybean meal, and it is an excellent source of protein for pigs. Cunha (1977) suggested that it is best to limit poultry by-product meal to 5 to 8% of the pig's diet because of the variability in the quality of the product available on the market.

J. Whey, Dried

1. Introduction

Leibbrandt and Benevenga (1991) provided background information on whey. Whey is the part of milk that separates from the curd during cheese manufacturing. Whey contains about 90% of the lactose, 20% of the protein, 40% of the Ca, and 43% of the P originally present in milk.

Dried whey should contain at least 65% lactose, which has been shown to be the best sugar for baby pigs (Cunha, 1977), and it normally contains about 13 to 17% of high-quality CP (Seerley, 1991). Generally, amino acid availability of milk products is considered high, but their quality can be impaired by overheating. Dried whey is an excellent source of B vitamins, most of which remain in the whey during cheese production, but it may be low in vitamins A and D, which are retained in the cheese (Cunha, 1977; Leibbrandt and Benevenga, 1991; Seerley, 1991). Season, type of cheese produced, and geographic locations can have an effect on the mineral content (Leibbrandt and Benevenga, 1991). The type of cheese produced and the addition of salt-laden press drippings influence the salt content of whey (Leibbrandt and Benevenga, 1991). (See Chapter 31 for more information.)

2. Feeding Dried Whey to Pigs

The efficacy of high-quality dried whey in enhancing growth performance of weanling pigs has been well established over the years (e.g., Graham et al., 1981; Cera et al., 1988). Tokach et al. (1995) reported that feeding milk product has beneficial effects in pigs during not only the starter phase, but also in the subsequent grower-finisher phase. Pancreatic enzyme activities in the digestive system seem to be higher in pigs fed diets containing dried whey (Graham et al., 1981; Lindemann et al., 1986), and consequently it is highly digestible and can be utilized efficiently (Cera et al., 1988).

In addition to its positive effects on digestive enzymes and/or high nutrient digestibility, other factors in dried whey may be responsible for the beneficial effects on weanling pig performance. By including either lactalbumin or lactose in the diet, Tokach et al. (1989) concluded that both the protein and carbohydrate fractions of dried whey are important. Lepine et al. (1991) and Mahan et al. (1993), however, reported that the protein fraction was not a limiting factor in weanling pig diets. After evaluating the efficacy of lactalbumin and lactose components of dried whey, Mahan (1992) concluded that the lactose component of dried whey was primarily responsible for the beneficial effects of dried whey. It has been shown that edible-grade deproteinized whey and crystalline lactose can replace the lactose provided by high-quality dried whey without affecting pig performance (Nessmith et al., 1997).

Dried whey can be fed to all classes of pigs, but it is primarily used for weanling pigs. As indicated by Seerley (1991), the inclusion rate of 10 to 30% is commonly used, though 30 to 45% can be included without any adverse effects. The optimum inclusion rate of dried whey in pig diets should be determined mostly on economical considerations.

REFERENCES

Adams, K. L., and A. H. Jensen. 1985. Effect of dietary protein and fat levels on the utilization of the fat in sunflower seeds by the young pig, *Anim. Feed Sci. Technol.*, 13:159.

Aherne, F. X., and J. M. Bell. 1990. Canola seed: full-fat. In *Nontraditional Feed Sources for Use in Swine Production*, Thacker, P. A., and R. N. Kirkwood, Eds., Butterworths, Boston, 79.

Aherne, F. X., and J. J. Kennelly. 1985. Oilseed meals for livestock feeding. In *Recent Developments in Pig Nutrition*, Cole, D. J. A., and W. Haresign, Eds., Butterworths, London, 278.

Allee, G. L. 1977. Using dehydrated alfalfa to control intake of self-fed sows during gestation, *Feedstuffs*, 49:20.

Anderson, R. L., J. J. Rackis, and W. H. Tallent. 1979. Biologically active substances in soy products. In *Soy Protein and Human Nutrition*, Wilcke, H. L., D. T. Hopkins, and D. H. Waggle, Eds., Academic Press, New York, 209.

Anonymous. 1994. Feed ingredient definitions, *Feedstuffs*, 66(30):145.

Baidoo, S. K., M. K. McIntosh, and F. X. Aherne. 1986. Selection preference of starter pigs fed canola meal and soybean meal supplemented diets, *Can. J. Anim. Sci.*, 66:1039.

Baird, D. M. 1981. Sunflower meal as partial and total supplement for finishing pigs, *J. Anim. Sci.*, 53(Suppl. 1):81 (Abstr.).

Balogun, T. F., and B. A. Koch. 1979a. Influence of trypsin inhibitor level and processing on the nutritional value of groundnuts for finishing pigs, *Trop. Agric.*, 56:245.

Balogun, T. F., and B. A. Koch. 1979b. Raw or roasted groundnuts as a partial protein and energy source in rations for growing pigs, *Trop. Agric.*, 56:135.

Batterham, E. S., R. E. Darnell, L. S. Herbert, and E. J. Major. 1986a. Effect of pressure and temperature on the availability of lysine in meat and bone meal as determined by slope-ratio assays with growing pigs, rats and chicks and by chemical techniques, *Br. J. Nutr.*, 55:441.

Batterham, E. S., R. F. Lowe, R. E. Darnell, and E. J. Major. 1986b. Availability of lysine in meat meal, meat and bone meal and blood meal as determined by the slope-ratio assay with growing pigs, rats and chicks and by chemical techniques, *Br. J. Nutr.*, 55:427.

Batterham, E. S., L. M. Anderson, D. R. Baigent, S. A. Beech, and R. Elliot. 1990. Utilization of ileal digestible amino acids by pigs, *Br. J. Nutr.*, 64:679.

Batterham, E. S., L. M. Anderson, D. R. Baigent, and A. G. Green. 1991. Evaluation of meals from Linola® low-linolenic acid linseed and conventional linseed as protein sources for growing pigs, *Anim. Feed Sci. Technol.*, 35:181.

Bell, J. M. 1984. Nutrients and toxicants in rapeseed meal: a review, *J. Anim. Sci.*, 58:996.

Bell, J. M., and M. O. Keith. 1994. Effects of adding barley hulls and linseed meal to wheat and hulless barley diets fed to growing pigs, *Anim. Feed Sci. Technol.*, 45:177.

Bergström, J. R., J. L. Nelssen, M. D. Tokach, R. D. Goodband, S. S. Dritz, K. Q. Owen, and W. B. Nessmith, Jr. 1997. Evaluation of spray-dried animal plasma and select menhaden fish meal in transition diets of pigs weaned at 12 to 14 days of age and reared in different production systems, *J. Anim. Sci.*, 75:3004.

Bowland, J. P. 1990. Linseed meal. In *Nontraditional Feed Sources for Use in Swine Production*, Thacker, P. A., and R. N. Kirkwood, Eds., Butterworths, Boston, 213.

Brooks, C. C., and H. R. Thomas. 1959. Supplements to peanut oil meal protein for growing fattening swine, *J. Anim. Sci.*, 18:1119.

Caldwell, R. W. 1958. Sesame meal. In *Processed Plant Protein Foodstuffs*, Altschul, A. M., Ed., Academic Press, New York, 535.

Campbell, J. M. 1998. The use of plasma in swine feeds, *Discoveries. A Quarterly Tech. Update*, American Protein Corp., Ames, 4.

Cera, K. R., D. C. Mahan, and G. A. Reinhart. 1988. Effects of dietary dried whey and corn oil on weanling pig performance, fat digestibility and nitrogen utilization, *J. Anim. Sci.*, 66:1438.

Chang, C. J., T. D. Tanksley, Jr., D. A. Knabe, and T. Zebrowska. 1987. Effects of different heat treatments during processing on nutrient digestibility of soybean meal in growing swine, *J. Anim. Sci.*, 65:1273.

Chiba, L. I., H. W. Ivey, K. A. Cummins, and B. E. Gamble. 1995. Effects of hydrolyzed feather meal as a source of extra dietary nitrogen on growth performance and carcass traits of finisher pigs, *Anim. Feed Sci. Technol.*, 53:1.

Chiba, L. I., H. W. Ivey, K. A. Cummins, and B. E. Gamble. 1996. Hydrolyzed feather meal as a source of amino acids for finisher pigs, *Anim. Feed Sci. Technol.*, 57:15.

Church, D. C., and R. O. Kellems. 1998. Supplemental protein sources. In *Livestock Feeds and Feeding*, Kellems, R. O. and D. C. Church, Eds., Prentice-Hall, Upper Saddle River, NJ, 135.

Close, W. H., and V. R. Fowler. 1985. Energy requirements of pigs. In *Recent Development in Pig Nutrition*, Cole, D. J. A., and W. Haresign, Eds., Butterworths, London, 1.

Coffey, R. D., and G. L. Cromwell. 1995. The impact of environment and antimicrobial agents on the growth response of early-weaned pigs to spray-dried porcine plasma, *J. Anim. Sci.*, 73:2532.

Combs, G. E., W. L. Alsmeyer, and H. D. Wallace. 1958. Feather meal as a source of protein for growing-finishing swine, *J. Anim. Sci.*, 17:468.

Combs, G. E., F. L. Osegueda, H. D. Wallace, and C. B. Ammerman. 1963. Digestibility of rations containing different sources of supplementary protein by young pigs, *J. Anim. Sci.*, 22:396.

Crenshaw, M. A., and D. M. Danielson. 1985a. Raw soybeans for gestating swine, *J. Anim. Sci.*, 60:163.

Crenshaw, M. A., and D. M. Danielson. 1985b. Raw soybeans for growing-finishing pigs, *J. Anim. Sci.*, 60:725.

Creswell, D. C., and C. C. Brooks. 1971a. Composition, apparent digestibility and energy evaluation of coconut oil and coconut meal, *J. Anim. Sci.*, 33:366.

Creswell, D. C., and C. C. Brooks. 1971b. Effect of coconut meal on coturnix quail and of coconut meal and coconut oil on performance, carcass measurements and fat composition in swine, *J. Anim. Sci.*, 33:370.

Cromwell, G. L. 1998. Feeding swine. In *Livestock Feeds and Feeding*, 4th ed., Kellems, R. O., and D. C. Church, Eds., Prentice-Hall, Upper Saddle River, NJ, 354.

Cromwell, G. L., and R. D. Coffey. 1994. Nutritional methods to reduce nitrogen and phosphorus levels in swine waste. Presented at the Southern Section Mtg. of the Am. Soc. of Anim. Sci., Nashville, February 8.

Cromwell, G. L., T. S. Stahly, and H. J. Monegue. 1991. Amino acid supplementation of meat meal in lysine-fortified corn-based diets for growing-finishing pigs, *J. Anim. Sci.*, 69:4898.

Cunha, T. J. 1977. *Swine Feeding and Nutrition*, Academic Press, New York.

Cupo, M. A., and A. L. Cartwright. 1991. The effect of feather meal on carcass composition and fat pad cellularity in broilers: influence of the calorie:protein ratio of the diet, *Poult. Sci.*, 70:153.

Danielson, D. M., and J. D. Crenshaw. 1991. Raw and processed soybeans in swine diets. In *Swine Nutrition*, Miller, E. R., D. E. Ullrey, and A. J. Lewis, Eds., Butterworth-Heinemann, Boston, 573.

Danielson, D. M, and J. J. Noonan. 1975. Roughages in swine gestation diets, *J. Anim. Sci.*, 41:94.

Darroch, C. S. 1990. Safflower meal. In *Nontraditional Feed Sources for Use in Swine Production*, Thacker, P. A., and R. N. Kirkwood, Eds., Butterworths, Boston, 373.

de Lange, C. F. M., V. M. Gabert, D. Gillis, and J. F. Patience. 1998. Digestible energy contents and apparent ileal amino acid digestibilities in regular or partial mechanically dehulled canola meal samples fed to growing pigs, *Can. J. Anim. Sci.*, 78:641.

de Moura, M. P., and V. R. Fowler. 1983. Soyabean, fish meal and milk as protein sources in the diets of pigs weaned at 3 weeks, *Anim. Prod.*, 36:523 (Abstr.).

Dietz, G. N., C. V. Maxwell, and D. S. Buchanan. 1988. Effect of protein source on performance of early weaned pigs, *J. Anim. Sci.*, 66(Suppl. 1):314 (Abstr.).

Diggs, B. G., and B. Baker, Jr. 1972. Does sunflower meal offer an acceptable swine feed? *Miss. Farm Res.*, 35:4.

Dinusson, W. E. 1990. Sunflower meal. In *Nontraditional Feed Sources for Use in Swine Production*, Thacker, P. A., and R. N. Kirkwood, Eds., Butterworths, Boston, 465.

D'Mello, J. P. F. 1994. Amino acid imbalance, antagonisms and toxicities. In *Amino Acids in Farm Animal Nutrition*, D'Mello, J. P. F., Ed., CAB International, Wallingford, 63.

Dong, F. M., R. W. Hardy, N. F. Haard, F. T. Barrows, B. A. Rasco, W. T. Fairgrieve, and I. P. Forster. 1993. Chemical composition and protein digestibility of poultry by-product meals for salmonid diets, *Aquaculture*, 116:149.

Early, R. 1992. Milk powders. In *The Technology of Dairy Products*, Early, R., Ed., VCH Publishers, New York, 167.

Ermer, P. M., P. S. Miller, and A. J. Lewis. 1994. Diet preference and meal patterns of weanling pigs offered diets containing either spray-dried porcine plasma or dried skim milk, *J. Anim. Sci.*, 72:1548.

Evans, D. F., and J. Leibholz. 1979a. Meat meal in the diet of the early-weaned pig. I. A comparison of meat meal and soyabean meal, *Anim. Feed Sci. Technol.*, 4:33.

Evans, D. F., and J. Leibholz. 1979b. Meat meal in the diet of the early-weaned pig. II. Amino acid supplementation, *Anim. Feed Sci. Technol.*, 4:43.

Fan, M. Z., W. C. Sauer, and V. M. Gabert. 1996. Variability of apparent ileal amino acid digestibility in canola meal for growing-finishing pigs, *Can. J. Anim. Sci.*, 76:563.

FAO. 1997. *FAO Yearbook. Production*, Vol. 50, 1996, Food and Agriculture Organization of the United Nations, Rome.

Feggeros, K., G. Papadopoulos, and V. Kafantares. 1992. Amino acid digestibility of cottonseed meal in swine: improvement of protein with addition of lysine, threonine and tryptophan, *Epitheorese Zootech. Epistemes*, 16:5.

Fitzner, G. E., R. H. Hines, R. D. Goodband, R. C. Thaler, G. R. Stoner, and T. L Weeden. 1989. Effect of black sunflower oil seeds on weanling pig performance, *J. Anim. Sci.*, 67(Suppl. 2):111 (Abstr.).

Fuller, M. F., and A. G. Chamberlain. 1985. Protein requirements of pigs. In *Recent Developments in Pig Nutrition*, Cole, D. J. A., and W. Haresign, Eds., Butterworths, London, 85.

Gatnau, R., and D. R. Zimmerman. 1990. Evaluation of different sources of protein for weanling pigs, Iowa State Univ. Swine Res. Rep., Iowa State University, Ames, 14.

Gatnau, R., and D. R. Zimmerman. 1992. Determination of optimum levels of inclusion of spray-dried porcine plasma (SDPP) in diets for weanling pigs fed in practical conditions, *J. Anim. Sci.*, 70(Suppl. 1):60 (Abstr.).

Geurin, H. B., G. A. Kesel, W. T. Black, T. B. Hatfield, and C. N. Daniels. 1988. Effect of isolated protein and whey on replacing dried skim milk in a prestarter for weaned baby pigs, *J. Anim. Sci.*, 66(Suppl. 1):320 (Abstr.).

Gore, A. M., R. W. Seerley, and M. J. Azain. 1990. Menhaden fish meal and dried whey levels in swine starter diets, Special Publ. No. 67, Georgia Agric. Exp. Sta., Athens, 11.

Graham, P. L., D. C. Mahan, and R. G. Shields, Jr. 1981. Effect of starter diet and length of feeding regimen on performance and digestive enzyme activity of 2-week-old weaned pigs, *J. Anim. Sci.*, 53:299.

Hall, O. G. 1957. Value of feather meal with and without amino acid supplementation for growing-finishing swine, *J. Anim. Sci.*, 16:1076 (Abstr.).

Han, Y., and C. M. Parsons. 1991. Protein and amino acid quality of feather meals, *Poult. Sci.*, 70:812.

Hansen, B. C., E. R. Flores, T. D. Tanksley, Jr., and D. A. Knabe. 1987. Effects of different heat treatments during processing on nursery and growing pig performance, *J. Anim. Sci.*, 65:1283.

Hansen, J. A., D. A. Knabe, and K. G. Burgoon. 1993a. Amino acid supplementation of low-protein sorghum-soybean meal diets for 5- to 20-kilogram swine, *J. Anim. Sci.*, 71:452.

Hansen, J. A., D. A. Knabe, and K. G. Burgoon. 1993b. Amino acid supplementation of low-protein sorghum-soybean meal diets for 20- to 50-kilogram swine, *J. Anim. Sci.*, 71:442.

Hansen, J. A., J. L. Nelssen, R. D. Goodband, and T. L. Weeden. 1993c. Evaluation of animal protein supplements in diets of early-weaned pigs, *J. Anim. Sci.*, 71:1853.

Hartman, A. D., W. J. Costello, G. W. Libal, and R. C. Wahlstrom. 1985. Effect of sunflower seeds on performance, carcass quality, fatty acids and acceptability of pork, *J. Anim. Sci.*, 60:212.

Haught, D. G., T. D. Tanksley, Jr., J. H. Hesby, and E. J. Gregg. 1977. Effect of protein level, protein restriction and cottonseed meal in sorghum-based diets on swine reproductive performance and progeny development, *J. Anim. Sci.*, 44:249.

Haumann, B. F. 1997. Bioengineered oilseed acreage escalating, *INFORM*, 8:804.

Haydon, K. D., and Newton, G. L. 1987. Effect of whole-roasted peanuts fed in either simple or complex diets on starter pig performance, Swine Rep., Univ. of Georgia, Athens, Special Publ. No. 44:25.

Haydon, K. D., G. L. Newton, C. R. Dove, and S. E. Hobbs. 1990. Effect of roasted or raw peanut kernels on lactation performance and milk composition of swine, *J. Anim. Sci.*, 68:2591.

Herkelman, K. L., G. L. Cromwell, T. S. Stahly, T. W. Pfeiffer, and D. A. Knabe. 1992. Apparent digestibility of amino acids in raw and heated conventional and low-trypsin-inhibitor soybeans for pigs, *J. Anim. Sci.*, 70:818.

Hill, G., D. Rozeboom, N. Trottier, D. Mahan, L. Adeoli, T. Cline, D. Forsyth, and B. Richert. 1998. Tri-State Swine Nutrition Guide, Bulletin 869, Ohio State University, Columbus.

Ilori, J. O., E. R. Miller, D. E. Ullrey, P. K. Ku, and M. G. Hogberg. 1984. Combinations of peanut meal and blood meal as substitutes for soybean meal in corn-based growing-finishing diets, *J. Anim. Sci.*, 59:394.

Johnson, L. A., T. M. Suleiman, and E. W. Lusas. 1979. Sesame protein: a review and prospectus, *J. Am. Oil Chem. Soc.*, 56:463.

Kass, M. L., P. J. van Soest, W. G. Pond, B. Lewis, and R. E. McDowell. 1980. Utilization of dietary fiber from alfalfa by growing swine. 1. Apparent digestibility of diet components in specific segments of the gastrointestinal tract, *J. Anim. Sci.*, 50:175.

Kats, L. J., J. L. Nelssen, M. D. Tokach, R. D. Goodband, J. A. Hansen, and J. L. Laurin. 1994a. The effect of spray-dried porcine plasma on growth performance of the early-weaned pig, *J. Anim. Sci.*, 72:2075.

Kats, L. J., J. L. Nelssen, M. D. Tokach, R. D. Goodband, T. L Weeden, S. S. Drits, J. A. Hansen, and K. G. Friesen. 1994b. The effects of spray-dried blood meal on growth performance of the early-weaned pig, *J. Anim. Sci.*, 72:2860.

Kennedy, J. J., F. X. Aherne, D. L. Kelleher, and P. J. Caffrey. 1974a. An evaluation of the nutritive value of meat-and-bone meal. 1. Effects of level of meat-and-bone meal and collagen on pig and rat performance, *Ir. J. Agric. Res.*, 13:1.

Kennedy, J. J., F. X. Aherne, D. L. Kelleher, and P. J. Caffrey. 1974b. An evaluation of the nutritive value of meat-and-bone meal. 2. Effects of protein, ash and available lysine content on pig performance and nitrogen retention, *Ir. J. Agric. Res.*, 13:11.

Kepler, M., G. W. Libal, and R. C. Wahlstrom. 1982. Sunflower seeds as a fat source in sow gestation and lactation diets, *J. Anim. Sci.*, 55:1082.

Kim, I. B., I. K. Han, and Y. J. Choi. 1993. The determination of digestibility of amino acids in feedstuffs on cannulated pigs, *Korean J. Anim. Nutr. Feedstuffs*, 17:57.

Knabe, D. A. 1996. Optimizing the protein nutrition of growing-finishing pigs, *Anim. Feed Sci. Technol.*, 74:1635.

Knabe, D. A., T. D. Tanksley, Jr., and J. H. Hesby. 1979. Effects of lysine, crude fiber and free gossypol in cottonseed meal on the performance of growing pigs, *J. Anim. Sci.*, 49:134.

Knabe, D. A., D. C. LaRue, E. J. Gregg, G. M. Martinez, and T. D. Tanksley, Jr. 1989. Apparent digestibility of nitrogen and amino acids in protein feedstuffs by growing pigs, *J. Anim. Sci.*, 67:441.

Kornegay, E. T. 1996. Natuphos™ phytase in swine diets: digestibility, bone and carcass characteristics. In *Proc. BASF Technical Symposium: Use of Natuphos™ Phytase in Swine Nutrition and Waste Management*, Research Triangle Park, NC, 28.

Laksesvela, B. 1961. Graded levels of herring meal to bacon pigs, effect on growth rate, feed efficiency and bacon quality, *J. Agric. Sci.* (Cambridge), 56:307.

LaRue, D. C., D. A. Knabe, and T. D. Tanksley, Jr. 1985. Commercially processed glandless cottonseed meal for starter, grower and finisher swine, *J. Anim. Sci.*, 60:495.

Laudert, S. B., and G. L. Allee. 1975. Nutritive value of sunflower seed for swine, *J. Anim. Sci.*, 41:318 (Abstr.).

Leamaster, B. R., and P. R. Cheeke. 1979. Feed preferences of swine: alfalfa meal, low and high saponin alfalfa, and quinine sulfate, *Can. J. Anim. Sci.*, 59:467.

Leibbrandt, V. D., and N. J. Benevenga. 1991. Utilization of liquid whey in feeding swine. In *Swine Nutrition*, Miller, E. R., D. E. Ullrey, and A. J. Lewis, Eds., Butterworth-Heinemann, Boston, 559.

Leibholz, J. 1979. Meat meal in the diet of the early-weaned pig. III. Meat and meat quality and the processing of meat meals, *Anim. Feed Sci. Technol.*, 4:53.

Leibholz, J. 1982. Meat meal in the diet of the early-weaned pig. IV. The supplementation of diets with tryptophan, lysine and methionine, *Anim. Feed Sci. Technol.*, 7:27.

Lekule, F. P., T. Homb, and J. A. Katagile. 1982. Optimum inclusion of coconut meal in growing-finishing pig diets, *East Afr. Agric. For. J.*, 48:19.

Lepine, A. J., D. C. Mahan, and Y. K. Chung. 1991. Growth performance of weanling pigs fed corn–soybean meal diets with or without dried whey at various lysine hydrochloride levels, *J. Anim. Sci.*, 69:2026.

Lewis, A. J. 1991. Amino acids in swine nutrition. In *Swine Nutrition*, Miller, E. R., D. E. Ullrey, and A. J. Lewis, Eds., Butterworth-Heinemann, Boston, 147.

Li, D. F., J. L. Nelssen, P. G. Reddy, F. Blecha, J. D. Hancock, G. L. Allee, R. D. Goodband, and R. D. Klemm. 1990. Transient hypersensitivity to soybean meal in the early-weaned pig, *J. Anim. Sci.*, 68:1790.

Li, D. F., J. L. Nelssen, P. G. Reddy, F. Blecha, R. D. Klemm, D. W. Giesting, J. D. Hancock, G. L. Allee, and R. D. Goodband. 1991. Measuring suitability of soybean products for early weaned pigs with immunological criteria, *J. Anim. Sci.*, 69:3299.

Lindemann, M. D., S. G. Cornelius, S. M. El Kandelgy, R. L. Moser, and J. E. Pettigrew. 1986. Effect of age, weaning and diet on digestive enzyme levels in the piglet, *J. Anim. Sci.*, 62:1298.

Mahan, D. C. 1992. Efficacy of dried whey and its lactalbumin and lactose components at two dietary lysine levels in postweaning pig performance and nitrogen balance, *J. Anim. Sci.*, 70:2182.

Mahan, D. C., R. A. Easter, G. L. Cromwell, E. R. Miller, and T. L. Veum. 1993. Effect of dietary lysine levels formulated by altering the ratio of corn soybean meal with or without dried whey and lysine hydrochloric acid in diets for weanling pigs, *J. Anim. Sci.*, 71:1848.

Marchello, M. J., N. K. Cook, V. K. Johnson, W. D. Slanger, D. K. Cook, and W. E. Dinusson. 1984. Carcass quality, digestibility and feedlot performance of swine fed various levels of sunflower seed, *J. Anim. Sci.*, 58:1205.

McIntosh, M. K., S. K. Baidoo, F. X. Aherne, and J. P. Bolans. 1986. Canola meal as a protein supplement for 6 to 20 kilogram pigs, *Can. J. Anim. Sci.*, 66:1051.

Miller, E. R. 1990. Blood meal: flash-dried. In *Nontraditional Feed Sources for Use in Swine Production*, Thacker, P. A., and R. N. Kirkwood, Eds., Butterworths, Boston, 53.

NCR-42. 1993. Variability among sources and laboratories in selenium analysis of corn and soybean meal, *J. Anim. Sci.*, 71(Suppl. 1):67 (Abstr.).

NCR-42 and S-145. 1997. Variability in mixing efficiency and in laboratory analysis of diets at 25 experiment stations, *J. Anim. Sci.*, 75(Suppl. 1):96 (Abstr.).

Nessmith, W. B., Jr., J. L. Nelssen, M. D. Tokach, R. D. Goodband, and J. R. Bergström. 1997. Effects of substituting deproteinized whey and/or crystalline lactose for dried whey on weanling pig performance, *J. Anim. Sci.*, 75:3222.

Newport, M. J., and H. D. Keal. 1983. Effect of protein source on performance and nitrogen metabolism of pigs weaned at 21 days of age, *Anim. Prod.*, 37:395.

Newton, G. L., and K. A. Haydon. 1988. Raw or roasted peanuts in growing-finishing diets. Swine Rep., University of Georgia, Athens, Special Publ. No. 56:41.

Newton, G. L., O. M. Hale, and K. D. Haydon. 1990. Peanut Kernels. In *Nontraditional Feed Sources for Use in Swine Production*, Thacker, P. A., and R. N. Kirkwood, Eds., Butterworths, Boston, 285.

Noland, P. R., M. Funderburg, J. Atteberry, and K. W. Scott. 1968. Use of glandless cotton seed meal in diets for young pigs, *J. Anim. Sci.*, 27:1319.

Noland, P. R., D. R. Campbell, and Z. B. Johnson, 1980. Use of unextracted sunflower seeds as a protein source, *Anim. Feed Sci. Technol.*, 5:51.

NRC. 1988. *Nutrient Requirements of Swine*, 9th ed., National Academy Press, Washington, D.C.

NRC. 1998. *Nutrient Requirements of Swine*, 10th ed., National Academy Press, Washington, D.C.

Orok, E. J., J. P. Bowland, and C. W. Briggs. 1975. Rapeseed, peanut and soybean meals as protein supplements with or without added lysine: biological performance and carcass characteristics of pigs and rats, *Can. J. Anim. Sci.*, 55:135.

Papadopoulos, M. C. 1985. Processed chicken feathers as feedstuff for poultry and swine. A review, *Agric. Wastes*, 14:275.

Parsons, C. M. 1996. Digestible amino acids for poultry and swine, *Anim. Feed Sci. Technol.*, 59:147.

Parsons, M. J., P. K. Ku, and E. R. Miller. 1985. Lysine availability in flash-dried blood meals for swine, *J. Anim. Sci.*, 60:1447.

Partanen, K. 1998. Utilisation of reactive lysine from meat and bone meals of different ash content by growing-finishing pigs, *Agric. Sci. Fin.*, 7:1.

Partanen, K., and M. Nasi. 1994. Nutritive value of meat and bone meal for growing pigs, *Agric. Sci. Fin.*, 3:449.

Patience, J. F. 1996. Precision in swine feeding programs: an integrated approach, *Anim. Feed Sci. Technol.*, 59:137.

Peo, E. R., Jr., and D. B. Hudman. 1962. Effect of levels of meat and bone scraps on growth rate and feed efficiency of growing-finishing swine, *J. Anim. Sci.*, 21:787.

Pesti, G.M. 1986. Feeding value of several poultry by-product meals. In *Proc. 1986 Georgia Nutr. Conf. for the Industry*, University of Georgia, Athens, 106.

Pike, I. H., M. K. Curran, M. Edge, and A. Harvey. 1984. Effect of nutrient density, presence of fish meal and method of feeding of unmedicated diets on early-weaned pigs, *Anim. Prod.*, 39:291.

Pollmann, D. S., D. M. Danielson, M. A. Crenshaw, and E. R. Peo, Jr. 1981. Long-term effects of dietary additions of alfalfa and tallow on sow reproductive performance, *J. Anim. Sci.*, 51:294.

Powley, J. S., P. R. Cheeke, D. C. England, T. P. Davidson, and W. H. Kennick. 1981. Performance of growing-finishing swine fed high levels of alfalfa meal: effects of alfalfa level, dietary additives and antibiotics, *J. Anim. Sci.*, 53:308.

Prawirodigdo, S., E. S. Batterham, L. M. Anderson, F. R. Dunshea, and D. J. Farrell. 1997. Nitrogen retention in pigs given diets containing cottonseed meal or soybean meal, *Anim. Feed Sci. Technol.*, 67:205.

Ravindran, V. 1990. Sesame meal. In *Nontraditional Feed Sources for Use in Swine Production*, Thacker, P. A., and R. N. Kirkwood, Eds., Butterworths, Boston, 419.

Reese, D. E., R. C. Thaler, M. C. Brumm, C. R. Hamilton, A. J. Lewis, G. W. Libal, and P. S. Miller. 1995. Nebraska and South Dakota Swine Nutrition Guide. Nebraska Cooperative Extension EC 95–273-C, University of Nebraska, Lincoln.

Richter, G., and H. Kohler. 1997. Suitability of extracted linseed meal for feeding to the suckling pig, *Muhle Mischfuttertech.*, 134:776.

Ristic, M., S. Kormanjos, R. Curcic, and V. Pupavac. 1993. The influence of inedible raw material rendering method on meat meal quality, *Acta Vet. Hung.*, 41:33.

Rowan, T. G., and T. L. J. Lawrence. 1986a. Growth and metabolism studies in growing pigs given diets containing a low glucosinolate rapeseed meal, *J. Agric. Sci.* (Cambridge), 107:483.

Rowan, T. G., and T. L. J. Lawrence. 1986b. Growth, tissue deposition and metabolism studies in growing pigs given low glucosinolate rapeseed meal diets containing different amounts of copper and polyethylene glycol, *J. Agric. Sci.* (Cambridge), 107:505.

SCA. 1987. Feeding Standard for Australian Livestock Pigs, Commonwealth Scientific and Industrial Research Organization, East Melbourne.
Schone, F., U. Kirchheim, F. Tischendorf, and B. Rudolph. 1997. Evaluation of linseed feedstuffs (ground linseed, solvent extracted linseed meal) with growing pigs — feed value, thiocyanate and thyroid hormone status, *Fett-Lipid,* 99:15.
Seerley, R. W. 1991. Major feedstuffs used in swine diets. In *Swine Nutrition*, Miller, E. R., D. E. Ullrey, and A. J. Lewis, Eds., Butterworth-Heinemann, Boston, 451.
Seerley, R. W., and R. C. Wahlstrom. 1965. Dehydrated alfalfa meal in rations for confined brood sows, *J. Anim. Sci.,* 24:448.
Seerley, R. W., D. Burdick, W. C. Russom, R. S. Lowrey, H. C. McCampbell, and H. E. Amos. 1974. Sunflower meal as a replacement for soybean meal in growing swine and rat diets, *J. Anim. Sci.,* 38:947.
Sohn, K. S., C. V. Maxwell, D. S. Buchanan, and L. L. Southern. 1994a. Improved soybean sources for early-weaned pigs. I. Effects on performance and total tract amino acid digestibility, *J. Anim. Sci.,* 72:622.
Sohn, K. S., C. V. Maxwell, L. L. Southern, and D. S. Buchanan. 1994b. Improved soybean sources for early-weaned pigs. II. Effects on ileal amino acid digestibility, *J. Anim. Sci.,* 72:631.
Southern, L. L., J. E. Pontif, K. L. Watkins, and D. F. Combs. 1990. Amino acid-supplemented raw soybean diets for finishing swine, *J. Anim. Sci.,* 68:2387.
Squibb, R. L., and E. Salazar. 1951. Value of corozo palm nut and sesame oil meals, banana, A.P.F. and cow manure in rations for growing and fattening pigs, *J. Anim. Sci.,* 10:545.
Stahly, T. S., and G. L. Cromwell. 1986. Responses to dietary additions of fiber (alfalfa meal) in growing pigs housed in a cold, warm or hot thermal environment, *J. Anim. Sci.,* 63:1870.
Stoner, G. R., G. L. Allee, J. L. Nelssen, M. E. Johnston, and R. D. Goodband. 1990. Effect of select menhaden fish meal in starter diets for pigs, *J. Anim. Sci.,* 68:2729.
Tanksley, T. D., Jr. 1990. Cottonseed meal. In *Nontraditional Feed Sources for Use in Swine Production*, Thacker, P. A., and R. N. Kirkwood, Eds., Butterworths, Boston, 139.
Tanksley, T. D., Jr., A. E. Calvez, and J. H. Hesby. 1973. Cottonseed meal in swine gestation and lactation rations, *J. Anim. Sci.,* 37:291 (Abstr.).
Teague, H. S. 1955. The influence of alfalfa on ovulation rate and other reproductive phenomena in gilts, *J. Anim. Sci.,* 14:621.
Thacker, P. A. 1990a. Alfalfa meal. In *Nontraditional Feed Sources for Use in Swine Production*, Thacker, P. A., and R. N. Kirkwood, Eds., Butterworths, Boston, 1.
Thacker, P. A. 1990b. Canola meal. In *Nontraditional Feed Sources for Use in Swine Production*, Thacker, P. A., and R. N. Kirkwood, Eds., Butterworths, Boston, 69.
Thacker, P. A., and R. N. Kirkwood, Eds. 1990. *Nontraditional Feed Sources for Use in Swine Production*, Butterworths, Boston.
Thorne, P. J., D. J. A. Cole, and J. Wiseman. 1990. Copra meal. In *Nontraditional Feed Sources for Use in Swine Production*, Thacker, P. A., and R. N. Kirkwood, Eds., Butterworths, Boston, 123.
Tokach, M. D., J. L. Nelssen, and G. L. Allee. 1989. Effect of protein and/or carbohydrate fractions of dried whey on performance and nutrient digestibility of early weaned pigs, *J. Anim. Sci.,* 67:1307.
Tokach, M. D., J. E. Pettigrew, L. J. Johnston, M. Overland, J. W. Rust, and S. G. Cornelius. 1995. Effect of adding fat and/or milk products to the weanling pig diet on performance in the nursery and subsequent grow-finish stages, *J. Anim. Sci.,* 73:3358.
Tuitoek, K., L. G. Young, C. F. M. de Lange, and B. J. Kerr. 1997. The effect of reducing excess dietary amino acids on growing-finishing pig performance: an evaluation of the ideal protein concept, *J. Anim. Sci.,* 75:1575.
Viljoen, J., S. E. Coetzee, J. C. Fick, F. K. Siebrits, and J. P. Hayes. 1998. The ileal amino acid digestibility of different protein sources for early-weaned piglets, *Livest. Prod. Sci.,* 54:45.
Wahlstrom, R. C. 1985. Sunflowers in pig nutrition, *Pig News Info.,* 6:151.
Wahlstrom, R. C. 1990. Sunflower meal. In *Nontraditional Feed Sources for Use in Swine Production*, Thacker, P. A., and R. N. Kirkwood, Eds., Butterworths, Boston, 473.
Wahlstrom, R. C., and G. W. Libal. 1977. Dried blood meal as a protein source in diets for growing-finishing swine, *J. Anim. Sci.,* 44:778.
Wahlstrom, R. C., G. W. Libal, and R. C. Thaler. 1985. Efficacy of supplemental tryptophan, threonine, isoleucine and methionine for weanling pigs fed a low-protein, lysine-supplemented, corn-sunflower meal diet, *J. Anim. Sci.,* 60:720.

Walker, G. L., D. M. Danielson, E. R. Peo, Jr., and R. F. Mumm. 1993. Bioavailability of calcium in sun-cured alfalfa meal and effect of dietary calcium concentration on bone and plasma characteristics during two phases of gestation in gilts, *J. Anim. Sci.*, 71:124.

Walker, W. R., C. V. Maxwell, F. N. Owens, and D. S. Buchanan. 1986. Milk versus soybean protein sources for pigs: I. Effects of performance and digestibility, *J. Anim. Sci.*, 63:505.

Whittemore, C. T. 1993. *The Science and Practice of Pig Production*, Longman Scientific and Technical, Essex, U.K.

Williams, K. C., and L. J. Daniels. 1973. Decorticated safflower meal as a protein supplement for sorghum and wheat based pig diets, *Aust. J. Exp. Agric. Anim. Husb.*, 13:48.

Williams, K. C., and P. K. O'Rourke. 1974. Decorticated safflower meal as a protein supplement in diets fed either restrictively or *ad libitum* to barrow and gilt pigs over 45 kg live weight, *Aust. J. Exp. Agric. Anim. Husb.*, 14:12.

Wiseman, J., and D. J. A. Cole. 1985. Energy evaluation of cereals for pig diets. In *Recent Developments in Pig Nutrition*, Cole, D. J. A., and W. Haresign, Eds., Butterworths, London, 246.

Wiseman, J., S. Jagger, D. J. A. Cole, and W. Haresign. 1991. The digestion and utilization of amino acids of heat-treated fish meal by growing/finishing pigs, *Anim. Prod.*, 53:215.

Yen, J. T., G. L. Cromwell, G. L. Allee, C. C. Calvert, T. D. Crenshaw, and E. R. Miller. 1991. Value of raw soybeans and soybean oil supplementation in sow gestation and lactation diets: a cooperative study, *J. Anim. Sci.*, 69:656.

Yi, Z., E. T. Kornegay, V. Ravindran, M. D. Lindemann, and J. H. Wilson. 1996. Effectiveness of Natuphos® phytase in improving the bioavailabilities of phosphorus and other nutrients in soybean meal–based semipurified diets for young pigs, *J. Anim. Sci.*, 74:1601.

Zimmerman, D. R. 1987. Porcine plasma proteins in diets of weanling pigs, Iowa State Univ. Swine Res. Rep., Iowa State University, Ames, 12.

Zongo, D., and M. Couibaly. 1993. Glandless cottonseed meal: an important source of protein in swine production, *Tropicultura*, 11:95.

37 Miscellaneous Feedstuffs

Robert O. Myer and Joel H. Brendemuhl

CONTENTS

I. Introduction 840
II. Factors to Consider 840
   A. Gross Composition and Quality 840
   B. Nutrient Composition and Nutrient Availability 841
   C. Suitability and Palatability 841
   D. Freedom from Potential Health Hazards 841
   E. Special Handling, Processing, and Storage Requirements 841
   F. Availability and Consistency 841
   G. Perishability 841
   H. Effect on End Product 842
   I. Storage Space 842
   J. Cost 842
III. Determining the Value of an Alternative Feedstuff 842
IV. Miscellaneous Energy Feedstuffs 842
   A. Bananas 842
   B. Cane Molasses and Sugarcane Juice 842
   C. Cassava 843
   D. Citrus Pulp 843
   E. Cocoyams 843
   F. Grain Screenings 843
   G. Pearl Millet 844
   H. Potatoes and Potato By-Products 844
   I. Rice and Rice By-Products 844
   J. Sugar Beets, Sugar Beet Pulp, and Molasses 845
   K. Sweet Potatoes 845
   L. Triticale 845
   M. Yams 846
V. Miscellaneous Protein Feedstuffs 846
   A. Beans 846
   B. Canola Seeds 846
   C. Cull Eggs 847
   D. Faba Beans 847
   E. Fish Silage 847
   F. Lentils 848
   G. Lupins 848
   H. Mung Beans 848
   I. Peanut Kernels 849
   J. Peas 849
   K. Poultry Hatchery By-Product Meal 850

	L.	Shrimp Meal	850
	M.	Sunflower Seeds	850
	N.	Other Legume Seeds	851
	O.	Other Oilseed Meals	851
VI.		Crystalline (Synthetic) Amino Acids	851
VII.		Other Miscellaneous Feedstuffs	851
	A.	Forages	851
	B.	Liquid Whey	851
	C.	Restaurant Food Wastes	852
	D.	Other Feedstuffs	852
VIII.		Summary	852
		References	858

I. INTRODUCTION

Traditionally, feed for pork production in developed countries consists mainly of cereal grains and oilseed meals. Pigs, however, have and can utilize a wide range of feedstuffs. Many of these "alternative" feedstuffs that can be utilized are by-products (or co-products) and edible waste products from the food-processing, food preparation, and food service industries. Example industries include grain milling, brewing and distillation, baking, fruit and vegetable processing, meat, milk and egg processing, seafood processing, prepared food manufacturing, and retail food outlets. Other alternatives include feedstuffs not commonly fed to pigs but which may be fed during times of low prices and/or surpluses, or fed during shortages of traditional feedstuffs. Alternative feedstuffs may also include those available in many areas that can be economical substitutes for traditional feedstuffs not available locally.

In the future, the variety and quantity of by-products and edible wastes are expected to increase and disposal options for many of these wastes, such as landfills, will become more limited and costly. Thus, the role of pigs in recycling and "adding value" to many of these by-products and wastes will become increasingly important as a viable waste-management option.

The objective of this chapter is to identify, provide the nutritional information, and the best use of alternative feedstuffs for pig feeding. Most feedstuffs will not be discussed in detail. For more information, the reader is referred to publications by NRC (1973), Ensminger and Olentine (1978), Pond and Maner (1984), and Thacker and Kirkwood (1990). Additional information can also be obtained from the *Pork Industry Handbook* publication 108 (Miller et al., 1987). Most cereal grains, alternative cereal grains, cereal grain by-products, and new cultivars of cereal grains are discussed in Chapter 35. Many protein sources and alternative protein sources are discussed in Chapter 36. This chapter discusses miscellaneous feedstuffs that may be potential alternatives to traditional feedstuffs.

II. FACTORS TO CONSIDER

Before discussing individual miscellaneous feedstuffs, factors and questions that should be considered before an alternative feedstuff is utilized for pig feeding will be discussed.

A. GROSS COMPOSITION AND QUALITY

A visual gross appraisal of the potential alternative feedstuff should be made for identification purposes and to ensure consistency of composition. The Association of American Feed Control Officials (AAFCO) official publication gives detailed descriptions and nomenclature of many feedstuffs (AAFCO, 1999). This publication is updated annually.

B. Nutrient Composition and Nutrient Availability

The best advice is to have representative samples periodically analyzed for important nutrients. Feedstuff composition tables (e.g., NRC, 1982; 1998) can also be utilized, but be aware that these tables generally report only averages based on information on hand at the time of their publication. Also, nutrient composition of some feedstuffs has changed over time due to the introduction of different cultivars and/or changes in processing.

The desirable nutrient information for an alternative feedstuff includes contents of digestible energy (DE) or metabolizable energy (ME), essential amino acids, fiber, fat, Ca, P, Na, Cl, ash, and moisture. Minimum information would include contents of lysine, P, and energy. While it is best to do an amino acid analysis to obtain the lysine content, the content of this essential amino acid can be estimated from crude protein content. Similarly, direct determination of the energy content of a feedstuff is rather difficult, but it can be estimated from its composition. Relationships of protein to lysine content of many feedstuffs are given in NRC (1998). Equations are also given in NRC (1998), as well as in Chapter 5, to predict DE and ME from chemical composition. Processing, however, especially heat processing, and/or the presence of antinutritional factors can decrease nutrient availability, especially lysine availability. More information about the effects that processing and antinutritional factors may have on nutrient availability are presented in Chapters 21 and 25, respectively.

C. Suitability and Palatability

The suitability of an alternative feedstuff will depend on age and weight of the pig, production goal, production stage, and feeding method. Obviously, a feedstuff that might be suitable for a gestating sow may not be suitable for a young growing pig. Factors that affect feed intake (and palatability) include natural taste, presence of molds and mycotoxins, contaminates, spoilage and rancidity, bulk density, physical form, moisture content, and inclusion level in the diet.

D. Freedom from Potential Health Hazards

Many feedstuffs may contain toxic substances, disease organisms, or antinutritional factors. If present, the alternative feedstuff should not be used unless the deleterious factors can be eliminated or neutralized inexpensively. Mycotoxins and antinutritional factors that may be present in feedstuffs are discussed in Chapter 25.

E. Special Handling, Processing, and Storage Requirements

Many alternative feedstuffs may require special transport, handling, storage, processing, mixing, and feeding compared with traditional feedstuffs. These additional requirements may inhibit the use of the alternative feedstuff because of the cost, or the lack of special equipment to store, process, etc.

F. Availability and Consistency

The supply and quality of many alternative feeds is inconsistent and this should be taken into consideration before using. *In general, alternative feedstuffs are more variable in composition and quality than traditional feedstuffs like corn or soybean meal.*

G. Perishability

Various factors can influence shelf life and nutrient stability. These factors can include moisture content, fat content and type, physical form, storage method, storage management, storage time, and level of inclusion in mixed feed (feed stability).

H. Effect on End Product

The alternative feedstuff when included in the diet should not harm the end product, such as affect the taste and quality of the meat or compromise food safety.

I. Storage Space

An alternative feedstuff will usually require separate storage facilities.

J. Cost

Added costs associated with the utilization of the alternative feedstuff (i.e., extra storage, special processing, transportation) must also be evaluated.

III. DETERMINING THE VALUE OF AN ALTERNATIVE FEEDSTUFF

The major costs in a typical pig diet are ingredients that provide energy, lysine, and/or P. An alternative feedstuff should supply one or more of these nutrients. Equations have been developed to calculate the relative value of alternative feedstuffs for use in pig diets, and they are published in the *Pork Industry Handbook* publication 108 (Miller et al., 1987).

IV. MISCELLANEOUS ENERGY FEEDSTUFFS

A. Bananas

Banana (*Musa sapientum; M. cavendishii*) production is primarily confined to tropical regions. Appreciable quantities of reject and surplus bananas are available for livestock feeding. Fresh bananas are high in water and are low in protein. Bananas are usually harvested green, but both ripe and green bananas can be fed. Green bananas, however, usually have a lower feeding value than ripe bananas due to tannins, which decrease during ripening (Clavijo and Maner, 1975; Campabadal et al., 1988; Perez, 1997). Ripe bananas can be used to supply 50 to 75% of the total dry matter (DM) intake of growing–finishing pigs and gestating sows in combination with a protein, mineral, and vitamin supplement (Solis et al., 1988; Ravindran, 1990a; Perez, 1997). Because of their high moisture content, ripe bananas should not be used as the major source of energy for lactating sows or for starter pigs (Ravindran, 1990a; Perez, 1997). Plantains (*M. paradisiaca*), or cooking bananas, are somewhat similar to bananas in composition and feeding value (Ravindran, 1990a; Perez, 1997).

B. Cane Molasses and Sugarcane Juice

Molasses is a major by-product of sugar production and can be an economical source of energy for pigs in many tropical and subtropical regions. Molasses contains 15 to 25% moisture and 50 to 60% carbohydrate (mostly sugars). The protein content is low and the ash content is relatively high (6 to 10% for final molasses). Molasses has a laxative effect if included at high levels in the diet (>20%). This effect can be minimized by blending with a fibrous product (i.e., 4:1 ratio with bagasse, which is the fibrous residue of sugarcane after the juice has been squeezed out). Research suggests that levels of up to 20% molasses can be fed to pigs between 10 and 50 kg live weight and up to 40% for pigs over 50 kg (Combs and Wallace, 1973; Pond and Maner, 1984). The addition of molasses to the diet, however, has been observed to cause a reduction in apparent N digestibility and biological value (Combs and Wallace, 1973; Loeza et al., 1997).

Research from Cuba has shown that corn can be completely replaced in the diet with "high-test" molasses (low-ash) without affecting growth performance of pigs from 6 to 40 kg, and no diarrhea was observed (Mederos et al., 1989). Further information about feeding molasses can be found in publications by Pond and Maner (1984), Cuaron (1992), Perez (1997), and Diaz and Lon-Wo (1998).

Sugarcane (*Saccharum officinarum* L.) juice may be a viable alternative energy source for pigs in tropical regions when refined sugar prices are low. Sugarcane juice is the liquid fraction upon extraction from fresh sugarcane. This liquid fraction contains 15 to 20% solids, and it is mostly sucrose. Results of feeding trials conducted in Latin America and Africa indicate that sugarcane juice may be a satisfactory replacement for corn in pig diets (Mena, 1988; Speedy et al., 1991; Motta et al., 1994; Paula et al., 1994; Perez, 1997).

C. Cassava

Cassava (or tapioca, manioc; *Manihot esculentis* crantz) is a perennial woody shrub that is grown almost entirely in the tropics. The crop is quite productive and yields of 20 to 30 metric tons/ha of starchy tubers are possible (Oke, 1990). Fresh cassava contains about 65% moisture. The DM portion is high in starch and low in protein (2 to 3%). Cassava can be fed fresh, cooked, ensiled, or as dried chips or dried meal. Cassava meal, however, is quite powdery and tends to produce a powdery, dusty diet when included at high levels.

Fresh cassava contains cyanogenic glucosides, which can reduce pig growth. Boiling, roasting, soaking, ensiling, or sun-drying can reduce cyanide levels (Okeke et al., 1985). The residual levels can be further neutralized with methionine and iodine supplementation (Oke, 1990; Tewe, 1994). The normal range of cyanide in fresh cassava is about 15 to 500 mg/kg fresh weight. It is recommended that pig diets should contain no more than 100 mg HCN equivalent/kg (Tewe, 1994).

Research has shown that properly processed cassava can replace corn in pig diets (Oke, 1990; Wu, 1991; Tewe, 1994; Rantanen et al., 1995). However, because of its powdery nature, low levels of protein, and economics, the usual recommended maximum inclusion level is 40% of the diet, and this corresponds with the level commonly used by European countries that import cassava (Oke, 1990). More information about feeding cassava, including cassava by-products, can be found in publications by Ravindran (1995) and Perez (1997).

D. Citrus Pulp

Citrus pulp is a dried by-product of citrus juice processing. Because of its high fiber content and low energy density, citrus pulp is best utilized in diets for gestating sows and at low levels for finishing pigs (Pond and Maner, 1984). Citrus pulp is well utilized in ruminant diets and thus is generally too expensive for use in pig diets.

E. Cocoyams

Cocoyam (taro; *Colocasia esculenta*) is grown in tropical and subtropical regions throughout the world. The plant produces a large starchy corm beneath the ground. Cocoyams are grown primarily for human consumption, but surplus and reject corms may be available for pig feeding. Cocoyams should be cooked before feeding to pigs (Nwokolo, 1990; Perez, 1997).

F. Grain Screenings

Screenings are obtained in the cleaning of cereal grains, and they include light and broken grains, weed seeds, hulls, chaff, straw, mill dust, sand, and dirt. Grain screenings are defined as containing at least 70% or more material from grains including light and broken grains, and many contain wild oats and buckwheat (AAFCO, 1999). If the screenings contain more than 50% of a predominant grain, then it can be declared as the first word of the name (i.e., corn screenings). Grain screenings should not contain more than 6.5% ash (AAFCO, 1999). Elevator dust is that separated from grain in commercial grain cleaning and should contain less than 15% ash (AAFCO, 1999).

Grain screenings for the most part have feed value for growing-finishing pigs. Grain screenings from wheat have been estimated to have a feeding value similar to that of barley (Beames, 1990). Dust (elevator) has been shown to have no detrimental effect on growth when replacing corn at levels of up to 50% (Baird, 1980; Beames, 1990).

G. Pearl Millet

Pearl millet (or grain millet; *Pennisetum glaucum*) is a drought-tolerant, short-season cereal grain crop. It has been reported to have higher contents of protein, lysine and other essential amino acids, and crude fat compared with corn. Digestibility data indicate that these nutrients are well utilized by pigs (Haydon and Hobbs, 1991; Adeola and Orban, 1995; Lawrence et al., 1995). Results of feeding trials concluded that pearl millet grain could be used as a satisfactory substitute for corn and part of the soybean meal in pig diets (Dove and Myer, 1995; Lawrence et al., 1995).

H. Potatoes and Potato By-Products

Cull and surplus potatoes (*Solanum tuberosum*) are often available for pig feeding. Potatoes are high in moisture (65 to 72%), but on a dry weight basis, potatoes contain 6 to 12% crude protein and are high in starch with little fiber and ash.

For optimum utilization, potatoes should be cooked (100°C) before feeding. Cooking improves starch availability and denatures an alkaloid glycoside (solanine) and a protease inhibitor found in raw potatoes (Edwards and Livingstone, 1990). Cooked potatoes are readily accepted by pigs with the only drawback being their high moisture content, which reduces daily nutrient intake, especially in young growing pigs. Ensiling does little to improve the palatability and feeding value of raw potatoes (Edwards and Livingstone, 1990; Brzoska et al., 1997).

Potato pulp is a by-product of the potato starch industry and comprises the residue remaining after the starch has been extracted. This product is usually uncooked and thus is utilized poorly by pigs (Edwards and Livingstone, 1990). Potato meal made from raw cull potatoes is also not well utilized by pigs (Pond and Maner, 1984).

Dehydrated cooked potato flakes or flour is well utilized by pigs (Edwards and Livingstone, 1990; Michal et al., 1995). Waste or scrap potato chips and french fries, which have been cooked in vegetable oil for human consumption, are high in energy and are very palatable. These products contain about 30 to 35% fat and are well used by pigs (Miller et al., 1987; Rahnema et al., 1997). Potato chips, however, are high in salt, which may limit feed intake and their inclusion level in the diet.

I. Rice and Rice By-Products

The polished white rice (*Oryza sativa* L.) that is used in human diets is obtained by milling paddy rice. By-products produced by milling paddy rice can be used in pig diets. In addition, off-grade paddy rice may also be available for pigs. Paddy rice contains the hull, which is high in poorly digestible fiber, and, thus, paddy rice has about 75 to 85% of the energy value of corn. Brown rice is paddy rice with the hull removed, and has an energy value similar to corn (Farrell and Hutton, 1990). Rice bran is obtained when brown rice is milled. Rice bran is usually a mixture of bran, polishings, and hulls with a maximum fiber level of 13% (AAFCO, 1999). Rice bran is quite high in crude fat.

Rice bran is readily consumed by pigs when fed fresh. Because of its high oil content, which is 80 to 85% unsaturated, the oil undergoes oxidation rapidly and will become rancid upon storage. Previous research on the evaluation of rice bran as a feedstuff for pig diets has resulted in mixed results (Pond and Maner, 1984; Farrell and Hutton, 1990). This variation was probably due to the quantity of hulls present and the freshness of the rice bran. The high content of unsaturated fat can result in carcasses with soft fat. In general, good-quality fresh rice bran can have an inclusion rate of up to 30% in the diet of growing-finishing pigs (Campabadal et al., 1976; Pond and Maner, 1984; Farrel and Hutton, 1990).

The high value of rice oil for human consumption has resulted in the availability of defatted rice bran. This product contains less energy than the unextracted product, but it has a much longer shelf life. Solvent-extracted rice bran contains a minimum of 14% crude protein and a maximum of 14% crude fiber (AAFCO, 1999). The high fiber content and bulky nature of defatted rice bran would limit its inclusion level in typical pig diets. Dietary levels of 30% have been reported with little adverse effect on performance of growing-finishing pigs (Farrell and Hutton, 1990; Warren and Farrell, 1990).

Rice polishings and broken rice also may be available. Polishings are obtained in the milling operation of brushing the grain to polish the kernel (AAFCO, 1999). Chipped and broken polished rice are the small fragments of rice kernels that have been separated from the larger kernels of milled rice. Broken rice, also known as brewer's rice, has an energy value similar to corn for pigs (Farrell and Hutton, 1990).

J. Sugar Beets, Sugar Beet Pulp, and Molasses

Fresh sugar beet (*Beta vulgaris*) roots are sometimes utilized for pig feeding in some regions of the world. Because of their high moisture content, they are best utilized by finishing pigs and sows (Longland and Low, 1990). Dried sugar beet roots can be utilized at higher levels and also by younger pigs (Longland and Low, 1990).

Sugar beet pulp is the residue left after sugar extraction. It contains a high level of fiber and nonstarch polysaccharides, and therefore is best utilized in sow diets (Longland and Low, 1990; Brouns et al., 1995). Molassed sugar beet pulp is beet pulp with sugar beet molasses added, and it can be utilized by growing-finishing pigs as well as by sows. Inclusion levels of 30% supported similar growth in growing-finishing pigs compared with control diets (Longland and Low, 1989). However, inclusion levels of up to 20% are usually recommended for growing-finishing pigs (Longland and Low, 1990; Lee and Crawshaw, 1991). The composition of sugar beet molasses is similar to that of cane molasses (final molasses; Longland and Low, 1990).

K. Sweet Potatoes

Sweet potatoes (*Ipomoea batatas* L.) are grown in many tropical, subtropical, and some temperate regions for human consumption. Waste, reject, and surplus sweet potatoes may be available for pig feeding. Fresh sweet potatoes contain about 30% DM and are low in protein but high in carbohydrate. Sweet potatoes can be fed raw, cooked, or as a silage. They can also be dehydrated as chips or to form a meal. For best utilization, sweet potatoes should be cooked to improve carbohydrate availability and to denature naturally occurring protease inhibitors (Nwokolo, 1990; Ravindran, 1995).

Properly heat processed, dehydrated sweet potato meal can have an energy value similar to corn. Sun-dried chips have a lower energy value than corn (80 to 90%) due to residual protease inhibitor activity and lower starch availability (Nwokolo, 1990). By-products from sweet potato canning also may be available. A dehydrated by-product meal, made from sweet potato peels and reject sweet potatoes, has been reported to be an economical replacement for corn in growing-finishing pig diets (Tor-Agbidye et al., 1990).

L. Triticale

Triticale grain (*X Triticosecale* Wittmack) is a synthetic cereal grain derived by crossing wheat with rye. Triticale has been produced for many years. However, advances in plant breeding have made this a viable commercial feed grain crop in many parts of the world, such as Europe, South America, and Australia. Modern grain triticales are high yielding and have grain of heavier test weight and higher starch content than older cultivars (NRC, 1989; Myer et al., 1990a; Varnghese, 1996). Research has shown that triticale grain is a satisfactory replacement for corn, and because of its superior lysine content, it can replace part of the soybean meal in typical corn–soybean meal diets for starting and growing-finishing pigs (Hale et al., 1985; Coffey and Gerrits, 1988; Batterham et al., 1990b; Myer et al., 1990a; 1996; Leterme et al., 1991). Modern triticale grain contains 11 to 14% crude protein and 0.36 to 0.44% lysine, which are lower than in older cultivars due to the increased grain plumpness of the newer cultivars.

The relative energy value of triticale, based on results of the research mentioned above, is about 95 to 100% of corn. Various antinutritional factors (ANF) such as nonstarch polysaccharides (pentosans) and protease inhibitors, while higher than in most other cereal grains, seem to have no effect on growth of pigs (Batterham et al., 1990b; Boros and Rakowska, 1991; Myer, 1998). Ergot infection, while a potential problem for triticale grown under cool and wet conditions, seems to be much less in the new triticales than previously noted with the older cultivars (NRC, 1989).

M. Yams

The "true yam" (*Dioscorea* sp.) is a tropical or subtropical root crop. Fresh yams contain 60 to 80% moisture, with the DM portion being mostly starch. Yams are low in protein. They are used primarily for human consumption and are generally too expensive for livestock feeding. Yams should be cooked before use in pig feeds (Pond and Maner, 1984; Perez, 1997).

V. MISCELLANEOUS PROTEIN FEEDSTUFFS

A. Beans

The common dry bean (*Phaseolus vulgaris*) is a legume that is widely grown, in particular in Central and South America, for human consumption. Dry beans are also grown in the United States. Common varieties include the navy, pinto, great northern, kidney (white, red, or black), pink, and small red. Appreciable quantities of cull beans are usually available as feed for livestock. These cull beans contain about 22 to 30% crude protein but <2% fat. They are a good source of lysine, but they are deficient in the sulfur-containing amino acids. Raw beans, however, contain several ANFs. These include tannins, protease inhibitors, lectins, and the nonstarch polysaccharides (Liener, 1976; Myer et al., 1982; Huisman and Jansman, 1991; Weder et al., 1997). Unlike most legume seeds, the lectins in beans are quite toxic (Myer et al., 1982; Pusztai, 1989; Huisman et al., 1990). Tannins are concentrated in the seed coat and their concentration is lowest in white beans and highest in colored beans (Ma and Bliss, 1978; Huisman and Jansman, 1991). Heat processing, such as steaming or extrusion, greatly improves the feed value of dry beans primarily by denaturating the lectins and protease inhibitors (Myer and Froseth, 1983; Rodriguez and Bayley, 1987; van der Poel et al., 1991a). Properly heated processed cull beans can be used to supply up to one half of the supplemental protein for pigs greater than 40 kg live weight (Myer and Froseth, 1983; Rodriguez and Bayley, 1987).

B. Canola Seeds

Whole canola seed contains about 40% ether extract and thus could serve as a source of added fat in addition to a supplemental protein source. Canola is a term used in North America to distinguish low glucosinolate, low erucic acid cultivars of rapeseed (*Brassica napus* or *B. campestris*). Canola is sometimes referred to as "double low" or "double zero" rapeseed.

Previous research has shown that ground raw full-fat canola can be included in pig diets up to 15% without affecting rate of weight gain; however, improvement in feed efficiency has been inconsistent

(Aherne and Bell, 1990; Gipp and Swenson, 1996; Thacker, 1998). Reasons for the lack of an improvement in feed efficiency normally associated with fat supplementation may be due to the residual ANFs in raw canola seed, and to its relatively high crude fiber content. Even though its level is low compared with rapeseed, raw canola seed contains the enzyme myrosinase, which hydrolyzes glucosinolate producing potentially toxic compounds (Bell, 1984). Various processing techniques, such as extrusion and micronizing, lower myrosinase activity and improve the feeding value of full-fat canola (Aherne and Bell, 1990; Thacker, 1998). The oil in canola seed is highly unsaturated and can result in carcasses with soft fat if fed at high levels to finishing pigs (Aherne and Bell, 1990; Myer et al., 1992).

C. Cull Eggs

Blood-spotted eggs from egg candling stations are often available. Raw eggs contain about 10% high-quality protein. Raw eggs in the shell are best utilized by growing-finishing pigs and are not recommended for young growing pigs (<20 kg) or sows (Miller et al., 1987). A biotin deficiency may result from feeding high levels of cull eggs.

D. Faba Beans

The faba bean (*Vicia faba* L.), also known as horse bean and broad bean, is a annual legume well adapted to cool growing conditions. Faba beans contain 24 to 30% crude protein and <2% fat. The protein is high in lysine and, like most legume seeds, is low in the sulfur amino acids. Faba beans contain several ANFs such as tannins, protease inhibitors, and lectins. However, the levels of trypsin inhibitor and lectin activities are low compared with other legume seeds (Thacker, 1990a; Vidal-Valverde et al., 1997).

The ANF that is of most concern in faba beans for nonruminants are tannins (Marquardt, 1989; Jansman et al., 1989; Garrido et al., 1991; van der Poel et al., 1991b). Tannins in whole faba beans are associated with the seed coat (testa), and the tannin content is related to the color of the seed coat (and flowers). Tannins are lower in white than in the color-seeded varieties (Reddy et al., 1985; van der Poel et al., 1991b; 1992a). Ground raw faba beans (low-tannin varieties) can be utilized by pigs with maximum recommended dietary inclusion levels at 15% for starter pigs, 20% for growing-finishing pigs, and 10% for breeding animals (Thacker, 1990a).

E. Fish Silage

Silage made with fish is a semiliquid product made from minced whole fish and/or fish offal liquefied by the action of endogenous enzymes in the digestive system of the fish, and it is preserved by low pH (pH of 4.0 or less). There are two methods for the production of fish silage: (1) by adding one or more organic acids (acid preserved silage), which lowers the pH sufficiently to prevent spoilage; and (2) by bacterial fermentation initiated by mixing with a fermentable carbohydrate source (Raa and Gildberg, 1982; Winter and Feltham, 1983). The process of making fish silage offers the potential of utilizing wastes from fish processing in areas where the quantity of wastes is insufficient to justify the production of fish meal. Fish silage, as expected, is 70 to 80% water. The quantity and quality of the protein is usually quite high, but both will be reflective of the raw material used. Most silages contain between 40 and 75% crude protein on a water-free basis, and this protein has a good pattern of essential amino acids.

All classes of pigs can be fed diets containing fish silage; however, there are some limitations. Silages made with fish or fish offal with a high fat content may lead to problems with a "fishy taste" in the pork when fed to growing-finishing pigs. This off-flavor problem can be minimized or eliminated by restricting the amount of fish silage in the diet for finishing pigs. In general, whenever the total diet for the pig contains 1% or more of fish oil, an off-flavor problem can result. This off-flavor problem can also be minimized by removing fish silage from the diet 3 weeks before slaughter. Off-flavor is not usually a problem for silage made with low-fat fish or fish offal (Raa and Gildberg, 1982; Van Lunen, 1990).

The ensiling process also has been adopted to process other waste products into nutritious feedstuffs for use in pig diets. Examples include scallop viscera (Myer et al., 1990b), sea clam viscera (Wohlt et al., 1994), poultry offal (Tibbetts et al., 1987; Van Lunen et al., 1991; Lallo et al., 1997), and ruminant offal (Machin et al., 1986).

F. Lentils

Lentils (*Lens culinaris*) are grown primarily as a human food crop. They are grown worldwide either as a winter or spring crop. In North America, lentil production (spring) is confined primarily to Western Canada and the Northwestern United States. Surplus and cull lentils represent a potential source of protein and energy for pig diets. Lentils contain 20 to 35% crude protein and, like most legume seeds, are a good source of lysine but a poor source of the sulfur amino acids (Savage, 1988; Castell, 1990b). The ANFs in raw lentils seem to be lower than in most other raw legume seeds (Savage, 1988; Castell, 1990b). Data are limited to suggest optimum levels of inclusion in diets for various classes of pigs. Diets containing 40% ground lentils with added methionine supported growth performance of growing and finishing pigs similar to those fed a soybean meal–based diet (Castell and Cliplef, 1990).

G. Lupins

There are many species of lupins, however, only a few are suitable for pigs. The suitable species include *Lupinus albus* (white lupin), *L. angustifolius* (narrow leaf lupin or blue lupin), and to a lesser extent *L. luteus* (yellow lupin) and *L. mutabilis* (South American pearl lupin). These species, sometimes referred to as "sweet" lupins, differ from other lupin species in that the seeds are of low alkaloid content. Alkaloid content usually ranges from <0.1 to 0.3 g/kg in cultivars of these species (Batterham, 1989). The pig is particularly sensitive to the ill effects of alkaloids. Maximum tolerance level for growing pigs has been reported as 0.2 g/kg of diet (Godfrey et al., 1985; Cheeke and Kelly, 1989; King, 1990; Hill and Pastuszewska, 1993). The upper limit for commercial sweet lupin meal, ground seeds of the above species, is set at 0.03% alkaloids (AAFCO, 1999). Lupin seed meal is otherwise free of other ANFs common to other legume seeds, and it can be fed raw. Lupins, however, are high in nonstarch polysaccharides (oligosaccharides of the raffinose family), which may interfere with optimal protein digestion and may result in an enlarged digestive tract (Cheeke and Kelly, 1989; Gdala et al., 1997; Zdunezyk et al., 1997).

The crude protein of lupins ranges from 25 to 40% with the protein content of *L. angustifolius* usually slightly below that in *L. albus*. Lysine is usually slightly lower than in soybean meal on a g/100 g protein basis and the methionine content is low. Crude fiber tends to be high in *L. angustifolius* (12 to 15%) but lower in *L. albus* (3 to 9%) (Batterham 1989; King, 1990). *Lupinus albus* is a manganese accumulator with reported levels as high as 3400 mg/kg (Batterham, 1989; King, 1990).

Lupin seed meal has been reported to have a low availability of lysine for growing pigs (Batterham et al., 1986). However, recent research has indicated availability slightly higher than that noted for soybean meal (Fernandez and Batterham, 1995). Several feeding studies obtained normal growth performance of pigs with dietary inclusion levels of up to 40% *L. angustifolius* (Batterham, 1989; King, 1990; Fernandez and Batterham, 1995).

Lupin seed meal (sweet) has considerable potential as a feedstuff for pigs. Lupin seed meal is a common protein source in pig diets in Australia and New Zealand. Maximum inclusion levels of 10 to 15% for *L. albus* cultivars (white lupins) and 20 to 30% for *L. angustifolius* (narrow leaf lupins) are usually recommended (Batterham, 1989; King, 1990).

H. Mung Beans

The mung bean (*Phaseolus aureus*, *P. mungo*, *Vigna radiata*) is a large-seeded legume grown in many tropical and subtropical regions and in some temperate regions, primarily for human consumption. Cull and surplus mung beans may be available for pig feeds. Like most legume seeds, the protein in mung beans is high in lysine, but low in the sulfur amino acids. The common ANFs associated with raw legume seeds seems to be low in mung beans (Maxwell, 1990; Wiryawan et al., 1997). Research has shown that ground raw mung beans can replace up to 30% of the supplemental protein for growing pigs and up to 60% for finishing pigs without a negative effect on growth performance (Maxwell, 1990).

I. Peanut Kernels

Raw peanut seed (*Arachis hypogaea* L.) contains 40 to 55% oil. Thus, peanuts could be a fat source as well as a protein source for pigs. Unlike most other legumes, the protein in peanuts is low in lysine as well as low in the sulfur amino acids.

Typically, peanuts not suitable for human consumption (splits, damaged seed, small seed, shriveled seed, etc.) are utilized in the production of peanut oil. An alternative use of these "oil stock" peanuts is as a fat source in pig diets. In addition, peanuts deemed unsuitable by candy and peanut butter manufacturers may also be available.

Peanuts contain low levels of ANFs; the major one seems to be the tannins, which are concentrated in the peanut skins (testa). Various studies have shown that ground or rolled peanuts (raw or roasted) are well utilized in pig diets (Newton et al., 1990; Myer and Gorbet, 1998). Their use in pig diets, however, is limited by their amino acid composition, and by its high level of unsaturated fatty acids. Maximum inclusion has been suggested to be 10% for diets of growing and finishing pigs. Higher levels will result in pigs producing carcasses with soft fat (Newton et al., 1990; Myer and Gorbet, 1998). Peanut kernels are an excellent source of fat for sow diets (Haydon et al., 1990). For young growing pigs under 30 kg, peanuts should be roasted before inclusion in diets (Newton et al., 1990). A word of caution, peanuts are particularly susceptible to mycotoxin contamination (especially aflatoxins); thus, peanuts intended to be fed should be tested (D. W. Gorbet, personal communication).

J. Peas

Peas (*Pisum sativum* L.) are an excellent source of supplemental dietary protein for pigs. Peas are widely grown in Europe and Canada for use in livestock diets as well as for human consumption. Peas are also grown in the United States, primarily in the Pacific Northwest and Northern Plains, where they are grown for human consumption and, more recently, for animal feeding. Where peas are grown for human consumption, appreciable quantities of cull peas are available that can be utilized for livestock feeding.

Two subspecies of peas, *hortense* and *arvense*, are grown for livestock feeding. Subspecies *hortense* (garden pea) typically has white flowers and large green or yellow seeds, and it is grown for both human and livestock consumption. Subspecies *arvense* (field pea) is characterized by colored flowers and dark seeds, and it is used for animal feed. In addition to flower color and seed color, pea cultivars are usually further divided into smooth- and wrinkle-seeded cultivars, and spring and winter cultivars (Castell, 1990a; Gatel and Grosjean, 1990).

The average crude protein content of peas is 23%; however, the variation is wide. Wrinkled cultivars tend to have higher protein contents than smooth cultivars. Protein also tends to be higher for winter vs. spring cultivars (Gatel and Grosjean, 1990; Castell et al., 1996). Peas, on a gram per 100 g protein basis, are high in lysine content, but they are low in the sulfur amino acids and tryptophan. As with many other legume seeds, raw peas contain several ANFs that can interfere with nutrient availability. The major ANFs in peas include protease inhibitors and tannins. Typical levels of ANFs found in raw peas are much lower than usually noted with other raw legume seeds. For example, protease inhibitor activity in raw peas is about one fifth to one twentieth that usually found in raw soybeans (Castell, 1990; Gatel and Grosjean, 1990). Winter peas generally have greater protease inhibitor activities than spring varieties, and smooth peas more than wrinkled peas. Tannin content is related to seed coat color, with the darker seed coat having higher tannin content.

Generally, ground raw peas are palatable and can be fed to all classes of pigs with few problems. The exception is young growing pigs (<20 kg). Reductions in feed intake have been reported for young pigs fed diets containing ground raw peas as the only supplemental protein source (Myer and Froseth, 1978; 1993; Gatel et al., 1988; Castell, 1990; Gatel and Grosjean, 1990); however, Michal et al. (1996) noted no reduction in feed intake. The white-flowered cultivars of peas generally have higher energy and protein digestibilities than colored flower or dark-seeded varieties (71 to 80% vs. 83 to 90% for protein)(Hlodversson, 1987; Marquardt and Bell, 1988; Castell, 1990; Gatel and Grosjean, 1990; Gdala et al., 1992). The energy and protein digestibilities of the white-flowered peas have been reported to be similar to those of soybean meal. Heat processing, such as extrusion, toasting, or even steam pelleting, has been reported to improve the feeding value of peas (Castell, 1990; van der Poel et al., 1992b; Myer and Froseth, 1993; O'Doherty, 1996; Canibe and Eggum, 1997). The greatest response to thermal processing of peas was noted when they were included in diets for young growing pigs. This response is probably due in part to the high dietary level of peas required in the diet to meet the young pig's amino acid requirements. In most instances, thermal processing is usually not economical, especially thermal processing of white-flowered, spring cultivars.

Ground raw peas can be included as the only source of supplemental protein for pig diets with the exception of young pig diets (<20 kg). For young pigs, it is best that raw peas constitute only part of the supplemental protein (Myer and Froseth, 1978; Gatel et al., 1988; Gatel and Grosjean, 1990; Castell, 1990; Jaikaran et al., 1995; Kehoe et al., 1995; Castell et al., 1996; Michal et al., 1996). In addition, methionine and perhaps tryptophan supplementation would be required for diets containing peas that are fed to pigs weighing <50 kg (Myer and Froseth, 1978; 1993; Gatel et al., 1988; Gatel and Grosjean, 1990; Jaikaran et al., 1995). Because of the variability in both nutrient composition and content of various ANFs, one should know the variety of peas before feeding. If not available, the acceptable maximum for young pigs (<20 kg) would be 15%, for growing and finishing pigs levels up to 30% can be used, and for sows, 15%. In all cases, it is assumed that any necessary supplementation will be made to the pea diet to ensure that dietary guidelines are met (Castell, 1990; Castell et al., 1996).

K. Poultry Hatchery By-Product Meal

This product is a mixture of eggshells, infertile and unhatched eggs, and cull chicks. The mixture is cooked, dried, and ground with or without removal of part of the fat (AAFCO, 1999). While this product seems to have good nutritional value, the high calcium content would limit its use in pig diets (Vandepopuliere et al., 1976; Miller et al., 1987).

L. Shrimp Meal

Shrimp meal is the dried waste from shrimp processing and contains parts and whole shrimp. If the meal contains more than 3% salt, the salt content must be stated (AAFCO, 1999). Shrimp meal has a high content of nonprotein nitrogen compounds (chitin); thus, corrected protein content is only about 20 to 25%. In addition, its high ash and salt levels would limit the amount that could be used in typical diets (Pond and Maner, 1984). A "well-processed" shrimp meal has been reported to be a satisfactory replacement for soybean meal in diets for growing-finishing pigs (Amador and Egnaola, 1995).

M. Sunflower Seeds

Sunflower (*Helianthus annus*) seeds contain about 38% oil, but they are high in fiber and low in lysine. Ground sunflower seeds can be used by pigs if properly supplemented with lysine. The high fiber content, however, may negate the positive effect that the oil portion may have on improving feed efficiency (Pond and Maner, 1984; Wahlstrom, 1990; Perez, 1997; Rodriguez et al., 1998).

N. OTHER LEGUME SEEDS

Chick peas (*Cicer arietinum*), cow peas (*Vigna sinensis* or *V. unquiculata*), lima beans (*Phaseolus lunatus*), and pigeon peas (*Cajanus cajun* or *C. indicus*) are primarily grown for human consumption. All four resemble peas in composition and are best heat processed before feeding. Chick peas, however, can be fed raw (NRC, 1973; Kachare et al., 1988; Todorov, 1988; Batterham et al., 1990a; Savage and Thompson, 1993; Nestares et al., 1996; Perez, 1997).

O. OTHER OILSEED MEALS

Additional oilseed meals that can be fed to pigs include palm kernel (*Elaeis guineensis*) meal, babassu palm (*Obrignya martiana*) meal, niger seed (*Guizotia abyssinica*) meal, crambe seed (*Crambe abyssinica*) meal (detoxified), mustard seed (*Brassica hitra, campestris*) meal, and rubber seed (*Hevea brasiliensis*) meal (Babatunde et al., 1990; Bell, 1990; Nwokolo, 1990; Ravindran, 1990b).

VI. CRYSTALLINE (SYNTHETIC) AMINO ACIDS

Both lysine (as L-lysine·HCl) and methionine (as DL-methionine or DL-methionine hydroxy analog) have been available for some time, and thus used by the swine industry. Threonine (L-threonine) and tryptophan (L-tryptophan) are now available and may be economical at times for use in pig feeds. There is evidence, however, that there may be a limit to how much natural intact protein can be replaced by free amino acids from crystalline amino acids and still obtain optimum lean growth (Kephart and Sheritt, 1990; Cervantes-Ramirez et al., 1991; Davis et al., 1991; D'Mello, 1993; Hansen et al., 1993; Brudevold and Southern, 1994; Kerr et al., 1995; Cromwell et al., 1996; Smith et al., 1999). Cromwell (1996), after reviewing several studies, concluded that the maximum reduction of crude protein in corn–soybean meal diets upon supplementation of crystalline lysine, threonine, tryptophan, and methionine without affecting growth performance of growing-finishing pigs was found to be 4 percentage units (i.e., from 16 to 12%). Even though growth performance was not affected, carcass fat content increased slightly (Cromwell, 1996).

VII. OTHER MISCELLANEOUS FEEDSTUFFS

A. FORAGES

Forage sources include pasture, silage, haylage, and ground dried forages. Pasture was and still is an important component of extensive pig-feeding programs. The high fiber content and low energy density, however, limit the use of forages in most intensive pig-feeding programs. Forages have their best use in diets of gestating sows. More information about forages for pigs can be found in an excellent fact sheet (126; Kephart et al., 1998) published in the *Pork Industry Handbook*.

B. LIQUID WHEY

Liquid whey is the watery portion of milk that is left after the curd is formed during cheese making. Two different wheys are commonly available — sweet whey from making hard cheese and acid whey from making cottage cheese. Liquid whey is only 7% DM. As such, liquid whey has its best use for feeding of growing-finishing pigs (20 kg to market weight). Further information about the utilization of liquid whey in feeding pigs is detailed in Chapter 34 of the first edition of this book (Leibbrandt and Benevenga, 1991).

C. Restaurant Food Wastes

Restaurant food wastes,* or "garbage," consist primarily of food discarded from restaurants, hotels, households, and other food preparation and food service establishments. Restaurant food wastes are high in moisture (50 to 80%); however, on a DM basis, they are high in nutrients desirable for pig feeding. Typical analyses of food wastes previously reported have shown contents (DM basis) of crude protein of 15 to 23%, fat (ether extract) at 17 to 24%, and ash at 3 to 6% (Kornegay et al., 1970, Pond and Maner, 1984; Ferris et al., 1995; Westendorf et al., 1996; 1998; Myer et al., 1999). The range is due to the varied nature of these wastes. These food wastes also tend to be high in salt (NaCl) content (2 to 3%, DM basis) (Westendorf et al., 1998; Myer et al., 1999). Traditionally, much of this waste has been fed to pigs; however, for health and safety reasons, the Swine Health Protection Act (U.S. Congress, 1980) mandates that restaurant food wastes must be "cooked" before feeding (100°C for 30 min). Please note that some states have regulations more restrictive than the federal regulation, and some states have a complete ban on feeding food wastes to pigs. Restaurant food wastes that must be "cooked," according to the Swine Protection Act, are those wastes that contain meat or have been in contact with meat. Because of the regulation and the high labor costs involved, the feeding of these wastes to pigs has declined over the last few decades (Westendorf et al., 1996). In recent years, increasing requirements for environmental protection and high disposal costs have made recycling of these wastes into livestock feeding an attractive option. Research has shown that restaurant food waste does have nutritional value for pigs (Kornegay et al., 1970; Westendorf et al., 1998; Myer et al., 1999).

The major drawback of feeding restaurant food wastes to pigs is the high moisture content, resulting in a reduction in DM intake and thus slow growth when fed as the only feed. This drawback can be overcome by supplementation with a dry feed (primarily an energy feed) (Kornegay et al., 1970; Westendorf et al., 1998). Additional information about feeding restaurant food wastes can be found in a review by Westendorf et al. (1996).

D. Other Feedstuffs

Many other feeds, too numerous to list and discuss, may also be available. Some examples include salvage candy (Miller et al., 1987), buckwheat (Thacker, 1990), crab meal (Van Lumen and Anderson, 1990; Liu et al., 1994), sugar (Pond and Maner, 1984; Beech et al., 1990), palm kernel cake (Rhule, 1996), palm oil slurry (Perez, 1997; Fanimo and Fashina-Bombata, 1998), single cell protein (NRC, 1973; Waterworth, 1990; Perez, 1997), potato protein product (Edwards and Livingstone, 1990; Kerr et al., 1998), milk chocolate product (McNaughton et al., 1997; Yang et al., 1997), and wild oats (Thacker, 1990b; Thacker and Sosulski, 1994), to name a few. In addition, potential new feedstuffs are becoming available. Examples include dehydrated restaurant food waste products (Myer et al., 1999), spray-dried whole egg (Nessmith et al., 1995), and a dried meat solubles product (Ragland et al., 1998).

VIII. SUMMARY

A summary of nutrient compositions of many miscellaneous feedstuffs are given in Tables 37.1 and 37.2. Note that many of the values given are estimates. Note also that the composition of most of the miscellaneous feedstuffs varies greatly, for example, reported digestible energy values for rice bran varied from 2540 to 3880 kcal/kg of DM (Farrell and Hutton, 1990). Tables 37.3 and 37.4 give suggested maximum inclusion levels of many of the above feedstuffs in diets for various classes of pigs. Again, most are estimates and tend to be conservative. Higher dietary levels may be used but a decrease in growth performance may occur. *Again, to emphasize that because of the variable nature of most of the above miscellaneous feedstuffs, it is strongly recommended that each lot be analyzed before inclusion in the diet.*

---

* Proposed AAFCO (1999) definition.

Miscellaneous Feedstuffs

TABLE 37.1
Nutrient Composition of Miscellaneous Energy Feedstuffs for Use in Pig Diets (as-fed basis)

Feedstuff	DM (%)	ME (kcal/kg)	Protein (%)	Lysine (%)	Fat (%)	Fiber (%)	Ca (%)	P (%)	Relative Feeding Value vs. Corn (%)	Remarks
Corn (maize)	89	3400	8.3	0.26	3.9	2.2	0.03	0.25	100	High energy, low lysine
Banana, whole green	26	700	1.0	<0.10	0.1	0.5	0.01	0.03	15–20	High moisture content, some tannins
Banana, whole ripe	25	750	1.0	<0.10	0.1	0.5	0.01	0.03	20–25	High moisture content
Buckwheat	88	2700	11.0	0.60	2.0	10.0	0.10	0.30	70–90	High fiber, possible photosensitization
Cassava meal	89	3300	3.0	0.10	0.5	5.0	0.12	0.15	95–100	Possible residual HCN
Cassava, fresh	35	1200	1.0	<0.10	0.2	1.5	0.04	0.05	30–40	HCN in some varieties
Cocoyams (taro)	35	1100	2.0	0.10	0.2	1.0	0.02	0.05	25–30	High moisture content, cooking improves utilization
Millet, pearl (grain)	88	3200	13.0	0.40	4.0	3.0	0.05	0.30	90–100	Small seed
Molasses, sugarcane	80	2200	3.0	<0.10	0.1	0	0.70	0.08	60–70	Laxative effect
Potato chips or fries	90	4400	6.0	0.20	30.0	1.0	0.10	0.20	120–150	Very high energy, high fat, high salt
Potato pulp, dried	88	2200	6.0	0.20	0.3	9.0	0.10	0.20	60–70	Cooking improves utilization
Potato, boiled	22	700	2.4	0.10	0.1	0.5	0.02	0.05	15–25	High moisture, low protein
Potato, cooked flakes	92	3500	8.0	0.40	0.5	2.0	0.10	0.20	100	High energy, low protein
Potato, raw	20	500	2.0	0.10	0.1	0.5	0.02	0.05	10–15	High moisture, cooking improves utilization
Restaurant food waste	20	800	5.0	0.20	5.0	1.0	0.10	0.10	15–25	Variable nutritional value, high moisture content
Rice bran	90	3000	12.5	0.60	12.0	11.0	0.05	1.70	70–100	Bulky, potential rancidity
Rice bran, fat extracted	91	2600	14.0	0.65	1.5	13.0	0.10	1.40	60–80	Bulky, high fiber
Rice polishings	90	3300	13.0	0.50	13.0	2.0	0.10	1.20	95–100	High energy, potential rancidity
Rice, broken	89	3300	8.0	0.30	0.6	0.6	0.04	0.18	95–100	High energy, low lysine
Rice, paddy	89	2800	9.0	0.30	2.0	10.0	0.05	0.25	70–80	Possible aflatoxin contamination, high fiber
Sugar beet, dried	90	2900	4.0	0.20	0.4	5.0	0.15	0.15	70–90	Bulky
Sugar beet, dried pulp	90	2600	9.0	0.50	1.0	18.0	0.70	0.10	60–80	High nonstarch polysaccharides
Sugar beet, fresh	24	700	1.5	0.10	0.1	1.5	0.04	0.04	15–25	High moisture content
Sugar beet, molasses pulp	90	2500	9.0	0.40	0.5	14.0	0.70	0.10	60–80	High nonstarch polysaccharides

continued

TABLE 37.1 (CONTINUED)
Nutrient Composition of Miscellaneous Energy Feedstuffs for Use in Pig Diets (as-fed basis)

Feedstuff	DM (%)	ME (kcal/kg)	Protein (%)	Lysine (%)	Fat (%)	Fiber (%)	Ca (%)	P (%)	Relative Feeding Value vs. Corn (%)	Remarks
Sugarcane juice	18	700	<1.0	<0.10	<0.1	2.0	0.20	0.05	15–25	High moisture content
Sugarcane stalks	25	500	1.0	<0.10	0.5	8.0	0.10	0.05	10–20	Bulky, high moisture content
Sweet potatoes, dried	90	2900	3.0	0.10	1.5	3.0	0.10	0.15	70–90	Cooking improves utilization
Sweet potatoes, fresh	30	1000	1.0	0.10	0.5	1.0	0.03	0.50	20–30	Cooking improves utilization, high moisture content
Triticale	90	3200	12.0	0.40	1.8	3.0	0.05	0.32	95–100	High energy, low lysine

Sources: NRC (1982; 1998), Pond and Maner (1984), Mena (1988), and Thacker and Kirkwood (1990).

TABLE 37.2
Nutrient Composition of Miscellaneous Protein Feedstuffs for Use in Pig Diets (as-fed basis)

Feedstuff	DM (%)	ME (kcal/kg)	Protein (%)	Lysine (%)	Fat (%)	Fiber (%)	Ca (%)	P (%)	Relative Feeding Value vs. SBM (%)[a]	Remarks
Soybean meal (48%)	90	3300	48.0	3.0	0.9	3.4	0.3	0.7	100	Excellent protein source
Babassa meal	90	3000	24.0	1.0	6.0	15.0	0.1	0.5	25–35	High Mg, high fiber
Beans (*Phaseolus*)	89	3000	23.0	1.3	1.2	4.5	0.1	0.5	35–50	Requires heat processing
Canola seeds	90	4200	22.0	1.2	40.0	7.5	0.4	0.6	30–40	Heat processing improves utilization
Chickpeas	90	3200	25.0	1.6	5.0	4.0	0.2	0.3	45–55	Low sulfur amino acids

Miscellaneous Feedstuffs

Feedstuff	DM (%)	ME (kcal/kg)	CP (%)						Comments
Cowpeas	90	3000	24.0	1.5	1.5	4.0	0.1	0.4	40–50	Low sulfur amino acids; heat processing improves utilization
Crambe seed meal	90	2600	42.0	2.2	1.0	13.0	0.2	1.0	60–80	Detoxification needed
Crab meal	92	1300	31.0	1.4	2.0	10.0	15.0	1.6	30–40	High ash limits use, high nonprotein nitrogen
Faba beans	89	3000	26.0	1.6	1.0	8.0	0.1	0.5	45–50	Tannins in color-seeded varieties
Fish silage	25	700	18.0	1.2	1.5	1.0	1.0	0.5	30–45	High moisture content, variable quality
Eggs, cull	40	500	10.0	0.5	10.0	0	6.0	0.2	20	Possible biotin deficiency
Lentils	90	3300	25.0	1.6	1.0	4.0	0.1	0.4	45–55	Low sulfur amino acids
Lupins (*L. albus*)	88	3300	35.0	1.6	8.0	10.0	0.2	0.4	50–65	Mn accumulator, high nonstarch polysaccharides
Lupins (*L. angustifolius*)	89	3200	29.0	1.4	5.0	13.0	0.2	0.3	40–50	High nonstarch polysaccharides
Mung beans	90	3200	26.0	1.6	1.0	5.0	0.1	0.5	50–60	Low sulfur amino acids
Niger seed meal	90	2800	35.0	1.6	7.0	18.0	0.1	0.8	40–50	Low lysine, high fiber
Palm kernel meal	90	2200	19.0	0.7	2.0	16.0	0.2	0.3	15–25	Bulky, low palatability
Peanut kernels	95	5000	25.0	0.9	45.0	3.0	0.1	0.4	25–35	High in energy, low lysine
Peas, dark seeded	89	3000	23.0	1.5	1.0	5.0	0.1	0.4	35–45	Low sulfur amino acids, some tannins
Peas, white flowered	89	3200	23.0	1.5	1.0	5.0	0.1	0.4	45–55	Low sulfur amino acids
Pigeon peas	90	3000	22.0	1.4	1.5	4.0	0.1	0.4	35–45	Low sulfur amino acids, heat processing improves utilization
Poultry hatchery by-product	90	1800	22.0	1.2	10.0	0	24.0	0.3	30–40	Broiler type chick, high ash limits use
										Egg type chick, high ash limits use
Rubber seed meal	90	2200	32.0	1.8	18.0	0	17.0	0.6	40–50	Should be dehulled
	90	3000	30.0	1.5	12.0	8.0	0.3	0.6	40–50	High ash limits use, high nonprotein nitrogen
Shrimp meal	93	2100	39.0	2.0	4.0	0	10.0	2.0	50–60	
Sunflower seeds	92	3800	17.0	0.7	38.0	15.0	0.2	0.6	25–30	High fiber, low lysine

[a] SBM = soybean meal.

Sources: NRC (1982; 1998), Pond and Maner (1984), and Thacker and Kirkwood (1990).

TABLE 37.3
Suggested Maximum Dietary Inclusion Levels of Various Miscellaneous Energy Feedstuffs

	Suggested Maximum Amount in Diets (%)				
	Pigs			Sows	
Feedstuff	Starting (<20 kg)	Growing (20–50 kg)	Finishing (50–110 kg)	Gestating	Lactating
Corn (maize)	75	85	90	90	85
Buckwheat	0	50	50	80[a]	0
Cassava meal	40	40	40	40	40
Millet, pearl	50[b]	85	90	90	50[b]
Molasses, final	10	10	20	10	10
Potato chips or fries	10	30	20[c]	30	30
Potato pulp, dried	0	10	10	50	0
Potato flakes, cooked	30	30	—[d]	—	—
Rice, broken	30	30	30	30	30
Rice, bran	0	20	20[c]	50	0
Rice, bran, defatted	0	10	20	50	0
Rice, paddy	0	30	30	50	0
Rice, polishings	0	20	20	20	20
Sugar beet, dried pulp	0	10	10	40	10
Sugar beet, molasses pulp	10	10	20	40	10
Triticale	75	85	90	90	85

[a] For sows housed indoors.
[b] Higher levels may be fed if the grain is free from excessive trash (i.e., husks, straw pieces).
[c] High levels may result in soft carcass fat.
[d] Usually too expensive to feed.

Sources: Pond and Maner (1984), Miller et al. (1987), and Thacker and Kirkwood (1990).

TABLE 37.4
Suggested Maximum Percentage Dietary Inclusion Levels of Various Miscellaneous Protein Feedstuffs

	Suggested Maximum Amount in Diets (%)				
	Pigs			Sows	
Feedstuff	Starting (<20 kg)	Growing (20–50 kg)	Finishing (50–110 kg)	Gestation	Lactation
Soybean meal (48%)	30	30	25	20	30
Beans (*Phaseolus*), heat processed, ground	0	10	20	20	10
Canola seeds, raw, ground	15	15	10[c]	10	10
Crab meal	0	5	5	5	5
Faba beans, raw, ground, low tannin	15	20	20	10	10
Lupins (*L. albus*), raw, ground	10	15	15	15	15
Lupins (*L. angustifolius*), raw, ground	20	30	30	20	20
Mung beans, raw, ground	0	10	15	10	0
Peanuts, raw, rolled, or ground	0[a]	20	10[c]	20	20
Peas, raw, ground, dark seeded	5[b]	10	20	10	10
Peas, raw, ground, white flowered	15[b]	30	30	20	20
Poultry hatchery by-product meal	0	3	3	3	3
Shrimp meal	0	5	5	5	5
Sunflower seeds, raw, ground	10	10	10[c]	30	20

[a] 10% for roasted peanuts.
[b] Can double levels if heat processed.
[c] Can feed at higher levels, however, soft carcass fat may result.

Sources: Pond and Maner (1984), Miller et al. (1987), and Thacker and Kirkwood (1990).

REFERENCES

AAFCO. 1999. *Official Publication*, Association of American Feed Control Officials, P. O. Box 478, Oxford, IN.

Adeola, O., and J. I. Orban. 1995. Chemical composition and nutrient digestibility of pearl millet (*Pennisetum glaucum*) fed to growing pigs, *Cereal Sci.*, 22:177.

Aherne, F. X., and J. M. Bell. 1990. Canola seed: full-fat. In *Nontraditional Feed Sources for Use in Swine Production*, Thacker, P. A., and R. N. Kirkwood, Eds., Butterworths, Stoneham, MA, 79.

Amador, R., and M. A. Egnaola. 1995. Shrimp waste meal as protein supplement in diets for growing and finishing pigs, *J. Anim. Sci.*, 73(Suppl. 1):178.

Babatunde, G. M., W. G. Pond, and E. R. Peo, Jr. 1990. Nutritive value of rubber seed (*Hevea brasiliensis*) meal: utilization by growing pigs of semipurified diets in which rubber seed meal partially replaced soybean meal, *J. Anim. Sci.*, 68:392.

Baird, D. M., 1980. Feeding and energy value of elevator grain dust, *Feedstuffs*, 52(49):17.

Batterham, E. S. 1989. Lupin-seed meal for pigs, *Pig News Info.*, 10(3):323.

Batterham, E. S., L. M. Anderson, R. F. Lowe, and R. E. Darnell. 1986. Nutritional value of lupin (*Lupinus albus*) seed meal for growing pigs: availability of lysine, effect of autoclaving and net energy content, *Br. J. Nutr.*, 56:645.

Batterham, E. S., L. M. Anderson, H. S. Saini, and D. R. Baignent. 1990a. Tolerance of growing pigs to trypsin and chymotrypsin inhibitors in chickpea (*Cicer arietinum*) and pigeon pea (*Cajanus cajan*) meals, *Proc. Aust. Soc. Anim. Prod.*, 18:453.

Batterham, E. S., H. S. Saini, and D. R. Baigent. 1990b. The effect of rate of feeding on the nutritional value of three triticale cultivars for growing pigs, *Anim. Feed Sci. Technol.*, 27:317.

Beames, R. M. 1990. Screenings. In *Nontraditional Feed Sources for Use in Swine Production*, Thacker, P. A., and R. N. Kirkwood, Eds., Butterworths, Stoneham, MA, 391.

Beech, S. A., R. Elliott, and E. S. Batterham. 1990. Sucrose as an energy source for growing pigs: digestible energy content and energy utilization, *Anim. Prod.*, 51:343.

Bell, J. M., 1984. Nutrients and toxicants in rapeseed meal: a review, *J. Anim. Sci.*, 58:996.

Bell, J. M. 1990. Mustard meal. In *Nontraditional Feed Sources for Use in Swine Production*, Thacker, P. A., and R. N. Kirkwood, Eds., Butterworths, Stoneham, MA, 265.

Boros, D., and M. Rakowska. 1991. Chemical and biological evaluation of triticale cultivars released in Poland. In *Proc. Second Int. Triticale Symp.*, CIMMYT, D.F., Mexico, 523.

Brouns, F., S. A. Edwards, and P. R. English. 1995. Influence of fibrous feed ingredients on voluntary intake of dry sows, *Anim. Feed Sci. Technol.*, 54:301.

Brudevold, A. B., and L. L. Southern. 1994. Low-protein, crystalline amino acid-supplemented, sorghum-soybean meal diets for the 10- and 20-kilogram pig, *J. Anim. Sci.*, 72:638.

Brzoska, F., R. Gasior, J. Urbanczyk, and E. Hanczakowska. 1997. Nutritive value of cereal-potato silages for fatteners, *Rocn. Nauk. Zootech.*, 24(1):143.

Campabadal, C., D. Creswell, H. D. Wallace, and G. E. Combs. 1976. Nutritional value of rice bran for pigs, *Trop. Agric.* (Trinidad), 53:141.

Campabadal, C., J. E. Solis, and J. R. Molina. 1988. Evaluation of different forms of supplying bananas in the feeding of pigs during growing and fattening, *Agron. Costarricense*, 12(2):213.

Canibe, N., and B. O. Eggum. 1997. Digestibility of dried and toasted peas in pigs. 2. Ileal and total tract digestibilities of amino acids, protein and other nutrients, *Anim. Feed Sci. Technol.*, 64:311.

Castell, A. G. 1990a. Field Peas. In *Nontraditional Feed Sources for Use in Swine Production*, Thacker, P. A., and R. N. Kirkwood, Eds., Butterworths, Stoneham, MA, 481.

Castell, A. G. 1990b. Lentils. In *Nontraditional Feed Sources for Use in Swine Production*, Thacker, P. A., and R. N. Kirkwood, Eds., Butterworths, Stoneham, MA, 205.

Castell, A. G., and R. L. Cliplef. 1990. Methionine supplementation of barley diets containing lentils (*Lens culinaris*) or soybean meal: live performance and carcass responses by gilts fed *ad libitum*, *Can. J. Anim*, 70:329.

Castell, A. G., W. Guenter, and F. A. Igbasan. 1996. Nutritive value of peas for nonruminant diets, *Anim. Feed Sci. Technol.*, 60:209.

Cervantes-Ramirez, M., G. L. Cromwell, and T. S. Stahly. 1991. Amino acid supplementation of a low-protein, grain sorghum-soybean meal diet for growing pigs, *J. Anim. Sci.*, 69(Suppl. 1):364.

Cheeke, P. R., and J. D. Kelly. 1989. Metabolism, toxicity and nutritional implications of quinolizidine (lupin) alkaloids. In *Recent Advances of Research in Antinutritional Factors in Legume Seeds*, Huisman, J., A. F. B. van der Poel, and I. E. Leiner, Eds., Pudoc, Wageningen, The Netherlands, 189.

Clavijo, H., and J. Maner. 1975. The use of waste bananas for swine feed. In *Proc. Conf. Anim. Feeds of Trop. and Subtrop. Origin*, Tropical Products Institute, London, U.K., 99.

Coffey, M. T., and W. J. Gerrits. 1988. Digestibility and feeding value of B858 triticale for swine, *J. Anim. Sci.*, 66:2728.

Combs, G. E., Jr., and H. D. Wallace. 1973. Utilization of high dietary levels of cane molasses by young and by growing-finishing swine, *Anim. Sci.*, Res. Rep. 49, No. 73–1, Anim. Science Department, University of Florida, Gainesville.

Cromwell, G. L. 1996. Synthetic amino acids may improve performance, reduce nitrogen excretion, *Feedstuffs*, 68(49):12.

Cromwell, G. L., M. D. Lindemann, G. R. Parker, K. M. Laurent, R. D. Coffey, H. J. Monegue, and J. R. Randolph. 1996. Low protein, amino acid supplemented diets for growing-finishing pigs, *J. Anim. Sci.*, 74(Suppl. 1):174.

Cuaron, J. A. 1992. Sugarcane molasses in swine nutrition: physiological and feeding considerations. In *Proc. of the Maryland Nutr. Conf. for Feed Manufacturers*, Maryland Feed Industry Council, Inc., College Park, 54.

Davis, D. J., J. H. Brendemuhl, R. O. Myer, W. R. Walker, and G. E. Combs, Jr. 1991. Amino acid supplementation of low-protein corn–soybean meal diets for 7–25 kg swine, *J. Anim. Sci.*, 69(Suppl. 1):21.

Diaz, C. P., and E. Lon-Wo. 1998. Use of sugar cane in swine and poultry feeding in Cuba, *Cuban J. Agric. Sci.*, 32 (2):105.

D'Mello, J. P. F. 1993. Amino acid supplementation of cereal-based diets for non-ruminants, *Anim. Feed Sci. Technol.*, 45:1.

Dove, C. R., and R. O. Myer. 1995. Performance of swine fed pearl millet grain. In *Proc. First Natl. Grain Pearl Millet Symp.*, Coop. Ext. Ser., University of Georgia, Athens, 110.

Edwards, S. A., and R. M. Livingstone. 1990. Potato and potato products. In *Nontraditional Feed Sources for Use in Swine Production*, Thacker, P. A., and R. N. Kirkwood, Eds., Butterworths, Stoneham, MA, 305.

Ensminger, M. E., and C. G. Olentine. 1978. *Feeds and Nutrition*. Ensminger Publishing Company, Clovis, CA.

Fanimo, A. O., and H. A. Fashina-Bombata. 1998. The response of weaner pigs to diets containing palm oil slurry, *Anim. Feed Sci. Technol.*, 71:191.

Farrell, D. J., and K. Hutton. 1990. Rice and rice milling products. In *Nontraditional Feed Sources for Use in Swine Production*, Thacker, P. A., and R. N. Kirkwood, Eds., Butterworths, Stoneham, MA, 339.

Fernandez, J. A., and E. S. Batterham. 1995. The nutritive value of lupin-seed and dehulled lupin-seed meals as protein sources for growing pigs as evaluated by different techniques, *Anim. Feed Sci. Technol.*, 53:279.

Ferris, D. A., R. A. Flores, C. W. Shanklin, and M. K. Whitworth. 1995. Proximate analysis of food service wastes, *Appl. Eng. Agric.*, 11:567.

Garrido, A., A. Gomez-Cabrera, J. E. Guerrero, and R. R. Marquardt. 1991. Chemical composition and digestibility *in vitro* of *Vicia faba* L. cultivars varying in tannin content, *Anim. Feed Sci. Technol.*, 35:205.

Gatel, F., and F. Grosjean. 1990. Composition and nutritive value of peas for pigs: a review of European results, *Livest. Prod. Sci.*, 26:155.

Gatel, F., F. Grosjean, and M. Leuillet. 1988. Utilization of white-flowered smooth-seeded spring peas (*Pisum sativum hortense*, cv. Amino) by the breeding sow, *Anim. Feed Sci. Technol.*, 22:91.

Gdala, J., L. Burachzewska, and W. Grala. 1992. The chemical composition of different types and varieties of pea and the digestion of their protein in pigs, *J. Anim. Feed Sci.*, 1:71.

Gdala, J., A. J. M. Jansman, L. Buraczewska, J. Huisman, and P. van Leeuwen. 1997. The influence of α-galactosidase supplementation on the ileal digestibility of lupin seed carbohydrates and dietary protein in young pigs, *Anim. Feed Sci. Technol.*, 67:115.

Gipp, W. F., and C. K. Swenson. 1996. Influence of full fat canola seed in prestarter and starter pig diets, *J. Anim. Sci.*, 74(Suppl. 1):176.

Godfrey, N. W., A. R. Mercy, Y. Emms, and H. G. Payne. 1985. Tolerance of growing pigs to lupin alkaloids, *Aust. J. Exp. Agric.*, 25:791.

Hale, O. M., D. D. Morey, and R. O. Myer. 1985. Nutritive value of Beagle 82 triticale for swine, *J. Anim. Sci.*, 60:503.

Hansen, J. A., D. A. Knabe, and K. G. Burgoon. 1993. Amino acid supplementation of low-protein sorghum-soybean meal diets for 20- to 50-kilogram swine, *J. Anim. Sci.*, 71:442.

Haydon, K. D., and S. E. Hobbs. 1991. Nutrient digestibilities of soft winter wheat, improved triticale cultivars, and pearl millet for finishing pigs, *J. Anim. Sci.*, 69:719.

Haydon, K. D., G. L. Newton, C. R. Dove, and S. E. Hobbs. 1990. Effect of roasted or raw peanut kernels on lactation performance and milk composition of swine, *J. Anim. Sci.*, 68:2591.

Hill, G. D., and B. Pastuszewska. 1993. Lupin alkaloids and their role in animal nutrition. In *Recent Advances of Research in Antinutritional Factors in Legume Seeds*, van der Poel, A. F. B., J. Huisman, and H. S. Saini, Eds., Wageningen Pers, Wageningen, The Netherlands, 343.

Hlodversson, R. 1987. The nutritive value of white- and dark-flowered cultivars of peas for growing-finishing pigs, *Anim. Feed. Sci. Technol.*, 17:245.

Huisman, J., and A. J. M. Jansman. 1991. Dietary effects and some analytical aspects of antinutritional factors in peas (*Pisum sativum*), common beans (*Phaseolus vulgaris*) and soyabeans (*Glycine max* L.) in monogastric farm animals. A literature review, *Livest. Feeds Feeding*, 61:901.

Huisman, J., A. F. B. van der Poel, P. van Leeuwen, M. W. A. Verstegen. 1990. Comparison of growth, nitrogen metabolism and organ weights in piglets and rats fed on diets containing *Phaseolus vulgaris* beans, *Br. J. Nutr.*, 64:743.

Jaikaran, S., S. K. Baidoo, and F. X. Aherne. 1995. Methionine supplementation of grower and finisher swine diets containing two varieties of field peas, *J. Anim. Sci.*, 73(Suppl. 1):312.

Jansman, A. J. M., J. Huisman, and A. F. B. van der Poel. 1989. Faba beans with different tannin contents: ileal and faecal digestibility in piglets and growth in chicks. In *Recent Advances of Research on Antinutritional Factors in Legume Seeds*, Huisman, J., A. F. B. van der Poel, and I. E. Liener, Eds., Pudoc, Wageningen, The Netherlands, 176.

Kachare, D. P., J. K. Chavan, and S. S. Kadam. 1988. Nutritional quality of some improved cultivars of cowpea, *Plant Foods Hum. Nutr.*, 38:155.

Kehoe, C., S. Jaikaran, S. K. Baidoo, and F. X. Aherne. 1995. Evaluation of field peas as a protein supplement in diets for weaned pigs, *J. Anim. Sci.*, 73(Suppl. 1):313.

Kephart, K. B., and G. W. Sheritt. 1990. Performance and nutrient balance in growing swine fed low-protein diets supplemented with amino acids and potassium, *J. Anim. Sci.*, 68:1999.

Kephart, K. B., G. R. Hollis, and D. M. Danielson. 1998. Forages for swine, in *Pork Industry Handbook*, No. 126, Coop. Ext. Ser., Purdue University, West Lafayette, IN.

Kerr, B. J., F. K. McKeith, and R. A. Easter. 1995. Effect on performance and carcass characteristics of nursery to finisher pigs fed reduced crude protein, amino acid-supplemented diets, *J. Anim. Sci.*, 73:433.

Kerr, C. A., R. D. Goodband, J. W. Smith II, R. E. Musser, J. R. Bergstrom, W. B. Nessmith, Jr., M. D. Tokach, and J. L. Nelssen. 1998. Evaluation of potato proteins on the growth performance of early-weaned pigs, *J. Anim. Sci.*, 76:3024.

King, R. H. 1990. Lupins. In *Nontraditional Feed Sources for Use in Swine Production*, Thacker, P. A., and R. N. Kirkwood, Eds., Butterworths, Stoneham, MA, 237 pp.

Kornegay, E. T., G. W. Van der Noot, K. M. Barth, G. Graber, W. S. MaGrath, R. L. Gilbreath, and F. J. Bielk. 1970. Nutritive evaluation of garbage as a feed for swine, New Jersey Exp. Sta. Bull. No. 829, Rutgers University, New Brunswick.

Lallo, H. O. C., R. Singh, A. A. Donawa, and G. Madoo. 1997. The ensiling of poultry offal with sugarcane molasses and *Lactobacillus* culture for feeding to growing/finishing pigs under tropical conditions, *Anim. Feed Sci. Technol.*, 67:213.

Lawrence, B. V., O. Adeola, and J. C. Rogler. 1995. Nutrient digestibility and growth performance of pigs fed pearl millet as a replacement for corn, *J. Anim. Sci.*, 73:2026.

Lee, P., and R. Crawshaw. 1991. Molassed sugar beet feed for pigs, *Br. Sugar Beet Rev.*, 59(2):57.

Leibbrandt, V. D., and N. J. Benevenga. 1991. Utilization of liquid whey in feeding swine. In *Swine Nutrition*, Miller, E. R., D. E. Ulrey, and A. J. Lewis, Eds., Butterworth-Heinemann, Stoneham, MA, 559.

Leterme, P., A. Thewis, and F. Tahona. 1991. Nutritive value of triticale in pigs as a function of its chemical composition. In *Proc. Second Int. Triticale Symp.*, CIMMYT, D.F., Mexico, 442.

Liener, I. E. 1976. Legume toxins in relation to protein digestibility — a review, *J. Food Sci.*, 41:1076.

Liu, Y. G., A. Steg, B. Smits, and S. Tamminga. 1994. Crambe meal: removal of glucosinolates by heating with additives and water extraction, *Anim. Feed. Sci. Technol.*, 48:273.

Loeza, R., D. H. Beemann, X. G. Lei, K. Roneker, and R. W. Blake. 1997. Effect of cane molasses in diets for finishing pigs, *J. Anim. Sci.*, 75(Suppl 1):129.

Longland, A. C., and A. G. Low. 1989. Digestion of diets containing molassed or plain sugar-beet pulp for growing pigs, *Anim. Feed Sci. Technol.*, 23:67.

Longland, A. C., and A. G. Low. 1990. Sugar beet. In *Nontraditional Feed Sources for Use in Swine Production*, Thacker, P. A., and R. N. Kirkwood Eds., Butterworths, Stoneham, MA, 453.

Ma, Y., and F. A. Bliss. 1978. Tannin content and inheritance in common bean, *Crop Sci.*, 18:201.

Machin, D. H., D. E. Silverside, D. A. Hector, and W. H. Parr. 1986. The utilisation by growing pigs of ruminant offal hydrolised in formic acid, *Anim. Feed. Sci. Technol.*, 15:273.

Marquardt, R. R. 1989. Dietary effects of tannins, vicine, and convicine. In *Recent Advances of Research on Antinutritional Factors in Legume Seeds*, Huisman, J., A. F. B. van der Poel, and I. E. Liener, Eds., Pudoc, Wageningen, The Netherlands, 141.

Marquardt, R. R., and J. M. Bell. 1988. Future potential of pulses for use in animal feeds. In *World Crops: Cool Season Food Legumes*, Summerfield, R. J., Ed., Kluwer, London, U.K., 421.

Maxwell, C. V. 1990. Mung beans. In *Nontraditional Feed Sources for Use in Swine Production*, Thacker, P. A., and R. N. Kirkwood, Eds., Butterworths, Stoneham, MA, 255.

McNaughton, E. P., R. O. Ball, and R. M. Friendship. 1997. The effects of feeding a chocolate product on growth performance and meat quality of finishing swine, *Can. J. Anim. Sci.*, 77:1.

Mederos, C. M., V. Figueroa, A. Garcia, and L. M. Mora. 1989. Different substitution levels of maize by sugar cane high-test molasses in diets for weaned pigs, *Arch. Anim. Nutr.*, 39:715.

Mena, A. 1988. Sugarcane juice as animal feed: an overview. In *Sugarcane as Feed*, Sansoucy, R., G. Aarts, and T. R. Preston, Eds., FAO Animal Production and Health Paper No. 72, FAO, Rome, Italy.

Michal, J. J., M. S. Han, J. A. Froseth, and C. E. Hostetler. 1995. Substitution of a dehydrated potato by-product for barley and corn in starter and grower pig diets, *J. Anim. Sci.*, 73(Suppl. 1):311.

Michal, J. J., J. A. Froseth, N. O. Ankrah, and C. E. Hostetler. 1996. Substitution of yellow peas for soybean meal in complex nursery pig diets, *J. Anim. Sci.*, 74(Suppl. 1):195.

Miller, E. R., P. J. Holden, and V. D. Leibbrandt. 1987. By-products in swine diets. In *Pork Industry Handbook*, No. 108, Coop. Ext. Serv., Purdue University, West Lafayette, IN.

Motta, M., M. A. Esnaola, B. Murillo, and A. Gernat. 1994. Ad-lib sugar cane juice supplemented with different levels of protein for growing and finishing pigs, *J. Anim. Sci.*, 72(Suppl. 1):99.

Myer, R. O. 1998. Evaluation of triticale in nursery diets for early weaned pigs. In *Proc. Fourth Int. Triticale Symp.* (Vol. I), Huskiw, P., Ed., Alberta Agriculture, Food and Rural Development Center, Lacombe, Canada, 196.

Myer, R. O., and J. A. Froseth. 1978. Methionine supplementation and processing of cull peas for swine, *Proc. West. Sec. Amer. Soc. Anim. Sci.*, 29:182.

Myer, R. O., and J. A. Froseth. 1983. Heat processed small red beans (*Phaseolus vulgaris*) in diets for young pigs, *J. Anim. Sci.*, 56:1088.

Myer, R. O., and J. A. Froseth. 1993. Evaluation of two methods of heat processing for improving the nutritional value of peas for swine. In *Recent Advances of Research in Antinutritional Factors in Legume Seeds*, van der Poel, A. F. B., J. Huisman, and H. S. Saini, Eds., Wageningen Pers, Wageningen, The Netherlands, 441.

Myer, R. O., and D. W. Gorbet. 1998. Raw cull (oil stock) peanuts as a fat source in diets for swine, *Proc. Soil and Crop Sci. Soc. Fla.*, 57:92.

Myer, R. O., and J. A. Froseth, and C. N. Coon. 1982. Protein utilization and toxic effects of raw beans (*Phaseolus vulgaris*) for young pigs, *J. Anim. Sci.*, 55:1087.

Myer, R. O., G. E. Combs, and R. D. Barnett. 1990a. Evaluation of three triticale cultivars as potential feed grains for swine, *Proc. Soil Crop Sci. Soc. Fla.*, 49:155.

Myer, R. O., D. D. Johnson, W. S. Otwell, W. R. Walker, and G. E. Combs. 1990b. Evaluation of scallop viscera silage as a high-protein feedstuff for growing-finishing swine, *Anim. Feed Sci. Technol.*, 31:43.

Myer, R. O., J. W. Lamkey, W. R. Walker, J. H. Brendemuhl, and G. E. Combs. 1992. Performance and carcass characteristics of swine when fed diets containing canola oil and added copper to alter the unsaturated:saturated ratio of pork fat, *J. Anim. Sci.*, 70:1417.

Myer, R. O., J. H. Brendemuhl, and R. D. Barnett. 1996. Crystalline lysine and threonine supplementation of soft red winter wheat or triticale, low-protein diets for growing-finishing swine, *J. Anim. Sci.*, 74:577.

Myer, R. O., J. H. Brendemuhl, and D. D. Johnson. 1999. Evaluation of dehydrated restaurant food waste products as feedstuffs for finishing pigs, *J. Anim. Sci.*, 77:685.

Nessmith, W. B., Jr., M. D. Tokach, R. D. Goodband, J. L. Nelssen, J. R. Bergstrom, J. W. Smith II, K. Q. Owen, and B. T. Richert. 1995. The effects of substituting spray-dried whole egg from grading plants only for spray-dried animal plasma in phase I diets, *J. Anim. Sci.*, 73(Suppl. 1):171.

Nestares, T., M. Lopez-Frias, M. Barrionuev, and G. Urbano. 1996. Nutritional assessment of raw and processed chickpea (*Cicer arietinum* L.) protein in growing rats, *J. Agric. Food Chem.*, 44(9):2760.

Newton, G. L., O. M. Hale, and K. D. Haydon. 1990. Peanut kernels. In *Nontraditional Feed Sources for Use in Swine Production*, Thacker, P. A., and R. N. Kirkwood, Eds., Butterworths, Stoneham, MA, 285.

NRC. 1973. *Alternative Sources of Protein for Animal Production*, National Academy Press, Washington, D.C.

NRC. 1982. *United States — Canadian Tables of Feed Composition*, 3rd ed., National Academy Press, Washington, D.C.

NRC. 1989. *Triticale: A Promising Addition to the World's Cereal Grains*, National Academy Press, Washington, D.C.

NRC. 1998. *Nutrient Requirements of Swine*, 10th ed., National Academy Press, Washington, D.C.

Nwokolo, E. 1990a. Sweet potato. In *Nontraditional Feed Sources for Use in Swine Production*, Thacker, P. A., and R. N. Kirkwood, Eds., Butterworths, Stoneham, MA, 481.

Nwokolo, E. 1990b. Rubber seeds, oil and meal. In *Nontraditional Feed Sources for Use in Swine Production*, Thacker, P. A., and R. N. Kirkwood, Eds., Butterworths, Stoneham, MA, 355.

O'Doherty, J. V. 1996. The effects of extrusion on the nutritive value of peas for pigs, *J. Anim. Sci.*, 74(Suppl. 1):176.

Oke, O. L. 1990. Cassava meal. In *Nontraditional Feed Sources for Use in Swine Production*, Thacker, P. A., and R. N. Kirkwood, Eds., Butterworths, Stoneham, MA, 103.

Okeke, G. C., P. C. Obioha, and A. E. Udeagu. 1985. Processing of cassava, *Nutr. Rep. Int.*, 32:139.

Paula, G. M. F., J. L. Donzele, H. V. Melo, P. M. A. Costa, and M. L. Tafuri. 1994. Sugar cane juice as a source of energy for pregnant gilts, *Rev. Soc. Bras. Zootec.*, 23(4):623.

Perez, R. 1997. Feeding pigs in the tropics, FAO Animal Production and Health Paper No. 132, FAO, Rome, Italy.

Pond, W. G., and J. H. Maner. 1984. *Swine Production and Nutrition*, AVI Publishing, Westport, CT.

Pusztai, A. 1989. Biological effects of dietary lectins. In *Recent Advances of Research in Antinutritional Factors in Legume Seeds*, Huisman, J., A. F. B. van der Poel and I. E. Liener, Eds., Pudoc, Wageningen, The Netherlands, 17.

Raa, J., and A. Gildberg. 1982. Fish silage: a review, *CRC Crit. Rev. Food Sci. Nutr.*, 16:383.

Ragland, D., C. R. Thomas, B. G. Harmon, R. Miller, and O. Adeola. 1998. Nutritional evaluation of two agroindustrial by-products for ducks and pigs, *J. Anim. Sci.*, 76:2845.

Rahnema, S., M. A. Barrieklow, R. H. Ellis, and T. Meek. 1997. Potato chip scrap as a source of energy in the diet of nursery pigs, *J. Anim. Sci.*, 75(Suppl. 1):58.

Rantanen, M. M., R. H. Hines, J. D. Hancock, K. C. Behnke, M. R. Cabrera, and I. H. Kim. 1995. Effects of novel carbohydrate sources on growth performance of nursery pigs, *J. Anim. Sci.*, 73(Suppl. 1):179.

Ravindran, V. 1990a. Bananas. In *Nontraditional Feed Sources for Use in Swine Production*, Thacker, P. A., and R. N. Kirkwood, Eds., Butterworths, Stoneham, MA, 13.

Ravindran, V. 1990b. Minor oilseed meals. In *Nontraditional Feed Sources for Use in Swine Production*, Thacker, P. A., and R. N. Kirkwood, Eds., Butterworths, Stoneham, MA, 247.

Ravindran, V. 1995. Use of cassava and sweet potatoes in animal feeding, FAO Better Farming Series No. 46, FAO, Rome, Italy.

Reddy, N. R., M. D. Pierson, S. K Sathe, and D. K. Salunkhe. 1985. Dry bean tannins: a review of nutritional implications, *J. Am. Oil Chem. Soc.*, 62(3):541.

Rhule, S. W. A. 1996. Growth rate and carcass characteristics of pigs fed on diets containing palm kernel cake, *Anim. Feed Sci. Technol.*, 61:167.

Rodriguez, J. P., and H. S. Bayley. 1987. Steam-heated culled beans: nutritional value and digestibility for swine, *Can. J. Anim. Sci.*, 67:803.

Rodriguez, M. L., L. T. Ortiz, J. Trevino, A. Rebole, C. Alzueta, and C. Centeno. 1998. Studies on the nutritive value of full-fat sunflower seed in broiler chick diets, *Anim. Feed Sci. Technol.*, 71:341.

Savage, G. P. 1988. The composition and nutritive value of lentils (*Lens culinaris*), *Can. J. Anim. Sci.*, 58:319.

Savage, G. P., and D. R. Thompson. 1993. Effect of processing on the trypsin inhibitor content and nutritive value of chickpea (*Cicer arietnum*). In *Recent Advances of Research in Antinutritional Factors in Legume Seeds*, van der Poel, A. F. B., J. Huisman, and H. S. Saini, Eds., Wageningen Pers, Wageningen, The Netherlands, 435.

Smith, J. W., II, P. R. O'Quinn, R. D. Goodband, M. D. Tokach, and J. L. Nelssen. 1999. Effects of low-protein, amino acid-fortified diets formulated on a net energy basis on growth performance and carcass characteristics of finishing pigs, *J. Appl. Anim. Res.*, 15:1.

Solis, J. E., C. Campabadal, and J. R. Molina. 1988. Estimation of optimum initial weight for feeding pigs on ripe bananas, *Agron. Costarricense,* 12(2):209.

Speedy, A. W., L. Seward, N. Langton, J. Du Plessis, and B. Dlamini. 1991. A comparison of sugarcane juice and maize as energy sources in diets for growing pigs with equal supply of essential amino acids, *Livest. Res. Rural Dev.*, 3(1):65.

Tewe, O. 1994. Indices of cassava safety for livestock feeding. International Workshop on Cassava Safety, Ibdan, Nigeria, *Acta Hortic.*, 375:241.

Thacker, P. A. 1990a. Fababeans. In *Nontraditional Feed Sources for Use in Swine Production*, Thacker, P. A., and R. N. Kirkwood, Eds., Butterworths, Stoneham, MA, 175.

Thacker, P. A. 1990b. Wild oat groats. In *Nontraditional Feed Sources for Use in Swine Production*, Thacker. P. A., and R. N. Kirkwood, Eds., Butterworths, Stoneham, MA, 509.

Thacker, P. A. 1998. Effect of micronization of full-fat canola seed on performance and carcass characteristics of growing-finishing pigs, *Anim. Feed Sci. Technol.*, 71:89.

Thacker, P. A., and R. N. Kirkwood. 1990. *Nontraditional Feed Sources for Use in Swine Production*, Butterworths, Stoneham, MA.

Thacker, P. A., and F. W. Sosulski. 1994. Use of wild oat groats in starter diets for swine, *Anim. Feed Sci. Technol.*, 46:229.

Tibbetts, G. W., R. W. Seerley, and H. C. McCampbell. 1987. Poultry offal ensiled with *Lactobacillus acidophilus* for growing and finishing swine diets, *J. Anim. Sci.*, 64:182.

Todorov, N. A. 1988. Cereals, pulses and oilseeds, *Livest. Prod. Sci.*, 19:47.

Tor-Agbidye, Y., S. Gelaye, S. L. Louis, and G. E. Cooper. 1990. Performance and carcass traits of growing-finishing swine fed diets containing sweet potato meal or corn, *J. Anim. Sci.*, 68:1323.

Vandepopuliere, J. M., H. K. Kanungo, H. V. Walton, and O. J. Cotterill. 1976. Broiler and egg type chick hatchery by-product meal evaluated as laying hen feedstuffs, *Poult. Sci.*, 56:1140.

van der Poel, A. F. B, J. Blonk, J. Huisman, and L. A. Den Hartog. 1991a. Effect of steam processing temperature and time on the protein nutritional value of *Phaseolus vulgaris* beans for swine, *Livest. Prod. Sci.*, 28:305.

van der Poel, A. F. B., L. M. W. Dellaert, A. van Norel, and J. P. F. G. Helsper. 1991b. The digestibility in piglets of faba bean (*Vicia faba* L.) as affected by breeding towards the absence of condensed tannins, *Br. J. Nutr.*, 68:793.

van der Poel, A. F. B., S. Gravendeel, D. J. van Kleef, A. J. M. Jansman, and B. Kemp. 1992a. Tannin-containing faba beans (*Vicia faba* L.): effects of methods of processing on ileal digestibility of protein and starch for growing pigs, *Anim. Feed Sci. Technol.*, 36:205.

van der Poel, A. F. B., W. Stolp, and D. J. van Zuilichem. 1992b. Twin-screw extrusion of two pea varieties: effects of temperature and moisture level of antinutritional factors and protein digestibility, *J. Sci. Food Agric.*, 58:83.

Van Lunen, T. A. 1990. Fish silage. In *Nontraditional Feed Sources for Use in Swine Production*, Thacker, P. A., and R. N. Kirkwood, Eds., Butterworths, Stoneham, MA, 197.

Van Lunen, T. A., and D. M. Anderson. 1990. Crab meal. In *Nontraditional Feed Sources for Use in Swine Production*, Thacker, P. A., and R. N. Kirkwood, Eds., Butterworths, Stoneham, MA, 153.

Van Lunen, T. A., D. M. Anderson, A. M. St. Laurent, J. Barclay, and J. W. G. Nicholson. 1991. The utilization of acid-preserved poultry offal by growing-finishing pigs, *Can. J. Anim. Sci.*, 71:935.

Varnghese, G. 1996. Triticale: present status and challenges ahead. In *Triticale: Today and Tomorrow*, Guedes-Pinto, H., N. Darvey, and V. P. Carnide, Eds., Kluwer Academic, Dordrecht, The Netherlands, 13.

Vidal-Valverde, C., J. Frias, C. Diaz-Pollan, M. Fernandez, M. Lopez-Jurado, and G. Urbano. 1997. Influence of processing on trypsin inhibitor activity of faba beans and its physiological effect, *J. Agric. Food Chem.*, 45:3559.

Wahlstrom, R. C. 1990. Sunflower seeds. In *Nontraditional Feed Sources for Use in Swine Production*, Thacker, P. A., and R. N. Kirkwood, Eds., Butterworths, Stoneham, MA, 473.

Warren, B. E., and D. J. Farrell. 1990. The nutritive value of full-fat and defatted Australian rice bran. 2. Growth studies with chickens, rats and pigs, *Anim. Feed Sci. Technol.*, 27:229.

Waterworth, D. G. 1990. Single cell protein. In *Nontraditional Feed Sources for Use in Swine Production*, Thacker, P. A., and R. N. Kirkwood, Eds., Butterworths, Stoneham, MA, 429.

Weder, J. K. P., L. Telek, M. Vozari-Hampe, and H. S. Saini. 1997. Antinutritional factors in anasazi and other pinto beans (*Phaseolus vulgaris* L.), *Plant Foods Human Nutr.*, 51:85.

Westendorf, M. L., E. W. Zirkel, and R. Gordon. 1996. Feeding food or table waste to livestock, *Prof. Anim. Sci.*, 12:129.

Westendorf, M. L., Z. C. Dong, and P. A. Schoknecht. 1998. Recycled cafeteria food as a feed for swine: nutrient content, digestibility, growth and meat quality, *J. Anim. Sci.*, 76:2976.

Winter, K. A., and L. A. W. Feltham. 1983. Fish silage: the protein solution, Contribution 1983–6E, Agriculture Canada, Res. Branch, Charlottetown, Prince Edward Island, Canada.

Wiryawan, K. G., H. M. Miller, and J. H. G. Holmes. 1997. Mung beans (*Phaseolus aureus*) for finishing pigs, *Anim. Feed Sci. Technol.*, 66:297.

Wohlt, J. E., J. Petro, G. M. J. Horton, R. L. Gilbreath, and S. M. Tweed. 1994. Composition, preservation, and use of sea clam viscera as a protein supplement for growing pigs, *J. Anim. Sci.*, 72:546.

Wu, J. F. 1991. Energy value of cassava for young swine, *J. Anim. Sci.*, 69:1349.

Yang, H., J. A. Kerber, J. E. Pettigrew, L. J. Johnston, and R. D. Walker. 1997. Evaluation of milk chocolate product as a substitute for whey in pig starter diets, *J. Anim. Sci.*, 75:423.

Zdunczyk, Z., J. Juskiewicz, S. Frejnagel, and K. Gulewicz. 1997. Influence of alkaloids and oligosaccharides from white lupin seeds on utilization of diets by rats and absorption of nutrients in the small intestine, *Anim. Feed Sci. Technol.*, 72:143.

Part VI

Techniques in Swine Nutrition Research

38 Swine Modeling

Phillip S. Miller and Christopher C. Calvert

CONTENTS

I. Introduction 867
    A. Why Use Modeling...867
    B. Models Are Not Just for Mathematicians 868
    C. Model Classifications and Definitions..868
II. Description of Models with Specific Application to Swine Nutrition 870
    A. Swine Simulation Models...872
        1. Simulation of Energy and Amino Acid Utilization in the Pig.......................872
        2. Lactating Sow Metabolism Model..873
        3. Computer Simulation Model of Swine Production Systems 875
III. Future of Swine Modeling...877
    A. Barriers 877
    B. Advantages 877
    C. How Will Swine Nutritionists Benefit? 877
IV. Conclusions 878
References 878

I. INTRODUCTION

Models represent the understanding of a biological, production, and/or economic concept. Models can be represented simply with diagrams or a series of mathematical equations. Clearly, the objectives of the modeling experience vary dramatically and ultimately control the impact of the exercise. All models and modeling exercises described in this chapter are based (in some part) on the understanding of biological processes involved in pig production and how the description of biology is applied to swine production (Figure 38.1). It is not surprising that significant discussions have been generated, and will continue to be generated, regarding the "level of science" required to describe adequately growth, pregnancy, and lactation in the pig. The objective of this chapter is to explain some of the quantitative methods used to describe biological and nutritional impacts on swine production. For more-detailed discussions of biological modeling, the reader is encouraged to consult the following references: France and Thornley (1984), Whittemore (1986), Baldwin (1995), and Black (1995).

A. Why Use Modeling

There are existing models that predict pig performance well. Borrowing from Baldwin's modeling text (Baldwin, 1995), Box (1979) made the statement, "All models are wrong, but some are useful." In general, the developers of models have worthy objectives; however, the degree to which models use underlying biological phenomena to describe how nutrients are used for growth and reproduction varies significantly. Ultimately, models simplify the processes they describe, but, unfortunately, the

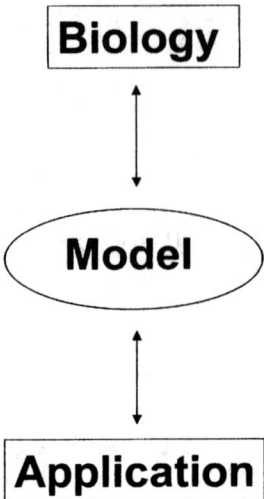

FIGURE 38.1 The application of biological concepts using models.

equations and technology used to implement models can be complicated. However, the potential degree of complexity is no reason to abandon the process (modeling exercise). Models can be the means by which knowledge of physiology and metabolism gained through studies of organ and cell function can be utilized to advance quantitative understanding of animal functions, sources of variation in animal performance, and, finally, effective utilization of this knowledge can help develop optimal animal production strategies.

There is a common tendency to identify which model is the best based on precision or accuracy, or the level of underlying mechanisms introduced and the model complexity; however, a simple model that describes reality is superior to complex models that confuse scientists. Model complexity must be justified in terms of the need for additional explanatory elements (i.e., the previous version did not predict pig performance) rather than, this level of complexity exists; therefore, it should be included in the model. Different models serve different purposes. The utility of a model can only be evaluated in the context of the modeling objectives. Therefore, some models are closely linked to research, whereas others can be applied directly to production settings.

B. Models Are Not Just for Mathematicians

Models are not constructed initially based on mathematical arguments. Biological concepts can be described mathematically, but are not, in themselves, mathematically derived. All models start with a plan or a road map (block diagram) that must be designed before equation forms can be discussed, or developed. Figure 38.2 represents the block diagram of a model of lactating sow metabolism (Pettigrew, 1992a). Although the equations describing the fluxes into and out of the various pools (state variables) are complex (see subsequent section), the block diagram helps capture the underlying mechanisms of the system. The block diagram does not require an extensive understanding of mathematics, but rather an understanding or knowledge of the system of interest.

C. Model Classifications and Definitions

Clearly, a great deal of swine nutrition research has been conducted using the model described in Figure 38.3. Classical input:output experiments cannot define and, indeed, do not lead to identification of the sources of variance in efficiencies of animal production. The limitation of this approach is that the inference space or potential for application is limited to the range of inputs used to define the

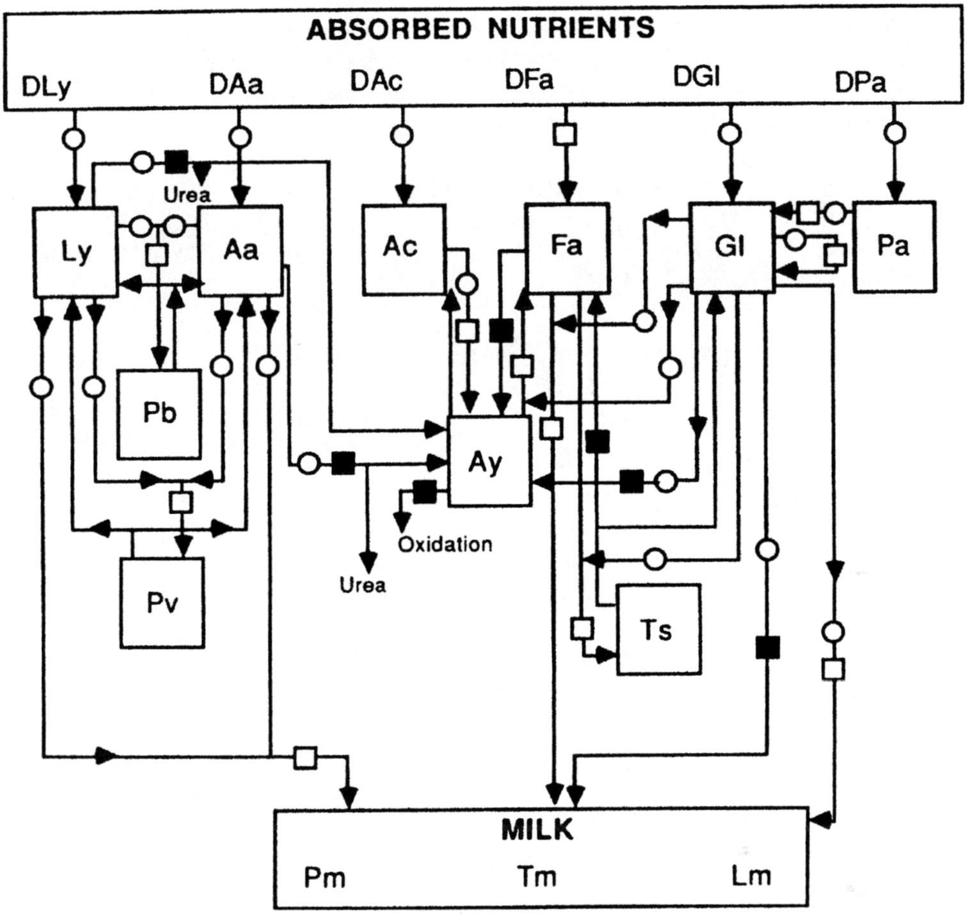

FIGURE 38.2 Schematic representation of a sow lactation model. State variables shown are lysine (Ly); other amino acids (Aa); acetic acid (Ac); fatty acids (Fa); glucose (Gl); propionic acid (Pa); acetyl-coenzyme A (Ay); protein in lean body (Pb); protein in viscera (Pv); storage triacylglycerol (Ts); and milk protein (Tm), fat (Tm), and lactose (Lm). Fluxes requiring/yielding adenosine triphosphate (ATP) indicated by □ (uses ATP in transport), ○ (uses ATP in reaction), and ■ (produces ATP in reaction). From Pettigrew, J. E. et al., *J. Anim. Sci.*, 70:3742, 1992. Reprinted with permission from the *Journal of Animal Science*.

model. Therefore, these models are referred to as *empirical-static models*. Empirical refers to developing equations that "best fit" the data. Often the parameters are estimated using statistical linear or nonlinear methods. In contrast, *mechanistic models* employ equation forms that provide insight into the biology of the process. A *static model* does not incorporate time as an implicit variable in the equations. On the other hand, *dynamic models* contain time as a variable in the equations. In addition, a model can provide an exact prediction or answer (*deterministic*) or output values can be associated

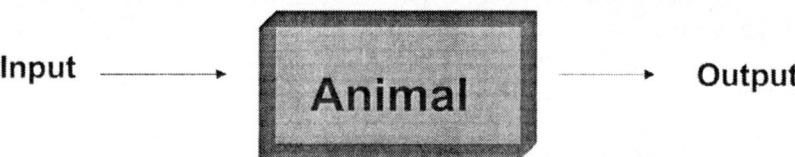

FIGURE 38.3 Input:output approach. This model views the animal (pig) as a "black box."

with a specific variance (stochastic). The variance of the output values are a function of the degree of probability associated with the equations in the model. The reader is encouraged to consult France and Thornley (1984) for an expanded description of model types and definitions.

The diagram represented in Figure 38.3 can be described mathematically according to the following differential equation:

$$d(\text{animal wt})/d(\text{time}) = \text{inputs} - \text{outputs} \tag{38.1}$$

The level of complexity describing the utilization of inputs (nutrient/energy intake) and the production of outputs can vary from:

$$d(\text{protein})/d(\text{time}) = \text{synthesis} - \text{degradation} \tag{38.2}$$

$$= \underbrace{(V_{max}/(1 + (K_s/(\text{amino acid}))))}_{(\textit{Michaelis–Menten kinetics})} - \underbrace{(\text{protein pool} \cdot K_d)}_{(\textit{Mass Action kinetics})} \tag{38.3}$$

where
- V_{max} = maximum velocity of protein synthesis
- K_s = amino acid concentration at which protein synthesis = $V_{max}/2$ (affinity constant)
- K_d = degradation rate concentration, to

$$d(\text{animal wt})/d(\text{time}) = Ae^{-kt}, \tag{38.4}$$

- A = constant
- k = rate constant
- t = time

Thus, the reader can appreciate that fitting differential equations ($d(\text{pool})/dt$) to a block diagram similar to the one represented in Figure 38.2 is an extensive endeavor. It is easy to see why static, empirical, deterministic models have been extensively used. There are a multitude of equation forms that can be used, all of which require parameterization (i.e., V_{max}, K_s, and K_d must be assigned unique and defendable values). Therefore, models can take on a number of forms and considerable time could be spent debating the utility of each approach; however, the focus of this chapter is to review past and current efforts in swine nutrition models.

II. DESCRIPTION OF MODELS WITH SPECIFIC APPLICATION TO SWINE NUTRITION

The deposition of muscle in the growing pig has been studied extensively (Campbell et al., 1984; Kerr, 1993; Bikker et al., 1994). Because the majority of pig marketing systems are based on the amount of lean in the carcass, the rate of lean growth and ultimate accumulation of muscle is critical to the pork producer. In addition to the pig's genetic potential to deposit lean, environmental effects (including nutrition) play a major role.

A number of approaches have been developed to model lean growth in the pig (Whittemore et al., 1988; Moughan, 1995; Schinckel et al., 1996). Schinckel and de Lange (1996) in their review described an approach (adopted from Whittemore et al., 1988) to estimate protein accretion (g/day, $d(\text{Pr})/dt$) using the following equation:

$$d(\text{Pr})/dt = d(\text{Wt})/dt \cdot d(\text{Pr})/d(\text{Wt}) \tag{38.5}$$

$d(\mathrm{Wt})/dt$ can be estimated using a number of different growth curve equations and $d(\mathrm{Pr})/d(\mathrm{Wt})$ can be estimated using an allometric function (e.g., $Y = aX^b$). Alternatively, protein accretion can be fit using the equation (Schinckel et al., 1996):

$$(d(\mathrm{Pr}))/(dt) = A + e^{(B \bullet \mathrm{Wt} + C/\mathrm{Wt} + D \bullet \mathrm{Wt}^2)} \qquad (38.6)$$

where A, B, C, and D are parameters and Wt is live weight in kilograms. Most important, is the behavior/shape of the lean-growth curve (Figure 38.4). Clearly, the work of Schinckel and others has highlighted the pattern of the lean-growth curve. In the recent National Research Council *Nutrient Requirements of Swine* (NRC, 1998), the lean-growth (fat-free lean; protein accretion) curve is used as the driving factor determining lysine (amino acid) requirements and ultimately the requirements for other nutrients. The reader is encouraged to review NRC (1998) for a complete description of the model (gestation and lactation models are also included). For reference, this model is considered to be empirical, static, and deterministic. The user is able to control inputs (e.g., temperature, space, and dietary energy concentration that may affect nutrient needs and feed intake). For the reader's reference, the screen for the growth program is provided in Figure 38.5.

The NRC model provides a flexible and progressive method to describe swine nutrient requirements. Using this interactive simulation model, with which the user can describe hundreds of different input scenarios, is superior to the previous approach of using "tables" to determine nutrient requirements for pigs. Although this recent version of the NRC nutrient requirements for swine is considerably more powerful than previous versions, several points of caution are provided:

1. The reader/user should be familiar with the assumptions underlying calculations of daily lysine requirements from lean-growth curves.
2. The program predicts nutrient requirements based on user inputs. For example, the requirements predicted by the model are a direct function of the adequacy of the protein accretion/fat-free lean-growth curve input to the model.

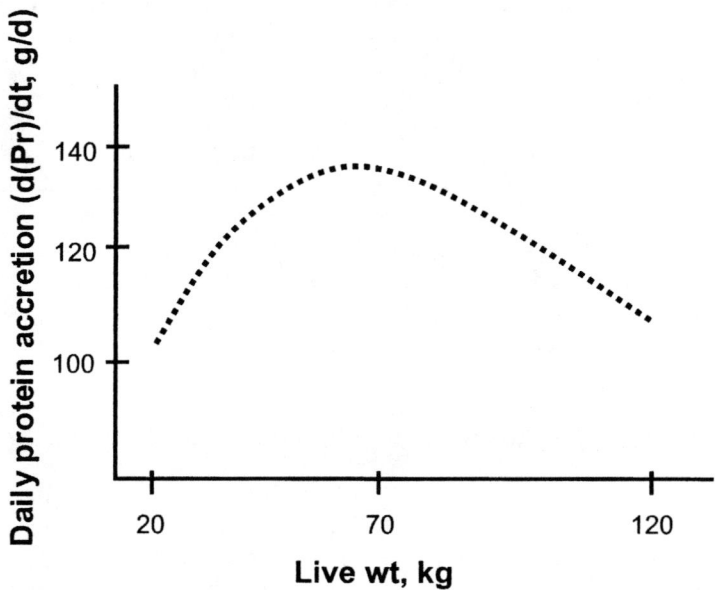

FIGURE 38.4 Example of a protein accretion vs. weight profile for growing-finishing pigs. (Adapted from NRC, 1998.)

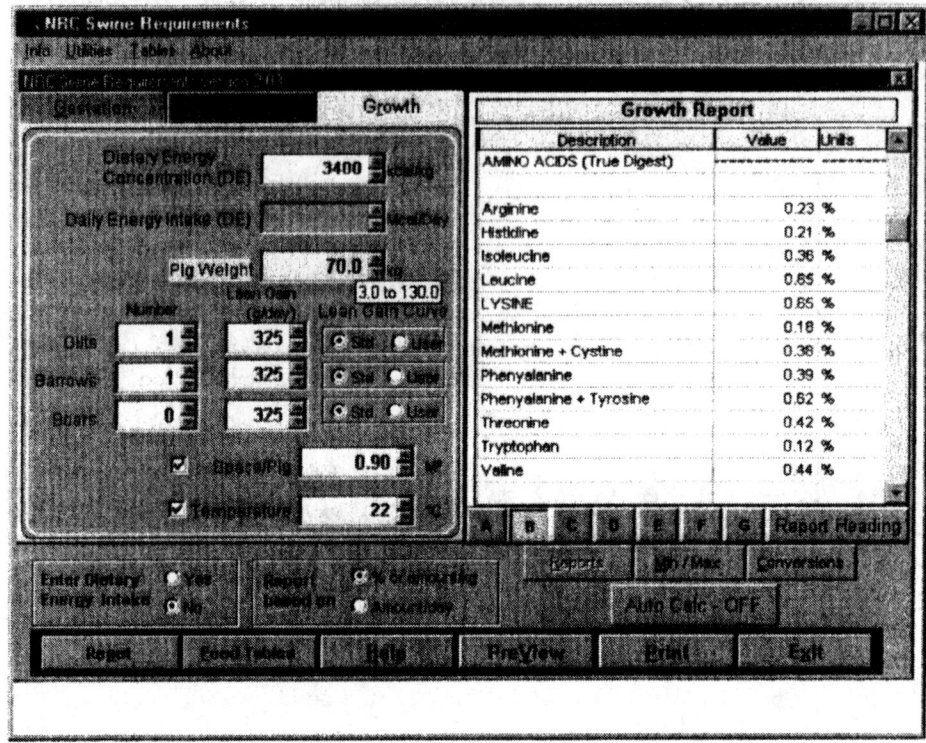

FIGURE 38.5 Screen for the NRC (1998) growth program. (From NRC, *Nutrient Requirements of Swine*, 10th ed., National Academy Press, Washington, D.C., 1998. With permission.)

3. Because only 40 to 50% of the variation in growth performance can be attributed to genetic effects (Hutchens and Hintz, 1981), other factors not considered by the model (e.g., animal interactions, disease, and other environmental stressors) may have pronounced effects on nutrient requirements, which cannot be predicted by the model.

A. Swine Simulation Models

In addition to the NRC growth model to predict swine nutrient requirements, a number of models have been developed to address how nutritional, environmental, and genetic variables affect pig and sow performance (Whittemore and Fawcett, 1976; Tess et al., 1983; Black et al., 1986; Moughan et al., 1987; Pomar et al., 1991a,b; Pettigrew et al., 1992a; Bastianelli et al., 1996). Three models will be discussed as examples in this section (those of Black et al., 1986; Pomar et al., 1991a,b,c; and Pettigrew et al., 1992a,b), but the reader is encouraged to consult other references cited above. An attempt has been made to identify unique features or principles from each of the models described.

1. Simulation of Energy and Amino Acid Utilization in the Pig

During the mid-1980s a simulation model (Black et al., 1986) was developed to predict the energy and amino acid needs of growing and reproducing pigs (gestation and lactation components are not covered here). Surprisingly, the program was originally based on a model developed for sheep (Black, 1984). The pig simulation model incorporated a number of empirical and mechanistic elements that were derived from pigs, sheep, and rats. A multitude of research from such workers as Campbell (Campbell et al., 1975; 1985), King (King et al., 1984; King and Dunkin, 1986), Close (Close and

Mount, 1978; Close and Stanier, 1984), and Mount (Mount, 1963; 1977), to name a few, helped provide the basis for model development and description, and evaluation of model behavior.

Feed intake, specifically nutrient needs, are determined from the estimated capacity to utilize nutrients. The biological needs for amino acids and energy drive feed intake; however, a provision is included within the model to predict feed intake. Estimates of feed intake are predicted from knowledge of the efficiency of the conversion of digestible energy (DE) to metabolizable energy (ME) and an estimate of digestibility. Thus, the pig's ME needs for

$$\text{maintenance + body growth + maintaining body temperature} \tag{38.7}$$

are used to calculate feed intake. Because environment plays a major role in affecting feed intake, equations were acquired from the literature that could be used to describe how energy is transferred between the pig and environment (see Bruce and Clark, 1979).

The amino acid requirements for growth are estimated by first predicting the potential rates of nitrogen (protein) deposition. The general equation form used to predict the potential rate of nitrogen deposition is:

$$\text{N retention, g/day} = k \cdot \text{Wt} \cdot ((N_{max} - N_t)/N_{max}) \tag{38.8}$$

where k, N_t, and N_{max} are the parameters describing the maximal rate of protein accretion, amount of nitrogen in the body at time t, and maximal amount of nitrogen in the body at maturity, respectively. The shape of this nitrogen retention curve is similar to the curve depicted for the relationship developed from the research of Schinckel et al. (1996; see Figure 38.4). However, the approach is different inasmuch as the rate of nitrogen deposition (at any specific time) is driven by the potential relative to the capacity to deposit nitrogen ($N_{max} - N_t$). Also, care must be taken in estimating the parameters k and N_{max}. Parameter estimates will differ or potentially differ for each genetic population of interest. There are other key factors that affect the maximal rate of nitrogen deposition. Specifically, the equation parameters used to predict the rate of nitrogen deposition are regulated by amino acid intake/balance, energy intake, sex, and stage of growth. These relationships were developed in part from the classical studies of Campbell et al. (1975), Dunkin et al. (1984), and Campbell et al. (1985).

The representation of how the model approached describing nitrogen retention in relation to body weight and ME intake is provided in Figure 38.6. The response of nitrogen retention to ME intake follows the two-slope model; however, because additional affecters can be considered simultaneously using this computer model, the response of nitrogen accretion vs. ME intake vs. body weight can be considered. The efficiency (Δ protein gain/Δ ME intake) of protein deposition relative to energy intake decreases as the pig develops from birth to market weight. In addition, the maximum rate of protein deposition follows a pattern similar to that depicted in Figure 38.4. Therefore, a distinct advantage of this modeling exercise (and others) is the ability to consider simultaneously multiple input variables when evaluating a particular output variable. The adjustment of how energy intake affects nitrogen retention (protein deposition) at various body weights was used in the current NRC (1998) model describing nutrient requirements of swine.

Although this model contains empirical as well as mechanistic elements, it did significantly build on the development of the system describing pig growth (e.g., describing patterns of lean growth and the effects of the physical environment on pig production). Thus, this model represented a substantial improvement in predicting swine growth compared with the factorial approaches commonly used previously.

2. Lactating Sow Metabolism Model

Pettigrew and co-workers (1992a,b) developed and evaluated a dynamic–mechanistic–deterministic model integrating energy and amino acid metabolism of the lactating sow. The concepts embodied

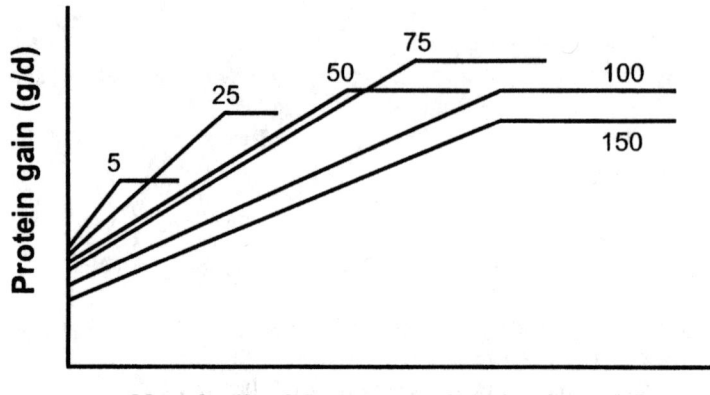

FIGURE 38.6 Protein accretion rate vs. energy intake at various body weights. Values shown refer to body weight (kg). (Adapted from Black et al., 1986.)

in the model are similar to those in the lactating cow model developed by Baldwin et al. (1987). The objective of this modeling exercise was to develop a mathematical model that represented the quantitative relationships between the metabolism of absorbed nutrients and milk production in the sow. A block diagram of the model is presented in Figure 38.2. The pools are represented by boxes, and transactions from pools are depicted with arrows. A simplified example of how rates entering and leaving pools in Figure 38.2 is depicted in Figure 38.7 and can be described according to the following differential equation:

$$d(\text{Pool } A)/dt = \text{Flux } A_1 - \text{Flux } A_2 \tag{38.9}$$

$$\text{Pool } A \text{ (at time } = t) = \int \text{Flux } A_1 - \text{Flux } A_2 \, dt \tag{38.10}$$

and (for example)

$$\text{Flux } A_1 = V/[1 + [k_1/S_1]\theta_1 + [k_2/S_2]\theta_2 + [I_3/J_3]\theta_3] \tag{38.11}$$

where
- V = maximum velocity per unit of Pool A
- k_1, k_2 = affinity constants for substrates
- S_1, S_2 = concentrations of substrates
- $\theta_1, \theta_2, \theta_3$ = steepness parameters, which help control the sensitivity of reactions within the physiological range of substrate concentrations
- I_3 = inhibitor concentration
- J_3 = inhibition constant

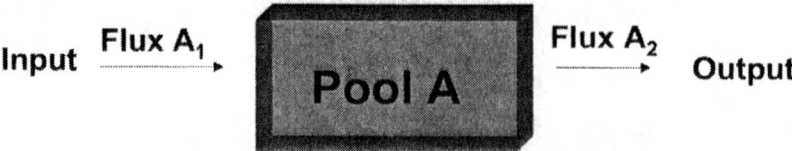

FIGURE 38.7 Block diagram of input and output fluxes for the hypothetical pool A.

$$\text{Flux } A_2 = k_3 \cdot S_A, \qquad (38.12)$$

where

- k_3 = affinity constant for substrate A
- S_A = concentration of substrate A

Although Equation 38.11 is provided as an example, the reader can appreciate not only the complexity of the equations used in this model, but also the data required to parameterize the equations. There must be a basis for parameterizing equations and defining model behavior. Parameter estimates are derived directly from experimental data or the literature and are often extrapolated from other species or from *in vitro* data. Therefore, as specific components of the model fail to predict reality (e.g., body protein and fat changes during lactation) additional data (preferably derived from swine) need to be acquired to reparameterize model equations.

The model performs well compared with actual performance data; however, equally important, the model highlights the lack of quantitative information describing the biochemistry and physiology of sow lactation (e.g., calculation of absorbed nutrients, predicting body protein changes during lactation, and/or changes in milk composition). Failures of the model will help identify key experiments that are needed to develop more knowledge about sow lactation (e.g., effects of circulating hormones on lactation performance). The advantage of this type of modeling exercise is that the model has the potential to apply in conditions (data inputs) outside the range of conditions used to parameterize the model.

The representation of the biology in the model is emphasized, in contrast to an attempt to identify the best "statistical" fit used in empirical models. Also, the development of this model illustrates the fundamental link of the modeling exercise to the scientific process. In this context, the model is referred to as a "research" model. The conceptual framework of the model must be challenged with existing data. This helps identify critical experiments and/or data required to refine the model. Thus, there is a cycle (scientific cycle) that continues with the advancement of the model (Figure 38.8). Model evaluation/challenge is accomplished by *direct comparison with data*, *behavior analysis* (i.e., does the biological response change appropriately according to the input variables?), and *sensitivity analysis* (do changes in key model parameters elicit changes in model pools, fluxes, or outputs?). Because of the difficulty and/or lack of data for the lactating sow, some key parameters were extrapolated from other species (e.g., ruminants or rats) or from swine in different physiological states (e.g., growth), thus increasing the potential for errors.

3. Computer Simulation Model of Swine Production Systems

Pomar and co-workers documented the development and application of a computer simulation model of swine production systems. The model incorporated theoretical elements that predicted

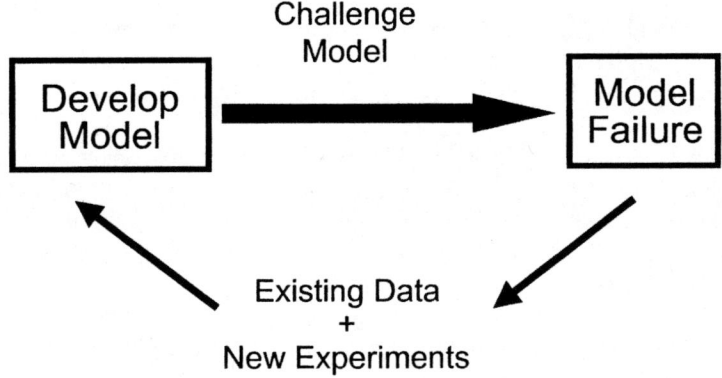

FIGURE 38.8 The scientific cycle.

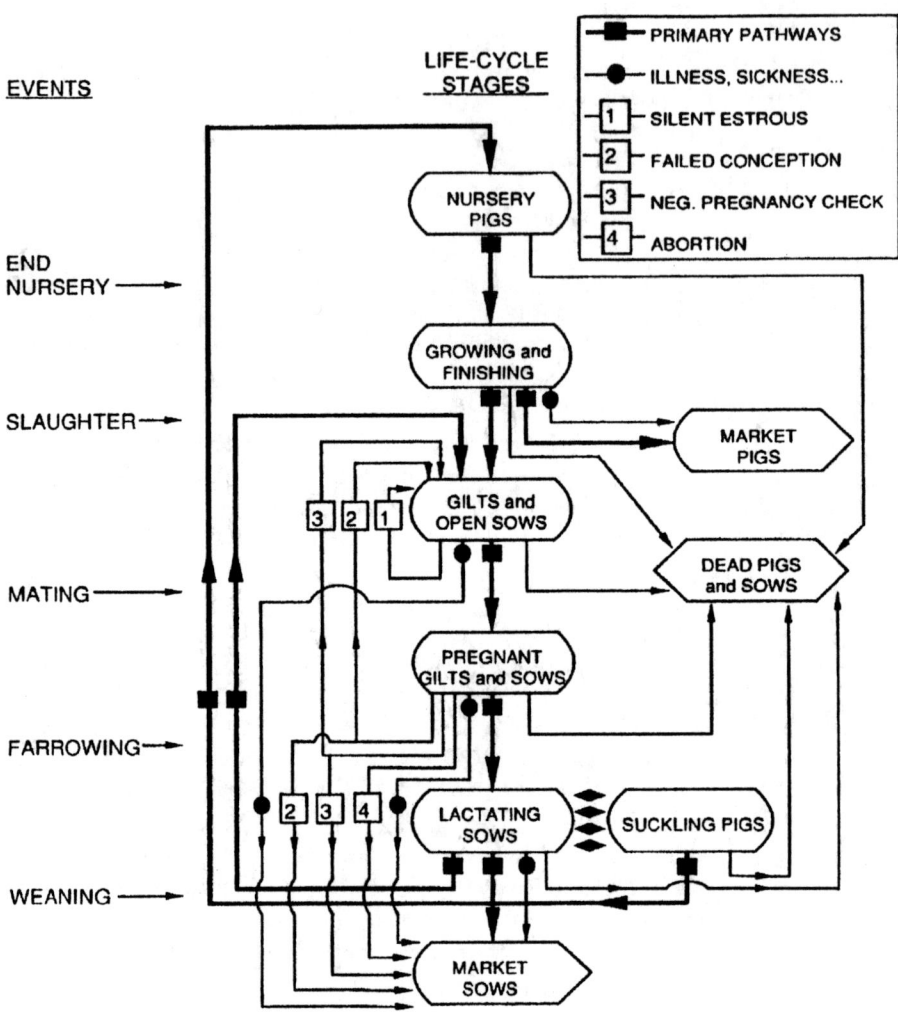

FIGURE 38.9 Diagram of animal flow through life-cycle stages and events. (From Pomar, C. et al., *J. Anim. Sci.*, 69:2822, 1991. With permission.)

pig growth and reproduction (Pomar et al., 1991a,b). Although the growth and reproduction elements of the simulation model have significant merit within the context of this chapter, the dynamic swine herd model (Pomar et al., 1991c) that describes pig movement/flow within and out of the herd is intriguing and will be highlighted. This portion of the modeling exercise incorporated deterministic, empirical, and mechanistic elements of growth and reproduction combined with stochastic components for culling and reproduction (e.g., death, mating, and conception/farrowing) to predict pig flow and dynamics within the herd. Figure 38.9 represents the flow diagram of pigs through the system. Performance and reproductive elements (e.g., gestational weight gain) are determined for individual pigs. The effects of illness/death, reproductive failure (e.g., failure to detect estrus, failed conception, or pregnancy check) randomly affect each animal using assumptions based on research literature or empirical extrapolations from the literature.

The authors have integrated key mechanistic and empirical elements of growth into a pig-flow production system. Because no data sets exist that completely define the range of inputs or the complete life cycle conditions described in the model, the model cannot be adequately challenged. However, the model did adequately predict growth and reproductive performance on an individual pig basis (Pomar et al., 1991a,b). There seem to be several potential benefits of using this approach:

1. The model contributes to explaining factors controlling pig flow within a production setting. For example, the model was able to describe the distribution of pigs within different production areas (gestation, lactation, suckling, nursery, and growing-finishing). In addition, the model predicted reproductive traits, death and culling losses, and herd output (total pig weight marketed, total protein marketed).
2. Although model accuracy and precision are relatively unchallenged, there is the potential to examine "what if?" scenarios (e.g., how will improving the rate of lean growth affect the flow of pigs through a specific production system).
3. A valuable template has been developed. Future efforts can build on the principles represented in this model. Too often, models are created, published, and returned to the shelves — never to be used or explored again.

III. FUTURE OF SWINE MODELING

A. Barriers

Knowledge of tissue and cellular nutrient utilization will need to be continually incorporated as mechanistic elements of swine simulation models. A formidable barrier to the modeling approach is that there continues to be a widening gap between production-oriented nutritionists and scientists working on the tissue, cellular, and/or molecular levels. Although the knowledge base of how nutrition affects pig performance continues to improve, little effort is being made to integrate this information into existing or new pig-production systems.

Also, there is a paucity of information available documenting how economic inputs are incorporated into swine simulation models. A number of least-cost diet formulation programs exist, but little progress has been made to evaluate how the biological/mechanistic behavior of models affect the economics of production. This is a significant limitation and must be addressed in future modeling efforts.

B. Advantages

Advantages to using a systems or modeling approach to swine nutrition/production problems exist in the context of the process. Instances where models fail to predict reality will help generate future needs for experiments and studies defining how pigs use nutrients for growth and reproduction.

Modeling should help improve understanding of swine nutrition by expanding the knowledge of how lower-level metabolism affects pig performance and, more importantly, improve the ability to describe biology quantitatively. Clearly, these models do not differ conceptually from other models that exist describing swine growth, gestation, and pregnancy. However, they do provide a distinct advantage over many models in that mathematical/computational methods are used to describe/simulate pig biology.

C. How Will Swine Nutritionists Benefit?

Qualitatively, there is an incredible amount of information describing how nutrients are supplied to the pig and digested and utilized by the pig. These relationships are extensively described for the neonate, growing-finishing, and reproducing pig. Unfortunately, outside the context of this text (and a few others), no means to integrate this information exists. For example, if a new metabolic mediator stimulating protein synthesis is discovered and described, there should be a means to determine (quantitatively) how the role of the metabolic mediator is impacted by nutritional status and physiological state, and its contribution to the overall process of growth.

The development of swine simulation models will help centralize critical information and it is hoped improve the quantitative understanding of how pigs use nutrients for growth and reproduction. Modeling will continue to help nutritionists better understand the systems they study by requiring the integration and synthesis of lower-level (e.g., cellular, molecular) mechanisms to describe whole-animal performance (e.g., daily weight gain, fat-free lean gain, feed intake, pigs weaned, etc.).

IV. CONCLUSIONS

Swine simulation models are potentially powerful tools to aid research scientists identify where critical gaps exist in the understanding of swine nutrition and physiology (Black et al., 1986; Pettigrew et al., 1992a). Also, simulation models have the potential to assist in making production decisions (Pomar et al., 1991c). Central to the potential of models to refine the scientific process and aid in production decisions will be the incorporation of advancing technologies. Promotion of the modeling approach will require a close linkage among scientists studying the pig at all levels, from the molecular to whole animal.

REFERENCES

Baldwin, R. L. 1995. *Modeling Ruminant Digestion and Metabolism*, Chapman & Hall, New York.
Baldwin, R. L., J. France, and M. Gill. 1987. Metabolism of the lactating cow. I. Animal elements of a mechanistic model, *J. Dairy Res.*, 54:77.
Bastianelli, D., D. Sauvant, and A. Rérat. 1996. Mathematical modeling of digestion and nutrient absorption of digestion and nutrient absorption in pigs, *J. Anim. Sci.*, 74:1873.
Bikker, P., M. W. A. Verstegen, and M. W. Bosch. 1994. Amino acid composition of growing pigs is affected by protein and energy intake, *J. Nutr.*, 124:1961.
Black, J. L. 1984. The integration of data for prediction of feed intake, nutrient requirements and animal performance. In *Herbivore Nutrition in the Subtropics and Tropics*, Gilchrist, I. M. C., and R. I. Mackie, Eds., Science Press, Craighall, South Africa, 648–671.
Black, J. L., R. G. Campbell, I. H. Williams, K. J. James, and G. T. Davies. 1986. Simulation of energy and amino acid utilization in the pig, *Res. Dev. Agric.*, 3:121.
Black, J. L. 1995. The evolution of animal growth models. In *Modelling Growth in the Pig*, Moughan, P. J., M. W. A. Verstegen, and M. I. Visser-Reyneveld, Eds., EAAP Publication No. 78, Wageningen Press, Wageningen, The Netherlands, 3–9.
Box, G. E. P. 1979. *Robustness in Statistics*, Academic Press, Washington, D.C., 201.
Bruce, J. M., and J. J. Clark. 1979. Models of heat production and critical temperature for growing pigs, *Anim. Prod.*, 78:353.
Campbell, R. G., M. R. Taverner, and P. D. Mullaney. 1975. The effect of dietary concentrations of digestible energy of the performance and carcass characteristics of early-weaned pigs, *Anim. Prod.*, 21:285.
Campbell, R. G., M. R. Taverner, and D. M. Curic. 1984. Effect of feeding level and dietary protein content on the growth, body composition and rate of protein deposition in pigs growing from 45 to 90 kg, *Anim. Prod.*, 38:233.
Campbell, R. G., M. R. Taverner, and D. M. Curie. 1985. The influence of feeding level on the protein requirement of pigs between 20 and 45 kg live weight, *Anim. Prod.*, 40:489.
Close, W. H., and L. E. Mount. 1978. The effects of plane of nutrition and environmental temperature on the energy metabolism of the growing pig. 1. Heat loss and critical temperature, *Br. J. Nutr.*, 40:433.
Close, W. H., and M. W. Stainer. 1984. Effects of plane of nutrition and environmental temperature on the growth and development of early-weaned pigs. 1. Growth and body composition, *Anim. Prod.*, 38:211.
Dunkin, A. C., J. L. Black, and K. J. James. 1984. Relationship between energy intake and nitrogen retention in the finisher pig, *Proc. Aust. Soc. Anim. Prod.*, 15:672.
France, J., and J. H. M. Thornley. 1984. *Mathematical Models in Agriculture*, Butterworths, Boston.
Hutchens, L. K. and R. L Hintz. 1981. A summary of genetic and phenotypic statistics for pubertal and growth characteristics in swine, Okla. State Univ. Agric. Exp. Sta. Tech. Publ. T-155.

Kerr, B. J. 1993. Optimizing lean tissue deposition in swine. BioKyowa Technical Review, Nutri-Quest, Chesterfield, MO.

King, R. H., and A. C. Dunkin. 1986. The effect of nutrition on the reproductive performance of first-litter sows. 3. The response to graded increases in feed intake during lactation, *Anim. Prod.*, 42:119.

King, R. H., I. H. Williams, and I. Barker. 1984. The effect of diet during lactation on the reproductive performance of first litter sows, *Proc. Aust. Soc. Anim. Prod.*, 15:412.

Moughan, P. J. 1995. Modelling protein metabolism in the pig — critical evaluation of a simple reference model. In *Modeling Growth in the Pig*, Moughan, P. J., M. W. A. Verstegen, and M. I. Visser-Royneveld, Eds., EAAP Publication No. 78, Wageningen Press, Wageningen, The Netherlands, 103–112.

Moughan, P. J., W. C. Smith, and G. Pearson. 1987. Description and validation of a model simulating growth in the pig (20–90 kg live weight), *N.Z. J. Agric. Res.*, 30:481.

Mount, L. E. 1963. The thermal insulation of the newborn pig, *J. Physiol.*, 168:698.

Mount, L. E. 1977. The use of heat transfer coefficients in estimating sensible heat loss from the pig, *Anim. Prod.*, 25:271.

NRC. 1998. *Nutrient Requirements of Swine*, 10th ed., National Academy Press, Washington, D.C.

Pettigrew, J. E., M. Gill, J. France, and W. H. Close. 1992a. A mathematical integration of energy and amino acid metabolism of lactating sows, *J. Anim. Sci.*, 70:3742.

Pettigrew, J. E., M. Gill, J. France, and W. H. Close. 1992b. Evaluation of a mathematical model of lactating sow metabolism, *J. Anim. Sci.*, 70:362.

Pomar, C., D. L. Harris, and F. Minvielle. 1991a. Computer simulation of swine production systems: I. Modeling the growth of young pigs, *J. Anim. Sci.*, 69:1468.

Pomar, C., D. L. Harris, and F. Minvielle. 1991b. Computer simulation model of swine production systems: II. Modeling body composition and weight of female pigs, fetal development, milk production and growth of suckling pigs, *J. Anim. Sci.*, 69:1487.

Pomar, C., D. L. Harris, and F. Minvielle. 1991c. Computer simulation model of swine production systems: III. A dynamic herd simulation model including reproduction, *J. Anim. Sci.*, 69:2822.

Schinckel, A. P., and C. F. M. de Lange. 1996. Characterization of growth parameters needed as inputs for pig growth models, *J. Anim. Sci.*, 74:2021.

Schinckel, A. P., P. V. Preckel, and M. E. Einstein. 1996. Prediction of daily protein accretion rates of pigs from estimates of fat-free lean gain between 20 and 120 kg live weight, *J. Anim. Sci.*, 74:498.

Tess, M. W., G. L. Bennett, and G. E. Dickerson. 1983. Simulation of genetic changes in life cycle efficiency of pork production. I. A bioeconomic model, *J. Anim. Sci.*, 56:336.

Whittemore, C. T. 1986. An approach to pig growth modeling, *J. Anim. Sci.*, 63:615.

Whittemore, C. T., and R. H. Fawcett. 1976. Theoretical aspects of a flexible model to simulate protein and lipid growth in pigs, *Anim. Prod.*, 22:87.

Whittemore, C. T., J. B. Tullis, and G. C. Emmans. 1988. Protein growth in pigs, *Anim. Prod.*, 46:437.

39 Statistical Techniques for the Design and Analysis of Swine Nutrition Experiments

Debra K. Aaron and Virgil W. Hays

CONTENTS

I. Introduction 882
II. Design of Experiments 882
    A. Importance of Planning...882
    B. Preexperiment Protocol..882
III. Some Basic Concepts 884
    A. Experimental Unit 884
    B. Sampling Unit 884
    C. Experimental Error..884
    D. Sensitivity..884
    E. Confounding..885
    F. Orthogonality 885
    G. Interaction..885
IV. Fundamentals of All Experiments 885
    A. Randomization 885
    B. Replication 886
    C. Error Control 886
V. Structures of All Experiments 886
    A. Treatment Structure...886
    B. Design Structure..887
        1. General Designs 887
        2. Extensions and Modifications..888
        3. Split-Plots and Repeated Measures 889
VI. Methods of Improving Precision of Designed Experiments...890
VII. Analysis of Data 893
    A. Analysis of Variance and Hypothesis Testing 893
    B. Designed Comparisons among Treatment Means..897
    C. Use and Misuse of Multiple Comparison Procedures 897
VIII. Interpretation and Presentation of Results 898
    A. Partitioning Treatment Effects..898
    B. Statistics in Manuscripts...898
IX. Role of the Statistician in Experimentation 899
References 900

I. INTRODUCTION

Statistical techniques should be considered as research tools that can produce meaningful, reliable, and unbiased results when properly applied to situations for which they are designed. However, no statistical technique can protect against poor planning, inaccuracies in the data, unsound analysis, or incorrect interpretation. High-quality research requires proper planning and careful execution of experiments, correct application of statistical techniques, and, finally, interpretation of results by one who understands not only the statistical techniques, but also the field to which they are applied.

The objectives of this chapter are to (1) review some basic statistical techniques that are useful in the design and analysis of swine nutrition experiments; (2) provide some guidelines for interpretation and presentation of results; and (3) examine the role of the statistician in experimentation. The statistical techniques discussed are not new and generally are no different from those used in other fields of biological research; therefore, basic biometrical or experimental design texts are recommended as references, for example, Cochran and Cox (1957), Gill (1978a,b), Snedecor and Cochran (1980), Steel and Torrie (1980), Damon and Harvey (1987), Lentner and Bishop (1993), and Hinkelmann and Kempthorne (1994). Also, it is assumed that readers are familiar with the basic features of experimental design and analysis, and with commonly used error terms.

II. DESIGN OF EXPERIMENTS

A. Importance of Planning

In planning experiments, the first consideration must be the availability of resources in terms of financial support, personnel, animals, equipment, and time. Then, within the restrictions imposed by the available resources, experiments should be designed to obtain unbiased estimates of treatment effects, treatment differences, and experimental error. Also, experiments should be designed and replicated in such a way that treatment effects will be estimated with adequate precision to detect differences, if they truly exist, at the desired probability level.

Careful planning and organization before an experiment is initiated can maximize the amount of information gained from the resources used. Also, careful planning will help protect against statistical problems associated with violation of the basic principles of experimental design. Mark Twain once observed, "Statistics are like garbage, one should have in mind what is to be done with the stuff before collecting it!" Similarly, researchers should have specific objectives in mind, and they should know how those objectives are to be resolved before experiments are initiated and data are collected.

B. Preexperiment Protocol

As part of the preexperiment protocol, six pertinent questions should be addressed. First, what is to be accomplished by the experiment? Objectives of the experiment should be stated definitely and concisely in terms of questions to be answered, hypotheses to be tested, or effects to be estimated. Second, how many treatments (factors) or treatment combinations are to be included in the experiment? The success of the experiment depends on the careful selection of treatments, the evaluation of which will resolve the initial objectives. Third, what is the experimental unit (an individual, a litter, a pen, etc.)? Also, what measurements will be made on the experimental units (how, when, where, and by whom)? Correct definition of the experimental unit is important because it is the variation among experimental units treated alike that provides the unbiased estimate of error for evaluating treatment effects. The objectives of the experiment should make clear whether a particular measurement will be a response variable (dependent variable) or a background variable (auxiliary variable or covariate). Fourth, how are the treatments or treatment combinations to be assigned to the experimental units? The randomization procedure used for assigning treatments to experimental units determines the design structure of the experiment, and it provides the mechanism that allows researchers to draw valid conclusions from the results. Fifth, how many times does each treatment need to be observed; that is, how much replication is necessary? The number of replications must be large enough to estimate treatment effects with the precision necessary to detect differences, if they truly exist, at the desired probability level. Sixth, and perhaps most importantly, can the resulting experimental design be analyzed? Also, can the desired comparisons be made? Sources of variation and appropriate degrees of freedom should be written out as part of the preexperiment protocol. Planned comparisons should be specified during this stage as well. Unfortunately, if too little time is spent in the planning stage of the experiment, researchers may find that no valid comparisons can be made, or that those that can be made do not resolve the objectives stated initially. The form presented in Table 39.1 can serve as a tool in the planning phase of experimentation, and it may serve as a summary of more extensive documentation and

TABLE 39.1
Form for Summarizing Preexperimental Protocol

I.	Experimental objective(s):		Enumerate definitely and concisely in terms of questions to be answered, hypotheses to be tested, or effects to be estimated.
II.	Background Information:		Summarize important results of literature review and/or prior research that have bearing on experiment being planned.
III.	Experimental Variables:		
	A.		
			Response Variables / **Measurement Technique**
		1.	Response variables (i.e., effects) are the outcomes of the experiment. They measure performance of the treatments (or treatment combinations). / How, when, where, and by whom will measurements be made?
		2.	
		etc.	
	B.		
			Factors (Treatments) and Classes (or Levels)
		1.	List each factor to be studied, and indicate the classes (or levels) each factor will take on. For example, the factor diet includes three classes: normal corn, normal corn plus lysine, high lysine corn.
		2.	
		etc.	
	C.		**Background Variables** / **Method of Control**
		1.	Background variables can affect responses but are not of interest as treatments. / Control by holding constant, using planned grouping (blocking), or treating as covariate.
		2.	
		etc.	
IV.	Experimental Unit:		Indicate whether an individual or a group (e.g., litter, pen, etc.)
V.	Replication:		Indicate number of times each treatment (or treatment combination) will be observed. Show how this number was estimated.
			Note: Each replication requires a separate experimental unit.
VI.	Experimental Design:		Describe treatment structure and design structure. Indicate randomization mechanism.
VII.	Data Collection Forms:		Attach copies. Forms should be designed for ease of recording, not for analysis. They should include space for recording significant events that happen during the course of the experiment.
VIII.	Planned Methods of Statistical Analysis:		Summarize planned methods of analysis. Include sources and degrees of freedom for the analysis of variance and the planned means separation procedure.
IX.	Schedule and Estimated Cost:		Attach copies of timelines and budgets.

Source: Adapted from Moen et al. (1999).

literature review. In addition, the completed form may be helpful in communicating to others the experimental plan and in certifying considerations given to the various tools of experimentation discussed in this chapter.

III. SOME BASIC CONCEPTS

A. EXPERIMENTAL UNIT

An *experimental unit* is the smallest division of experimental material to which a treatment (or treatment combination in factorial experiments) can be assigned in a single act of randomization. Correct definition of the experimental unit is important because it is the variation among experimental units treated alike that provides the unbiased estimate of error for evaluating treatment effects. An experimental unit may be an individual (e.g., pig) or a group of individuals (e.g., litter, pen). Whether an individual or a group of individuals, it is important that researchers understand the experimental unit is the smallest entity receiving a single treatment, provided two such entities could receive different treatments.

Consider the following example. An experiment is conducted to compare the effects of four different diets on performance of growing-finishing pigs. Four pens of the same size are available and each will house eight pigs of the desired age and weight. The investigator assigns eight pigs to each pen and then, randomly assigns diets to pens. The investigator believes pig is the experimental unit and that there are eight replications. However, because diets were assigned to pens, and all pigs in the same pen receive the same diet, pen constitutes the experimental unit. As a result, the experiment has no replication, and further assumptions are needed before valid conclusions can be drawn. More will be said about this later.

B. SAMPLING UNIT

The unit of experimental material on which an observation is recorded is referred to as the *sampling unit*. In some cases, the experimental unit and the sampling unit are the same. In others, the experimental unit may be divided into two or more sampling units. In the previous example, the pen of pigs represents the experimental unit. If the response variable is gain:feed, and pigs are group-fed, then pen is both the experimental unit and the sampling unit. On the other hand, if the response variable is average daily gain, and pigs are weighed individually, then pig is the sampling unit and there are eight sampling units per experimental unit (pen).

C. EXPERIMENTAL ERROR

Variation is a characteristic of all experimental material. Results of experiments are affected not only by the action of treatments but also by unexplained, random variation, which tends to mask treatment effects. The term *experimental error* refers to variation that exists among experimental units treated alike. This variation is the primary basis for deciding whether a treatment effect is real or due to chance. Clearly, every experiment must be designed to have a measure of experimental error.

In a pure or probabilistic sense, the term experimental error refers to the natural, random variation expected under repetition of the experiment. In a less restrictive sense, it is a collective term often used to describe variation resulting from all sources of variation unaccounted for in the experiment. For this reason, experimental error is frequently referred to as residual variation.

D. SENSITIVITY

Sensitivity refers to the ability of the experiment to detect real differences, if they exist, at the desired probability level. The terms *power*, *precision*, and *sensitivity* have very similar meanings.

Given two experiments, the one that can detect the smaller difference between two means has the greater sensitivity (power or precision).

Size of the experiment, as measured by the number of replications, is highly dependent on desired sensitivity. In turn, sensitivity depends on size of the difference to be detected and size of experimental error. The chance of detecting smaller differences is increased as sensitivity is increased, and this occurs when experimental error is decreased.

E. CONFOUNDING

The word *confounding* means the mixing together of effects. Effects of two independent variables (e.g., treatments, blocks, etc.) on a dependent (response) variable are said to be confounded when they cannot be distinguished from each other in the statistical analysis. Confounding may be partial or complete. In either case, it obscures the true effects of treatments on the response variable. It is sometimes a deliberate feature of the design structure but most often arises as a result of inadvertent imperfections, unequal replication, and/or improper randomization.

To illustrate the concept of confounding, recall the nutrition experiment (four diets, growing-finishing pigs) described previously. The lack of replication has already been discussed. Now, consider a second problem. It is unlikely that the four pens are exactly the same; thus, there would be some variation due to pen differences. If the experiment were to be analyzed, pen and treatment (diet) effects would be completely confounded. In other words, it would be impossible to separate pen differences from differences between diets. Therefore, should differences in response be observed, it would be just as easy to argue they were due to pen effects as it would be to argue they were due to treatment effects.

F. ORTHOGONALITY

The word *orthogonal* occurs in several distinct but related senses in statistics. It is often used to denote independence. In relation to linear functions of treatment means, two contrasts or comparisons are said to be orthogonal if they are statistically independent. In relation to an experimental design, the design is said to be orthogonal if there is no interaction between components of the design structure and components of the treatment structure.

G. INTERACTION

Interaction means the presence of joint factor effects. An interaction exists among two or more factors if the effect of one factor on response depends on the levels or classes of other factors. As this definition implies, the presence of interactions precludes an assessment of the effect of one factor without simultaneously assessing effects of other factors. This is the essence of an interaction effect; when interactions occur, factors involved cannot be evaluated individually (Mason et al., 1989).

IV. FUNDAMENTALS OF ALL EXPERIMENTS

A. RANDOMIZATION

Randomization refers to the assignment of treatments to experimental units so that all units have an equal chance of receiving a treatment. Randomization prevents systematic bias from being introduced into an experiment and ensures that estimates of treatment means and differences, as well as experimental error, are unbiased. Accordingly, Moen et al. (1999) compares randomization to insurance: "You only need it (insurance/randomization) when a problem arises. However, unlike insurance, when randomization is not done, the experimenter may not be aware of the impact of nuisance variables and might draw incorrect conclusions." As experimental designs are simply plans to be used for assigning treatments to experimental units, the manner in which the randomization is restricted is the key to the type of design structure. Design structures are addressed later in this chapter.

B. REPLICATION

Replication refers to the assignment of more than one experimental unit to the same treatment or treatment combination. Each replication of a treatment is an independent observation; thus, each replication involves a different experimental unit. The basic function of replication is to provide an estimate of experimental error. In general, increasing the number of replications results in a more accurate estimate of experimental error and more precise estimates of treatment effects. For a particular experiment, the number of replications depends on the magnitude of the difference to be detected, the sensitivity required, and the variability of the experimental material. Improving the precision of experiments by increasing the number of replications is discussed in a later section.

C. ERROR CONTROL

Error control, a collective term that refers to techniques used to reduce or control experimental error, is to a large extent what experimental design is all about. Error control may involve selection of more homogeneous (uniform) experimental material, stratification of experimental units into more homogeneous groups, use of concomitant observations as covariates, and/or choice of size and type of experimental units. Choice of the design structure (e.g., planned grouping to form blocks) is the primary statistical technique used to control experimental error. The design structure controls experimental error by grouping experimental units so variation among units within a group is less than that among units in different groups. Then, variation among groups is excluded from experimental error and precision of the experiment is improved. This is addressed in greater detail later in this chapter.

V. STRUCTURES OF ALL EXPERIMENTS

A. TREATMENT STRUCTURE

All experiments consist of two basic structures (Milliken and Johnson, 1984). The first is the treatment structure and consists of the set of treatments or treatment combinations that have been selected for evaluation. The term *treatment* refers to those factors (either qualitative or quantitative) to be compared as measured by their effect on given response traits. The term may be used to denote imposed or controllable factors such as types or levels of protein in the diet or uncontrollable factors such as sexes or breeds of pigs (Gill, 1978a). The most common types of treatment structures are the one-way classification and the factorial arrangement.

The one-way treatment classification consists of t treatments, which may be structured (those treatments having a gradient or grouped composition) or unstructured (those treatments that are unrelated). With respect to treatments, observations are classified on the basis of a single factor. As an example of a one-way treatment classification, consider comparing growth rates of pigs fed two types of corn (e.g., normal and high-lysine). The two groups (normal and high-lysine) are referred to as classes of the main classification, type of corn. This is the simplest treatment structure. It may be used in conjunction with a completely randomized design, which results in the basic one-way analysis of variance, or it can be used in association with either a randomized complete block design or a Latin square design. These are discussed in more detail later in this chapter.

The factorial treatment arrangement consists of a set of treatment combinations constructed by combining the classes (or levels) of two or more different types of treatments (often called factors). Every class (or level) of one factor occurs in combination with every class (or level) of each other factor in the experiment. Factorial treatment arrangements provide information about each factor included in the experiment and also information about interactions among the different factors. Suppose the normal and high-lysine corn of the previous example had been stored by two different methods, dry and high-moisture. Thus, each of the two types of corn occurs in combination with each of the two storage methods, giving four treatment combinations in all. With this 2×2 factorial treatment arrangement, observations are classified by both type of corn and storage method. Experiments involving factorial treatment arrangements are often referred to as "factorial" experiments; however, it should be emphasized that factorial refers to the treatment structure and not the design structure of the experiment. Like the one-way treatment classification, a factorial arrangement may be used with any of the general design structures.

B. Design Structure

1. General Designs

The second structure common to all experiments is the design structure. This refers to the method of grouping experimental units into homogeneous groups or blocks, that is, the way in which the randomization is restricted. One of the primary objectives in choosing a design structure is to reduce experimental error. There are three general types of design structures: (1) completely randomized (CR); (2) randomized complete block (RCB); and (3) Latin square (LS). Most other design structures can be considered to be modifications or extensions of these three. The treatment structures previously described can be used in conjunction with any of the three general design structures. For example, an experimental design might consist of a one-way treatment classification in a CR, RCB, or LS design, or treatments could have a factorial arrangement in any one of the three general design structures.

The CR design is the simplest design structure possible because treatments (or treatment combinations in the case of factorial experiments) are assigned to experimental units completely at random. Thus, randomization is not restricted, and the only criterion for grouping experimental units is treatment (or treatment combination). Use of this design is appropriate when experimental units are relatively homogeneous (uniform), or when there are no identifiable criteria for arranging the units into more homogeneous groups. As pointed out by Hinkelman and Kempthorne (1994), however, the word *homogeneous* in this context should not be interpreted too narrowly. Identical experimental units do not exist in nature, and, thus, homogeneous here means "alike to the extent possible." Even this phrase is relative. For example, the variability that arises naturally among pigs of a given gender or within a certain age (or weight) range will be much higher than the variability among experimental units manufactured and manipulated under controlled laboratory situations (such as test tubes, petri dishes, etc.). Yet, in both situations, a CR design may be appropriate.

Although the CR design provides the maximum number of degrees of freedom for estimating experimental error, it is often inefficient. In many cases, there are identifiable sources of variation among the experimental units other than treatments. However, because randomization is unrestricted in the CR design, all variation among experimental units except that due to treatments is included in the experimental error. When other sources of variation can be identified before the allocation of treatments, it may be possible to group experimental units so that the variation among units within a group is less than that among units in different groups. Then, randomization is done within each group rather than overall. Design structures that take advantage of this grouping will exclude variation among groups from the experimental error and, as a result, increase sensitivity of the experiment.

In the RCB design, experimental units are arranged in homogeneous groups (blocks) on the basis of a single source of extraneous variability; that is, there is one restriction on the randomization. The extraneous source of variability may be a management factor such as time or location (e.g., different farms, buildings, sites within a single building, etc.) or an animal factor such as litter, breed, or gender. In some situations, blocks may be formed by combining two or more sources of extraneous variability, such as time–location, gender–weight, location–weight, or litter–gender combinations. Ott (1975) referred to such block effects as "chunk-type factors" because differences attributed to the combined effect of the different sources will be partitioned out of the experimental error in one "chunk" of variation.

Once blocks are formed, treatments are assigned randomly to experimental units within a block, and an independent randomization is carried out for each block. Every treatment occurs the same number of times, usually once, within each block and each block contains each treatment; therefore, each block is complete with respect to the whole set of treatments. The objective of the RCB design is to have units within a block as uniform as possible with regard to the blocking factor so that observed differences within blocks will be largely due to treatments. Ideally, variation not due to treatments is minimized within blocks and maximized among blocks. The variation among blocks is then arithmetically removed from the experimental error, thus improving sensitivity of the experiment. If there is no appreciable variability among blocks, the RCB design will not increase the precision of detecting treatment differences over that of the CR design. In fact, if the reduction in experimental error does not compensate for the loss in error degrees of freedom, blocking may actually reduce the power of the experiment. Also, as block size increases, variability within blocks not brought about by treatment tends to increase as well, causing a larger experimental error. Finally, an important assumption of the RCB design is that block and treatment effects are additive; that is, there is no interaction between blocks and treatments. Violation of this assumption results in an inflated experimental error and inaccurate estimates of treatment differences.

The LS design arises from blocking in two different ways; that is, there are two restrictions on the randomization. This double blocking makes it possible to remove two independent, extraneous sources of variability from the experimental error. Generally, *rows* and *columns* are the terms used to refer to the two blocking factors. They may refer to the sequence in which treatments are applied or to the spatial distribution of experimental units. Often in swine nutrition experiments, columns refer to individual pigs and rows refer to time periods. Each row and each column is a complete replicate or block. As a result, randomization is more complicated than in the RCB design. Treatments are randomly allotted to experimental units such that each treatment occurs once and only once in each row and once and only once in each column. The number of rows, columns, and treatments must be equal, and this is a major disadvantage associated with the LS design. The most commonly used squares range from 5×5 to 8×8. Squares smaller than 5×5 provide few degrees of freedom for experimental error, whereas squares larger than 8×8 may encounter the same problem as the RCB design in that experimental error may increase with size of the square. Because there are many possible configurations of squares, it is necessary to select the one to be used by some random method. One method of randomization is presented by Cochran and Cox (1957).

Use of the LS design will result in more precise estimates of treatment means and differences than the RCB design only when there is appreciable variation associated with the second blocking factor. Also, an important assumption of the LS design is that rows and columns do not interact with each other or with treatments. Violation of this assumption will result in an inflated experimental error and inaccurate estimates of treatment effects.

2. Extensions and Modifications

There are often situations that require extending or modifying the general RCB and LS design structures. A commonly used extension of the RCB design involves the use of b blocks of size ct, where c is a positive integer ≥ 2 and t is the number of treatments. Called a *generalized* RCB design, each treatment is randomly allotted to c experimental units per block, and randomization is done anew within each block. The primary advantage of the generalized RCB design is that it permits investigation of block × treatment interaction. Each block–treatment combination defines a population of observations; thus, when each treatment occurs c times within each block, estimates of block × treatment interaction and experimental error can be estimated and will be orthogonal. The generalized RCB may be the most appropriate design structure when block × treatment interaction is strongly suspected *a priori*, and where such interaction may be a major focus of the experiment. This may occur, for example, when a blocking factor is introduced to broaden the inference from the experiment (e.g., different genetic types, locations, laboratories).

The primary disadvantage of the general LS design is that it requires an equal number of rows, columns, and treatments. When a small number of treatments are involved, there may be few degrees of freedom for experimental error and, thus, low precision. Modifying the basic LS design by increasing one of the blocking factors (either the number of rows or the number of columns) will increase experimental error degrees of freedom and, ultimately, precision of the experiment. To maintain the necessary balance characteristics of the general LS design, the one blocking factor must be increased by some multiple of the number of treatments. For example, the number of column blocks might be increased to give a rectangular arrangement of experimental units of size $t \times mt$. Then, the t treatments would be randomly allocated to experimental units such that every treatment occurs once in every column and m times in every row. This arrangement is referred to as a Latin *rectangle*.

Both the LS and the Latin rectangle control for two independent sources of extraneous variation, but the Latin rectangle may be the design structure of choice because it provides more degrees of freedom for experimental error. However, in some situations, time restrictions, laboratory space, animal housing, quantity of experimental material, or personnel limitations may make it impossible to conduct an experiment larger than the general LS design. It is common, in such situations, to use more than one Latin square. The same treatments are used in each square, but each square involves new experimental material and a separate randomization. Rows and/or columns may be different in each square (nested), or they may be common to all squares (cross-classified). Like the Latin rectangle, the multiple (or repeated) LS design increases the degrees of freedom available for estimating experimental error. Advantages and disadvantages of Latin rectangle and multiple (or repeated) LS designs are discussed in detail by Lentner and Bishop (1993).

3. Split-Plots and Repeated Measures

In addition to the three general design structures (CR, RCB, and LS) and their extensions, two other design structures are often useful in swine nutrition experiments. These are split-plot (SP) and repeated measures (RM) designs. Sometimes RM designs are referred to as *split-plots in time*, although *repeated measures* is a more accurate term. These two designs have identical structures, and both involve more than one size of experimental unit. However, the RM design differs from the SP design in that the former involves a stage where there is no randomization of treatment levels and the latter involves randomization at all stages. Both are considered classes of designs in which treatments have a factorial arrangement.

The basic SP design involves assigning treatments of one factor to main plots according to the randomization procedure for a CR, RCB, or LS design. The treatments of the second factor are assigned randomly to subplots within each main plot. This design usually sacrifices precision in estimating the average effects of the main plot treatments, but it often improves the precision for comparing the average effects of the subplot treatments as well as the interaction. This occurs because the experimental error for main plots is usually larger than the experimental error used to compare subplot treatments. Also, the number of degrees of freedom available for experimental error is usually smaller for main plot comparisons than for subplot comparsions.

The primary advantage of the SP design is that it enables factors that require relatively large amounts of experimental material and factors that require small amounts to be combined in the same experiment. If the experiment is planned to investigate the first factor, so that large amounts of experimental material are going to be used anyway, the second factor often can be included at little extra cost, and some additional information is obtained. Sometimes, in factorial experiments, the nature of the experimental material or the operations involved simply makes it difficult to handle all treatment combinations in the same manner, and an SP design is required. As an example, consider an experiment investigating the effects of environmental temperature and diet on growth performance of pigs. Two temperatures (10 and 35°C) and three corn-based diets (normal corn, normal corn plus lysine, and high-lysine corn) are used in the experiment. Temperatures are randomly allotted to main plots consisting of environmental chambers (the larger experimental unit), and diets are randomly allotted to subplots consisting of either individually fed or group-fed pigs (the smaller experimental unit) within each main plot.

The RM design is appropriate for experiments in which treatments are assigned to animals according to the randomization procedure of the CR, RCB, or LS design and animals are measured for trend at several sampling times (i.e., nonrandom, repeated sampling). For example, suppose an experiment is conducted to evaluate the effect of increasing levels of dietary protein on pig performance and plasma urea nitrogen. Levels of dietary protein are assigned to pigs at random, and plasma urea nitrogen is measured on each pig at several sampling times. Thus, time of sampling is one of the factors in the treatment structure of the experiment. By measuring the same animal at different sampling times, the animal is essentially "split" into parts (time periods), and the response is measured on each part. The animal is the larger experimental unit (which corresponds to the main plot), and the time period is the smaller experimental unit (which corresponds to the subplot). However, because the levels of time cannot be assigned at random to the time periods, time is considered a nonrandom, repeated factor. Gill and Hafs (1971) provided an early discussion of appropriate statistical techniques for experiments that involve repeated measurements in animals. More recently, Littell (1989) discussed mathematical conditions required for validity of the SP type of analysis for RM experiments, and Littell et al. (1998) compared several statistical methods for analyzing such data. Analysis of RM designs is addressed in more detail later in this chapter.

VI. METHODS OF IMPROVING PRECISION OF DESIGNED EXPERIMENTS

The precision (sensitivity) of an experiment refers to its ability to detect true treatment differences at a given significance level (Little and Hills, 1978). Generally, the smaller the variability among experimental units treated alike, the more precise the experiment will be in detecting treatment differences. Also, as the number of replications increases, the variance of the difference between two means decreases, and the precision of the experiment increases. Therefore, statistical techniques used to improve the precision of an experiment involve either an increase in the number of replications or a reduction in the magnitude of the experimental error. In some cases, refinement of nonstatistical techniques, such as procedures for administration of treatments or collection of data, may improve precision more than statistical techniques. The discussion here is limited to improving precision by statistical means.

Increasing the number of replications is probably the statistical technique first thought of as a means of improving precision of designed experiments. Although additional replications generally will improve the precision with which treatment means and differences are estimated, the extent of improvement declines as the number of replications increases. For example, if a difference in rate of gain of 40 g/day can be detected with four replicates, an experiment of approximately 16 replicates will be needed to detect half this difference, or 20 g/day, because the standard errors are in the ratio of 2:1 (assuming the same variance). However, if the difference is halved again, to 10 g/day, approximately 64 replicates will be necessary to detect this difference.

The number of replications needed depends on the magnitude of the difference to be detected, the desired precision, and the variability of the experimental material. For a specific situation, this number can be estimated using procedures described by Cochran and Cox (1957) or Berndtson (1991). Estimates of the number of replications needed to detect differences of various sizes at several levels of variability and selected significance levels (1, 5, 10%) are presented for sow reproduction experiments and growing-finishing pig experiments in Tables 39.2 and 39.3, respectively. In both tables, estimates are based on an 80% chance of obtaining a significant result.

TABLE 39.2
Estimated Number of Replications Needed in Sow Reproduction Experiments[a]

Significance Level (%)[c]	Average Coefficient of Variation[d]	Expected Difference in Litter Size (% mean)[b]					
		2	4	6	8	10	12
1	40	9343	2336	1039	584	374	260
	35	7154	1788	795	448	287	199
	30	5256	1314	584	329	211	146
	25	3650	913	406	229	146	102
	20	2336	584	260	146	94	67
5	40	6280	1570	698	393	252	175
	35	4808	1202	533	301	193	134
	30	3533	883	393	221	142	99
	25	2453	614	273	154	99	69
	20	1570	393	175	99	63	45
10	40	4946	1237	550	310	197	138
	35	3787	947	421	237	152	106
	30	2782	696	310	174	112	78
	25	1932	483	215	121	78	55
	20	1237	310	138	78	50	36

[a] Assumes a completely randomized design with two treatments, two-tailed test of significance, and an 80% chance of detecting a significant result (i.e., probability of accepting the null hypothesis when it is false is 20%).
[b] A 10% difference in litter size represents approximately 1 and 0.8 live pigs at birth and weaning, respectively.
[c] Probability of rejecting the null hypothesis when it is true.
[d] Average coefficient of variation = (pooled standard deviation/mean) × 100.

For the sow reproduction experiments (Table 39.2), a CR design with two treatments was assumed because it is common to assign treatments completely at random to individually fed sows. For the growing-finishing pig experiments (Table 39.3), an RCB design with four treatments was assumed because this design is commonly applied in such experiments. In both cases, the estimates of error available in the literature are based largely on these designs (CR in sow experiments and RCB in growing-finishing pig experiments). Although estimates of the number of replications are presented for various levels of experimental error (expressed as the coefficient of variation) and differences of several sizes (expressed as percent of the mean of the experiment), levels selected are within realistic ranges. The average coefficients of variation for total number of pigs born, number of live pigs at birth, and number of live pigs at 21 days are 28, 29, and 36%, respectively (Hays and Aaron, unpublished results). These values are based on five different estimates involving 7925 litters. Among these five studies, the estimates ranged from 26 to 28%, 28 to 33%, and 29 to 39% for the three reproductive traits, respectively. The average coefficients of variation for rate of gain and feed efficiency are approximately 4.5 and 5%, respectively (Hays and Aaron, unpublished results). These are based on data combined from several experiments and involve 3425 group-fed pigs (four to eight pigs per group).

Realistically, the prospective improvement in precision, as the number of replications is increased, must be balanced with increases in cost and time. As research is expensive, it is important not to replicate more than is necessary. At the same time, experiments with inadequate replication are of little value.

Another factor that affects the precision of an experiment is the choice of experimental unit. As discussed earlier, the experimental unit may be an individual animal, a litter, or a pen of animals. It is the smallest unit receiving a single treatment, provided two such units could receive different treatments. Correct definition of the experimental unit is important because it is the variation among

TABLE 39.3
Estimated Number of Replications (blocks) Needed in Growing-Finishing Pig Experiments[a]

Significance Level (%)[b]	Average Coefficient of Variation[c]	Expected Difference in Rate of Gain or Feed Efficiency (% mean)					
		2.5	5.0	7.5	10.0	12.5	15.0
1	15.0	842	211	97	54	35	25
	12.5	583	146	67	38	25	18
	10.0	374	97	43	25	17	12
	7.5	210	54	25	15	10	7
	5.0	97	25	12	7	5	4
	2.5	25	7	4	3	3	3
5	15.0	565	141	64	36	23	17
	12.5	393	99	44	26	17	12
	10.0	252	64	29	17	11	8
	7.5	142	36	17	10	7	5
	5.0	64	17	8	5	4	3
	2.5	17	5	3	3	2	2
10	15.0	445	111	51	29	19	13
	12.5	309	73	35	20	13	10
	10.0	198	51	23	13	9	7
	7.5	112	29	13	8	6	4
	5.0	51	13	7	4	3	3
	2.5	13	4	3	2	2	2

[a] Assumes a randomized complete block design with four treatments, two-tailed test of significance, and an 80% chance of detecting a significant result (i.e., probability of accepting the null hypothesis when it is false is 20%).
[b] Probability of rejecting the null hypothesis when it is true.
[c] Average coefficient of variation = (pooled standard deviation/mean) × 100. For growing-finishing pigs (group-fed, 4 to 8 pigs/group), values range from 2.5 to 10%; for very young pigs, values range from 7.5 to 15%.

experimental units treated alike that provides the unbiased estimate of error for evaluating treatment effects. Failure to recognize the appropriate experimental unit, and to replicate it, is a common mistake in animal experiments. As illustrated by the nutrition experiment (four diets, growing-finishing pigs) described previously, this mistake often occurs because pen effects are ignored when animals are treated in groups. In some experiments, pen is correctly recognized as the experimental unit for a response variable such as gain:feed, which is measured on the pen of pigs, but not for traits such as loin eye area or plasma urea nitrogen, which are measured on the individual pig. Pen is both the experimental unit and the sampling unit for gain:feed, but for loin eye area and plasma urea nitrogen pen is the experimental unit and pig the sampling unit. In either case, replication involves increasing the number of pens per treatment. Increasing the number of pigs per experimental unit will increase precision up to a point, but if a given number of pigs can be fed individually, precision may be increased more by using the individual pig as the experimental unit and having more replications than by using the same number of pigs in fewer experimental units. Treating pigs individually maximizes the use of animals, but maximizing the efficiency of total resources may necessitate the grouping of pigs. Also, pigs treated individually may or may not respond to treatment in the same manner as pigs treated in groups.

Although the number of replications and the choice of experimental unit are both important factors, the primary statistical technique used to improve precision of designed experiments is to group experimental units into homogeneous groups or blocks; that is, to choose an efficient design structure. General design structures and their roles in error control were discussed in the preceding section. Generally, as experimental error is reduced, efficiency is increased. Thus, the more efficient the design structure, the more precise the experiment will be for estimating treatment effects. Relative efficiencies of the basic designs can be estimated using procedures described in the references suggested earlier. Basically, estimates of relative efficiency involve comparison of the relative size of the error term, with and without the blocking component included.

Another statistical technique for improving precision of designed experiments is to take additional quantitative measurements on the experimental units. These additional measurements are referred to as *auxiliary variables* or *covariates*. Suppose that in the experiment designed to compare growth rates of pigs fed two types of corn (normal and high-lysine) there is considerable variation in weight from pig to pig at the start of the experiment. Treatment effects may be estimated with more precision if differences associated with initial weight are removed from the total variability in growth rate. As discussed earlier, blocking (in this case by weight class) is one way this can be accomplished; however, in some cases use of a covariate will be more effective in reducing experimental error and at the same time will preserve more degrees of freedom for estimating error. Generally, the use of a covariate will be most effective when the primary and auxiliary variables are closely related in a linear manner, or if the auxiliary variable is responsible for a large portion of the total variation in the primary variable. Also, the use of an auxiliary variable as a covariate may allow the use of another factor for blocking. As an example, a littermate set of pigs may serve as a factor for blocking and initial weight may be used as a covariate. Damon and Harvey (1987) and Lentner and Bishop (1993) provide more detailed discussions of the analysis of covariance.

VII. ANALYSIS OF DATA

A. Analysis of Variance and Hypothesis Testing

The analysis of variance (Fisher, 1935) is a powerful and efficient statistical technique for partitioning the total variability within an experiment into orthogonal components resulting from recognizable sources of variation. There are three general components of the analysis of variance: (1) a component representing the treatment structure; (2) a component representing the design structure (blocks, rows, columns, etc.); and (3) a component resulting from unknown or uncontrollable causes generally referred to as the experimental error. The first two components are sometimes referred to collectively as the model component. Once the treatment and design structures have been specified, the statistical model and its associated analysis of variance also have been specified. Thus, the time to ask, "How should the data be analyzed?" is before, not after, data have been collected. Unfortunately, this question is often asked too late.

One of the primary functions of the analysis of variance is to test hypotheses about the equality of treatment means and the presence of interactions among the treatment factors. Generally, hypotheses are stated in a form that is believed to be untrue (null hypotheses), and data from the experiment are used to reject or disprove this hypothesis. In this way, the null hypothesis acts as a base from which an alternate hypothesis may deviate. For the swine nutrition experiment described previously, a null hypothesis might be stated as, "The growth rate of pigs fed the normal corn diet is equal to the growth rate of pigs fed the high-lysine diet." The corresponding alternate hypothesis might be, "The growth rate of pigs fed the high-lysine corn diet is different than the growth rate of pigs fed the normal corn diet." Evidence in favor of the alternate hypothesis is found by rejecting or disproving the null hypothesis.

The decision to reject the null hypothesis in favor of the alternate is based on a statistical test of significance, in this case an F test, which has some measure of confidence associated with it, based on the laws of probability. This measure of confidence is the chosen probability of rejecting the null hypothesis when it is really true, and it is referred to as the probability of a type I error. The most commonly chosen probability levels are $P < 0.10$, $P < 0.05$, $P < 0.01$, and $P < 0.001$. The choice of the level of probability should be based on the relative consequences of rejecting the null hypothesis when it is true (type I error) and accepting the null hypothesis when it is false (type II error).

Another basic function of the analysis of variance is to estimate the residual variability among experimental units treated alike. Throughout this chapter, this has been referred to as the experimental error. Sometimes this quantity is referred to as an estimate of the "common" variance. As indicated previously, the experimental error includes variation from all uncontrolled sources of variation. It may be a result of naturally inherent differences among experimental units, faulty experimental techniques, and other extraneous variation such as variation resulting from using an incomplete statistical model for the analysis. With proper experimental design and careful experimental technique, the two latter components should be negligible. The magnitude of the experimental error provides a measure of the precision of the experiment for evaluating treatment effects.

Each time an analysis of variance is conducted, certain assumptions about the data are made. The first major assumption involves the experimental error terms and is really a series of assumptions. The error terms are assumed to be normally and independently distributed with zero mean and a common (homogeneous) variance. Violation of these assumptions may affect both probability levels and precision; however, minor violations are usually not serious. As a precaution, however, assumptions should be checked to ensure that major violations do not exist in the data being analyzed.

The first of this series of assumptions, that of normality, does not affect the estimation of treatment means and differences; however, it can be critical to probability statements and hypothesis tests. Fortunately, means from all but very small samples are at least approximately normally distributed. Also, the F test of the hypothesis of treatment effects is not greatly affected by moderate departures from normality. In experiments from which data are obviously non-normal, transformations (e.g., square root for data consisting of rare events, arc sine for data expressed as percentages or proportions, and logarithmic for data where standard deviations are proportional to means) will ensure approximate normality for the transformed variable (Little and Hills, 1978).

The second of this series of assumptions, that of independence, is usually not a problem if proper randomization has been followed. Exceptions are experiments that involve repeated measurement. Ignoring the correlation of errors induced by the nonrandom, repeated measurement is a common mistake made in experiments in which animals are measured at several different times. When this correlation is ignored, inferences about the repeated factor (time) and associated interactions may be distorted.

The last of this series of assumptions, that of a common or homogeneous variance, is the one most frequently violated in animal experiments. In these types of experiments, it is not unusual for the mean and variance to be related; that is, groups with large means tend to have large variances and those with smaller means tend to have smaller variances. A typical example of heterogeneity of variances is found in experiments dealing with the effect of dietary copper levels on liver copper stores. As the dietary level of copper increases from a low level (approximately 10 ppm) to a high level (approximately 250 ppm), the mean and the variance of liver copper stores remain low up to a point and then increase rapidly at higher levels. Although the F test is only slightly affected by mild departures from homogeneous variances, it is always advisable to check this assumption. Several test procedures for homogeneity of variances are available. Two of the most commonly used are Hartley's maximum F test (Hartley, 1950) and Bartlett's test statistic (Bartlett, 1957). Both of these procedures are described in detail by Gill (1978a). In cases where the experimental error is heterogeneous, the error component can be divided into components that are homogeneous as described by Cochran and Cox (1957).

The second major assumption is that the three general components of an analysis of variance are additive. For example, in an RCB design, an experimental observation may be thought of as comprising the overall mean plus a treatment effect plus a block effect plus a random error effect. Note that all terms are added; thus, the term *additivity*. This implies that a treatment effect is the same for all blocks and that the block effect is the same for all treatments; that is, blocks and treatments are independent. This was one of the assumptions made earlier about the RCB design.

The final major assumption associated with the analysis of variance is that treatments or treatment combinations are randomly assigned to experimental units within a homogeneous group. As discussed earlier, randomization prevents systematic bias from being introduced into an experiment and ensures that estimates of treatment means and differences, as well as experimental error, are unbiased. Often, this last assumption is not stressed as much as it should be.

The General Linear Models (GLM) program in SAS (SAS, 1989a) is commonly used to compute analyses of variance for most experimental designs. Analysis of variance plans (sources of variation and degrees of freedom) for the three general design structures (CR, RCB, and LS), a generalized RCB design and a SP design are shown in Tables 39.4, 39.5, and 39.6, respectively. Plans for the general design structures (Table 39.4) are based on an experiment involving four treatments and four replications, giving a total of 16 experimental units. The plan for the generalized RCB (Table 39.5) is based on an experiment with four treatments with two replications in each of four blocks. The plan for the SP design (Table 39.6) is based on an experiment with two levels of factor A (main plot treatment), three levels of factor B (subplot treatment), and five replications. Levels of factor A are assigned to main plots according to the randomization for the CR design. If factor A refers to environmental temperature (10 and 35°C) and factor B refers to diet (normal corn, normal corn plus lysine, and high-lysine corn), then this experiment corresponds to the SP example presented earlier.

TABLE 39.4
Analysis of Variance Plans for the Three General Design Structures[a]

Design Structure[b]					
CR		RCB		LS	
Source of Variation	df	Source of Variation	df	Source of Variation	df
				Rows	3
		Blocks	3	Columns	3
Treatments	3	Treatments	3	Treatments	3
Experimental error	12	Experimental error	9	Experimenal error	6
Total	15	Total	15	Total	15

[a] Assumes an experiment involving four treatments and four replications, giving a total of 16 experimental units.
[b] *Abbreviations:* CR, completely randomized; RCB, randomized complete block; LS, Latin square.

TABLE 39.5
Analysis of Variance Plan for a Generalized Randomized Complete Block Design Structure[a]

Source of Variation	df
Blocks	4 − 1 = 3
Treatments	4 − 1 = 3
Block × Treatment[b]	(4 − 1)(4 − 1) = 9
Experimental error	(4)(4)(2 − 1) = 16
Total	(4)(4)(2) − 1 = 31

[a] Assumes an experiment involving four treatments and four blocks, with two replications per block, giving a total of 32 experimental units.
[b] Error term for testing treatment effects if blocks are considered random; otherwise, treatment effects are tested using experimental error. If blocks are random and the block × treatment interaction is nonsignificant, the sum of squares for this interaction can be pooled with the residual (experimental error) sum of squares for an error term. If blocks are fixed, then block × treatment interaction is neither pooled with the residual, nor is it used as an error term.

TABLE 39.6
Analysis of Variance Plan for a Split-Plot Design[a]

Source of Variation	df
Main plot analysis	
Factor A (environmental temperature)	2 − 1 = 1
Main plot error (error a)[b]	2(5 − 1) = 8
Main plot total	(2)(5) − 1 = 9
Subplot analysis	
Factor B (diet)	3 − 1 = 2
A × B interaction	(2 − 1)(3 − 1) = 2
Subplot error (error b)[c]	2(5 − 1)(3 − 1) = 16
Subplot total	(2)(5)(3 − 1) = 20
Total	(2)(3)(5) − 1 = 29

[a] Based on an experiment with two levels of factor A, three levels of factor B, and five replications. Levels of factor A are assigned to main plots according to the randomization plan for the completely randomized design.
[b] Error term for testing factor A.
[c] Error term for testing factor B and the A × B interaction.

Analysis of variance plans for the Latin rectangle and multiple (or repeated) LS experiments are not presented here. With appropriate modifications of degrees of freedom, the analysis of variance, tests, and inferences for the Latin rectangle are otherwise the same as for the basic LS design. The analysis of variance for multiple (or repeated) LS experiments is a straightforward extension of that for a single square. However, analyses will differ depending primarily on whether squares are considered to be fixed or random effects, and also, in the latter case, whether there is a significant interaction between squares and treatments. Readers can refer to Damon and Harvey (1987) and Lentner and Bishop (1993) for more detailed information on the analysis of multiple (or repeated) LS experiments.

As noted previously, one of the usual assumptions in the analysis of variance is that random error terms are uncorrelated across measures. When measurements are taken over time on the same experimental unit, this assumption is likely to be false. Thus, analysis of RM designs is more complex than for the other designs discussed in this chapter. In the past, the approach most commonly taken was to treat repeated measures data as an SP over time and analyze using PROC GLM of SAS. The main plot portion of the analysis would be an "among-animals" analysis and the subplot portion would be a "within-animals" analysis with time as the subplot treatment. The problem with this approach, referred to as a "univariate repeated measures analysis of variance," is that measurements taken on the same animal are correlated. Furthermore, measurements taken close together in time are likely to be more highly correlated than measurements taken far apart in time. As a result, the power or sensitivity of the data analysis may be decreased and invalid conclusions may be drawn.

An approach that requires no special methodology for repeated measures involves conducting a separate analysis at each time period. If differences among treatments at each collection time are of intrinsic interest, analysis by time period is a simple, acceptable method of analysis that can be conducted using the GLM procedure of SAS. Often, however, RM experiments are conducted with the objective of comparing trends over time. To satisfy this objective, the kind of "mixed model" methodology developed by animal breeders is required. The MIXED procedure of SAS (SAS, 1996) enables researchers to model the covariance structure of the data, and, as a result, it provides valid standard errors and efficient statistical tests for repeated measures data. For further information and guidance in analyzing repeated measures data, readers are referred to SAS (1996) and Littell et al. (1998), who discuss and compare several methods of analyzing repeated measures data, and/or a consulting statistician.

B. DESIGNED COMPARISONS AMONG TREATMENT MEANS

Designed comparisons (sometimes referred to as planned F tests) should be based on the initial objectives of the experiment and identified during the planning stage. Carefully selected comparisons can answer as many independent questions as there are degrees of freedom for treatments. Contrary to popular belief, a significant overall F test for treatments is not a prerequisite for partitioning degrees of freedom into single degree of freedom contrasts. In fact, Chew (1976) stressed that the overall F test need not and should not be carried out at all. In comparing t treatments with $(t-1)$ degrees of freedom, the overall F test is averaged over $(t-1)$ orthogonal contrasts. If only one of these $(t-1)$ contrasts is significant, the overall F test is weakened by the $(t-2)$ nonsignificant contrasts and as a result may give a nonsignificant overall F value.

There are two types of designed comparisons among treatment means: (1) class comparisons (orthogonal contrasts) and (2) trend comparisons (orthogonal polynomials). Class comparisons are used when a set of treatments consists of several qualitative classes. For comparisons of this type, single degree of freedom F tests are the most sensitive of techniques for comparing means. This technique enables researchers to answer specific meaningful questions about the treatment effects in a way that is both simple and powerful. Methods of constructing orthogonal coefficients and calculations for component sums of squares are outlined by Little and Hills (1978).

Trend comparisons are used when the set of treatments consists of quantitative levels of some factor, that is, dose–response experiments. For comparisons of this type, regression analysis or curve fitting is the most appropriate technique. By using orthogonal polynomials, treatment sum of squares and degrees of freedom are partitioned into linear and curvilinear regression components. If the levels are equally spaced and replicated, the computations for obtaining the linear, quadratic, cubic, etc. components are simple. Coefficients of orthogonal polynomials for most equally spaced levels, and selected unequally spaced levels, can be found in Gill (1978c) as well as most other experimental design textbooks. Also, orthogonal polynomials can be constructed using SAS/IML (SAS, 1989b). For further details about polynomial coefficients and computations, readers should refer to one of the biometrics references cited at the beginning of this chapter.

C. USE AND MISUSE OF MULTIPLE COMPARISON PROCEDURES

Whenever possible, specific contrasts should be planned before the experiment is conducted rather than selecting comparisons after the data have been collected. This will help guard against ambiguous comparisons and will ensure maximum sensitivity for comparisons that are meaningful. For the few situations in which an experiment consists of a set of treatments that are unrelated, unstructured, or undifferentiated by prior experience or theory (e.g., experiments to evaluate different varieties of feedstuffs), all possible pairwise comparisons among the observed treatment means may be appropriate. Several pairwise multiple comparison procedures (Duncan's Multiple Range Test, Tukey's Honestly Significant Difference, Student–Newman–Kuel's Test, Fisher's Least Significant Difference) are available for such cases. Of these procedures, Fisher's Least Significant Difference, or LSD, is the test recommended when comparisons each involve only two of the treatment means. Carmer and Walker (1985) presented an excellent review of the properties of these and other multiple comparison tests.

There are three specific situations where pairwise multiple comparisons should not be used: (1) comparing treatments to a control, (2) comparing treatments factorial in nature, and (3) comparing levels of a quantitative factor (dose–response experiments). In the first situation, the goal is to detect treatments that are different from a standard or a control and the problem is to compare the mean of each treatment group with the mean of the control group. A more appropriate procedure than any of the pairwise multiple comparison procedures is Dunnett's t-like test (Dunnett, 1955). In the second situation, the effects and relationships of the factors used in the experiment can best be evaluated by partitioning the treatment sum of squares into main effects and interactions. This approach provides the experiment with the most powerful method of evaluating interaction effects or main effects if the interaction is absent or weak. Pairwise multiple comparison techniques provide no direct tests of these effects. In the third situation, the objective should be to characterize the nature of the response (linear or some degree of curvilinear) to the level or dose of treatment imposed. As pointed out by Chew (1976), if the linear regression is significant, no pairwise multiple comparison procedure is necessary because all treatments are significantly different in their effects.

VIII. INTERPRETATION AND PRESENTATION OF RESULTS

A. Partitioning Treatment Effects

Although the purpose of an experiment is to answer specific questions, results are often presented and interpreted with little reference to either the initial objectives of the experiment or the treatment structure. This is especially true of dose–response and factorial experiments (Little, 1981).

As indicated earlier, dose–response experiments measure the response to quantitative levels of some treatment factor, for example, concentrations of dietary protein, levels of growth hormone, percentages of oats in the diet. The objective of these types of experiments is to characterize the nature of the response curve. This can be stated in one simple question: What is the relationship between dose level and response? Orthogonal polynomials can be used to answer this question. This is the correct approach regardless of whether the overall treatment effect was significant or not.

In some cases, orthogonal polynomials were used in the analysis; however, when results were presented in manuscripts, superscripts indicating statistical significance among all possible pairs of means were used to summarize results. This dual approach is neither correct nor useful. A more meaningful method of summarization would be to show the partitioned treatment sum of squares and the percentages of the variability among responses accounted for by linear and curvilinear components. If there is evidence of a significant linear relationship, pairwise tests of significance are unnecessary, and, in fact, provide no useful information. Even if the observed differences between two levels is determined to be "nonsignificant" by a pairwise test, the regression already implies that an increment in dosage may be expected to effect a response.

Experiments involving factorial treatment structures constitute the second class of experiments that frequently is interpreted and presented poorly. For these types of experiments, logical questions arise: What is the effect of each factor? Does the response to one factor depend on the class (or level) or another factor, or, in other words, are there any interactions?

In factorial experiments, when the factors are not independent (interaction is present), considerable caution must be exercised in drawing conclusions about the overall main effects. The presence of the interaction means the response to different classes (or levels) of one factor changes (in either rank or magnitude) according to the class (or level) of another factor. If the interaction is one of rank, and, thus, considered moderate to strong, treatment combination (or subclass) means should be presented instead of main effect means. If the interaction is one of magnitude, and, thus, considered weak to moderate, the interaction should be acknowledged, but main effect means may still provide meaningful information.

Graphs are often an effective means of summarizing the results of factorial experiments. For example, simple response plots, which illustrate the relationship between the response and important factors in an experiment, can be used to show various degrees of interaction and, thus, provide insight into cause-and-effect relationships when interactions are present. Construction of such plots involves only simple arithmetic and is described in detail by Moen et al. (1999).

B. Statistics in Manuscripts

When experimental results are reported in scientific manuscripts, the statistical methods should be summarized in a clear and concise manner that can be easily understood. Obviously, the biology should be emphasized, but a clear account of the way the experiment was conducted and how the results were analyzed assures readers that proper design and analysis were used. Ashton and McMillan (1981) presented a useful list of suggestions for the presentation of statistics in scientific manuscripts. Although primarily directed toward medical researchers, Byrne (1998) provides a discussion of the importance of statistics in manuscripts that is worthwhile reading for researchers in any field, including swine nutrition.

Stating only the computer software package used to analyze data is not, in itself, a sufficient description of the statistical analysis. User's manuals for computer software packages generally are not adequate references for statistical methods. Analysis of standard designs should be described by name and size. For a factorial experiment in an RCB design, an adequate description of the analysis might be, "Data were analyzed as a randomized complete block design with a 2 × 3 factorial arrangement of treatments in five blocks." Also, the experimental unit should be defined. In cases in which the usual experimental error is not the term used for testing treatment differences, such as in SP or RM designs, the error term that was used should be identified. Finally, contrasts used to answer specific questions should be identified. If the contrasts were nonorthogonal, the test procedure should be referenced as well.

Significance levels associated with specific tests provide measures of reliability and should be identified in text, tables, and figures. The most commonly reported significance levels are $P < 0.10$, $P < 0.05$, $P < 0.01$, and $P < 0.001$. An alternative is to state exact probabilities for each comparison and let the reader decide what to reject; however, this tends to clutter a paper with numerous probability levels. Whatever level of significance is chosen by researchers, the choice should be based on the relative consequences of rejecting the null hypothesis when it is true (type I error) and accepting the null hypothesis when it is false (type II error). Because significance is implied when a probability statement is used, it is redundant to use any form of the word *significance* in the same sentence.

Regardless of the method of presentation or whether the results are statistically significant, some measure of residual variation (e.g., error mean square, pooled standard deviation, pooled standard error, coefficient of variation) should be reported with treatment means. Giving results of significance tests does not eliminate the need to present some measure of variability. As pointed out by Morse and Thompson (1981), this is so for several reasons. First, a measure of residual variability (experimental error) is required if a reader wants to consider a hypothesis other than the stated one or to combine subsets of published results with those from other sources. Second, a measure of the inherent variability in the experimental material may be valuable for researchers designing similar experiments. Third, a measure of variability will give an idea of the precision and power of the experiment. Fourth, estimation of treatment effects is often as important as hypothesis testing, and reliability of such estimates can be assessed if some measure of variability is presented.

Generally, either a pooled standard deviation (square root of the error mean square) or a pooled standard error (pooled standard deviation divided by the square root of the number of replications) will suffice. Unless there is heterogeneity of variances, standard errors should not be presented for individual means. In some situations, researchers may choose to report the coefficient of variation (pooled standard deviation multiplied by 100 and divided by the mean); however, the use of the coefficient of variation generally is confined to giving a subjective measure of the efficiency of the experimental techniques or to comparing the relative variation among experiments.

IX. ROLE OF THE STATISTICIAN IN EXPERIMENTATION

Including a statistician as a member of the research team will circumvent many potentially serious statistical problems. The statistician's role should begin during the planning stage of the experiment. Later, the statistician can be involved in data analysis, and finally, in interpretation and presentation of results. It is beneficial for the statistician on the team to have some training and expertise in the research field of interest. Similarly, it is beneficial for other team members to have some biometrical training to comprehend the potentials as well as the limitations of statistics as a research tool. Obviously, the degree to which a statistician is needed in the experiment will depend on the biometrical training of the primary researcher. If approached as a cooperative effort, the association between biologists and statistician can be of mutual benefit. As pointed out by Van Vleck and Henderson (1965), although statistical techniques should be considered as research tools, the statistician is not such a tool. As an active member of the research team, the statistician's contribution should be recognized just as any other team member's contribution would be recognized.

REFERENCES

Ashton, G. C., and I. McMillan. 1981. *A Medley of Statistical Techniques for Researchers*, Kendall/Hunt, Dubuque, IA.
Bartlett, M. S. 1937. Some examples of statistical methods of research in agriculture and biology, *J. R. Stat. Soc.*, 4(Suppl.):137.
Berndtson, W. E. 1991. A simple and reliable method for selecting or assessing the number of replicates for animal experiments, *J. Anim. Sci.*, 69:67.
Byrne, D. W. 1998. *Publishing Your Medical Research Paper*, Williams & Wilkins, Baltimore.
Carmer, S. G., and W. M. Walker. 1985. Pairwise multiple comparisons of treatment means in agronomic research, *J. Agron. Educ.*, 14:19.
Chew, V. 1976. Comparing treatment means: a compendium, *HortScience*, 11:348.
Cochran, W. G., and G. M. Cox. 1957. *Experimental Designs*, 2nd ed., John Wiley & Sons, New York.
Damon, R. A., Jr., and W. R. Harvey. 1987. *Experimental Design, ANOVA and Regression*, Harper & Row, New York.
Dunnett, C. W. 1955. A multiple comparison procedure for comparing several treatments with a control, *J. Am. Stat. Assoc.*, 50:1096.
Fisher, R. A. 1935. *The Design of Experiments*, Oliver and Boyd, London.
Gill, J. L. 1978a. *Design and Analysis of Experiments in the Animal and Medical Sciences*, Vol. 1, Iowa State University Press, Ames, IA.
Gill, J. L. 1978b. *Design and Analysis of Experiments in the Animal and Medical Sciences*, Vol. 2, Iowa State University Press, Ames, IA.
Gill, J. L. 1978c. *Design and Analysis of Experiments in the Animal and Medical Sciences*, Vol. 3, Iowa State University Press, Ames, IA.
Gill, J. L., and H. D. Hafs. 1971. Analysis of repeated measurements of animals, *J. Anim. Sci.*, 33:331.
Hartley, H. O. 1950. The maximum F-ratio as a short-cut test for heterogeneity of variance, *Biometrika*, 37:308.
Hinkelmann, K., and O. Kempthorne. 1994. *Introduction to Experimental Design*, Vol. I of *Design and Analysis of Experiments*, John Wiley & Sons, New York.
Lentner, M., and T. Bishop. 1993. *Experimental Design and Analysis*, 2nd ed., Valley Book Co., Blacksburg, VA.
Littell, R. C. 1989. Statistical analysis of experiments with repeated measurements, *HortScience*, 24:37.
Littell, R. C., P. R. Henry, and C. B. Ammerman. 1998. Statistical analysis of repeated measures data using SAS procedures, *J. Anim. Sci.*, 76:1216.
Little, T. M. 1981. Interpretation and presentation of results, *HortScience*, 16:19.
Little, T. M., and F. J. Hills. 1978. *Agricultural Experimentation*, John Wiley & Sons, New York.
Mason, R. L., R. F. Gunst, and J. L. Hess. 1989. *Statistical Design and Analysis of Experiments with Applications to Engineering and Science*, John Wiley & Sons, New York.
Milliken, G. A., and D. E. Johnson. 1984. *Designed Experiments*, Vol. 1 of *Messy Data*, Van Nostrand Reinhold, New York.
Moen, R. D., T. W. Nolan, and L. P. Provost. 1999. *Quality Improvement through Planned Experimentation*, 2nd ed., McGraw-Hill, New York.
Morse, P. M., and B. K. Thompson. 1981. Presentation of experimental results, *Can. J. Plant. Sci.*, 61:799.
Ott, E. R. 1975. *Process Quality Control*, McGraw-Hill, New York.
SAS. 1989a. *SAS/STAT Users Guide* (Version 6, 4th ed.), SAS Inst. Inc., Cary, NC.

SAS. 1989b. *SAS/IML Software: Usage and Reference* (Version 6), SAS Inst. Inc., Cary, NC.
SAS. 1996. *SAS System for Mixed Models*, SAS Inst. Inc., Cary, N.C.
Snedecor, G. W., and W. G. Cochran. 1980. *Statistical Methods*, 7th ed., Iowa State University Press, Ames, IA.
Steel, R. G. D., and J. H. Torrie. 1980. *Principles and Procedures of Statistics: A Biometrical Approach*, 2nd ed., McGraw-Hill, New York.
Van Vleck, L. D., and C. R. Henderson. 1965. Statistics in the design and analysis of physiology experiments, *J. Anim. Sci.*, 24:559.

40 Digestion and Balance Techniques in Pigs

Olayiwola Adeola

CONTENTS

I. Introduction 903
II. Methodological Considerations 904
    A. Quantitative Feed and Feces (Total Collection) Method 904
    B. Index Method 906
    C. Direct and Difference (Indirect) Approaches 906
    D. Total Collection vs. Index Methods 907
III. Energy Digestibility and Balance 909
    A. Cereal Grains, Protein Supplements, Fats, and Oils 909
    B. Energy Retention and Heat Production 910
        1. Comparative Slaughter Technique 911
        2. Carbon–Nitrogen Balance Technique 911
        3. Direct Calorimetry 912
        4. Indirect Calorimetry 912
IV. Nitrogen Digestibility and Balance 912
    A. Apparent Nitrogen Digestibility and Balance 912
    B. Estimating Endogenous Nitrogen Loss 913
References 915

I. INTRODUCTION

The information presented by Young et al. (1991) in the previous edition of this book served as a foundation for the contents of this chapter. The textbooks by Schneider and Flatt (1975), McLean and Tobin (1987), and Whittemore (1990) provide detailed discussion of several procedures for conducting digestion and balance studies. These studies are essentially relationships between input and output of nutrients. A digestion study involves quantifying the intake of a specific component of a feedstuff, the fecal output from the undigested portion of that component of the feedstuff, and the difference between intake and output. Component of a feedstuff as used throughout this chapter refers to energy or nutrients such as nitrogen, amino acids, and minerals. A balance study, as well as quantifying intake and fecal output, also involves quantifying the excretion of the component of interest, or its derivative, in urine, gases, products of conception (in gestating pigs), or milk (in lactating pigs). The procedures for conducting energy and nitrogen digestibility and balance are discussed in this chapter. Chapter 9 of this book gives a detailed discussion on amino acid digestibility.

II. METHODOLOGICAL CONSIDERATIONS

Pigs, similar in weight and in age, are selected and moved into crates that allow for separate collection of feces and urine. The crates are designed in such a way that they are fully adjustable to accommodate pigs of different sizes, and to permit feces to drop into trays behind the pigs rather than through perforated floors. It is also essential that the crates are equipped with feed troughs that minimize spillage, as well as trays underneath the troughs for collecting spilled feed. Males are normally used, which makes the separate collection of feces and urine easier. It is imperative that pigs are given adequate time to adapt to the crates and the feed being evaluated. In this regard, an adaptation period of 3 to 7 days and a collection period of 4 to 6 days will suffice. Expeditious adaptation to crates and feed is facilitated by holding off feed, but providing a generous supply of water on the day pigs are moved into crates.

In a standard study to determine the digestibility of a component of a test feedstuff, the requirement is to measure the intake of that component and the fecal output of the component belonging to the measured intake. The quantitative feed and feces (total collection) method requires meticulous records of feed intake and output of feces together with chemical analysis of the feed and feces. The index method avoids the need for quantitative records of feed intake and feces output, but relies heavily on accurate chemical analyses of index compounds in feed and feces.

A. QUANTITATIVE FEED AND FECES (TOTAL COLLECTION) METHOD

The quantitative feed and feces method of determining the digestibility of a component of a given feedstuff is essentially a record-keeping operation. It requires an accurate record of feed intake for determining the amount of the component ingested, as well as an accurate record of the output of feces for determining the amount of component voided via the feces. A satisfactory measure of the feces belonging to the measured feed intake presents a technical problem during a digestion study. Feces belonging to a given feed are usually identified by the use of markers, which are colored compounds consumed as a part of the first meal marking the beginning of the collection period of the digestion study, and consumed a second time as a part of the meal marking the end of the collection period of the digestion study. The marker colors the feces, and fecal collection starts with the appearance of the first colored feces. The color tails off as fecal collection progresses. Fecal collection stops with the second appearance of the colored feces. The quantity of feces collected is taken to represent the fecal output from the diet consumed from when the first marker was fed to the last unmarked meal (before the second marker was fed). Substances commonly used as markers are ferric oxide, chromic oxide, carmine red, or indigo carmine. The fundamental assumption in the use of a marker is that the marker moves with the digesta in the lumen of the gastrointestinal tract and that it does not diffuse into adjacent unmarked digesta. Sometimes the assumption does not hold true and consequently the separation of feces is not accurate. However, with timed feeding and a constant daily intake over a sufficiently long adaptation period, the daily fecal output should remain relatively constant.

Once pigs are in crates, it is essential that they are adequately adapted to the crates and feed being given. The adaptation period, which is usually 3 to 7 days, is followed by a collection period of 4 to 6 days. At Purdue University, an adaptation period of 5 days followed by a collection period of 5 days is usually practiced.

The objectives of a particular experiment, the nature of the diets, and the acceptability of the diet by the pigs will have effects on the level of feeding. In general, the adaptation period is used to establish the level of feeding that will be maintained throughout the collection period. The minimum level of feeding should be maintenance (110 kcal digestible energy × body weight in kilograms$^{0.75}$). Feeding at four times maintenance is desirable, but may not be practical because of the possibility of feed refusal. Feed refusal creates more work in collecting and weighing the refused feed (orts) and conducting a chemical analysis of the refused feed to account for possible changes in dry matter content, selection, and contamination with saliva. For feeds without unusual ingredients that could present palatability or acceptability problems, a level of feeding at 3.5 times maintenance, or approximately 4% of body weight per day, should suffice. As body weight increases above 50 kg, the level of feeding is reduced to between 2.7 and 4% of body weight or 2.5 and 3.5 times maintenance. In lieu of unrestricted access to water, 2 to 2.5 l/kg of dry feed is appropriate.

In an experiment consisting of an adaptation period of 5 days followed by a collection period of 5 days, a marker (to color the feces) is added to approximately 100 g of feed during the morning feeding on day 6 (reckoning the day pigs are moved into crates as day 1) to start as the collection period. After pigs have consumed the marker and the feed, the remainder of the feed allotment for that mealtime is offered. On day 11, the marker is fed, as was done on day 6, for a second time to end the collection period. For pigs up to 50 kg body weight, 1 g of ferric oxide added to 100 g of feed on day 6 and 11 should suffice; 2 g of ferric oxide added to 100 g of feed should be adequate for pigs heavier than 50 kg. Amounts when carmine red is used as a marker are 0.25 and 0.5 g for pigs under and over 50 kg body weight, respectively. It is assumed that, as the marker passes through the gut, there is very little mixing of the marker with digesta from adjacent meals. The feces voided and collected between the first and second appearances of the marker are assumed to originate from the feed consumed between the administration of the two markers during the 5-day collection period. Because colored feces may not appear until 18 to 36 h after the marker is fed, it is important to maintain the same level of feeding through the second appearance of colored feces, at which time the collection of feces ends. In a balance study, which requires quantitative collection of urine, the accumulation of urine in bladder and periodic voiding make it difficult to identify urine as originating from specific meals. It is usual to start quantitative collection of urine at the start of the collection period when the marker is first fed in the morning on day 6 and to stop urine collection when the marker is fed a second time in the morning on day 11.

Feces are collected at meal times, weighed, sealed in plastic bags, and stored in a freezer at $-18°C$. Feces from each day are combined, mixed thoroughly, sampled, weighed, and dried. For a balance study, urine is collected over preservatives, which also trap ammonia. These preservatives include formaldehyde, hydrochloric acid, and sulfuric acid. Preservatives are added to collection receptacles in sufficient amounts at collection times to acidify (bring the pH down to approximately 5) the urine. The volume of urine is measured at meal times, sampled (10 to 30% aliquot) and stored in a freezer at $-18°C$. Urine samples from each day are combined and strained through glass wool to remove particulate matter. For feces and urine, lyophilization (freeze-drying) or drying in a forced-draft oven at 55 to 60°C gives similar results with minimal loss of volatile compounds. Drying in a forced-draft oven at temperatures over 70°C results in significant loss of volatile compounds. In classical experiments designed to examine the effects of storage on nitrogen and energy losses from pig feces and urine after collection, Fuller and Cadenhead (1965) demonstrated that storage of feces and urine for 8 days at 1°C did not result in any significant losses of nitrogen and energy when compared with feces and urine processed immediately after they were voided. In another study examining the method of preparation of feces on nitrogen digestibility, Jørgensen et al. (1984) demonstrated that oven-drying or freeze-drying did not affect nitrogen digestibility when compared with wet feces. Thus, once adequate care is taken to freeze feces and acidify urine, the losses of nitrogen and energy should be minimal.

Digestibility is calculated as follows:

$$\text{Digestibility, \%} = 100 \times \left[\frac{\text{amount of component consumed} - \text{amount of component voided in feces}}{\text{amount of component consumed}} \right] \quad (40.1)$$

B. Index Method

The need for quantitative records of feed intake and for quantitative collection of feces can sometimes be avoided by the use of index compounds. Index compounds should have the following attributes: chemically easily to analyze for, nonabsorbable, nonessential, nontoxic, completely inert (indigestible), regularly and completely voided in the feces, and uniformly mixed with the feed and feces. Thus, the amount of the index compound in the feed and the amount voided in the feces should be similar over equal periods of time. Chromic oxide or acid insoluble ash uniformly mixed in the diet at 0.1 to 0.5% are commonly used as index compounds. Other index compounds that have been evaluated include dysprosium (Kennelly et al., 1980), rare earth metals (Pond et al., 1986), and titanium oxide (Jagger et al., 1992). The use of the index method does not require housing pigs in digestion crates; however, care must be exercised to ensure that the index compound is not recycled through coprophagy. Samples collected are processed as described in the total collection methods section above. In addition, the feed and the feces are chemically analyzed for their concentrations of the index compound.

With the index method, digestibility is calculated as follows:

$$\text{Digestibility, \%} = 100 - \left[100 \times \left(\frac{\text{concentration of index compound in feed} \times \text{concentration of component in feces}}{\text{concentration of index compound in feces} \times \text{concentration of component in feed}} \right) \right] \quad (40.2)$$

C. Direct and Difference (Indirect) Approaches

The digestibility of a component of a test feedstuff is determined either by the direct or the difference (indirect) approach.

With the direct approach, the diet is formulated such that all of the component of interest is supplied by the test feedstuff alone. In other words, no other feedstuffs in the diet (except the test feedstuff) supply the component. Diets formulated as such are offered to pigs, and digestibility of the component is determined using either the total collection or index methods described above.

In some instances of feedstuff evaluation, the test feedstuff cannot be fed for a long enough period of time to determine the digestibility of the component of interest. Also, it may be impossible, with the feedstuffs available, to formulate the diet with the test feedstuff alone supplying all the component of interest. The diets are therefore formulated with other feedstuffs, in addition to the test feedstuff, also supplying the component of interest. These diets are offered to pigs in a digestion study using either the total collection or index methods described above. However, because feedstuffs other than the test feedstuff supply the component of interest in the diet, digestibility for the component of interest in the test feedstuff is calculated using the difference (indirect) approach. Digestibility determined using the difference approach assumes that the feedstuffs supplying the same component in the total diet do not interact with one another to enhance or depress the digestibility of that component, i.e., there are no associative effects among feedstuffs supplying the same component in the total diet.

One of three methods is frequently used in the difference approach. One method is to feed a basal diet to group of pigs and determine the digestibility of this basal diet. Simultaneously, another group of pigs is fed the basal diet plus a known quantity of the test feedstuff and to determine the digestibility of the mixture. The digestibility of the component in the test feedstuff is calculated as follows:

$$\text{Digestibility of the component in the test feedstuff, } A, \% = 100 \times \left[\frac{(T \times t) - (B \times b)}{a} \right] \quad (40.3)$$

where: T is the digestibility, %, of the component in the total diet (basal diet plus the test feedstuff); t is the amount of the component in the total diet (basal diet plus the test feedstuff) consumed; B is the digestibility, %, of the component in the basal diet; b is the amount of the component in the basal diet consumed; and a is the amount of the component in the test feedstuff added to the basal diet $t = b + a$. The digestibilities of the basal diet, B, and the total diet (basal diet plus the test feedstuff), T are determined using either the total collection or the index methods described above.

Another method is to feed a basal diet to a group of pigs and simultaneously feed another group of pigs a diet that has a proportion of the basal diet replaced by the test feedstuff. The digestibility of the component in the test feedstuff is calculated as follows:

$$\text{Digestibility of the component in the test feedstuff, } A, \% = 100 \times \left[\frac{(T \times T_p) - (B \times B_p)}{A_p} \right] \quad (40.4)$$

where A, T, and B are as defined above; B_p is the proportion, %, of the component in the total diet contributed by the basal diet; A_p is the proportion, %, of the component in the total diet contributed by the test feedstuff; $T_p = B_p + A_p = 100\%$. Again, the digestibilities B and T are determined using either the total collection or the index methods as described.

The third method is to feed a basal diet to a group of pigs and simultaneously feed another groups of pigs diets that have at least two proportions of the component in the basal diet replaced by the test feedstuff. Regression of the digestibility of the component against proportions of the component replaced and extrapolation to 100% replacement is used to estimate digestibility. There is always a danger in extrapolating outside the range of tested replacement levels, and the errors associated are inversely related to the level of the basal diet replaced by the test feedstuff.

D. TOTAL COLLECTION VS. INDEX METHODS

The use of index methods to determine digestibility avoids the need for quantitative records of feed intake and feces output. The question then arises whether both methods of determining digestibility give similar values. The question was addressed in the experiments reported by Jørgensen et al. (1984), Adeola et al. (1986a), Jagger et al. (1992), Mroz et al. (1996), and Thompson and Wiseman (1998). For diets composed of corn, cornstarch, or soybean meal, the use of chromic oxide as an index compound gave dry matter digestibility values similar to those obtained by total collection (Figure 40.1). For soybean

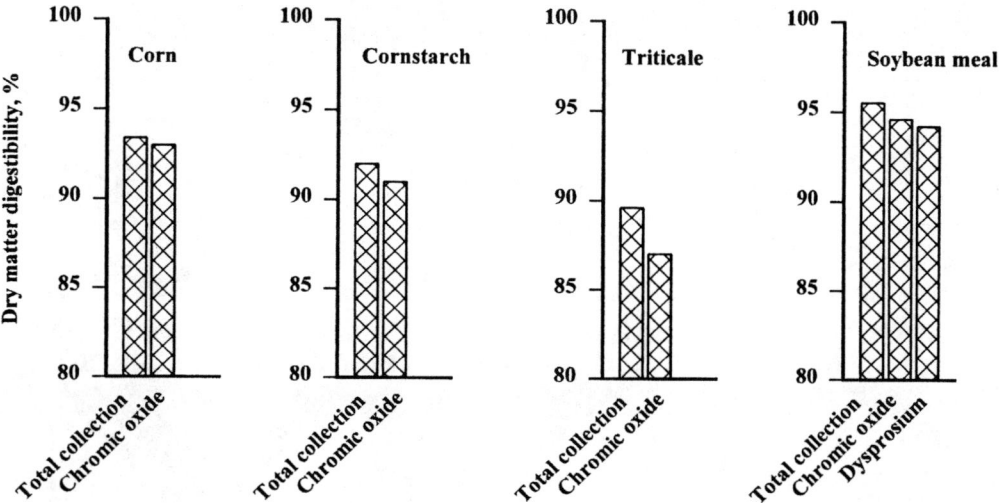

FIGURE 40.1. Comparison of total collection and index methods in the determination of dry matter digestibility of feeds for pigs. The corn and triticale data were taken from Adeola et al. (1986a); cornstarch and soybean meal data were taken from Jørgensen et al. (1984).

meal, dysprosium as an index compound also gave a similar dry matter digestibility value to total collection. However, for diets composed of triticale, the chromic oxide index underestimated dry matter digestibility (Figure 40.1).

The use of chromic oxide as an index also underestimated energy digestibility compared with total collection in a diet composed of triticale (Figure 40.2). For a corn diet or complete feed (wheat, wheat feed, soybean meal, and fish meal), the use of chromic oxide or titanium oxide as index compounds gave similar energy digestibility values to total collection (Figure 40.2). As shown in Figure 40.3, total collection and index methods gave similar nitrogen digestibility values

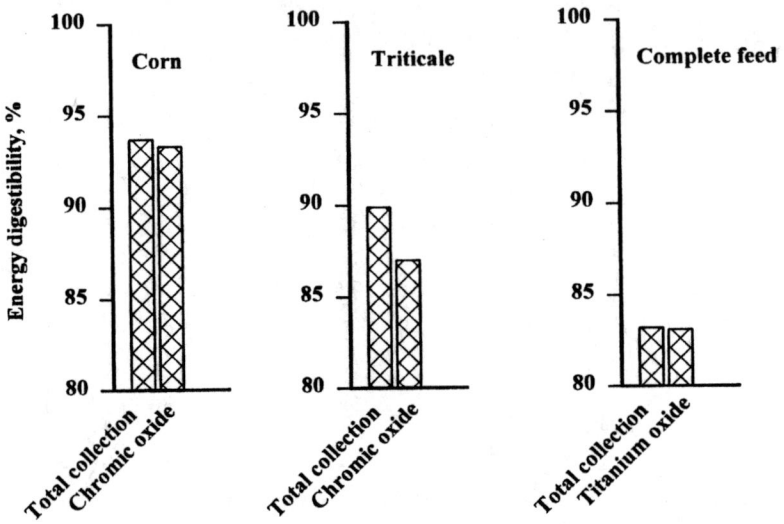

FIGURE 40.2. Comparison of total collection and index methods in the determination of energy digestibility of feeds for pigs. The corn and triticale data were taken from Adeola et al. (1986a); complete feed data were taken from Thompson and Wiseman (1998).

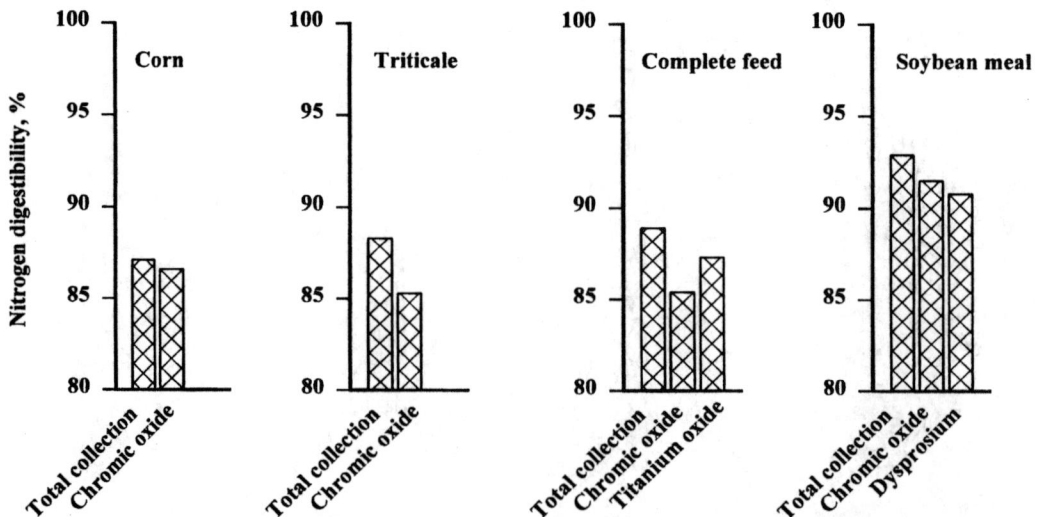

FIGURE 40.3. Comparison of total collection and index methods in the determination of nitrogen digestibility of feeds for pigs. The corn and triticale data were taken from Adeola et al. (1986a); complete feed data were taken from Jagger et al. (1992); soybean meal data were taken from Jørgensen et al. (1984).

except for chromic oxide in diets composed of triticale and dysprosium in diets composed of soybean meal as its only nitrogen source. Triticale inherited the sticky characteristics of its rye parent in producing viscous digesta. Therefore, chromic oxide may not mix uniformly with the digesta as it passes through the digestive tract, which could account for the lower estimate of digestibility relative to total collection. From the foregoing, it would appear that the nature of the feed has important consequences on the choice of using the index (using chromic oxide) or total collection methods.

III. ENERGY DIGESTIBILITY AND BALANCE

The energy digestibility of a feed and energy balance in pigs may be determined by feeding the pigs over a period of time and collecting the feces and urine voided as described above. Feces and urine are each dried as described above. Samples of feed and dried feces are ground to pass through a 1-mm screen and analyzed for energy by bomb calorimetry. For urine, drying a known volume (200 to 300 ml) in a shallow, wide container (to give a high ratio of surface area to volume) placed in a forced-draft oven at 55°C works well. The dry urine, which is crisp (not gummy) like corn chips, is weighed and quickly transferred to airtight polythene bags (Whirl-Pak) and stored in the freezer until analysis by bomb calorimetry. Each dry, crispy urine sample is taken out of the freezer minutes before it is weighed into crucibles and combusted in a bomb calorimeter. The procedure described above for determining the energy content of urine by bomb calorimetry works very well and is used routinely at Purdue University.

Table 40.1 shows for a pig, an example calculation of energy balance taken from an experiment reported previously (Adeola and Bajjalieh, 1997). In the example, the dry matter (%) of feces is obtained in a two-staged drying process. In the first stage, the wet feces is homogenized and dried at 55°C in a forced-draft oven to obtain a sample preparation dry matter, DM_1 (e.g., 32.3%). The dried feces is ground through a 1-mm screen and an analytical dry matter, DM_2 (e.g., 94.6%), is determined in triplicate using approximately 2-g subsamples. The product of DM_1 and DM_2 (0.323 × 94.6% = 30.6%) gives the dry matter of feces. As shown in Table 40.1, 100 × (GEI − GEO) ÷ GEI gives the percentage energy digestibility and (GEI − GEO) ÷ DMI or FI gives the digestible energy content of the feed on a dry matter or an as-fed basis, respectively. GEI is gross energy intake, GEO is gross energy output in the feces, DMI is dry matter intake, and FI is feed intake.

The digestibility calculation shown in Table 40.1 is termed *apparent* because all the energy in the feces is not of feed origin. Spent digestive enzymes, secretions of the bile, sloughed-off cells lining the gastrointestinal tract, and intestinal microbial activity products are collectively termed *endogenous losses*. These products are not directly of feed origin, but they contribute to the energy in feces. Correcting the energy in feces for these endogenous losses gives true energy digestibility. True energy digestibility is always greater than or equal to apparent digestibility, and while apparent energy digestibility is affected by the dietary energy level, true energy digestibility is not. In pigs, however, the determination of endogenous energy losses is not practicable.

A. CEREAL GRAINS, PROTEIN SUPPLEMENTS, FATS, AND OILS

The digestibility of energy in a cereal grain of reasonable protein level may be determined by feeding the cereal grain supplemented with a small amount of vitamins and minerals. In this case, a feed with approximately 97% cereal grain and 3% vitamins and minerals is formulated and fed, and the digestibility is determined using the direct approach. In situations where it is not possible to use cereal grains at 97% of the diet (due to palatability or formulation restriction), the difference approach may be used. The determination of energy digestibility and balance in protein supplements such as fish meal or soybean meal and in fats and oils such as tallow or soybean oil present other

TABLE 40.1
Example Calculation of Energy Balance

Pig weight (kg)		24.5
Feed intake (FI) (kg/day)		1.0
Dry matter (DM) (%)		88
Dry matter intake (DMI) (kg/day)	(88/100) × 1.0	0.88
Gross energy of feed (kcal/kg DM)		4390
Gross energy intake (GEI) (kcal/d)	4,390 × 0.88	3863
Weight of feces collected over a 5-day collection period (kg)		1.89
Dry matter of feces, % (see text)		30.6
Dry feces output (kg/day)	(30.6/100) × 1.89 ÷ 5	0.116
Gross energy of feces (kcal/kg DM)		4955
Gross energy output in feces (GEO) (kcal/day)	4,955 × 0.116	575
Volume of urine collected over a 5-day collection period (l)		6.76
Dry matter of urine (kg/l)		0.02
Dry urine output (kg/day)	0.02 × 6.76 ÷ 5	0.027
Gross energy of urine (kcal/kg DM)		3075
Gross energy output in urine (GEU) (kcal/day)	3,075 × 0.027	83
Energy digestibility (%)	100 × (GEI − GEO) ÷ GEI	
	100 × (3863 − 575) ÷ 3863	85
Digestible energy content of feed (kcal/kg DM)	(GEI − GEO) ÷ DMI	
	(3863 − 575) ÷ 0.88	3736
Digestible energy content of feed (kcal/kg as fed)	(GEI − GEO) ÷ FI	
	(3863 − 575) ÷ 1.0	3288
Energy metabolizability (%)	100 × (GEI − GEO − GEU) ÷ GEI	
	100 × (3863 − 575 − 83) ÷ 3863	83
Metabolizable energy of feed (kcal/kg DM)	(GEI − GEO − GEU) ÷ DMI	
	(3863 − 575 − 83) ÷ 0.88	3642
Metabolizable energy of feed (kcal/kg as fed)	(GEI − GEO − GEU) ÷ FI	
	(3863 − 575 − 83) ÷ 1.0	3205

considerations. As these feedstuffs cannot be fed alone, digestibility is determined in a diet that includes other energy-supplying feedstuffs as described in the difference approach above. The difference approach is illustrated with the following example. A nutrient-adequate basal diet is formulated and fed to a group of 25-kg pigs at 0.85 kg/day. To the 0.85 kg of basal diet, 0, 0.05, 0.1, or 0.15 kg of the test feedstuff is added. Thus, each of four groups of 25-kg pigs simultaneously receive 0.85, 0.9, 0.95, or 1.0 kg of basal diet plus the test feedstuff. The digestible energy (difference between gross energy in feed and in feces) intake is regressed against feed intake to obtain the graph shown in Figure 40.4. The constant at zero added test feedstuff represents the digestible energy value of the basal diet (2975 kcal in 0.85 kg or 3500 kcal/kg) and the slope of the regression plane represents the digestible energy value of the test feedstuff (3800 kcal/kg).

B. ENERGY RETENTION AND HEAT PRODUCTION

Metabolizable energy is the gross energy of feed minus the energy in feces and urine as illustrated in Table 40.1. Studying the utilization of metabolizable energy requires the measurement of either the energy retained in the animal's tissues or the animal's heat production. The difference between metabolizable energy intake and energy retention is heat production. Heat production may be measured by direct or indirect calorimetry. Energy retention, the actual part of feed energy retained by the animal, may be measured either by the comparative slaughter technique or by carbon–nitrogen balance.

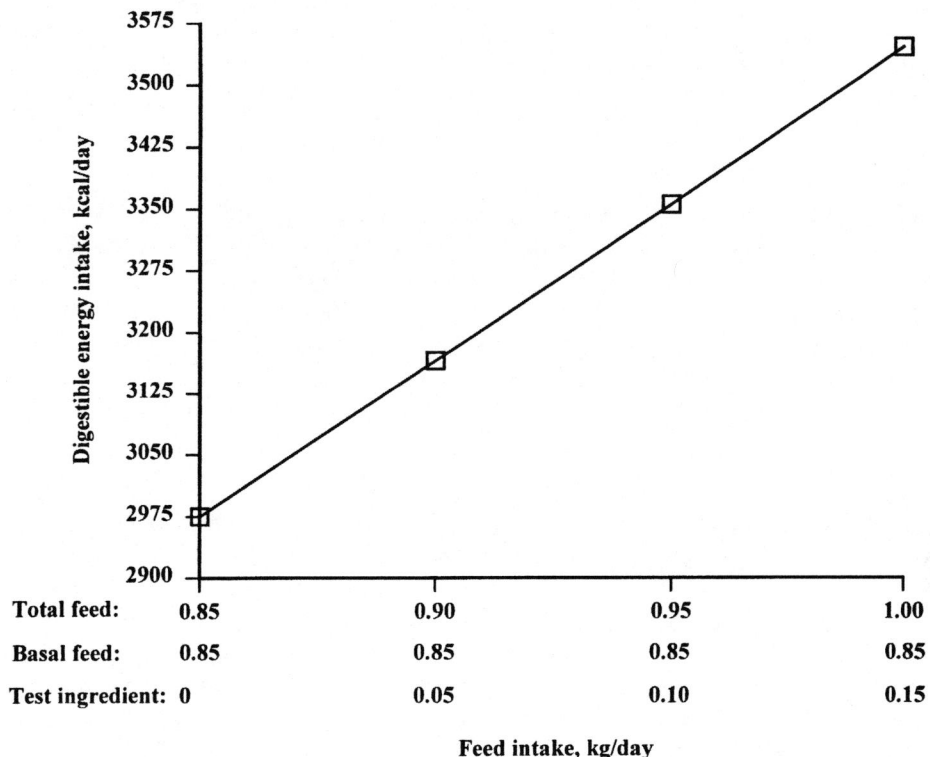

FIGURE 40.4. Illustration of the difference approach for determining digestibility by regression analysis. A nutrient-adequate basal diet is fed at 0.85 kg/day; and 0, 0.05, 0.1, or 0.15 kg of the test ingredient is added. Thus, each of four groups of 25-kg pigs simultaneously receive 0.85, 0.9, 0.95, or 1.0 kg of basal diet plus the test ingredient. The digestible energy (difference between gross energy in feed and in feces) intake is regressed against feed intake. The constant at zero added test feedstuff represents the digestible energy value of the basal diet (2975 kcal in 0.85 kg or 3500 kcal/kg) and the slope of the regression plane [(3545 − 2975) ÷ (0.15 − 0)] represents the digestible energy value of the test ingredient (3800 kcal/kg).

1. Comparative Slaughter Technique

Pigs (four to six) are killed, ground, and dried as an initial slaughter group. The energy content of the carcasses is measured by bomb calorimetry. Pigs, similar in age and weight to those used as the initial slaughter group, are fed for a specific period on a diet the metabolizable energy content of which has been determined as described in the preceding sections. After the feeding period, the pigs are killed as a final slaughter group and the energy content of carcasses determined as described for the initial slaughter group. Energy retention is the difference between the carcass energy contents of the final and initial slaughter groups.

2. Carbon–Nitrogen Balance Technique

Energy is stored in a growing pig mainly as protein and fat. Reserves of carbohydrate (as glycogen) are very low. Carbon–nitrogen balance technique requires knowing the intake of carbon and nitrogen from measuring feed intake, and the output of carbon and nitrogen from measuring feces, urine, and gases (carbon dioxide and methane) voided. Thus, carbon and nitrogen retention are calculated as the difference between intake and output. Body protein is assumed to contain 16% nitrogen; thus, the amount of protein stored in the retained nitrogen can be calculated. Furthermore, body protein is assumed to contain 51.2% carbon; thus, the amount of carbon in the stored protein can be calculated and subtracted from the total carbon to obtain carbon retained as fat. The remainder of the carbon is fat and is assumed to contain 74.6% carbon; thus, the amount of stored fat can be calculated. The protein and fat stored in the body are multiplied by 5.65 and 9.13 kcal/g, respectively, and summed to give an estimate of energy retention.

3. Direct Calorimetry

The routes of heat loss from the body of a pig include conduction, convection, evaporation of water from skin and lungs, radiation, and excretion in feces and urine. To determine heat loss, the pig is enclosed in an adequately insulated chamber where heat loss can be measured. Heat loss is measured as it passes through the wall of the chamber. Due to the prohibitive costs of building, maintaining, and operating chambers for measuring heat production by direct calorimetry, this method is rarely used to measure heat production in pigs.

4. Indirect Calorimetry

Heat production is closely correlated to oxygen consumption and carbon dioxide production. Therefore, by measuring oxygen consumption and production of carbon dioxide and methane, it is possible to estimate heat production. Respiratory intake and output of gases may be measured in closed- or open-circuit respiration chambers. In the closed-circuit respiration chamber, the air and respiratory gases are recirculated, and it is therefore less suitable for pigs kept for several days. It is more common to use open-circuit respiration chambers where outside air is passed continuously through the chamber. The amount of ingoing and outgoing air is measured and sampled for analyses of oxygen, carbon dioxide, and methane. In addition to measurements of respiratory gases, urine is also collected, measured, and analyzed for nitrogen. Heat production is calculated from respiratory gas exchanges and nitrogen loss in urine using the equation proposed by Brouwer (1965):

$$\text{Heat production, kcal} = (3.866 \times \text{oxygen}) + (1.2 \times \text{carbon dioxide}) - (0.518 \times \text{methane}) - (1.431 \times \text{nitrogen}) \tag{40.5}$$

where oxygen represents the liters of oxygen consumed, carbon dioxide represents the liters of carbon dioxide produced, methane represents the liters of methane produced, and nitrogen represents the grams of urinary nitrogen produced.

In a well-planned and carefully conducted study, Noblet et al. (1987) presented strikingly similar values for heat production of pigs that were determined by indirect calorimetry (open-circuit) or by comparative slaughter techniques; 201 and 217 kcal per day/body weight, $kg^{0.75}$, respectively.

An example of the method of calculating heat production for a pig raised from 20 to 100 kg body weight is illustrated in Table 40.2. The empty body weight and the energy therein at 20 kg are the mean values obtained from six pigs killed as an initial slaughter group. The metabolizable energy intake is calculated as the product of total feed intake (over the 94 days it took to reach 100 kg body weight) and metabolizable energy content of the diet (215.7 kg × 3276 kcal/kg = 706,633 kcal). Total heat production over the 20- to 100-kg weight interval is the difference between metabolizable energy intake and body energy retention (706,633 − 228,208 = 478,425 kcal). Mean daily heat production per unit metabolic body weight is 478,425 kcal ÷ 94 days ÷ 60 $kg^{0.75}$ = 236. The 60 kg represents the midpoint between 20 and 100 kg body weight.

IV. NITROGEN DIGESTIBILITY AND BALANCE

A. Apparent Nitrogen Digestibility and Balance

The digestibility of nitrogen in a feed and nitrogen balance in pigs may be determined by feeding the pigs over a period of time and collecting the feces and urine voided as described above. Feces

TABLE 40.2
Example Calculation of Heat Production from Energy Retention Obtained Using the Comparative Slaughter Technique and Metabolizable Energy Intake

Initial body weight (kg)		20.0
Empty body weight (kg)[a]		19.4
Final body weight (kg)		100.0
Empty body weight (kg)		95.0
Days from 20 to 100 kg body weight (days)		94.0
Metabolizable energy intake from 20 to 100 kg body weight (kcal)[b]		706,633
Energy in 19.4 kg empty body (kcal)[a]		45,408
Energy in 95 kg empty body (kcal)		273,616
Energy retention from 20 to 100 kg body weight (kcal)	273,616 – 45,408	228,208
Heat production from 20 to 100 kg body weight (kcal)	706,633 – 228,208	478,425
Mean heat production (kcal/day)	478,425 ÷ 94	5,090
Mean heat production (kcal/day/body weight in $kg^{0.75}$)[c]	$5,090 \div 60^{0.75}$	236

[a] Empty body weight and energy at 20 kg are the mean values obtained from six pigs killed as an initial slaughter group.
[b] The 20-kg pigs consumed 215.7 kg feed in the 94 days it took to reach a body weight of 100 kg. The metabolizable energy content of the diet was 3276 kcal/kg giving a metabolizable energy intake of 215.7 × 3276 = 706,633 kcal.
[c] 60 represents the midpoint between 20 and 100 kg body weight.

and urine are each processed as described above. Samples of feed and dried feces are ground to pass through a 1-mm screen and analyzed for nitrogen using the Kjeldahl or combustion procedure. Samples of the liquid urine (approximately 5 ml, depending on nitrogen concentration) are also analyzed for nitrogen.

Table 40.3 shows a sample calculation of nitrogen balance taken from the same pig as the example presented for energy balance in Table 40.1. As shown in Table 40.3, 100 × (NI – NOF) ÷ NI gives the percentage nitrogen digestibility and (NI – NOF – NOU) gives the nitrogen balance (NB) or retention. NI is nitrogen intake, NOF is nitrogen output in the feces, and NOU is nitrogen output in the urine. The proportion of nitrogen intake that is retained in the body is the net protein utilization (100 × NB ÷ NI). The biological value of the protein is the proportion of the digested and absorbed nitrogen that is retained in the body (100 × NB ÷ (NI – NOF)). The calculations shown in Table 40.3 are termed apparent because all the nitrogen in the feces is not of feed origin. Spent digestive enzymes, secretions of the bile, sloughed-off cells lining the gastrointestinal tract, and intestinal microbial activity products are collectively termed endogenous losses. These products are not directly of feed origin, but they contribute to the nitrogen in feces. Correcting the nitrogen in feces for these endogenous losses gives true nitrogen digestibility. Some of the methods that may be used to estimate endogenous losses of nitrogen are discussed in the next section.

B. ESTIMATING ENDOGENOUS NITROGEN LOSS

Apparent digestibility estimates do not differentiate between endogenous nitrogen and undigested and unabsorbed nitrogen of feed origin. Endogenous protein and amino acids consist of protein from gastric, pancreatic, and biliary secretions, sloughed-off mucosal cells, and endogenous ammonia and urea. Obtaining true nitrogen digestibility requires the correction of feces nitrogen for endogenous nitrogen. In a 30-kg pig, approximately 90% of the endogenous nitrogenous compounds secreted into the lumen of the gastrointestinal tract is digested and absorbed, leaving only a small fraction lost in the feces (Fuller and Reeds, 1998). Endogenous nitrogen losses are affected by dietary protease inhibitors (e.g., trypsin inhibitor), and fat, fiber, pectin, and protein levels.

TABLE 40.3
Example Calculation of Nitrogen Balance

Pig weight (kg)		24.5
Feed intake (FI) (g/day)		1000
Dry matter (DM) (%)		88
Dry matter intake (DMI) (g/day)	(88/100) × 1000	880
Nitrogen in feed (% on a DM basis)		1.44
Nitrogen intake (NI) (g/day)	(1.44/100) × 880	12.67
Weight of feces collected over a 5-day collection period (g)		1890
Dry matter of feces (%)		30.6
Dry feces output (g/day)	(30.6/100) × 1890 ÷ 5	116
Nitrogen in feces (% on a DM basis)		2.49
Nitrogen output in feces (NOF) (g/day)	(2.49/100) × 116	2.89
Volume of urine collected over a 5-day collection period (ml)		6760
Nitrogen in urine (g/100 ml)		0.046
Nitrogen output in urine (NOU) (g/day)	(0.046/100) × 6760	3.11
Nitrogen digested (NA) (g/day)	NI − NOF	
	12.67 − 2.89	9.78
Nitrogen digestibility (%)	100 × (NI − NOF) ÷ NI	
	100 × (12.67 − 2.89) ÷ 12.67	77.1
Nitrogen balance (NB) (g/day)	NI − NOF − NOU	
	12.67 − 2.89 − 3.11	6.67
Net protein utilization (%)	100 × NB ÷ NI	
	100 × 6.67 ÷ 12.67	52.6
Biological value of feed protein (%)	100 × NB ÷ NA	
	100 × 6.67 ÷ 9.78	68.2

The methods that may be used for estimating endogenous nitrogen include the following:

1. In the direct method, animals are fed a nitrogen-free diet and the feces are collected and analyzed for nitrogen. Implicit in the use of a nitrogen-free diet to estimate endogenous nitrogen loss is the assumption that nitrogen in the diet does not affect the recovery of endogenous nitrogen. The assumption, of course, is contradicted by strong evidence that diets with greater nitrogen levels have greater endogenous nitrogen losses (Letterme et al., 1996). Using the direct method of feeding a nitrogen-free diet to estimate endogenous nitrogen in the feces, Adeola et al. (1986b) reported a value of 0.0012 g nitrogen/g of dry matter intake. In the example calculation shown in Table 40.3, the daily nitrogen intake of 12.67 g translates to 0.0144 g nitrogen/g of dry matter intake (12.67 ÷ 880), and the daily nitrogen output in feces of 2.89 g translates to 0.0033 g nitrogen/g of dry matter intake (2.89 ÷ 880). Correcting this daily output of nitrogen in the feces for endogenous nitrogen loss in the feces gives 0.0021 g nitrogen/g of dry matter intake (0.0033 − 0.0012). Therefore, true nitrogen digestibility in this example is 100 × (0.0144 − 0.0021) ÷ 0.0144 = 85.4%, compared with apparent nitrogen digestibility of 77.1% (Table 40.3).

True nitrogen digestibility is always greater than or equal to apparent digestibility; while apparent nitrogen digestibility is affected by the dietary nitrogen level, true nitrogen digestibility is not.

2. The regression method involves feeding three or more levels of dietary nitrogen and regressing the concentration of nitrogen in the feces (expressed per unit of dry matter intake) against concentration of dietary nitrogen (expressed per unit of dry matter intake). Endogenous nitrogen in the feces is obtained by extrapolating to zero dietary nitrogen. Just as in the feeding of a nitrogen-free diet, this method also assumes that nitrogen content in the diet does not affect the recovery of endogenous nitrogen, or that there is a constant output of endogenous nitrogen regardless of dietary protein intake.

3. Guanidination involves treating dietary protein with *O*-methylisourea for the conversion of the lysine residues into homoarginine (Hagemeister and Erbersdobler, 1985; Schmitz et al., 1991). Assumptions in the use of guanidinated proteins to estimate endogenous nitrogen losses are that modification of the protein has no effect on digestion, there is no selective endogenous secretion of homoarginine into the lumen, and homoarginine is absorbed in the same proportion as other nitrogen constituents of the diet and thus serves as an index of undigested nitrogen. The guanidination method may be useful for digestibility determined at the end of the ileum, but the exposure of homoarginine to metabolism by hindgut microbes renders the method unsuitable for digestibility determined by collection of the feces.

4. Completely digestible protein may be fed to pigs. All the nitrogen in the feces collected is thus assumed to be of endogenous origin.

Because of its relative simplicity, the direct method of feeding a nitrogen-free diet still remains the most commonly used method for estimating endogenous losses of nitrogen.

REFERENCES

Adeola, O., and N. L. Bajjalieh. 1997. Energy value of high-oil corn for pigs, *J. Anim. Sci.*, 75:430.

Adeola, O., L. G. Young, E. G. McMillan, and E. T. Moran, Jr. 1986a. Comparative protein and energy value of OAC Wintri triticale and corn for pigs, *J. Anim. Sci.*, 63:1854.

Adeola, O., L. G. Young, E. G. McMillan, and E. T. Moran, Jr. 1986b. Comparative availability of amino acids in OAC Wintri triticale and corn for pigs, *J. Anim. Sci.*, 63:1862.

Brouwer, E. 1965. Report of sub-committee on constants and factors. In *Energy Metabolism*, Blaxter, K. L., Ed., Academic Press, London, 441–443.

Fuller, M. F., and A. Cadenhead. 1965. The preservation of feces and urine to prevent losses of energy and nitrogen during metabolism experiments. In *Energy Metabolism of Farm Animals*, Blaxter, K. L., J. Kielanowski, and G. Thorbek, Eds., Oriel Press, Newcastle-upon-Tyne, England, 455.

Fuller, M. F., and P. J. Reeds. 1998. Nitrogen cycling in the gut, *Annu. Rev. Nutr.*, 18:385.

Hagemeister, H., and H. F. Erbersdobler. 1985. Chemical labeling of dietary protein by transformation to homoarginine: a new technique to follow intestinal digestion and absorption, *Proc. Nutr. Soc.*, 44:133A (Abstr.).

Jagger, S., J. Wiseman, D. J. A. Cole, and J. Craigon. 1992. Evaluation of inert markers for the determination of ileal and fecal apparent digestibility values in the pig, *Br. J. Nutr.*, 68:729.

Jørgensen, H., W. C. Sauer, and P. A. Thacker. 1984. Amino acid availabilities in soybean meal, sunflower meal, fish meal and meat and bone meal fed to growing pigs, *J. Anim. Sci.*, 58:926.

Kennelly, J. J., F. X. Aherne, and M. J. Apps. 1980. Dysprosium as an inert marker for swine digestibility studies, *Can. J. Anim. Sci.*, 60:441.

Leterme, P., T. Monmart, A. Thewis, and P. Morandi. 1996. Effect of oral and parenteral N nutrition vs. N-free nutrition on the endogenous amino acid flow at the ileum of the pig, *J. Sci. Food Agr.*, 71:265.

McLean, J. A., and G. Tobin. 1987. *Animal and Human Calorimetry*, Cambridge University Press, Cambridge, U.K.

Mroz, Z., G. C. M. Bakker, A. W. Jongbloed, R. A. Dekker, R. Jongbloed, and A. van Beers. 1996. Apparent digestibility of nutrients in diets with different energy density, as estimated by direct and marker methods for pigs with or without ileo-cecal cannulas, *J. Anim. Sci.*, 74:403.

Noblet, J., Y. Henry, and S. Dubois. 1987. Effect of protein and lysine levels in the diet on body gain composition and energy utilization in growing pigs, *J. Anim. Sci.*, 65:717.

Pond, W. G., K. R. Pond, W. C. Ellis, and J. H. Matis. 1986. Markers for estimating digesta flow in pigs and the effects of dietary fiber, *J. Anim. Sci.*, 63:1140.

Schmitz, M., H. Hagemeister, and H. F. Erbersdobler. 1991. Homoarginine labeling is suitable for determination of protein absorption in miniature pigs, *J. Nutr.*, 121:1575.

Schneider, H., and W. P. Flatt. 1975. *The Evaluation of Feeds through Digestibility Experiments*, University of Georgia Press, Athens, GA.

Thompson, J. E., and J. Wiseman. 1998. Comparison between titanium oxide as an inert marker and total collection in the determination of digestible energy of diets fed to pigs, *Proc. Br. Soc. Anim. Sci.*, 67:157.

Whittemore, C. T. 1990. *Elements of Pig Science*, Longman Scientific and Technical, Harlow, Essex, U.K.

Young, L. G., A. G. Low, and W. H. Close. Digestion and metabolism techniques. In *Swine Nutrition*, Miller, E. R., D. E. Ullrey, and A. J. Lewis, Eds., Butterworth-Heinemann, Boston, MA, 623–630.

41 Techniques for Measuring Body Composition of Swine*

A. D. Mitchell and Armin M. Scholz

CONTENTS

I. Introduction	918
II. Factors that Influence Body Composition	919
III. Physical and Chemical Basis for Composition Measurement	919
IV. Methods of Analysis	921
A. Subjective Methods	921
B. Physical and Chemical Methods	922
1. Weight	922
2. Linear Measurements	922
3. Densitometry (Specific Gravity)	922
4. Dissection and Chemical Analysis	923
5. Models	924
C. Dilution Methods	926
1. Deuterium Oxide	927
2. Urea	928
D. Metabolic Analysis	928
1. Creatinine Excretion	928
E. Tissue Interaction (Molecular Level)	929
1. Bioelectrical Impedance	929
2. Total-Body Electrical Conductivity	931
3. X-Ray Absorptiometry	932
4. Near-Infrared Interactance	934
5. Nuclear Magnetic Resonance Spectroscopy	935
F. Atomic Analysis	936
1. Total-Body Potassium	936
2. Neutron Activation	936
G. Image Analysis	937
1. Magnetic Resonance Imaging	938
2. X-Ray Computed Axial Tomography	942
3. Ultrasound	945
4. Video Imaging and Three-Dimensional Topometry	946
V. Summary	946
References	947

---

* The contents of this publication do not necessarily reflect the views or policies of the U.S. Department of Agriculture, nor does mention of trade names, commercial products, or organizations imply endorsement from the U.S. Government.

I. INTRODUCTION

Nutritional status (feed intake) and diet composition, in addition to environmental conditions, gender, and the genetic background of pigs, affect every aspect of the body composition and/or body compartment composition during growth, maturity and/or pregnancy, and following lactation (Bastianelli and Sauvant, 1997; Lobley, 1998; Nuernberg et al., 1998). During growth as well as during the different reproductive cycles, the muscle, fat, and bone compartments undergo alterations in the absolute amounts and relative proportions of lipid, protein, water, and minerals. However, Susenbeth and Keitel (1988) demonstrated that pigs exceeding 60 kg body weight have a relatively constant protein content within the fat-free fraction "empty body minus carcass" of 17.6%, and within fat-free lean of 21.8%.

Body composition, (metabolic) body weight, and the distribution of fat (and protein) depots affect both maintenance requirements for basic metabolic processes and requirements for different performance characteristics. These requirements finally determine the feed efficiency (Luiting, 1993). Changes in the fat and/or water content are especially highly correlated to changes in the total body weight (mass), which can be easily measured. However, only measurement of the *in vivo* body composition provides detailed information about nutritional and/or health status because the body composition compartments are indicative of the different energy stores: fat, protein, carbohydrate (glycogen), or fat- and fat-free mass components in swine. Body weight can be used only as an approximate indicator of body composition in one population or one herd, because body weight does not reveal whether an individual pig is obese or well muscled, healthy or sick, mal- or overnurished. Exact *in vivo* body composition measurements have to be applied or developed to be able to monitor and understand the body composition alterations resulting from new emerging technologies for nutritional manipulation, and genetic engineering of livestock (Wray-Cahen et al., 1998).

There are a number of criteria for an "ideal" method for measuring body composition:

1. *Rapid:* Depends on the application (i.e., only a few seconds for online carcass evaluation, <1 min for evaluation of market animals, to <20 min for selection of breeding stock);
2. *Nondestructive:* And preferably noninvasive;
3. *Accurate:* >95% accuracy;
4. *Easy to operate:* Minimal animal handling and restraint, no anesthesia, user-friendly instrumentation and data processing;
5. *Economical:* Includes both initial and operating costs, the cost per measurement could depend on application and might range from a few cents for market animals to a few dollars for breeding animals; and
6. *Real time measurement:* Minimal data manipulation and processing, ideally, results are immediately available.

To achieve a suitable level of accuracy, the method will likely need to provide a direct measure of one or more of the major determinants of body composition, at the tissue level (muscle, fat), chemical level (protein, lipid, water), or elemental level (carbon, hydrogen, nitrogen). Furthermore, the measurement should be based on the total-body rather than a localized sampling approach.

In recent years, various instruments have been used to penetrate the animal in an attempt to gather information on body composition. These include the use of ultrasound, x-rays, γ-rays, near-infrared rays, nuclear magnetic resonance, electrical impedance, electromagnetic conductivity, and neutron activation. Many of these approaches are capable of providing accurate and useful information, but fail to meet the criteria for practical application, primarily the combination of accuracy and economy.

II. FACTORS THAT INFLUENCE BODY COMPOSITION

The body composition of meat-producing animals varies as a result of breeding (including transgenic manipulation), sex, age (stage of growth or reproduction), nutritional status, environment (temperature), and the use of metabolic modifiers (repartitioning agents). An illustration of the wide variation in body composition that can be observed in growing pigs as a result of these factors is shown in Figure 41.1.

Changes in body or carcass composition as a result of all of the above factors are manifested primarily as an alteration the fat:lean ratio. To provide consumers with a more healthful product, the livestock industry is striving to produce animals that have less fat and more lean. Thus, accurate measurement of body composition is needed to select superior animals for breeding stock, to optimize feeding programs, to establish the efficacy of metabolic modifiers or other treatments, and to determine the value of animals going to slaughter.

III. PHYSICAL AND CHEMICAL BASIS FOR COMPOSITION MEASUREMENT

Why is the body composition of the live animal so difficult to measure accurately? The answer, no doubt, lies within the complex heterogeneity of the living system. At the atomic level, >95%

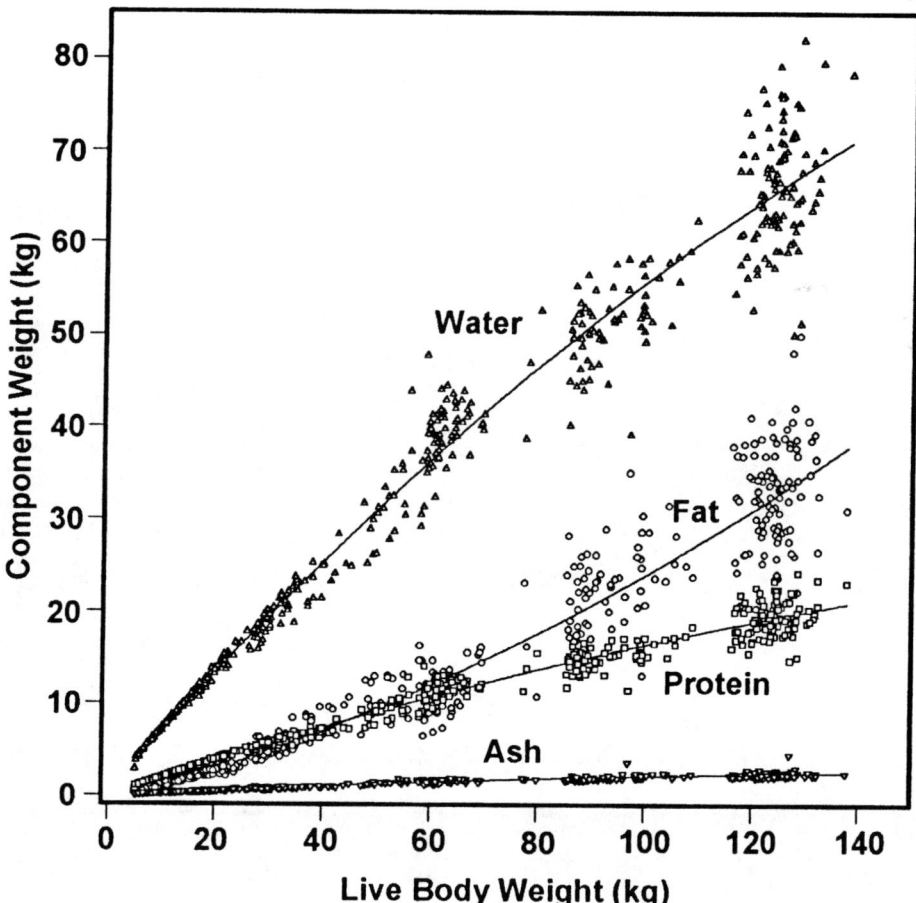

FIGURE 41.1 Analysis (by dual energy X-ray absorptiometry) of differences in body composition of growing pigs at weights ranging from 5 to 138 kg. Other variables included breed, halothane genotype, transgenic manipulation, and dietary manipulation (energy and protein intake). (Mitchell and Scholz, unpublished data.)

of the body mass consists of four elements: O, C, H, and N. The inclusion of an additional seven elements — Na, K, P, Cl, Ca, Mg, and S — brings the total to over 99.5% (Wang et al., 1992). At the molecular level, these elements are organized into hundreds of different compounds, but for the purpose of body composition, they are generally classified as lipid, water, protein, glycogen, and "ash," which together account for >99% of the body mass. At the tissue–organ level, in addition to meat (skeletal muscle) and fat (which can be subcutaneous, internal, or inter- and intramuscular), the body also contains variable amounts of bone; blood; connective tissue and skin; hair, hooves, organs of the cardiovascular, respiratory, nervous, reproductive, and urinary systems; and the gastrointestinal tract containing variable amounts of digesta.

Techniques for body composition measurement are based on a variety of physical and chemical constants. In addition, certain constant physiological relationships are necessary to measure accurately the composition of the pig or its carcass, especially by the more indirect methods. In the young pig, the relationship among the dissectable components (adipose tissue, lean, and bone) and the chemical components (lipid, water, protein, and water) is not constant. During the first few weeks following birth, the protein content of the fat-free body of the pig increases rapidly, accompanied by a rapid decrease in water content (Figure 41.2). This trend continues on a more gradual basis until "chemical maturity" is achieved somewhere between 150 and 300 days of age (Moulton,

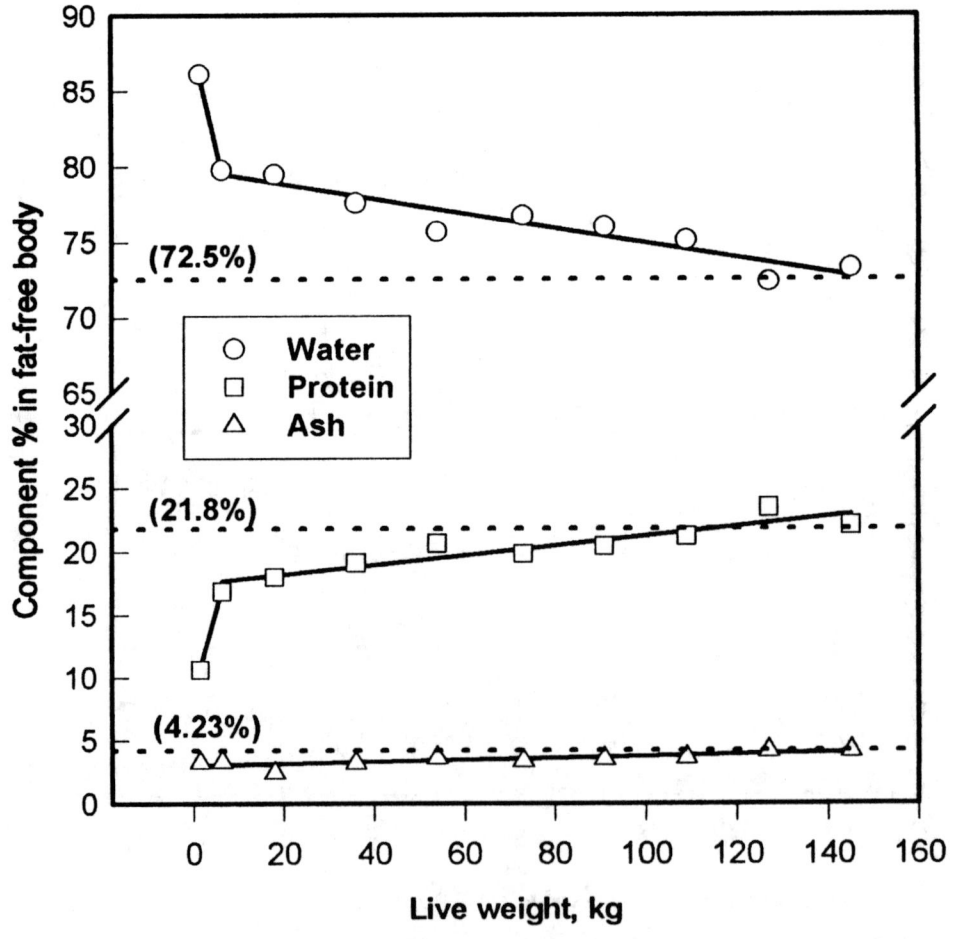

FIGURE 41.2 Relationship between live weight and the water, protein, and ash content of the fat-free body of growing pigs. (Adapted from Shields et al., 1983c; Gnaedinger et al., 1963; and Susenbeth and Keitel, 1988.)

TABLE 41.1
Physical and Chemical Properties Useful for Body Composition Measurement

Electrical conductivity of fat and lean (water)
X-ray attenuation of fat, lean, and bone
Nuclear magnetic resonance properties of protons in fat and water
Near-infrared reflectance or interactance of fat and water
Energy spectra of γ-rays emitted by N, C, and O, following neutron activation
Diffraction of ultrasonic waves at tissue boundaries
Densities (specific gravity) of fat, lean, and bone
Nitrogen content of protein
Carbon content of fat
Potassium content of cells
Water and protein content of the fat-free carcass of the mature pig

1923). As a result, the protein–water ratio of pork muscle increases from 0.156 at birth to 0.296 at 6 to 7 months of age (Kauffman et al., 1964). The water and lipid content of adipose tissue also changes. The adipose tissue (backfat) of the newborn pig contains ~85% water and 6% lipid — by 28 weeks of age the water content has dropped to ~5% and the lipid content has increased to 93% (McMeekan, 1940a). The water and lipid content of adipose tissue is also related to the total fat content of the pig. In fact, Aberle et al. (1977) proposed that a measure of either the water or lipid content of adipose tissue could be used to predict carcass composition ($r \cong 0.8$) of market-weight pigs. A list of the properties that are commonly exploited for body composition measurement are shown in Table 41.1. The accuracy of any given method will depend on how well it is able to measure one or more of these properties.

IV. METHODS OF ANALYSIS

A. Subjective Methods

Visual and tactile assessment (condition or conformation scoring in terms of fatness or leanness/muscling) were the only means for selection and/or body composition evaluation in pig production for centuries, starting with domestication (Figure 41.3). These assessments resulted in

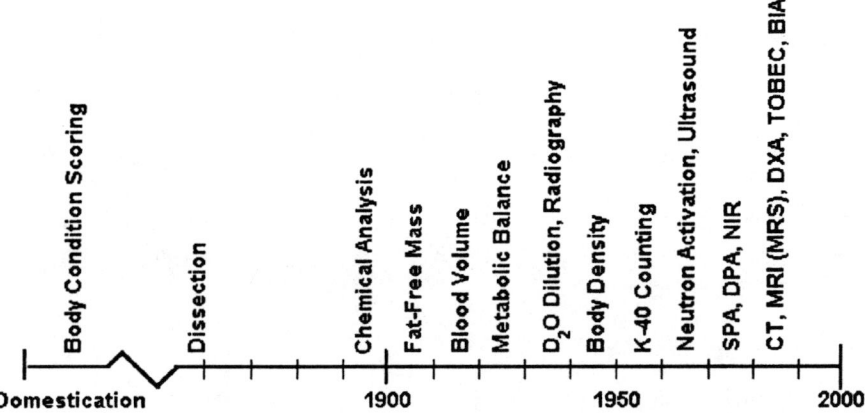

FIGURE 41.3 History of body composition assessment in livestock. (Modified from Forbes, 1999.)

a large number of pig breeds with a wide variation in their body composition, with the extremely muscled Pietrain breed on one side and the very fertile but fat Chinese breeds on the other side. The characteristic shape of meaty pig strains can be described as short and blocky with well-filled rounded hams and a more Ω-shaped than n-shaped rear view (Whittemore, 1987). However, exterior traits describing size and structure of the body are no longer relevant for growth performance (body composition) estimation (van Steenbergen, 1990), because several techniques for application on live animals enable objective and more accurate measurements of body composition. In many cases, highly correlated body composition indicators such as backfat thickness or area and longissimus muscle area are being measured *in vivo* to estimate the whole-body composition. These *indirect* methods are still difficult to implement on large-scale farms. Charette et al. (1996) describe the evaluation of the porcine body condition (sows) by a body scoring technique as an alternative to *in vivo* body composition measurements predicted from body morphology.

The combination of linear measurements (WIDTH across the rear hams, pelvic HEIGHT) with semiquantitative scores (visual and palpation scores for THORAX morphology, and TAIL setting) has a higher reproducibility coefficient (ratio of variance due to animals to total variance) than the body condition SCORE (Patience and Thacker, 1989) has (0.9137 vs. 0.7726). The difference was caused by the higher OBSERVER effect for the body condition SCORE indicating a very subjective evaluation technique. Both methods described by Charette et al. (1996) were not validated on objective reference data such as chemical body composition. Generally, subjective body condition scoring cannot contribute to an already sufficient evaluation of the animal's actual body composition.

B. Physical and Chemical Methods

1. Weight

As shown in Figure 41.1, as pigs grow larger, the proportion of fat in the body increases. This results in a high positive correlation between body weight and percentage fat (Bush et al., 1969). However, in this same figure it can be seen that within a given weight class there can be a large variation in fat content, especially by the time pigs reach market weight. Thus, weight alone is a poor predictor of composition. In developing and evaluating various techniques for predicting body or carcass composition, weight is often included as a variable in regression equations. When studies include a wide range of body weights, weight is highly correlated with measurements such as fat or lean mass. Therefore, when comparing the relative merits of different techniques for assessing body composition it is always best to be able to evaluate the ability of each technique to predict composition independent of body weight.

2. Linear Measurements

The body or carcass of the pig lends itself to a variety of possible linear measurements, including body length, circumference, depth, width, foreleg and hindleg length and circumference, etc. For the most part, such measurements have been found to be of little value for predicting composition (Houseman and McDonald, 1976). However, two measurements, backfat depth and longissimus muscle area, are useful for estimating fat and lean content (Mersmann, 1982a). Both measurements can easily be performed on the carcass using a ruler and longissimus muscle tracing and on the live animal using ultrasonics.

3. Densitometry (Specific Gravity)

Specific gravity analysis, commonly performed by underwater weighing, has been used extensively in human body composition studies (Lukaski, 1987), and has been studied as a method of measuring the carcass composition of pigs (Brown et al., 1951; Kraybill et al., 1953; Whiteman et al., 1953), cattle

(Kraybill et al., 1952; Kelly et al., 1968; Garrett and Hinman, 1969), and lambs (Kirton and Barton, 1958; Field et al., 1963). Specific gravity determinations have also been made on wholesale cuts of pork (Price et al., 1957), beef (Ledger et al., 1973; Mata-Hernandez et al., 1981), and lamb (Field et al., 1963; Timon and Bichard, 1965; Latham et al., 1966; Pradham et al., 1966). Because underwater weighing cannot be performed on the live animal, various volumetric techniques have been tested.

Compositional analysis by densitometry or specific gravity is based on a two-component model involving differences in the density of fat and fat-free components, with water and bone assumed to be a constant portion of the fat-free mass. The commonly reported densities of fat, lean, and bone are 0.9, 1.1, and 1.8, respectively. Once the specific gravity has been determined by either underwater weighing or derived from volumetric analysis, the estimation of composition is generally based on an experimentally derived regression equation. Kraybill et al. (1953) proposed the following empirical relationship between percentage of body fat and whole animal specific gravity: % body fat = 100 [(5.405 ÷ Sp. Gr.) − 4.914]. This method is reported to be more accurate in carcasses containing ≥20% fat (Hedrick, 1983) and is not applicable to young animals, where the water content of the fat-free body is not constant (Pearson et al., 1968; Shields et al., 1983c).

The correlation (r) between the specific gravity of pork carcasses and extractable lipid content was reported to be −0.75 (Brown et al., 1951), −0.86 (Kelly, 1955), and −0.95 (Doornenbal et al., 1962); for specific gravity and percentage lean cuts it was 0.67 (Brown et al., 1951), and for protein 0.91 (Doornenbal et al., 1962). The specific gravity of the ham is highly correlated (0.93, Pearson et al., 1956; 0.94, Whiteman et al., 1953) with that of the carcass. Despite these correlations, the prediction of body composition based on specific gravity is subject to considerable error (Shields and Mahan, 1983; Shields et al., 1983a.), probably because of lack of a constant composition of the fat-free mass and variation in the muscle/bone ratio. In addition, the procedure is too slow for most applications.

4. Dissection and Chemical Analysis

One of the traditional methods of carcass analysis is that of physical dissection. The use of dissection to determine whole-body composition of the pig dates to the mid-19th century (Lawes and Gilbert, 1859). Dissection along with chemical analysis has been the cornerstone of much of the present knowledge of the composition of the pig and continues to serve as the standard by which other methods are measured. However, these procedures are very time-consuming and difficult to perform without error. A detailed quantitative dissection procedure described by Cuthbertson and Pomeroy (1962) required an average of 110 h per half-carcass. The other obvious disadvantage is that it can only be performed on the carcass — not the live animal. Examples of extensive studies based on dissection are those of McMeekan (1940a,b,c; 1941), which also included chemical analysis, and that of Walstra (1980).

There are many ways that the carcass can be analyzed by dissection. These range from a simple separation into wholesale or lean cuts, separation of organs and tissues, a dissection of the half-carcass or sections into fat, lean, and bone, to a detailed separation of individual muscles or bones. Chemical analysis generally refers to a proximate analysis of fat (ether extract), protein (nitrogen × 6.25), water, and ash. The chemical analysis can be performed on the whole body, empty body, half-carcass, any of the individually dissected parts or on samples obtained by coring, cross-sectional slicing, or the tissue sawdust obtained by cross-sectional slicing. Always of concern are adequate homogenization, representative sampling, and various losses that can occur.

Most of the studies based on dissection and chemical analysis have been descriptive in nature. These techniques have been used to describe the composition of the pig at various stages of growth and development (Manners and McCrea, 1963; Elsley, 1963a; Wood and Groves, 1965; Stant et al., 1968; Shields et al., 1983c; Hiner, 1971; Susenbeth and Keitel, 1988; Ellowson and Carlsten, 1997), composition of the market-weight pig (Elsley, 1963b; Gnaedinger et al., 1963), to describe dietary effects (McMeeKan, 1940a,b; Richmond and Berg, 1971), and to describe the relative or allometric changes that occur during growth and development (Davies, 1974a,b;

1975; Walstra, 1980; Tess et al., 1986). Although very important to the understanding of growth and development of the pig, much of the data is only applicable to specific situations. Other studies have attempted to provide information that could be used to predict carcass composition. It has been demonstrated that there is a high correlation between the amount of dissectable fat or lean (Cross et al., 1970; Smith and Carpenter, 1973) or the chemical determination of protein (Doornenbal, 1971) or fat (Doornenbal, 1972) in the ham, loin, shoulder, and belly when compared with the whole carcass. The study by Smith and Carpenter (1973) also found that the separable tissue percentages for a small section of the loin accounted for >80% of the variation in separable lean content of the half-carcass.

5. Models

For an appropriate use of the techniques for *in vivo* body composition analysis it is necessary to know, on one hand, the physical and chemical principles of the techniques and, on the other hand, the basic biological models of body composition (Pietrobelli et al., 1996). While human body composition or fat content assessment (*in vivo*) can only be based on various model assumptions (Pietrobelli et al., 1996, Butte et al., 1997, Goran et al., 1998, Wang et al., 1998a,b), in swine (livestock) this is not the main problem. For swine, reference values for the content or mass of fat, protein, glycogen, soft tissue minerals, water, and bone minerals (six-compartment model) can be relatively easily determined chemically from whole carcasses provided that soft tissue and bone are analyzed separately after dissection and homogenization (Elowsson et al., 1998). In humans, the problem is being solved by performing reference studies on deceased human bodies or body parts (Lloyd and Mays, 1987; Mitsiopoulus et al., 1998), by using model animals, or by reference phantoms. The main animal model for reference studies related to human body composition is the pig (Sheng et al., 1988; Fowler et al., 1992; Brunton et al., 1993; 1997; Svendson et al., 1993; Ellis et al., 1994; Fuller et al., 1994; Jebb et al., 1995; Mitchell et al., 1996a; Picaud et al., 1996; Pintauro et al., 1996; Elowsson et al., 1998). Therefore, some general aspects from human body composition assessment, which are related to porcine body composition research, will be discussed in addition to "pure" swine or livestock body composition.

Wang et al. (1998a) divide the methods of estimating total body fat (body composition) *in vivo* into two main groups. The first group, statistically derived or *descriptive fat estimation* methods depend on a reference method and subsequent statistical data analysis for the development of a prediction formula. The second group, model-dependent or *mechanistic fat determination* methods are based on established "constant" body composition component relationships (Table 41.2). Both

TABLE 41.2
Methods of Estimating Total Body Fat *in Vivo*

Descriptive Methods (using prediction formulas based on chemical reference values or model assumptions)	Model-Dependent (*mechanistic*) Methods (assuming "body composition constants" for the prediction equations)
Magnetic resonance imaging	^{40}K counting — total-body potassium
Computer assisted tomography	Deuterium or tritium dilution[a] — total-body water
Ultrasound (A- and B-mode)	Neutron activation and inelastic neutron scattering — total-body nitrogen, calcium, carbon, and oxygen
Video imaging (anthropometry)	
Bioelectrical impedance analysis	Single and dual photon absorptiometry
Total body electrical conductivity	Dual (triple) energy X-ray absorptiometry[a]
Near infrared interactance	Whole-body density (underwater weighing, acoustic plethysmography)
Creatinine excretion	

[a] These methods can also make use of prediction equations based on chemical reference values, since especially dual energy X-ray absorptiometry raw fat estimates differed significantly from carcass lipid content (Mitchell et al., 1996a; 1998a).

groups belong to static models as opposed to dynamic models applied for modeling (prediction) of growth responses — growth models (e.g., Baldwin and Sainz, 1995; Bastianelli and Sauvant, 1997; Emmans and Kyriazakis, 1997).

Most mechanistic methods of *in vivo* body composition (total body fat) assessment available measure whole-tissue compartments using a two-compartment or three-compartment model (Roubenoff and Kehayias, 1991; Pietrobelli et al., 1996; Bastianelli and Sauvant, 1997; Zemel et al., 1997; Heymsfield et al., 1997; Tölli et al., 1998; Forbes, 1999). Figure 41.4 gives an overview for the different body composition compartments being used to estimate the total-body fat content in livestock, fish, and humans. The simple two-compartment model, introduced by Magnus-Levy in 1906 (Forbes, 1999), distinguishes only between fat mass and fat-free mass (or lean body mass, Roubenoff and Kehayias, 1991) for the total body assuming constant densities of fat (≈ 0.9 g/ml) and of the fat-free body (≈ 1.1 g/ml) for all individuals, whereas the now more often used three-compartment model divides the total body mass (body weight) into fat, lean body mass (or soft lean tissue), and bone (minerals). Chemically, the two-compartment model is based on the division of the mammalian body into fat on one side and protein, ash (mineral), and water on the other side (Keys and Brozek, 1953), actually leading to a four-compartment model (Hörnicke, 1962; Emmans and Kyriazakis, 1997; Roemmich et al., 1997; Goran et al., 1998). All physically based body composition methods were developed upon the basis of these two models (Lukaski, 1987). Another four-compartment model — mainly focused on the metabolically active *body cell mass* — consists of the following compartments: (1) *fat* (covering adipose tissue, brain, membranes, connective tissue, and adipocytes); (2) *body cell mass* (covering connective tissue, adipocytes, cell solids, and intracellular water); (3) *extracellular fluid* (covering plasma volume, interstitial water, and transcellular water); and (4) *skeletal tissue* (covering connective tissue and bone) (Pierson et al., 1997).

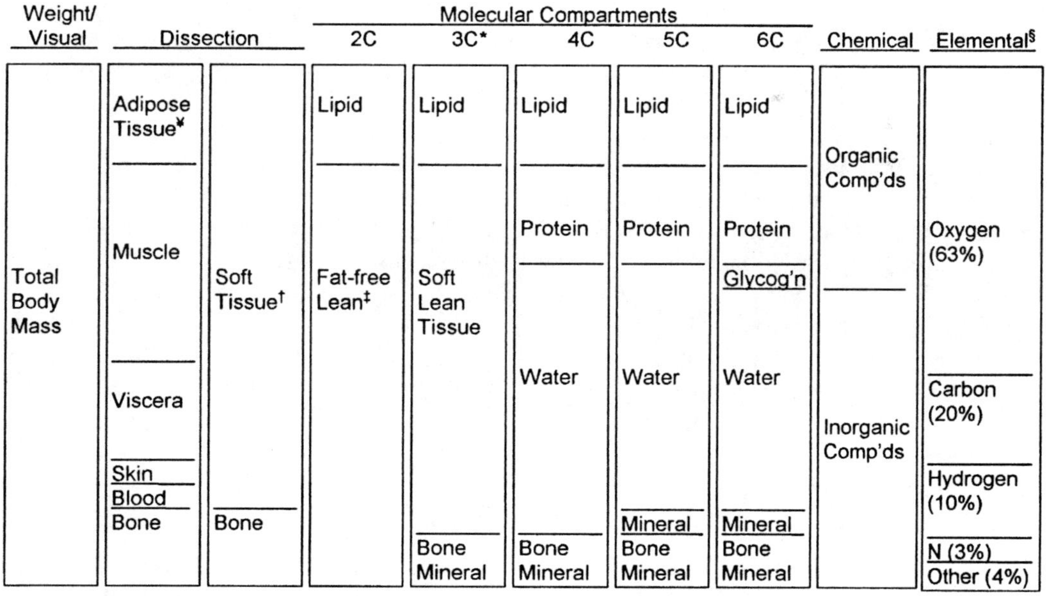

Weight/Visual	Dissection	Molecular Compartments					Chemical	Elemental[§]
		2C	3C*	4C	5C	6C		
Total Body Mass	Adipose Tissue[¥]	Lipid	Lipid	Lipid	Lipid	Lipid	Organic Comp'ds	Oxygen (63%)
	Muscle	Soft Tissue[†]	Fat-free Lean[‡]	Soft Lean Tissue	Protein	Protein		
						Protein		
						Glycog'n		
	Viscera			Water	Water	Water	Inorganic Comp'ds	Carbon (20%)
	Skin							Hydrogen (10%)
	Blood					Mineral	Mineral	
	Bone	Bone		Bone Mineral	Bone Mineral	Bone Mineral	Bone Mineral	N (3%) / Other (4%)

* Different 3C models, I: fat + mineral + other, II: fat + water + solids.
§ Sajonski and Smollich (1981).
¥ Main fat depots: subcutaneous, inter- and intramuscular, perinephric, and internal.
† Soft lean tissue + lipids.
‡ Soft lean tissue + bone ; fat-free tissue is not totally identical with lean tissue.

FIGURE 41.4 Models of body composition compartments combining atomic, molecular, cellular, tissue-system, and whole-body levels. (Modified from Hornicke, 1962; Wang et al., 1992; Pietrobelli et al., 1996; and Heymsfield et al., 1997.)

The theoretical pitfall of the two-compartment model results from the assumption that the proportions of minerals, water, and proteins in the fat-free mass are (relatively) constant independent of differences in age, body weight, body composition, and sex (Susenbeth and Keitel, 1988; Fogelholm and van Marken Lichtenbelt, 1997; Forbes, 1999) and that individuals differ only in their percentage of fat by weight provided the fat-free mass is estimated from a single measurement (Mackie et al., 1989). In terms of the pig, especially during the growth period or in extreme pig breeds (very obese or very lean) the above assumption is not suitable. Only recent technological developments apply more complex five- or six-compartment models on the molecular level (Ryde et al., 1993; Heymsfield et al., 1997; Wang et al., 1998a). Depending on the assessment technique, Wang et al. (1992) distinguish among models on the atomic level (dividing the body into its atomic elements), molecular level (dividing the body into chemically different compartments, such as lipid, protein, carbohydrates, water, mineral), cellular level (cell mass, extracellular fluid, and extracellular solids), tissue system level (adipose tissue, skeletal muscle tissue, viscera, skin tissue, bone tissue), and whole-body level (body weight or body volume), although most body composition models combine at least two body component levels. On the molecular level, fat, water, protein, cell mineral, and bone mineral account for approximately 96% of the porcine body weight (Shulman, 1993; Scholz, unpublished; see Figure 41.17). Often, the carbohydrate content (i.e., glycogen, glucose) of the body is simply ignored, leading to a slight overestimation of at least one of the above-mentioned components, fat, protein, or water (not including cell and bone mineral).

The higher level always consists of components from the lower level. A second — more questionable — concept assumes the existence of a "body-composition steady state," meaning (relatively) constant ratios among body components as long as body weight or hydration status does not change (Fogelholm and van Marken Lichtenbelt, 1997; Heymsfield et al., 1997; Wang et al., 1998b). One example is the assumed constant ratio of 4:5 between fat mass on the molecular level and adipose tissue mass on the tissue-system level. This ratio does not take into account the possible different proportions of so-called empty fat cells and the significant change of the proportion of nontriglyceride lipids within the total-body lipid fraction, especially during situations with a negative energy balance resulting from absolute or relative food intake restrictions and/or exercise (Comizio et al., 1998).

Since calibration (reference) data for regression equations are often derived and cross-validated from a specific population, these data may not be applicable to individuals of a different population. Multicomponent models that consider individual variation in the water and mineral compartments of the fat-free body should be applied to quantify differences in fat-free body composition due to differences among breeding lines, extreme diets, gender, or age groups so that accurate prediction equations can be developed for the various body composition assessment techniques. To achieve the most accurate body composition estimates, it is necessary to reduce all error sources such as reference method error (chemical analysis) or model assumption error and measurement error (Guo et al., 1996; Atkinson and Nevill, 1998).

C. Dilution Methods

Dilution techniques for body composition analysis are based on the principle that water occupies a relatively fixed fraction (74.5%; see Figure 41.2) of the fat-free mass. The dilution technique involves the introduction of a known amount of a tracer that will then equilibrate throughout a given compartment (i.e., total-body water) in the animal body. A sample of the compartment is then taken and the concentration of the tracer is measured. It is assumed that the tracer has the same distribution volume as the compartment, is nontoxic, and in the case of water is exchanged by the body in a similar manner. The most common tracers that have been tested in animals include deuterium oxide, tritiated water, and urea. Other include oxygen-18 labeled water ($H_2^{18}O$), antipyrine, and N-acetyl-1,4-aminoantipyrine. The main advantage of the dilution technique is that it can be used on any size of animal.

1. Deuterium Oxide

Measurement of body water content has been shown to be an acceptable method for determination of body composition of many animal species (Sheng and Huggens, 1979). The *in vivo* dilution of either tritiated water (^3H_2O) or deuterium oxide (D_2O) has been used extensively for this purpose. Groves and Wood (1965) used D_2O in suckling pigs, tritiated water (Kay et al., 1966) and D_2O (Wood and Groves, 1963; Houseman et al., 1973; Shields et al., 1983b; 1984; Ferrell and Cornelius, 1984) have been used in growing pigs, and Shields et al. (1984), Knudson (1986), and Rozeboom et al. (1994) used D_2O in sows. Although both forms of isotopically labeled water seem to be appropriate for use in swine, each has some inherent disadvantages (i.e., radioactivity in the case of ^3H_2O and time-consuming sample preparation in the case of D_2O). Both ^3H_2O (Aschbacher et al., 1965) and D_2O (Byers, 1979; Odwongo et al., 1984; Arnold et al., 1985) have been used to measure total-body water and body composition in cattle, sheep (Foot and Greenhalgh, 1970), goats (Treitl, 1996), and chickens (Farrell and Balnave, 1977; Johnson and Farrell, 1988).

Although D_2O is routinely administered orally in human studies, with animals it is generally given by intravenous infusion to ensure complete dosage and rapid equilibration. The time and frequency of collection of blood samples for D_2O vary among studies. The equilibration time of D_2O throughout the body was reported to be complete after 110 min in sows (Knudson, 1986) or within 120 min in 84-kg pigs (Houseman et al., 1973). By the collection of a series of blood samples, regression equations can be used to derive intercept values for D_2O space, which can be used in a two-compartment kinetic model (Figure 41.5) to estimate both empty-body water and water in the digestive tract (Shields et al., 1983b; 1984; Ferrell and Cornelius, 1984). The studies by Shields et al. (1983b, 1984) found that D_2O space overestimated total-body water in growing-finishing and reproducing swine by as much as 18 to 20%.

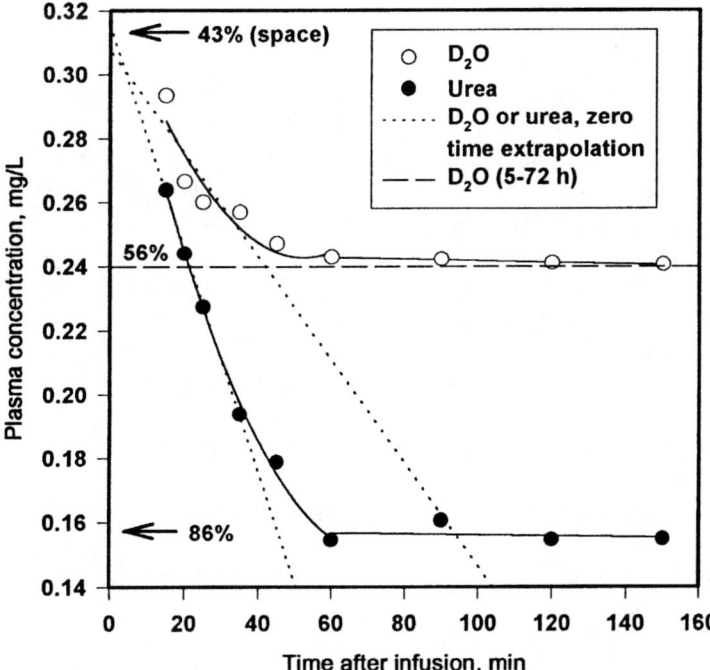

FIGURE 41.5 Decline in plasma D_2O and urea concentrations as a function of time after infusion in a 90-kg pig. The percentage figures indicated along the *Y* axis refer to the corresponding urea or D_2O space values at the zero time intercepts. (Adapted from Mitchell and Steele, 1987.)

In a study with growing pigs, Houseman et al. (1973) reported that total-body water, lipid, and protein could be estimated from D_2O space with coefficients of variation (CV) of 1.9, 6.7, and 5.6%. Likewise, Shields et al. (1983b) found that D_2O space could predict chemical components of body composition with CVs of <5% and $R^2 \geq 0.90$. On the other hand, when using pigs of diverse body type, Ferrell and Cornelius (1984) found that, although relationships between D_2O space and chemical composition were highly significant, they were influenced by body type and were little better than body weight for the estimation of body composition.

2. Urea

Urea dilution has been used to estimate body water space in some species, but has not been studied extensively in the pig (Stansbury et al., 1985; Mitchell and Steele, 1987; Chiba et al., 1990). The potential advantages of urea dilution as a method for measuring body composition include lower cost and ease of analysis. The rapid distribution of urea throughout the body water compartments was described by Donovan and Brenner (1930). Urea space was found to be equivalent to total-body water in the dog (Painter, 1940) and D_2O space in the human (San Pietro and Rittenberg, 1953). Urea dilution has been evaluated for estimating body composition in steers (Preston and Kock, 1973; Kock and Preston, 1979; Hammond et al., 1984), bulls (Meissner et al., 1980), and sheep (Meissner, 1976; Jones et al., 1982). Variations in the level of endogenous urea present a potential problem for the urea dilution method; however, it does not seem to have been a source of significant error in the ruminant species.

The urea space technique involves preinjection blood sampling to establish a baseline level of plasma urea, followed by infusion of a flooding dose of urea and subsequent blood sampling at various times to determine the extent of urea dilution. Infusion of urea increases urea entry, excretion, and turnover rates, but does not affect urea space (Mosenthin et al., 1992a). However, the presence of starch in the lower intestine can reduce the plasma urea level (Mosenthin et al., 1992b). Thus, variation in equilibration time, sampling time, diet, and the determination of baseline urea concentration are all possible sources of error with this technique.

Regression coefficients (R^2) for the relationship between urea space and empty body protein (kg) range from 0.52 (Stansbury et al., 1985) and 0.60 (Mitchell and Steele, 1987) to 0.80 (Chiba et al., 1990). For kilograms of empty body fat, R^2 values were 0.58 (Stansbury et al., 1985) and 0.29 to 0.76 (Chiba et al., 1990) and for percentage of empty body fat the R^2 was 0.42 (Mitchell and Steele, 1987). In the study by Mitchell and Steele (1987), the feasibility of urea space measurement for estimation of body composition in swine was evaluated by comparison with simultaneous measurement of D_2O space and with chemical analysis of the carcass. Urea was cleared from the plasma pool more rapidly than D_2O and seemed to equilibrate at a relative concentration that was lower than that of D_2O (see Figure 41.5). Consequently, urea and D_2O space values were closest when extrapolated to zero time values. Correlations between urea space and D_2O space were highest at 15 min postinfusion ($R^2 = 0.75$) or between urea space at 15 min and D_2O at equilibrium ($R^2 = 0.86$). Urea space at 15 min and D_2O space at 35 min most closely approximated total-body water, whereas D_2O space at 15 min was nearly equivalent to empty-body water. Overall, D_2O space at equilibrium had the highest correlations with carcass values of water, lipid, and protein and seems to be preferable to urea space for estimating carcass composition of pigs.

D. Metabolic Analysis

1. Creatinine Excretion

Creatinine is produced by the nonenzymatic hydrolysis of free creatine resulting from the dephosphorylation of creatine phosphate (Borsook and Dubnoff, 1947). Most of the creatine (98%) in the body is located in skeletal muscle, predominately as creatine phosphate. Thus, the amount of creatinine excreted from the body should be proportional to the muscle mass (Folin, 1905; Hoberman et al., 1948). Human studies have shown that urinary creatinine excretion is related to muscle mass or fat-free mass (Talbot, 1938; Cheek, 1968; Forbes and Bruining, 1976; Boileau et al., 1972); however, considerable individual variation in daily creatinine excretion has been reported. Physiological factors such as age, sex, and exercise may affect the relationship between fat-free mass and the amount of creatinine excreted (Boileau et al., 1972). Also, factors such as diet and complete and timely urine collection can be problematic. A study by Aulstad (1970) found that there was too much variation in creatinine excretion for it to be considered a reliable method for estimation of body composition.

E. Tissue Interaction (Molecular Level)

1. Bioelectrical Impedance

The use of bioelectrical impedance analysis (BIA) to measure the fat-free mass in humans was described by Lukaski et al. (1985). The system is portable, inexpensive, rapid, and simple to operate. In limited studies, BIA has been used to predict the fat-free mass of live pigs and carcasses (Swantek et al., 1992) and the Boston butt portion of pork carcasses (Marchello and Slanger, 1992). It has also been tested for measuring the fat-free mass of lambs and lamb carcasses (Berg and Marchello, 1994; Berg et al., 1996; 1997; Hegarty, 1998), the retail cuts from lamb carcasses (Slanger et al., 1994), and the composition of steer carcasses (Velazco et al., 1999).

When a low-level alternating electrical current is applied to a biological system, a voltage drop or impedance to the electrical flow is detected. Conductance, which is the opposite of impedance, is greatest in the electrolyte-rich body water and is lower in lipids and bone mineral. The impedance (Z) and its main components, resistance (Rs) and reactance (Xc) are dependent on geometric configuration and the volume of conductor in the biological system and the signal strength and frequency of the applied current. If the geometry is relatively constant, then the impedance would be a function of the electrical potential of the mass and could be calculated as $Z = (Rs^2 + Xc^2)^{0.5}$. The impedance is also related to the volume of the conductor, thus, $Z = \rho L^2/V$, where Z is in ohm, ρ is volume resistivity in ohm-cm, L is conductor length in cm, and V is volume in cm^3.

The BIA procedure consists of placing two sets of electrodes at defined locations on either the live pig or carcass (Figure 41.6). Once the electrodes are in place, the impedance readings (Rs and Xc) are taken. In addition, body weight and the distance between detector electrodes are measured. The study by Swantek et al. (1992) reported correlations of –0.56 and –0.63 between Rs and fat-free mass (FFM) and 0.64 and 0.70 between Rs and % fat for live and carcass measurements, respectively. The correlations were not as good for Xc (–0.11, –0.08, –0.11, and 0.17, respectively). The same study reported regression models that included Rs, Xc, weight, and length for the prediction of FFM in both the live pig and cold carcass (carc):

FFM (live) = 0.486 live wt – 0.881 Rs + 0.480 length + 0.860 Xc + 7.959

FFM (carc) = 0.326 half carc wt – 0.081 Rs + 0.239 length + 0.060 Xc + 9.945

The regression coefficients (R^2) for these equations were 0.817 (live) and 0.844 (carcass). In a later study (Swantek et al., 1999), the use of the above (live) prediction equation resulted in a consistent 9-kg underestimation of the FFM of pigs weighing between 50 and 130 kg. The correlation (r) between predicted and actual FFM was approximately 0.67; however, the regression intercept was found to be 17.159 rather than the 7.959 shown above. Although more studies are needed, it would seem that this could be a useful technique for both live animal and carcass evaluation.

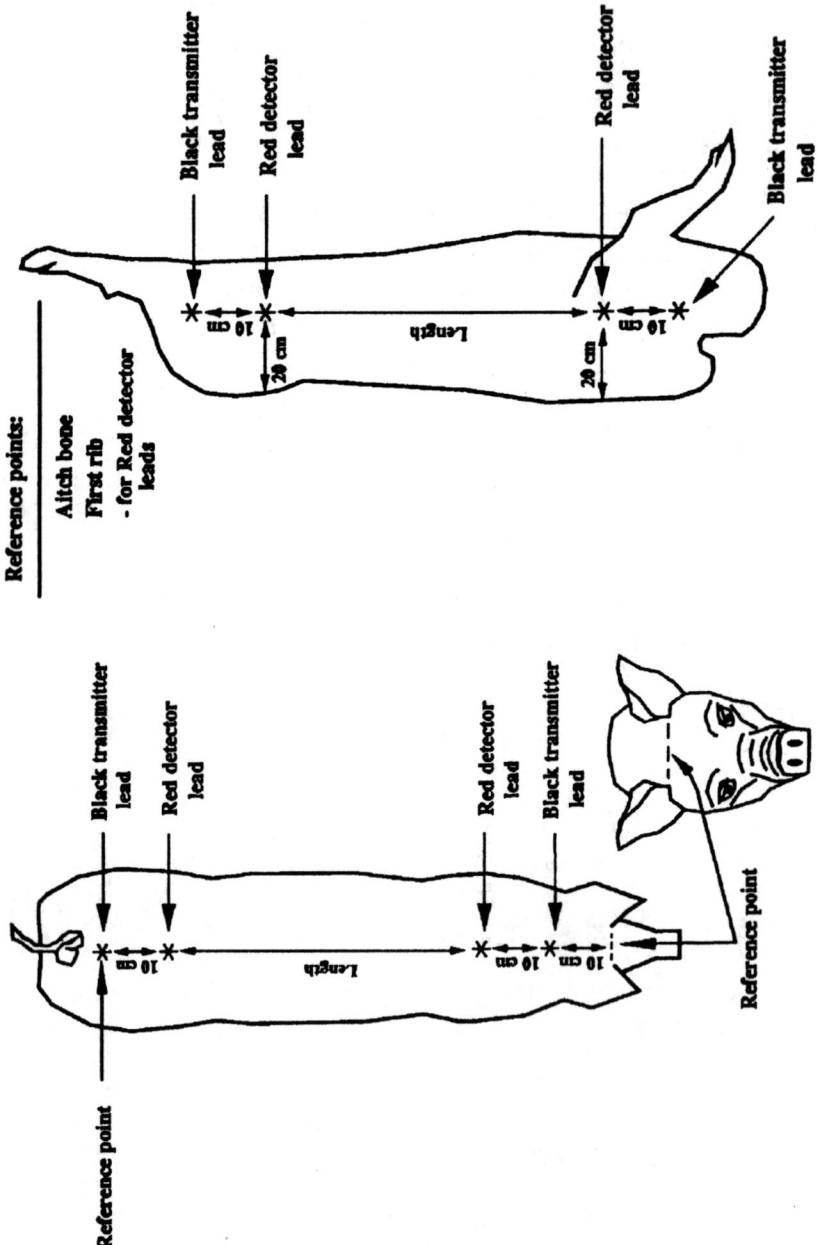

FIGURE 41.6 Reference points, position of electrodes, and terminal attachments for bioelectrical impedance analysis of the live pig or carcass. For the live pig, the cranial reference point was the anterior baseline of the ears (dashed line) and the caudal reference point was the second caudal vertebra. For the carcass, the cranial reference point was opposite the first rib and the caudal reference point was opposite the aitch bone. Electrodes (denoted by asterisks) were placed along the dorsal axis of the live pig and on the outside of the carcass. (From Swantek, P. M. et al., *J. Anim. Sci.*, 77:893, 1992. With permission.)

2. Total-Body Electrical Conductivity

The use of total-body electrical conductivity (TOBEC), also known as electromagnetic scanning, for measuring the lean content of the four lean cuts of pork carcasses was first described by Domeruth et al. (1973). Over the years, several TOBEC systems have been developed. Because of the importance of size and geometry, specific electromagnetic coils have been designed for the various applications. The TOBEC method is rapid (a few seconds) and easy to operate; however, it is moderately expensive, and there are a number of variables that can affect the readings. The TOBEC method can be used to measure both live pigs (Domermuth et al., 1976; Fredeen et al., 1979; Mersmann et al., 1984, Keim et al., 1988) and pig cacasses (Domermuth et al., 1973; Mersmann et al., 1984; Forrest et al., 1989; Akridge et al., 1992; Berg et al., 1994b; 1998). In addition, TOBEC has been used to measure beef carcasses (Koch and Varnadore, 1976), lamb carcasses (Berg et al., 1994a; Wishmeyer et al., 1996), rats (Baer et al., 1993; Bell et al., 1994), poultry (Staudinger et al., 1995; Danicke et al., 1997), and used in a number of human studies (see reviews by Lukaski, 1987 and Boileau, 1988).

The principles for the use of TOBEC for measuring body composition are similar to those of BIA, one of the main differences is that the electrodes used in BIA are replaced by an electromagnetic coil (Figure 41.7). The measurement obtained with TOBEC is actually energy absorption (E) rather than impedance or conductivity. When the subject is placed within the electromagnetic field, the amount of energy absorbed is a function of the area (A^2), the magnetic field strength (B), the conductivity per unit volume at a specific frequency (c), and a series of constants (k), such that $E = A^2 \cdot B \cdot c \cdot k$. The energy absorption signal produced by the TOBEC is primarily a function of the volume of the FFM and is measured as the difference between the coil impedance when empty and that when the subject is inside.

Depending on the instrument design, measurements may be taken with the subject stationary within the coil (measures E value) or scanned as it passes through the coil (measures phase average).

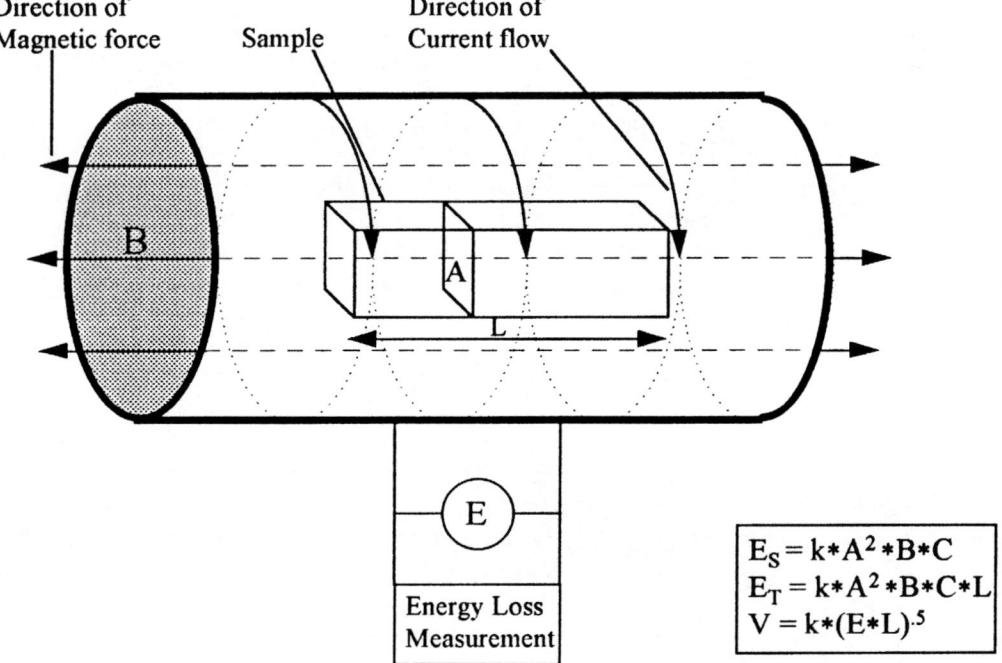

FIGURE 41.7 Diagram of a total-body electrical conductivity coil. (Adapted from EM-SCAN, 1992.)

Calibration using subjects of similar geometry and known composition is necessary to predict accurately the FFM. A measure of the weight of the subject is also required. For live animal measurements, TOBEC readings can be affected by movement and position; for carcass measurements, temperature can also be an important variable.

Two early studies involving TOBEC measurements of live pigs by Domermuth et al. (1976) reported correlations (r) of 0.87 and 0.68 between TOBEC and carcass water. Fredeen et al. (1979) and Mersmann et al. (1984) reported variable results with generally low correlation between the TOBEC readings and subsequent carcass information. A later study by Keim et al. (1988) in which sedated live pigs were scanned with a newer model instrument resulted in high correlations (r) between TOBEC and empty body water (0.979), empty body FFM (0.980), and empty-body crude protein (0.962).

Similarly, the early carcass TOBEC measurements reported by Mersmann et al. (1984) had low correlation with carcass measurement, such as backfat, longissimus muscle area, percentage fat, and percentage protein. Forrest et al. (1989) developed a multiple regression equation with an R^2 of 0.89 to predict the weight of total dissected lean based on the TOBEC scan, carcass length, and carcass temperature. Berg et al. (1994b) evaluated TOBEC scanning of pork carcasses in an online industrial configuration. They developed prediction equations based on TOBEC scan results at two different processing plants. One set of equations, based on chilled carcass weight, length, temperature, and a portion of the TOBEC phase curve, predicted total lean with an R^2 of 0.830 and percentage lean with an R^2 of 0.820. The other set of equations, based on hot carcass weight, the TOBEC peak reading, and a portion of the TOBEC phase curve, predicted total lean with an R^2 of 0.904 and percentage lean with an R^2 of 0.863. A study by Akridge et al. (1992) found the TOBEC scan to be superior to either an optical probe or a real-time ultrasound scan for determining the value of pork carcasses. The use of a neural network model in place of regression equations reportedly improves TOBEC prediction of total carcass lean by 0.31 kg (Berg et al., 1998).

3. X-Ray Absorptiometry

Early attempts at using X-ray technology to measure the carcass composition of pigs included measurements of the variation in the shape of hams (Kronacher and Hogreve, 1936) and the thickness of subcutaneous fat and belly fat (Hogreve, 1938a,b). X-ray attenuation or absorptiometry is the basis for a commonly used instrument (Anyl-Ray) for measuring the lean/fat ratio of meat products. In principle, the measurement of fat or lean by X-ray absorptiometry is based on the greater attenuation of the X-rays by lean (water and protein) than by fat. Furthermore, the X-ray is greatly attenuated by bone or ash, and, for that reason, the Anyl-Ray is used only for ground meat with little or no bone present. On the other hand, dual-energy X-ray absorptiometry (DXA) scans the sample at two different X-ray energy levels (i.e., 38 and 70 keV), providing a two-dimensional image and measurements of bone mineral, fat and lean content, and total tissue mass. The DXA technique has been used to measure the body composition of live pigs (Svendsen et al., 1993; Brunton et al., 1993; Pintauro et al., 1996; Mitchell et al., 1996a,b; 1998a,b; Mitchell and Scholz, 1998) and pig carcasses (Mitchell et al., 1998c). Also, DXA has been used to measure the composition of chickens (Mitchell et al., 1997a) and beef carcass rib sections (Mitchell et al., 1997b). Even though a two-dimensional image is generated as a result of the DXA scan (see Figure 41.8), quantitative analysis does not rely on image analysis per se. In contrast, composition analysis by computerized X-ray tomography (CT) is based on image analysis and is discussed elsewhere in this chapter.

The DXA method evolved from a similar technique known as dual-energy photon absorptiometry (DPA). The DPA was originally developed for the measurement of bone mineral mass and density in humans (Peppler and Mazess, 1981). The basic theory and methodology for measuring body composition by DXA is similar to that for DPA, which has been described in detail (Peppler and Mazess, 1981; Gotfredsen et al., 1984). The measurement of body composition by DXA is

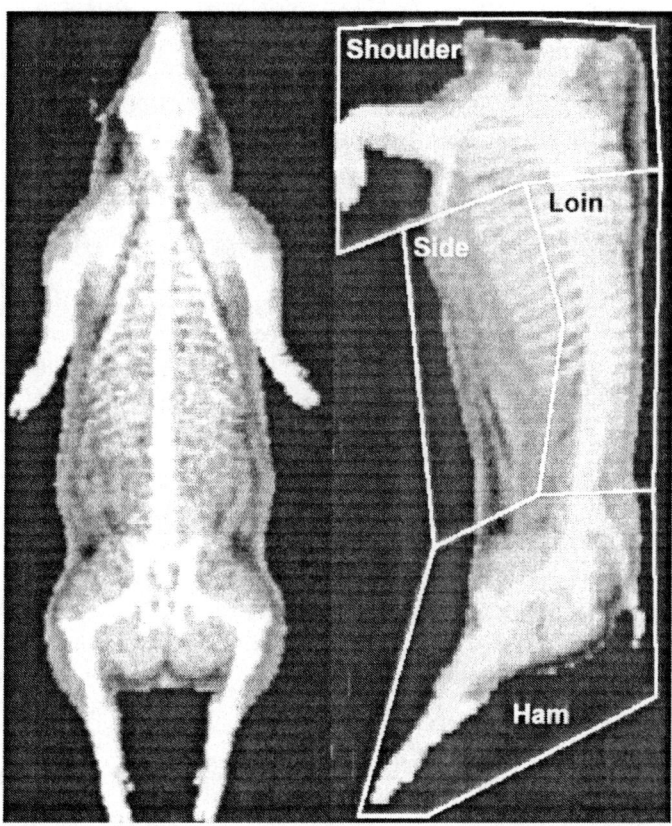

FIGURE 41.8 Dual energy X-ray absorptiometry scans of a live pig and a pork half-carcass. Manually defined regions of interest are shown on the half-carcass.

based on the differential attenuation of low- (38 keV) and high-energy (70 keV) X-rays by fat and other soft tissues. The fat and lean content is determined for each pixel (0.46 cm^2) of a total-body scan that does not overlie bone and is reported to be virtually independent of tissue thickness (Mazess et al., 1990). The soft tissue attenuation ratio (R_{st}) is the ratio of the mass attenuation coefficients (μ) (Gotfredsen et al., 1986) at 38 and 70 keV. Calibration studies at DXA energies of 38 and 70 keV report that R_{st} values range from 1.2 for fat to 1.4 for 100% lean. In addition to whole-body composition values for fat and lean content, DXA measurement also estimates bone mineral content (BMC), total mass of soft tissues (TMST), and, by analyzing only those pixels within a defined area, composition can be determined on a regional basis. Because of the low radiation dose and the ability to detect the differential attenuation of the radiation by bone, fat, and lean tissue, both DPA and DXA have received considerable attention for the measurement of human body composition (Heymsfield et al., 1989; Mazess et al., 1990; Lukaski, 1993).

Because it is necessary that the pig remain motionless during the DXA scan (which may take anywhere from 5 to 35 min, depending on the type of instrument, size of the pig, and scan mode selected), the pig must be anesthetized before placing it on the scan table. Once the scan is completed, the analysis requires only a few minutes and provides readings of percent fat, total fat, lean mass, bone mineral content, bone mineral density, and total tissue mass. No input of external measurements (i.e., weight or length) is needed.

The DXA measurement of fat content of the live pig is highly correlated to fat content ($r = 0.915$ for percentage fat and 0.989 for fat weight) of the chemically analyzed carcass (Mitchell et al., 1996b). However, there is a negative bias for smaller percentages that seems to be related to body weight, which if not corrected results in an underestimation of the fat content of smaller pigs (Mitchell et al., 1998a). This bias also seems to be related to instrument manufacturer and software, because other studies have reported both an overestimation and underestimation of fat in small pigs (Brunton et al., 1993; Ellis et al., 1994; Picaud et al., 1996; Pintauro et al, 1996; Brunton et al., 1997; Elowsson et al., 1998; Rigo et al., 1998). The DXA method seems to provide accurate measurements of total-body fat, lean, and bone mineral mass in market-weight pigs (Svendsen et al., 1993; Mitchell et al., 1996a,b). Regression equations have been developed for the prediction of fat, protein, and water content of the live pig (see Figure 41.1).

In addition, DXA can be used to scan and analyze pork half-carcass (Mitchell et al., 1998c). These scans can be analyzed for specific regions (e.g., shoulder, ham, loin, and belly; see Figure 41.8). As with smaller pigs, DXA was found to underestimate percentage fat, but was highly correlated ($r = 0.90$) with chemical analysis. Region of interest analysis of the carcass scans indicated that the inaccuracy was primarily due to underestimation of fat in the loin and belly regions.

4. Near-Infrared Interactance

Compositional analysis by near-infrared (NIR) spectroscopy is based on the detection of definitive transmission or reflectance characteristics of radiation in the 850 to 2600 nm region by the major components (i.e., water, fat, or protein) of the sample in question (Figure 41.9). The NIR method is widely used to predict the composition or quality of various plant materials (Norris, 1983). This technique has also been studied as a method for compositional analysis of homogeneous samples of animal tissues (Kruggel et al., 1981; Lanza 1983) or whole-carcass composition of homogeneously prepared mouse (Eisen et al., 1984) or chicken (Renden et al., 1986) carcasses. Slaughter

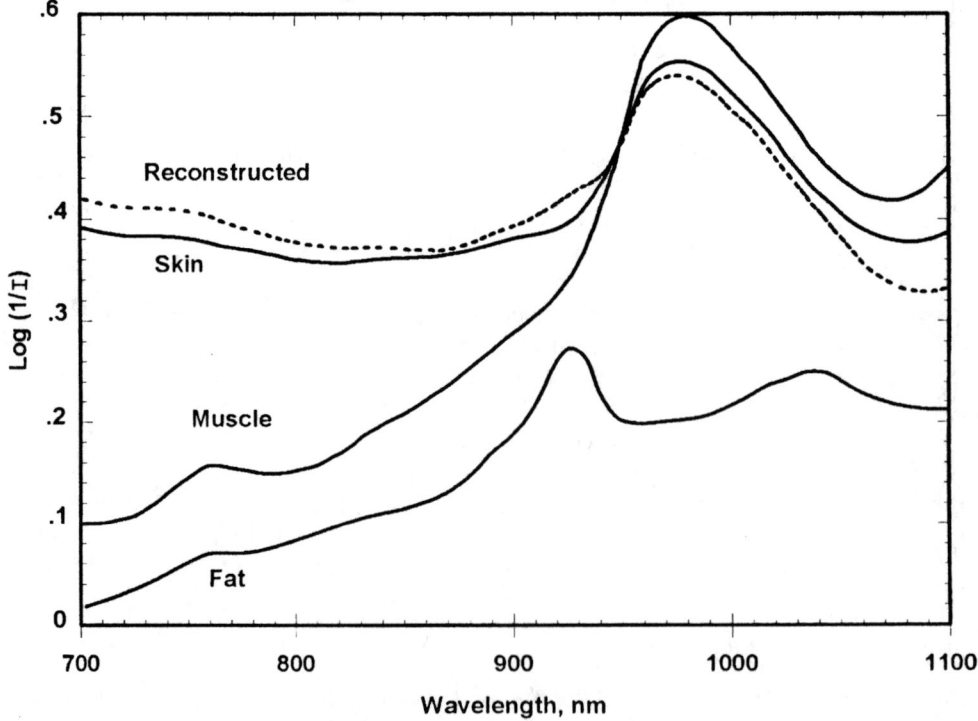

FIGURE 41.9 Near-infrared interactance spectra of pork tissues. (Mitchell, unpublished data.)

et al. (1989) used NIR to measure the fat and protein content of samples of ground hog carcasses. The use of NIR spectroscopy in the 1100 to 2500 nm region has also been evaluated for measuring the tenderness of beef longissimus muscle (Park et al., 1998).

In humans, NIR has received considerable attention as a possible technique for predicting body composition. In the initial study involving adult females, Conway et al. (1984) reported correlation coefficients (r) of 0.94, 0.90, and 0.89 when NIR alone was compared with D_2O dilution, skinfold, and ultrasound measurements. However, subsequent studies have either suggested the method to be invalid (Israel et al., 1989; Elia et al., 1990; Heyward et al., 1992; McLean and Skinner, 1992; Eaton et al., 1993; Wilmore et al., 1994) or that the instrument manufacturer's prediction equation needed refinement (Haddock et al., 1990; Klimis-Tavantzis et al., 1992; Nielsen et al., 1992).

In a test of the NIR technique for predicting the body composition of both live pigs and pork carcasses, Mitchell et al. (1986) utilized a fiber-optic probe for multiple site measurements on the body. When compared with chemical analysis, NIR alone gave correlation coefficients (r) of no better than approximately 0.75 for either the live pig or carcass. Although the estimation with the pig could be improved by including live body weight in the equation, NIR alone is a better indicator of the value of the method. Potential problems with this technique include skin color, thickness of both the skin and adipose tissue, and choice of the appropriate sites. With a penetration depth of only about 1 cm, readings taken from most locations on the pig would include only skin and fat. However, this may still be of value for estimating the composition of growing pigs, because as animals become fatter the chemical composition of the adipose tissue changes. Adipose tissue from fatter animals contains more lipid and less water and protein (Lush, 1926; Callow, 1948). Aberle et al. (1977) reported a correlation coefficient of 0.85 for log% lipid in ham and % lipid in the adipose tissue (data from 25 carcasses weighing between 68 and 82 kg).

5. Nuclear Magnetic Resonance Spectroscopy

The phenomenon of nuclear magnetic resonance (NMR) is the basis for both spectroscopy and imaging techniques. A brief description of the NMR principle is presented later in this chapter (see Section IV.G.1). Spectroscopic applications focus mainly on components of metabolic processes — as does positron emission tomography (e.g., Hsu et al., 1996; Müller et al., 1997) — such as glycogen and glucose with ^{13}C NMR spectroscopy; or phosphocreatine, ATP, and inorganic phosphate with ^{31}P NMR spectroscopy (Scholz et al., 1998). For *in vivo* body composition studies, Mitchell et al. (1991b,c) applied ^1H NMR spectroscopy to quantify the lipid and water content in lean and obese mice yielding a correlation of 0.92 between percent water or lipid in the body and the NMR ratio of water and lipid hydrogen areas. However, whole-body spectroscopy and/or imaging for (body) composition studies would be limited to either relatively small animals (e.g., <120-kg pigs) or sections of large animals (e.g., beef carcass parts) (Groeneveld, 1985; Mitchell et al., 1991a).

Geers et al. (1995) and Villé et al. (1997) measured *in vivo* the intramuscular fat (IMF) content of the longissimus dorsi muscle in pigs by ^1H NMR spectroscopy comparing these measurements with chemical (gravimetric) analysis and Fourier transform infrared spectroscopy (both *in vitro*). In both studies there were significant differences between the *in vitro* IMF% content(s) and the NMR IMF%. Especially large differences appeared in a genetic line with the highest chemical IMF% of 1.76 vs. 1.11 NMR IMF% (Villé et al., 1997). The relationship between gravimetry IMF% and NMR IMF%, with a R^2 of 0.41, indicates a still relatively low reliability for measuring body tissue components that represent only small proportions (e.g., IMF < 1.5%) of the total tissue amount (Geers et al., 1995). Improving the resolution with the latest NMR/MRI technology and/or selecting a larger volume of interest (VOI) by using a larger surface coil will also increase the accuracy for minor tissue components.

F. Atomic Analysis

1. Total-Body Potassium

The determination of total-body potassium based on a total body count of naturally occurring ^{40}K can be used to estimate total-body cell mass or lean mass. Whole-body counters used in this procedure were first tested in humans (Forbes et al., 1961). With proper calibration, shielding of background radiation, and correction for body geometry, an accurate measurement of total-body potassium can be obtained. However, the equipment is expensive and is available at only a few locations. In animal studies, this technique has been tested with live pigs and pork carcasses (Mullins et al., 1969; Stant et al., 1969; Schmidt et al., 1974; Siemens et al., 1991), live lambs and lamb carcasses (Judge et al., 1963), cattle (Johnson and Ward, 1966), steer carcasses (DiCostanzo et al., 1995), and rats (Pommer and Lakshmanan, 1975).

Potassium is essentially an intracellular cation, with approximately 95% of it located in the cell mass, but not in triglycerides. The potassium content of pork muscle varies somewhat with age and breed, but is approximately 2.8 g/kg (Stant et al., 1969). Most of the naturally occurring potassium is nonradioactive ^{39}K; however, a virtually constant 0.0118% consists of radioactive ^{40}K (half-life of 3×10^9 years). The 1.46-MeV γ-decay of ^{40}K can be detected by whole-body counters of various designs. The typical whole-body counter consists of one or more thallium-activated sodium iodide crystals positioned near the subject and a large cylinder (4π) or half cylinder (2π) containing a liquid or plastic scintillator. The detection may be from a stationary placement or scanning mode. The entire unit is contained within a heavily shielded compartment to reduce background radiation. The animal must be restrained but does not necessarily have to be sedated.

The potassium content of ground pork (Kirton and Pearson, 1963) and pork carcasses (Kirton et al., 1963) is highly correlated with the water, fat, and protein content. The relationships between the ^{40}K content of pork hams and composition were demonstrated by Kulwich et al. (1958; 1960; 1961) and Pfau et al. (1961). Kirton et al. (1961) found a high correlation between the ^{40}K content and chemical composition of ground pork. In studies by Schmidt et al. (1974) and Siemens et al. (1991), ^{40}K was measured in both live pigs and their carcasses over a wide range in live body weight (13.5 to 135.5 kg). These studies reported regression coefficients (R^2) between ^{40}K and carcass chemical analysis, i.e., fat (%) 0.70, fat (kg) 0.80, protein or nitrogen (%) 0.63 to 0.71, and water (%) 0.75 to 0.87. Lower correlations were reported for pigs measured at 98 kg (Mullins et al., 1969). However, similar measurements by Stant et al. (1969) reported higher correlations for heavier pigs than for lighter-weight groups. As pigs grow (between 23 and 91 kg), there is a small but significant decrease in the potassium content (mg/g protein) in muscle (Stant et al. 1969); however, with increasing weight a higher proportion of the total-carcass potassium is found in the muscle. These changes can contribute to variations in the accuracy of this method for estimating carcass composition.

2. Neutron Activation

Neutron activation (NA) analysis is the only method available for multielemental analysis of the total body. This technique is capable of quantifying all of the major elements found in the body: hydrogen, carbon, nitrogen, oxygen, calcium, phosphorus, sodium, and chlorine. Total-body potassium can be measured by whole-body ^{40}K counting as discussed separately. Unfortunately, NA is quite expensive, requires considerable expertise, and is fairly slow (15 to 60 min). Only a few instruments are currently available, although efforts are being made for commercial development of a unit suitable for large-animal measurements (Wolff et al., 1996; Mitra et al., 1998). Although NA has been used in a number of studies for the measurement of human body composition (see reviews by Lukaski, 1987 and Heymsfield et al., 1997), there have been relatively few animal studies. Animal studies involving NA include pigs (Preston et al., 1985a), sheep (Wolff et al., 1996), rats (Preston et al., 1985b; Yasumura et al., 1998), fish (Talbot et al., 1986), and ground meat (Mitra et al., 1995a).

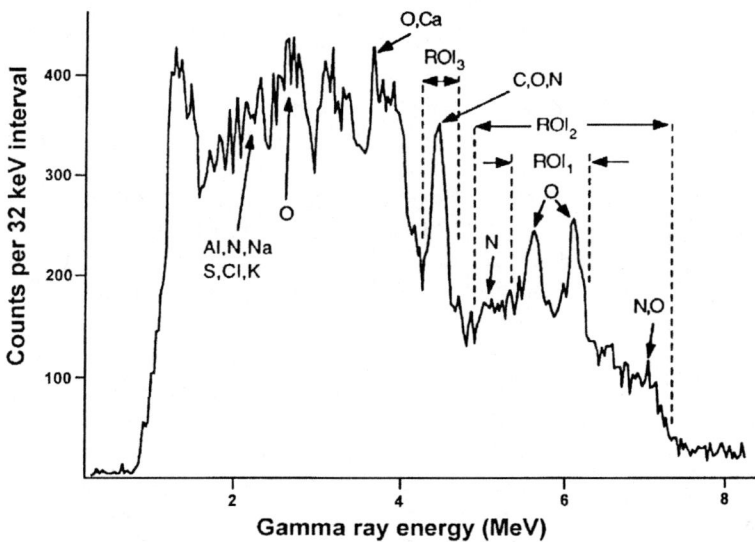

FIGURE 41.10 A time-gated γ-ray spectrum following neutron activation of a meat phantom showing the different regions of interest for extracting γ-rays due to C, N, O and other major energy peaks of activated elements. (From Mitra, S. et al., *Phys. Med. Biol.*, 40:1045, 1995a. With permission.)

Neutron activation analysis consists of irradiating the subject with fast neutrons during a total-body scan. The neutrons are captured by elements within the body, resulting in unstable isotopes. When these isotopes return to a stable condition, they emit one or more γ-rays at specific energy levels (Figure 41.10). Various techniques have been developed for measuring elements of interest. Total-body nitrogen can be measured by the prompt-γ technique (Ellis, 1992). By this procedure ^{14}N is activated by ~3.5 MeV neutrons to ^{15}N which quickly reverts to ^{14}N, releasing a characteristic 10.83 MeV γ-ray. The spectra also includes a hydrogen peak at 2.223 MeV, which is used as a standard. Sodium iodide detectors are used to quantify the γ-rays. The accuracy and precision of nitrogen analysis by this method is 3% (Vartsky et al., 1984).

Neutron inelastic scatter can be used to measure carbon and oxygen content (Kyere et al., 1982; Kehayias et al., 1991; Kehayias and Zhuang, 1993). By this procedure fast neutrons are generated as the subject passes over an accelerator/neutron source during a whole-body scan. The fast neutrons interact with matter by inelastic collisions resulting in prompt nuclear deexcitation and release of γ-rays ($n, n'\gamma$). The 4.44 MeV-rays produced from carbon are detected by bismouth germanate or sodium iodide crystals placed on each side of the subject. The reproducibility for carbon determination is approximately 3% (Kehayias et al., 1991). Total-body fat can be calculated using empirical formulas for the carbon content of protein, fat, glycogen, and bone. An oxygen peak appears at 6.13 MeV on the spectra. The carbon-to-oxygen ratio is used to calculate the axial distribution of fat (Kehayias and Zhuang, 1993).

Another neutron activation technique useful for body composition studies is the associated particle technique (Garrett and Mitra, 1991; Mitra et al., 1995a,b; 1998; Wolff et al., 1996). This procedure uses 14 MeV neutrons and sodium iodide detectors to produce a γ-ray spectra containing peaks for carbon, oxygen, and nitrogen. Based on the scans of 41 kg of ground sheep meat, this elemental analysis can be used to measure the content of protein, fat, and water with precisions of 4.1, 5.4, and 1.2% (Mitra et al., 1995b).

G. IMAGE ANALYSIS

Body composition cannot only be defined from absolute or relative proportions of fat or lean within the porcine body. It is also of significant interest to know the distribution of the different fat depots or muscle groups within the body. Especially different distributed fat depots may affect the nutritional status of an animal (Luiting et al., 1995; Kolstad, 1996; Kolstad and Vangen, 1996; Kolstad et al., 1996). Only imaging technology can provide *in vivo* (or post-mortem) insight into the spatial anatomy of the porcine body (Leymaster, 1986; Baulain, 1997; Mitchell et al., 1998d). The first successful attempts to make the pig's fat and muscle depots visible noninvasively were made by Hogreve (1938b) using X-ray radiography. Later followed ultrasound, X-ray computer axial tomography (CAT; Skjervold et al., 1981; Leymaster, 1986; Jopson et al., 1995), and magnetic resonance imaging (MRI; Groeneveld, 1985; Griep, 1991; Kallweit, 1993). Another approach to predict porcine body composition noninvasively just from the body contour or body shape was made using stereophotogrammetry and the computer-aided video image analysis. Imaging technologies share only the procedures to analyze the two-dimensional or three-dimensional information provided by the image data (signal intensities) in the form of gray values. However, they are based on completely different physical principles. The most common statistical procedures to differentiate among signal classes for measuring or calculating the size of fat depots, muscle bundles, or organs include area, distance, and volume measurements based on the manual, semiautomatic, or automatic (computer-aided) definition of regions of interest (ROI) or volumes of interest (VOI). Each image consists of a matrix of picture elements (pixels) or actually for MRI and CAT of volume elements (voxels), because one slice (image) is defined by height × width × depth. Therefore, it is possible to calculate (measure) the actual volume of body tissues (adipose tissue, skeletal muscle, connective tissue, bone), internal organs (liver, heart, skin, gastrointestinal tract), body parts, or the volume of the total body. Another approach is histogram analysis, which divides the signal intensities into a defined number of "tissue" classes resulting in frequencies (proportions) of the different body tissue classes for fat, muscle, lean, and bone in a certain body region or of the whole body (Leymaster, 1986; Baulain, 1994a,b). The disadvantage of this procedure lies in overlapping tissue classes, which makes it difficult to define fixed thresholds between two separate tissues. Other imaging procedures apply texture analysis (Ehricke and Laub, 1990; Kolb, 1991), cluster analysis (Scholz et al., 1993; Scholz, 1997), correlation analysis, genetic or other "self-learning" algorithms within artificial neural networks (Figure 41.11).

- Area, distance, and volume measurements within defined regions or volumes of interest
- Threshold analysis (using fixed or fuzzy thresholds depending on target tissue) grey value (signal intensity) profiles
- Histogram analysis (one and/or multidimensional) classes of grey value frequencies or "mixture distribution" technique (Luiting et al., 1995)
- Texture analysis relationship among neighborhood pixels
- Correlation analysis
- Cluster analysis object attributes (e.g., time array of subsequent signal intensities) within one pixel or voxel vector
- Neural network analysis (using different "self learning" algorithms — e.g., genetic algorithms

FIGURE 41.11 Statistical procedures for quantitative image analysis. (Modified from Scholz, 1994.)

Most important for the image quality is the performance of the signal (image) acquisition itself. In addition, preprocessing algorithms (e.g., filtering) can enhance the image quality by reducing the noise level or by automated edge and area (volume) detection (Baulain and Scholz, 1996).

1. Magnetic Resonance Imaging

The phenomenon of magnetic resonance (MR) is based on the magnetic spin that atomic nuclei with an odd number of protons and/or neutrons possess (Figure 41.12). In static magnetic fields combined with special gradient coils (Figure 41.13), some of the nuclei advance from their basic energy state to a higher energy state — the "excitation" state — after the body was exposed to a high-frequency pulse exactly on the Larmor (resonance) frequency of the nuclei in interest (e.g., protons for ^{1}H MR imaging; Table 41.3). After completion of the high-frequency pulse (or during

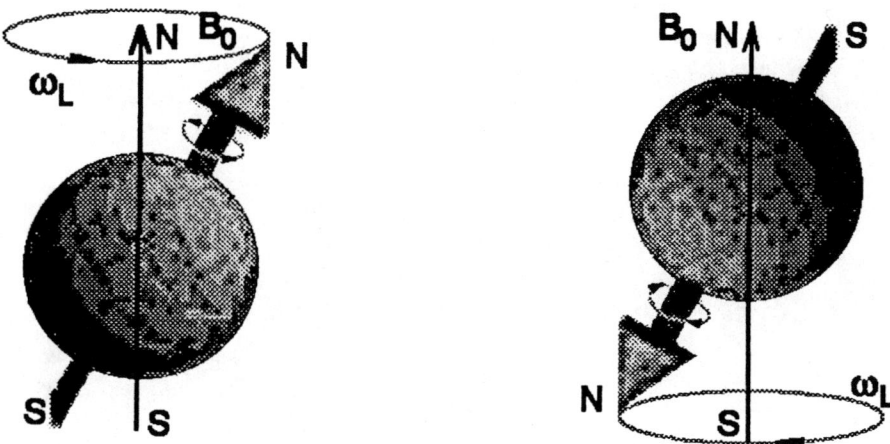

FIGURE 41.12 Nuclei precessing in a magnetic field after RF pulse stimulation (left: parallel; right: antiparallel — characterizing the higher energy level which causes a new transversal magnetization and a decreased magnetization in the direction of the fixed magnetic field).

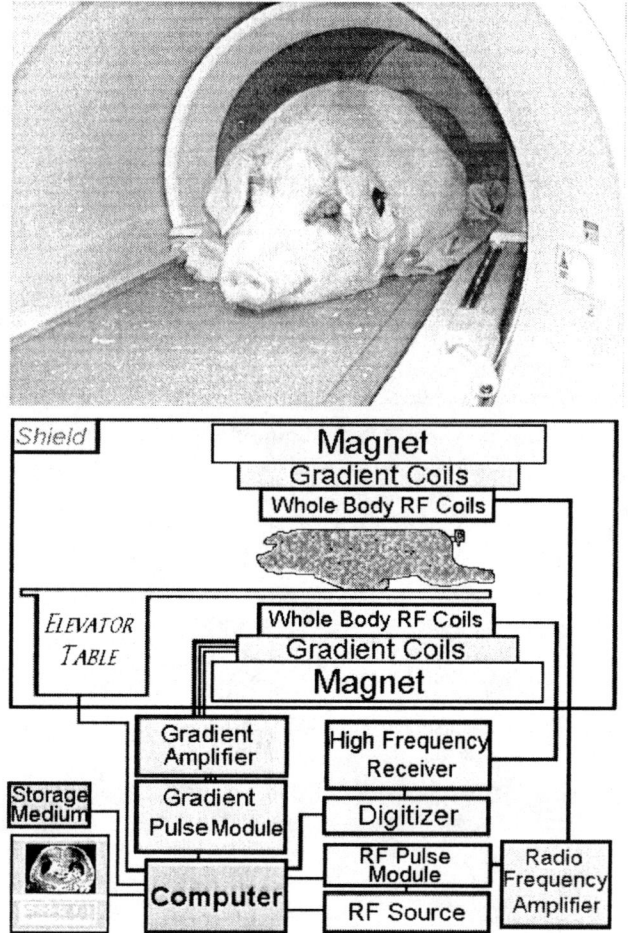

FIGURE 41.13 Positioning of a 90-kg pig in a whole-body magnetic resonance imaging tomograph (bottom scheme) for body composition analysis.

TABLE 41.3
Characteristics of Important Nuclei

Isotope Frequency	Spin	Resonance Frequency at 4.7 T (MHz)	Natural Occurrence (%)	Relative Sensitivity (%)
^{1}H[a]	1/2	200.11	99.985	100
^{2}H	1	30.72	0.015	0.96
^{3}H	1/2	213.45	—	121.36
^{12}C	0	—	98.89	0
^{13}C	1/2	50.33	11.11	1.59
^{31}P	1/2	80	100	6.63

[a] ^{1}H = resonance frequency at 1.5 T = 63.87 MHz.

the interval between the excitation waves) the nuclei return to their basic energy level emitting the absorbed energy, which can be detected by receiver coils. These (magnetization) signals can be transformed from spectral data into image data (gray values) by a Fourier transformation. The signal intensity of each pixel depends on its underlying tissue (water/muscle, fat, or bone). For a given magnetic field strength (e.g., 1.5 or 4.7 tesla), depending on the high-frequency pulse sequence (e.g., a 90° pulse followed by 180° pulse), the signal intensity is affected by T1 (spin-lattice or longitudinal), T2 (spin-spin or transversal) relaxation times (T1 > T2) and the proton density. Adipose tissue is characterized by short T1 and long T2 proton relaxation times, resulting in high signal intensities (bright pixels or voxels) on T1-weighted images — in contrast to muscle tissue (water) with low signal intensities (see Figures 41.15 and 41.16).

Magnetic resonance imaging for the determination of the porcine body composition belongs to the "descriptive" methods using prediction formulas based on chemical reference values. Based on known constants for body tissue densities, MRI provides also direct measurements of anatomical defined body part weights by determining the respective volumes via three-dimensional image analysis. In a study by Scholz and Mitchell (1996), 45 pigs in three weight groups of 30, 60, and 90 kg live weight were scanned *in vivo* in a 1.5-tesla, 1-m horizontal bore magnet at 63 MHz using a whole-body coil. Two MRI/body regions (Figures 41.14, 41.15, and 41.16) contributed a total of 25 images (slices): (1) the region of the longissimus dorsi muscles starting at 14th vertebra in the cranial direction with ten slices (cm) and (2) the ham region starting at the first coccygeal vertebra in the cranial direction (with back legs extended in the caudal direction) with 15 slices (cm). Following the MRI procedure, the pigs were slaughtered, dissected, and chemically analyzed for their fat, lean (protein + water), and ash content. Figure 41.17 demonstrates that a combination of two body sections — as expected — results in a higher precision (R^2 and standard error of estimation,

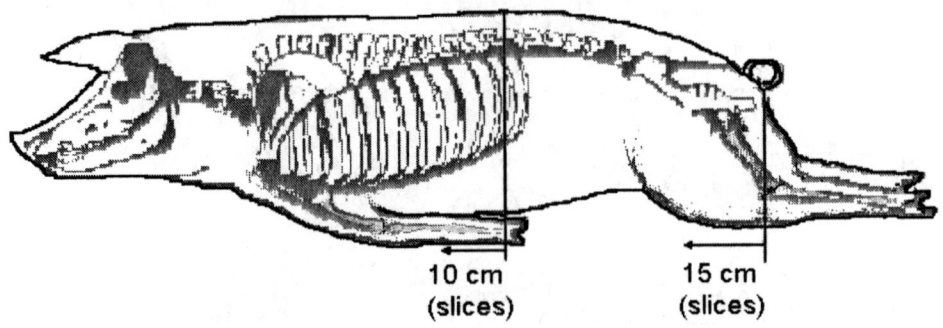

FIGURE 41.14 Definition of possible volumes of interest for body composition assessment using magnetic resonance imaging or X-ray CAT.

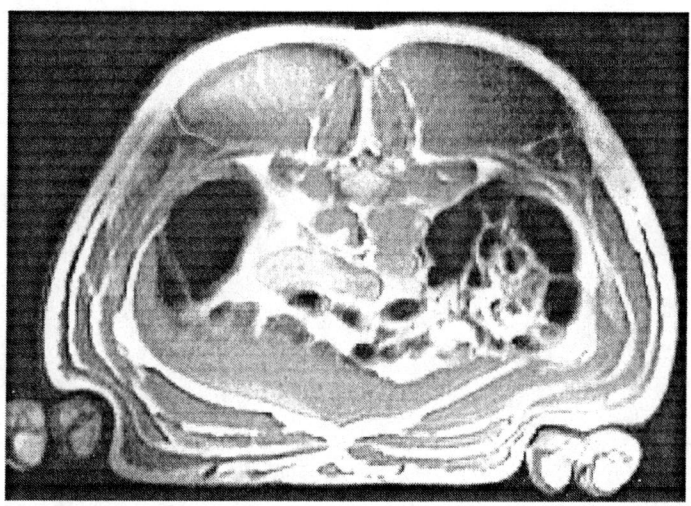

FIGURE 41.15 Example of one magnetic resonance imaging axial slice from the thoracic region.

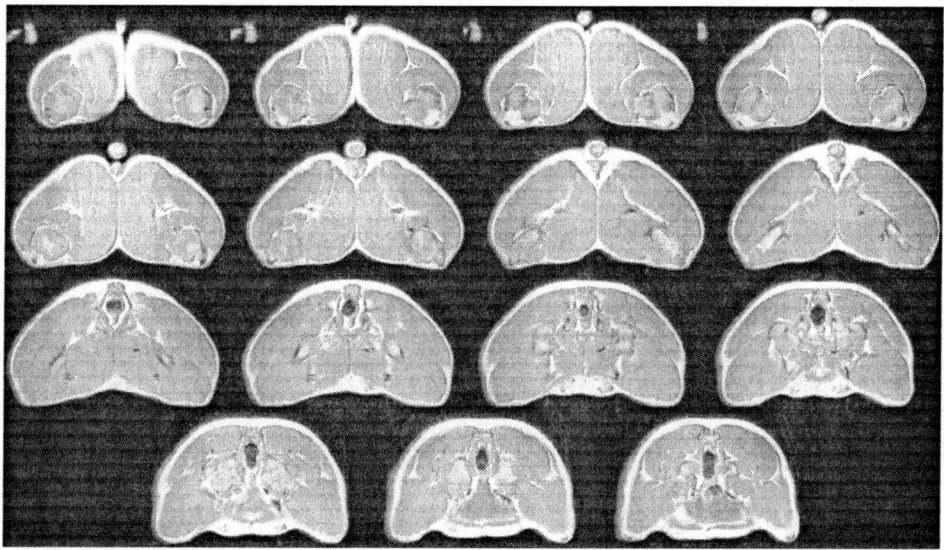

FIGURE 41.16 Example of 15 contiguous slices within the ham region of a 90-kg pig, which can be used for the volume calculation of fat tissue, lean tissue, or of special muscle groups.

SEE) for estimating the body composition than does just the imaging of one section (ham or longissimus dorsi muscle). A combination of up to five body sections may yield even better conformity between the results of MRI and chemical analysis or dissection (Baulain et al., 1996). Actually, the highest accuracy — defined as a measure of the performance of a prediction equation applied to an independent sample (Guo et al., 1996) — would result from a whole-body MRI analysis. However, so far, whole-body MRI is only applicable for research and validation purposes because of the very comprehensive data-processing requirements (Fowler et al., 1992; Fuller et al., 1994). In a whole-body MRI study, Mitchell et al. (1991b; 1993) traced main muscle groups (longissimus dorsi, shoulder, ham, psoas), subcutaneous fat layers (jowl and back fat), internal organs (heart, liver, kidneys, brain), and the entire outline of 21 pigs (8 to 60 kg) for volume calculations finding very high correlations between MRI volume and dissected weight measurements — with an average correlation coefficient of $r = 0.92$. The protein and lipid content determined

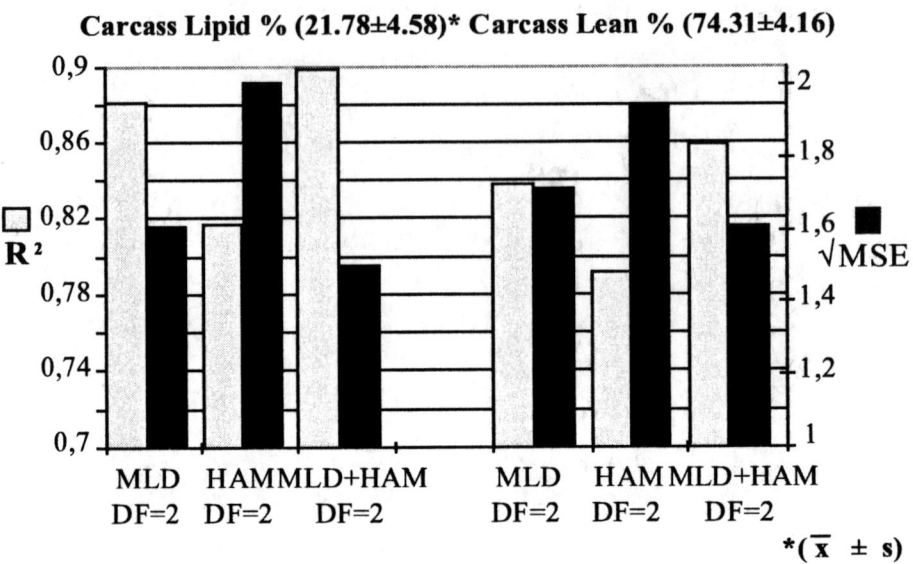

FIGURE 41.17 Coefficients of determination and root mean square errors for predicting carcass lipid % and carcass lean % (carcass water % + carcass protein %) comparing different sources (longissimus dorsi muscle area, MLD, or ham muscle area, HAM) of information from *in vivo* MRI (p ≤ 0.05).

by chemical analysis agreed highly with the MRI predicted amounts (r^2 = 0.98 and r^2 = 0.94 for protein and lipid, respectively). Correspondingly, Table 41.4 summarizes prediction accuracy from *in vivo* body composition studies on pigs using MRI. In most cases, carcass fat percentage can be predicted with a higher accuracy than carcass lean (muscle) percentage. Generally, the prediction accuracy increases with the number of scan positions and with higher body weights mainly because of a larger variation within the population studied (e.g., Baulain, 1994b; 1997; Baulain et al., 1996).

2. X-Ray Computed Axial Tomography

As an alternative to magnetic resonance imaging or spectroscopy, Vangen and Enting (1990) studied the potential of computerized tomography (CT) to determine the intramuscular fat content in pigs with different proportions of Duroc genes (0, 25, and 50%). At that time, their results indicated a low accuracy (R^2 ≤ 0.33; residual standard deviation, RSD ≥ 0.79; n = 823) for predicting IMF%. Generally, CT or X-ray computed axial tomography (CAT) delivers images of the body's interior that are quite similar to those obtained by MRI. The CT image produces good contrast between fat and lean tissue, but lacks the ability of MRI to provide detailed contrast among or within various tissues and organs in the lean tissue category. However, CT is based on a completely different physical principle. The images are derived from transmission data created by a rotating X-ray tube as described by Leymaster (1986). This technique uses, as does dual-energy X-ray absorptiometry, the different attenuation of X-rays in separate body tissues such as muscle (water + protein), fat, or bone caused by the different (assumed) densities of 0.993 g/cm^3 for water, 1.34 g/cm^3 for protein, 0.9 g/cm^3 for fat, and 3.075 g/cm^3 for (bone) minerals at 37°C (Sutcliffe, 1996). The linear attenuation coefficients are transformed into Hounsfield units (HU) or CT values ranging from +1023 (complete absorption) for bone and other dense material to –1024 (no absorption) for air; with protein at 349 HU, water at 7.5 HU, and lipid at –191 HU. Adipose tissue has approximate values of –30 to –190 HU, while soft lean tissue (mainly muscle) can be classified between –29 and 150 HU (Baulain, 1994a; Luiting et al., 1995). However, the estimated fat and muscle distributions may overlap around the zero HU level, although theoretically fat (lipid) has only negative values and muscle (protein + water) has only positive values (Vangen, 1992). Horn et al. (1997)

TABLE 41.4
Precision of *in vivo* Body Composition Estimation in Swine Using Magnetic Resonance Imaging

Population(s)	Weight Group (kg range)	n	Reference Trait	R^2	$RSD = \frac{\sqrt{MSE}}{SD}$	Number of Scan Positions	Ref.
German Landrace	90	75	Carcass fat %	0.66	0.60	2 (5 slices)	Henning et al. (1991)
			Carcass lean % (dissection)	0.64	0.63	2 (7 slices) (shoulder and ham)	
	90	75	Carcass fat %	0.75	0.52	1 (3 slices)	Scholz et al. (1993)
			Carcass lean % (dissection)	0.76	0.50	1 (3 slices) (loin)	
Crossbred pigs	76–79 (lean and obese)	12	Carcass lipid % (chemical)	0.96	0.24	13	Fowler et al. (1992)
			Adipose tissue % (dissection)	0.96	0.22	13 (shoulder to ham)	
Duroc, Landrace, Spotted Poland China × Landrace, Hampshire	30–90	45	Carcass lipid % (chemical)	0.90	0.33	2	Scholz and Mitchell (1996)
			Carcass lean % (chemical — protein % + water %)	0.86	0.39	2 (loin and ham — 25 slices)	
German Landrace	20	43	Carcass fat %	0.68	0.59	≤5	Baulain et al. (1996)
			Carcass lean %	0.55	0.73	≤5	
	50	40	Carcass fat %	0.80	0.46	≤5	
			Carcass lean %	0.83	0.46	≤5	
	90	60	Carcass fat %	0.89	0.36	≤5	
			Carcass lean % (all by dissection)	0.87	0.38	≤5 (shoulder to ham)	

defined density ranges for fat between −10 and −150 HU, water between −10 and +10, muscle between +10 and +150, and bone between +250 and +1000 HU. Based on this classification, various computer programs written for semiautomated or fully automated tissue separation in digital CT images, respectively, quantify the weights of the different body components of interest such as subcutaneous fat, inter/intramuscular fat, noncarcass fat, total-body fat, lean tissue, nonfat visceral, bone, and total-body tissue, independent of prediction equations (Thompson and Kinghorn, 1992; Jopson et al., 1995). Regression equations using chemical or dissection data as independent variables and CT data as dependent variables are being used commonly to evaluate the accuracy of the new techniques. In addition to R^2 and RSD as precision measures, the accuracy can be expressed as percentage ratio between the standard error of prediction (SEP) and the standard deviation (SD) of the dependent variable. Measurements of the fat content (kg) of live pigs produces RSD values as low as 18.6% in gilts and 27.1% in boars, while estimation of the protein content (kg) results in slightly higher prediction errors with 31.8% in gilts and 27.7% in boars (Vangen, 1988a,b; Baulain, 1994a). In the first *in vivo* CT study on 23 pigs, Skjervold et al. (1981) published R^2 values of 0.89 for percentage fat in the carcass, 0.83 for percentage protein in the carcass, and 0.85 for the energy content in the carcass. A lower accuracy resulted from measurements of a lean line of pigs, with $R^2 = 0.73$ for the energy content in the carcass. Jopson et al. (1995) found an R^2 of 0.93 and an RSD of 0.32 for carcass fat weight (kg) measured post-mortem by CT using a combination of NIR spectroscopy and dissection to determine the reference fat weight. Correspondingly, carcass lean weight measured by CT showed an R^2 of 0.86 and an RSD of 0.63 in addition to a systematic overestimation of the "CT carcass lean" by an average of 3.44 kg. The differences between these techniques depend on the accuracy of the dissection itself (e.g., separating lean totally from bone and fat), on the exact truncation point dividing lean from bone (Jopson et al., 1995), on inaccuracies caused by a lower relationship between Hounsfield units and the tissue density especially for high-density tissues, and on different definitions for each tissue measured by CT, dissection, or NIR, respectively. Using chemical body analysis on 20 pigs (10 gilts and 10 barrows) at 105 kg live weight as reference, Szabo et al. (1998) found lower relationships between *in vivo* CT-derived lean or fat tissue volumes and body protein or body fat content with maximum R^2 values of 0.51 and 0.8, respectively. Alone, the body weight (carcass) combined with the gender effect of the animals explained 44 or 37% of the variation in protein or fat content, respectively.

Allen and Leymaster (1985) studied the basic machine error sources in X-ray CT. The lowest noise level (best two-dimensional or three-dimensional image quality) results from combining the higher voltage (e.g., 150 kV), the wider slice thickness (e.g., 8 mm), and the highest current (with the highest number of projections). As hardware and software for X-ray CT (or CAT) steadily improve, the latest stage in the development of X-ray tomography consists of "spiral" CAT scanners where object (animal) translation and data acquisition take place simultaneously using continuously rotating gantry and a high-heat-capacity X-ray tube (Horn et al., 1997). Spiral CAT scanning actually allows volumetric imaging, which *in vivo* results in high estimation accuracy: for ham muscle mass, an R^2 value of 0.92 and an RSD (SEE/SD) of 0.30; for ham + bone mass, an R^2 value of 0.91 and an RSD of 0.33; for longissimus dorsi muscle mass, an R^2 value of 0.96 and an RSD of 0.19; for longissimus dorsi mass + bone mass, an R^2 value of 0.91 and an RSD of 0.27; for total muscle mass (longissimus dorsi + psoas major + ham + bacon side meat), an R^2 value of 0.9 and an RSD of 0.34; and for total subcutaneous fat + skin on the carcass mass, an R^2 value of 0.92 and an RSD of 0.34. Slightly higher accuracy (R^2 and RSD) can be expected from post-mortem (spiral) CAT or CT measurements (e.g., Sehested and Vangen, 1988; Jopson et al., 1995; Horn et al., 1997).

A strong relationship exists between volumetric spiral CAT measurements and traditional (planar) CAT image parameters. Horn et al. (1997) reported R^2 values between 0.93 and 0.99 for fat tissue distances and surfaces on various parts of the scans (9th, 11th, 13th thoracic vertebra, 2nd, 4th, 6th lumbar vertebra, and the head of the femur including the bacon side), and R^2 values between 0.87 and 0.97 for muscle tissue distances and surfaces on the same anatomical positions of the scans.

In general, despite the higher price, volumetric spiral CAT imaging has a number of advantages compared with the traditional CT (or CAT) imaging for *in vivo* body composition measurements, which are elimination of motion artifacts and low radiation dose due to very short scanning times (120 s for 110 scans with a slice thickness of 10 mm), and (almost) no limitations for two- and three-dimensional reconstruction with a high resolution of 1024×1024 pixels/slice compared with the conventional 256×256 pixel matrix (Baulain, 1994a).

3. Ultrasound

Because of the technological development of real-time linear array ultrasonic transducers and scanners in the medical field during the last decade, this technique has become the most common *in vivo* technology in swine body composition assessment, ranging from simple distance to area measurements using A-mode, B-mode, or M-mode devices (Kliesch et al., 1957; Lauprecht et al., 1957; Stouffer et al., 1961; 1991; Horst, 1964; 1971; Busk, 1989). Two-dimensional ultrasound images provide information about adipose tissue depots and cross-sectional areas of muscles (Busk, 1989). The simple probes were used to measure backfat depths in swine as early as the 1950s and 1960s (DePape and Whatley, 1956; Hazel and Kline, 1959; Urban and Hazel, 1965). Mersmann (1982a,b; 1984) evaluated the use of ultrasound backfat depth and longissimus muscle area (LMA) measurements for live swine for estimating carcass composition. Subsequently, this technology has been used extensively worldwide for live animal and carcass evaluation of swine, cattle, and sheep (see the following reviews: Topel and Kauffman, 1988; O'Grady, 1988; Houghton and Turlington, 1992; Kauffman and Warner, 1993).

In principle the ultrasound device uses a probe to convert electronic energy to high-frequency ultrasonic energy, which is capable of penetrating the body in short pulses. When these ultrasonic waves encounter an interface between two tissues that differ in acoustical properties, part of the ultrasonic energy is reflected back to the receiver probe. The received signal is transformed to electrical energy, amplified, and displayed on an oscilloscope. Variations in tissue depths result in time differences in reflected signals. Real-time images are made possible by rapid electronic switching or linear array transducers. Once a suitable image is displayed on screen, it can be captured and analyzed. With the aid of a computer, an area (e.g., LMA) within the on-screen image can be traced with a cursor to yield an area measurement, and tissue depths (e.g., backfat depth) can be measured as the distance between two points on the image. For a more-detailed description, see Houghton and Turlington (1992).

In general, the results of ultrasound studies with live pigs indicate a good agreement between ultrasound measurements of backfat depth or LMA and actual carcass measurements. Results will vary depending on the skill of the operator as well as such factors as the range of size and composition of the animals included in the study. From studies conducted over a period of 30 years, using a variety of instruments, the correlation (r) between ultrasound and carcass measurements of LMA range from 0.27 to 0.93, with an average of approximately 0.67. For most studies the correlation between ultrasound and carcass measurements of fat depth are usually higher, ranging from 0.2 to 0.94, with and average of approximately 0.78. Aside from the accuracy of the ultrasound measurements, its usefulness in predicting carcass composition ultimately depends on the relationship between the measurements of either LMA or backfat and carcass component of interest, such as lean yield. These relationships are further influenced by factors such as breed, gender, and age. The correlations between lean percentage and ultrasound fat depth readings range from -0.44 to -0.63 (Isler and Swiger, 1968; Anderson and Wahlstrom, 1969). Several studies have reported equations for the prediction of percentage lean or lean cuts utilizing ultrasound measurements of live pigs (Terry et al., 1989; Gresham et al., 1992; 1994; Cisneros et al., 1996). These equations, based on transverse or longitudinal scans, include anywhere from one to four fat depth readings from a variety of locations; most include either LM depth or area and some include body weight. The reported accuracy of these equations range from an R^2 of 0.36 and an RSD of 3.17 to an R^2 of 0.83 and an RSD of 1.67. Similar equations have been derived from carcass measurements (Terry et al., 1989; Gresham et al., 1992; 1994), with accuracy ranging from an R^2 of 0.41 and an RSD of 3.05 to an R^2 of 0.82 and an RSD of 1.68.

The practical application of ultrasound measurements of the live animal and carcass are being extended to genetic selection programs (Wilson, 1992; Lo et al., 1992; Moeller et al., 1998; Moeller and Christian, 1998) and online carcass evaluation (Liu and Stouffer, 1995; Brøndum et al., 1998). In a review by Wilson (1992) it was noted that for percentage lean, there is a strong negative genetic correlation with backfat depth and positive correlation with LMA. Automated ultrasound systems have been developed that are applicable to online processing of pork carcasses. A scan system described Liu and Stouffer (1995) used longitudinal average fat depth and muscle depth to predict percentage carcass lean with an R^2 of 0.78 and an RSD of 1.50. The online system described by Brøndum et al. (1998) was reported to be capable of scanning up to 1150 carcasses per hour while predicting percentage lean with an accuracy of 1.58 to 1.95%.

4. Video Imaging and Three-Dimensional Topometry

Recent developments in computer technique and digital camcorders provide the opportunity to evaluate the *in vivo* body conformation as an indicator of the actual body composition in swine. This technique most likely cannot result in accurate estimates of the body composition in terms of lipid, protein, water, or ash content. However, it should be possible to calculate accurately the body volume using three-dimensional topometry (Tschümperlin, 1996). This result, in combination with some linear measurements such as wither height, hip height, thorax width, and ham width, could provide "objective conformation scoring" that would give precise estimates for the carcass value, assuming that meat quality is not the main criterion (Patterson, 1990). So far, video image analysis — partly in conjunction with probe fat depth measurements — is being used routinely only for post-mortem beef or pork classification to predict conformation, fat class, or percentage saleable yield with R^2 values ranging from 0.30 to 0.90 and RSDs from 1.52 to 0.52% (Allen and Walstra, 1996; Stanford et al., 1998).

The main advantages of all *in vivo* noninvasive imaging (or spectroscopic) methods (1) are easily standardized repeated measurements, (2) enable large volumes of interest of the whole body, body tissues, or body parts to be studied separately, and (3) cause no damage or specific suffering to the animals. Magnetic resonance, ultrasound, and video imaging have an advantage over X-ray techniques because of the absence of nonionizing radiation, while especially "spiral" CAT has an enormous advantage regarding the scanning time for similar body parts, sections, or tissues.

V. SUMMARY

Advances in techniques for body/carcass composition analysis are based on the development of electronic/computer-based methods, thus avoiding destructive, labor-intensive, or subjective approaches. A comparison of instrument-based techniques used for body composition measurements is shown in Table 41.5. In general, the choice of a particular technique depends on the purpose or application, i.e., research, production (breeding and selection), or processing (carcass evaluation). Beyond that, selection is based on both technical and practical aspects of the technique. Technical aspects include accuracy, reliability, and the type of information needed (live or carcass, whole body, or specific area, fat, bone, lean muscle, protein, organs, total-body water). Practical aspects include cost (to purchase and operate), portability, need for restraint or anesthesia, speed (sampling or scan time + analysis time), ease of use or training required, safety (i.e., exposure to X-rays), and size of the animal to be measured.

TABLE 41.5
A Comparison of Instrumentation Techniques Used for Body Composition Measurements

Method[a]	Reference Body Component, Body Part	Precision in 90-kg Pigs (average published)		Scanning Time for the Whole Body	Radiation Exposure (mrem)
		R2	RSD		
CT	Body fat and lean tissue content (%)	0.87	0.35	15–20 min	200
CAT	Body fat and lean tissue content (%)	0.92	0.29	10 s	9
MRI	Body fat and lean tissue content (%)	0.82	0.42	25–30 min	None
NMRS	Local fat content (IMF)	0.41	—	5–10 min	None
DXA (DPA)	Body fat and lean tissue content (%)	0.81	—	5–35 min	0.03–0.06
NAA (NIS)	Single atom content: total body C, O, and N	≈0.98	—	20–30 min	6–20
40K	Body fat tissue (%)	0.70	—	5–15 min	None
TOBEC	Fat-free mass (weight)	0.90	—	<5 min	None
US	Backfat depth	0.78	—	<5 min	None
	Loin eye area	0.27	—		
	Percentage lean cuts	0.63	2.04		
NIR	Body fat tissue (%)	<0.55	—	<1 min	None
BIA	Fat-free mass (weight)	0.82	—	2–5 min	None

[a] CT = X-ray computer tomography, CAT = X-Ray computer axial tomography, MRI = magnetic resonance imaging, NMRS = nuclear magnetic resonance spectroscopy, DPA = dual photon absorptiometry, DXA = dual energy X-ray absorptiometry, NAA = neutron activation analysis, NIS = neutron inelastic scattering, 40K = total-body potassium (^{40}K) counting, TOBEC = total-body electrical conductivity, US = ultrasound, NIR = near-infrared interactance, BIA = bioelectrical impedance.

REFERENCES

Aberle, E. D., T. D. Etherton, and C. E. Allen. 1977. Prediction of carcass composition using adipose tissue moisture or lipid concentration, *J. Anim. Sci.*, 45:449.

Akridge, J. T., B. W. Brorsen, L. D. Whipker, J. C. Forrest, C. H. Kuei, and A. P. Schinckel. 1992. Evaluation of alternative techniques to determine pork carcass value, *J. Anim. Sci.*, 70:18.

Allen, P., and K. A. Leymaster. 1985. Machine error in X-ray computer tomography and its relevance to prediction of *in vivo* body composition, *Livest. Prod. Sci.*, 13:383.

Allen, P., and P. Walstra. 1996. Non-invasive techniques for carcass assessment-grading applications, presented at 47th Annual Meeting of the EAAP, Lillehammer, Norway, 18 pp.

Anderson, L. M., and R. C. Wahlstrom. 1969. Ultrasonic prediction of swine carcass composition, *J. Anim. Sci.*, 28:593.

Arnold, R. N., E. J. Hentges, and A. Trenkle. 1985. Evaluation of the use of deuterium oxide dilution techniques for determination of body composition of beef cattle, *J. Anim. Sci.*, 60:1188.

Aschbacher, P. W., T. H. Kamal, and R. G. Cragle. 1965. Total body water estimations in dairy cattle using tritiated water, *J. Anim. Sci.*, 24:430.

Atkinson, G., and A. M. Nevill. 1998. Statistical methods for assessing measurement error (reliability) in variables relevant to sports medicine, *Sports Med.*, 26:217.

Aulstad, D. 1970. *In vivo* estimation of carcass composition in young boars. III. The use of urinary creatinine, total protein and total plasma cholesterol, *Acta Agric. Scand.*, 20:65.

Baer, D. J., W. V. Rumpler, R. E. Barnes, L. L. Kressler, J. C. Howe, and T. E. Haines. 1993. Measurement of body composition of live rats by electromagnetic conductance, *Physiol. Behav.*, 53:1195.

Baldwin, R. L., and R. D. Sainz. 1995. Energy partitioning and modeling in animal nutrition, *Annu. Rev. Nutr.*, 15:191.

Bastianelli, D., and D. Sauvant. 1997. Modelling the mechanism of pig growth, *Livest. Prod. Sci.*, 51:97.

Baulain, U. 1994a. Bestimmung der Körperzusammensetzung landwirtschaftlicher Nutztiere mit Hilfe der Röntgen-CT [Body composition assessment in livestock by X-ray computer tomography], *Landbauforsch. Völkenrode Sonderh.*, 145:110.

Baulain, U. 1994b. MR-Imaging zur Erfassung der Körperzusammensetzung *in vivo* [MR Imaging for body composition assessment *in vivo*], *Landbauforsch. Völkenrode, Sonderh.*, 145:119.

Baulain, U. 1997. Magnetic resonance imaging for the *in vivo* determination of body composition in animal science, *Comp. Elec. Agric.*, 17:189.

Baulain, U., and A. Scholz. 1996. Image evaluation for different acquisition techniques in animal production, 47th Annual Meeting of the EAAP, Lillehammer, Norway, Book of Abstracts No. 2, Wageningen Pers, 269 (PS5.5).

Baulain, U., M. Henning, and E. Kallweit. 1996. Bestimmung der Körperzusammensetzung von Landrasse-Schweinen unterschiedlichen Alters mittels MRI. [Determination of body composition in German Landrace pigs of various age by means of MRI], *Arch. Tierz.* (Dummerstorf), 4:431.

Bell, R. C., A. J. Lanou, E. A. Frongillo, D. A. Levitsky, and T. C. Campbell. 1994. Accuracy and reliability of total body electrical conductivity (TOBEC) for determining body composition of rats in experimental studies, *Physiol. Behav.*, 56:767.

Berg, E. P., and M. J. Marchello. 1994. Bioelectrical impedance analysis for the prediction of fat-free mass in lambs and lamb carcasses, *J. Anim. Sci.*, 72:322.

Berg, E. P., J. C. Forrest, D. L. Thomas, N. Nusbaum, and R. G. Kauffman. 1994a. Electromagnetic scanning to predict lamb carcass composition, *J. Anim. Sci.*, 72:1728.

Berg, E. P., J. C. Forrest, and J. E. Fisher. 1994b. Electromagnetic scanning of pork carcasses in an on-line industrial configuration, *J. Anim. Sci.*, 72:2642.

Berg, E. P., M. K. Neary, J. C. Forrest, D. L. Thomas, and R. G. Kauffman. 1996. Assessment of lamb carcass composition from live animal measurement of bioelectrical impedance or ultrasonic tissue depths, *J. Anim. Sci.*, 74:2672.

Berg, E. P., M. K. Neary, J. C. Forrest, D. L. Thomas, and R. G. Kauffman. 1997. Evaluation of electronic technology to assess lamb carcass composition, *J. Anim. Sci.*, 75:2433.

Berg, E. P., B. A. Engel, and J. C. Forrest. 1998. Pork carcass composition derived from a neural network model of electromagnetic scans, *J. Anim. Sci.*, 76:18.

Boileau, R. A. 1988. Utilization of total body electrical conductivity in determining body composition. In *Designing Foods: Animal Product Options in the Marketplace*, National Academy Press, Washington, D.C., 251.

Boileau, R. B., D. H. Horstman, E. R. Buskirk, and J. Mendez. 1972. The usefulness of urinary creatinine excretion in estimating body composition, *Med. Sci. Sports*, 4:85.

Borsook, H., and J. W. Dubnoff. 1947. The hydrolysis of phospho-creatine and the origin of urinary creatinine, *J. Biol. Chem.*, 168:493.

Brøndum, J., M. Egebo, C. Agerskov, and J. Busk. 1998. On-line pork carcass grading with the Autofom ultrasound system, *J. Anim. Sci.*, 76:1859.

Brown, C. J., J. C. Hillier, and J. A. Whatley. 1951. Specific gravity as a measure of the fat content of the pork carcass, *J. Anim. Sci.*, 10:97.

Brunton, J. A., H. S. Bayley, and S. A. Atkinson. 1993. Validation and application of dual-energy x-ray absorptiometry to measure bone mass and body composition in small infants, *Am. J. Clin. Nutr.*, 58:839.

Brunton, J. A., H. A. Weiler, and S. A. Atkinson. 1997. Improvement in the accuracy of dual energy X-ray absorptiometry for whole body and regional analysis of body composition: validation using piglets and methodologic considerations in infants, *Pediatr. Res.*, 41:590.

Bush, D. A., C. A. Dinkel, and J. A. Minyard. 1969. Body measurements, subjective scores and estimates of certain carcass traits as predictors of edible portion in beef cattle, *J. Anim. Sci.*, 29:557.

Busk, H. 1989. Applications of ultrasound imaging in animal science. In *Application of NMR Techniques on the Body Composition of Live Animals*, Kallweit, E., M. Henning, and E. Groeneveld, Eds., Elsevier Applied Science, New York, 75.

Butte, N. F., J. M. Hopkinson, K. J. Ellis, W. W. Wong, and E. O. Smith. 1997. Changes in fat-free mass and fat mass in postpartum women: a comparison of body composition models, *Int. J. Obes. Relat. Metab. Disord.*, 21:874.

Byers, F. M. 1979. Measurement of protein and fat accretion in growing beef cattle through isotope dilution procedures, Ohio Agric. Res. Dev. Center, Anim. Sci., Ser. 79–1, p. 36.

Callow, E. H. 1948. Comparative studies of meat; the changes in the carcass during growth and fattening and their relation to the chemical composition of the fatty and muscular tissues, *J. Agric. Sci.*, 38:174.

Charette, R., M. Bigras-Poulin, and G.-P. Martineau. 1996. Body condition evaluation in sows, *Livest. Prod. Sci.*, 46:107.

Cheek, D. B. 1968. *Human Growth: Body Composition, Cell Growth, Energy, and Intelligence*, Lea and Febiger, Philadelphia.

Chiba, L. I., A. J. Lewis, and E. R. Peo, Jr. 1990. Efficacy of the urea dilution technique in estimating empty body composition of pigs weighing 50 kilograms, *J. Anim. Sci.*, 68:372.

Cisneros, F., M. Ellis, K. D. Miller, J. Novakofski, E. R. Wilson, and F. K. McKeith. 1996. Comparison of transverse and longitudinal real-time ultrasound scans for prediction of lean cut yields and fat-free lean content of live pigs, *J. Anim. Sci.*, 74:2566.

Comizio, R., A. Pietrobelli, Y. X. Tan, Z. M. Wang, R. T. Withers, S. B. Heymsfield, and C. N. Boozer. 1998. Total body lipid and triglyceride response to energy deficit: relevance to body composition models, *Am. J. Physiol.*, 274:E860.

Conway, J. M., K. H. Norris, and C. E. Bodwell. 1984. A new approach for the estimation of body composition: infrared interactance, *Am. J. Clin. Nutr.*, 40:1123.

Cross, H. R., J. W. Carpenter, and A. Z. Palmer. 1970. Pork carcass muscling: fat, lean and bone ratios, *J. Anim. Sci.*, 30:866.

Cuthbertson, A., and R. W. Pomeroy. 1962. Quantitative anatomical studies of the composition of the pig at 50, 68 and 92 kg carcass weight. I. Experimental material and methods, *J. Agric. Sci.*, 59:207.

Danicke, S., I. Halle, and H. Jeroch. 1997. Evaluation of the non invasive TOBEC (total body electrical conductivity) procedure for prediction of chemical components of male broilers with special consideration of dietary protein level, *Arch. Tierernähr.*, 50:137.

Davies, A. S. 1974a. A comparison of tissue development in Pietrain and Large White pigs from birth to 64 kg live weight. 1. Growth changes in carcass composition, *Anim. Prod.*, 19:367.

Davies, A. S. 1974b. A comparison of tissue development in Pietrain and Large White pigs from birth to 64 kg live weight. 2. Growth changes in muscle distribution, *Anim. Prod.*, 19:377.

Davies, A. S. 1975. A comparison of tissue development in Pietrain and Large White pigs from birth to 64 kg live weight. 3. Growth changes in bone distribution, *Anim. Prod.*, 20:45.

DePape, J. G., and J. A. Whatley, Jr. 1956. Live hog probes at various sites, weights and ages as indicators or carcass merit, *J. Anim. Sci.*, 15:1029.

DiCostanzo, A., R. J. Lipsey, M. G. Siemens, J. C. Meiske, and H. B. Hedrick. 1995. Prediction of carcass and empty body composition of steers by ^{40}K emission detection, *J. Anim. Sci.*, 73:2882.

Domermuth, W. F., T. L. Vaum, H. B. Alexander, H. B. Hedrick, and J. L. Clark. 1973. Evaluation of EMME for swine, *J. Anim. Sci.*, 37:259.

Domermuth, W., T. L. Veum, M. A. Alexander, H. B. Hedrick, J. Clark, and D. Eklund. 1976. Prediction of lean body composition of live market weight swine by indirect methods, *J. Anim. Sci.*, 43:966.

Donovan, H., and O. Brenner. 1930. The influence of the intravenous injection of urea on the exchange of substances between the blood and the tissue, *Br. J. Exp. Pathol.*, 11:419.

Doornenbal, H. 1971. Growth, development and chemical composition of the pig. I. Lean tissue and protein, *Growth*, 35:281.

Doornenbal, H. 1972. Growth, development and chemical composition of the pig. II. Fatty tissue and chemical fat, *Growth*, 36:185.

Doornenbal, H., G. H. Wellington, and J. R. Stouffer. 1962. Comparison of methods used for carcass evaluation in swine, *J. Anim. Sci.*, 21:464.

Eaton, A. W., R. G. Israel, K. F. O'Brien, T. Hortobagyi, and M. R. McCammon. 1993. Comparison of four methods to assess body composition in women, *Eur. J. Clin. Nutr.*, 47:353.

Ehricke, H. H., and G. Laub. 1990. Tissue discrimination in three-dimensional imaging by texture analysis. In *Tissue Characterization in MR Imaging*, Higer, H. P., and G. Bielke, Eds., Springer-Verlag, Berlin, 149.

Eisen, E. J., T. R. Bandy, W. F. McClure, and G. Horstgen-Schwark. 1984. Estimating body composition in mice by near-infrared spectrophotometry, *J. Anim. Sci.*, 58:1181.

Elia, M., S. A. Parkinson, and E. Diaz. 1990. Evaluation of near infrared interactance as a method for predicting body composition, *Eur. J. Clin. Nutr.*, 44:113.

Ellis, K. J. 1992. Measurement of whole-body protein content *in vivo*. In *Modern Methods in Protein Nutrition and Metabolism*, Nissen, S., Ed., Academic Press, New York, 195.

Ellis, K. J., R. J. Shypailo, J. A. Pratt, and W. G. Pond. 1994. Accuracy of dual-energy X-ray absorptiometry for body-composition measurements in children, *Am. J. Clin. Nutr.*, 60:660.

Elowsson, P., and J. Carlsten. 1997. Body composition of the 12-week-old pig studied by dissection. *Lab. Anim. Sci.*, 47:200.

Elowsson, P., A. H. Forslund, H. Mallmin, U. Feuk, I. Hansson, and J. Carlsten. 1998. An evaluation of dual-energy X-ray absorptiometry and underwater weighing to estimate body composition by means of carcass analysis in piglets, *J. Nutr.*, 128:1543.

Elsley, F. W. 1963a. Studies of growth and development in the young pig. Part I. The carcass composition at 56 days of age of pigs reared along different growth curves, *J. Agric. Sci.*, 61:233.

Elsley, F. W. 1963b. Studies of growth and development in the young pig. Part II. A comparison of the performance to 200 lb of pigs reared along different growth curves to 56 days of age, *J. Agric. Sci.*, 61:243.

Emmans, G. C., and I. Kyriazakis. 1997. Models of pig growth: problems and proposed solutions, *Livest. Prod. Sci.*, 51:119.

EM-SCAN. 1992. Information Bulletin: EM-SCAN Small Animal TOBEC Body Composition Analyzer Technical Brief, EM-SCAN, Inc., Springfield, IL.

Farrell, D. J., and D. Balnave. 1977. The *in vivo* estimation of body fat content of laying hens, *Br. Poult. Sci.*, 18:381.

Ferrell, C. L., and S. G. Cornelius. 1984. Estimation of body composition of pigs, *J. Anim. Sci.*, 58:903.

Field, R. A., J. D. Kemp, and W. Y. Varney. 1963. Indices for lamb carcass composition, *J. Anim. Sci.*, 22:218.

Fogelholm, M., and W. van Marken Lichtenbelt. 1997. Comparison of body composition methods: a literature analysis, *Eur. J. Clin. Nutr.*, 51:495.

Folin, O. 1905. Laws governing the chemical composition of urine, *Am. J. Physiol.*, 13:66.

Foot, J. Z., and J. F. D. Greenhalgh. 1970. The use of deuterium oxide space to determine the amount of body fat in pregnant Blackface ewes, *Br. J. Nutr.*, 24:815.

Forbes, G. B. 1999. Body composition: overview, *J. Nutr.*, 129:270S.

Forbes, G. B., and G. J. Bruining. 1976. Urinary creatinine excretion and lean body mass, *Am. J. Clin. Nutr.*, 29:1359.

Forbes, G. B., J. Gallup, and J. B. Horst. 1961. Estimation of total body fat from potassium-40 content, *Science*, 133:101.

Forrest, J. C., C. H. Kuei, M. W. Orcutt, A. P. Schimckel, J. R. Stouffer, and M. D. Judge. 1989. A review of potential new methods of on-line pork carcass evaluation, *J. Anim. Sci.*, 67:2164.

Fowler, P. A., M. F. Fuller, C. A. Glasbey, G. G. Cameron, and M. A. Foster. 1992. Validation of the *in vivo* measurement of adipose tissue by magnetic resonance imaging of lean and obese pigs, *Am. J. Clin. Nutr.*, 56:7.

Fredeen, H. T., A. H. Martin, and A. P. Sather. 1979. Evaluation of an electronic technique for measuring lean content of the live pig, *J. Anim. Sci.*, 48:536.

Fuller, M. F., P. A. Fowler, G. McNeill, and M. A. Foster. 1994. Imaging techniques for the assessment of body composition, *J. Nutr.*, 124:1546S.

Garrett, R., and S. Mitra. 1991. A feasibility study of *in vivo* 14-MeV neutron activation analysis using the associated particle technique, *Am. Assoc. Phys. Med.*, 18:916.

Garrett, W. N., and N. Hinman. 1969. Re-evaluation of the relationship between carcass density and body composition of beef steers, *J. Anim. Sci.*, 28:1.

Geers, R., C. Decanniere, H. Villé, P. Van Hecke, and L. Bosschaerts. 1995. Variability within intramuscular fat content of pigs as measured by gravimetry, FTIR and NMR spectroscopy, *Meat Sci.*, 40:373.

Gnaedinger, R. W., A. M. Pearson, E. P. Reineke, and V. M. Hix. 1963. Body composition of market weight pigs, *J. Anim. Sci.*, 22:495.

Goran, M. I., M. J. Toth, and E. T. Poehlman. 1998. Assessment of research-based body composition techniques in healthy elderly men and women using the 4-compartment model as a criterion method, *Int. J. Obes.*, 22:135.

Gotfredsen, A., J. Borg, C. Christiansen, and R. B. Mazess. 1984. Total body bone mineral *in vivo* by dual photon absorptiometry. I. Measurement procedures, *Clin. Physiol.*, 4:343.

Gotfredsen, A., J. Jensen, J. Borg, and C. Christiansen. 1986. Measurement of lean body mass and total body fat using dual photon absorptiometry. *Metabolism*, 35:88.

Gresham, J. D., S. R. McPeake, J. K. Bernard, and H. H. Henderson. 1992. Commercial adaptation of ultrasonography to predict pork carcass composition from live animals and carcass measurements, *J. Anim. Sci.*, 70:631.

Gresham, J. D., S. R. McPeake, J. K. Bernard, M. J. Riemann, R. W. Wyaatt, and H. H. Henderson. 1994. Prediction of live and carcass characteristics of market hogs by use of a single longitudinal ultrasonic scan, *J. Anim. Sci.*, 72:1409.

Griep, W. 1991. [Estimation of Carcass Composition of Pigs at Different Ages with Magnetic-Resonance-Tomogarphy (MRT)], Thesis, Georg-August-University, Göttingen, 118 pp.

Groeneveld, E. 1985. Schätzung der Schlachtkörperzusammensetzung lebender Tiere mit neueren Verfahren [Estimation of the carcass composition in live animals with new technologies], *Tierzüchter*, 37:305.

Groves, T. D. D., and A. J. Wood. 1965. Body composition studies on the suckling pig. II. The in-vivo determination of total body water, *Can. J. Anim. Sci.*, 45:14.

Guo, S. S., W. C. Chumlea, and D. B. Cockram. 1996. Use of statistical methods to estimate body composition, *Am. J. Clin. Nutr.*, 64(Suppl.):428S.

Haddock, B. L., S. A. Tan, and L. S. Berk. 1990. Body composition assessment with near infrared interactance, *Med. Sci. Sports Exerc.*, 22:S111.

Hammond, A. C., T. S. Rumsey, and G. L. Haaland. 1984. Estimation of empty body water in steers by urea dilution, *Growth*, 48:29.

Hazel, L. N., and E. A. Kline. 1959. Ultrasonic measurements of fatness in swine, *J. Anim. Sci.*, 18:815.

Hedrick, H. B. 1983. Methods of estimating live animal and carcass composition, *J. Anim. Sci.*, 57:1316.

Hegarty, R. S., J. J. McPhee, V. H. Oddy, B. J. Thomas, and L. C. Ward. 1998. Prediction of the chemical composition of lamb carcasses from multi-frequency impedance data, *Br. J. Nutr.*, 79:169.

Henning, M., E. Hüster, U. Baulain, and E. Kallweit. 1991. Evaluation of porcine body composition during growth by means of magnetic resonance tomography (MRT), presented at 42nd Annual Meeting of the EAAP, Berlin, Germany.

Heymsfield, S. B., J. Wang, S. Hesjka, J. J. Kehayias, and R. N. Pierson. 1989. Dual-photon absorptiometry: comparison of bone mineral and soft tissue mass measurements *in vivo* with established methods, *Am. J. Clin. Nutr.*, 49:1283.

Heymsfield, S. B., Z. M. Wang, R. N. Baumgartner, and R. Ross. 1997. Human body composition: advances in models and methods, *Annu. Rev. Nutr.*, 17:527.

Heyward, V. H., K. L. Cook, V. L. Hicks, K. A. Jenkins, J. A. Quatrochi, and W. L. Wilson. 1992. Predictive accuracy of three field methods for estimating relative body fatness of nonobese and obese women, *Int. J. Sports Nutr.*, 2:75–86.

Hiner, R. L. 1971. Growth effects on compositional changes in the carcass and tissues of growing-finishing swine, *J. Anim. Sci.*, 32:1113.

Hoberman, H. D., E. A. H. Sims, and J. H. Peters. 1948. Creatine and creatinine metabolism in the normal male adult studied with the aid of isotopic nitrogen, *J. Biol. Chem.*, 172:45.

Hogreve, F. 1938a. Ausbau eines neuen Forschungsweges zur Bestimmung der Fettwüchsigkeit und Fettleistung in verschiedener Mastabschnitten beim lebenden Schwein verschiedener Rassenzugehörigkeit [A new experimental method for determining fat deposition and fat production at different stages of fattening in live pigs of various breeds], *Z. Zücht. B*, 40:377.

Hogreve, F. 1938b. Untersuchungen über die Fettbildung wachsender Mastschweine mittels der Röntgendurchleuchtung [Fat deposition in growing pigs studied by X-ray graphy], *Züchtungskunde*, 13:178.

Horn, P., G. Kövér, I. Repa, E. Berényi, and G. Kovách. 1997. The use of spiral CAT for volumetric estimation of body composition of pigs, *Arch. Tierz. (Dummerstorf)*, 40:445.

Hörnicke, H. 1962. Methoden zur Bestimmung der Körperzusammensetzung lebender Tiere unter besonderer Berücksichtigung des Schweines. V. Die Körperzusammensetzung normal ernährter Schweine im Verlauf des Wachstums, *Z. Tierernähr. Futtermittelkd.*, 17:28.

Horst, P. 1964. Entwicklung eines Verfahrens zur Durchführung von Ultraschallmessungen beim lebenden Schwein, *Z. Tierz. Züchtungsbiol.*, 80:341.

Horst, P. 1971. Erste Untersuchungsergebnisse über den Einsatz des "Vidoson"-Schnittbildgerätes beim Schwein, *Züchtungskunde*, 43:208.

Houghton, P. L., and L. M. Turlington. 1992. Application of ultrasound for feeding and finishing animals: a review, *J. Anim. Sci.*, 70:930.

Houseman, R. A., and I. McDonald. 1976. The comparative precision of estimates of body composition in living pigs, obtained from numerous different predictors applied severally or jointly, *J. Agric. Sci.* (Cambridge), 87:499.

Houseman, R. A., I. McDonald, and K. Pennie. 1973. The measurement of total body water in living pigs by deuterium oxide dilution and its relation to body composition, *Br. J. Nutr.*, 30:149.

Hsu, H., M. Yu Yong, J. W. Babich, J. F. Burke, E. Livni, R. G. Tompkins, V. R. Young, N. M. Alpert, and A. J. Fischman. 1996. Measurement of muscle protein synthesis by positron emission tomography with L-[methyl-^{11}C] methionine, *Proc. Natl. Acad. Sci. U.S.A.*, 93:1841.

Isler, G. A., and L. A. Swiger. 1968. Ultrasonic prediction of lean cut percent in swine, *J. Anim. Sci.*, 27:377.

Israel, R. G., J. A. Houmard, K. F. O'Brien, M. R. McCammon, B. S. Zamora, and A. W. Eaton. 1989. Validity of a near-infrared spectrophotometry device for estimating human body composition, *Res. Q. Exerc. Sport*, 60:379.

Jebb, S. A., G. R. Goldberg, G. Jennings, and M. Elia. 1995. Dual-energy X-ray absorptiometry measurements of body composition: effects of depth and tissue thickness, including comparisons with direct analysis, *Clin. Sci.*, 88:319.

Johnson, J. E., and G. M. Ward. 1966. Body composition of live animals as determined by ^{40}K. I. A crystal-type, whole-body counter for determining body composition of live animals, *J. Dairy Sci.*, 49:1163.

Johnson, R. J., and D. J. Farrell. 1988. The prediction of body composition in poultry by estimation *in vivo* of total body water with tritiated water and deuterium oxide, *Br. J. Nutr.*, 59:109.

Jones, S. D. M., J. S. Walton, J. W. Wilson, and J. E. Szkotnicki. 1982. The use of urea dilution and ultrasonic backfat thickness to predict the carcass composition of live lambs and cattle, *Can. J. Anim. Sci.*, 62:371.

Jopson, N. B., K. Kolstad, E. Sehested, and O. Vangen. 1995. Computed tomography as an accurate and cost effective alternative to carcass dissection, *Proc. Aust. Assoc. Anim. Breed. Genet.*, 11:635.

Judge, M. D., M. Stob, W. V. Kessler, and J. E. Christian. 1963. Lamb carcass and live lamb evaluation by potassium-40 and carcass measurements, *J. Anim. Sci.*, 22:418.

Kallweit, E. 1993. Methodical development of growth analysis up to magnetic resonance imaging, *Anim. Res. Dev.*, 37:79.

Kauffman, R. G., and R. D. Warner. 1993. Evaluating pork carcasses for composition and quality. In *Growth of the Pig*, Hollis, G. H., Ed., CAB International, Wallingford, U.K., 141.

Kauffman, R. G., Z. L. Carpenter, R. W. Bray, and W. G. Hoekstra. 1964. Interrelationships of gross chemical components of pork muscle, *Agric. Food Chem.*, 12:102.

Kay, M., A. S. Jones, and R. Smart. 1966. The use of tritiated water, 4-aminoantipyrene and *N*-acetyl-4-aminoantipyrene for the measurement of body water in living pigs, *Br. J. Nutr.*, 20:439.

Kehayias, J. J., and H. Zhuang. 1993. Measurement of regional body fat *in vivo* in humans by simultaneous detection of regional carbon and oxygen, using neutron inelastic scattering at low radiation exposure. In *Human Body Composition*, Ellis, K. J., and J. D. Eastman, Eds., Plenum Press, New York, 49.

Kehayias, J. J., S. B. Heymsfield, A. F. LoMonte, J. Wang, and R. N. Pierson, Jr. 1991. *In vivo* determination of body fat by measuring total body carbon, *Am. J. Clin. Nutr.*, 53:1339.

Keim, N., L. P. L. Mayclin, S. J. Taylor, and D. L. Brown. 1988. Total-body electrical conductivity method for estimating body composition: validation by direct carcass analysis of pigs, *Am. J. Clin. Nutr.*, 47:180.

Kelly, R. F. 1955. The Influence of Crystalline Aureomycin Supplementation of the Ration on Distribution, Quantity and Quality of Fat Deposited in Swine, Ph.D. thesis, University of Wisconsin, Madison.

Kelly, R. F., J. P. Fontenot, P. P. Graham, W. S. Wilkinson, and C. M. Kincaid. 1968. Estimates of carcass composition of beef cattle fed at different planes of nutrition, *J. Anim. Sci.*, 27:620.

Keys, A., and J. Brozek. 1953. Body fat in adult man, *Physiol. Rev.*, 33:245.

Kirton, A. J., and R. A. Barton. 1958. Specific gravity as an index of the fat content of mutton carcasses and various joints, *N.Z. J. Agric. Res.*, 1:633.

Kirton, A. H., and A. M. Pearson. 1963. Comparison of methods of measuring potassium in pork and lamb and prediction of their composition from sodium and potassium, *J. Anim. Sci.*, 22:125.

Kirton, A. H., A. M. Pearson, R. W. Porter, and R. H. Nelson. 1961. The use of natural gamma activity to measure the composition of pork and lamb samples, *J. Food Sci.*, 26:475.

Kirton, A. H., R. H. Gnaedinger, and A. M. Pearson. 1963. Relationship of potassium and sodium content to the composition of pigs, *J. Anim. Sci.*, 22:904.

Kliesch, J., U. Neuhaus, E. Silber, and H. Kostzewske. 1957. Versuche zur Messung der Speckdicke am lebenden Tier mit Hilfe des Ultraschalls [Studies of measurement of fat depth of live animals by means of ultrasound], *J. Anim. Breed. Genet.*, 70:29.

Klimis-Tavantzis, D., M. Oulare, H. Lehnhard, and R. A. Cook. 1992. Near infrared interactance: validity and use in estimating body composition in adolescents, *Nutr. Res.*, 12:427.

Knudson, B. J. 1986. Estimation of *in Vivo* Body Composition in Sows Following Weaning, M.S. thesis, University of Minnesota, St. Paul.

Koch, R. M., and W. L. Varnadore. 1976. Use of electronic meat measuring equipment to measure cut out yield of beef carcasses, *J. Anim. Sci.*, 43:108.

Kock, S. W., and R. L Preston. 1979. Estimation of bovine carcass composition by the urea dilution technique, *J. Anim. Sci.*, 48:319.

Kolb, R. 1991. Analyse digitalisierter Ultraschallbilder an lebenden Schweinen zur Abschätzung des Fleischanteils im Bauch und des intramuskulären Fettgehaltes im Rückenmuskel, Ph.D. thesis, University of Hohenheim, Hohenheim.

Kolstad, K. 1996. Genetic differences in fat mobilisation of growing pigs fed at maintenance, and the use of blood components as indicators of changes in body composition, 47th Annual Meeting of the EAAP, Lillehammer, Norway, Book of Abstracts No. 2:276.

Kolstad, N., and O. Vangen. 1996. Breed differences in maintenance requirements of growing pigs when accounting for changes in body composition, *Livest. Prod. Sci.*, 47:23.

Kolstad, N., N. B. Jopson, and O. Vangen. 1996. Breed and sex differences in fat distribution and mobilization in growing pigs fed at maintenance, *Livest. Prod. Sci.*, 47:33.

Kraybill, H. F., H. L. Bitter, and O. G. Hankins. 1952. Body composition of cattle. II. Determination of fat and water content from measurement of body specific gravity, *J. Appl. Physiol.*, 4:575.

Kraybill, H. F., E. R. Goode, R. S. B. Robertson, and H. S. Sloane. 1953. *In vivo* measurement of body fat and body water in swine, *J. Appl. Physiol.*, 6:27.

Kronacher, C., and F. Hogreve. 1936. Beiträge zur Kenntnis der Grundlagen der Beckenformen bei verschiedenen Schweinerassen, gewonnen an Hand röntgenologischer Studien [Investigations on the causes of rump shape in different breeds of pigs from X-ray studies], *Z. Zücht. B*, 35:161.

Kruggel, W. G., R. A. Field, M. L. Riley, H. D. Radlof, and K. M. Horton. 1981. Near-infrared reflectance determination of fat, protein and moisture in fresh meat, *J. Assoc. Off. Anal. Chem.*, 64:692.

Kulwich, R., L. Feinstein, and E. C. Anderson. 1958. Correlation of potassium-40 concentration and fat-free lean content of hams, *Science*, 127:338.

Kulwich, R., L. Feinstein, and C. Golumbic. 1960. Beta radioactivity of the ash in relation to the composition of ham, *J. Anim. Sci.*, 19:119.

Kulwich, R., L. Feinstein, T. L. Hiner, W. R. Seymour, and W. R. Kauffman. 1961. Relationship of gamma-ray measurements to the lean content of hams, *J. Anim. Sci.*, 20:497.

Kyere, K., B. Oldroyd, C. B. Oxby, L. Burkinshaw, R. E. Ellis, and G. L. Hill. 1982. The feasibility of measuring total body carbon by counting neutron inelastic scatter gamma rays, *Phys. Med. Biol.*, 27:805.

Lanza, E. 1983. Determination of moisture, protein, fat, and calories in raw pork and beef by near infrared spectroscopy, *J. Food Sci.*, 48:471.

Latham, S. D., W. G. Moddy, and J. D. Kemp. 1966. Techniques for estimating lamb carcass composition, *J. Anim. Sci.*, 25:492.

Lauprecht, E., J. Scheper, and J. Schröder. 1957. Messungen der Speckdicke lebender Schweine nach dem Echolotverfahren [Measurements of fat thickness of live pigs with the echo-ranging technique], *Mitt. Dtsch. Landwirtsch. Ges.*, 72:881.

Lawes, J. B., and J. H. Gilbert. 1859. Experimental inquiry into the composition of some of the animals fed and slaughtered as human food, *Philos. Trans. B*, 1859:494.

Ledger, H. P., B. Gilliver, and J. M. Robb. 1973. An examination of sample joint dissection and specific gravity techniques for assessing the carcass composition of steers slaughtered in commercial abattoirs, *J. Agric. Sci.* (Cambridge), 80:381.

Leymaster, K. A. 1986. Tomography to estimate changes in body tissues, *J. Anim. Sci.*, 63(Suppl. 2):89.

Liu, Y., and J. R. Stouffer. 1995. Pork carcass evaluation with an automated and computerized ultrasonic system, *J. Anim. Sci.*, 73:29.

Lloyd, R. D., and C. W. Mays. 1987. A model for human body composition by total body counting, *Hum. Biol.*, 59:7.

Lo, L. L., D. G. McLaren, F. K. McKeith, R. L. Fernando, and J. Novakofski. 1992. Genetic analyses of growth, real-time ultrasound, carcass, and pork quality traits in Duroc and Landrace pigs: I. Breed effects, *J. Anim. Sci.*, 70:2373.

Lobley, G. E. 1998. Nutritional and hormonal control of muscle and peripheral tissue metabolism in farm species, *Livest. Prod. Sci.*, 56:91.

Luiting, P. 1993. The biological nature of genetic variation in net feed efficiency, presented at 44th Annual Meeting of the EAAP, Aarhus, Denmark, 9 pp.

Luiting, P., K. Kolstad, H. Enting, and O. Vangen. 1995. Pig breed comparison for body composition at maintenance: analysis of computerized tomography data by mixture distributions, *Livest. Prod. Sci.*, 43:225.

Lukaski, H. C. 1987. Methods for the assessment of human body composition: traditional and new, *Am. J. Clin. Nutr.*, 46:537.

Lukaski, H. C. 1993. Soft tissue composition and bone mineral status: evaluation by dual-energy X-ray absorptiometry, *J. Nutr.*, 123:438.

Lukaski, H. C., P. E. Johnson, W. W. Bolonchuk, and G. I. Lykken. 1985. Assessment of fat-free mass using bioelectrical impedance measurements of the human body, *Am. J. Clin. Nutr.*, 41:810.

Lush, J. L. 1926. Practical methods for estimating the proportions of fat and bone in cattle slaughtered in commercial packing plants, *J. Agric. Res.*, 32:727.

Mackie, A., W. J. Hannan, and P. Tothill. 1989. An introduction to body composition models used in nutritional studies, *Clin. Phys. Physiol. Meas.*, 10:297.

Manners, M. J., and M. R. McCrea. 1963. Changes in the chemical composition of sow-reared piglets during the 1st month of life, *Br. J. Nutr.*, 17:495.

Marchello, M. J., and W. D. Slanger. 1992. Use of bioelectrical impedance to predict leanness of Boston butts, *J. Anim. Sci.*, 70:3443.

Mata-Hernandez, A., J. A. Marchello, C. B. Roubicek, M. F. Ochoa, J. A. Bennett, and W. D. Gorman. 1981. Quantitative estimates of beef carcass composition from specific gravity measurements and certain carcass traits of feedlot steers, *J. Anim. Sci.*, 53:1246.

Mazess, R. B., H. S. Barden, J. P. Bisek, and J. Hanson. 1990. Dual energy X-ray absorptiometry for total-body and regional bone-mineral and soft-tissue composition, *Am. J. Clin. Nutr.*, 51:1106.

McLean, K. P., and J. S. Skinner. 1992. Validity of Futrex-5000 for body composition determination, *Med. Sci. Sports Exerc.*, 24:253.

McMeekan, C. P. 1940a. Growth and development in the pig, with special reference to carcass quality characters. Part I, *J. Agric. Sci.*, 30:276.

McMeekan, C. P. 1940b. Growth and development in the pig, with special reference to carcass quality characters. Part II. The influence of the plane of nutrition on growth and development, *J. Agric. Sci.*, 30:387.

McMeekan, C. P. 1940c. Growth and development in the pig, with special reference to carcass quality characters. Part III. Effect of plane of nutrition on the form and composition of the bacon pig, *J. Agric. Sci.*, 30:511.

McMeekan, C. P. 1941. Growth and development in the pig, with special reference to carcass quality characters. Part IV. The use of sample joints and of carcass measurements as indices of the composition of the bacon pig, *J. Agric. Sci.*, 31:1.

Meissner, H. H. 1976. Urea space versus tritiated water space as an *in vivo* predictor of body water and body fat, *S. Afr. J. Anim. Sci.*, 6:171.

Meissner, H. H., J. H. van Staden, and E. Pretorius. 1980. *In vivo* estimation of body composition in cattle with tritium and urea dilution. I. Accuracy of prediction equations for the whole body, *S. Afr. J. Anim. Sci.*, 10:165.

Mersmann, H. J. 1982a. Ultrasonic determination of backfat depth and loin area in swine, *J. Anim. Sci.*, 54:268.

Mersmann, H. J. 1982b. The utility of ultrasonic measurements in growing swine, *J. Anim. Sci.*, 54:276.

Mersmann, H. J. 1984. Accretion of fat and muscle in growing swine as assessed by ultrasonic methods, *J. Anim. Sci.*, 58:324.

Mersmann, H. J., L. J. Brown, E. Y. Chai, and T. J. Fogg. 1984. Use of electronic meat measuring equipment to estimate body composition in swine, *J. Anim. Sci.*, 58:85.

Mitchell, A. D., and A. M Scholz. 1998. Energy deposition and body composition measurement of pigs of different ryanodine receptor genotypes by dual energy X-ray absorptiometry. In *Energy Metabolism of Farm Animals*, McCracken, K. J., E. F. Unsworth, and A. R. G. Wylie, Eds., CAB International, Wallingford, 249.

Mitchell, A. D., and N. C. Steele. 1987. Comparison of urea space, deuterium oxide space and body composition in growing pigs, *Growth*, 51:118.

Mitchell, A. D., K. H. Norris, H. H. Klueter, N. C. Steele, and M. B. Solomon. 1986. Estimation of live body and carcass composition of pigs by near-infrared reflectance, *J. Anim. Sci.*, 63 (Suppl. 1):234.

Mitchell, A. D., P. C. Wang, and C. M. Evock. 1991a. Body composition analysis of control and pGH treated pigs by NMR imaging, *J. Anim. Sci.*, 69(Suppl. 1):308.

Mitchell, A. D., P. C. Wang, T. H. Elsasser, and W. F. Schmitt. 1991b. Application of NMR spectroscopy and imaging for body composition analysis as related to sequential measurement of energy deposition. In *Energy Metabolism of Farm Animals, Proc. 12th Symposium*, Kartause Ittingen, Switzerland, 222.

Mitchell, A. D., P. C. Wang, and T. H. Elsasser. 1991c. Determination of fat and water content *in vitro* and *in vivo* by proton nuclear magnetic resonance, *J. Sci. Food Agric.*, 56:265.

Mitchell, A. D., J. M. Conway, and W. J. E. Potts. 1996a. Body composition analysis of pigs by dual-energy X-ray absorptiometry, *J. Anim. Sci.*, 74:2663.

Mitchell, A. D., J. M. Conway, and A. M. Scholz. 1996b. Incremental changes in total and regional body composition of growing pigs measured by dual-energy X-ray absorptiometry, *Growth Dev. Aging*, 60:95.

Mitchell, A. D., R. W. Rosebrough, and J. M. Conway. 1997a. Body composition analysis of chickens by dual-energy X-ray absorptiometry, *Poult. Sci.*, 76:1746.

Mitchell, A. D., M. B. Solomon, and T. S. Rumsey. 1997b. Compositional analysis of beef 9,10,11-rib sections by dual-energy x-ray absorptiometry, *Meat Sci.*, 47:115.

Mitchell, A. D., A. M. Scholz, and J. M. Conway. 1998a. Body composition analysis of small pigs by dual-energy X-ray absorptiometry, *J. Anim. Sci.*, 76:2392.

Mitchell, A. D., A. M. Scholz, and J. M. Conway. 1998b. Body composition analysis of pigs from 5 to 95 kg by dual energy X-ray absorptiometry. In International Symposium on *in Vivo* Body Composition Studies, Alpsten, M., and S. Mattsson, Eds., *Appl. Radiat. Isot.*, 49:521.

Mitchell, A. D., P. C. Wang, H. F. Song, and W. F. Schmidt. 1993. Body composition analysis of the pig by magnetic resonance imaging. In *Human Body Composition*, Ellis, K. J., and J. D. Eastman, Eds., Plenum Press, New York, 105.

Mitchell, A. D., A. M. Scholz, V. G. Pursel, and C. M. Evock-Clover. 1998c. Composition analysis of pork carcasses by dual-energy X-ray absorptiometry, *J. Anim. Sci.*, 76:2104.

Mitchell, A. D., P. C. Wang, H. F. Song, J. M. Conway, and A. M. Scholz. 1998d. Application of magnetic resonance imaging and dual-energy X-ray absorptiometry for the measurement of body composition of pigs. In *8th World Congress on Anim. Prod.*, Seoul, Korea, 1:150.

Mitra, S., J. E. Wolff, R. Garrett, and C. W. Peters. 1995a. Application of the associated particle technique for the whole-body measurement of protein, fat and water by 14 MeV neutron activation analysis — a feasibility study, *Phys. Med. Biol.*, 40:1045.

Mitra, S., J. E. Wolff, R. Garrett, and C. W. Peters. 1995b. Whole body measurement of C, N, and O using 14 MeV neutrons and the associated particle time-of-flight technique, *Asia Pac. J. Clin. Nutr.*, 4:187.

Mitra, S., J. E. Wolff, and R. Garrett. 1998. Calibration of a prototype *in vivo* total body composition analyzer using 14 MeV neutron activation and the associated particle technique. In International Symposium on *in Vivo* Body Composition Studies, Alpsten, M., and S. Mattsson, Eds., *Appl. Radiat. Isot.*, 49:537.

Mitsiopoulos, N., R. N. Baumgartner, S. B. Heymsfield, W. Lyons, D. Gallagher, and R. Ross. 1998. Cadaver validation of skeletal muscle measurement by magnetic resonance imaging and computerized tomography, *J. Appl. Physiol.*, 85:115.

Moeller, S. J., and L. L. Christian. 1998. Evaluation of the accuracy of real-time ultrasonic measurements of backfat and loin muscle area in swine using multiple statistical analysis procedures, *J. Anim. Sci.*, 76:2503.

Moeller, S. J., L. L. Christian, and R. N. Goodwin. 1998. Development of adjustment factors for backfat and loin muscle area from serial real-time ultrasonic measurements on purebred lines of swine, *J. Anim. Sci.*, 76:2008.

Mosenthin, R., W. C. Sauer, and C. F. M. deLange. 1992a. Tracer studies of urea kinetics in growing pigs: I. The effect of intravenous infusion of urea on urea recycling and the site of urea secretion into the gastrointestinal tract, *J. Anim. Sci.*, 70:3458.

Mosenthin, R., W. C. Sauer, H. Henkel, F. Ahrens, and C. F. M. deLange. 1992b. Tracer studies of urea kinetics in growing pigs: II. The effect of starch infusion at the distal ileum on urea recycling and bacterial nitrogen excretion, *J. Anim. Sci.*, 70:3458.

Moulton, C. R. 1923. Age and chemical development of mammals, *J. Biol. Chem.*, 57:79.

Müller, M. J., O. Selberg, and W. Burchert. 1997. Use of positron emission tomography (PET) in the assessment of skeletal muscle glucose metabolism, *Z. Ernährungswiss.*, 36:359.

Mullins, M. F., H. B. Hedrick, S. E. Zobrisky, W. J. Coffman, and C. W. Gehrke. 1969. Comparison of potassium and other chemical constituents as indices of pork carcass composition, *J. Anim. Sci.*, 28:192.

Nielsen, D. H., S. L. Cassady, L. M. Wacker, A. K. Wessels, B. J. Wheelock, and R. A. Oppliger. 1992. Validation of the Futrex-5000 near-infrared spectrophotometer analyzer for assessment of body composition, *J. Orthop. Sports Phys. Ther.*, 16:281.

Norris, K. H. 1983. Instrumental techniques for measuring quality of agricultural crops. In *Post-Harvest Physiology and Crop Preservation*, Lieberman, M., Ed., Plenum Press, New York, 84.

Nuernberg, K., J. Wegner, and K. Ender. 1998. Factors influencing fat composition in muscle and adipose tissue of farm animals, *Livest. Prod. Sci.*, 56:145.

Odwongo, W. O., H. R. Conrad, and A. E. Staubus. 1984. The use of deuterium oxide for the prediction of body composition in live dairy cattle, *J. Nutr.*, 114:2127.

O'Grady, J. F., compiler. 1989. New Techniques in Pig Carcass Evaluation, Proceedings of the EAAP Symposium of the Commission on Pig Production, Helsinki, Finland.

Painter, E. 1940. Total body water in the dog, *Am. J. Physiol.*, 129:744.

Park, B. Y., R. Chen, W. R. Hruschka, S. D. Shackelford, and M. Koohmaraie. 1998. Near-infrared reflectance analysis for predicting beef longissimus tenderness, *J. Anim. Sci.*, 76:2115.

Patience, J. F., and P. A. Thacker. 1989. *Swine Nutrition Guide*, Prairie Swine Center, Saskatoon, Canada, 260.

Patterson, D. L. 1990. Obtaining objective measurements of animal conformation by video image analysis. In *Proc. 4th World Congress on Genetics Applied to Livestock Production*, Edinburgh, 15:295.

Pearson, A. M., L. J. Bratzler, R. J. Deans, J. F. Price, J. A. Hoefer, E. P. Reineke, and R. W. Luecke. 1956. The use of specific gravity of certain untrimmed pork cuts as a measure of carcass value, *J. Anim. Sci.*, 15:86.

Pearson, A. M., R. W. Purchas, and E. P. Reineke. 1968. Theory and potential usefulness of body density as a predictor of body composition. In *Body Composition in Animals and Man*, National Academy of Sciences, Washington, D.C., 153.

Peppler, W. W., and R. B. Mazess. 1981. Total body bone mineral and lean body mass by dual-photon absorptiometry. I. Theory and measurement procedure, *Calcif. Tissue Int.*, 33.353.

Pfau, A., G. Kallistratrs, and J. Schroder. 1961. Zur Bestimmung des Fleischgehaltes im Schweineschinken mit Hilfe von 40K-Gammaaktivitätsmessungen, *Atompraxis*, 7:279.

Picaud, J. C., J. Rigo, K. Nyamugabo, J. Milet, and J. Senterre. 1996. Evaluation of dual-energy X-ray absorptiometry for body-composition assessment in piglets and term human neonates, *Am. J. Clin. Nutr.*, 63:157.

Pierson, R. N., J. Wang, and J. C. Thornton. 1997. Measurement of body composition: applications in hormone research, *Horm. Res.*, 48(Suppl. 1):56.

Pietrobelli, A., C. Formica, Z. M. Wang, and S. B. Heymsfield. 1996. Dual-energy X-ray absorptiometry body composition model: review of physical concepts, *Am. J. Physiol.*, 271:E941.

Pintauro, S. J., T. R. Nagy, C. M. Duthie, and M. I. Goran. 1996. Cross-calibration of fat and lean measurements by dual-energy X-ray absorptiometry to pig carcass analysis in the pediatric body weight range, *Am. J. Clin. Nutr.*, 63:293.

Pommer, A. M., and F. L. Lakshmanan. 1975. Estimation of body fat in rats by whole-body counting, *J. Appl. Physiol.*, 39:150.

Pradham, S. L., W. R. McManus, C. L. Goldstone, R. F. Hart, V. N. Khandekar, and G. W. Arnold. 1966. Indices of the carcass composition of Dorset Horn top-cross lambs. 3. Relationships between chemical composition, specific gravity and weight of carcasses and joints, *J. Agric. Sci.* (Cambridge), 66:41.

Preston, R. L., and S. W. Kock. 1973. *In vivo* prediction of body composition in cattle from urea space, *Proc. Soc. Exp. Biol. Med.*, 143:1057.

Preston, T., M. F. Fuller, B. W. East, and I. Bruce. 1985a. Preliminary experiments to assess the suitability of whole body neutron activation for body composition analysis in 70 kg pigs, *Proc. Nutr. Soc.*, 44:109A.

Preston, T., P. J. Reeds, B. W. East, and P. H. Holmes. 1985b. A comparison of body protein determination in rats by *in vivo* neutron activation and carcass analysis, *Clin. Sci.*, 68:349.
Price, J. F., A. M. Pearson, and E. J. Benne. 1957. Specific gravity and chemical composition of the untrimmed ham as related to leanness of pork carcasses, *J. Anim. Sci.*, 16:85.
Renden, J. A., S. S. Oates, and R. B. Reed. 1986. Determination of body fat and moisture in dwarf hens with near-infrared reflectance spectroscopy, *Poult. Sci.*, 65:1539.
Richmond, R. J., and R. T. Berg. 1971. Tissue development in swine as influenced by liveweight, breed, sex and ration, *Can. J. Anim. Sci.*, 51:31.
Rigo, J., K. Nyamugabo, J. C. Picaud, P. Gerard, C. Pieltain, and M. D. Curtis. 1998. Reference values of body composition obtained by dual energy X-ray absorptiometry in preterm and term neonates, *J. Pediatr. Gastroenterol. Nutr.*, 27:184.
Roemmich, J. N., P. A. Clark, A. Weltman, and A. D. Rogol. 1997. Alterations in growth and body composition during puberty. I. Comparing multicompartment body composition models, *J. Appl. Physiol.*, 83:927.
Roubenoff, R., and J. J. Kehayias. 1991. The meaning and measurement of lean body mass, *Nutr. Rev.*, 49:163.
Rozeboom, D. W., J. E. Pettigrew, R. L. Moser, S. G. Cornelius, and S. M. El Kandelgy. 1994. *In vivo* estimation of body composition of mature gilts using live weight, backfat thickness, and deuterium oxide, *J. Anim. Sci.*, 72:355.
Ryde, S. J. S., J. L. Birks, W. D. Morgan, C. J. Evans, and J. Dutton. 1993. A five-compartment model of body composition of healthy subjects assessed using *in vivo* neutron activation analysis, *Eur. J. Clin. Nutr.*, 47:863.
Sajonski, H., and A. Smollich. 1981. *Zelle und Gewebe* [*Cell and Tissue*], S. Hirzel Verlag, Leipzig, 278.
San Pietro, A., and D. Rittenberg. 1953. A study of the rate of protein synthesis in humans. I. Measurement of the urea pool and urea space, *J. Biol. Chem.*, 201:445.
Schmidt, M. K., J. L. Clark, T. L. Veum, and G. F. Krause. 1974. Prediction of composition of crossbred swine from birth to 136 kg live weight via the liquid scintillation whole body counter, *J. Anim. Sci.*, 39:855.
Scholz, A. 1994 [Quantitative analysis of MR-images to determine the body composition of living pigs], *Landbauforsch. Völkenrode Sonderh.*, 145:38.
Scholz, A. 1997. [Determining the degree of marbling in the loin eye area by Video Image Analysis using different SAS procedures] 1. Konferenz der SAS-Benutzer in Forschung und Entwicklung (KSFE), Humboldt-University, Berlin, 295, available at http://www.hu-berlin.de/inside/rz/ksfe.
Scholz, A. M., and A. D. Mitchell. 1996. Accuracy of *in vivo* body composition measurements comparing magnetic resonance imaging and dual energy X-ray absorptiometry, *J. Anim. Sci.*, 74(Suppl. 1):152.
Scholz, A., U. Baulain, and E. Kallweit. 1993 [Multivariate statistical analysis of images from magnetic-resonance-tomography on living pigs], *Züchtungskunde*, 65:206.
Scholz, A. M., A. D. Mitchell, H. Song, and P. C. Wang. 1998. *In vivo* glycogen and phosphate metabolism in relation to body composition in young pigs of different genotypes studied by nuclear magnetic resonance techniques. In *Proc. of the 6th World Congress on Genetics Appl. to Livestock Prod.*, Armidale, NSW, Australia, 25:125.
Sehested, E., and O. Vangen. 1988. Computer tomography, a non-destructive method of carcass evaluation, presented at VI World Conference on Animal Production, Helsinki, Finland, 5 pp.
Sheng, H.-P., and R. A. Huggins. 1979. A review of body composition studies with emphasis on total body water and fat, *Am. J. Clin. Nutr.*, 32:630.
Sheng, H.-P., A. L. Adolph, E. O'Brien Smith, and C. Garza. 1988. Body volume and fat-free mass determinations by acoustic plethysmography, *Pediatr. Res.*, 24:85.
Shields, R. G., Jr., and D. C. Mahan. 1983. Evaluation of ground carcass, sawdust residue and specific gravity methods for estimating body composition of reproducing swine, *J. Anim. Sci.*, 57:604.
Shields, R. G., Jr., D. C. Mahan, and V. R. Cahill. 1983a. A comparison of methods for estimating carcass and empty body composition in swine from birth to 145 kg, *J. Anim. Sci.*, 57:55.
Shields, R. G., D. C. Mahan, and F. M. Byers. 1983b. Efficacy of deuterium oxide to estimate body composition of growing swine, *J. Anim. Sci.*, 57:66.
Shields, R. G., Jr., D. C. Mahan, and P. L. Graham. 1983c. Changes in swine body composition from birth to 145 kg, *J. Anim. Sci.*, 57:43.
Shields, R. G., D. C. Mahan, and F. M. Byers. 1984. *In vivo* body composition estimation in nongravid and reproducing first-litter sows with deuterium oxide, *J. Anim. Sci.*, 59:1239.

Shulman, R. J. 1993. The piglet can be used to study the effects of parenteral and enteral nutrition on body composition, *J. Nutr.*, 123:395.

Siemens, A. L., R. J. Lipsey, W. M. Martin, M. G. Siemens, and H. B. Hedrick. 1991. Composition of pork carcasses by potassium-40 liquid scintillation detection: estimation and validation, *J. Anim. Sci.*, 69:47.

Skjervold, H., K. Grønseth, O. Vangen, and A. Evensen. 1981. In vivo estimation of body composition by computerized tomography, *Z. Tierz. Züchtungsbiol.*, 98:77.

Slanger, W. D., M. J. Marchello, J. R. Busboom, H. H. Meyer, L. A. Mitchell, W. F. Hendrix, R. R. Mills, and W. D. Warnock. 1994. Predicting total weight of retail-ready lamb cuts from bioelectrical impedance measurements taken at the processing plant, *J. Anim. Sci.*, 72:1467.

Slaughter, D. C., H. H. Klueter, A. D. Mitchell, and K. H. Norris. 1989. Near infrared reflectance of ground hog carcass composition. In *Proc. 2nd Int. NIR Spectra Conf.*, Osaka, Japan.

Smith, G. C., and Z. L. Carpenter. 1973. Evaluation of factors associated with the composition of pork carcasses, *J. Anim. Sci.*, 36:493.

Stanford, K., R. J. Richmond, S. D. M. Jones, W. M. Robertson, M. A. Price, and A. J. Gordon. 1998. Video image analysis for on-line classification of lamb carcasses, *Anim. Sci.*, 67:311.

Stansbury, W. F., R. L. Preston, C. B. Ramsey, and L. F. Tribble. 1985. Urea as a body water dilutent to determine body composition of swine, *J. Anim. Sci.*, 61(Suppl. 1):302.

Stant, E. G., T. G. Martin, M. D. Judge, and R. B. Harrington. 1968. Physical separation and chemical analysis of the porcine carcass at 23, 46, 68 and 91 kilograms liveweight, *J. Anim. Sci.*, 27:636.

Stant, E. G., Jr., T. G. Martin, and W. V. Kessler. 1969. Potassium content of the porcine body and carcass at 23, 46, 68 and 91 kilograms live weight, *J. Anim. Sci.*, 29:547.

Staudinger, F. B., R. P. Rorie, and N. B. Anthony. 1995. Evaluation of a noninvasive technique for measuring fat-free mass in poultry, *Poult. Sci.*, 74:271.

Stouffer, J. R. 1991. Using ultrasound to objectively evaluate composition and quality of livestock. In *21st Century Concepts Important to Meat-Animal Evaluation*, University of Wisconsin, Madison, 49.

Stouffer, J. R., M. V. Wallentine, G. H. Wellington, and A. Diekmann. 1961. Development and application of ultrasonic methods for measuring fat thickness and rib-eye area in cattle and hogs, *J. Anim. Sci.*, 20:759.

Susenbeth, A., and K. Keitel. 1988. Partition of whole body protein in different body fractions and some constants in body composition in pigs, *Livest. Prod. Sci.*, 20:37.

Sutcliffe, J. F. 1996. A review of in vivo experimental methods to determine the composition of the human body, *Phys. Med. Biol.*, 41:791.

Svendsen, O. L., J. Haarbo, C. Hassager, and C. Christiansen. 1993. Accuracy of measurement of body composition by dual-energy X-ray absorptiometry in vivo, *Am. J. Clin. Nutr.*, 57:605.

Swantek, P. M., J. D. Crenshaw, M. J. Marchello, and H. C. Lukaski. 1992. Bioelectrical impedance: a nondestructive method to determine fat-free mass of live swine and pork carcasses, *J. Anim. Sci.*, 70:169.

Swantek, P. M., M. J. Marchello, J. E. Tilton, and J. D. Crenshaw. 1999. Prediction of fat-free mass of pigs from 50 to 130 kilograms live weight, *J. Anim. Sci.*, 77:893.

Szabo, Cs., M. W. Verstegen, L. Babinszky, A. J. M. Jansman, O. Vangen, E. Kanis, P. Horn, R. Romvari, and I. Takacs. 1998. The possibility to estimate protein and fat content of pigs by computer tomography, *J. Anim. Sci.*, 76(Suppl. 1):167.

Talbot, C., T. Preston, and B. W. East. 1986. Body composition of Atlantic salmon (*Salmo salar* L.) studied by neutron activation analysis, *Comp. Biochem. Physiol.*, A85:445.

Talbot, N. B. 1938. Measurement of obesity by the creatinine coefficient, *Am. J. Dis. Child.*, 55:42.

Terry, C. A., J. W. Savell, H. A. Recio, and H. R. Cross. 1989. Using ultrasound technology to predict pork carcass composition, *J. Anim. Sci.*, 67:1279.

Tess, M. W., G. E. Dickerson, J. A. Nienaber, and C. L. Ferrell. 1986. Growth, development and body composition in three genetic stocks of swine, *J. Anim. Sci.*, 62:968.

Thompson, J. M., and B. P. Kinghorn. 1992. CATMAN — A program to measure CAT-scans for prediction of body composition in live animals. In *Proc. of the 10th Conf. of Aust. Assoc. of Anim. Breeding and Genetics*, Rockhampton, Australia, 5 pp.

Timon, V. M., and M. Bichard. 1965. Quantitative estimates of lamb carcass composition. 2. Specific gravity determination, *Anim. Prod.*, 7:183.

Tölli, J., B.-Å. Bengtson, I. Bosaeus, G. Johansson, and M. Alpstein. 1998. A comparison of different methods to measure body composition in patients. In International Symposium on *in Vivo* Body Composition Studies, Alpsten, M., and S. Mattsson, Eds., *Appl. Radiat. Isot.*, 49:469.

Topel, D. G., and R. Kauffman. 1988. Live animal and carcass composition measurement. In *Designing Foods: Animal Product Options in the Marketplace*, National Research Council, National Academy Press, Washington, D.C., 258.

Treitl, U. 1996. Applicability of the dilution method using D_2O to determine body composition of growing kids, 47th Annual Meeting of the EAAP, Lillehammer, Norway, 277.

Tschümperlin, K. 1996. Schätzung der Körperzusammensetzung am lebenden Rind [Estimation of Body Composition in Live Beef], Thesis, No. 11447, ETH, Zürich.

Urban, W. E., and L. N. Hazel. 1965. Ultrasonic measurement of fattening rate in swine, *J. Anim. Sci.*, 24:830.

van Steenbergen, E. J. 1990. Relevance of Exterior Appraisal in Pig Breeding, Ph.D. thesis, Wageningen, The Netherlands.

Vangen, O. 1988a. X-Ray CT for body composition. In *Application of NMR Techniques on the Body Composition of Live Animals*, Kallweit, E., M. Henning, and E. Groeneveld, Eds., EC-Seminar, Mariensee, Elsevier Applied Science, New York, p. 91.

Vangen, O. 1988b. Experience from several years of using computerized tomography (CT) in animal breeding research. In *VI World Conference on Animal Production*, Helsinki, Finland, 4.37.

Vangen, O. 1992. Assessing body composition of pigs by computer assisted tomography, *Pig News Info.*, 13:159.

Vangen, O., and H. Enting. 1990. Intramuscular fat in different Duroc-crosses estimated by computerized tomography (CT). In *Proc. Seminar on Meat Quality in Slaughter Animals*, NJF Seminar, 183:243.

Vartsky, D., K. J. Ellis, A. N. Vaswani, S. Yasumura, and S. H. Cohn. 1984. An improved calibration for the *in vivo* determination of body nitrogen, hydrogen and fat, *Phys. Med. Biol.*, 29:209.

Velazco, J., J. L. Morril, and K. K. Grunewald. 1999. Utilization of bioelectrical impedance to predict carcass composition of Holstein steers at 3, 6, 9, and 12 months of age, *J. Anim. Sci.*, 77:131.

Villé, H., G. Rombouts, P. Van Hecke, S. Perremans, G. Maes, G. Spincemaille, and R. Geers. 1997. An evaluation of ultrasound and nuclear magnetic resonance spectroscopy to measure *in vivo* intramuscular fat content of longissimus muscle of pigs, *J. Anim. Sci.*, 75:2942.

Walstra, P. 1980. Growth and Carcass Composition from Birth to Maturity in Relation to Feeding Level and Sex in Dutch Landrace Pigs, Ph.D. dissertation, Communications Agricultural University, Wageningen, The Netherlands.

Wang, Z. M., R. N. Pierson, Jr., and S. B. Heymsfield. 1992. The five level model: a new approach to organizing body composition research, *Am. J. Clin. Nutr.*, 56:19.

Wang, Z. M., P. Deurenberg, S. S. Guo, A. Pietrobelli, J. Wang, R. N. Pierson, Jr., and S. B. Heymsfield. 1998a. Six-compartment body composition model: inter-method comparisons of total body fat measurement, *Int. J. Obes.*, 22:329.

Wang, Z. M., P. Deurenberg, W. Wang, R. N. Pierson, Jr., and S. B. Heymsfield. 1998b. Fraction of carbon-free body mass as oxygen is a constant body composition ratio in men, *J. Nutr.*, 128:1008.

Whiteman, J. V., J. A. Whatley, and J. C. Hillier. 1953. A further investigation of specific gravity as a measure of pork carcass value, *J. Anim. Sci.*, 12:859.

Whittemore, C. T., 1987. *Elements of Pig Science*, Longman Handbooks in Agriculture, Longman Scientific and Technical, Harlow, U.K.

Wilmore, K. M., P. J. McBride, and J. H. Wilmore. 1994. Comparison of bioelectric impedance and near-infrared interactance for body composition assessment in a population of self-perceived overweight adults, *Int. J. Obes.*, 18:375.

Wilson, D. E. 1992. Application of ultrasound for genetic improvement, *J. Anim. Sci.*, 70:973.

Wishmeyer, D. L., G. D. Snowder, D. H. Clark, and N. E. Cockett. 1996. Prediction of live lamb chemical composition utilizing electromagnetic scanning (ToBEC), *J. Anim. Sci.*, 74:1864.

Wolff, J. E., S. Mitra, R. Gaarrett, and P. A. Webb. 1996. Measuring body composition by fast neutron activation analysis, *Proc. N.Z. Soc. Anim. Prod.*, 56:212.

Wood, A. J., and T. D. D. Groves. 1963. Changes in body composition of the pig during early growth based on deuterium oxide dilution technique, *Ann. N.Y. Acad. Sci.*, 110:349.

Wood, A. J., and T. D. D. Groves. 1965. Body composition studies on the suckling pig I. Moisture, chemical fat, total protein, and total ash in relation to age and body weight, *Can. J. Anim. Sci.*, 45:8.

Wray-Cahen, C. D., D. E. Kerr, C. M. Evock-Clover, and N. C. Steele. 1998. Redefining body composition: nutrients, hormones, and genes in meat production, *Annu. Rev. Nutr.*, 18:63.

Yasumura, S., I. E. Stamatelatos, C. N. Boozer, R. Moore, and R. Ma. 1998. *In vivo* body composition in rats: assessment of total body protein. In International Symposium on *in Vivo* Body Composition Studies, Alpsten, M., and S. Mattsson, Eds., *Appl. Radiat. Isot.*, 49:731.

Zemel, B. S., E. M. Riley, and V. A. Stallings. 1997. Evaluation of methodology for nutritional assessment in children: anthropometry, body composition, and energy expenditure, *Annu. Rev. Nutr.*, 17:211.

42 Blood Sampling and Surgical Techniques*

Jong-Tseng Yen

CONTENTS

I.	Introduction	962
II.	Acute Venipuncture	962
	A. Venipuncture of Anterior Vena Cava	962
	B. Venipuncture of Brachiocephalic Vein	963
	C. Venipuncture of Jugular Vein	964
	D. Venipuncture of Cephalic Vein	964
	E. Venipuncture of Ear Veins	964
	F. Venipuncture of Miscellaneous Blood Vessels	965
III.	Chronic Catheterization of Blood Vessels	965
	A. External Jugular Vein-Vena Cava Catheterization by Cutaneous Puncture	965
	B. Catheterization of Jugular Veins or Carotid Artery via Cut-Down Methods	966
	C. Cephalic Vein Catheterization	967
	D. Abdominal Aorta Catheterization via Saphenous Artery	967
	E. Catheterization of Femoral Artery or Vein	968
	F. Portal and Ileal Vein Catheterization	968
	G. Mammary Vein Catheterization	969
IV.	Care and Use of Swine in Experimental Surgery	969
V.	Preparation for Aseptic Surgery	970
VI.	Presurgical Care of the Animal	970
VII.	Anesthesia	970
VIII.	Monitoring the Animal during and after Surgery	971
IX.	Surgical Techniques for Selected *in Vivo* Nutrition Studies	972
	A. Nutrient Digestibility Studies	972
	B. Net Portal Nutrient Absorption	974
	C. Salivary Secretion	975
	D. Gastric Secretion	976
	E. Pancreatic Secretion	977
	F. Bile Secretion	979
	G. Gastrointestinal Lymph	980
References		980

---

* The contents of this publication do not necessarily reflect the views or policies of the U.S. Department of Agriculture, nor does mention of trade names, commercial products, or organizations imply endorsement from the U.S. Government.

I. INTRODUCTION

Blood is a transport medium of nutrients, metabolites, hormones, and other substances in the pig. Properly obtained blood samples offer a means for accurately monitoring the response of blood constituents to dietary factors and the nutritional status of a pig. Blood samples can be collected from a pig by acute venipuncture or chronic catheterization.

Surgically prepared pigs provide a powerful tool for investigating digestion and absorption of nutrients in swine. They are particularly useful for studies relating to the kinetics of nutrient digestion and absorption. The use of surgically prepared pigs indicates an intensive type of research and limits the number of animals that can be employed for the experiment. Because of their capacity for control observations and repeat measurements of the phenomenon under investigation, less surgically prepared animals are needed as compared with intact animals.

This chapter provides a brief description of blood sampling and surgical techniques for nutritional studies in the pig. The information should be used only as a guide. The surgical techniques may have to be modified in most cases to accommodate the objectives of certain research, the availability of surgical equipment and supplies, the variation in the size of animals, and the unavoidable anatomical deviation among pigs even of the same breed, sex, and size. Nevertheless, the surgically prepared pig is an extremely valuable tool for nutritional research, and, in some cases, the use of such pig is the only way to obtain certain types of nutritional data.

II. ACUTE VENIPUNCTURE

The pig lacks superficial blood vessels for easy blood sampling. Many different techniques of venipuncture have been described for acutely obtaining blood samples from various sites in the pig. The location of some of the major blood vessels in the ventral cervical region of a pig in dorsal recumbency are shown in Figure 42.1, and that of a standing pig are depicted in Figure 42.2.

A. Venipuncture of Anterior Vena Cava

The method for sampling blood from anterior vena cava has been used widely since it was first described by Carle and Dewhirst (1942). An experienced person can obtain a desirable quantity of blood repeatedly from the anterior vena cava of a pig of any size. The procedures provided below are based on those described by Schwartz and Smallwood (1977), Straw and Meuten (1992), and Swindle (1998).

In a pig weighing <20 kg, the animal is restrained in a dorsal recumbent position, with its front legs pulled back along the body and the head extended fully. A 3.8-cm, 20-gauge needle is used. Because severe respiratory distress in the pig can be caused by damage to the left phrenic or vagus nerve, which is more prone to injury by the needle, insertion of the needle into the right rather than left side of the neck is recommended. The needle is inserted slowly at a point in the right jugular groove on a line drawn from the manubrium sterni to the base of the right ear. The needle is directed inward, downward, and at a 30 to 45° angle toward the dorsal border of the left shoulder until its point is within the arch between the two first ribs. With a slight vacuum applied to the syringe as the needle is advanced, blood will flow into the syringe when the needle enters the vena cava. If no blood is obtained after the first insertion, the needle should be slowly withdrawn before being redirected to prevent lacerating the blood vessels. As the needle is withdrawn, blood may sometimes begin to enter the syringe if the needle had initially penetrated completely through the opposite wall of the vein.

With a larger pig, the animal is restrained in a standing position by a nose snare. The body of the standing pig should be straight and its front legs well back. The pig's head should be elevated so that its manubrium sterni can be reached easily. The thumb or fingers are used to trace the right jugular groove to its caudal end just anterior to the thoracic inlet. A 6.5-cm, 18-gauge needle is used for pigs weighing ≤120 kg, and a 16-gauge needle with longer length may be needed in large breeding swine. The needle is inserted at the caudal end of the right jugular groove and directed

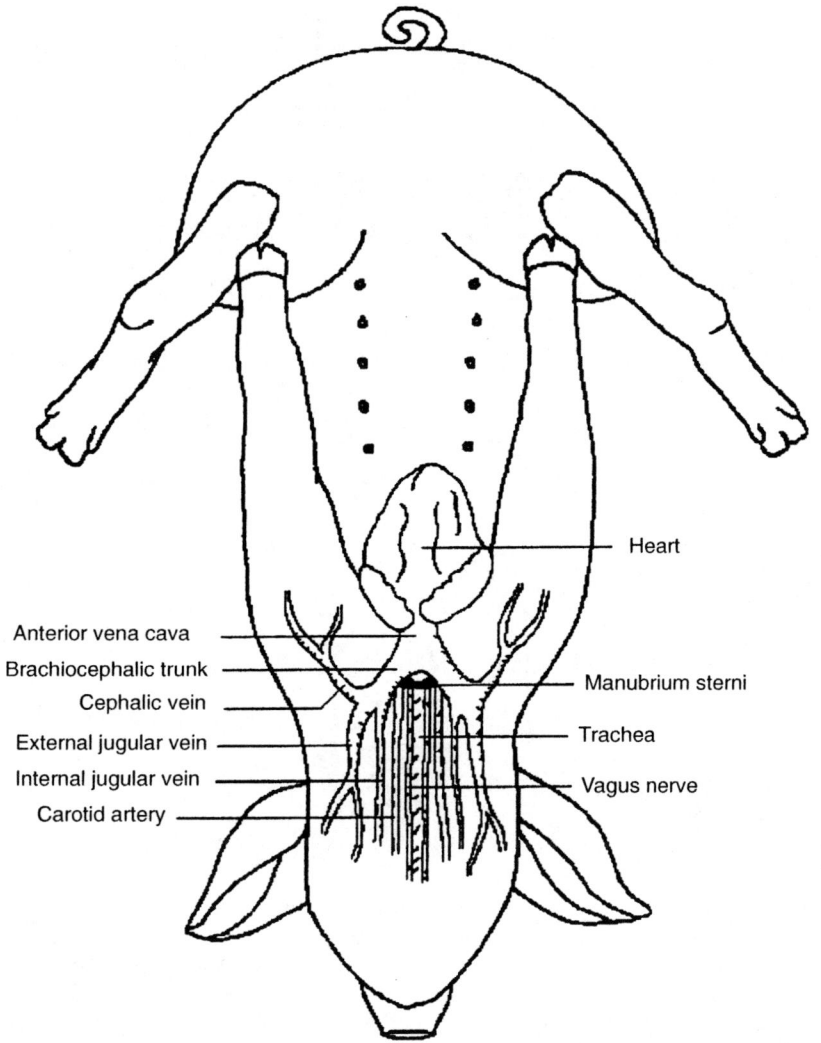

FIGURE 42.1 Major blood vessels in the ventral cervical region. The pig is shown in dorsal recumbancy. This position works well for blood sampling of young pigs (<20 kg).

toward the dorsal border of the left shoulder, with the needle tip remaining anterior to the first pair of ribs. As the needle is slowly advanced and a slight vacuum is applied to the syringe, blood will flow into the syringe when the vena cava is penetrated.

B. Venipuncture of Brachiocephalic Vein

A modification of the anterior vena cava technique has been described by Lawhorn (1988) for obtaining blood from the brachiocephalic vein. The pig is restrained standing, with its head held firmly forward and in a raised position. A 3.8-cm, 16-, or 18-gauge needle is used. The needle is inserted into the right jugular groove at the point where an imaginary transverse line that is between the manubrium sterni and shoulders, and parallel to the ground, intersects a second imaginary line originating from the manubrium sterni and projecting dorsolaterally toward the right scapula at a 45° angle with the transverse line. The needle is inserted perpendicularly to the ventral surface of the extended neck and advanced in a caudodorsal direction.

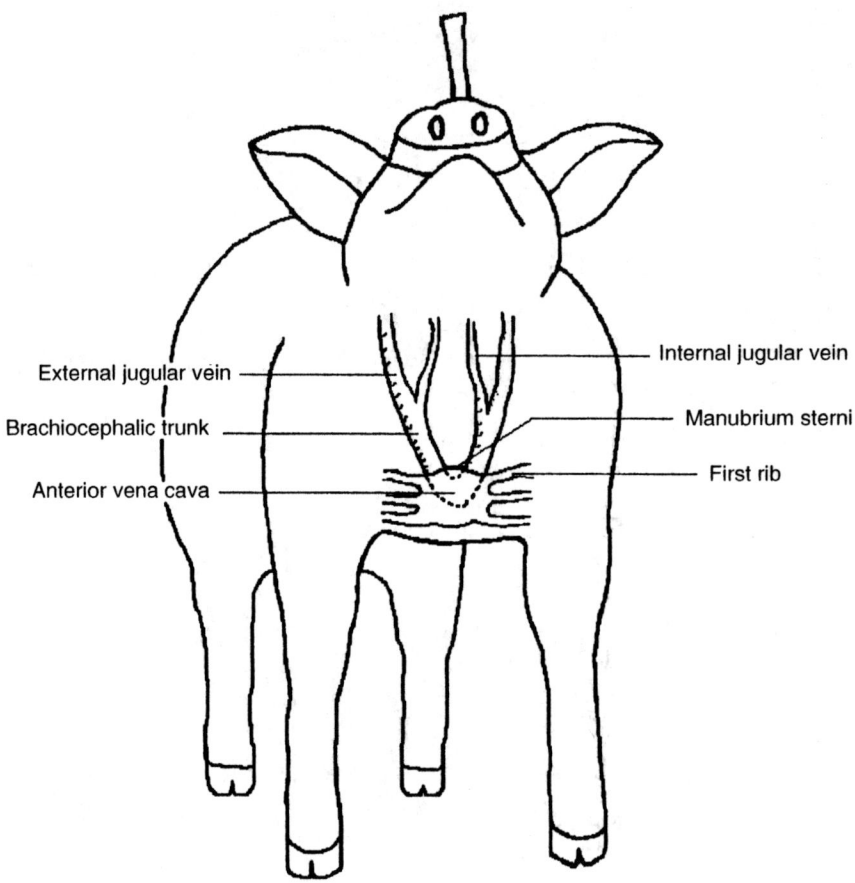

FIGURE 42.2 Major blood vessels in the ventral cervical region. The pig is shown in a standing position with the head restrained by a nose snare. This position works well for blood sampling of pigs >20 kg and for adult sows and boars.

C. Venipuncture of Jugular Vein

Blood can also be withdrawn from a pig via the jugular vein. The pig is restrained as for blood sampling from the anterior vena cava. A 3.8-cm, 20-gauge needle is used for pigs of any age. Depending upon the size of the pig, the needle is inserted in the jugular groove about 3 to 5 cm cranial to the thoracic inlet. The needle is directed dorsally and slightly medially when advancing.

D. Venipuncture of Cephalic Vein

Blood samples can be collected from cephalic vein, which is smaller than anterior vena cava, brachiocephalic vein, and jugular vein. After restraining the pig on its back with its front legs stretched back and slightly outward from the body, the cephalic vein is readily observed under the skin and is raised with digital pressure. With a 3.8-cm, 20-gauge needle, 5 to 10 ml of blood can be obtained from pigs weighing between 9 to 23 kg.

E. Venipuncture of Ear Veins

The ear veins of a pig are generally located in three sites of the ear and are readily visible in a white-eared pig. One vein coursing along the outer edge and another in the middle of the ear are more useful than the third about 2 cm from the medial margin or top of the ear. Because repeated venipuncture is difficult, ear veins of a pig are normally used for injection rather than for blood sampling. An amount of 1 to 2 ml of blood may be collected from ear veins with a 2.5-cm, 20-gauge needle.

F. Venipuncture of Miscellaneous Blood Vessels

Blood can be sampled from tail veins of a large pig whose tail has not been docked. The tail vein is located in the ventral surface of the tail. A 20- or 22-gauge needle is inserted and directed toward the junction of the tail with the body.

The orbital venous sinus may also be a site for blood sampling (Friend and Brown, 1971). However, the method is unaesthetic and blood flow is slow compared with venipuncture at other sites.

III. CHRONIC CATHETERIZATION OF BLOOD VESSELS

Chronic indwelling catheters allow repeated sampling from and long-term infusion to well-buried blood vessels of an unrestrained pig, minimize excitement and stress of the animal, and present the investigator with a more physiologically representative blood sample.

Catheters can be constructed from various materials that are chemically inert and nontoxic. Commonly used catheter materials are medical-grade polyvinyl chloride (e.g., Tygon microbore tubing), polyurethane (e.g., Micro-Renathane tubing), and silicon rubber (e.g., Silastic medical-grade tubing). The size of the catheter depends on the size of the blood vessel.

Peripheral veins that are commonly catheterized include the external and internal jugular veins, cephalic vein, and femoral vein. Peripheral arterial catheterization is generally performed in the common carotid artery, femoral artery, and saphenous artery. Catheterization of peripheral blood vessels is a relatively simple procedure. Through peripheral vessels, the central vascular system can be catheterized (e.g., anterior vena cava via external or internal jugular vein; abdominal aorta via saphenous or femoral artery; and the brachiocephalic trunk and aorta via the common carotid artery). Deep-body blood vessels such as portal vein, ileal vein, and other abdominal veins and arteries can also be catheterized following a laparotomy.

Carotid artery catheterization is the preferred procedure for obtaining systemic arterial blood. Compared with catheterization of the saphenous or femoral artery, catheterization of the carotid artery is simpler to perform because of the direct and easy access to the blood vessel and the use of a larger catheter. Because of adequate collateral circulation and its anastomosis with the vertebral artery, the occlusion of one of two carotid arteries should not cause any physiological detriment to the pig.

A. External Jugular Vein-Vena Cava Catheterization by Cutaneous Puncture

An example of catheterization of the anterior vena cava through cutaneous puncture of the external jugular vein in pigs weighing 140 to 220 kg has been described by Ford and Maurer (1978). Polyvinyl tubing (Tygon microbore tubing, 1.27 mm inside diameter, 2.29 mm outside diameter) is cut in 100-cm length with an end cut at a 30° angle. The inside lumen of the catheter is treated with a TDMAC (tridodecylmethyl-ammonium chloride)–heparin complex and the catheter is gas-sterilized with ethylene oxide. The anesthetized pig is placed in a dorsal recumbent position. At a point 4 to 8 cm anterior to the manubrium sterni and 4 to 5 cm lateral to the ventral midline, an 11-gauge, thin-walled needle with a short bevel and a 10-ml syringe attached is inserted into the external jugular vein by cutaneous puncture. The syringe is removed, and the bevel end of the heparinized saline solution–filled catheter is inserted through the needle and passed 25 to 30 cm into the vein. The needle is removed after a 1-cm skin incision is made adjacent to the needle. A 30-cm long steel trocar and cannula is inserted into this incision, passed subcutaneously and dorsally to a point midway toward the back, and exteriorized through a second 1-cm incision. After removing the trocar, the free end of the catheter is passed through the cannula and the cannula is removed. The process is repeated so that the free end of the catheter is exteriorized through a third 1-cm incision located immediately anterior to the scapula and 10 to 20 cm posterior to the ears. Each of the three incisions is closed with a single suture. The catheter is anchored to animal's back with a collar. The collar is prepared by inverting a 2.54-cm length rubber tubing back onto itself and placing a 20-cm length of nonabsorbable surgical suture between the two layers of tubing. After sliding over the catheter, the collar is sutured to the skin directly over the final point of catheter exteriorization and adhered to the catheter with silicone adhesive. The external end of the catheter is reduced to a length of 12 cm, fitted with a female luer adapter (16-gauge needle adapter) and stoppered. The catheter is then attached to the animal's back with tag cement and elastic adhesive tape. The catheter can be functional for >46 days.

The catheterization technique of Ford and Maurer (1978), with different sizes of thin-wall needle and catheter, can be used in pigs 40 to 250 days of age (Allrich et al., 1982). The method has also been modified for pigs without a general anesthesia and for short-term blood sampling and administering test substances (Kraeling et al., 1982; Barb, 1993). The pig is restrained with a snout snare and held in standing position. The ventral cervical area of the pig is disinfected with a povidone iodine solution. Following a cutaneous puncture of the external jugular vein, the catheter is passed through the 11-gauge, thin-walled needle and placed into the vena cava. After its external end is fitted with a female luer adapter and stoppered, the catheter is secured on the outside of the neck by a 7.62-cm-wide elastic bandage wrapped around the neck and shoulder area. A 10.2-cm-wide duct tape is placed over the elastic bandage to protect the catheter.

B. Catheterization of Jugular Veins or Carotid Artery via Cut-Down Methods

Through a minor surgical cut-down, a catheter can be placed easily in the external or internal jugular vein and into the vein cava, as well as in the carotid artery and into the brachiocephalic trunk (Yen and Killefer, 1987; Swindle, 1998). By placing the anesthetized pig (20 to 40 kg) in a dorsal recumbent position and drawing its front legs caudally along the body, the jugular groove can be visualized as a line slightly medial from the point of the shoulder to the point of the jaw. After making a 7- to 8-cm paramedian skin incision in the jugular groove over the larynx and incising subcutaneous tissue and cutaneous colli muscle, the external jugular vein, which locates between the scalenus medius and the sternohyoideus and sternothyroideus muscles, can be exposed by blunt dissection. A 2- to 3-cm segment of the external jugular vein is then isolated for catheterization. Through this paramedian incision, the internal jugular vein and the common carotid artery can also be isolated. The internal jugular vein and carotid artery, in company with vagus nerve, are medial than the external jugular vein and lie side by side along the ventral surface of the cervical vertebrae parallel to the trachea. After dissecting bluntly the dorsal fascia of the sternohyoideus muscle, the carotid pulse can be palpated easily. The carotid artery, internal jugular vein, and vagus nerve can then be exposed, and a 2- to 3-cm segment of each blood vessel can be isolated for catheterization.

For pigs weighing 20 to 40 kg, polyurethane catheter (1.68 mm inside diameter, 2.41 mm outside diameter) or similar-sized polyvinyl tubing can be used to catheterize either external or internal jugular vein or carotid artery. To prevent vasospasm during catheterization, several drops of antispasmatic agents such as lidocaine or procaine are applied to the isolated segment of the blood vessel. Three ligatures of 2/0 nonabsorbable suture are placed loosely around the blood vessel, two caudally and one cranially from the intended insertion site. After the connective tissue is cleared, a puncture in the blood vessel is made with a blood vessel punch or a small cut is made in the blood vessel with a pair of fine iris scissors. With the aid of a catheter introducer placed in the puncture or the cut, the catheter is inserted into the blood vessel. The catheter is inserted into external or internal jugular vein about 12 cm, so its tip is well situated in the vena cava. A length of 15 cm of catheter is inserted into the carotid artery toward the aorta; thus, the tip of the catheter is located in the brachiocephalic trunk. To avoid serious loss of blood caused by the strong arterial blood pressure, the arterial catheter should be clamped immediately after its insertion into the artery. Upon completion of catheter insertion, the three ligatures around the blood vessel are tied and the catheter is secured with the aid of the retention nylon mesh, cuffs, or beads prebonded to the catheter. The catheter is exteriorized to the right side of the neck before the skin incision is closed. The distal end of the catheter is tunneled subcutaneously and exteriorized 2 to 3 cm lateral to the dorsal mid-line. The catheter is threaded through a protective sleeve made of silicon rubber tubing with inside diameter slightly larger than the outside diameter of the catheter. The catheter with its protective sleeve are then threaded through two pieces of catheter collars made of thick-wall silicon rubber or polyvinyl tubing. Two segments of nonabsorbable surgical suture are placed between the protective sleeve and the catheter collars. By loosely stitching the surgical suture to animal's skin, the catheter is anchored and secured on the pig. The catheter is fitted with tubing adaptor, filled with heparinized saline, and stopped with male luer locking cap. The adapter and cap are wrapped with elastic bandage to prevent damage.

C. Cephalic Vein Catheterization

The cephalic vein can be catheterized on the anterior surface of the foreleg or the ventral aspect of the neck near the thoracic inlet (Tilton et al., 1993; Swindle, 1998). The anesthetized pig is placed in lateral recumbent position. The cephalic vein is located by applying finger pressure into the thoracic inlet and watching for subcutaneous dilation of the vein along its course from the leg through the neck. A 7-cm skin incision over the cephalic vein is made about 2 cm anterior to the foreleg and 14 cm lateral to the fore-point of sternum. The external cephalic vein lies in an adipose layer beneath the skin incision and can be exposed by removing all extraneous fat. Two ligatures (2/0 suture) are placed around the vein. The posterior ligature is tied tightly to restrain blood flow. A small cut is made on the vein between the ligatures and the catheter is inserted into the vessel. The catheter is made of polyvinyl tubing (Tygon microbore tubing, 1.02 mm inside diameter and 1.78 mm outside diameter) and its lumen is pretreated with a heparin complex. Two pieces of 1-mm segments of polyvinyl tubing (1.27 mm inside diameter, 2.29 mm outside diameter) are placed over the catheter to serve as vein anchors. After inserting both anchors into the vein, the anterior ligature is tied between the anchors and around the vein. The vein is circled with the anterior suture and the suture is then stitched to the adipose layer. The posterior suture is tied loosely around the catheter. Before the skin incision is closed with 2/0 suture, the free end of the catheter is exteriorized to the shoulder and then to the dorsal midline of the pig. The catheter is held on the animal's back by two nonabsorbable skin sutures.

D. Abdominal Aorta Catheterization via Saphenous Artery

A procedure for catheterizing the abdominal aorta through the saphenous artery in pigs weighing between 20 and 40 kg has been described by Yen and Killefer (1987). The anesthetized pig is placed in a dorsal recumbent position and its rear leg is retracted caudally. The saphenous artery descending superficially from the distal end of the femoral canal and appearing on the medial surface of the leg can be located by palpating for a pulse. A 5-cm skin incision, 6 to 7 cm cephalad to the anterior end of the tibia and perpendicular to the artery, is made. By using blunt dissection, the saphenous artery along with the medial saphenous vein and saphenous nerve are exposed. Saphenous artery is identified by its pulsation and isolated. Several drops of lidocaine or procaine are applied to the artery to prevent the blood vessel from spasm and to facilitate the insertion of the catheter. Three 2/0 sutures are placed loosely around the artery, two proximally and one distally from the intended nicking site on the artery. The artery is nicked with a pair of iris scissors, and the catheter is inserted. Care should be taken to ensure that the intima of the artery is not pushed ahead of the catheter to occlude the lumen of the artery and prevent the insertion of the catheter. The catheter is made of polyvinyl (0.71 mm inside diameter, 1.17 outside diameter) or polyurethane (0.65 mm inside diameter, 1.02 mm outside diameter) tubing and has a piece of nylon mesh bonded 27.5 cm posterior to the tip. The lumen of the catheter is treated with a heparin complex. The catheter is inserted cranially for 27.5 cm, so its tip travels from the saphenous artery through femoral and external iliac arteries and, eventually, rests within the abdominal aorta. After tying off the three ligatures, the saphenous artery is severed. The catheter is secured *in situ* by, first, tying the remaining strand of the second proximal ligature to the nylon mesh and, then, suturing the nylon mesh to the adjacent previously separated connective tissue. Immediately distal to the nylon mesh, a loop for making a 180° change in the direction of the distal end of the catheter is made. The loop is tucked inside a subcutaneous pocket formed by blunt dissection and is secured to the adjacent tissue with two 2/0 sutures. Before closing the skin incision, the distal end of the catheter is exteriorized dorsally through the subcutaneous tunnel and exits near the fold of the flank of the pig.

E. CATHETERIZATION OF FEMORAL ARTERY OR VEIN

Swindle (1998) has provided a description of catheterization of femoral blood vessels. The anesthetized pig is placed in dorsal recumbency and its rear leg retracted caudally. By following the pulsation of the superficial saphenous artery cranially to the level of the thigh, a fascial division of the sartorius and gracilis muscles can be located as the arterial pulse disappears. The femoral artery, vein, and nerve are situated below the edge of the body of the gracilis muscle. The blood vessels can be reached by making a longitudinal surgical incision over the fascial division of the sartorius and gracilis muscles on the medial surface of the thigh. Both the artery and vein have lateral and deep branches. To avoid their rupture, which can lead to vasoconstriction, these branches should be ligated during the isolation of the blood vessels. With the technique similar to that described for catheterizing the saphenous artery, the catheter can be inserted into the femoral blood vessel and secured to the adjacent tissue. The distal end of the catheter is then exteriorized to the dorsal midline of the animal. For 20- to 40-kg pigs, the femoral catheter can be made of polyvinyl or polyurethane tubing (1.02 mm inside diameter, 2.03 mm outside diameter) with its lumen treated with a heparin complex.

F. PORTAL AND ILEAL VEIN CATHETERIZATION

Various techniques have been published for catheterizing the portal vein of pigs (Rerat et al., 1980; Yen and Killefer, 1987; Ten have et al., 1996; Swindle, 1998). The procedure reported by Yen and Killefer (1987), with slight modification, is described in this section. The anesthetized pig (20 to 40 kg) is placed in left lateral recumbency. A 15- to 20-cm incision is made 2 to 3 cm behind and parallel to the last rib on the right side of the animal. The portal vein is brought toward the incision by inserting the middle finger into the space between the pig's portal vein and posterior vena cava. The gastroduodenal vein entering the portal vein and a cluster of lymph nodes lying caudal to the gastroduodenal vein are located. The connective tissue and outer sheet of a 1-cm segment of the portal vein cranial to the gastroduodenal vein are separated to reveal clearly the portal vein. Three ligatures (3/0 nonabsorbable suture) are placed on the separated connective tissue and outer sheet of the exposed segment of the portal vein, with one ligature cranial and two ligatures lateral to the intended puncture site in the portal vein. A puncture is made in the portal vein cranial to the gastroduodenal vein. Any hemorrhage from the puncture on the portal vein is removed by aspiration. The catheter is inserted into the portal vein toward the hilum of the liver. The portal vein catheter is made of polyurethane tubing (1.68 mm inside diameter, 2.41 mm outside diameter) and its lumen is treated with a heparin complex. Two pieces of nylon mesh are bonded to the catheter, with the first one 5 cm and the second one 27.5 cm posterior to the tip of the catheter. By suturing the first piece of nylon mesh to the two lateral ligatures on the connective tissue and the outer sheet of the veins and then tying up the anterior ligature, the catheter is secured to the portal vein with no occlusion of the blood vessel.

The ileal vein of the pig can be approached from the same abdominal incision made for the portal vein catheterization. Through this same incision, the segment of terminal ileum having a mass of clusters of lymph nodes and network of mesenterium veins is brought toward the incision and the ileal vein is located. The surrounding connective tissue of the intended puncture site in the ileal vein is carefully separated. Three ligatures (3/0 nonabsorbable suture) are placed on the separated connective tissue, with one ligature cranial and two ligatures lateral to the intended puncture site. A small puncture is made and the catheter is inserted cranially into the ileal vein for 10 cm. The ileal vein catheter is made of polyurethane tubing (0.65 mm inside diameter, 1.02 mm outside diameter) and its lumen is treated with heparin complex. The catheter has a bonded piece of nylon mesh 10 cm posterior to the catheter tip and another piece of nylon mesh 17.5 cm posterior to the first mesh. By suturing the anterior piece of nylon mesh to the two lateral ligatures on the connective tissue and then tying up the anterior ligature, the catheter is secured to the ileal vein in a fashion similar to that for the portal vein.

The portal vein catheter is exteriorized and exits 2 to 3 cm dorsal and anterior to the abdominal incision, and the ileal vein catheter exits dorsal and posterior to the incision. After suturing the second nylon mesh of each catheter to the body wall and sealing off the pierced wound, the abdominal incision is closed with 2/0 absorbable suture in four layers: the peritoneum, two muscle layers, and the skin. The distal end of each catheter is exteriorized subcutaneously to dorsal midline and anchored to the skin, using the same technique as described for the jugular vein or carotid artery catheter.

G. Mammary Vein Catheterization

A technique for the catheterization of the mammary vein in the lactating sow has been described by Trottier et al. (1995). The anesthetized sow is positioned in left lateral recumbency. An incision is made 4 to 5 cm above the plica lateralis, between the first and second anterior mammary gland. After dissecting the fat and connective tissue, a venous branch draining the skin and running dorsal to ventral is exposed. An opening through the fascia of the vein is created by the insertion of a 16-gauge needle. The catheter is inserted into the vein for a length of 16 cm or until its tip reaches the most anterior point of the mammary vein. The 110-cm catheter is made of polyvinyl microbore tubing (0.96 mm i.d, 1.68 mm outside diameter) and its lumen is treated with a heparin complex. Six, 5-mm rings made of silicon rubber are bonded to the catheter in pairs to form three cuffs starting 32 cm anterior to the distal end of the catheter. Each pair of rings is placed 1 cm apart and has a 12-cm suture (3/0) tied between the rings. The catheter is secured in position by suturing the cuffs to the connective tissue underlying the vein. The distal end of the catheter is exteriorized subcutaneously to the dorsal midline 10 cm anterior to the point of the shoulder. The free end of the mammary vein catheter is fitted with a blunt 18-gauge needle fixed with a luer-lock injection cap and placed, along with the carotid artery catheter, in a protective purse, which is glued to the skin.

IV. CARE AND USE OF SWINE IN EXPERIMENTAL SURGERY

It cannot be overemphasized that routine care and management of pigs for experimental surgery should carefully adhere to the regulations specified in the Animal Welfare Act and amendments, as well as the guidelines established under the Public Health Service Policy and the Health Research Extension Act. These regulations and guidelines can be found in the policies and procedures manual for the use of animals prepared by the Institutional Animal Care and Use Committee at every research and teaching institution, as well as in the training manual for the use of animals in research by Bennett et al. (1990) and the special report on guidelines for animal surgery in research and teaching by Brown et al. (1993). The Federation of Animal Science Societies (FASS, 1999) has recently published a first revised edition of the *Guide for the Care and Use of Agricultural Animals in Agricultural Research and Teaching*, that provides information on the requirements and recommendations for operating institutional animal facilities and programs concerning animals residing in simulated or actual production agricultural settings. If the surgically prepared pigs are used as models for biomedical research projects, the care and use of these animals should also meet the requirements and recommendations given in the *Guide for the Care and Use of Laboratory Animals*, published by the Institute for Laboratory Animal Resources (ILAR, 1996). It should be realized that all proposed activities regarding the care and use of swine in any experimental surgery must be reviewed and approved by the Institutional Animal Care and Use Committee.

V. PREPARATION FOR ASEPTIC SURGERY

The use of rigid aseptic technique in swine surgery is mandatory. The common misconception that pigs are not especially susceptible to postsurgical infection is a fallacy arising from the short-term use of the surgically prepared animals, and from the fact that casualties in the operated animals are soon forgotten. The routine, indiscriminate administration of antibiotics to the animal following surgery tends to cover the trails of poor technique.

The preparation for aseptic surgery includes as least four areas: sterilization of instruments and supplies needed to perform surgery; aseptic preparation of the surgical site on the animal; aseptic preparation of the surgeon and assistants; and aseptic draping of the animal. Detailed information and general principles regarding the preparation for aseptic surgery in swine are readily available and can be found in textbooks, such as that by Swindle (1983) on basic surgical exercises with pigs and those on large animal surgery by Oehme (1988), Turner et al. (1989), and Hickman et al. (1995).

VI. PRESURGICAL CARE OF THE ANIMAL

To obtain meaningful information from surgically prepared swine, the animals need to be trained properly, so their normal physiological functions and behavior will not be altered under the experimental conditions. For experiments in which pigs have to be housed individually in specially designed cages or crates for continuous infusion and repeated sampling, proper training of the animals is needed before surgery. In the studies with pigs having their portal vein, ileal vein, and carotid artery catheterized permanently, the animals were housed in individual pens, measuring 1.2 × 1.2 m, and trained to adapt to rectangular crates designed for infusion and sampling study. Usually within 3 to 4 days, the animals were well adapted and were willing to enter the rectangular crates, consume their daily feed allowance, and rest inside the crates until they were put back into the pens (Yen and Killefer, 1987).

Before surgery, the pigs should be fasted for 12 to 24 h to prevent vomiting or severe gaseous gastrointestinal distention (Thurmon et al., 1996). Water should be available to the pig until the time of surgery with the exception of gastrotomy, in which case water should be withheld for at least 6 h (Swindle, 1998).

VII. ANESTHESIA

It is beyond the scope of this chapter to provide detailed information of anesthesia in swine. Individuals interested in the principles and techniques of anesthesia should consult textbooks and

Blood Sampling and Surgical Techniques

TABLE 42.1
Selected Agents in Swine Anesthesia

Drug	Route of Administration	Dose	Purpose
Preanesthetics			
Atropine	IM	0.04 mg/kg	Reduce saliva and prevent bradycardia
Azaperone	IM	1–8 mg/kg	1–2 h sedation
Injectable anesthetics			
Ketamine	IM	20 mg/kg	20–30 min immobilization
Tiletamine/zolazepam (Telazol)	IM	2–8.8 mg/kg	20–30 min immobilization
Xylazine + ketamine	IM	2 + 20 mg/kg	30–45 min anesthesia
Xylazine + Telazol	IM	2.2 + 4.4 mg/kg	30–50 min anesthesia (juvenile pigs)
Xylazine + ketamine + Telazol	IM	2.2 + 2.2 + 4.4 mg/kg	45–60 min anesthesia
Pentobarbital	IV	10–30 mg/kg	15–45 min induction
Thiamylal	IV	6–18 mg/kg	10–20 min induction
Thiopental	IV	10–20 mg/kg	10–20 min induction
Inhalant anesthetics			
Halothane	Inh.	4–5%	Induction
		1–2%	Maintenance anesthesia
Isoflurane	Inh.	3–5%	Induction
		1.5–2.5%	Maintenance anesthesia

Abbreviations: IM, intramuscularly; IV, intravenously; Inh., inhalation.

references of veterinary anesthesia such as those by Riebold et al. (1995) and Thurmon et al. (1996). Excellent overviews of anesthesia in swine have also been published by Moon and Smith (1996), Thurmon et al. (1996), Smith et al. (1997), and Swindle (1998). A list of selected preanesthetics, intramuscularly and intravenously injectable anesthetics, and inhalation anesthetics for swine is given in Table 42.1.

The preferred inhalant anesthetic for the author's swine surgery is isoflurane. Compared with halothane, isoflurane costs more currently but it has a greater safety margin and allows a more rapid induction and recovery of the pig (Thurmon et al., 1996). The use of isoflurane rather than halothane can minimize adverse side effects on the animal and reduce personnel risks from chronic exposure to inhalant anesthetics (Stimpfel and Gershey, 1991; Swindle, 1998).

Using a nose cone or face mask, anesthesia of the pig can be safely induced with 3 to 5% of isoflurane in oxygen delivered from a closed-circle anesthetic machine. Anesthesia during the surgery is maintained with 2% (ranges from 1.5 to 2.5%) of isoflurane in oxygen flowing at a rate of 1 to 2 l/min. Induction of anesthesia can also be accomplished by restraining the pig with a snout snare and injecting intravenously sodium thiopental (10 to 20 mg/kg body weight as a 2.5 or 5% solution) into the external jugular vein or the ear vein.

VIII. MONITORING THE ANIMAL DURING AND AFTER SURGERY

Because ocular reflexes are not reliable in anesthetized pigs (Riebold et al., 1995; Swindle, 1998), the depth of anesthesia in pigs is best monitored by the degree of muscle relaxation and respiratory movement. A practical guide to muscle relaxation in pigs is the absence of withdrawal reflex of the legs when a pinch is applied between the hooves. In anesthetized pigs, the normal respiration rate is 10 to 25 breaths/min and heart rate is 80 to 130 beats/min (Riebold et al., 1995). Loss of withdrawal reflex to painful stimulus and full, rhythmic respiration indicate the surgical plane of anesthesia. To minimize shock due to surgery trauma and to hasten recovery from surgery, the pigs should be given a continuous, intravenous drip of isotonic, balanced electrolyte solutions, such as lactated Ringer's solution, during the surgery. The solution can be administered at a rate of 10 ml/kg/h (Riebold et al., 1995) into a ear vein, through an infusion set with a 21-gauge needle or via a 22-gauge intravenous catheter. The rate should be increased if blood loss occurs.

Postoperative administration of antibiotics to the animals is not necessary when strict aseptic surgery is conducted. If it is needed, an antibiotic can be given intramuscularly to the pig after surgery once daily for 3 days. After surgery, the pig should be monitored daily for appetite, bowel movement, urinary output, and behavior. The length of recovery after surgery depends on the type of surgery. A good indication of recovery is the restoration of normal appetite.

IX. SURGICAL TECHNIQUES FOR SELECTED *IN VIVO* NUTRITION STUDIES

This section describes a few surgical techniques that are valuable for *in vivo* nutrition studies in the pig. Information about surgical procedures for organ systems other than the digestive system in the pig has been published in two monographs by Swindle (1983, 1998) and a book chapter by Pond and Houpt (1978).

A. Nutrient Digestibility Studies

The digestibility of a nutrient in swine is traditionally estimated by the disappearance of that nutrient from the gastrointestinal tract (GIT). Recognition of the occurrence of substantial modification of carbohydrate, protein, and fats by microflora in the large intestine has led to the general acceptance of ileal digestibility, which measures the disappearance of ingested nutrients when digesta reach the terminal ileum in pigs.

Numerous methodologies have been developed to intercept digesta before they enter the cecum in conscious swine (Fuller, 1991; Sauer and de Lange, 1992; Batterham, 1994). The simplest technique to collect digesta is by the use of a T-cannula inserted in the distal ileum. An example of implanting a simple T-cannula in the ileum of 30- to 35-kg pigs has been described by Gargallo and Zimmerman (1980). A laparotomy incision is made in the right abdominal wall 4 cm below the transverse process of the fifth lumbar vertebra. The terminal ileum is located using the cecum as anatomical reference. A longitudinal incision is made on the antimensenteric surface 10 cm cranial to the ileo-cecal junction. The cannula is inserted into the lumen of the ileum. A purse string is placed around the barrel of the cannula. The cannula is exteriorized through a stub wound made through the right body wall. It is essential that the flanges of the cannula bring the ileum in close contact with the body wall so good adhesion can take place. A simple T-cannula for ileal cannulation in preweaned pigs has been described by Walker et al. (1986). Stein et al. (1998) have recently reported a technique for implanting a simple T-cannula in the ileum of pregnant sows. Simple T-cannulation does not allow total collection of digesta, and the digestibility must be calculated from the change in the concentrations of an indigestible marker (Sauer and Ozimek, 1986).

Collection of the entire ileal digesta flow can be accomplished with the use of reentrant cannulas that allow digesta to be collected and sampled from the proximal cannula and then returned to the pig through the distal cannula. The distal cannula can be placed either in the terminal ileum or in the cecum. Procedures for reentrant cannulation that bypasses the ileo-cecal valve and allows digesta to flow through externally connected cannulas in pigs have been reported by Easter and Tanksley (1973). This and other conventional reentrant cannulas have two main drawbacks (Fuller, 1991). One drawback is blockage of digesta, especially when pigs are fed diets that contain fibrous ingredients. Another problem relates to the complete transection of the small intestine that interrupts the transmission of normal migrating myoelectric complex needed for normal gut motility and function.

The integrity of the small intestine can be preserved by the use of the ileo-colic post-valvular (ICPV) reentrant cannulation introduced by Darcy et al. (1980). The approach involves resecting the cecum and placing the proximal cannula immediately behind the ileo-cecal valve. The reentrant distal cannula is implanted in the proximal colon. The two cannulas are not connected as the conventional reentrant cannulations. The proximal cannula is used to collect digesta continuously and the distal one is for intermittent return of digesta. This technique is surgically more difficult and it still cannot avoid the problem of blockage of the proximal cannula when pigs are given coarsely ground or fibrous diets.

These problems of reentrant cannulation may be solved partially by the postvalvular T-cecum (PVTC) cannula described by Van Leeuwen et al. (1988). In this approach, a para-costal laparotomy is made 10 cm above the mammary tissue in the right abdominal wall. The cecum along with the terminal portion of the ileum is exteriorized. The cecum is removed and replaced with a simple T-cannula made of silicon rubber. The T-cannula is placed directly opposite to the ileo-cecal valve that protrudes into the cecum. The inside and outside diameters of the cannula are 19 and 24 mm, respectively, for 10-kg pigs, and 25 and 30 mm for 40-kg pigs. The cannula flange is made rigid by a nylon strap placed around the cannula. The cannula is anchored to the body wall with a plastic ring. A silicon stopper is used to close the lumen of the cannula. When the cannula is closed, the digesta flows directly from the ileum into the colon. When the stopper is removed, the pressure in the abdomen causes the ileo-cecal valve to move into the cannula. As a consequence, the colon is closed and the digesta flows from the ileum into the cannula. The PVTC cannulation maintains the integrity of the small intestine as does the ICPV reentrant cannulation. However, the PVTC cannulation is surgically simpler than the ICPV reentrant cannulation. The relatively large size of its T-cannula also allows the PVTC cannulation to be used in the study of normal, non-reground feed ingredients or fibrous diets without the problem of blockage proximal to the cannula as commonly encountered with conventional reentrant cannulations.

A major concern with the PVTC cannulation relates to the possible physiological effect of cecectomy on ileal digestibility. A modified version of the PVTC technique has been proposed by Mroz et al. (1996). The technique, steered ileo-cecal-valve (SICV) cannulation, does not involve the removal of the cecum but use a two-ring, valve-steering system to steer the ileo-cecal valve toward the cecal cannula when digesta are collected. The inner ring of the steering system is introduced via a small incision into the lumen of the distal-ileum about 15 cm from the ileo-cecal valve. The outer ring, which is slightly smaller than the inner ring, is placed around the terminal ileum close to the ileo-ceco-colonic junction. The inner ring is connected with a nylon cord, led outside the pig through a silicon T-cannula placed in the cecum. By pulling the nylon cord, the ileo-cecal valve is steered into the T-cannula to discharge the digesta.

An alternative technique to ileal cannulation is the ileo-rectal anastomosis (IRA; Green et al., 1987; Laplace et al., 1989). The IRA method allows the digesta to bypass the large intestine and be excreted via the anus for collection. The technique involves making a 15-cm laparotomy incision in the ventral abdominal wall 15 cm caudal to the base of the sternum and dextral to the midline. The terminal ileum is transected 10 cm cranial to the ileo-cecal junction. The caudal end of the ileum is closed using a purse-string suture and then reinforced by an oversew suture. The open cranial end of the cut ileum is packed with gauze to prevent digesta contamination and tissue drying. The descending colon is located. A 3-cm longitudinal incision is made on the antimesenteric surface of the colon 12 cm cranial to the anus. The open cranial end of the ileum is sutured on the colon over the incision to form a T-shaped ileo-colonic junction. The colon loop immediately cranial to the newly formed junction is then transected 2 cm cranial to the junction. The two transected ends are closed with the purse-string and oversew sutures. The colon is then isolated completely from the rest of the GIT. A 2-cm longitudinal incision is made on the antimesenteric surface of the isolated colon 5 cm cranial to the caudal end of the colon. A simple T-cannula is inserted into the lumen of the colon and a purse-string suture is placed around the barrel of the cannula. The cannula is exteriorized through a stab wound in the left dorsal flank 15 cm caudal to the last rib to allow products of residual fermentation to escape from the isolated colon. The absence of colonic function causes IRA pigs to have frequent discharge of liquid and acidic digesta from the anus, and greater losses of water and electrolytes. The IRA pigs thus require larger dietary supplementation of sodium, other mineral elements, and vitamins to compensate for their losses. Furthermore, the digestion of organic matter in the IRA pig may be affected, because its ileum could adapt to make up some of the functions of bypassed large intestine (Fuller, 1991). The considerable discomfort associated with frequent outpouring of digesta from the anus makes the IRA technique undesirable from the animal welfare standpoint.

B. Net Portal Nutrient Absorption

Concentration difference of a nutrient between the efferent (portal venous) and afferent (systemic arterial) blood of the GIT reflects the net uptake from, or loss to, the GIT and is a more critical measurement of nutrient availability than is the disappearance of a nutrient from the GIT. By multiplying concentration differences of a nutrient between the portal and arterial blood by the simultaneously determined portal blood flow rate, the net nutrient absorption into the portal vein per unit of time can be estimated (Rerat et al., 1980; 1984a,b; Yen and Killefer, 1987; Yen et al., 1989; 1991; Yen and Pond, 1990; Yen and Nienaber, 1992; 1993).

Techniques have been developed to collect blood samples from the portal vein and the systemic artery, and to measure portal vein blood flow in conscious swine (Rerat et al., 1980; Yen and Killefer, 1987). The principles for quantifying the net portal absorption as adopted by Rerat et al. (1980) and by Yen and Killefer (1987) are similar. However, the techniques for cannulating blood vessels and for estimating the portal vein blood flow rate are different between the two laboratories. A constant infusion of P-aminohippuric acid (PAH) into the ileal vein was used by Yen and Killefer (1987) to provide an indicator-dilution method for estimating the portal vein blood flow rate, and an electromagnetic probe was used by Rerat et al. (1980).

Surgical procedures developed by Yen and Killefer (1987) to catheterize the carotid artery as well as the portal vein and ileal vein of pigs weighing 20 to 40 kg are described in Sections III.B and III.F of this chapter. Figure 42.3 shows the placement of these three catheters in a pig. The approach with PAH as the indicator to estimate the portal blood flow rate and net portal flux of nutrients in pigs as described by Yen and Killefer (1987) has also been used by other researchers. However, rather than ileal vein, a mesenteric vein was used by Van der Meulen et al. (1997) for infusing PAH. In the studies of Ten have et al. (1996) and Deutz and Soeters (1997), PAH was infused into the distal end of the splenic vein.

Rerat et al. (1980) have described a method of placing an electromagnetic flow probe to measure portal vein blood flow and for cannulating the portal vein in pigs weighing 41 to 63 kg. To place the flow probe, a 20-cm incision is made along the right upper lateral region of the abdomen, behind the last rib. The portal vein between the convergence of mesenteric veins and its entrance into the hepatic hilum is exposed. A 1- to 1.5-cm peritoneal tunnel is made between the portal vein and the mesentery. The probe is placed around the portal vein, and the opening of the tunnel is closed. The probe wire is fastened to the parietal peritoneum and then exteriorized near the upper angle of the margins of the incision. To cannulate the portal vein, a purse-string suture is placed on the portal vein between the flow probe and the liver. A hole in the center of the purse-string suture is made with a special needle containing the cannula over two thirds of its length. The needle will split lengthwise into two parts and yet is hinged to permit opening. The cannula is pushed inside the portal vein and the needle is withdrawn, opened, and removed from the cannula. The purse-string suture is tightened and the cannula is thus fastened directly in the portal vein. The cannula is exteriorized through an abdominal wound at the top of the right side of the body along the edge of the lumbar muscles.

Bajjalieh et al. (1981) also described procedures for placing an electromagnetic blood flow probe around the portal vein in 12- to 15-kg pigs. A mechanical, hydraulically activated sample needle is attached to the portal vein for obtaining blood samples. A cannula is placed in the vena cava for sampling systemic blood. Rerat et al. (1980) showed that the concentrations of reducing

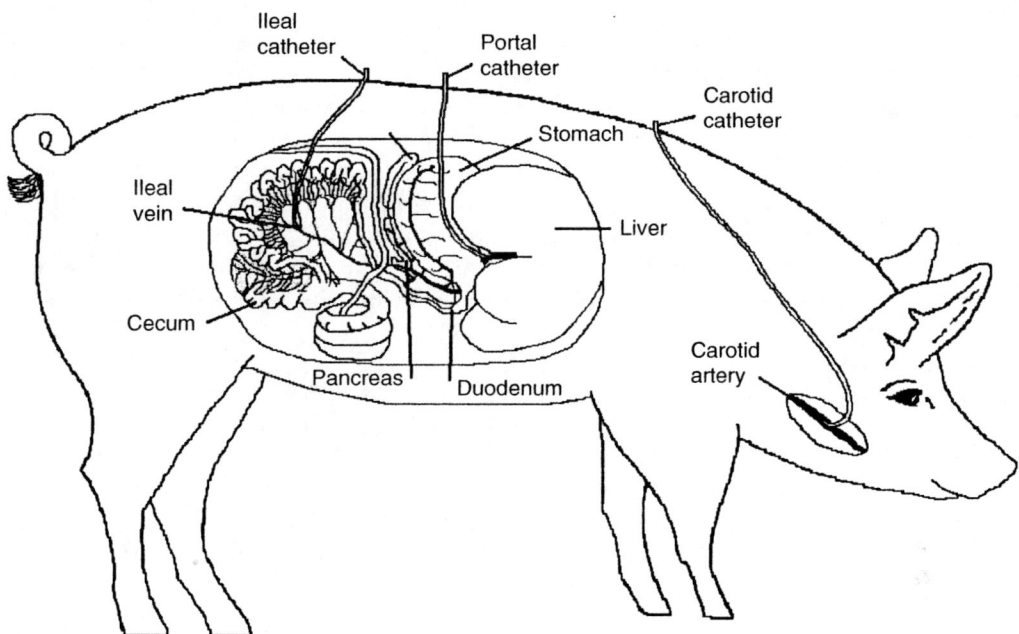

FIGURE 42.3 Placement of chronic indwelling catheters in the carotid artery and the portal and ileal veins.

sugars and amino acids in the pig are lower in the vena cava blood than in the arterial blood. Thus, a systematic error would exist if the porto-venal instead of the porto-arterial difference were used for estimating net portal absorption.

The measurement of net portal nutrient absorption can be expanded to include the subsequent hepatic metabolism of the absorbed nutrient by further catheterizing a hepatic vein in pigs infused continuously with PAH (Ten have et al., 1996). In pigs fitted with a flow probe around the portal vein, in addition to catheterizing a hepatic vein, a second flow probe should be placed around the hepatic artery if both determinations of net portal absorption and hepatic metabolism are to be conducted (Rerat, 1993).

C. Salivary Secretion

The saliva in a pig's mouth is a composite contributed by all salivary glands (Moran, 1982). The salivary glands of the pig consist of three major pairs of glands (parotid, mandibular, and sublingual) and small glands of the oral cavity such as buccal, labial, and lingual glands (Schummer et al., 1979). The number and various locations of salivary glands make it almost impossible to cannulate all the glands for a complete collection of saliva. Corring (1980) reported the use of an esophageal fistula to study the entire saliva collected during consumption of feed. However, no description of surgical procedures was given. Techniques for preparing esophageal fistulas in ruminants have been reviewed by Dougherty (1981) and may be useful to individuals interested in fistulating the esophagus of the pig. Denny and Messervy (1972) have described surgical techniques for the translocation of the parotid salivary duct and the cannulation of the parotid and submandibular salivary ducts in the pig. The translocation of the salivary duct provides a longer period for salivary collection than does the cannulation but can only be used for the parotid salivary duct.

To translocate the parotid salivary duct in a 1-year-old pig, a 12-cm skin incision is made over the ventral border of the lower jaw, beginning on a level with the eye and ending on a level with the ear. The subcutaneous fat and platysma muscle are incised to expose the mandibular part of the parotid gland, which is attached to the masseter muscle by a fascial sheet. The parotid duct lies dorsally within the fascial sheet. A 5-cm segment of the parotid duct is isolated. The duct is severed and its anterior end is brought out through the skin. The sheet of fascia is reattached to the masseter muscle and the incision of subcutaneous fat and platysma muscle is closed. A 1-cm longitudinal incision is made in the end of the parotid duct and the edge of the duct is sutured to the skin and the incision closed. Parotid saliva can be collected 2 days after surgery and for up to 2 months.

To cannulate the parotid duct, the duct is exposed as for translocation. A 2-cm length of the parotid duct is isolated. Through an incision in the duct, a 1.5-mm cannula is inserted caudally for 14 cm and secured by two ligatures tied around the duct. The fascial sheet is reattached to the masseter muscle and the cannula is anchored to the fascia to avoid kinking. The cannula is exteriorized through the subcutaneous tissue to exit 8 cm behind the ear. It is then anchored to the neck with a collar of adhesive tape.

For the cannulation of the submandibular duct, a 12-cm incision is made cranial to the angle of the jaw and parallel to the vertical ramus. The platysma muscle is incised and retracted caudally along with the adherent parotid gland to show a sheet of fascia attached to the caudal border of the vertical ramus. The fascia is incised and retracted to expose the submandibular salivary gland and its duct, which is cranial to the gland. A 7-cm segment of the duct is isolated, severed cranially, and brought out through the incision. A 1.5-mm cannula is inserted into the lumen of the duct and secured to the duct by two ligatures. The cannula is exteriorized to exit behind the ear and anchored to the neck.

D. Gastric Secretion

Gastric secretion in the pig has been studied with the use of a Heidenhain pouch or gastric cannula. Because both the pH and pepsin activity of the gastric secretion obtained from a Heidenhain pouch are significantly lower than those from a gastric cannula, the use of a Heidenhain pouch to study the gastric secretion has been questioned (Corring, 1980). Besides permitting study of gastric secretion, gastric cannulas also provide a convenient tool for administering a gastric load.

A technique for gastric cannulation in the pig has been described by Abel and Buck (1967). A 13-cm anterioventral laparotomy is made caudal to the 12th rib. The stomach is located, and two intestinal clamps that have been covered with surgical tubing are used to isolate the portion of the stomach intended for cannulation. Around the intended incision site, a purse-string suture is placed. An incision with the length equal to the diameter of the cannula and parallel to the greater curvature of the stomach is made. The flange of the cannula is inserted into the lumen of the stomach. After inverting the stomach wall, the purse-string suture is tied off around the cannula and a second purse-string suture is placed peripheral to the first one. The cannula is exteriorized through a second abdominal incision, dorsal to the first one and between the distal ends of the last two ribs. The stomach is pulled up against the abdominal peritoneum, and the washer of the cannula is positioned to hold the cannula in place.

Gastric cannulas can also be prepared with the technique described by Decuypere et al. (1977). The technique employs two types of cannulas made of disposable plastic syringes. For pigs weighing 3 to 10 and 10 to 20 kg, syringes of 2- and 5-ml capacity, respectively, are used as the insertion cannulas. Depending on the size of the animal, syringes of 5- or 10-ml capacity are used as the replacement cannulas. For gastric cannulation, a 5- to 7-cm midline incision is made cranial to the navel. A purse-string suture is placed in the lateroventral fundus region of the stomach. The insertion cannula is inserted into the stomach through an incision in the center of the suture. The stomach is drawn around the barrel of the cannula after the stomach wall is properly inverted. The cannula is placed in the cranial end of the midline incision and the incision is closed. The first replacement cannula is installed 7 to 8 days after surgery. If necessary, the animal is sedated or anesthetized. The insertion cannula is removed. The internal washer of the replacement cannula is introduced through the fistula and into the stomach. The barrel of the replacement cannula with its external washer in place is then inserted, and the internal washer is pulled on the barrel. By knotting the nylon strings that thread through the internal and external washers, the cannula is secured against the abdominal wall.

This technique described by Decuypere et al. (1977) can also be adopted for duodenal, ileal, and cecal cannulations in the pig. Björnhag and Jonsson (1984) have also described one type of replaceable gastrointestinal cannula for 12- to 40-kg pigs.

A surgical technique for installing a flexible, T-shaped gastric cannula in pregnant (85 ± 5 days of gestation), multiparous sows weighing 200 to 225 kg has been reported by Matzat et al. (1990). Sows were placed in right lateral recumbency. A 20-cm incision is made in the 11th intercostal space, beginning 20 cm from the dorsal midline. The ribs are separated with a rib spreader. After moving the spleen caudally, the stomach is located and brought toward the incision. The exposed portion of the stomach is packed with towels soaked with normal saline solution. A purse-string suture (4 cm in diameter) is placed in an avascular area of the dorsal greater curvature of the stomach. Within the purse-string suture, a 3-cm incision is made through the wall of the stomach. The base of the flexible, T-shaped cannula (16 mm inside diameter, 22 mm outside diameter) is folded, and both ends of the base are inserted simultaneously into the incision. The pursestring suture is tied off, and a second purse-string suture is placed in the stomach wall around the barrel of the cannula. The cannula is then manipulated to extend the base to its original T-shape. Through a stab incision in the 10th intercostal space, the cannula is exteriorized. The stomach is pulled up against the abdominal peritoneum, and the cannula is positioned to form an upward angle at approximately 45°. To prevent the cannula from being pulled into the abdominal cavity, the exteriorized cannula is wrapped with adhesive tape to 2-cm thickness.

E. Pancreatic Secretion

The exocrine pancreatic secretion in the pig can be collected by direct cannulation of the pancreatic duct (Pekas, 1965; Corring et al., 1972; Pierzynowski et al., 1988) or a duodenal pouch (Zebrowska et al., 1983; Hee et al., 1985). Direct cannulation allows collections for ≤45 days (Corring et al., 1972; J. T. Yen and A. H. Jensen, unpublished data), whereas a duodenal pouch may allow the collection to last several months (Corring, 1980). However, the secretion collected from a duodenal pouch may be contaminated with duodenal secretions, and the technique is more stressful to the animal because of the transection of the duodenum.

Corring (1974) demonstrated that the exocrine pancreatic secretion in the pig is regulated by a negative feedback mechanism. To avoid hypersecretion and to obtain a normal physiological response in the pancreatic secretion, it is imperative that the collected pancreatic secretion be returned to the duodenum of the animal. The reintroduction of the pancreatic secretion also prevents dehydration, acidosis, and eventual death in the pig (Wass, 1965).

A method for direct cannulation of the pancreatic duct and reintroduction of the pancreatic secretion into the duodenum in 4-week-old pigs has been described by Pekas (1965). A 10-cm incision is made parallel to the caudal-ventral margin of the rib cage on the right side of the animal. A rubber cannula (size, French 8) with a polyethylene nipple (PE 90) is inserted into the pancreatic duct toward the pancreas and 1 to 2 mm from the entrance of the duct into the intestine. A slightly larger rubber cannula is inserted into the duodenum in the area adjacent to the entrance of the pancreatic duct. The duodenum cannula is secured to the duodenum with a purse-string suture. The two cannulas are exteriorized, 14 cm apart and through stab wounds, to the back of the body and behind the last rib. A one-way valve, which allows a flow only from the pancreas to the duodenum and thus prevents the duodenal-pancreatic reflux, is used to connect the two cannulas. The ends of the one-way valve are secured to the skin of the pig by intradermal sutures. A two-way stopcock at the entrance of the one-way valve provides a simple means of collecting the pancreatic secretion.

Corring et al. (1972) have described another method for reentrant cannulating the pancreatic duct and duodenum in the pig weighing 35 to 45 kg. A 15-cm incision is made parallel to and behind the last rib on the right side of the animal. A 5-mm segment of the pancreatic duct is exposed. A polyethylene cannula (1.2 mm inside diameter, 1.7 mm outside diameter) with two polyethylene cuffs bonded to its proximal end is inserted into the duct and toward the pancreas for 1 to 2 cm. The cuff closest to the tip of the cannula is also inserted, and a ligature is placed between the two cuffs and toward the pancreas to tie off the duct around the cannula. The cannula is further fixed to the duodenum at the second cuff by a ligature. The duodenal cannula (1.5 mm inside diameter, 2.0 mm outside diameter) is then inserted into the duodenum near the entrance of the pancreatic duct with the first polyethylene cuff remaining in the lumen of the duodenum. The duodenal cannula is also secured to the duodenum by the cuff with two ligatures. The two cannulas are exteriorized to the right side of the body. The part of the duodenum where two cannulas are attached is brought up against the peritoneum. The incision is closed and the cannulas are anchored to the skin. The two cannulas are connected in such a way to return the pancreatic secretion immediately to the animal. Because no duodenal-pancreatic reflux has been noted, the one-way valve is not needed between the two cannulas. The pancreatic secretion can be collected continuously in a fraction collector with collection tubes maintained at 2°C. After being sampled, the secretion is brought to 38°C and reintroduced to the animal with a variable-rate peristaltic pump.

In pigs between 3 days and 9 weeks of age, procedures for direct cannulation of the pancreatic duct have been reported by Pierzynowski et al. (1988). A 4- to 5-cm incision is made between the two most caudal ribs on the right side of the pig. The head of the pancreas is identified and the pancreatic duct is dissected free. A silicon rubber catheter (0.3 to 0.64 mm inside diameter, 0.64 to 1.19 mm outside diameter, depending on the age of the pig) is inserted at 2 to 5 mm from the duodenal entrance and into the pancreatic duct for 5 to 10 mm. A cuff bonded to the catheter 10 mm from the tip is tied loosely to the securely ligated distal pancreatic duct. Anterior to the entry point of the catheter, a ligature is tied tightly around the inserted catheter and the pancreatic duct. A 3- to 4-cm segment of duodenum immediately distal to the entrance of the pancreatic duct is isolated, using two intestinal clamps. Between the clamps, two nonpenetrating purse-string sutures, 10 and 15 mm wide, are placed, one within the other. A reentrant, perforated T-cannula made of silicone tubing is inserted into the duodenum through an incision inside the purse-string sutures. The duodenal T-cannula and the pancreatic duct cannula are exteriorized between the ribs. The duodenal cannula is exteriorized directly through stab wound, whereas the pancreatic duct cannula is exteriorized through an additional abdominal cannula placed between the parietal peritoneum and the muscle layers in the dorsal part of the incision. The duodenal and abdominal cannulas are anchored on the body of the pig by retaining external cuffs. This surgical procedure allows exocrine pancreatic secretion to be collected for 1 to 2 weeks from animals operated at 3 days of age and for 6 to 8 weeks from those operated at 2 weeks of age.

Techniques for collecting pancreatic secretion through a duodenal pouch in pigs weighing 30 kg have been described by Hee et al. (1985). A 15-cm incision is made parallel and caudal to the last rib on the right side of the animal. A 4- to 6-cm segment of the duodenum that receives the pancreatic duct is isolated. Two intestinal clamps are placed on the duodenum 2 to 3 cm caudal to the pancreatic duct. The duodenum is transected between the two clamps, and the cranial end is closed by a Parker–Kerr oversew to form the bottom of the pouch. Another pair of clamps is applied to the duodenum 2 to 3 cm cranial to the pancreatic duct. The duodenum is transected between the clamps and a purse-string suture is placed around the opening of the pouch. The draining arm of the silicon rubber cannula with its perforated basket at the tip is inserted and secured. After the remaining duodenum is anastomosed, the silicon rubber reentrant arm of the cannula is inserted into the duodenum through the antimesenteric side 1 cm cranial to the anastomosis and secured by a purse-string suture. The draining and reentrant arms are exteriorized and exit 15 cm apart and dorsal to the costochondral junction of the right side of the animal. They are connected by stainless steel tubing and secured to the body with rigid polyvinyl chloride washers and silicon rubber retaining rings. For collecting pancreatic secretion, the reentrant cannula is disconnected and an extension tubing is attached. Pancreatic secretion is reintroduced to the animal by gravity flow.

F. Bile Secretion

To study bile secretion in the pig with little interruption of the enterohepatic circulation of bile salt, the bile has to be reintroduced to the animal. A bile duct reentrant cannulation technique in pigs of 25 to 30 kg has been described by Sambrook (1981). A 25-cm midline incision is made. After separating the bile duct from the adjacent tissue, an incision is made at the midpoint of the duct. An exit cannula and then entry cannula are inserted and ligated in place. The cannulas are made of 30-cm-long silicon rubber tubing (2 mm inside diameter, 4 mm outside diameter) with a 2-cm-long rigid nylon tip. The bile duct is transected between the two cannulas. The two cannulas are sutured to the parietal peritoneum and exteriorized to the right flank of the animal. After suturing the entry cannula to the pylorus, the midline incision is closed. The two exteriorized cannulas are connected with curved stainless steel tubing and covered with adhesive tape. For bile flow measurement and sampling, a small Perspex dropchamber with a three-way stopcock is connected to the cannulas by silicon rubber tubing. A photoelectric counting system is used to record drops of bile.

Juste et al. (1983) have described an automated system in which bile is returned to the pig at a rate directly corresponding to its secretion rate. In the pig weighing 50 kg, a silicone rubber cannula (2.65 mm inside diameter, 4.88 mm outside diameter) is inserted through an incision into the bile duct toward the liver and ligated in place. A second silicon rubber cannula (1.57 mm inside diameter, 3.18 mm outside diameter) is inserted between the first cannula and the sphincter of Oddi and toward the duodenum without reaching the sphincter muscle. The two cannulas are exteriorized to the right flank of the animal. For measurement and sampling of bile, the exit cannula is connected to the plastic container of the automated system and the entry cannula to a peristaltic pump. The system also consists of a glass container having two platinum wire electrodes, an electronic relay, an electric stop valve, a recorder pen, a bile sampling tube, and two nitrogen caps. Bile is reintroduced automatically in a volume determined by the position of one of the two electrodes. The system records bile flow and continuously samples bile for analysis.

The direct cannulation of bile duct, described by Sambrook (1981) and Juste et al. (1983), allows bile to be collected from the pig for <40 days. Symonds and Charmley (1990) have reported a surgical method that provides the collection of bile in pigs of 30 to 40 kg for up to 11 months. The technique, however, is more complex and may cause the collected bile to be contaminated with jejunal secretion, because it uses two isolated lengths of jejunum with one to divert bile from the bile duct and one to return bile to the duodenum. The surgery involves making an incision parallel to and 3 cm behind the last rib, and from 5 cm below the transverse processes to near the xiphisternum on the right flank of the pig. The bile duct is dissected before its attachment to the duodenum. A single length of jejunum, about twice the length from the entry of the bile duct to halfway up the flank, is isolated. The rest of the jejunum is joined by an end-to-end anastomosis. The ampulla of Vater, the site where bile duct enters the duodenum, is excised with a 1- to 2-mm margin of duodenal wall around it. The ampulla is stitched into the cranial end of the isolated segment of jejunum. The caudal end of the isolated jejunal segment is anastomosed to the duodenum over the stoma at the site of excision of Vater's ampulla. The jejunal segment is then divided into two equal sections, and each cut end is closed by an inversion suture. Into the side of each jejunal section near its inverted distal end, a T-cannula made of glass fiber reinforced nylon is inserted through an incision and a purse-string suture. The stem length of the T-cannula is made less than the thickness of the body wall to prevent the cannula from being pulled out or pushed in. After each cannula is brought through the peritoneum, a outer ring containing circular holes is passed over the stem of the cannula and positioned between the peritoneum and the body wall. A thin washer of silicone rubber is placed between the fixed inner flange of the cannula and the peritoneum. A silicone rubber extension tubing is inserted through a stab incision in the right body wall from the exterior, pushed over and tied to the stem of each cannula to hold the outer ring firmly in place. The two cannulas are not connected for 2 days after surgery to prevent formation of fistula from possible leakage of bile through sutures.

Supplements of electrolytes and protein are given to the pig during the first few days after surgery. For bile collection, the pig is not restrained. Bile is collected from the proximal cannula into plastic bottles held on pig's back by adhesive tape. After sampling for analysis, the remaining bile is returned to the duodenum of the pig through the distal cannula.

G. Gastrointestinal Lymph

Long-chain fatty acids absorbed from the GIT are transported by the lymphatic system. Cisterna chyli, the dilated sac at the lower end of the thoracic duct, receives lymph from the visceral and lumbar lymphatic trunks (Schummer et al., 1981).

Techniques for the cannulation of the cisterna chyli of the pig weighing 45 kg have been described by Manolas et al. (1983). A laparotomy is made 3 cm beneath and parallel to the costal margin and extends from the lateral end of the costal margin to the midline on the left side of the pig. An incision is made in the caudal peritoneum above the left kidney and 4 cm from the midline. A 5- to 10-cm cisterna chyli is exposed by pulling the left kidney toward the midline and separating the celiac aortic wall from the left psoas muscle with a very gentle blunt dissection. An incision is made in the lymph vessel wall and a T-shaped cannula (1.6 mm inside diameter, 2.7 mm outside diameter) is inserted into the lumen of the cisterna chyli. The caudal peritoneum is closed after returning the left kidney to its normal position. The cannula is exteriorized below the left kidney and through the abdominal wall. In ten pigs so prepared, the cannula was found to be patent for only 2 to 7 days.

REFERENCES

Abel, M., and W. B. Buck. 1967. A technic for gastric cannulation of swine, *Cornell Vet.*, 57:383.

Allrich, R. D., R. K. Christenson, J. J. Ford, and D. R. Zimmerman. 1982. Pubertal development of the boar: testosterone, estradiol-17β, cortisol and LH concentrations before and after castration at various ages, *J. Anim. Sci.*, 55:1139.

Bajjalieh, N. L., A. H. Jensen, G. R. Frank, and D. E. Brown. 1981. A technique for monitoring nutrient absorption in the conscious, unrestrained pig, *J. Anim. Sci.*, 52:101.

Barb, C. R. 1993. Technique for chronic catheterization of the jugular vein in swine. In *Handbook of Methods for Study of Reproductive Physiology in Domestic Animals*, Section VIIIA2A and IXA1, Dziuk, P. J., Ed., University of Illinois, Urbana.

Batterham, E. S. 1994. Ileal digestibilities of amino acids in feedstuffs for pigs. In *Amino Acids in Farm Animal Nutrition*, D'Mello, J. P. F., Ed., CAB International, Edinburgh, U.K., 113, chap. 6.

Bennett, B. T., M. J. Brown, and J. C. Schofield. 1990. Essentials for Animal Research, A Primer for Research Personnel, USDA, National Agricultural Library, Beltsville, MD.

Björnhag, G., and E. Jonsson. 1984. Replaceable gastro-intestinal cannulas for small ruminants and pigs, *Livest. Prod. Sci.*, 11:179.

Brown, M. J., P. T. Pearson, and F. N. Tomson. 1993. Guidelines for animal surgery in research and teaching, *Am. J. Vet. Res.*, 54:1544.

Carle, B. N., and W. H. Dewhirst. 1942. A method for bleeding swine, *J. Am. Vet. Med. Assoc.*, 101:495.

Corring, T. 1974. Feed-back regulation of pancreatic secretion in the pig, *Ann. Biol. Anim. Bioch. Biophys.*, 14:487.

Corring, T. 1980. Endogenous secretions in the pigs. In Current Concepts of Digestion and Absorption in Pigs, Low, A. G., and I. G. Partridge, Eds., Technical Bulletin 3, National Institute for Research in Dairying, Reading, U.K., 136.

Corring, T., A. Aumaitre, and A. Rérat. 1972. Permanent pancreatic fistulation in the pig: secretory response to meal ingestion, *Ann. Biol. Anim. Bioch. Biophys.*, 12:109.

Darcy, B., J. P. Laplace, and P. A. Villiers. 1980. Digestion dans l'intestin grele chez le porc. 2. Cinetique comparee de passage des digesta selon le mode de fistulation, ileo-caecale ou ileo-colique post-valvulaire, dans diverses conditions d'alimentation, *Ann. Zootech.*, 29:147.

Decuypere, J. A., I. J. Vervaeke, H. K. Henderickx, and N. A. Dierick. 1977. Gastro- intestinal cannulation in pigs: a simple technique allowing multiple replacements, *J. Anim. Sci.*, 45:463.

Denny, H. R., and A. Messervy. 1972. Surgical techniques for the extirpation of the submandibular salivary glands and the collection of salivary secretions in the pig, *Vet. Rec.*, 90:650.

Deutz, N.E.P., and P. B. Soeters. 1997. Intestinal metabolism and absorption during enteral nutrition in the pig. In *Digestive Physiology in Pigs*, Laplace, J.-P., C. Fevrier, and A. Barbeau, Eds., Proc. VIIth International Symposium on Digestive Physiology in Pigs, INRA, St. Malo, France, EAAP Publ. No. 88, 41.

Dougherty, R. W. 1981. *Experimental Surgery in Farm Animals*, Iowa State University Press, Ames.

Easter, R. A., and T. D. Tanksley. 1973. A technique for reentrant ileo-caecal cannulation of swine, *J. Anim. Sci.*, 36:1099.

Federation of Animal Science Societies. 1999. *Guide For the Care and Use of Agricultural Animals in Agricultural Research and Teaching*, rev. ed., FASS, Savoy, IL.

Ford, J. J., and R. R. Maurer. 1978. Simple technique for chronic venous catheterization of swine, *Lab. Anim. Sci.*, 28:615.

Friend, D. W., and R. G. Brown. 1971. Blood sampling from suckling pigs, *Can. J. Anim. Sci.*, 51:547.

Fuller, M. F. 1991. Methodologies for the measurement of digestion. In *Digestive Physiology in Pigs*, Verstegen, M. W. A., J. Huisman, and L. A. den Hartog, Eds., Proc. Vth International Symposium on Digestive Physiology in Pigs, Purdoc, Wageningen, The Netherlands, EAAP Publ. No. 54, 273.

Gargallo, J., and D. R. Zimmerman. 1980. A simple intestinal cannula for swine, *Am. J. Vet. Res.*, 41:618.

Green, S., S. L. Bertrand, M.J.C. Duron, and R. A. Maillard. 1987. Digestibility of amino acids in maize, wheat and barley meals, measured in pigs with ileo-rectal anastomosis and isolation of the large intestine, *J. Sci. Food Agric.*, 41:29.

Hee, J. H., W. C. Sauer, R. Berzins, and L. Ozimek. 1985. Permanent re-entrant diversion of porcine pancreatic secretions, *Can. J. Anim. Sci.*, 65:451.

Hickman, J., J. Houlton, and B. Edwards. 1995. *An Atlas of Veterinary Surgery*, 3rd ed., Blackwell Science, Osney Mead, Oxford, U.K.

ILAR (Institute for Laboratory Animal Resources). 1996. *Guide for the Care and Use of Laboratory Animals*, National Research Council, Washington, D.C.

Juste, C., T. Corring, and Y. Le Coz. 1983. Bile restitution procedures for studying bile secretion in fistulated pigs, *Lab. Anim. Sci.*, 33:199.

Kraeling, R. R., G. B. Rampacek, N. M. Cox, and T. E. Kiser. 1982. Prolactin and luteinizing hormone secretion after bromocryptine (CB-154) treatment in lactating sows and ovariectomized gilts, *J. Anim. Sci.*, 54:1212.

Laplace, J. P., B. Darcy-Vrillon, J. M. Pérez, Y. Henry, S. Giger, and D. Sauvant. 1989. Associative effects between two fibre sources on ileal and overall digestibilities of amino acids, energy and cell-wall components in growing pigs, *Br. J. Nutr.*, 61:75.

Lawhorn, B. 1988. A new approach for obtaining blood samples from pigs, *JAVMA*, 192:781.

Manolas, K. J., H. M. Farmer, M. Cussen, and R. B. Welbourn. 1983. An experimental model for simultaneous chronic sampling of portal and systemic blood and gastrointestinal lymph via cannulae in conscious swine, *Cornell Vet.*, 73:333.

Matzat, P. D., N. K. Ames, and M. G. Hogberg. 1990. Gastric cannulation of pregnant sows, *Am. J. Vet. Res.*, 51:2031.

Moon, P. F., and L. J. Smith. 1996. General anesthetic techniques in swine. In *The Veterinary Clinics of North America, Food Animal Practice*, Anesthesiology Update, Vol. 12, No. 3, Swanson, C. R., Ed., W. B. Saunders, Philadelphia, 663.

Moran, E. T., Jr. 1982. *Comparative Nutrition of Fowl and Swine — The Gastrointestinal Systems*, University of Guelph, Guelph, Ontario, Canada.

Mroz, Z., G. C. M. Bakker, A. W. Jongbloed, R. A. Dekker, R. Jongbloed, and A. van Beers. 1996. Apparent digestibility of nutrients in diets with different energy density, as estimated by direct and marker methods for pigs with or without ileo-cecal cannulas, *J. Anim. Sci.*, 74:403.

Oehme, F. W. 1988. *Textbook of Large Animal Surgery*, 2nd ed., Williams & Wilkins, Baltimore, MD.

Pekas, J. C. 1965. Permanent physiological fistula of the pancreas and other digestive glands, *J. Appl. Physiol.*, 20:1082.

Pierzynowski, S. G., B. R. Weström, B. W. Karlsson, J. Svendsen, and B. Nilsson. 1988. Pancreatic cannulation of young pigs for long-term study of exocrine pancreatic function, *Can. J. Anim. Sci.*, 68:953.

Pond, W. G., and K. A. Houpt. 1978. *The Biology of the Pig*, Cornell University Press, Ithaca, NY, 203–237.

Rerat, A. A. 1993. Nutritional supply of proteins and absorption of their hydrolysis products: consequences on metabolism, *Proc. Nutr. Soc.*, 52:335.

Rerat, A. A., P. Vaissade, and P. Vaugelade. 1984a. Absorption kinetics of some carbohydrates in conscious pigs, 1. Qualitative aspects, *Br. J. Nutr.*, 51:505.

Rerat, A. A., P. Vaissade, and P. Vaugelade. 1984b. Absorption kinetics of some carbohydrates in conscious pigs, 2. Quantitative aspects, *Br. J. Nutr.*, 51:517.

Rerat, A., P. Vaugelade, and P. Villiers. 1980. A new method for measuring the absorption of nutrients in the pig: Critical examination. In *Current Concepts of Digestion and Absorption in Pigs*, Low, A.G. and I.G. Partridge, Eds., National Institute for Research in Dairying, Reading, England, Hannah Research Institute, Ayre, Scotland, Tech. Bull. 3, p. 117.

Riebold, T. W., D. R. Geiser, and D. O. Goble. 1995. *Large Animal Anesthesia — Principles and Techniques*, 2nd ed., Iowa State University Press, Ames.

Sambrook, I. E. 1981. Studies on the flow and composition of bile in growing pigs, *J. Sci. Food Agric.*, 32:781.

Sauer, W. C., and C. F. M. de Lange. 1992. Novel methods for determining protein and amino acid digestibilities in feedstuffs. In *Methods in Protein Nutrition and Metabolism*, Nissen, S., Ed., Academic Press, San Diego, CA.

Sauer, W. C., and L. Ozimek. 1986. Digestibility of amino acids in swine: results and their practical applications. a review, *Livest. Prod. Sci.*, 15:367.

Schummer, A., R. Nickel, and W. O. Sack. 1979. The viscera of the domestic mammals. In *The Anatomy of the Domestic Animals*, Vol. 2, 2nd rev. ed., Springer-Verlag, New York.

Schummer, A., H. Wilkens, B. Vollmerhaus, K.-H. Habermehl, W. G. Siller, and P. A. L. Wight. 1981. The circulatory system, the skin, and the cutaneous organs of the domestic mammals. In *The Anatomy of the Domestic Animals*, Vol. 3, 2nd rev. ed., Springer-Verlag, New York.

Schwartz, W. L., and J. E. Smallwood. 1977. Collection of blood from swine, *Tex. Vet. Med. J.*, 39(3):6.

Smith, A. C., W. J. Ehler, and M. M. Swindle. 1997. Anaesthesia and analgesia in swine. In *Anesthesia and Analgesia in Laboratory Animals*, Kohn, D. H., S. K. Wixson, W. J. White, and G. J. Benson, Eds., Academic Press, New York, 313.

Stein, H. H., C. F. Shipley, and R. A. Easter. 1998. Technical Note: A technique for inserting a T-cannula into the distal ileum of pregnant sows, *J. Anim. Sci.*, 76:1433.

Stimpfel, T. M., and E. L. Gershey. 1991. Selecting anesthetic agents for human safety and animal recovery surgery, *FASEB J.*, 5:2099.

Straw, B. E., and D. J. Meuten. 1992. Physical examination. In *Diseases of Swine*, 7th ed., Leman, A. D., B. E. Straw, W. L. Mengeling, S. D'Allaire, D. J. Taylor, Eds., Iowa State University Press, Ames, 793.

Swindle, M. M. 1983. *Basic Surgical Exercises Using Swine*, Praeger Publishers, New York.

Swindle, M. M. 1998. *Surgery, Anesthesia, and Experimental Techniques in Swine*, Iowa State University Press, Ames.

Symonds, H. W., and L. L. Charmley. 1990. A surgical technique for the long term collection of bile in the pig and measurement of the biliary excretion of copper and zinc, *Res. Vet. Sci.*, 48:28.

Ten have, G. A. M., M. C. F. Bost, J. C. A.W. Suyk-Wierts, A. E. J. M. van den Bogaard, and N. E. P. Deutz. 1996. Simultaneous measurement of metabolic flux in portally-drained viscera, liver, spleen, kidney and hindquarter in the conscious pig, *Lab. Anim.*, 30:347.

Thurmon, J. C., W. J. Tranquilli, and G. J. Benson. 1996. *Lumb & Jones' Veterinary Anesthesia*, 3rd ed., Williams & Wilkins, Baltimore, MD.

Tilton, J. E., K. Plaine, and R. M. Weigl. 1993. Cephalic vein cannulation of the pig. In *Handbook of Methods for Study of Reproductive Physiology in Domestic Animals*, Section VIII A2C, Dziuk, P. J., Ed., University of Illinois, Urbana.

Trottier, N. L., C. F. Shipley, and R. A. Easter. 1995. A technique for the venous cannulation of the mammary gland in the lactating sow, *J. Anim. Sci.*, 73:1390.

Turner, A. S., C. W. McIlwraith, and B. L. Hull. 1989. *Techniques in Large Animal Surgery*, 2nd ed., Lea & Febiger, Philadelphia.

van Leeuwen, P., J. Huisman, M. W. A. Verstegen, M. J. Baak, D. J. van Kleef, and L. A. den Hartog. 1988. A new technique for collection of ileal chyme in pigs. In *Digestive Physiology in the Pig, Proc. IVth International Symposium*, Buraczewska, K., S. Buraczewski, B. Pastuszewska, and T. Zebrowska, Eds., Polish Academy of Sciences, Jablonna, Poland, 289.

Van der Meulen, J., G. C. M. Bakker, J. G. M. Bakker, H. de Visser, A. W. Jongbloed, and H. Everts. 1997. Effect of resistant starch on net portal-drained viscera flux of glucose, volatile fatty acids, urea, and ammonia in growing pigs, *J. Anim. Sci.*, 75:2697.

Walker, W. R., G. L. Morgan, and C. V. Maxwell. 1986. Ileal cannulation in baby pigs with a simple T-cannula, *J. Anim. Sci.*, 62:407.

Wass, W. M. 1965. The collection of porcine pancreatic juice by cannulation of the pancreatic duct, *Am. J. Vet. Res.*, 26:1106.

Yen, J. T., and J. Killefer. 1987. A method for chronically quantifying net absorption of nutrients and gut metabolites into hepatic portal vein in conscious swine, *J. Anim. Sci.*, 64:923.

Yen, J. T., and J. A. Nienaber. 1992. Influence of carbadox on fasting oxygen consumption by portal-drained organs and by the whole animal in growing pigs, *J. Anim. Sci.*, 70:478.

Yen, J. T., and J. A. Nienaber. 1993. Effects of high-copper feeding on portal ammonia absorption and on oxygen consumption by portal vein-drained organs and by the whole animal in growing pigs, *J. Anim. Sci.*, 71:2157.

Yen, J. T., J. A. Nienaber, D. A. Hill, and W. G. Pond. 1989. Oxygen consumption by portal vein-drained organs and by whole animal in conscious growing swine, *Proc. Soc. Exp. Biol. Med.*, 190:393.

Yen, J. T., J. A. Nienaber, D. A. Hill, and W. G. Pond. 1991. Potential contribution of absorbed volatile fatty acids to whole-animal energy requirement in conscious swine, *J. Anim. Sci.*, 69:2001.

Yen, J. T., and W. G. Pond. 1990. Effect of carbadox on net absorption of ammonia and glucose into hepatic portal vein of growing pigs, *J. Anim. Sci.*, 68:4236.

Zebrowska, T., A. G. Low, and H. Zebrowska. 1983. Studies on gastric digestion of protein and carbohydrate, gastric secretion and exocrine pancreatic secretion in the growing pigs, *Br. J. Nutr.*, 49:401.

Index

A

AA, *see* Amino acids
AAFCO (Association of American Feed Control Officials), 823
Abdominal aorta catheterization, 967–968
Absorption efficiency of minerals
    calcium, 357
    chloride, 360
    copper, 361
    iodine, 361
    iron, 363
    magnesium, 360
    manganese, 363
    phosphorus, 359
    potassium, 360–361
    selenium, 363–364
    sodium, 360
    zinc, 364–365
Acetic acid, 50, 95–97
Acromegaly, 10
Acid detergent fiber (ADF), 108
α-Acid glycoprotein (AGP), 549
Active oxygen method test (AOM), 98
Acute-phase proteins, 549
Acute venipuncture
    anterior vena cava, 962–963
    brachiocephalic vein, 963
Additives to feed, *see* Protein supplements
Adenosine diphosphate (ADP), 632
Adenosine triphosphate (ATP), 632–633
ADF (acid detergent fiber), 108
Adipose tissue
    nutrient partitioning and, 428–429
    porcine somatotropin and, 430
ADP (adenosine diphosphate), 632
Adrenaline and muscle metabolism, 633–634
α-Adrenergic agonists, 7
Adrenergic agonists, 433–435
Aflatoxin, 563, 564, 565–566
Agalactia, 757
AGP (α-acid glycoprotein), 549
Alcoholism research using pigs, 9
Alfalfa (*Medicago* sp.), 110, 809–810
Alkaloids, 577
Alternative feedstuffs, *see also* Feed
    crystalline amino acids, 851
    energy feedstuffs
        bananas, 842
        cane molasses, 842–843
        cassava, 843
        citrus pulp, 843
        cocoyams, 843
        grain screenings, 843–844
        pearl millet, 844
        potatoes, 844
        rice, 844–845
        sugar beets, 845
        sugarcane, 843
        sweet potatoes, 845
        triticale, 845–846
        yams, 846
    factors to consider, 840–842
    forages, 851
    liquid whey, 851
    maximum dietary inclusion suggestions, 856, 857
    nutrient compositions table, 853–855
    protein feedstuffs
        beans, 846
        canola seed, 846–847
        cull eggs, 847
        faba beans, 847
        fish silage, 847–848
        legumes, 851
        lentils, 848
        lupins, 848
        mung beans, 848–849
        oilseed meals, 851
        peanuts, 849
        peas, 849–850
        poultry hatchery by-product meal, 850
        shrimp meal, 850
        sunflower seeds, 850–851
    restaurant food waste, 852
    value determination, 842
Alumino silicate, 572
Ambient temperature (Ta), *see* Thermal environment
Amine/diamine oxidases, 236–237
Amines, 596–597
Amino acids
    absorption and intestinal bacteria, 595
    balance and protein quality
        disproportions, 136–137
        ideal protein, 135–136
    bioavailability, *see* Bioavailability of amino acids
    catabolites and intestinal bacteria
        amines, 596–597
        ammonia, 597
        phenols and indoles, 597–598
    in cereal grains, 137–138, 792–794
    crytalline use
        as alternative feedstuff, 851
        frequency of feeding, 141–142
        isomers, 141
        nutraceuticals, 142
        as supplements, 142

dietary requirements, 77
diet formulation based on, 139
digestion and endogenous losses factors
    antibiotics, 176
    dietary fat, 172
    dry matter intake, 169–170
    fiber in diet, 173–174
    ingredient and feed processing, 170–171
    lectins, 175
    organic acids, 176–177
    phytates, 174
    protein level in diet, 171–172
    tannins, 175–176
    trypsin inhibitors, 174–175
energy relationships, 140
essentiality of, 133–135
genetic modifications to improve, 800
ileal digesta collection, 163–166
immune function and, 551–553
lactating sows requirement, 750–752, 753, 755
limitations in feeds
    cereal grains, 137–138
    complete diets, 139
    protein supplements, 138–139
nitrogen excretion and, 616–617
preslaughter intake manipulation, 641–642
protein requirements with metabolic enhancers, 440–441
proteins and nonprotein nitrogen
    crude and true, 132
    nonprotein nitrogen use, 132–133
requirements, 143
simulation of use model, 872–873
sulfur and, 224–225
transport systems, 53–54
true ileal digestibilities
    definition and significance, 166
    endogenous losses measurement, 166–169
weanling pig requirements, 693–694
Ammonia
    emission and NSPs, 123–124
    emission and odor reduction strategies, 624
    intestinal bacteria and, 597
    protein digestion and, 54
Ammonia salts, 132–133
Amylase, 42
Amylopectin, *see also* Carbohydrates
    described, 46
    genetic modifications to improve, 799–800
Amylose, *see also* Carbohydrates
    described, 46
    genetic modifications to improve, 799–800
Analysis of variance
    assumptions, 894–895
    components, 893
    functions of, 893–894
    plans, 895–896
7-α-Androstenone, 12
Anemia studies, 11, 245
Anesthesia for swine, 970–971
Animal activity and energy maintenance, 73–74

ANOVA, *see* Analysis of variance
Antibiotics, *see also* Antimicrobial agents
    for growing-finishing pigs, 720–721
    ileal AA digestibilities influenced by, 176
    resistance from pork consumption, 14
    supplementation effects on NSP, 117
    in weanling pig diet, 702–703
Antigenic proteins, 576
Antimicrobial agents, *see also* Antibiotics
    background on use, 402–404
    definition, 401
    economic benefits, 402, 417
    efficacy as growth promoters
        benefits, 405–407
        copper use, 407–408
        studies results, 405
        zinc use, 408
    efficacy on reproductive efficiency, 409
    mode of action
        disease control effect, 412–413
        metabolic role, 409, 411
        nutritional effect, 411–412
    proper usage, 413–414
    safety of, 414–417
Antinutritional factors, *see also* Mycotoxins
    alkaloids, 577
    antigenic proteins, 576
    glucosinolates, 577
    lectins, 574–575
    protease inhibitors, 573–574
    reducing, 577–578
    tannins, 575–576, 577
Antioxidants functions, 292
AOM (active oxygen method test), 98
Arachidonic acid and prostaglandin metabolism, 294
Arachis hypogaea (peanuts), 816–817, 849
Arginine
    function and uses, 134
    immune function and, 551
Arsenic (As), 253
Artificial insemination, 28
Artificial rearing
    advantages, 672–673
    disadvantages, 673
    performance after, 681–682
As (arsenic), 253
Ascorbic acid
    deficiency/toxicity symptoms, 342
    history, 340
    metabolism, 340–341
    nutritional requirements, 341–342
    status and sources, 342
    structure, 340
Ash
    association with protein, 67
    percent composition of pigs, 66
    skeletal composition and, 191
Aspergillus and penicillium
    aflatoxin, 565–566
    citrinin, 567
    ochratoxins, 566–567

Index

Association of American Feed Control Officials (AAFCO), 823
Atherosclerosis research using pigs, 9
Atomic analysis of body composition
    neutron activation, 936–937
    total-body potassium, 936
ATP (adenosine triphosphate), 632–633
Auxiliary variables, 893

B

Babassu palm (*Obrignya martiana*), 851
Bacillus subtilis, 418
Bacteroides spp. in GI tract, 55, 588, 592
Bananas (*Musa* spp.), 842
Barley
    amino acid content, 792–794
    energy content, 788–792
Barrows lean and fat deposition pattern, 718
Basal metabolic rate, 73–74
Beans (*Phaseolus vulgaris*), 573–575, 846, 848–849, 851
Beta-adrenergic agonists
    lipolysis and, 7
    nutritional requirements during use, 441
    performance enhancing substances, 433–435
Betaine, 435
Beta vulgaris (sugar beets), 845
BHA (butylated hydroxy anisole), 98
BHT (butylated hydroxy toluene), 98
BIA (bioelectrical impedance analysis), 929–930
Bifidobacterium in GI tract, 588
Bile
    acids
        biotransformation, 598–599
        digestion and absorption, 55
    salts, 40–42
    secretion *in vivo* study techniques, 979
    secretions, 40–42
Bioavailability of amino acids
    apparent ileal digestibilities determination
        analytical considerations, 162
        difference method, 160
        direct method, 159–160
        marker method, 162–163
        rapid measurement, *161–162*
        regression method, 160–161
        total collection method, 162
    in cereal grains, 792–794
    determination methods, 139–140, 153–154
    digestibility analysis, 152–153
    estimation of, 152
    ileal digestibilities determinations
        definitions, 154–155
        factors involved, 156–158
Bioavailability of minerals
    calcium, 357
    chloride, 360
    copper, 361
    iodine, 361
    iron, 361–363
    magnesium, 360
    manganese, 363
    phosphorus, 359–360
    potassium, 360–361
    selenium, 282–283, 363–364
    sodium, 360
    zinc, 364–365
Bioavailability of vitamins
    bioassay methodology, 365
    biotin, 367–368
    folacin/folic acid, 369
    niacin, 370
    pantothenic acid, 370
    riboflavin, 370–371
    thiamin, 371
    vitamin A, 365–366
    vitamin B_{12}, 372
    vitamin B_6, 371–372
    vitamin C, 372
    vitamin D, 366
    vitamin E, 367
    vitamin K, 367
Bioelectrical impedance analysis (BIA), 929–930
Biotin
    bioavailability, 367–368
    for breeding boars, 780
    deficiency/toxicity symptoms, 320
    history, 317
    metabolism, 318–319
    nutritional requirements, 319
    status and sources, 320
    structure, 318
Bite drinkers, 387
Blood meal as protein supplement, 823–824
Blood sampling
    acute venipuncture
        anterior vena cava, 962–963
        blood vessels, 965
        brachiocephalic vein, 963
        cephalic vein, 964
        ear veins, 964–965
        jugular vein, 964
    chronic catheterization
        abdominal aorta, 967–968
        cephalic vein, 967
        external jugular vein-vena cava, 965–966
        femoral artery/vein, 968
        jugular vein via cut-down, 966–967
        mammary vein, 969
        overview, 965
        portal and ileal vein, 968–969
Boars
    energy intake effects, adults, 775–777
    energy requirements assessment
        growth, 778
        maintenance, 777–778
        reproduction, 778–779
        total requirements, 779
    odor problem, 12
    protein and energy intake effects, developing, 772–773
    protein intake effects, adults, 773–775

reproductive performance characteristics, 771–772
Se and vitamin E deficiency effects, 303
thermal environment and, 778
vitamin and mineral needs
    biotin, 780
    calcium and phosphorus, 779–780
    selenium, 303, 779
    vitamin A, 780
    vitamin E, 779
    zinc, 780
water use, 387
Body composition
    atomic analysis
        neutron activation, 936–937
        total-body potassium, 936
    basis for measurement
        elemental percentage in body, 920
        physical and chemical constants, 920–921
    chemical and physical, 66–68
    dilution methods of analysis
        deuterium oxide, 927–928
        overview, 926
        urea, 928
    elemental percentages, 214
    environmental stresses, 78
    factors influencing, 919
    growth patterns
        curve development and use, 68–69
        curve establishment methods, 71–72
        mathematical functions applications, 70
    image analysis
        background, 937–938
        MRI, 938–942
        ultrasound, 945–946
        video imaging, 946
        X-ray computed axial tomography, 942, 944–945
    measurement techniques
        accuracy need, 918
        ideal method characteristics, 918
    metabolic analysis, 928–929
    mineral chemistry, 214
    nutrient and energy intake, 77–78
    physical and chemical analysis
        modeling, 924–926
        overview, 922–924
    similarity to humans, 7
    subjective analysis methods, 921–922
    techniques comparison table, 947
    tissue interaction analysis
        bioelectrical impedance, 929–930
        near-infrared interactance, 934–935
        nuclear magnetic resonance, 935
        total-body electrical conductivity, 929–932
        X-ray absorptiometry, 932–934
    weight gain and composition determinants
        body protein deposition, 74
        chemical/physical components relationship, 77
        energy intake/PDmax relationship, 74–76
        maintenance energy/nutrient requirements, 73–74
        pig genotype, 72
        voluntary feed intake, 76

Body energy reserves, 523–524
Body fat association with protein, 67
Body protein deposition (PDmax), 74–76, 78
Bones, see Skeletal tissue
Boron (B), 254
Bowl drinkers, 387
Bowman-Birk inhibitors, 573–574
Brachiocephalic vein, 963
Brassica sp. (canola, mustard, rapeseed), 810, 846–847, 851
Breeding facilities, 28
Brunner's glands, 45
Brush border digestion, 48, 49, 52
Butylated hydroxy anisole (BHA), 98
Butylated hydroxy toluene (BHT), 98
Butyric acid, 50
Butyrivibrio in GI tract, 588

C

Ca, see Calcium
Cajanus cajun (pigeon peas), 851
Calcitonin (CT), 188, 195, 203
Calcium (Ca)
    absorption of, 193, 194, 357
    bioavailability, 357
    body composition and compartments, 189–191
    for breeding boars, 779–780
    deficiency symptoms, 197–198
    excretion, 194
    extracellular concentrations, 193
    functions of, 196–197
    for growing-finishing pigs, 720
    homeostatic mechanisms, 192–193
    interdependence with other minerals, 188
    in lactating sow diet, 757
    physical and chemical properties, 192
    regulation, 195
    requirements for, 189, 197
    requirements with metabolic enhancers, 441
    skeletal tissue and, 189, 191–192, 196–197
    skeleton storage and mobilization, 195–196
    sources and availability, 198
    toxicity, 198
    vitamin D and, 203
Calcium phosphate, 192
Calorimetry use, 912
Cancer research using pigs, 9
Cane molasses, 842–843
Cannulation, 56–57, 164–165, 972–974
Canola seed (*Brassica* sp.), 810–812, 846–847
Carbohydrases, 42, 49
Carbohydrates
    digestive system and
        absorption of digestion products, 49
        absorption of VFA, 50–51
        digestion and fermentation, 46–47
        digestion in large intestine, 49–50
        digestion in small intestine, 47–49
        gastric emptying, 47

Index

microbial activity in small intestine, 49
starch oral digestion, 46
neonatal development and, 678–679
preslaughter intake manipulation, 640–641
in weanling pig diet, 698
Carbon-nitrogen balance technique, 911–912
γ-Carboxylation reactions, 206–207
Cardiovascular disease research using pigs, 9
Carnitine, 436, 680
β-Carotene, 267, 366
Carotenoids, *see also* Vitamin A
absorption of, 269–270
bioavailability, 366
storage, transport, interactions, 271–272
Carthamus tictorius (safflower meal), 817–818
Casein diets, 167, 677–678
Cassava (*Manihot esculentis*), 843
Catheterization
abdominal aorta, 967–968
cephalic vein, 967
external jugular vein-vena cava, 965–966
femoral artery/vein, 968
jugular vein via cut-down, 966–967
mammary vein, 969
portal and ileal vein, 968–969
CCK (cholecystokinin), 41, 43, 448
Cecum, 38
Cephalic vein catheterization, 967
Cephalic vein venipuncture, 964
Cereal grains, *see also* Feed
amino acids limitations, 137–138
digestibility analysis, 909–910
energy and nutrient content
amino acid bioavailability, 792–794
antinutritive factors, 796, 798
diversity of, 787
energy-yielding constituents, 788–792
minerals, 794–795
variability in, 796, 797
vitamins, 795–796
genetic modifications to improve
amino acid content, 800
oil concentration, 800–801
overview, 798–799
phosphorus bioavailability, 801
starch form and availability, 799–800
grain production, 785–787
hybrid grain marketing and handling, 801
palatability of, 801
processing, 486–488, 798
production sustainability, 801–802
quality standards, 786
Cerebrovascular arteriosclerosis research using pigs, 9
Ceruloplasmin (Cp), 236
CHD (coronary heart disease), 637
Chicken egg albumen effect on neonatal growth, 678
Chick peas (*Cicer arietinum*), 851
Chloride (Cl), *see also* Chlorine
bioavailability, 360
chemistry, 214
elemental percentage in body, 214

Chlorine (Cl), *see also* Chloride
assay, 219
deficiency symptoms, 218
dietary sources, 218
function of, 217–218
metabolism, 217
requirements for, 218
toxicity, 218
Chlortetracycline, 409
Cholecalciferol, *see* Vitamin D
Cholecystokinin (CCK), 41, 43, 448
Cholesterol
in bile, 40–42
digestion and absorption, 55
Choline
bioavailability, 368–369
deficiency/toxicity symptoms, 322
history, 320
metabolism, 321
nutritional requirements, 321–322
pig vs. human need for, 8
status and sources, 322
structure, 321
Chromic oxide, 163, 907–909
Chromium (Cr)
function and uses, 233–234
as a growth enhancer, 435
in lactating sow diet, 757–758
muscle conversion and, 647, 654
pig vs. human need for, 8
Chylomicrons, 291
Chymosin, 37, 51
Chymotrypsin, 42, 573–574
Cicer arietinum (chick peas), 851
Cimaterol, 433, 434
Citrinin, 567
Citrus pulp, 843
Cl, *see* Chloride; Chlorine
CLA, *see* Conjugated linoleic acid
Clays (phyllosilicates), 572
Clenbuterol, 433, 434
Clostridium in GI tract, 588
Cobalt (Co), 234
Coconut meal (*Cocos nucifera*), 812–813
Cocoyams (*Colocasia esculenta*), 843
Colostrum
biomedical research using pigs, 9
composition, 747
neonatal development and, 294, 674, 679
thermal environment effects on, 524
Comparative slaughter technique, 911
Competitive exclusion strategy, 590
Completely randomized (CR) design, 887
Complex IV, 654
Computerized tomography (CT), 944–945
Conditionally essential amino acids, 133–134
Confounding in statistics, 885
Conjugated linoleic acid (CLA)
described, 96, 436
dietary factors in muscle conversion and, 644–645
PPAR and, 664–665

Consumers, *see also* Human diet
    interest in nutrition, 12
    preference for lean pork, 24
Copper (Cu)
    absorption, 235
    bioavailability, 361
    deficiency symptoms
        blood, 239–240
        growth, 239–240
        reproduction, 240–241
        tissue function, 240
    in excretion, 616
    functions
        amine/diamine oxidases, 236–237
        ceruloplasmin, 236
        cytochrome *c* oxidase, 237–238
        growth stimulants, 238–239
        immunity, 238
        superoxide dismutase, 237
        tyrosinase, 238
    as a growth enhancer, 435
    growth rate response to, 407–408
    immune function and, 555
    muscle conversion and, 654
    toxicity, 241
    transport systems, 235–236
    in weanling pig diet, 701, 703
Corn, *see also* Cereal grains
    amino acid content, 792–794
    energy content, 788–792
Coronary heart disease (CHD), 637
Cottonseed meal (*Gossypium* spp.), 813–815
Covariates, 893
Cow peas (*Vigna sinensis*), 851
Crambe seed (*Crambe abyssinica*), 851
Crates for pigs, 26
C-reactive protein (CRP), 549
Creatine phosphate (CP), 632
Creatinine excretion analysis, 928–929
Cu, *see* Copper
Cull eggs as alternative protein feedstuff, 847
Cystines, 134
Cytochrome *c* oxidase, 237–238
Cytoplasmic peptidases, 52

D

Dark, firm, and dry (DFD) pork, 637–638, 639, 641
DE, *see* Digestible energy
Denaturing gradient gel electrophoresis (DGGE), 601
Dent corn, 796; *see also* Cereal grains
Deoxynivalenol (DON), 563, 564, 568–569
Deoxyribonucleic acid (DNA), 659
Detergent methods of fiber analysis, 108–109
Deuterium oxide use in body composition analysis, 927–928
DFD (dark, firm, and dry) pork, 637–638, 639, 641
Diabetes research using pigs, 9
Diacetoxyscirpenol (DAS), 569
Diarrhea and neonatal development, 680–681

Diet, *see* Feed intake
Dietary electrolyte balance (DEB), 216
Dietary fat
    biological effects, 100–101
    ileal AA digestibilities influenced by, 172
    for lactating sows, 758–759
    lipid metabolism pathways, 101
    performance affected by, 101–103
    physical and chemical properties, 95–97
    quality of, 98
    specific uses of fat, 99–100
    vitamin E absorption and, 289–290
Dietary fiber
    feed content and energy utilization, 90
    feeding management, 122–123
    ileal AA digestibilities influenced by, 173–174
    in lactating sow diet, 755–757
    nonstarch polysaccharides
        ambient temperature interactions, 116–117
        ammonia emission and, 123–124
        antibiotics interactions, 117
        concentrations in feed, 109–110, 111
        described, 108
        dietary nutrient metabolism affected by, 114–115
        digestion of, 110, 112–114
        feeding considerations, 122–123
        growth performance and body composition effects, 115–116
        health affected by, 117
        quantifying, 108–109
        sows affected by, 118–122
    oligosaccharides
        benefits of, 419, 420
        concentrations in feed, 109–110, 111
        described, 108
        dietary nutrient metabolism affected by, 114–115
        digestion of, 110, 112–114
        growth performance and body composition effects, 115–116
        health affected by, 117
        quantifying, 109
Dietary undetermined anion (dUA), 216
Digestible energy (DE)
    in cereal grains, 788–792
    content determination procedures, 909
    definition, 86
    energy retention/heat production measurement, 910–912
    feedstuffs, 909–910
Digestion and balance techniques
    energy digestibility
        content determination procedures, 909
        energy retention/heat production measurement, 910–912
        feedstuffs, 909–910
    methodology
        comparison of methods, 907–909
        direct and difference approaches, 906–907
        general considerations, 904
        index method, 906
        quantitative collection method, 904–905

Index

nitrogen digestibility
    apparent, 912–913
    endogenous loss estimation, 913–915
Digestive system
  amino acids and
    antibiotics, 176
    dietary fat, 172
    dry matter intake, 169–170
    fiber in diet, 173–174
    ingredient and feed processing, 170–171
    lectins, 175
    organic acids, 176–177
    phytates, 174
    protein level in diet, 171–172
    tannins, 175–176
    trypsin inhibitors, 174–175
  anatomy and histology
    diagram of, 33
    large intestine, 38
    liver, 34, 35
    mouth and salivary glands, 32
    pancreas, 34, 36
    pharynx and esophagus, 34
    small intestine, 36–38
    stomach, 34
  antibody absorption, 56
  carbohydrates and
    absorption of digestion products, 49
    absorption of VFA, 50–51
    digestion and fermentation, 46–47
    digestion in large intestine, 49–50
    digestion in small intestine, 47–49
    gastric emptying, 47
    microbial activity in small intestine, 49
    starch oral digestion, 46
  fat digestion and absorption
    gastric digestion, 54
    in large intestine, 55
    in small intestine, 54–55
  intestinal bacteria and, *see* Intestinal bacteria
  neonatal development and enzymes
    enzyme system overview, 675
    intestinal enzymes, 676
    pancreatic enzymes, 675–676
  nonstarch polysaccharides and
    degradation products, 110
    energy value of VFA, 113–114
    fermentation, 112–113
    gastric emptying, 112
    gastrointestinal tract affected by, 112
  nutrient digestion and absorption measurements, 56–57
  protein digestion and absorption
    absorption of products, 53–54
    gastric digestion, 51–52
    in large intestine, 52–53
    in small intestine, 52
  secretions
    bile, 40–42
    gastric, 37–40
    pancreatic exocrine, 42–45
    salivary, 38–37
    small intestine, 45–46
  similarity to humans, 6–7
  water and electrolyte absorption, 55–56
Dilution methods of body composition analysis
  deuterium oxide, 927–928
  overview, 926
  urea, 928
Dioscorea sp. (yams), 846
Direct-fed microbials, *see* Promicrobial agents
Diurnal patterns and eating behavior, 500–501
DNA (deoxyribonucleic acid), 659
DON (deoxynivalenol), 563, 564, 568–569
Dopamine β-hydroxylase, 237
DPA (dual-energy photon absorptiometry), 932–934
Dried skim milk effect on neonatal growth, 677
Drinker design/location and feed intake
  extraneous voltage, 509–510
  medication dosage estimations and, 509
  nipple drinker use, 387, 508, 680
  spacing recommendation, 508
Dry matter intake and ileal AA digestibilities, 169–170; *see also* Feed intake
Dual-energy photon absorptiometry (DPA), 932–934
Dual-energy X-ray absorptiometry (DXA), 932–934
Duroc pigs, 67

E

EAA (essential amino acids), 133; *see also* Amino acids
Ear veins venipuncture, 964–965
Eating behavior
  characteristics of
    diurnal patterns, 500–501
    eating speed and duration, 501
    feed restriction, 501–502
    meal frequency, 500
    post-weaning, 502
  drinker design/location and feed intake
    extraneous voltage, 509–510
    medication dosage estimations and, 509
    nipple drinker use, 387, 508, 680
    spacing recommendation, 508
  feeder design and feed intake
    feed wastage, 504–505
    number of feeding spaces, 502–503
    quality of feeding spaces, 503–504
    social facilitation, 506–507
    wet and wet/dry feeders, 505–506, 719–720
  space allocation and group size
    diet and space interaction, 513–514
    pigs per social group, 512–513
    prediction equations, 510–511
    recommendations, 510
    stocking density, 510
Economics
  antimicrobial agents use, 402, 417
  costs of P and Ca in feed, 189
  feed costs, 85
  feeding program considerations, 759
  feed wastage cost, 620–<u>621</u>

profitability of pork production, 5
value of swine industry, 23
Eicosanoids, 99
Elaeis guineenis (palm kernel), 851
Embryo survival, 733
Endogenous amino acid losses, 166–169
Energy
   digestibility analysis
      content determination procedures, 909
      energy retention/heat production measurement, 910–912
      feedstuffs, 842–846, 909–910
   digestible
      in cereal grains, 788–792
      content determination procedures, 909
      definition, 86
      energy retention/heat production measurement, 910–912
      feedstuffs, 909–910
   gross, 85–86
   metabolizable
      in cereal grains, 787, 788–792
      definition, 86
      required for maintenance, 91
   net
      amino acids and, 140
      definition, 86
      evaluation of feed ingredients, 87–88
   nutrient requirements and
      activity and, 73–74
      intake effects, 77–78
   requirement modeling for lactation, 752–754
   retained, 87–88
   utilization
      efficiency of, 88–89
      energy requirements, 91–92
      evaluation of feed ingredients, 87–88
      factors affecting, 90–91
      from feed, 86
      nutrient-to-energy ratios, 89
      TDN system, 85
Englyst and Cummings procedure, 109
Enterocytes, neonatal, 56
Environmental pollution and odor control
   ammonia emission and, 123–124
   manure management, 610–611
   modern production facilities, 609–610
   nutrition and feeding strategies
      diet formulation, 614
      excess nutrients reduction, 614–616
      feed intake and efficiency enhancement, 617–619
      feed waste reduction, 620–621
      genetically modified feedstuff use, 619
      knowledge of nutrient requirements, 614
      phase feeding, 619–620
      principle of diminishing returns, 621–622
      protein reduction/amino acid supplementation, 616–617
      split-sex feeding, 620
   odor reduction strategies
      diet manipulation, 624
      manure components, 622–623, 624
      microbes manipulation, 624–625
      nitrogen level reduction, 623–624
   percent of consumed nutrients used, 611, 613
   pork industry and, 14–15
   summary of nutritional means, 625–626
Environmental stresses on body composition, 78
Enzootic ataxia, 240
Enzymatic-gravimetric method, 109
Enzymes, digestive
   in neonatal development, 675–676
   supplements in weanling pig diet, 703–704
Epinephrine, 433, 633–634
Error control in statistics, 886
Escherichia in GI tract, 588
Essential amino acids (EAA), 133; *see also* Amino acids
Estrogen, 237
Ethoxyquin, 98
Eubacterium in GI tract, 587
Eutrophication and phosphorus in animal manure, 10
Exocrine pancreatic components, 34, 36
Exogenous nutrients, 524
Experimental error in statistics, 884
Experimental unit in statistics, 884
External jugular vein-vena cava catheterization, 965–966
Extrusion of feed
   cereals and complete diets, 486–488
   soybeans, 488–490, 491

F

Faba beans (*Vicia faba*), 847
Farrowing facilities
   pigs produced per litter, 26–27
   types, 25–26
Fast-twitch MHC isoforms, 635
Fat
   association with protein, 67
   content in newborn pigs, 7
   content in pork, 12, 636–637
   dietary
      biological effects, 100–101
      ileal AA digestibilities influenced by, 172
      for lactating sows, 758–759
      lipid metabolism pathways, 101
      performance affected by, 101–103
      physical and chemical properties, 95–97
      quality of, 98
      specific uses of fat, 99–100
      vitamin E absorption and, 289–290
   digestibility analysis, 909–910
   digestion and absorption
      gastric digestion, 54
      in large intestine, 55
      in small intestine, 54–55
   muscle conversion to meat and
      CLA and, 644–645
      process of, 642–644
   neonatal development and, 679–680
   percent composition of pigs, 24, 66

Index

in weanling pig diet, 698–699
Fatty acids
    dietary fat quality and, 98
    dietary requirements for, 99
    function and uses, 95–97
    from luminal lipid digestion, 55
    profile alteration, 99
Fatty acid synthase, 662
Feather meal as protein supplement, 824–825
Feed, *see also* Cereal grains
    additives in weanling pig diet, 702–704
    alternative, *see* Alternative feedstuffs
    amino acids limitations
        cereal grains, 137–138
        complete diets, 139
        protein supplements, 138–139
    bioavailability of amino acids, *see* Bioavailability of amino acids
    bioavailability of mineral, *see* Bioavailability of minerals
    bioavailability of vitamins, *see* Bioavailability of vitamins
    energy evaluation of ingredients, 87–88
    energy utilization by pigs, 86
    intake
        dry matter and body weight, 169–170
        eating behavior, *see* Eating behavior
        in lactating sows, 743–744
        nutrient and energy intake, 77–78
        relationship to growth rate, 115–116
        thermal environment effects, 454–456, 527–529
        voluntary, 76
    possible contaminants, 470
    processing, *see* Feed manufacturing processes
    supplements, *see* Protein supplements
Feeder design and feed intake
    feed wastage, 504–505
    number of feeding spaces, 502–503
    quality of feeding spaces, 503–504
    social facilitation, 506–507
    wet and wet/dry feeders, 505–506
Feed intake
    drinker design/location and
        extraneous voltage, 509–510
        medication dosage estimations and, 509
        nipple drinker use, 387, 508, 680
        spacing recommendation, 508
    feeder design and
        feed wastage, 504–505
        number of feeding spaces, 502–503
        quality of feeding spaces, 503–504
        social facilitation, 506–507
        wet and wet/dry feeders, 505–506, 719–720
    gestating sows
        feeding program considerations, 759–760
        feeding program objectives, 735
        feeding strategies, 736–738
        feeding systems, 735
    growing-finishing pigs, *see* Feed intake in growing-finishing pigs
    lactating sows
        feed and diet composition, 754–757
        feeding program considerations, 759–760
        feeding program objectives, 742
        feeding strategies, 743–744
    neonatal pigs
        artificial rearing, 672–673, 681–682
        carbohydrate sources and use, 678–679
        diarrhea and nutrition, 680–681
        digestive enzyme system, 675–676
        environmental requirements, 673–674
        fat sources and use, 679–680
        liquid diets for SEW, 681
        management, 680
        nutrient requirements, 674
        passive immunity, 674
        performance after artificial rearing, 681–682
        protein sources and use, 677–678
        selenium and, 297–298
        weaning strategies, 671–672
    photoperiod and, 456
    thermal environment influence on, 454–456
    voluntary, 76
    weanling pigs
        energy sources, 697–699
        feed additives, 702–704
        minerals, 694, 701–702
        protein sources, 699–701
        vitamins, 702
Feed intake in growing-finishing pigs
    animal factors influencing
        breed differences, 451–452
        growth stage, 454
        selection strategies in research, 452–453
        sex differences, 453–454
    environmental factors influencing
        climatic, 454–456
        disease, 457
        living conditions, 457
        photoperiod, 456
        temperature, 529–531
    feeding behavior
        day-to-day variation, 461
        diurnal pattern, 460–461
        feeder design and, 461–462
        studies on, 458–460
    measuring and predicting, 462–463
    nutritional factors influencing
        energy level of diet, 448–450
        vitamin/mineral content of diet, 450
    physiological control, 447–448
Feed manufacturing processes
    extrusion
        cereals and complete diets, 486–488
        soybeans, 488–490, 491
    grinding feedstuffs
        efficiency of gain studies, 471–472
        nutrient digestibility and, 470–471, 472–474
        production rates and, 471
    ileal AA digestibilities influenced by, 170–171
    mill type, 474–476
    mixers, 476–479

pelleting
    binders, 485–486
    feed efficiency and, 721
    mill conditioners, 483–485
    pellet quality, 483
    pellet size, 481–483
    process and benefits, 480–481
    for weanling pig diet, 706
    procurement quality control, 470
    stomach morphology considerations, 490, 492
Feed wastage
    costs of, 620–621
    feeder design and, 504–505
    management considerations, 719–720
Femoral artery/vein catheterization, 968
Fermentation of carbohydrates in stomach, 46–47
Ferritin, 244
Fiber in diet, see Dietary fiber
Fibrobacter succinogenes, 112
Fish meal/silage
    as alternative protein feedstuff, 847–848
    effect on neonatal growth, 678
    as protein supplement, 825–826
    weanling pig diet source, 700
Flax (*Linum usitatissimum*), 815–816
Floor area recommendations for pigs, 29
Flushing, 733
Folacin bioavailability, 369
Folate
    bioavailability, 369
    deficiency/toxicity symptoms, 325
    history, 323
    metabolism, 323–324
    nutritional requirements, 324–325
    status and sources, 325
    structure, 323
Follicle-stimulating hormone (FSH), 733
Food and Drug Administration, U.S., 11
Forage grasses
    as alternative feedstuffs, 851
    vitamin E content of, 286
Fructo-oligosaccharides (FOS), 108, 419, 420
Fructose, 49
FSH (follicle-stimulating hormone), 733
Fusarium toxins
    fumonisins, 563, 564, 570–571
    occurrence of, 567–568
    trichothecenes, 568–569
    zearalenone, 563, 564, 569–570
Fusobacterium in GI tract, 587

G

α-Galacto-oligosaccharides (GOS), 108
Galactose, 49
Gamma irradiation, 14
Gastricsin, 37
Gastric system, see Stomach
Gastric ulcers research using pigs, 9
Gastrin, 675

Gastrointestinal system
    intestinal bacteria and, see Intestinal bacteria
    NSPs and, 112
    similarity to humans, 6–7
GE (gross energy), 85–86
Gene expression and nutrition
    carbohydrate example, 662
    lipid example, 663
    mineral example, 661–662
    overview, 659
    post-translational protein modification, 661
    transcription, 659–661
    translation, 661
General Agreements on Trade and Tariffs (GATT), 24
General Linear Models (GLM) program, 895
Genetic engineering
    clinical applications of pig-derived knowledge, 10
    genetically modified plants, 798–799
    recombinant DNA-derived products, 11
Gestating sows
    efficiency of energy utilization, 89
    energy requirements, 92
    estimated nutrient requirements, 742
    facilities for, 29
    feeding program considerations, 759–760
    feeding program objectives, 735
    feeding strategies
        constant level, 736
        interval feeding, 737–738
        metabolic disorders, 738
        phase feeding, 736–737
    feeding systems, 735
    mammary development, 738–739
    modeling of nutrient requirements
        fetal growth, 740
        maintenance levels determination, 739–740
        maternal weight gain, 740–742
        usefulness of approach, 739
    thermal environment effects on, 534
    water use, 386–387
Gilts
    feeding program objectives, 726
    lean and fat deposition pattern, 718
    nutrition and longevity
        feeding recommendations, 729–730
        lean and fat accretion, 727
        locomotor problems, 728–729
        practical considerations, 733–734
        pre- and postmating, 733
        puberty occurrence, 730–733
        reproductive performance factors, 727–728
Glands
    mammary
        development, 738–739
        gland nutrient uptake, 749–750
    mouth and salivary, 32, 38–37
    stomach, 34
    study techniques, 975–976
GLM (general Linear Models) program, 895
β-Glucan, 800
Glucose, 49, 114

Index

Glucose transporter (GLUT4), 663
Glucosinolates, 577
GLUT4 (glucose transporter), 663
Glutamine, 135, 551–552
Glycine max (soybeans), 819–821
Glycogen stores, 523–524, 632
Glycolysis, 632
Goblet cells, 45
Gossypium spp. (cottonseed meal), 813–815
Gravimetric analysis, 108–109
Grinding of feedstuffs
    efficiency of gain studies, 471–472
    nutrient digestibility and, 470–471, 472–474
    production rates and, 471
Gross energy (GE), 85–86
Growing-finishing pigs
    facilities for, 27–28
    feeding management considerations
        antibiotics use, 720–721
        budgeting methods, 721
        calcium and phosphorus, 720
        feed wastage, 719–720
        processing and pelleting, 721
        specialty grains, 720
    feed intake, *see* Feed intake in growing-finishing pigs
    nutrient requirements factors
        environmental temperature and, 719
        genetics, 717–718
        herd health, 719
        selenium and, 299–300
        sex, 718
        stage of maturity, 718–719
    thermal environment effects on
        carcass composition, 532–533
        feed intake, 529–531
        growth rate and feed efficiency, 531–532
    water use, 385
Growth
    efficiency of energy utilization, 88–89
    energy requirements, 91–92
    enhancers, *see* Performance-enhancing substances
    NSPs and, 115–116
    patterns
        curve development and use, 68–69
        curve establishment methods, 71–72
        mathematical functions applications, 70
    selenium effect on, 299–300
GSH-Px, 292–293
Guizotia abyssinica (niger seed), 851

H

HA (homoarginine method), 168–169
Hammermills, 472–474
Hand mating, 28
Haptoglobin, 549
Heat increment (HI), 86
Heat of combustion, 85–86
Helianthus annus (sunflower seeds), 821–823, 850–851
Hemagglutinins, 574

Hepatic lobule, 34
Hevea brasiliensis (rubber seed), 851
HI (heat increment), 86
High-oil corn for growing-finishing pigs, 720;
    see also Cereal grains
Histidine, 134, 138
Homoarginine method (HA), 168–169
Horizontal mixers, 476, 478
Human diet
    nutrient requirements of pig vs. humans, 7–8
    nutrition research using pigs, 9
    pork in
        acceptability, 12–14
        composition, 12, 13
        consumption worldwide, 5–6
        nutritional quality, 11–12, 636–637
        profitability of production, 5
        quality relation to Se and vitamin E, 300
        societal issues, 14–15
Hungate's Principles, 587
Huts for pigs, 26
Hydroxyapatite, 191
Hypertension research using pigs, 9
Hypocalcemia, 757

I

IgA, 593–594, 747
IGF-I (insulin-like growth factor I)
    biomedical research using pigs, 9
    porcine somatotropin and, 431
IgG, 747
IgM, 747
Ileal amino acid digestibilities
    antibiotics influence on, 176
    collection of digesta, 163–166
    determination considerations
        definitions, 154–155
        factors involved, 156–158
    determination of apparent
        analytical considerations, 162
        difference method, 160
        direct method, 159–160
        marker method, 162–163
        rapid measurement, 161–162
        regression method, 160–161
        total collection method, 162
    digestibility values, 56–57
    of grains, 792–794
    true
        definition and significance, 166
        endogenous losses measurement, 166–169
    trypsin inhibitors and, 574
Ileo-rectal anastomosis (IRA), 164–165
Image analysis for body composition
    background, 937–938
    MRI, 938–942
    ultrasound, 945–946
    video imaging, 946
    X-ray computed axial tomography, 942, 944–945

Immune exclusion, 594
Immune function and nutrition
   colostrum's importance to survival, 674
   cytokines
      impact on nitrogen metabolism, 548–549
      metabolism altered by, 547–548
   interaction applications, 557
   intestinal bacteria benefits
      epithelium, 592
      hosts defense stimulation, 590–591
      lamina propria, 592–593
      mucus layer, 591–592
      physiological characteristics, 591
      secretory IgA, 593–594
      T lymphocytes, 593
   nutrient requirements
      amino acids, 551–553
      copper, 555
      deficiency effects, 550–551
      iron, 555
      lipids, 553–554
      selenium, 556
      vitamin A, 556–557
      vitamin E, 556
      zinc, 554–555
   performance enhancing substances and, 436, 438
   porcine immunology concepts, 546–547
   relationship between, 545
Immunity, 238, 547
Indoles, 597–598
Ingredient and feed processing, see Feed manufacturing processes
Innate immunity, 547
Inositol acid, 8
Insulin-like growth factor I (IGF-I)
   biomedical research using pigs, 9
   porcine somatotropin and, 431
Interaction in statistics, 885
Intestinal bacteria
   autochthonous vs. allochthonous, 587
   colonization resistance benefits, 589–590
   competitive/negative effects
      amino acid catabolites, 596–598
      bile acid biotransformation, 598–599
      cost–benefit analysis, 595–596
      mucin degradation, 599–600
   GI tract characteristics, 586
   growth efficiency and, 586
   immune system benefits
      epithelium, 592
      hosts defense stimulation, 590–591
      lamina propria, 592–593
      mucus layer, 591–592
      physiological characteristics, 591
      secretory IgA, 593–594
      T lymphocytes, 593
   location in digestive system, 588–589
   major bacterial groups, 587–588
   management practices influence, 602
   molecular ecology
      described, 600
      DGGE approach, 601
      probe use, 601–602
      sequency analysis, 600
   nutritional contributions, 594–595
   protective features, 602
Iodine (I)
   bioavailability, 361
   function and uses, 241–242
Ipomoea batatas (sweet potatoes), 845
Iron (Fe)
   absorption, 242–243
   bioavailability, 361–363
   classifications, 242
   deficiency symptoms, 245
   functions, 244
   as a growth enhancer, 435
   immune function and, 555
   interrelationships, 243
   requirements, 244
   storage, 244
   toxicity, 245, 298
   transport, 243–244
Islets of Langerhans, 36
Isoleucine, 139
Isoproterenol, 433

J

Jugular vein venipuncture, 964
Jugular vein via cut-down catheterization, 966–967

K

Kidneys and water excretion, 382
KOH test, 161
Kunitz protease inhibitors, 573–574
Kwashiorkor/marasmus research using pigs, 9

L

Lactating sows
   amino acids requirement modeling, 750–752, 753, 755
   body weight
      composition of, 745
      net fat loss considerations, 744
      nutrient and reproduction interaction, 745–746
   dietary fat, 758–759
   efficiency of energy utilization, 89
   energy requirement modeling, 752–754
   energy requirements, 92, 121
   feed and diet composition
      dietary fiber use, 755–757
      feed ingredients, 754–755
   feeding program considerations, 759–760
   feeding program objectives, 742
   feeding strategies
      feed intake factors, 743
      feed intake maximization, 744
      postfarrow appetite depression, 743

Index

metabolism simulation model, 873–875
milk production
    mammary development, 738–739
    mammary gland nutrient uptake, 749–750
    nutrient composition, 746–748
mineral nutrition
    calcium and magnesium, 757
    calcium and phosphorus, 757
    chromium, 757–758
    selenium, 758
    vitamin E, 758
porcine somatotropin effects, 432–433
Se and vitamin E deficiency and, 301–302
thermal environment effects on, 534–535
Lactic acid
    in muscle, 632
    production of, 46
Lactobacillus acidophilus, 404, 417
Lactobacillus in GI tract, 587, 676
Lactoferrin, 243
Lactose
    hydrolysis of, 48
    in weanling pig diet, 697–698
Lameness in gilts, 728
Lamina propria, 592–593
Landrace pigs, 67
Large intestine
    anatomy and histology, 38
    digestion and fermentation of carbohydrates, 49–50
    fat digestion and absorption in, 55
    intestinal bacteria in, 588
    protein digestion and absorption in, 52–53
    water and electrolyte absorption in, 56
Latin square (LS) design, 888
LCT (lower critical temperature), 520, 537–538
Lean tissue growth curves, 69
Least Significant Difference, 897
Lectins
    antinutritional factors, 574–575
    ileal AA digestibilities influenced by, 175
Legumes in diet, 851
Lentils (*Lens culinaris*), 848
Leptin, 436, 448
Leukocytes and immune function, 546–547
Leukopenia, 239
LH (luteinizing hormone), 733
Libido, 771–772
Light:dark sequences and eating behavior, 500–501
Lignin, 108
Lima beans (*Phaseolus lunatus*), 851
Limit feeding, 428–429
Linoleic acid, 99
Linseed meal (*Linum usitatissimum*), 815–816
Linseed oil, 99–100
Lipases, 42
Lipids
    digestion and absorption, 55
    metabolism of
        fat digestion and, 55
        immune function and, 553–554
        pathways, 101
        in pigs vs. humans, 7
        NSPs effect on metabolism of, 114
        percent composition of pigs, 66
        peroxisome proliferator-activated receptors
            overview, 663
            regulation of differentiation, 663
            role in nutritional regulation, 663–665
Lipogenesis, 101
Liquid whey as alternative feedstuffs, 851
Litters
    average annual, 26–27
    lysine and size, 745–746
    Se and vitamin E deficiency effects on size, 301
Liver
    anatomy and histology, 34, 35
    bile secretions, 40–42
    glycogen stores in, 632
    vitamin A uptake and storage, 270–271
Locomotor problems of gilts, 728–729
Lower critical temperature (LCT), 520, 537–538
Low phytic acid corn (LPA), 619
LS (Latin square) design, 888
Luminal digestion, 47–48, 52
Lupins (*Lupinus albus*), 848
Luteinizing hormone (LH), 733
Lymphocytes and immune function, 546–547
Lysine, *see also* Amino acids
    animal use of isomers, 141
    bioavailability determination, 153–154
    dietary requirements, 77
    immune function and, 553
    lactating sows requirement, 750–752, <u>753</u>
    limitations in feeds, 138
    litter size and, 745–746
    need during lactation, 739
    nitrogen excretion and, 616–617
    weanling pig requirements, 693–694
Lysyl oxidase, 237, 240

M

Magnesium (Mg)
    bioavailability, 360
    chemistry, 214
    elemental percentage in body, 214
    function and uses, 219–220
    in lactating sow diet, 757
    muscle conversion and, 647, 653
Magnetic resonance imaging (MRI), 938–942
Major histocompatibility complex (MHC), 592
Maltose, 48
Maltotriose, 48
Mammary glands
    development, 738–739
    gland nutrient uptake, 749–750
Mammary vein catheterization, 969
Mandibular glands, 32
Manganese (Mn)
    bioavailability, 363
    function and uses, 245–247

Manihot esculentis (cassava), 843
Mannan-oligosaccrides (MOS), 419
Marker method, ileal digestibility, 162–163
Mastitis, metritis, and agalactia (MMA), 302–303
Maternal weight gain, 740–742
Mating options, 28
*m*ATPase (myofibrillar actomyosin adenosine triphosphatase), 632, 634
MCT (medium-chain triglycerides), 523
ME, *see* Metabolizable energy
Meat and bone meal protein supplements, 826–828
Medicago sp. (alfalfa), 110, 809–810
Medication dosage estimations for drinkers, 509
Medium-chain triglycerides (MCT), 523
Menadione, 204
Menaquinones, 204–206
Messenger ribonucleic acid (mRNA), 659
Metabolic modifiers, *see* Performance enhancing substances
Metabolizable energy (ME)
    in cereal grains, 787, 788–792
    definition, 86
    required for maintenance, 91
Metallothionein, 252–253, 661–662
Methanogenesis, 49
Methionine
    absorption of, 289
    animal use of isomers, 141
    essentiality of, 134, 138, 139
    immune function and, 551
Mg, *see* Magnesium
MHC (major histocompatibility complex), 592
MHC (myosin heavy-chain isoforms), 635
Microbial supplements in weanling pig diet, 703
Migrating myoelectric complex (MMC), 47
Milk
    dried, as protein supplement, 828
    importance to neonatal pigs, 674, 679
    production
        mammary development, 738–739
        mammary gland nutrient uptake, 749–750
        nutrient composition, 746–748
    proteins effect on neonatal growth, 677
    proteins in weanling pig diet, 700
    from sows
        digestibility of fat in, 100
        neonatal development and, 679
Mills, 474–476
Minerals, *see also* specific minerals
    absorption efficiency
        calcium, 357
        chloride, 360
        copper, 361
        iodine, 361
        iron, 363
        magnesium, 360
        manganese, 363
        phosphorus, 359
        potassium, 360–361
        selenium, 363–364
        sodium, 360
        zinc, 364–365
    bioavailability
        calcium, 357
        chloride, 360
        copper, 361
        iodine, 361
        iron, 361–363
        magnesium, 360
        manganese, 363
        phosphorus, 359–360
        potassium, 360–361
        selenium, 363–364
        sodium, 360
        zinc, 364–365
    in cereal grains, 794–795
    chemistry, 215
    chlorine
        assay, 219
        deficiency symptoms, 218
        dietary sources, 218
        function of, 217–218
        metabolism, 217
        requirements for, 218
        toxicity, 218
    elemental percentages in body, 214
    general functions
        acid-base homeostatsis, 216
        mineral-enzyme relationships, 217
        nutrients and, 216–217
        signal transduction, 217
        water homeostatsis, 215–216
    magnesium, 219–220, 360
    muscle conversion and, 645
    NSPs effect on metabolism of, 115
    potassium, 220–222
    sodium, 222–224
    sulfur, 224–225
    weanling pig requirements, 694, 701–702
Mixers, 476–479
MMA (mastitis, metritis, and agalactia), 302–303
MMC (migrating myoelectric complex), 47
Mobile nylon bag technique (MNBT), 154–155, 161
Modeling of swine, *see also* Statistical techniques
    advantages, 877
    barriers to, 877
    block diagram basis, 868
    body composition, 924–926
    classifications and definitions, 868–870
    reasons to use, 867–868
    specific application models
        approaches, 870–872
        energy/amino acid use simulation, 872–873
        lactating sow metabolism, 873–875
        production systems, 875–877
    uses for, 877–878
Molybdenum (Mo), 253
Monoglycerides digestion, 55
Mortality, neonatal, 672
MOS (mannan-oligosaccrides), 419
Mouth and salivary glands
    anatomy and histology, 32

Index

secretions, 38–37
MRI (magnetic resonance imaging), 938–942
mRNA (messenger ribonucleic acid), 659
Mucosal digestion
  described, 48–49, 52
  lactase activities, 676
  mucus layer
    bacterially mediated degradation, 599–600
    functions, 34, 40
    intestinal bacteria and, 591–592
Mung beans (*Phaseolus* spp.), 848–849
Musa spp. (bananas), 842
Muscle conversion to meat
  biochemical factors, 632–633
  dietary factors
    chromium, 647, 654
    copper, 654
    magnesium, 647, 653
    source and profile of fat, 642–645
    vitamin D, 645–646
    vitamin E, 646–647, 648–652
    vitamins and minerals, 645
  feeding strategies for quality
    preslaughter carbohydrate intake manipulation, 640–641
    preslaughter feed restriction, 640
    preslaughter feed withdrawal, 639–640
    preslaughter protein/amino acid manipulation, 641–642
  molecular factors, 633
  percent composition of muscles in pigs, 66
  physiological factors
    muscles, 634–635
    stress, 633–634
  post-mortem conditioning effects, 637
  structural factors
    fat, 636–637
    protein, 635–636
    protein-water interactions, 636
Mustard seed (*Brassica hitra*), 851
Mycotoxins, *see also* Antinutritional factors
  aspergillus and penicillium
    aflatoxin, 565–566
    citrinin, 567
    ochratoxins, 566–567
  control strategies, 572
  description and impact, 563–564
  fusarium toxins
    fumonisins, 563, 564, 570–571
    occurrence of, 567–568
    trichothecenes, 568–569
    zearalenone, 563, 564, 569–570
  interactions, 571
Myeloperoxidase, 244
Myofibrillar actomyosin adenosine triphosphatase (*m*ATPase), 632, 634
Myosin, 634
Myosin heavy-chain isoforms (MHC), 635

N

NAFTA (North American Free Trade Association), 24
NDF (neutral detergent fiber), 108, 800
NE, *see* Net energy
NEAA (nonessential amino acids), 133
Near-infrared interactance (NIR), 934–935
Neonatal pigs
  biomedical research using, 9
  calcium recovered from, 189
  colostrum's importance to survival, 294, 674, 679
  enterocytes and antibody absorption, 56
  feeding
    artificial rearing, 672–673, 681–682
    carbohydrate sources and use, 678–679
    diarrhea and nutrition, 680–681
    digestive enzyme system, 675–676
    environmental requirements, 673–674
    fat sources and use, 679–680
    liquid diets for SEWs, 681
    management, 680
    nutrient requirements, 674
    passive immunity, 674
    performance after artificial rearing, 681–682
    protein sources and use, 677–678
    selenium and, 297–298
    weaning strategies, 671–672
  nursery facilities, 27
  thermal environment effects on
    cold stress role, 526
    energy provision, 523–525
    heat production mechanisms, 523
    microenvironment provision, 525–526
    neonatal mortality, 522
    newborn susceptibility to cold, 522–523
    suckling period remainder, 526–527
Net energy (NE)
  amino acids and, 140
  definition, 86
  evaluation of feed ingredients, 87–88
Neutral detergent fiber (NDF), 108, 800
Neutron activation (NA) analysis, 936–937
Newborn pigs, *see* Neonatal pigs
Niacin
  bioavailability, 370
  deficiency/toxicity symptoms, 327
  history, 325–326
  metabolism, 326–327
  nutritional requirements, 327
  status and sources, 327–328
  structure, 326
Nickel (Ni), 253
Niger seed (*Guizotia abyssinica*), 851
Nipple drinkers, 387, 508, 680
NIR (near-infrared interactance), 934–935
Nitrates in water, 393
Nitric oxide and immune function, 551
Nitrogen (N)
  amino acid digestibility and NSP, 115
  digestibility analysis
    apparent, 912–913

endogenous loss estimation, 913–915
excretion and amino acids, 616–617
high-fiber diets and excretion of, 123–124
manure management and, 611
protein content calculated from, 132
protein digestion and, 53
reduction for odor management, 623–624
NMR (nuclear magnetic resonance), 935
Nonessential amino acids (NEAA), 133
Nonprotein nitrogen (NPN), 132–133
Nonstarch polysaccharides (NSP)
    ambient temperature interactions, 116–117
    ammonia emission and, 123–124
    antibiotics interactions, 117
    concentrations in feed, 109–110, 111
    described, 108
    dietary nutrient metabolism affected by
        glucose, 114
        lipids, 114
        minerals, 115
        protein, 114–115
    digestion of
        degradation products, 110
        energy value of VFA, 113–114
        fermentation, 112–113
        gastric emptying, 112
        gastrointestinal tract affected by, 112
    feeding considerations
        diet formulation, 122–123
        physical limitations, 123
    growth performance and body composition effects, 115–116
    health affected by, 117
    quantifying, 108–109
    sows affected by
        behavior, 121–122
        reproductive performance, 118–121
        source effects on reproductive performance, 121
Noradrenaline, 633–634
Norepinephrine, 433, 633–634
North American Free Trade Association (NAFTA), 24
NPN (nonprotein nitrogen), 132–133
NSP, *see* Nonstarch polysaccharides
Nuclear magnetic resonance (NMR), 935
Nucleases, 42
Nursery facilities, 27
Nursing pigs, *see* Suckling pigs
Nutraceuticals, 142, 435–436
Nutrient partitioning, 428–429
Nutrient-to-energy ratios, energy utilization, 89

O

Oats
    amino acid content, 792–794
    energy content, 788–792
Obesity
    in humans
        biomedical research using pigs, 9
        fat in diet and, 637
    in pigs, 7
Obrignya martiana (babassu palm), 851
Ochratoxins, 566–567
Odor reduction strategies, *see also* Environmental pollution and odor control
    diet manipulation, 624
    manure components, 622–623, 624
    microbes manipulation, 624–625
    nitrogen level reduction, 623–624
Oils digestibility analysis, 909–910
Oilseed meals, 807–809, 851
Oleic acid, 637
Olestra, 269
Oligosaccharides
    benefits of, 419, 420
    concentrations in feed, 109–110, 111
    described, 108
    dietary nutrient metabolism affected by
        glucose, 114
        lipids, 114
        minerals, 115
        protein, 114–115
    digestion of
        degradation products, 110
        energy value of VFA, 113–114
        fermentation, 112–113
    growth performance and body composition effects, 115–116
    health affected by, 117
    quantifying, 109
Oral cavity, *see* Mouth and salivary glands
Organic acids
    benefits of, 420, 421
    ileal AA digestibilities influenced by, 176–177
    in weanling pig diet, 704
Orthogonality in statistics, 885
Ortho-phosphates, *see* Phosphorus (P)
Oryza sativa (rice), 844–845
Osteocalcin, 207
Osteochondrosis in gilts, 728
Osteomalacia, 197
Osteoporosis research using pigs, 9

P

P, *see* Phosphorus (P)
Pairwise multiple comparisons, 897
Pale, soft, and exudative (PSE) pork, 637–638, 639, 641
Palmitate, 95–97
Palm kernel (*Elaeis guineenis*), 851
Palmitic acid, 637
Pancreas
    anatomy and histology, 34, 36
    enzymes in, 675–676
    pancreatic exocrine secretions
        age and diet factors, 43
        enzyme classes, 42
        hormone regulation, 43–44
        patterns of development, 42–43
        preprandial basal outflow, 44

Index

responses to diet composition changes, 44–45
study techniques, 977–978
Pantothenic acid
  bioavailability, 370
  deficiency/toxicity symptoms, 329
  history, 328
  metabolism, 328–329
  nutritional requirements, 329
  status and sources, 329–330
  structure, 328
Para-amino-benzoic acid, 8
Parakeratosis, 554
Parathyroid hormone (PTH), 188, 195, 203
Parotid glands, *see* Mouth and salivary glands
PDmax (body protein deposition), 74–76, 78
Peanuts (*Arachis hypogaea*), 816–817, 849
Pearl millet (*Pennisetum glaucum*), 844
Peas (*Pisum sativum*), 849–850
Pelleting
  binders, 485–486
  feed efficiency and, 721
  mill conditioners, 483–485
  pellet quality, 483
  pellet size, 481–483
  process and benefits, 480–481
  for weanling pig diet, 706
Penicillin, 411; *see also* Antimicrobial agents
Pennisetum glaucum (pearl millet), 844
Pens for pigs, 26
Pepsin A, 37, 51
Pepsin B, 37
Peptide hormones
  similarity to humans, 6–7
  transport systems, 53–54
Peptostreptococcus in GI tract, 588
Performance-enhancing substances
  beta-adrenergic agonists, 433–435
  challenge for nutritionists, 428
  interactions with immune functions, 436, 438
  leptin, 436
  nutraceuticals, 435–436
  nutrient partitioning, 428–429
  nutrient requirements impacted by
    amino acid needs, 440–441
    energy, 441
    factors involved, 439
    mineral and vitamins, 441
  porcine somatotropin
    growth effects, 429–432
    history of use, 429
    lactation effects, 432–433
  prolactin, 436
Periparturient hypogalactic syndrome (PHS), 738, 756
Peroxidase, 244
Peroxisome proliferator-activated receptors (PPAR)
  overview, 663
  regulation of differentiation, 663
  role in nutritional regulation, 663–665
Peyer's patches, 593–594
Pharynx and esophagus, 34
Phaseolus beans, 573–575, 846, 848–849, 851

Phenols and indoles, 597–598
Phenylalanine, 134
pH in water, 392
Phospholipids in bile, 40–42
Phosphorus (P)
  absorption and excretion, 199
  absorption interferences, 199–200
  bioavailability, 359–360
  for breeding boars, 779–780
  chemical and physical properties, 198–199
  deficiency symptoms, 200
  excretion and, 617
  function of, 200
  genetic modifications to improve bioavailability, 801
  interdependence with other minerals, 188
  in lactating sow diet, 757
  manure management and, 610–611
  reducing for growing-finishing pigs, 720
  requirements for, 10, 189, 200
  requirements with metabolic enhancers, 441
  skeletal tissue and, 191–192
  sources and availability, 201
  toxicity, 200
Photoperiod and feed intake, 456
Phylloquinones, 204–206
Phyllosilicates (clays), 572
Phytase
  clinical applications of pig derived knowledge, 10–11
  phosphorus reduction and, 720
Phytates
  ileal AA digestibilities influenced by, 174
  mineral bioavailability affected by, 359–360
  phosphorus bioavailability and, 200
  phytase supplementation, 617–619
Pietrain pigs, 67
Pigeon peas (*Cajanus cajun*), 851
Pigs and humans
  anatomical/physiological similarities
    body composition, 7
    gastrointestinal system, 6–7
    nutrient requirements, 7–8
  biomedical research and
    general considerations, 9
    nutrition, 9
    physiology and pathophysiology, 9–10
  clinical applications of knowledge
    genetic engineering, 10
    phytase and mineral-related metabolic disorders, 10–11
    recombinant DNA-derived products, 11
    xenotransplantation, 10
  demographic relationships, 4–6
  pig domestication, 3–4
  pigs' scavenger nature, 4–5
  pork in human diet
    acceptability, 12–14
    composition, 12, 13
    nutritional quality, 11–12, 636–637
    societal issues, 14–15
Pisum sativum (peas), 849–850
Plantains (*Musa paradisiaca*), 842

Plasma protein, 699–700, 828–829
Pollution, *see* Environmental pollution and odor control
Polyamines, 675
Polyunsaturated fatty acids (PUFAs), 553–554
Porcine somatotropin (pST), *see also* Performance enhancing substances
    growth effects, 11
        adipose tissue, 430
        development stages, 431–432
        mechanism, 429–430
        muscle metabolism, 430–431
    history of use, 429
    lactation effects, 432–433
Porcine stress syndrome, 11
Pork industry, *see* Swine industry
Pork in human diet, *see also* Swine industry
    acceptability, 12–14
    annual consumption worldwide, 5–6
    composition, 12, 13
    desirable qualities, 637–638, 639, 641
    nutritional quality, 11–12, 636–637
    profitability of production, 5
    quality relation to Se and vitamin E, 300
    societal issues, 14–15
Portal and ileal vein catheterization, 968–969
Postvalvular T-cecum cannulation (PVTC), 165
Postweaning reproductive performance, 760
Potassium (K)
    bioavailability, 360–361
    in body mass estimation, 936
    chemistry, 214
    elemental percentage in body, 214
    function and uses, 220–222
Potatoes (*Solanum tuberosum*), 844
Poultry
    by-product meal as protein supplement, 829, 850
    mineral bioavailability
        calcium, 357
        copper, 361
        iron, 362
        manganese, 363
        phosphorus, 359
        zinc, 364–365
    promicrobial agent studies, 418–419
PPAR, *see* Peroxisome proliferator-activated receptors
Pregnant sows, *see* Gestating sows
Prochymosin, 51
Production systems for swine
    breeding facilities, 28
    farrowing facilities, 25–26
    gestation facilities, 29
    growing-finishing facilities, 27–28
    nursery facilities, 27
    overview, 24–25
    recommended floor area, 29
    recommended thermal conditions, 28
Prolactin, 436
Proline, 134
Promicrobial agents
    background on use, 404–405
    definition, 401
    efficacy of, 417–418
    mode of action, 418–419
    other beneficial organisms, 419–420
    uses of, 417
Propionic acid, 50
Prostaglandin metabolism, 294
Protease inhibitors, 573–574
Proteases, 37, 42
Protein
    alternative feedstuffs
        beans, 846
        canola seed, 846–847
        cull eggs, 847
        faba beans, 847
        fish silage, 847–848
        legumes, 851
        lentils, 848
        lupins, 848
        mung beans, 848–849
        oilseed meals, 851
        peanuts, 849
        peas, 849–850
        poultry hatchery by-product meal, 850
        shrimp meal, 850
        sunflower seeds, 850–851
    cytokines and synthesis of, 549
    digestion and absorption
        absorption of products, 53–54
        gastric digestion, 51–52
        in large intestine, 52–53
        in small intestine, 52
    feed content and energy utilization, 90
    growth curves for, 69
    ileal AA digestibilities influenced by, 171–172
    intake effects on boars
        adult, 773–775
        developing, 772–773
    main tissues, 67
    muscle conversion to meat and, 635–636
    myosin, 634
    neonatal development and, 677–678
    nitrogen excretion and, 616–617
    nonprotein nitrogen and
        crude and true, 132
        nonprotein nitrogen use, 132–133
    NSPs effect on metabolism of, 114–115
    percent composition of pigs, 66
    preslaughter intake manipulation, 641–642
    requirements with metabolic enhancers, 440–441
    sources, 172
    supplements, *see* Protein supplements
    weanling pig diet sources
        dried porcine solubles, 700
        fish meal, 700
        milk, 700
        plasma, 699–700
        spray-dried protein products, 701
Protein deposition (PD), 88
Protein supplements
    amino acid limitations, 138–139

Index

animal sources
  benefits of, 823
  blood meal, 823–824
  feather meal, 824–825
  fish meal, 825–826
  meat and bone meal, 826–827
  meat meal, 827–828
  milk, dried, 828
  plasma, 828–829
  poultry by-product meal, 829
  whey, dried, 829–830
benefits of efficient feed use, 805
diet formulation
  goal of, 805, 807
  nutrient availability considerations, 807
digestibility analysis, 909–910
feeding values and incorporation rates, 805, 806
plant sources
  alfalfa meal, 809–810
  canola seed, 810–812
  coconut meal, 812–813
  cottonseed meal, 813–815
  linseed meal, 815–816
  oilseed meals, 807–809
  peanuts, 816–817
  safflower meal, 817–818
  sesame meal, 819
  soybeans, 819–821
  sunflower seeds, 821–823
PSE (pale, soft, and exudative) pork, 637–638, 639, 641
pST, *see* Porcine somatotropin
PTH (parathyroid hormone), 188, 195, 203
Puberty in gilts
  age range, 730
  dietary nutrient supply, 732–733
  nutrition and hormone interactions, 731–732
  thresholds, 731
PUFAs (polyunsaturated fatty acids), 553–554

R

Ractopamine, 433, 435, 441
Randomization in statistics, 885–886
Randomized complete block (RCB) design, 887–888
Rapeseed (*Brassica* sp.), 810
Recombinant DNA-derived products, 11
Reentrant cannulation, 164
Regression method for endogenous AA losses estimation, 167–168
Rendement Napole (RN) gene, 639
Repeated measures (RM) designs, 889–890
Replication in statistics, 886
Reproduction
  antibiotic use during cycle, 409
  copper requirement, 240–241
  performance characteristics of boars, 771–772
  Se and vitamin E needs for
    boars, 303
    sows, 300–303
  vitamin A role, 273–274, 276

  zinc requirement, 252
Restaurant food waste as alternative feedstuffs, 852
Retained energy, 87–88
Riboflavin
  bioavailability, 370–371
  deficiency/toxicity symptoms, 331–332
  function and uses, 293
  history, 330
  metabolism, 330–331
  nutritional requirements, 331
  sources and availability, 332
  structure, 330
Rice (*Oryza sativa*), 844–845
Rickets, 197
Roller mills, 472–474
Rubber seed (*Hevea brasiliensis*), 851
Rumen microbial ecosystems, 586
Ruminococcus flavefaciens, 112

S

Saccaromyces cerevisiae, 116, 418
Saccharum officinarum (sugarcane), 843
Safflower meal (*Carthamus tictorius*), 817–818
Salbutamol, 433, 435
Salinomycin, 117
Salivary glands
  anatomy and histology, 32
  secretions, 38–37
  in vivo study techniques, 975–976
Sampling unit in statistics, 884
Secretin, 41, 43
Segregated early weaning (SEW), 20
  neonatal development and, 681
  weanling pig lysine requirements, 693–694
Selenide, *see* Selenium (Se)
Selenium (Se)
  absorption, 289
  bioavailability, 363–364
  blood and tissue distribution, 290–291
  for breeding boars, 779
  commercial sources, 286–287
  deficiency onset and symptoms
    clinical symptoms, 296
    tissue responses, 295–296
  dietary requirements, 304–305
  excess effects, 303–304
  excretion, 294–295
  factors contributing to deficiency, 296–297
  in fetal and neonatal pigs
    condition at birth, 297–298
    iron toxicity, 298
  growing-finishing period
    growth, 299–300
    pork quality affected by, 300
  immune function and, 293–294, 556
  iron toxicity and, 298
  in lactating sow diet, 301–302, 758
  metabolic role, 292–293
  nursing and postnatal pigs, 298–299

plant and grain sources, 283–284
reproduction and, 300–303
role in animal nutrition, 282
soil supply of bioavailable, 282–283
toxicity to humans, 283
Selenocysteine, *see* Selenium (Se)
Selenomethionine, *see* Selenium (Se)
Selenomonas in GI tract, 588
Selenoproteins, 293
Selenosis, 304
Sensitivity in statistics, 884–885
Sesame meal (*Sesamum indicum*), 819
Set point theory of feed control, 448
SEW, *see* Segregated early weaning
Shrimp meal, 850
Silicon (Si), 8, 253
Simple T-cannulation, 164
Skatole, 598
Skeletal tissue
    calcium contained in, 189
    calcium functions, 191–192, 196–197
    calcium storage and mobilization, 195–196
    function of, 67–68
    percent composition of pigs, 66
Skim milk effect on neonatal growth, 677
Skin percent composition of pigs, 66
Slaughter method to collect ileal digesta, 163–164
Slope-ratio assay for AA bioavailability, 153–154
Slow-twitch MHC isoforms, 635
Small intestine
    absorption of digestion products, 49
    anatomy and histology, 36–38
    digestion of carbohydrates
        luminal, 47–48
        mucosal, 48–49
    fat digestion and absorption in, 54–55
    intestinal bacteria in, 588
    microbial activity in, 49
    protein digestion and absorption in, 52
    secretions, 45–46
    water and electrolyte absorption in, 55–56
Social facilitation and eating behavior, 506–507, 512–513
Societal issues and pork consumption, 14
SOD (superoxide dismutase), 237, 292
Sodium (Na)
    bioavailability, 360
    chemistry, 214
    elemental percentage in body, 214
    function and uses, 222–224
Solanum tuberosum (potatoes), 844
Sorghum
    amino acid content, 792–794
    energy content, 788–792
Sows
    fat in diet and nutrition, 102
    gestating, *see* Gestating sows
    lactating, *see* Lactating sows
    milk from
        digestibility of fat in, 100
        neonatal development and, 679
    NSPs effect on

    behavior, 121–122
    reproductive performance, 118–121
    source effects on reproductive performance, 121
    Se and vitamin E and
        diseases, 302–303
        gestation, 300–301
        lactation, 301–302
    thermal environment effects on, 534–535
    water use, 386–387
Soybeans (*Glycine max*)
    effect on neonatal growth, 677
    extrusion uses and benefits, 488–490, 491
    in feed, 110
    as protein supplement, 819–821
Split-plot (SP) design, 889–890
Spray-dried plasma protein, 699–700, 701
Starch, 799–800; *see also* Carbohydrates
Statistical techniques, *see also* Modeling of swine
    analysis of variance
        assumptions, 894–895
        components, 893
        functions of, 893–894
        plans, 895–896
    basic concepts, 884–885
    designed comparison among treatment means, 897
    design of experiments
        planning/organization importance, 882
        preexperiment protocol, 882–884
    design structure of experiments
        extensions and modifications, 888–889
        repeated measures, 889–890
        split-plots, 889–890
        types, 887–888
    error control, 886
    multiple comparison procedures, 897–898
    precision improvement methods
        design structure efficiency, 892–893
        experimental unit choice, 891–892
        replication increase, 890–891
    randomization, 885–886
    replication, 886
    results interpretation/presentation
        partitioning treatment effects, 898
        reporting results, 898–899
    statisticians' role, 899–900
    treatment structure of experiments, 886–887
Stearate, 95–97
Stearic acid, 637
Steered ileo-cecal valve cannulation (SICV), 165
Stereotypic behavior and diet, 121–122
Sterols and digestion, 55
Stocking density, 510
Stomach
    anatomy and histology, 34
    carbohydrates digestion and fermentation, 46–47
    fat digestion and absorption, 54
    gastric secretions, 37–40, 976–977
    gastrointestinal system
        intestinal bacteria and, *see* Intestinal bacteria
        NSPs and, 112
        similarity to humans, 6–7

Index

intestinal bacteria in, 588
protein digestion and absorption, 51–52
similarity to humans, 6–7
Stray voltage and eating behavior, 509–510
Streptococcus faecium, 418
Streptococcus in GI tract, 587
Streptomyces aureofaciens, 402
Streptomycin, 411; *see also* Antimicrobial agents
Sublingual glands, 32
Suckling pigs
    digestibility of sow's milk fat, 100
    gastric secretions, 37–40
    lactase activity, 48
    lactose fermentation, 46
    pancreatic exocrine secretions, 42–45
    Se and vitamin E needs for, 298–299
    water use, 383–385
Sucrose hydrolysis, 48
Sufamethazine, 413–414
Sugar beet pulp, 122
Sugar beets (*Beta vulgaris*), 845
Sugarcane (*Saccharum officinarum*), 843
Sulfates in water, 393
Sulfur (S)
    amino acids and, 224–225
    chemistry, 214
    elemental percentage in body, 214
Sunflower seeds (*Helianthus annus*), 821–823, 850–851
Superoxide dismutase (SOD), 237, 292
Supplements, *see* Protein supplements
Surgical techniques
    anesthesia, 970–971
    care and use of swine during, 969–970
    monitoring during and after, 971–972
    preparation for aseptic surgery, 970
    presurgical care, 970
    in vivo studies
        bile secretion, 979
        gastric secretion, 976–977
        gastrointestinal lymph, 980
        net portal nutrient absorption, 974–975
        nutrient digestibility, 972–974
        pancreatic secretion, 977–978
        salivary secretion, 975–976
Sweet potatoes (*Ipomoea batatas*), 845
Swine industry, *see also* Pork in human diet
    carcass variables, 24
    economic value, 23
    evolution from generalized to specialized, 20
    feed-efficiency, 21
    future of
        global economy pressures, 23
        vertically coordinated operations, 24
        world market, 24
    historical background, 19
    number of hog farms, 20, 22
    post-mortem conditioning effects on quality, 637
    production systems
        breeding facilities, 28
        farrowing facilities, 25–26
        gestation facilities, 29
        growing-finishing facilities, 27–28
        nursery facilities, 27
        overview, 24–25
        recommended floor area, 29
        recommended thermal conditions, 28
    societal issues, 14

T

T-4 toxin, 563, 564, 569
Ta (ambient temperature), *see* Thermal environment
Tannins
    antinutritional factors, 575–576, 577
    ileal AA digestibilities influenced by, 175–176
Taro (*Colocasia esculenta*), 843
TCA (tricarboxylic acid), 632
T-cannula, 56–57, 972–974
TDF (total dietary fiber), 109
TDN (total digestible nutrient) system, 85
TDS (total dissolved solids) in water, 391–392
Teeth in swine, 32
Testosterone derivatives and pork quality, 12
Tetracycline, 411; *see also* Antimicrobial agents
Thermal environment
    critical temperatures, 520
    energy exchanges, 520
    energy requirements for boars and, 778
    energy utilization and, 90–91
    extra thermoregulatory heat production, 521
    feed intake influenced by, 454–456
    growing-finishing pigs and Ta
        carcass composition, 532–533
        feed intake, 529–531, 719
        growth rate and feed efficiency, 531–532
    lactating sows and Ta, 534–535
    neonatal/young pigs affected by
        cold stress role, 526
        energy provision, 523–525
        heat production mechanisms, 523
        microenvironment provision, 525–526
        neonatal mortality, 522
        newborn susceptibility to cold, 522–523
        suckling period remainder, 526–527
    NSP and, 116–117
    nutritional interactions with Ta
        amino acid needs, 536–537
        dietary energy concentration, 535–536
        optimal temperature significance, 537–538
    pregnant sows and Ta, 534
    recommended conditions, 28
    water functions, 381
    weanlings affected by
        ambient temperature factors, 527–529
        relative humidity and ventilation, 529
Thermic effect of feed, 535
Thiamin
    bioavailability, 371
    deficiency/toxicity symptoms, 334
    history, 332
    metabolism, 333

nutritional requirements, 333–334
status and sources, 12, 334–335
structure, 332–333
Thin sow syndrome, 122
Thioredoxin reductase, 293
Three-dimensional topometry, 946
Threonine, see also Amino acids
    animal use of isomers, 141
    essentiality of, 139
    lactating sows requirement, 750–752
    limitations in feeds, 138
Thymulin, 554–555
Thyroid hormone, 293
Tissue interaction analysis for body composition
    bioelectrical impedance, 929–930
    near-infrared interactance, 934–935
    nuclear magnetic resonance, 935
    total-body electrical conductivity, 929–932
    X-ray absorptiometry, 932–934
Titanium oxide, 163
Titer, 98
T lymphocytes and intestinal bacteria, 593
α-Tocopherol, see Vitamin E
Tocopherols, see Vitamin E
Tocotrienols, see Vitamin E
Total-body electrical conductivity (TOBEC), 929–932
Total collection method, ileal digestibility, 162
Total dietary fiber (TDF), 109
Total digestible nutrient (TDN) system, 85
Total dissolved solids (TDS) in water, 391–392
Trace elements, see also specific elements
    analysis, 232–233
    arsenic, 253
    boron, 254
    chromium, 233–234
    cobalt, 234
    copper
        absorption, 235
        deficiency symptoms, 239–241
        functions, 236–239
        toxicity, 241
        transport systems, 235–236
    essentiality and toxicity, 230–231
    interactions, 231–232
    iodine, 241–242
    iron
        absorption, 242–243
        classifications, 242
        deficiency symptoms, 245
        functions, 244
        interrelationships, 243
        requirements, 244
        storage, 244
        toxicity, 245
        transport, 243–244
    manganese, 245–247
    molybdenum, 253
    nickel, 253
    silicon, 253
    vanadium, 253
    zinc
        absorption, 247–249
        deficiency symptoms, 251–253
        functions, 250–251
        toxicity, 253
        transport, 249–250
Trans fatty acids, 96
Trehalose, 48
Tricarboxylic acid (TCA), 632
Trichinella spiralis, 14
Trichinosis, 12
Trichothecenes, 568–569
Triglycerides, 54, 95
Triticale (X Triticosecale), 845–846
Trypsin, 42
Trypsin inhibitor activity (TIA), 573–574
Trypsin inhibitors
    antinutritional factors, 573–574
    ileal AA digestibilities influenced by, 174–175
Tryptophan
    animal use of isomers, 141
    essentiality of, 139
    limitations in feeds, 138
    nutraceutical properties, 142
Tyrosinase, 238
Tyrosine, 134

U

Ulcers in pigs, 490, 492
Ultrasound, 945–946
Unsaturated fatty acids in pork, 12
Upper critical temperature (UCT), 520
Upstream stimulatory factors (USF), 662
Urea
    in body composition analysis, 928
    as NPN feed additive, 132–133
USDA, 12

V

Valine, 139
Vanadium (V), 8, 253
Vegetable oils, 98
Venipuncture
    acute, 962–963
    blood vessels, 965
    cephalic vein, 964
    ear veins, 964–965
    jugular vein, 964
    vena cava, 962–963
Vertical screw mixer, 476, 478
VFA, see Volatile fatty acids
Vicia faba (faba beans), 847
Video imaging, 946
Vigna sinensis (cow peas), 851
Virginiamycin, 117; see also Antimicrobial agents
Visceral organs
    function of, 67–68

Index

percent composition of pigs, 66
Vitamin A
    absorption, 268–269
    bioavailability, 265–266, 365–366
    biological functions
        cell proliferation and differentiation, 273
        gene regulation, 273
        immunity and health, 275
        reproductive role, 273–274
        vision role, 272–273
    for breeding boars, 780
    carotenoids
        absorption of, 269–270
        bioavailability, 366
        storage, transport, interactions, 271–272
    deficiencies
        clinical symptoms, 275
        factors causing, 276–277
        immune function effects, 276
        reproductive performance and, 276
    dietary requirements, 267–268
    immune function and, 556–557
    metabolism, 272
    nomenclature and occurrence, 263–265
    nutrient interactions, 268
    retinol binding proteins and transport, 271
    toxicities associated with, 277–278
    uptake and storage by liver, 270–271
Vitamin B_6
    bioavailability, 371–372
    deficiency/toxicity symptoms, 336–337
    history, 335
    metabolism, 335–336
    nutritional requirements, 336
    status and sources, 337
    structure, 335
Vitamin B_{12}
    antimicrobial agents use and, 402
    bioavailability, 372
    cobalt and, 234
    deficiency/toxicity symptoms, 339
    history, 337
    metabolism, 338
    nutritional requirements, 339
    status and sources, 339–340
    structure, 337–338
Vitamin C
    bioavailability, 372
    pig vs. human need for, 8
Vitamin D
    bioavailability, 366
    calcium absorption and, 193
    deficiency symptoms, 204, 208–209
    forms and derivatives
        absorption and synthesis, 201–202
        chemical structure, 201
    muscle conversion and, 645–646
    physiological action, 203
    requirements for, 203–204, 208
    requirements with metabolic enhancers, 441
    status assessment, 207–208

toxicity, 204, 209
Vitamin E
    absorption, 289–290
    arachidonic acid and prostaglandin metabolism, 294
    bioavailability, 367
    blood and tissue distribution, 291–292
    for breeding boars, 779
    commercial sources, 287–288
    deficiency onset and symptoms
        clinical symptoms, 296
        tissue responses, 295–296
    dietary requirements, 304–305
    excess effects, 304
    excretion, 295
    factors contributing to deficiency, 296–297
    in fetal and neonatal pigs
        condition at birth, 297–298
        iron toxicity, 298
    growing-finishing period
        growth, 299–300
        pork quality affected by, 300
    immune function and, 293–294, 556
    iron toxicity and, 298
    in lactating sow diet, 758
    metabolic role, 293
    muscle conversion and, 646–647, 648–652
    nursing and postnatal pigs, 298–299
    plant and grain sources, 284–286
    reproduction and
        boars, 303
        sows, 300–303
    role in animal nutrition, 282
Vitamin K
    absorption and synthesis, 204–206
    bioavailability, 367
    chemical structure, 204
    physiological action, 206–207
Vitamins, *see also* specific vitamins; Water-soluble vitamins
    bioavailability
        bioassay methodology, 365
        biotin, 367–368
        folacin/folic acid, 369
        niacin, 370
        pantothenic acid, 370
        riboflavin, 370–371
        thiamin, 371
        vitamin A, 365–366
        vitamin B_6, 371–372
        vitamin B_{12}, 372
        vitamin C, 372
        vitamin D, 366
        vitamin E, 367
        vitamin K, 367
    in cereal grains, 794–795
    choline, 368–369
    in weanling pig diet, 702
    weanling pig requirements, 694
Volatile fatty acids (VFA)
    energy value of, 113–114
    feed content and energy utilization, 90

fermentation of carbohydrates and, 50–51
similarity to humans, 6–7
Vomitoxin, 563, 564, 568–569

W

Water
  association with protein, 67
  balance, 382, 383
  consequences of inadequate intake, 389–390
  delivery system
    amount and placement, 388–389
    types, 387–388
  electrolyte absorption, 55–56
  excretion, 382–383
  functions and content, 381–382
  in lactating sow diet, 755
  percent composition of pigs, 66
  protein interactions in muscle conversion, 636
  quality determinants
    allowable pathogen content, 391
    hardness, 392
    nitrates, 393
    other contaminants, 393
    pH, 392
    sulfates, 393
    total dissolved solids, 391–392
  quality improvement guidelines, 393–394
  requirements summary, 387
  sources for swine, 382
  use by classes
    boars, 387
    gestating sows, 386–387
    growing-finishing pigs, 385
    lactating sows, 387
    suckling pigs, 383–385
    weanling pigs, 385, 694–695
  waste reduction in operations, 390–391
Water-soluble vitamins, *see also* specific vitamins; Vitamins
  ascorbic acid
    deficiency/toxicity symptoms, 342
    history, 340
    metabolism, 340–341
    nutritional requirements, 341–342
    status and sources, 342
    structure, 340
  biotin
    deficiency/toxicity symptoms, 320
    history, 317
    metabolism, 318–319
    nutritional requirements, 319
    sources and availability, 320
    status assessment, 320
    structure, 318
  choline
    deficiency/toxicity symptoms, 322
    history, 320
    metabolism, 321
    nutritional requirements, 321–322
    status and sources, 322
    structure, 321
  folate
    deficiency/toxicity symptoms, 325
    history, 323
    metabolism, 323–324
    nutritional requirements, 324–325
    status and sources, 325
    structure, 323
  niacin
    deficiency/toxicity symptoms, 327
    history, 325–326
    metabolism, 326–327
    nutritional requirements, 327
    status and sources, 327–328
    structure, 326
  pantothenic acid
    deficiency/toxicity symptoms, 329
    history, 328
    metabolism, 328–329
    nutritional requirements, 329
    status and sources, 329–330
    structure, 328
  riboflavin
    deficiency/toxicity symptoms, 331–332
    history, 330
    metabolism, 330–331
    nutritional requirements, 331
    sources and availability, 332
    structure, 330
  thiamin
    deficiency/toxicity symptoms, 334
    history, 332
    metabolism, 333
    nutritional requirements, 333–334
    status and sources, 334–335
    structure, 332–333
  vitamin B_6
    deficiency/toxicity symptoms, 336–337
    history, 335
    metabolism, 335–336
    nutritional requirements, 336
    status and sources, 337
    structure, 335
  vitamin B_{12}
    deficiency/toxicity symptoms, 339
    history, 337
    metabolism, 338
    nutritional requirements, 339
    status and sources, 339–340
    structure, 337–338
Weanling pigs
  changes in carbohydrases from weaning, 49
  diet composition
    energy sources, 697–699
    feed additives, 702–704
    minerals, 694, 701–702
    protein sources, 699–701
    vitamins, 702
  diet forms, 706
  digestive capacity/enzyme activity, 692

Index

factors affecting nutrient requirements
    antigen exposure, 695–696
    sex and genotype, 696
    summary table, 695
    thermal environment, 527–529
    weaning age, 695
nutrient requirements
    amino acids, 693–694
    energy, 693
    minerals, 694
    vitamins, 694
    water, 694–695
performance estimates, 704–705
phased program recommendation, 705–706
postweaning reproduction performance, 760
water use, 385, 694–695

Weight gain and composition determinants
    body protein deposition, 74
    chemical/physical components relationship, 77
    energy intake/PDmax relationship, 74–76
    maintenance energy/nutrient requirements, 73–74
    pig genotype, 72
    voluntary feed intake, 76
Wet and wet/dry feeders, 505–506, 719–720
Wheat
    amino acid content, 792–794
    energy content, 788–792
Whey, dried
    as alternative feedstuffs, 851
    as protein supplement, 829–830
White grease, 98

X

Xenotransplantation, 10
X-ray absorptiometry, 932–934
X-ray computed axial tomography, 942, 944–945
X Triticosecale (triticale), 845–846

Y

Yams (*Dioscorea* sp.), 846
Yellow grease, 98
Yorkshire pigs, 67

Z

Zearalenone, 563, 564, 569–570
Zeolites, 572
Zinc (Zn)
    absorption, 247–249
    bioavailability, 364–365
    for breeding boars, 780
    deficiency symptoms, 251–253
    effects of high dietary content, 408
    in excretion, 616
    functions, 250–251
    as a growth enhancer, 435
    immune function and, 554–555
    toxicity, 253
    transport, 249–250
    in weanling pig diet, 702, 703
Zoonosis, 10